Early Visual Development
Normal and Abnormal

Early Visual Development
Normal and Abnormal

Edited by
Kurt Simons

Committee on Vision
Commission on Behavioral and Social Sciences
and Education
National Research Council

NEW YORK   OXFORD
OXFORD UNIVERSITY PRESS
1993

Oxford University Press

Oxford   New York   Toronto
Delhi   Bombay   Calcutta   Madras   Karachi
Kuala Lumpur   Singapore   Hong Kong   Tokyo
Nairobi   Dar es Salaam   Cape Town
Melbourne   Auckland   Madrid

and associated companies in
Berlin   Ibadan

Library of Congress Cataloging-in-Publication Data
Early Visual Development, Normal and Abnormal /
edited by Kurt Simons ;
Committee on Vision, Commission on Behavioral and Social Sciences
and Education, National Research Council.
p.   cm   Includes bibliographical references and index.
ISBN 0-19-507721-0
1. Vision in infants.   2. Pediatric ophthalmology.
3. Eye—Growth.   I. Simons, Kurt.
II. National Research Council (U.S.), Committee on Vision.
[DNLM: 1. Vision—in infancy & childhood
2. Vision Disorders—in infancy & childhood
WW 600 I43]   RE48.2.C5I54   1993
612.8′4′0832—dc20   DNLM/DLC   for Library of Congress   92-42966

9   8   7   6   5   4   3   2   1
Printed in the United States of America
on acid-free paper

Foreword

This volume celebrates a wonderful fact—"baby vision" has come of age! The developmental study of human vision is now a fully mature field with a large body of well-established findings and well-reasoned models to explain them. Infant vision is as diverse a field as its elder parent. Thus, the chapters in this volume cover developmental aspects of the same topics found in comparable volumes on adult vision—optics, oculomotor behavior, psychophysics, and neurophysiology. In addition, because of the need of pediatric ophthalmologists to assess the functional integrity of infants' visual systems, they have long had a special interest in infant vision research, and so this volume also includes several chapters (Section VI) on particular clinical issues in visual development.

How did infant vision reach its current mature status? Psychologists have studied human development since the inception of the science, and techniques for measuring the visual capabilities of infants and children were available by the 1960s. Nevertheless, for me and many other American psychophysicists, infant vision began with Davida Teller's presentation of the forced-choice preferential looking technique at a meeting of the Association for Research in Vision and Ophthalmology (ARVO) in 1974. Davida had made a minor modification of Fantz's preferential looking technique, but it was a change that brought the full rigor of adult psychophysics to infant visual studies. Fantz had discovered that infants would stare preferentially at some visual displays, indicating not just a preference, but some capacity to discriminate among displays. There were weaknesses in Fantz's technique: If an infant stared for 10 seconds at one target and for 5 seconds at the other, did the difference in fixation duration indicate something about the difficulty of the discrimination? Were first fixations more important than subsequent gaze shifts? Davida converted preferential looking into a simple two-alternative forced-choice judgment, a judgment that was largely unaffected by experimenter bias or expectations. The experimenter made the choice by watching the behavior of the infant. If the experimenter could correctly identify the spatial location of test target on a criterion percentage of trials, then the infant must be able to discriminate between the stimuli.

As Davida herself related in the twenty-fifth anniversary edition of *Vision Research* (No. 9, 1986), in the early 1970s four different laboratories began doing infant psychophysics almost simultaneously: her own laboratory at the University of Washington, Dick Held's

group at the Massachusetts Institute of Technology, Janette Atkinson and Oliver Braddick at the University of Cambridge, and Marty Banks in Phil Salapatek's laboratory at the University of Minnesota. I note that these same researchers have all contributed chapters to this volume, which suggests that infant vision is an enduring passion. These high-power laboratories initiated a shift from intriguing studies on infant cognition (face preferences and the like) to the more "boring" studies of the stimulus dimensions used in conventional adult psychophysics. Studies on acuity, luminance sensitivity, color vision, flicker, contrast sensitivity, and refractive development all appeared within a decade of Davida's ARVO presentation. This shift in research strategy meant that the physiologically based explanations for the limitations of adult vision could now be applied to the developing visual system. For example, recent models of infant psychophysical data have incorporated Anita Hendrickson's anatomical findings on the changes in the retinal mosaic that occur over the first 5 years of life to explain the development of acuity, hyperacuity, and contrast sensitivity; see the chapters by Banks, Wilson, and Hendrickson.

Nowhere is the value of basic studies on visual development more evident than in the clinic. Eye care specialists want to know if their infant patients are "normal." This requires two things: a well-researched definition of what is normal and some means of measuring infant patients in a clinical setting. Over the past two decades, careful studies on the normal development of acuity and constant sensitivity have provided a sturdy yardstick for judging abnormality in these important functions. By sheer ingenuity, the Atkinson-Braddick team and Howard Howland and his collaborators were able to measure normal refractive development—another important clinical yardstick. The results in the chapters by Shimojo, Held, and Birch on the development of normal binocular vision may prove clinically useful in the future. Studies on the normal development of the oculomotor system described here in chapters by Dick Aslin and by Karen Preston and Dom Finocchio may also provide important benchmarks for the clinical assessment of strabismus.

The normative data for all these functions was accumulated from many laboratories over several years. How do you measure an infant patient within the brief time allotted for a clinical examination? A laboratory estimate of acuity based on FPL is both time-consuming and labor intensive, so Davida and her associates designed an abbreviated screening technique, the Teller acuity cards, to discriminate between "probably normal" and "probably abnormal" acuity. We must applaud the tireless efforts of Velma Dobson and her colleagues in standardizing and testing this valuable screening technique; see the chapter by Dobson. The demand for rapid clinical assessment was partially responsible for the development of VEP techniques in infant vision. Although several infant laboratories had made desultory use of the VEP, much credit must be given to Christopher Tyler and Tony Norcia for converting the VEP into a standard procedure of infant visual research.

How did the Committee on Vision of the National Research Council come to initiate a meeting on infant vision which led to this volume? During my membership on this committee, we held a number of workshops to respond to inquiries from our sponsors. Frequently, these workshops addressed visual problems in a military context (contact lens wear under adverse conditions, motion sickness in tanks, etc.). While these workshops often expanded into basic visual questions, their primary function was to solve practical defense-related problems. Anne Fulton, a former member of the committee, called me and also the senior staff officer, Pamela Ebert-Flattau, to request a workshop devoted to a clinical question ("something besides tanks"). Pam and I asked David Guyton, a committee member who is an ophthalmologist, if he would organize a conference on infant vision because of its clinical relevance. He persuaded Kurt Simons to run the conference, and Kurt decided to hold the "best infant vision meeting ever."

It is hard to overestimate Kurt's contribution to this meeting. It was his foresight, organization, and hard work that made the Symposium on Infant Vision Research held on March 7–9, 1991, such a phenomenal success. We thank the sponsors of the Committee on Vision for their enthusiastic support of this endeavor and The Smith-Kettlewell Eye Research Institute, which provided additional support and cosponsored the meeting. During the meeting, the William A. Kettlewell Lecture, in honor of one of Smith-Kettlewell's founders, was given by Creig S. Hoyt.

From the beginning, Kurt insisted that the end product of this symposium should be a volume that would summarize the state of the science, a book of sufficient breadth that it could serve as a developmental text. All speakers were persuaded to submit a review chapter of their field. Kurt pushed and prodded, cajoled and demanded, and assembled this remarkable collection of manuscripts. The Committee on Vision offers special thanks to him, and to all the authors who worked so hard to produce this volume.

Suzanne P. McKee, *Chair*
Committee on Vision (1989–1991)

Acknowledgments

No volume the scope of this one is compiled without the input of many people. At the head of the list here are the chapter and introduction authors, whose common vision of the need of a reference text on early visual development made this book possible. The Editor would like to thank some others as well, however, beginning with Tom Bower, Bob Reinecke and Sheldon White, who first introduced me to the tangled fascination of visual development, in both its normal and clinical aspects. Marty Banks, David Guyton and Suzanne McKee all provided astute advice during the gestation of the book itself, and Genie Grohman and Elaine McGarraugh of the NRC staff provided the endless logistic support essential to delivering a finished work to the publisher.

Kurt Simons, *Editor*

Contents

I REFRACTIVE DEVELOPMENT

Introduction 3
Howard C. Howland

1. **Early Refractive Development 5**
Howard C. Howland

   Early Infancy: Normal Development 5
   Early Infancy: Prematurity 7
   Refractive Development From 3 Months to 1 Year
   of Age 8
   Refractive Development From 1 to 5 Years of
   Age 9
   General Aspects of Early Refractive
   Development 10
   Conclusions 11

2. **Visually Guided Control of Refractive
   State: Results From Animal Models 14**
Frank Schaeffel

   Variability of Optical Components in the Eye and
   Refractive Errors 14
   Refractive Errors: Genetically Determined or
   Inappropriately Triggered Feedback Loops? 14
   Experimental Evidence for Visually Guided Eye
   Growth: Results From Refractive Development
   Under Open Loop Conditions: "Deprivation
   Myopia" 15
   Emmetropization Under Closed-Loop
   Conditions 17
   Possible Mechanisms for Control of Refractive State
   and Eye Growth 19
   Why do Refractive Errors Develop Despite Two
   Visually Guided Feedback Loops? 20
   Targets for Future Research 24
   Conclusions: What Can be Learned From Animal
   Models Regarding Human Refractive
   Development? 26

3. **Infant Accommodation and
   Convergence 30**
Richard N. Aslin

   Accommodation 30
   Convergence 33
   Accommodation–Convergence Interactions 36
   Summary and Conclusions 37

II OCULOMOTOR FUNCTION

Introduction 39
Clifton M. Schor

4. **Conjugate Eye Movements of Infants 47**
Louise Hainline

   Classes of Conjugate Eye Movements 47
   Neural Mechanisms Controlling Conjugate Eye
   Movements 48
   Developmental Data on Saccades 53
   Developmental Data on Fixation 59
   Developmental Data on Pursuit 62
   Developmental Data on Oculomotor
   Interactions 66
   Developmental Considerations in Oculomotor
   Behavior 67
   Methodological Considerations 70
   Critique of Infant Eye Movement Studies 75

5. **Development of the Vestibuloocular and
   Optokinetic Reflexes 80**
Karen L. Preston and Dom V. Finocchio

   Development of the VOR 81
   Optokinetic Response 83
   Discussion 85

III SPATIAL AND CHROMATIC VISION

Introduction 89
Martin S. Banks

6. **Front-end Limitations to Infant Spatial
   Vision: Examination of Two Analyses 91**
Martin S. Banks and James A. Crowell

   Filtering and Sampling by the Optics, Receptors, and
   Neural Transfer Function 91
   Pupil, Media Transmittance, and Receptor
   Efficiency 92
   Optics 94
   Receptor Aperture 94
   Receptor Spacing 94
   Neural Transfer Function 95
   Predicting Adult Data 97
   Banks and Bennett Analysis of Development 98
   Wilson Model of Development 104
   Differences Between the Approaches 109
   Modified Version of Wilson's Model 112
   Conclusion 115

7. **Development of the Human Visual
   Field 117**
D. Luisa Mayer and Anne B. Fulton

   Methods to Assess Visual Fields of Infants 117
   Maturation of the Infant Visual Field 123

Summary of Maturation of Infant Visual Fields and Implications 126

8. Development of Scotopic Retinal Sensitivity 130
   Ronald M. Hansen and Anne B. Fulton

   Specification of Retinal Illuminance for Infant Eyes 130
   Light Losses in the Ocular Media 130
   Measurements of Dark-Adapted Sensitivity 130
   Mechanisms of Increased Sensitivity: Changes in Quantal Catch 133
   Axial Density of Rhodopsin in Rod Outer Segments 133
   Temporal Summation Functions 135
   Postreceptoral Pooling: Spatial Processing 136
   Background Adaptation in Infants 136
   Dynamics of Bleaching Adaptation 139
   Summary 139

9. Infant Color Vision: OKN Techniques and Null Plane Analysis 143
   Davida Y. Teller and Delwin T. Lindsey

   Three-Dimensional Color Spaces 144
   Moving Stimuli and Optokinetic Nystagmus 152
   Experiments with Infant Subjects 155
   Summary and Conclusions 160

10. Orientation- and Motion-Selective Mechanisms in Infants 163
    Oliver Braddick

    Development of Orientation Selectivity 163
    Motion-Selective Mechanisms 170
    Motion-Selectivity: Discussion 173

11. Intrinsic Noise and Infant Visual Performance 178
    Angela M. Brown

    Infant Rod Vision and the Contribution of Hansen and Fulton 179
    Infant Color Vision and the Contribution of Teller and Lindsey 182
    Ideal Observer Theory and the Contribution of Banks and Crowell 183
    Contrast Discrimination Experiment 187
    Conclusions 192
    Appendix 193

IV BINOCULAR VISION

    Introduction 197
    Eileen E. Birch

12. Development of Interocular Vision in Infants 201
    Shinsuke Shimojo

    Onset of Binocular Functions 201
    Prestereoptic Visual System 202

Interocular Vision and Occlusion Constraints 214
Concerning Acquisition of Interocular Visual Functions 221

13. Stereopsis in Infants and its Developmental Relation to Visual Acuity 224
    Eileen E. Birch

    Paradigms for Assessment of Stereopsis in Human Infants 224
    Onset of Stereopsis in the Human Infant 225
    Factors That May Determine Age of Onset 225
    What Are Infants Discriminating? 227
    Stereoacuity Development During Infancy 228
    Hyperacuity 228
    Simultaneous Perception, Fusion, and Stereopsis 229
    Acuity and Stereopsis 229
    Neural Mechanisms of Binocular Development 231
    Stereopsis and Acuity in Infantile Esotropia 232
    Summary and Conclusions 234

14. Sensorimotor Adaptation and Development of the Horopter 237
    Clifton M. Schor

    Binocular Disparity 237
    Theoretical Longitudinal Horopter 238
    Theoretical Vertical Horopter 238
    Empirical Longitudinal Horopter 240
    Empirical Vertical Horopter 242
    Development of Ocular Parameters 242
    Influence of Growth Parameters on the Empirical Horopter 243
    IPD 244
    Hering's Law of Yoked Versional Eye Movements 246

15. Two Stages in the Development of Binocular Vision and Eye Alignment 250
    Richard Held

    Onset of Stereopsis 250
    Further Tests of the Two-Stage Model 252
    Clinical Relevance 253
    Conclusions 255

16. On the Development of the Threshold Nonlinearity, Peripheral Acuity, Binocularity, and Complex Stereoscopic Processing 258
    Christopher W. Tyler

    Nature of Sensory Threshold in Infants 258
    Visual Processing in the Infant Periphery 261
    Development of Stereopsis 263
    Modes of Binocular Processing 267
    Proposed Experiments for Infant Binocular Vision 278

V RETINAL AND CORTICAL DEVELOPMENT

Introduction 285
Michael P. Stryker

17. Morphological Development of the Primate
    Retina **287**
    Anita E. Hendrickson

    Development of Cell Populations in Primate
        Retina 287
    Development of the Fovea 287
    Development of Peripheral Retina 291
    Relation of Foveal Maturation and Spatial Visual
        Acuity Development 293

18. Biological Limits on Visual Development in
    Primates **296**
    J. Anthony Movshon and Lynne Kiorpes

    Development of Spatial Vision 296
    Limits on Normal Visual Development 297
    Environmental Influences on Visual
        Development 300
    Limits on Visual Performance After Visual
        Deprivation 301
    Conclusions 303

VI ABNORMAL VISUAL DEVELOPMENT

Introduction 307
Mark J. Greenwald

19. Clinical Examination of Infant Visual
    Status **309**
    Anne B. Fulton, Ronald M. Hansen,
    D. Luisa Mayer, and Dorothy W. Rodier

    Patients 309
    Office Examination by Pediatric
        Ophthalmologist 311
    Clinical Measures of Visual Function 312
    Summary 315

20. Visual Acuity Testing in Infants: From
    Laboratory to Clinic **318**
    Velma Dobson

    Acuity Card Procedure 318
    Research Base 319
    Acuity Card Studies 321
    Limitations of the Acuity Card Procedure 329
    Nonscientific Considerations Related to Transition
        from Laboratory to Clinic 330
    Summary and Speculation about Transition of
        Acuity Cards from Laboratory to Clinic 331

21. Infant Vision Screening: Prediction and
    Prevention of Strabismus and Amblyopia
    from Refractive Screening in the
    Cambridge Photorefraction Program **335**
    Janette Atkinson

    Review of Screening Procedures 336
    New Screening Techniques 338
    Cambridge Infant Screening Program 340
    Meridional Amblyopia 344
    Accommodative Ability in Children with Refractive
        Errors 345
    Summary and Conclusions 346

22. Detection and Treatment of Congenital
    Esotropia **349**
    Steven M. Archer

    Detection of Congenital Esotropia 349
    Treatment of Congenital Esotropia 353
    Summary 359

23. Motion Sensitivity and the Origins of
    Infantile Strabismus **364**
    Lawrence Tychsen

    Onset of Eye Alignment During the First Year of
        Life 364
    Possible Visual Signals Guiding Eye Alignment 365
    Methods That Probe Motion Pathways of the Visual
        Cortex 365
    Nasotemporal Biases of Motion Processing in
        Strabismus 366
    Nasal Motion Bias and Interruptions of Binocularity
        During the Critical Period 367
    Nasotemporal Inputs to the Primary Visual Cortex:
        Example of Nasal Dominance 371
    Topographical Distortions of the Motion Pathway in
        Strabismus 372
    Codevelopment of Motion Processing, Stereopsis,
        and Eye Alignment 374
    Vicious Cycle: Visual Motion Pathway in
        Immaturity and Esotropia 375
    Esotropia as a Motor Adaptation to a Visual
        Bias 376
    Genetic and Environmental Factors That May
        Retard Motion Pathway Development and
        Promote Esotropia 376
    Schematic for the Topographical Abnormalities of
        Nasally Biased Motion Processing 377
    Movement Detector Model for Nasally Directed
        Bias 379
    Binocular Motion Processing Inputs to
        Vergence 381
    Experiments Necessary to Validate the Model 382
    Historical Notions of the Cause of Infantile
        Strabismus 384

24. Amblyopia: A Consequence of Abnormal
    Visual Development **391**
    Dennis M. Levi and Andrew Carkeet

    Visual Function in Amblyopia 391
    Visual Function in Infants 395
    Susceptibility to Abnormal Visual Input: "Detroit
        Model" 398
    Does the Infant Visual System Provide a Reasonable
        Model for Amblyopia? 399

"Natural History" of Amblyopia Development   401
Summary   405

25.   Stereoscopic Neurontropy and the Origins
      of Amblyopia and Strabismus   409
      Kurt Simons

      Visual Development: Biocularity to Binocular
         Stereopsis   409
      Binocular versus Monocular Vision in
         Development   413
      Risk Factors for Spatial Mapping Distortions in
         Strabismic Amblyopia   415
      Optomotor and Fusion Defects   426
      Neurontropy Model of Mapping Distortion
         Origins   427
      Fusion versus Stereopsis in Strabismogenesis   435
      Conclusions: Clinical and Research
         Implications   438

26.   Visual Outcomes After Infantile
      Cataract   454
      Daphne Maurer and Terri L. Lewis

      Grating Acuity   455
      Linear Letter Acuity   463
      Contrast Sensitivity   466
      Fusion and Stereopsis   472
      Symmetry of OKN   474
      General Discussion   477

27.   Prematurity and Visual Development   485
      Alistair R. Fielder, Nigel Foreman,
      Merrick J. Moseley, and Judith Robinson

      Premature Population   486
      Neonatal Eye   486
      Ophthalmology of the Preterm Infant   489
      Environment   490
      Attention   492
      Electroretinography   496
      Visually Evoked Potentials   496
      Behavioral Tests   497
      Visual Field and Color Vision   497
      Innate versus Environmental Influences   497
      Refractive Status   498
      Clinical Issues   498

28.   Visual Factors in Developmental Delay and
      Neurological Disorders in Infants   505
      Creig S. Hoyt and William V. Good

      Electrophysiological and Psychophysical
         Studies   506
      Pathogenesis of Delayed Visual Maturation During
         Infancy   507
      Neuroradiological Considerations   508
      Discussion and Conclusions   510

VII   WHAT NEXT IN INFANT RESEARCH?

      Introduction   513
      Kurt Simons

29.   Use of Models to Improve Hypothesis
      Delineation: A Study of Infant
      Electroretinography   517
      Donald C. Hood, David G. Birch, and
      Eileen E. Birch

      Neonatal Electroretinogram   517
      Simple, Static, Two-Stage Model of the Adult
         ERG   519
      Measuring the Parameters of the Receptors (σ_{P3} and
         Rm_{P3})   521
      Need for a Dynamic Model of the ERG   524
      Dynamic Model of the ERG   526
      Dynamic Model and Hypotheses About
         Development   526
      Summary of the Modeling of the Infant ERG   531
      Delineating Hypotheses About Mechanisms of
         Development and a Comparison to Anatomical
         Data   531
      Comparison to Psychophysical Data and
         Consideration of General Problems With
         Psychophysical Models   532
      Comments on Behavioral Models   532
      Summary   533

30.   Improving Infant Evoked Response
      Measurement   536
      Anthony M. Norcia

      Special Challenges of Pediatric Low-Vision
         Assessment   536
      Quantitative Assessment of Vision Using the Sweep
         VEP   537
      Threshold Assumption   538
      Modern Signal Processing Methods Applied to the
         SSVEP   539
      Improving Measurements Through Multichannel
         Recording   541
      Improved Detection of Small VEPs by Recording
         Multiple Response Harmonics   543
      Frequency Diversity Methods for VEP
         Detection   544
      Improving Measurements Through Judicious Choice
         of Stimuli   544
      Improving Grating Acuity Measurement   545
      Alternative VEP Resolution Measures   545
      Multiinput Stimulation/Analysis Paradigms   548
      Conclusion   550

31.   Whither Infant Psychophysics?   553
      Israel Abramov

      Who Are the Subjects?   553
      Stimulus Variables   554
      Methods for Testing Infants   555

Psychophysiological Linking Hypotheses 557
Conclusions 558

32. Theories of Infant Visual
     Development 560
     Hugh R. Wilson
     Infant Retinal Anatomy 560
     Effect of Reduced Outer Segment Length 561

Effect of Reduced Foveal Cone Density 561
Mathematical Development 563
Infant Acuity and Contrast Sensitivity 565
Flicker Sensitivity 568
Cortical Development 569
Conclusions and Conjectures 569

Index 573

Contributors

ISRAEL ABRAMOV
Infant Study Center, Brooklyn College, City
    University of New York

STEVEN M. ARCHER
W.K. Kellogg Eye Center, University of Michigan

RICHARD N. ASLIN
Center for Visual Science, University of Rochester

JANETTE ATKINSON
Visual Development Unit, University of Cambridge,
    U.K.

MARTIN S. BANKS
School of Optometry and Department of Psychology,
    University of California, Berkeley

DAVID G. BIRCH
Retina Foundation of the Southwest, Dallas

EILEEN E. BIRCH
Retinea Foundation of the Southwest, Dallas, Texas,
    and Department of Ophthalmology, University
    of Texas Southwestern Medical Center

ANGELA M. BROWN
College of Optometry, Ohio State

OLIVER BRADDICK
Department of Experimental Psychology, University
    of Cambridge, U.K.

ANDREW CARKEET
College of Optometry, University of Houston

JAMES A. CROWELL
School of Optometry and Department of Psychology,
    University of California, Berkeley

VELMA DOBSON
Departments of Psychiatry and Psychology, University
    of Pittsburgh

ALISTAIR R. FIELDER
Department of Ophthalmology, University of
    Birmingham Medical School, U.K.

DOM V. FINOCCHIO
Department of Psychology, University of Washington

NIGEL FOREMAN
Department of Psychology, University of Leicester,
    U.K.

ANNE B. FULTON
Department of Ophthalmology, Children's Hospital,
    Boston, and Harvard Medical School

WILLIAM V. GOOD
Department of Ophthalmology, University of
    California, San Francisco

MARK J. GREENWALD
Children's Memorial Hospital, Chicago

LOUISE HAINLINE
Infant Study Center, Brooklyn College, City
    University of New York

RONALD M. HANSEN
Department of Ophthalmology, Children's Hospital,
    Boston, and Harvard Medical School

RICHARD HELD
Infant Vision Laboratory, Massachusetts Institute of
    Technology

ANITA E. HENDRICKSON
Departments of Biological Structure and
    Ophthalmology, University of Washington

DONALD C. HOOD
Department of Psychology, Columbia University

HOWARD C. HOWLAND
Section of Neurobiology and Behavior, Cornell
    University

CREIG S. HOYT
Department of Ophthalmology, University of
    California, San Francisco

LYNNE KIORPES
Center for Neural Science, and Department of
    Psychology, New York University

DENNIS M. LEVI
College of Optometry, University of Houston

TERRI L. LEWIS
McMaster University and The Hospital for Sick
    Children, Ontario

DELWIN T. LINDSEY
Department of Psychology, University of Washington

DAPHNE MAURER
McMaster University and The Hospital for Sick
    Children, Ontario

D. LUISA MAYER
Department of Ophthalmology, Children's Hospital,
    Boston

MERRICK J. MOSELEY
Department of Ophthalmology, University of
    Birmingham Medical School, U.K.

J. ANTHONY MOVSHON
Howard Hughes Medical Institute, and Department
    of Physiology and Biophysics, New York
    University

ANTHONY M. NORCIA
Smith-Kettlewell Eye Research Institute, San
    Francisco

KAREN L. PRESTON
Department of Psychology, University of Washington

JUDITH ROBINSON
Department of Ophthalmology, University of
    Birmingham Medical School, U.K.

DOROTHY W. RODIER
Department of Ophthalmology, Children's Hospital,
    Boston, and Harvard Medical School

FRANK SCHAEFFEL
Department of Experimental Ophthalmology,
    University Eye Hospital, Tübingen, Germany

CLIFTON M. SCHOR
School of Optometry, University of California,
    Berkeley

SHINSUKE SHIMOJO
Department of Psychology, University of Tokyo

KURT SIMONS
The Wilmer Ophthalmological Institute, The Johns
    Hopkins University School of Medicine

MICHAEL P. STRYKER
Department of Physiology, University of California,
    San Francisco

DAVIDA Y. TELLER
Department of Physiology and Biophysics, University
    of Washington

LAWRENCE TYCHSEN
Departments of Ophthalmology, Anatomy and
    Neurobiology, Washington University School of
    Medicine, St. Louis

CHRISTOPHER W. TYLER
Smith-Kettlewell Eye Research Institute, San
    Francisco

HUGH R. WILSON
Visual Sciences Center, University of Chicago

Early Visual Development
Normal and Abnormal

I. Refractive Development Introduction

HOWARD C. HOWLAND

How does the image come to be focused on the retina, and how can our two eyes point so precisely at the same object of regard? These central questions are addressed in this first section on refractive development.

We accept the incredible competence of adult vision as a given of our sensory world. However, anyone who has attempted to attract the attention of a newborn infant knows that infant motor control of fixation is uncertain at best. The same may be said for neonatal focusing, as is shown in Chapter 2. How then does the competent binocular vision of adults develop from the uncertain fixation and focusing of infancy? How indeed do we answer such a question?

As at the beginning of all investigations, we must first describe what happens before we can discover how and why it happens. Chapter 1, on early refractive development, is largely devoted to a description of various techniques for measuring refractive state and focusing as well as the measurements obtained with these techniques of the eyes of infants and young children. Ophthalmologists have long used cycloplegic drugs to paralyze the accommodation of the eye to fix it in a constant optical state. Developmental studies, however, have concentrated on the focusing and fixation abilities of infants under normal viewing conditions. This change has come about because it is now known that both the quality and the alignment of images in the two eyes determine whether a child will become amblyopic or develop normal binocular vision.

The hope of many developmental studies of focusing and refractive state has been to relate early findings to later visual problems. To use this technique requires long-term, longitudinal studies that are generally difficult to conduct, especially in the United States, which has a mobile population. However, several studies, reviewed in Chapter 1, have begun to produce useful data on the fate of astigmatism, on the genesis of myopia and hyperopia, and on the association of early refractive and focusing conditions with later development of strabismus and amblyopia.

Another finding that has arisen from the review of developmental refractive studies is the importance of genetic background on the prevalence of refractive anomalies. It is clear that descriptions of normal refractive development must take into account the racial and genetic composition of the groups studied.

The kinds of experimental intervention prevented in humans by ethical considerations are still possible in animal studies. During the 1980s and early 1990s experimental animal research has begun to provide us with a picture of the mechanisms and feedback loops that guide refractive development. As is seen in Frank Schaeffel's review, both primates and birds have supplied us with models of myopia induced by environmental interventions—generally, growing eyes with sutured lids or covered by translucent occluders. In addition, it has been possible to demonstrate in chickens that emmetropization (growth such that the image falls on the retina) can be modified by lenses. These studies have opened the door to biochemical investigations of the regulation of eye growth and hold out the hope that the growth of human eyes may one day be manipulated therapeutically with pharmacological means.

Although chicks provide a good model for emmetropization, they fail as models for the development of frontal, binocular vision. Here we must turn again to human developmental data as outlined in the third chapter of this section.

Aslin gives four general categories of explanation of the maturation of the accommodative and convergence systems. They involve changes in (1) motivation, (2) sensory capacity, (3) motor capacity, and (4) coordination between sensory and motor mechanisms. The relative contributions of these four factors to development is still a matter of research.

During the first year of life, accommodative and convergence behavior are changing along with visual acuity. How are these three linked? Aslin shows that both accommodative and convergence behavior mature rapidly over the first 3 *months* of life, whereas visual acuity matures slowly over the first *year* of life. Parallel to this slow improvement of acuity is a corresponding improvement in the *accuracy* of vergence movement.

Aslin suggests that the first 3 months of life, when development is so rapid, afford a fertile area for research, provided we can bring to it instruments that have suitable dynamic capabilities for measuring accommodation and convergence. In addition, he shows that we need new animal models for the development of binocular vision.

Taken together, these chapters should convince the reader that the growth and emmetropization of the eye, the development of focusing mechanisms, and the development of the interacting feed back and feed-forward loops of accommodation and convergence are intertwined and that any difficulty encountered in any one of them has the potential of derailing the development of all of them. The elements of these interactions are expanded upon in many of the subsequent chapters of this book.

1 | Early refractive development

HOWARD C. HOWLAND

When discussing the refractive development of infants and young children, one must distinguish among the various measures of refraction. By *cycloplegic refraction*, we mean the refractive state of the eye after it has been instilled with drugs that paralyze the muscles of accommodation. In this situation, the visual scene at which the eye is directed plays no role in the measured refractive state. By *noncycloplegic* or *manifest refraction*, we mean the refractive state of the eye as measured without drugs. In this situation, the visual conditions under which the eye is refracted may play a significant role in the resulting refraction. For example, the eye may be examined while the fellow eye views a scene through a positive or "fogging" lens, a procedure designed to relax the accommodation. Often this measure is referred to simply as a noncycloplegic refraction. However, because there are several kinds of noncycloplegic refractions, it might more properly be called a *fogged refraction*. Alternatively, the eye may be refracted in near total darkness, in which case it would be logical to refer to the result as a "dark" refraction, although this measure has come to be known in the literature as a *near refraction* (Mohindra, 1977). In this situation, the eye is assumed to revert to a resting state of refraction, often slightly myopic. Still other refractive measurements may be made while the infant or child is fixated, and presumably attempting to focus, on a target at a finite distance. Such a situation is typical of photorefractive measurements (Howland and Howland, 1974; Howland et al., 1983; Howland, 1985). Clearly, in young accommodating eyes, such measurements can tell nothing about the degree of hyperopia that other refractive methods might measure. Such a procedure, however, would reveal myopias where the eye was focused in front of the visual target and, depending on the type of measurement, astigmatisms. For the sake of the following discussions, we may term such a procedure a *finite focus refraction*.

It is important to note that each refractive procedure has certain advantages. Whereas it is of interest to measure the most hyperopic position of focus of the eye as induced by drugs, it is also of interest to know how the undrugged eye behaves in the presence of normal visual stimuli.

Insofar as we broaden our discussion beyond cycloplegic refractions, we must include some consideration of accommodation in our review. It is particularly true of photorefractive studies of infants in whom the ability to accommodate to targets at finite distances is not fully developed.

Another aspect of refractive studies to which we must devote some attention is the method of subject or patient selection and the nature of the population under study. It is known that there are significant differences in refraction among the races (Curtin, 1985). It is also clear that particular patient groups (premature or mentally deficient patients) may show significantly augmented refractive errors (Howland and Sayles, 1983).

The reader may also wish to consult earlier reviews that bear on the subject handled here. Particularly to be recommended is that of Banks (1980). I have also written two short reviews on this topic (Howland, 1982a, 1988), and a useful refractive bibliography has been provided by Baldwin (1990).

In the following review, I have first treated those studies that could conveniently be grouped as covering one of three age groups: (1) neonates; (2) 1 month to 1 year; and (3) 1–5 years. Net spherical refraction and astigmatism in particular are treated in this manner. I then consider individual topics that did not seem to fit well into this age classification. They include biometric components of refraction, anisometropia, and the implications of early refractive states for later refractive development.

EARLY INFANCY: NORMAL DEVELOPMENT

Many workers have commented on the difficulty of refracting newborn infants. The neonates' lids may have to be held open, their pupils are small, and their gaze wanders erratically. The last factor must contribute considerable variance to the data because of the inability to precisely control which axis is being refracted.

5

Net Spherical Defocus: Cycloplegic and Noncycloplegic Findings

Early in the study of infant refraction, data were collected that indicated a large difference between cycloplegic and noncycloplegic refractions. Jaeger (1861), as cited by Goldschmidt (1969), found that the eyes of 78 of 100 infants in Copenhagen were myopically focused when examined without atropine; and in New York City, Ely (1880) found that 72 of 100 infants' eyes that he examined with atropine were hyperopic. Herrnheiser (1892) examined 1920 atropinized eyes of neonates, all of which were hyperopic, in German clinics. In all of the above studies, the refraction was determined with an ophthalmoscope.

Cook and Glasscock (1951) examined by retinoscopy 1000 eyes of neonates in Little Rock, Arkansas. The population studied included a high percentage of blacks (63%). The authors found that approximately 75% of the eyes were hyperopic and 25% myopic. The early data of cycloplegic refractions, obtained from primarily European white populations and summarized by Goldschmidt (1969), show an average cycloplegic refraction of between 2.2 and 4.4 diopters (D) hyperopia.

Mehra et al. (1965) examined 100 term infants in Benares, India. They found that 79 were hyperopic, 9 were myopic, and 12 had astigmatisms greater than 2.0 D.

Santonastaso (1930), using retinoscopy, found a large difference between cycloplegic and noncycloplegic refraction in infants. Using his data from an Italian population, it may be calculated that for 19 infants during the first 15 days of life (cases 1–8 and 26) there was a mean ($\pm$ SD) net spherical noncycloplegic refraction of -7.03 ± 3.53 D. Cycloplegic refractions for the same infants yielded a mean of $+0.98 \pm 2.65$ D.

Santonastaso's cycloplegic refractions were generally less hyperopic than those reported by earlier workers, as were those of Goldschmidt (1969). Goldschmidt, who examined 356 infants 2–10 days of age in Copenhagen, found a mean ($\pm$ SD) refraction of 0.62 ± 2.24 D with no difference between males and females. Neither Goldschmidt nor this reviewer could determine whether the wide variation seen in cycloplegic refractions of newborns is due to differences in technique or genetic differences between groups of infants. From observations on nonhuman primates, I know that atropinized eyes may exhibit large pupils even though the accommodation is not paralyzed. Thus it may well be that with procedures where the examination was made at a considerable time after the instillation of atropine (e.g., Goldschmidt, who examined the infants 24 hours after atropine instillation), it was not an effective cycloplegic. With ophthalmoscopy, it is possible that the observer accommodates, thus requiring the use of more negative power than otherwise would be necessary. It would of course bias the results toward myopia. Because the early ophthalmoscopic examinations on atropinized eyes showed a predominant hyperopia, it is unlikely that this potential error played much of a role in their results.

On the other hand, there is much evidence to suggest racial differences in refractions (Curtin, 1985), and one should perhaps not be surprised that international comparisons of data sets should yield discrepant values of net sphere. Thus if forced to a single opinion, I would incline to the view that the differences seen in net spherical refractions of atropinized eyes of infants are due to genetic differences among the populations studied.

Mohindra and Held (1981) reported net spherical refractions for 48 neonates between birth and 4 weeks of age obtained by noncycloplegic "near" retinoscopy (Mohindra, 1977) in Boston area hospitals. The distribution of refractive errors for this age group was compared to the data of Cook and Glasscock (1951) and found to be similar, but more myopic by several diopters. Their average ($\pm$ SE) refraction was -0.7 ± 0.46 D. The reader should be aware that in this study, although the working distance was 0.5 meter, only 1.25 D was subtracted from the neutralizing net sphere to obtain the reported refractions. This "correction" was discussed further by Mohindra (1977).

In summary, it is clear from the above studies that neonates are generally myopically focused when not cyclopleged. Moreover, they exhibit, on average, somewhat hyperopic refractions under cycloplegia.

Artifact of Retinoscopy

Glickstein and Millodot (1970) have suggested that the apparent hyperopia of small mammals may be the result of the retinoscopic reflex being reflected from the retinal vitreous border approximately 135 μm in front of the photoreceptor layer of the retina. They evidently averaged data from Cook and Glasscock (1951) for human neonates to arrive at a value of 1.75 D hyperopia, which they then combined with data from 23 other mammals to obtain a regression relation between apparent hyperopia and eye diameter. Their regression relation is:

$$\text{Apparent hyperopia (D)} = k/x^2 \qquad (1)$$

where k = a constant whose whose units are meters; and x = the diameter of the eye, also in meters. Unfortunately, Glickstein and Millodot did not give the value of x; however, from their Figure 2, it may be inferred to be 2.571×10^{-4} in Eq. (1). If we assume that the axial diameter of a neonate's eye is 18 mm, Eq. (1) gives a value of 0.8 D hyperopia, in agreement with the calculations of Banks (1980). It should be noted that, however likely in theory the existence of such an artifact may be, to my knowledge there is no direct evidence of one in human eyes as there is, for example, in the eyes of flying foxes (Murphy et al., 1983).

Astigmatism During Early Infancy

Relatively few workers have examined astigmatism during early infancy. Cook and Glasscock (1951) reported that 29% of their hyperopes and 27% of they myopes were astigmatic, with mixed astigmatism present in only 3% of their subjects. Unfortunately, the criteria for the presence of astigmatism are not given, nor are any further data on its severity.

Santonastaso (1930) reported refractions in both the vertical and horizontal meridians for both cycloplegic and noncycloplegic refractions from which minimum values of astigmatism may be calculated. Using his neonatal data (19 infants), I find a mean absolute difference ($\pm$ SE) in vertical and horizontal meridians to be 1.13 $\pm$ 0.17 D for noncycloplegic refractions and 0.95 $\pm$ 0.11 D for cycloplegic refractions. He saw a large difference in the astigmatism under these two conditions. It may be calculated that the average absolute value of this difference between astigmatisms measured under these two conditions on the same eyes is 1.3 D. Neither group exhibits significantly more astigmatism, nor does there appear to be a systematic change in astigmatism with the application of atropine.

Using 93 children from birth to 1 year in Cambridge, England, Howland et al. (1978) and Braddick et al. (1979) examined the astigmatism of early infancy using noncycloplegic orthogonal (Howland and Howland, 1974) and isotropic (Howland et al., 1983) photorefraction. These techniques refract orthogonal axes simultaneously and hence are not subject to errors of fluctuation of accommodation when estimating astigmatisms. They found that approximately half of the neonates had astigmatisms of between 0.75 and 2.00 D. Using the same techniques, they found that only 10% of mothers of the infants they studied were astigmatic, and these women exhibited astigmatisms of 1.0 D or less.

Mohindra et al. (1978), using near retinoscopy, found a smaller proportion of neonates (20%) to be astigmatic; however, their proportions during subsequent weeks rose to approximately the levels of Howland et al. (1978) for comparable age groups. The astigmatisms reported by Mohindra et al. (1978) were generally more severe than those of Howland et al. (1978), but this difference is doubtless due to the limits of measurement of orthogonal photorefraction.

There seems to be little doubt that a considerable proportion of neonates exhibit astigmatisms that would be of clinical significance in adults and that, as will be seen, generally diminish over the first few years of life.

Infant Astigmatism: Not an Artifact of Off-Axis Refractions

Banks (1980) considered the argument that infant astigmatism may be an artifact of off-axis refractions. He noted that the eye should exhibit against-the-rule astigmatism in the horizontal meridian as it is refracted off-axis, and that either failure to refract the correct axis or the large angle alpha of infants (the angle between the optic axis and the visual axis) could result in the large astigmatisms seen during infancy.

However, there are now three arguments against this hypothesis. First, Howland and Sayles (1987) showed that, with their photorefractive procedures conducted on 360 volunteers in central New York, infants fixated their cameras with a standard deviation of 2.3 degrees, which implies that more than 95% of photorefractions were within 5 degrees of the visual axis. Hence it is unlikely that the observed astigmatisms are due to refractions far from the visual axis. It is further unlikely that the astigmatism is due to large separation of the visual and optic axes and therefore reflects the off-axis astigmatism of a simple optical system. It is because the off-axis astigmatism of the human eye within 25 degrees of the optic axis is generally less than 1.0 D (Dunne and Barnes, 1987). Lastly, we have shown that a great proportion of infant astigmatism is corneal in nature (Howland and Sayles, 1985).

EARLY INFANCY: PREMATURITY

Net Spherical Defocus: Cycloplegic Refractions

Gleiss and Pau (1952) studied the cycloplegic refractions of 23 premature German infants and divided them into three groups: hyperopes ($n = 12$); myopes that emmetropized or became hyperopic ($n = 7$); and myopes that remained myopic ($n = 4$). In all but one infant, the trend of subsequent refractions was toward increased hyperopia. In Israel, Scharf et al. (1975) found a strongly bimodal distribution of net spherical refractions in 180 premature infants with peaks at -4.0 and $+1.0$ D. They found no relation between birth weight and degree of myopia. After 6 months there appeared to be a general trend toward emmetropia in both myopic and hyperopic infants. In a later study, these authors found that 7 years after the initial examination 54% of 67 premature infants who were followed retained their myopia, though generally in lesser degrees than they had exhibited at birth. Unfortunately, the authors did not follow a control group for comparison.

Working with the charts of 233 infants in two Boston hospitals, Dobson et al. (1981) found higher levels of myopia and anisometropia in a population of 146 premature infants than in a control group. They found a significant correlation between myopia and prematurity. The bimodality seen by Scharf et al. (1975) was not evident in their data. Subsequent studies have tended to confirm the picture described above (Gerhard, 1983; Grose and Harding, 1990).

Astigmatism in Premature Infants

Dobson et al. (1981) found that more than 70% of their premature infants showed an astigmatism of 1.0 D or more, and that the magnitude of cylindrical error was inversely correlated with gestational age. These amounts of astigmatism were much higher than reported by other workers in premature infants, as reviewed by Dobson et al. (1981), and larger than are generally reported for cycloplegic refractions of normal infants.

REFRACTIVE DEVELOPMENT FROM 3 MONTHS TO 1 YEAR OF AGE

By about 3 months after birth, infants can hold up their heads and direct their gaze fairly reliably and accurately, making it possible to refract them using a variety of methods. From 3 to 6 months, the infant's ability to fixate and focus a target at 1.5 meters improves dramatically (Braddick et al., 1979).

Net Spherical Defocus: Cycloplegic Findings

Santonastaso (1930) found a peak mean net spherical refraction of almost 3.0 D in 1-month-old infants that declined gradually to less than 2.0 D by 12 months. Dobson et al. (1981) examined 5042 consecutive charts of children examined in the Boston Children's Hospital Medical Center and determined the distribution of refractive errors for normal, esotropic, and amblyopic patients. They reported that distributions for the age classes of the first 3 years were similar. The mean refraction was 1.27 D for normal children, with 90% of the children exhibiting a refraction between 0 and 2.25 D.

In Cambridge, England, Atkinson et al. (1984) screened 1096 infants between 6 and 9 months of age with cyclopentolate cycloplegia and isotropic photorefraction. They found 55 infants to have hyperopia of more than 3.5 D, 45 infants to have myopias greater than 1.33 D, 14 anisometropes, and 3 strabismics. Eighty-nine percent of their infants showed none of the above characteristics and were therefore classified as "normal."

Net Spherical Defocus: Noncycloplegic Findings

Mohindra and Held (1981), examining a Boston metropolitan population of volunteers, found that the net spherical refraction ($\pm$ SE) as measured by near retinoscopy increased from -0.5 ± 0.25 D in infants aged 9–16 weeks to 0.8 ± 0.15 D in infants aged 33–64 weeks. At the same time, the standard deviations of their distributions decreased from 2.0 D to 1.0 D.

Howland and Sayles (1987) observed a similar sharpening in the distribution of net spherical defocus of two groups of infants focusing a photographer's face at 1.5 meters distance. The mean ages of the two groups were 0.3 and 0.7 years. In the first group, 95% of the infants exhibited a defocus of between -1.7 and $+2.4$ D, whereas in the second group these limits were -0.8 and $+1.2$ D. Their 360 subjects were recruited from a university community in central New York State.

The similarity of reduction in refractive and focusing errors over the first year of life raises the possibility that the two techniques are, in fact, measuring the same thing: that is, either that near retinoscopy is measuring the focusing error of infants, or photorefraction is measuring the refractive error of infants. The first possibility suggests that the retinoscope presents a good accommodative target. However, this point was shown not to be so by Owens et al. (1980). Somewhat more likely is the possibility that, during the first half year of life, photorefraction is measuring the noncyclopleged refractive state of some infants, as the ability to focus a target at 1.5 meters is imperfect in 2- to 3-month-old infants (Braddick et al., 1979). Be that as it may, there is no reason to suppose that emmetropization and increased focusing ability occur with the same time course over the first year of life.

Reduction of Astigmatism During the First Year(s) of Life

Dobson et al. (1984) reported on the astigmatism seen in a retrospective study of 5042 cyclopleged infants and young children in Boston Children's Hospital. They showed a slight increase in the percentage of astigmatics when groups of infants 0–6 months of age and 6–18 months were compared. However, it is difficult to interpret this increase because this clinical sample is from a children's hospital.

Various noncycloplegic studies of infant astigmatism have shown that the defect reduces over time but that there are different courses for its reduction. Studying 62 children between 9 and 39 months old in Cambridge, England, Atkinson et al. (1980) showed that individual infants exhibit a strong tendency toward the reduction of astigmatism over the first year of life, estimating that it returned to adult levels within 1.5 years. In a population of 312 children in central New York State, Howland and Sayles (1984) found that this reduction was slower and estimated that it occurred over the first 5 years of life. Gwiazda et al. (1984), in their study of 1000 Boston area children at birth to age 6 years, showed a still slower time course, with significant amounts of astigmatism remaining at 6 years.

All three of the above studies reported a prevalence of against-the-rule astigmatism (negative cylinder axis within 15 degrees of vertical meridian) during early infancy and a reduction of this against-the-rule astigmatism by school age; all were based on samples of primarily caucasian infants from the eastern United States. Evidently, the axis of infant astigmatism (with- or against-the-rule) is racially determined. Thorn et al. (1987) found in a study of 23 Chinese and 22 caucasian infants that, although most caucasian infants had against-the-rule astigmatism, most of the Chinese infants had with-the-rule astigmatism.

As noted before, Howland and Sayles, in a study of 90 infants and young children in central New York State, showed by photokeratometry that the astigmatism of infancy is primarily corneal in nature (Howland and Sayles, 1985).

Consequences of Early Astigmatism

In a study of 89 infants 7–53 weeks old in the Boston area, Gwiazda et al. (1985) have shown that there is no evidence for the development of meridional amblyopia in infant astigmatics during the first year of life. When infants undergo optical correction for their astigmatism, their preferential looking behavior to striped acuity targets is indistinguishable from that of nonastigmatic infants.

Elsewhere I have speculated that the astigmatism of infancy might be useful for improving the accuracy of accommodation to complex targets in that the overlap of the zones of high contrast with respect to focus is greatly narrowed with astigmatism (Howland, 1982b). If this hypothesis is true, it must be that astigmatic infants focus a complex target within the interval of Sturm, and that they exhibit less net spherical defocus than nonastigmatic infants. A somewhat cursory inspection of data in our longitudinal photorefractive study (Howland, unpublished data) shows that this possibility indeed may be the case. For a group of 40 infants (20 < 1.5 D cylinder, 20 > 1.5 D cyl, mean age 140 days), the net spherical defocus of astigmatics and nonastigmatics attempting to focus the face of the photographer differed by approximately 0.5 D, with the astigmatics defocused on the average by 0.5 D and the nonastigmatics by 1.0 D. It will be interesting to see if a more complete analysis of our data bears out the significance of this preliminary result.

If astigmatism does indeed improve the accuracy of accommodation, it might explain why Gwiazda et al. (1985) did not detect a difference in visual acuity between astigmatic and nonastigmatic infants at 1 year of age. The blur induced by astigmatism may have been compensated for by the reduction in blur due to more accurate focusing.

It is also important to note that accommodation not only improves the sharpness of images transmitted to the brain but also serves to steer convergence (Carpenter, 1988). Despite these considerations, why some infants are astigmatic and some are not remains an open question.

REFRACTIVE DEVELOPMENT FROM 1 TO 5 YEARS OF AGE

Net Spherical Defocus: Cycloplegic Findings

Herrnheiser (1892) reported that of 534 young children in a German kindergarten, 72% were hyperopic, 24% emmetropic, and 4% myopic. Brown (1938) conducted a longitudinal study designed to reveal the changes in refraction for subjects examined two times or more. Basing his results on more than 1600 "retinoscopic computations" done on children in the Chicago area, he reported that the average annual increases in hyperopia over the first 7 years of life were 0.41, 0.43, 0.27, 0.21, 0.13, and 0.02. The alert reader may note that there are only six values—not seven. Be that as it may, it is also clear that as time progresses the increase in hyperopia decreases. Indeed, Brown found that it decreases for the subsequent 26 years of life.

Slataper (1950), using longitudinal and cross-sectional techniques, reported a gradual increase in average hyperopia from 2.3 D at birth to 3.5 D at 5 years of age. Ingram and Barr (1979) also reported an increase in hyperopia from ages 1.0 to 3.5 years, results obtained from a study of 148 children in Kettering, England.

Net Spherical Defocus: Noncycloplegic Findings

Mohindra and Held (1981), using near retinoscopy, found no increases in hyperopia between the first and fifth years of life, their measurements of net spherical defocus averaging approximately 0.75 D of hyperopia. Using similar techniques, but substituting "distance retinoscopy" for near retinoscopy for children over 3 years of age, Gwiazda et al. (1990) noted that children tend to converge on a slight degree of hyperopia. (As we will see, these authors reported that only after the first 5 years of life do infant refractions apparently affect subsequent refractive states.)

Howland and Sayles (1987), using a variety of photorefractive techniques, noted a steady decrease in the net spherical defocus of infants and children's eyes focusing the face of a photographer from the first to the fifth year of life. This decrease had a different (slower) time course than that of the standard deviation of dark retinoscopy reported by Mohindra and Held, presumably indicating that the infants were not focusing during dark retinoscopy and were focusing during photorefraction.

Net Spherical Refractions of Premature Infants

Shapiro et al. (1980) examined the refraction of 198 premature children in Jerusalem with birth weights of 2000 g or less. They reported that "between the ages of 6.0 months to 3.5 years these children had a mild hypermetropia." They found no changes of refraction over this period, and they noted that the refractions were similar to those of normal children.

Astigmatism

We have already reported that infant astigmatism lessens with age (Atkinson et al., 1980; Dobson et al., 1984; Gwiazda et al., 1984; Howland and Sayles, 1984). Most authors find that it reduces to adult levels in 5-year-olds.

GENERAL ASPECTS OF EARLY REFRACTIVE DEVELOPMENT

Biometric Components of Refractive State

For a general study of the ocular components of the eye and their development, the reader should consult Sivak and Bobier (1990). The relation between particular optical components and the refraction of the eye was examined by Stenstrom (1946), who studied 1000 adults between 20 and 35 years of age. He showed that the refractive state of the eye is most strongly correlated with the axial length of the eye ($r = -0.76$) and less strongly correlated with anterior chamber depth ($r = -0.34$) and corneal curvature ($r = -0.18$). The refractive state was not correlated at all with the refractive power of the lens.

In light of these findings, it is not surprising that the principal factor in both anisometropia (Sorsby et al., 1962) and myopia (Tokoro and Suzuki, 1968) is the axial length. In both these studies (the former using 68 patients at the Royal Eye Hospital in London and the latter 18 patients at the Tokyo Medical and Dental University), the power of the cornea and the lens were found to play minor roles.

Larsen, in a series of four ultrasonographic studies on 896 infants and children in Norway, showed that with regard to axial length (Larsen, 1971d) there are three growth phases: (1) a rapid postnatal growth from birth to 1.5 years; (2) a slower infantile phase lasting to 5 years; and (3) a yet slower increase to adult values from 5 to 13 years. The negative correlation between axial length and refraction can be observed by the first year of life. With regard to the anterior chamber Larsen (1971a) again identified three growth phases with decreasing rapidity, but with termination of the juvenile phase between 7 and 8 years. The negative correlation between anterior chamber depth and refraction can be observed by the end of the second year of life. Similar observations were made on the growth of the lens (Larsen, 1971b) and the depth of the vitreous chamber (Larsen, 1971c). The former is not correlated with refraction; and the latter, like the axial length, is strongly correlated with refraction.

We have already noted above that infantile astigmatism is corneal in nature (Howland and Sayles, 1985). It should also be remarked that Yankov (1982) provided biometric data for 100 Bulgarian neonates. In all biometric studies, most components of female eyes of all ages average slightly smaller than corresponding components of male eyes, a not surprising result as this observation could also be made of most other parts of the human body.

Anisometropia

Of all the refractive techniques currently in use, only photographic or video techniques permit simultaneous measurement of the focus of both eyes. If there is any possibility of a change of focus between measurements, a simultaneous method is to be preferred. Howland and Sayles (1987), using several methods of photorefraction in a study of 360 normal infants and children, described the limits of the distribution of net spherical anisometropic refractions that circumscribed 95% of the subjects examined for several age classes. For the years 0–1, 1–2 . . . 4–5, these limits were 0.97 for the first year, then 0.54, 0.34, 0.40, and 0.34, respectively. On a longitudinal sample of subjects who could be followed for several years taken from the same (augmented) sample population, Almeder et al. (1990) found that none of the subjects initially identified as being anisometropic—i.e., falling outside the 95% limits of Howland and Sayles (1987)—retained the anisometropia. These findings are similar to those of Abrahamsson et al. (1990), who examined 310 astigmatic children in Sweden; 19 of the 33 children who were anisometropic at their first visit at 1 year of age were no longer anisometropic at 4 years, and 14 children who were not anisometropic at the first visit were anisometropic at the last. Unlike Almeder et al. (1990), they did find persistent anisometropia in almost half of their subjects, at least over the 3-year study period.

Implications of Early Refractive State for Later Refractive and Visual Development

A number of workers have studied the early refractive state with a view toward either predicting or preventing certain visual conditions, such as myopia, strabismus, and amblyopia. We began our studies on the assumption that early anisometropia was a significant cause of amblyopia (Howland and Sayles, 1987; Almeder et al., 1990). Our strategy was to detect anisometropes and refer them for correction. We believed that not all subjects would in fact wear refractive corrections, for a variety of reasons; and that if we were able to follow a sufficient number of subjects, we would be able to assess the influence of anisometropia on the generation of amblyopia. To date (Almeder et al., 1990) we have not found sufficient numbers of persistent anisometropes to test this hypothesis, and we are beginning to suspect that anisometropia, at least in the population we studied, may be more often a result than a cause of amblyopia.

Ingram et al. (1986), in a screening study of 795 infants at 1 year of age in Northamptonshire, England, found that 48% of those children who had a cyclopleged refraction of more than 3.5 D hyperopia in any meridian became amblyopic. Furthermore, 45% of these hyperopes became strabismic, although 66% of those children who were strabismic did not have more than 3.5 D of hyperopia. Interestingly, these authors noted that of the 38 children identified as having definite or possible amblyopia only 18% (seven children) were "straight eyed." This finding, as in our study (Almeder et al., 1990), suggested that many adult straight-eyed, anisometropic amblyopes were either not straight-eyed or not anisometropic as young children.

Ingram et al. (1986) noted that "astigmatism is common in infancy," but they did not find 1.5 D or more astigmatism significantly with strabismus, amblyopia, or a combination of the two. Dobson et al. (1981) also found no predictive value of infant astigmatism. However, these authors failed to find a significant relation between hyperopia or anisometropia on the one hand and strabismus or amblyopia on the other, as Ingram (1977) had earlier reported. They remarked that "this limits the efficacy of cycloplegic refraction as a screening measure." Atkinson et al. (personal communication) note that the Dobson et al. study looked at associations between refraction and strabismus at the time of presentation of strabismus, whereas Ingram's study concerned the prediction of strabismus.

Finally, we may cite two interesting studies that to date have appeared only in abstract form. Atkinson et al. (1990) have screened more than 6000 infants 6–9 months of age in Cambridge and Bristol (England) using cyclopentolate cycloplegia. Five percent of the screened population showed hyperopia of more than 4 D. In those infants whose hyperopia was not corrected, 25% developed strabismus. In addition, of those infants who were found to be both hyperopic and astigmatic at 6–9 months, 60% showed a meridional amblyopia at 4 years if their astigmatism was not corrected.

Gwiazda et al. (1990), in a study of 1500 Boston area children, looked at the refractive fate of 72 who had been refracted repeatedly from birth to 7–15 years. Although both myopic and hyperopic infants tend to emmetropize, their infantile spherical refractive errors were found to reappear after 7 years of age. Furthermore, the strength of this "reappearance" was found to be correlated with the nature of the subjects' infant astigmatisms. They found a difference between with-the-rule and against-the-rule astigmatics. The former tended to become emmetropic, whereas the latter tended to return with greater frequency to their infantile refractive errors. This finding is reminiscent of similar data reported by Atkinson et al. (1990), who found that children who had with-the-rule infantile astigmatism lost this condition more rapidly than those who had against-the-rule astigmatism.

CONCLUSIONS

It is impossible to review the literature of refractive development without gaining some impressions of what the underlying causes of diversity in results might be and how we should treat those of methodological origin. In the first place, it seems clear that there are significant genetic differences among groups of infants and children that are reflected in differences in refractive development. The different sign of infantile astigmatism in orientals and whites living in the eastern United States is probably the best example. The presence or absence of infantile astigmatism is probably also genetically based, but with no obvious correlation to other phenotypic features. Recognizing the importance of genetic background for refractive development means that we researchers should make some effort to characterize the genetic background of the populations we study. I make this statement with no practical suggestion as to how it might be done. However, I feel confident that as the importance of genetic counseling in the prevention of inheritable diseases becomes more developed and sophisticated there may become available simple to use and socially acceptable techniques for characterizing the racial and genetic background of individuals.

In the meantime we must be wary of applying Procrustean filters to data of diverse origins. The same caution applies to refractive data gleaned with different techniques. Fixed focus photorefractive techniques may have little power to predict the net spherical atropine refraction, and the latter may tell little about the actual focus of the eyes in a normal visual task. The two techniques provide useful information about refractive development, however, and we should resist the temptation to "standardize" our procedures by eliminating one or the other.

The facts are that we do not yet know for sure what aspects of infant focusing and refraction we must measure or when we must measure them in order to predict and prevent such damaging conditions as amblyopia, myopia, and strabismus. What are lacking are longitudinal data that span the age range treated in this review and a bit beyond, i.e., birth to 7–8 years of life. I cite 7 or 8 years because I would like to be sure of the diagnosis of amblyopia based on acuity charts.

It is to be regretted that in this age of ubiquitous computers and networked data transmission we cannot devise a medical records-keeping scheme that would allow longitudinal studies on our highly mobile national population. I believe that if we had any hope of following infants and young children as they moved from place to place we would rapidly enough find agreement on what tests to perform and what data to record in their records.

Acknowledgments. I wish to thank Leilani Peck for editorial assistance with the manuscript and Yasmine Iqbal for help with the bibliography. This work was supported in part by NIH grant EY02994.

REFERENCES

ABRAHAMSSON, M., FABIAN, G., AND SJOSTRAND, J. (1990). A longitudinal study of a population based sample of astigmatic children. II. The changeability of anisometropia. *Acta Ophthalmol (Copenh.)* 68, 435–440.

ALMEDER, L. M., PECK, L. B., AND HOWLAND, H. C. (1990). Prevalence of anisometropia in volunteer laboratory and school screening populations. *Invest. Ophthalmol. Vis. Sci.* 31, 2448–2455.

ATKINSON, J., BRADDICK, O., AND FRENCH, J. (1980). Infant astigmatism: its disappearance with age. *Vision Res.* 20, 891–893.

ATKINSON, J., BRADDICK, O. J., DURDEN, K., WATSON, P. G., AND ATKINSON, S. (1984). Screening for refractive errors in 6–9 month old infants by photorefraction. *Brt. J. Ophthalmol.* 68, 105–112.

ATKINSON, J., BRADDICK, O., WATTAM-BELL, J., DURDEN, K., BOBIER, W., POINTER, J., AND ATKINSON, S. (1990). Photorefractive screening of infants and effects of refractive correction. *Invest. Ophthalmol. Vis. Sci.* 28, 399.

BALDWIN, W. (1990) Refractive status of infants and children. In *Principles and Practice of Pediatric Ophthalmology*. Philadelphia: Lippincott. Ch. 6.

BANKS, M. (1980). Infant refraction and accommodation. *Int. Ophthalmol. Clin.* 20, 205–232.

BRADDICK, O., ATKINSON, J., FRENCH, J., AND HOWLAND, H. C. (1979). A photorefractive study of infant accommodation. *Vision Res.* 19, 1319–1330.

BROWN, E. V. L. (1938). Net average yearly changes in refraction of atropinized eyes from birth to beyond middle life. *Arch. Ophthalmol.* 19, 719–734.

CARPENTER, R. H. S. (1988). *Movements of the Eyes*. London: Pion.

COOK, R. C., AND GLASSCOCK, R. E. (1951). Refractive and ocular findings in the newborn. *Am. J. Ophthalmol.* 34, 1407–1413.

CURTIN, B. J. (1985). *The Myopias: Basic Science and Clinical Management*. Philadelphia: Harper & Row.

DOBSON, V., FULTON, A. B., MANNING, K., SALEM, D., AND PETERSEN, R. A. (1981). Cycloplegic refractions of premature infants. *Am. J. Ophthalmol.* 91, 490–495.

DOBSON, V., FULTON, A., AND SEBRIS, S. (1984). Cycloplegic refractions of infants and young children: the axis of astigmatism. *Invest. Ophthalmol. Vis. Sci.* 25, 83–87.

DUNNE, M. C. M., AND BARNES, D. A. (1987). Schematic modelling of peripheral astigmatism in real eyes. *Ophthalmic Physiol. Opt.* 3, 235–239.

ELY, E. T. (1880). Beobachtungen mit dem Augenspiegel bezüglich der Refraction der Augen neugeborener. *Arch. Augenheilkd.* 9, 431–442.

GERHARD, J. P. (1983). A propos de la myopie du premature. *Bull. Soc. Ophthalmol. Fr.* 83, 221–223.

GLEISS, J., AND PAU, H. (1952). Die entwicklung der Refraktion vor der Geburt. *Klin. Monatsbl. Augenheilkd.* 121, 440–445.

GLICKSTEIN, M., AND MILLODOT, M. (1970). Retinoscopy and eye size. *Science* 168, 605–606.

GOLDSCHMIDT, E. (1969). Refraction in the newborn. *Acta Ophthalmol. (Copenh.)* 47, 570–578.

GROSE, J., AND HARDING, G. (1990). The development of refractive error and pattern visually evoked potentials in pre-term infants. *Clin. Vis. Sci.* 5, 375–382.

GWIAZDA, J., SCHEIMAN, M., MOHINDRA, I., AND HELD, R. (1984). Astigmatism in children: changes in axis and amount from birth to six years. *Invest. Ophthalmol. Vis. Sci.* 25, 88–92.

GWIAZDA, J., MOHINDRA, I., BRILL, S., AND HELD, R. (1985). Infant astigmatism and meridional amblyopia. *Vision Res.* 25, 1269–1276.

GWIAZDA, J., THORN, F., BAUER, J., AND HELD, R. (1990). Prediction of school age myopia from infant refractive errors. *Invest. Ophthalmol. Vis. Sci.* 31, 233.

HERRNHEISER, J. (1892). Die Refractionsentwicklung des menschlichen Auges. *Z. Heilkunde* 13, 342–377.

HOWLAND, H. C. (1982a). Infant eye: optics and accommodation. *Curr. Eye Res.* 2, 217–224.

HOWLAND, H. C. (1982b). Optical techniques for detecting and improving deficient vision. In G. von Bally and P. Greguss (eds.): *Optics in Biomedical Sciences*. Berlin: Springer-Verlag.

HOWLAND, H. C. (1985). Optics of photoretinoscopy: results from ray tracing. *Am. J. Optom. Physiol. Opt.* 62, 621–625.

HOWLAND, H. C. (1988). Visual development: optical aspects of the eye. In E. Meisami and P. S. Timiras (eds): *Handbook of Human Growth and Developmental Biology*. Boca Raton; FL: CRC Press, pp. 155–162.

HOWLAND, H. C., AND HOWLAND, B. (1974). Photorefraction, a technique for the study of refractive state at a distance. *J. Opt. Soc. Am.* 64, 240–249.

HOWLAND, H. C., AND SAYLES, N. (1983). Photorefractive studies of normal and handicapped infants and children. *Behav. Brain Res.* 10, 81–85.

HOWLAND, H. C., AND SAYLES, N. (1984). Photorefractive measurements of astigmatism in infants and young children. *Invest. Ophthalmol. Vis. Sci.* 25, 93–102.

HOWLAND, H. C., AND SAYLES, N. (1985). Photokeratometric and photorefractive measurements of astigmatism in infant and young children. *Vision Res.* 25, 73–81.

HOWLAND, H. C., AND SAYLES, N. (1987). A photorefractive characterization of focusing ability of infants and young children. *Invest. Ophthalmol. Vis. Sci.* 28, 1005–1015.

HOWLAND, H. C., ATKINSON, J., BRADDICK, O., AND FRENCH, J. (1978). Infant astigmatism measured by photorefraction. *Science* 202, 331–333.

HOWLAND, H. C., BRADDICK, O., ATKINSON, J., AND HOWLAND, B. (1983). Optics of photorefraction: orthogonal and isotropic methods. *J. Opt. Soc. Am.* 73, 1701–1708.

INGRAM, R. (1977). Refraction as a basis for screening children for squint and amblyopia. *Brt. J. Ophthalmol.* 61, 8–15.

INGRAM, R., AND BARR, A. (1979). Changes in refraction between the ages of 1 and 3.5 years. *Brt. J. Ophthalmol.* 63, 339–342.

INGRAM, R., WALKER, C., WILSON, J., ARNOLD, P., AND DALLY, S. (1986). Prediction of amblyopia and squint by means of refraction at age 1 year. *Brt. J. Ophthalmol.* 70, 12–15.

JAEGER, E. (1861). *Ueber die Einstellung des dioptrischen Apparates im menschlichen Auge.* Vienna: Verlag Weissnichtwem.

LARSEN, J. S. (1971a). The sagittal growth of the eye. I. Ultrasonic measurement of the depth of the anterior chamber from birth to puberty. *Acta Ophthalmol. (Copenh.)* 49, 939–969.

LARSEN, J. S. (1971b). The sagittal growth of the eye. II. Ultrasonic measurement of the axial diameter of the lens and the anterior segment from birth to puberty. *Acta Ophthalmol. (Copenh.)* 49, 427–440.

LARSEN, J. S. (1971c). The sagittal growth of the eye. III. Ultrasonic measurement of the posterior segment (axial length of the vitreous) from birth to puberty. *Acta Ophthalmol. (Copenh.)* 49, 441–453.

LARSEN, J. S. (1971d). The sagittal growth of the eye. IV. Ultrasonic measurement of the axial length of the eye from birth to puberty. *Acta Ophthalmol. (Copenh.)* 49, 873–886.

MEHRA, K. S., KHARE, B. B., AND VAITHILINGAM, E. (1965). Refraction in full-term babies. *Brt. J. Ophthalmol.* 49, 276–277.

MOHINDRA, I. (1977). Comparison of "near retinoscopy" and subjective refraction in adults. *Am. J. Optom. Physiol. Opt.* 54, 319–322.

MOHINDRA, I., AND HELD, R. (1981). Refraction in humans from birth to five years. *Doc. Ophthalmol.* 28, 19–27.

MOHINDRA, I., HELD, R., GWIAZDA, J., AND BRILL, S. (1978). Astigmatism in infants. *Science* 202, 329–330.

MURPHY, C. J., HOWLAND, H. C., KWIECINSKI, G. G., KERN, T., AND KALLEN, F. (1983). Visual accommodation in the flying fox (*Pteropus giganteus*). *Vision Res.* 23, 617–620.

OWENS, D. A., MOHINDRA, I., AND HELD, R. (1980). The effectiveness of a retinoscope beam as an accommodative stimulus. *Invest. Ophthalmol. Vis. Sci.* 19, 942–949.

SANTONASTASO, A. (1930). La refrazione oculare nei primi anni di vita. *Ann. Ottalmol. Clin. Ocul.* 58, 852–885.

SCHARF, J., ZONIS, S., AND ZELTZER, M. (1975). Refraction in Israeli premature babies. *J. Pediatr. Ophthalmol.* 12, 193–196.

SHAPIRO, A., YANKO, L., NAWRATSKI, I., AND MERIN, S. (1980). Refractive power of premature children at infancy and early childhood. *Am. J. Ophthalmol.* 90, 234–238.

SIVAK, J. G., AND BOBIER, W. R. (1990). Optical components of the embryology and postnatal development. In A. A. Rosenbloom (ed.). *Principles and Practice of Pediatric Optometry.* Philadelphia: Lippincott, pp. 31–45.

SLATAPER, F. J. (1950). Age norms of refraction and vision. *Arch. Ophthalmol.* 43, 466–481.

SORSBY, A., LEARY, G. A., AND RICHARDS, M. J. (1962). The optical components in anisometropia. *Vision Res.* 2, 43–51.

STENSTROM, S. (1946). Untersuchungen uber die Variation und Kovariation der optischen Elemente des menschlichen Auges. *Acta Ophthalmol. Suppl 26 (Copenh.)* 24, 1–103.

THORN, F., HELD, R., AND FANG, L. (1987). Orthogonal astigmatic axes in Chinese and caucasian infants. *Invest. Ophthalmol. Vis. Sci.* 28, 191–194.

TOKORO, T., AND SUZUKI, K. (1968). Significance of changes of refractive components to development of myopia during seven years. *Acta Soc. Ophthalmol. Jpn.* 72, 1472–1477.

YANKOV, L. (1982). Ocular biometry in neonates. *J. Fr. Ophthalmol.* 5, 237–241.

2 | Visually guided control of refractive state: results from animal models

FRANK SCHAEFFEL

The vertebrate eye is an optical instrument of impressive precision. Although the images provided by modern camera lenses are of higher quality, the optics of eyes in humans and some higher vertebrates can provide a spatial resolution that is ultimately limited by physical parameters. In humans, at a pupil size of about 2.4 mm, diffraction of light at the pupil aperture limits further improvement of the retinal image quality (Campbell and Gubisch, 1966). In foveate eyes, some optical weaknesses may be obvious in the off-axis imagery. Human eyes are known to be astigmatic in the periphery and tend to have a hyperopic refractive error (Millodot, 1981). These factors are not important, however, because the peripheral visual acuity is low.

It is possible to calculate how precisely the retinal plane must be matched to the focal length of the eye. The required precision is determined by the depth of focus, which in turn is closely related to visual acuity (Green et al., 1980). In a human eye, the depth of focus is about 0.4 diopters (D) (Campbell, 1957). If the retinal plane in an emmetropic eye moves posteriorly from its optimal position by more than 100 μm, the resulting refractive error is greater than the depth of focus, causing a noticeable decline in visual acuity.

It must be remembered that a shift of 100 μm is less than 1% of the total axial length of the eye. Considering this precision, it is difficult to understand how eye growth can be so precise if it is controlled solely by genetic factors. It also seems unlikely that gradients of different growth factors in the eye can interact such that growth control is accurate to 0.1 mm for an eye of diameter 24 mm. From these observations one would suspect that there is a growth-regulating mechanism guided by additional information from outside.

VARIABILITY OF OPTICAL COMPONENTS IN THE EYE AND REFRACTIVE ERRORS

If the factors contributing to the refractive power of an eye are examined in a large human population, it can be seen that corneal radius of curvature, power of the lens, and anterior chamber depth are normally distributed (Stentstrom, 1946, cited by McBrien and Barnes, 1984) [standard deviation (SD) is approximately 2 D for both corneal power and lens, and approximately 1 D for anterior chamber depth]. By contrast, the distribution of axial length has more points at the mean than would be expected for a normal distribution; but plotted as dioptric equivalents, it still displays more variability than the other parameters. Strikingly, the distribution of ocular refractive states is much more finely tuned than would be expected if the different factors were randomly combined. The fine tuning of refractive state near emmetropia suggests regulatory mechanisms that can match the focal length to the length of the eye. It cannot be concluded, however, that these mechanisms are visually guided. Previous works (for a review see Curtin, 1985) have described a number of "mechanisms" that produce significant correlations among the various refracting elements contributing to emmetropia. How this enormous precision is achieved remains unclear.

REFRACTIVE ERRORS: GENETICALLY DETERMINED OR INAPPROPRIATELY TRIGGERED FEEDBACK LOOPS?

Although there is some indirect evidence for control of refractive state by exogenous factors, Sorsby (1967) did not come to this conclusion after his extensive study of the components of refraction in a large population. The differences arise partly because refractive errors can be grouped into several categories. Genetic factors are probably responsible if one or several of the refractive components fall far outside the normal range. If a feedback loop controls normal refractive development, it may not be able to deal with this disturbance because it creates conditions outside its operating range. This situation may be the case, for example, with the pathological forms of myopia that develop early in life (early-onset myopia). The moderate types of myopia (school myopia, or late-onset myopia), however, could be a physiological adaptation to a change in the average viewing distance. Until now, this assumption could not be proved from studies on human refractive development. In humans, many factors not directly related to the question (ocular motor problems, anisometropia) may also influence refractive development, so a direct conclusion becomes more difficult. On the other hand, experimental manipulations of refractive development in animal models are more promising because the cause-and-effect relation can be examined under controlled conditions.

The findings from these animal studies are described in detail in this chapter. Although not all the conclusions can be directly applied to humans, the studies showed the mechanisms for guiding refractive development that are acting in the model eye and those that conceivably exist in biological systems.

EXPERIMENTAL EVIDENCE FOR VISUALLY GUIDED EYE GROWTH: RESULTS FROM REFRACTIVE DEVELOPMENT UNDER OPEN LOOP CONDITIONS: "DEPRIVATION MYOPIA"

In terms of feedback regulation of eye growth and refractive state, deprivation would provide open-loop conditions. If normal refractive development is dependent on visual experience, removal of appropriate visual information should result in less precisely tuned refractions. The first such observation was made by Hubel and Wiesel (cited in Raviola and Wiesel, 1985). They noted that, in young monkeys, a lid suture lasting several months resulted in increased axial eye growth with a myopic refractive error (Wiesel and Raviola, 1977). They further demonstrated that the change in eye growth was not the result of changes in metabolic or thermal conditions under the closed eyelids but, rather, of changes in visual input (Raviola and Wiesel, 1978; Wiesel and Raviola, 1979). A similar conclusion could be drawn from the observation (Oishi and Lauber, 1988) that no deprivation myopia could be induced in chickens after the photoreceptor function was abolished by formoguanamine. Manipulation of retinal image is now the most frequently used technique to study experimental myopia. Image degradation by lid suture, by applying translucent occluders or goggles, or even by raising chickens in a featureless environment (Nickla et al., 1989) has been found to be an efficient way to produce variable degrees of refractive errors in a number of species (e.g., monkeys: Smith et al., 1987; marmosets: Troilo et al., 1990; tree shrews: McKanna and Casagrande, 1978, Norton, 1990; cats: Gollender et al., 1979, Kirby et al., 1982; chickens: Wallman et al., 1978, Yinon et al., 1980, Hodos and Kuenzel, 1984). The striking observation is that degradation of the retinal image need only be subtle to produce prominent effects on eye growth. Opaque occluders are no more efficient than

translucent ones (Sivak, personal communication 1988; Norton, personal communication 1990). This result is not surprising, as a mechanism capable of extracting small amounts of optical defocus from the retinal image to trigger an appropriate growth response should be sensitive to small changes.

Myopia as a result of image degradation is referred to below as "deprivation myopia," although the deprivation is moderate.

Comparison of Deprivation Myopia in Humans and Animal Models

If deprivation myopia results from removing correct visual control of eye growth, human eyes should also be affected. The major problem is that the required deprivation cannot be induced intentially in humans, so one must rely on results from naturally occurring "visual deprivation." Such cases include congenital cataracts, ptosis, and blepharospasm. However, in those cases the eyes may be affected by nonvisual problems that could also influence refractive development and may well be genetically preprogrammed. It is therefore difficult to isolate the effects of pure visual deprivation, making a higher variability more likely.

A number of studies do show that deprivation myopia occurs in humans (e.g., O'Leary and Millodot, 1979; Hoyt et al., 1981; Rabin et al., 1981; Johnson et al., 1982), although other studies (e.g., Awaya et al., 1979; Merriam et al., 1980; von Noorden and Lewis, 1987) have shown that deprivation myopia does not develop in all cases of visual deprivation. The statement does not conflict with the assumption of visually guided eye growth because one would expect an increase in variability.

Features of Deprivation Myopia in Monkeys, Tree Shrews, and Chickens

Role of Accommodation. After "form deprivation myopia" was observed for the first time, a large number of studies focused on the question of whether excessive accommodation could be the result of exaggerated axial eye growth (e.g., McKanna and Casagrande, 1981a; Wallman et al., 1981). Pharmacological paralysis of accommodation (mainly by atropine) was frequently used to elucidate the role of accommodation (e.g., tree shrew: McKanna and Casagrande, 1981b; monkey: Raviola and Weisel, 1985). The assumption is largely based on the observation that near work can produce myopia in humans (Curtin, 1985), and because the accommodative effort is increased during such work it may indeed be one of the factors responsible for the development of myopia. Also, the average level of accommodation would be a perfect sensor for the current refractive state because the two are directly proportional, and it would fit well for a closed-loop model of emmetropization. This view changed, however, when deprivation myopia was also found to develop in chicks without functional accommodation (Troilo, 1989) and even after the optic nerve had been cut (Troilo et al., 1987; Wildsoet and Pettigrew, 1988a). Furthermore, Hodos and Kuenzel (1984) suspected and Wallman et al. (1987) later showed that deprivation myopia could be induced in local retinal areas. The observation of local myopia precludes a role for accommodation because no study has shown that the process of accommodation can selectively focus local retinal areas. There is also clear evidence in mammals that the development of deprivation myopia does not depend on functional accommodation. Raviola and Wiesel (1985) noted that in one monkey species (*Macaca mulatta*) the development of deprivation myopia was not suppressed by lesioning the accommodation pathways. Cutting the optic nerve also failed to prevent the development of myopia. Because deprivation myopia can be induced monocularly in monkeys without affecting the contralateral eye, accommodation cannot be responsible because it cannot be uncoupled in the two eyes. Norton et al. (1989) found that, in tree shrews, depletion of retinal ganglion cells by tetrodotoxin did not inhibit myopia. With no visual output to the brain, it is improbable that there was a consistent increase in accommodative tonus. There is no evidence, then, that accommodation plays a direct role during development of deprivation myopia.

Nature of the Visual Signal that Produces Deprivation Myopia.

It is important to note that during visual deprivation a mechanism controlling eye growth and refractive state is triggered under open-loop conditions. The removal of high contrast and higher spatial frequencies also provides a real error signal for the eye. This point can be demonstrated most easily in young chicks. Here, deprivation myopia develops rapidly with up to 2 D a day if the animals are deprived of sharp vision and are kept in normal white light. By contrast, the refractive state changes little or not at all within the same period of time if the animals are kept under low light levels or under ultraviolet light where the visual acuity is low (Rohrer et al., 1992). The growing chick is able to maintain almost normal refraction for at least a week, even if no appropriate visual information is provided on the refractive state. Therefore the idea of an open loop acting alone is insufficient, and one must postulate that image degradation also produces a clear error signal for the eye to grow in axial length and become more myopic. There is a second argument that deprivation myopia is not just the lack of the appropriate visual information but, rather, the result of a real error signal

for a high acuity system. If one compares different animal species with different visual acuity (monkeys and chicks versus cats), it appears that myopia develops more readily in eyes with high visual acuity than in eyes optimized for light sensitivity (cats).

Recovery from Deprivation Myopia.

Whereas it was difficult to show (Troilo et al., 1990) that mammalian eyes can recover from deprivation myopia (Norton, 1990), a fast recovery has been observed in chickens (Wallman and Adams, 1987). In fact, myopia disappears in chicks almost as fast as it develops. This observation certainly supports the idea of active emmetropization. Here eye growth no longer occurs under open-loop conditions, and from a closed-loop model one would expect the refractive error to be corrected. The speed of recovery depends on the current growth rate of the eye. Because chicken eyes grow almost linearly over a period of at least 50 days (Hayes et al., 1986; Schaffel and Howland, 1988a) and deprivation myopia can reach high levels after only a week, the working time is extended. It is more difficult in mammals, and only careful determination of the sensitive periods made it possible to detect recovery (Norton, 1990). In chicks recovery occurs mainly by a change in the speed of axial eye growth (Wallman and Adams, 1987; Troilo, 1989) (Fig. 2-1). In tree shrews, some changes were also observed in the refractive power of the cornea (Norton, 1990). Recovery from deprivation myopia has not yet been observed in monkeys. Here changes in eye growth during deprivation are slow, and recovery is probably so slow that the eyes reach their final length before recovery can occur. Eyes have never been known to shrink once they become too long.

If a retinal image that does not contain higher spatial frequencies results in deprivation myopia, recovery should be possible only if enough high spatial frequencies are present in the retinal image upon removal of the occluder. If the myopic defocus is so severe that an image degradation remains for all viewing distances, the eye should remain myopic without recovery. This situation was, in fact, the case with chickens, where the amount of myopia exceeded about 15 D (Fig. 2-1) or 20 D (Wallman and Adams, 1987).

In conclusion, the studies of recovery from form deprivation myopia suggest that an inappropriate refractive state can be corrected by an active mechanism sensitive to either defocus or abnormal eye shape.

Chickens as a Model for Experimental Myopia

There are two basic questions one hopes to answer in the experiments on animal models: How is the refractive state normally regulated in the growing eye? Why do refractive errors develop in humans? On the one hand, it seems appropriate to use an animal model closely

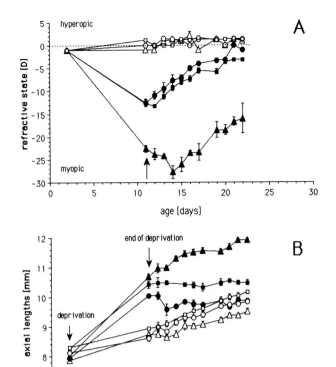

FIG. 2-1. If young chickens are deprived of sharp vision when translucent occluders are placed over the eyes, they quickly develop considerable amounts of axial myopia. Open symbols = control eyes; closed symbols = treated eyes. (A) Refractive development in three chicks. Treatment started monocularly at day 2 after hatching. Occluders were removed at day 11. If refractive errors were less than about 15 D, the eyes recovered quickly. If myopia exceeded 15 D (arrow), recovery was inhibited because the myopic refractive error was a deprivation by itself. In this chick, myopia worsened for 3 more days. (B) Axial eye growth in the same chicks as in (A). Upon removal of the occluders, axial eye growth stopped in order to correct for the refractive error, except in the chick with myopia exceeding 15 D. Here the difference in axial lengths in the two eyes remained constant (about 2 mm) for the entire period of observation. Examples are from a larger sample of chickens (n = 11).

related to humans, such as monkeys. On the other hand, because results can be obtained only slowly and the number of individuals that can be used is low, chickens have proved to be more valuable: Their eyes grow rapidly, and their excellent optical quality throughout post-hatching development points to a precise regulation of the refractive state. They also have an impressive accommodative range of about 20 D (Schaeffel et al., 1986, additional personal observations), which allows one to study the effects of accommodation on refractive development. Finally, because chicks are inexpensive and small at the age of the experiments (first 4 weeks after hatching), large numbers can easily be housed in the laboratory. With these advantages, it is not surprising that most of the results came originally from the

chicken studies and were subsequently reproduced in mammals. At this time, several conclusions derived from the chicken model (described in detail below) appear valid for mammals. Nevertheless, chickens also pose some problems. There are interactions between refractive development and general light conditions (light cycle and light levels). Most importantly, chicks develop the so-called avian buphthalmos under dim light and a light-induced avian glaucoma under continuous illumination, with considerable changes in intraocular pressure and increased globe sizes (for a review see Lauber, 1987). Continuous dim blue light produces myopic refractive errors after prolonged exposure (Bercowitz et al., 1971). These problems can be avoided if light cycle and light levels are carefully controlled (Oishi and Murakami, 1985).

EMMETROPIZATION UNDER CLOSED-LOOP CONDITIONS

Recovery from Refractive Errors

As discussed earlier, recovery from deprivation myopia in itself does not prove visual guidance of the refractive state. The picture becomes clearer, however, if eyes can be shown to recover from both hyperopia and myopia. These experiments, performed in the chicken by Troilo (1989), became possible because hyperopia could be produced by dark rearing of both chickens and monkeys (Greene et al., 1989; Guyton et al., 1989). In the chicken, the hyperopic refractive error was not the result of a shorter eye but, rather, of a flatter than normal cornea. The eyes were actually larger than normal, but the loss of refractive power of the cornea overcompensated for the expected myopia. The growth response of the eyes after they were returned to normal light conditions is particularly interesting. Because of the hyperopic refractive error, one would expect the axial growth to increase to correct for hyperopia. The eyes were already longer than normal, however, so such a growth response would carry the eyes even farther out of the normal range. What happened was that the eyes did in fact grow longer. Simultaneously, corneal refractive power increased rather than decreased, as should happen normally. The two factors combined resulted in a rapid recovery until near-emmetropic refraction was regained. Chicks accommodate in part by changing their corneal curvature (Schaeffel and Howland, 1987; Troilo and Wallman, 1987). Therefore the increase in corneal refractive power must not be a growth process but, rather, a result of regained accommodative tonus.

The observation that chicks can recover from both myopia and the hyperopia clearly indicates visually guided regulation of refractive state.

Results from Lens Experiments

Possibly the strongest evidence for active regulation of the refractive state comes from experiments with defocusing lenses. Here the assumed emmetropizing mechanisms are presented with a defined error signal; and if they are present, they should respond with a defined compensatory growth. The optical quality in the retinal image must be good at all times because, as described above, deprivation myopia also develops with little deterioration in the retinal image. A reduction in the high spatial frequency content also occurs if the power of the lenses used is exaggerated enough to keep the image seriously defocused at all times.

Results from Cats and Monkeys. There is still no definite evidence that the eyes in cats and monkeys respond in a predictable way to treatment with a defocusing lens. The result seems to be contrary to what would be expected from the above arguments. The observations must be analyzed with care, however, as a number of explanations are possible for the failure. First, because accommodation in the eyes is tightly coupled in humans (Campbell, 1960), monkeys (personal observation by infrared photoretinoscopy), and cats (personal observation by infrared photoretinoscopy), monocular treatment with a defocusing lens is not appropriate. One eye probably guides the accommodative tonus, and the other remains permanently defocused by the amount of power in the lens. As a result, this eye should always develop deprivation myopia independent of the sign of the lens. Another problem is the absolute power of the lens. If it exceeds the amplitude of accommodation, particularly for negative lenses, the retinal image is permanently defocused for all viewing distances, resulting again in deprivation myopia. The most important, and still missing, experiment would therefore be to raise monkeys with weak ophthalmic lenses but with the same lens in both eyes. Although a control eye is missing during this procedure, the development of a refractive state should provide enough information.

Few studies have used lenses. Crewther et al. (1988) used contact lenses in monkeys, but there was no consistent correlation between lens powers and refractions after treatment. Ni and Smith (1989) applied lenses monocularly in cats and found only myopia but with a correlation between absolute lense power and degree of refractive error. Maguire et al. (1982) used powerful lenses in cats. The authors did not record the refractive state after the treatment but tested visual function behaviorally and found amblyopia. Finally, a similar experiment was performed by Hendrickson (1987), who applied radial radiokeratotomy in cats and claimed to find increased axial eye growth that corrected for the induced hyperopia.

Lens Experiments in Chickens. Chickens have uncoupled accommodation and pupillary responses (Schaeffel et al., 1986), making asymmetrical treatment of both eyes possible. This option is particularly valuable if the changes in eye growth are small. If a young chicken eye is treated with a moderately powered lens (i.e., -4 D) for complete compensation of the lens, the expected increase in axial eye growth is approximately 250 μm. The difference in axial length between the treated eye and the control eye can be measured with sensitive A-scan ultrasonography, such as the 3M "Echo Rule," with minor modifications (Schaeffel and Howland, 1991). The changes in refractive state can be easily recorded by infrared photoretinoscopy (Schaeffel et al., 1987). Corneal power is affected only slightly by the lens treatment, and the power of the crystalline lens is unaffected. The main factor responsible for the compensatory change in refractive state is the change in axial eye length (Schaffel and Howland, 1988a).

Raising chickens with lenses is a time-consuming task but is acceptable because the experiment lasts only about 10 days. The lenses can either be attached to small leather hoods with Velcro and removed frequently for cleaning (Schaeffel et al., 1988), or soft contact lenses can be applied directly to the eye (Callender et al., 1989). However, soft contact lenses abolish corneal accommodation in the chick and also provide a direct mechanical influence to the eye. The magnitude of the observed effects may therefore differ.

In contrast to the results from cats and monkeys, lenses induce consistent changes in axial eye growth and refractive state. After only about 3–4 days of treatment, both parameters change in a highly predictable fashion, such that the imposed refractive error is largely compensated. The experiment therefore provides the most direct evidence for active regulation of refractive state during eye growth. Furthermore, the experiment allows one to study the system properties in an elegant way. It was found that the feedback regulation of the refractive state is highly nonlinear (Fig. 2-2) because positive lenses have a much stronger effect on eye growth and refractive state than negative lenses. Furthermore, positive lenses make the eye shorter than normal, untreated eyes, showing that no effects of deprivation (which would produce eye enlargement) were superimposed on the effects of the lenses. Because a negative lens can largely be compensated for by accommodation whereas a positive lens cannot, it would be plausible if positive lenses more efficiently trigger a compensatory growth response. The closed-loop model also provides more information on the nature of the visual stimuli involved

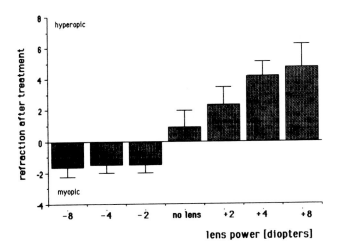

FIG. 2-2. Effect of spectacle lenses on development of refractive state in chickens. Positive lenses induce hyperopia, and negative lenses induce myopia but with a lower gain in the feedback loop for visual control of refractive state. Averages from 8–18 chicks for each group. (Redrawn from Schaeffel and Howland, 1988b, with data added.)

in guiding axial eye growth and refractive state (see below).

POSSIBLE MECHANISMS FOR CONTROL OF REFRACTIVE STATE AND EYE GROWTH

In an eye with a strong decline in visual acuity in the periphery, such as a primate eye, emmetropization need be precise only in the central area. By contrast, in a chicken or pigeon eye, where refractive state, visual acuity, and ganglion cell density (Ehrlich, 1981; Morris, 1987) vary little across the visual field, it is necessary to match the photoreceptor plane to the entire image plane. It therefore appears reasonable to assume that a local emmetropizing mechanism is acting in addition to a central one.

Evidence for Local Control of Eye Growth

The most compelling evidence in the chicken that there are local growth-promoting mechanisms sensitive to visual experience was provided by Wallman et al. (1987), who found that partial occlusion results in myopia only in the deprived fractions of the visual field. Similarly, Troilo et al. (1987) and Wildsoet and Pettigrew (1988a) found that deprivation myopia can be induced after the optic nerve had been cut or after the oculomotor nuclei driving accommodation (Edinger-Westphal nucleus) had been lesioned (Troilo, 1989). To demonstrate that there is closed-loop regulation of the refractive state by visual experience, one must show that compensatory changes in refractive state can be induced by a defined imposed defocus. Part of the argument for this concept rests with the observations that the eye recovers from deprivation myopia even after accommodation had been destroyed by lesioning the Edinger-Westphal nucleus or cutting the optic nerve (Troilo, 1989, 1990). Because no one has yet shown that the eye can also recover from hyperopia, the evidence is incomplete. Schaeffel and Howland (1991) found that recovery from deprivation myopia also occurs in chicks even if the refractive error has been corrected by appropriate lenses. It must be assumed that an additional nonvisual mechanism, possibly sensitive to abnormal eye shape, is involved in the recovery. Therefore recovery from deprivation myopia is not in itself final proof of visually guided regulation of refractive state.

Another approach was chosen by Schaeffel et al. (1990). In this study, chickens with lesions in the Edinger-Westphal nuclei were treated with lenses. Despite the lack of functional accommodation, there was a compensatory change in axial eye growth and refraction. Although it is safe to conclude that functional accommodation is not obligatory for emmetropization in the chick, the possibility remains that other signals from the brain—perhaps by efferent fibers from the isthmooptic tract—control refractive development. There is extensive evidence for efferent innervation of the retina in the chick with fibers ending in the amacrine cell layer (Miles, 1972). To prove that a local mechanism can emmetropize the eye, Miles and Wallman (1990) raised chickens under a low ceiling to shorten the average viewing distance. Compared to a control group raised under a high ceiling, relative myopia should develop in the upper visual field. Although the chicks raised under a low ceiling had generally smaller eyes than the controls, for which the authors had no explanation, the overall result was in agreement with the expectations. There is some evidence that local emmetropization also occurs under natural conditions. Several authors (e.g., Fitzke et al., 1985a) have described a so-called lower field myopia in the pigeon, which is considered an adaptation to "keep the ground in focus," although sharp distance vision is also possible (Hodos and Erichson, 1990). Fitzke et al. (1985b) used a technique to refract the pigeon based on electroretinography, which is not subject to the "small eye artifact" (Glickstein and Millodot, 1970). It is more difficult to use optical techniques to measure the real refractive state far away from the optical axis because the small eye artifact cannot be easily quantified and because optical aberrations make the refractions more difficult.

There is some evidence that local emmetropization occurs in the chicken and pigeon and that it is guided visually by the current refractive error. Such a mechanism is fascinating because it can apparently extract both amount and sign of defocus locally and transmit an appropriate growth command to the underlying sclera. It therefore has stimulated a number of new investigations, described later in the chapter.

Evidence for Control of Eye Growth and Refractive State by Central Mechanisms

Not all results can be explained by the action of local growth-controlling mechanisms. One problem is obvious: If chicken eyes are treated with weak ophthalmic lenses, the animals immediately compensate for the lenses by accommodation. Schaffel et al. (1988) have shown that chicks have enough accommodative power to compensate for a negative lens by positive accommodation; and for near-viewing distances, there are also high spatial frequencies in the retinal image even if the chick is made nearsighted by a positive lens. As a result, no consistent defocus is present in the retinal image that could trigger a local mechanism. Because accommodation was used to remove the defocus caused by the lens, it would also make sense to measure the power of the lens. The plausibility of such a feedback loop make its assumption tempting, although there is still no clear proof for its presence. The evidence that has accumulated is more indirect. First, lowering the accommodative tonus by ciliary ganglion lesions always produces more hyperopic refractions than normal (Troilo, personal communication; Wildsoet and Howland, personal communication). Also Edinger-Westphal lesions resulted initially in a considerable amount of hyperopia, although the eyes recovered to more normal refractions later (Schaeffel et al., 1990; Troilo, 1990). Second, experiments with defocusing lenses worked well in chicks even if they were carried out in the monochromatic light of low pressure sodium lamps (Schaeffel and Howland, 1991). Because it is difficult to understand how a local mechanism in the retina could determine the sign of defocus without chromatic cues, a central mechanism would seem more plausible. Finally, there is some support here for the old hypothesis that near work produces myopia in humans because of the increased accommodative effort. If the eyes were focused on the target, no defocus was present in the retinal image that could drive a local emmetropizing mechanism. Emmetropia must then be triggered centrally and may in fact be the result of an accommodative feedback loop. An entirely different interpretation was presented by Wallman et al. (1987), who pointed out that a printed text provides information with a restricted spatial frequency pattern. They assumed that this condition can be considered as a kind of deprivation that ultimately produces myopia.

Many studies in which accommodation has been par-alyzed pharmacologically (mainly by atropine) have investigated possible effects of accommodation on refractive development (for a summary see Curtin, 1985, pp. 221–225). The interpretations are more difficult, however, because atropine has a number of side effects other than on accommodation (McBrien et al., 1991). The studies all involve mammals, including humans. The overall pattern of results is complex, and a role for accommodation in refractive development cannot be deduced. In birds, cycloplegia is not as easily obtained owing to the fast aqueous outflow and striated nature of the ciliary muscles.

Mathematical Model for Emmetropization with Two Feedback Loops

The above considerations show that two mechanisms for control of the refractive development must be postulated if all experimental results are to be explained. A simple mathematical model to simulate the experiments has been described by Schaeffel and Howland (1988b). The model includes two feedback loops that use the current defocus in the retinal image to trigger a change in axial eye growth to minimize the error signal. The gains in both loops have been multiplied by the first derivate of axial eye growth to consider the experimental observation that all manipulation becomes less efficient if the genetically predetermined eye growth slows when maturity is reached. One loop uses the accommodative effort as a sensor, and the other acts directly in the eye (Fig. 2-3A). After appropriate adjustment of the time constants and gains in the loops, the output of the model could be well matched to the experimental results (Fig. 2-3B,C)

WHY DO REFRACTIVE ERRORS DEVELOP DESPITE TWO VISUALLY GUIDED FEEDBACK LOOPS?

At this point, it is particularly important to separate refractive errors into different groups. Not all refractive errors that develop early in life, such as early-onset myopia (McBrien and Barnes, 1984) or those that affect the two eyes asymmetrically (anisometropia), can be easily explained by the action of visual feedback loops for control of refractive state, as they are probably genetically predetermined. However, the results from animal models allow one to speculate why refractive errors develop later in life after an emmetropic refraction had already been reached and maintained for some time (late-onset myopia). One hypothesis is that the gains in the visual feedback loops vary among individuals.

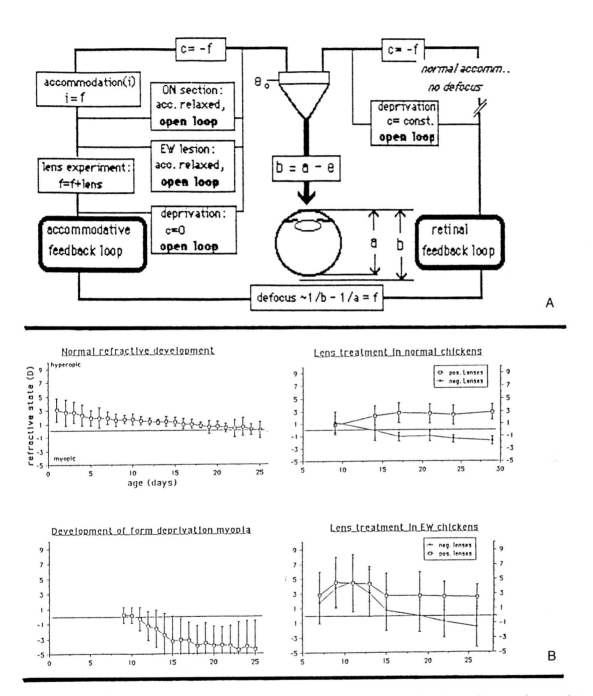

FIG. 2-3. (A) Flow chart of a simple mathematical model designed to simulate the experimental results of chicken refractive development under various treatments, as indicated in (B). The simulation showed that two feedback loops are necessary to describe the results of the experiments, a local "retinal" one, and a central "accommodative" one. (B) Experimental results to be described by the model. (C) Results of the simulation. (After Schaeffel and Howland, 1988b.)

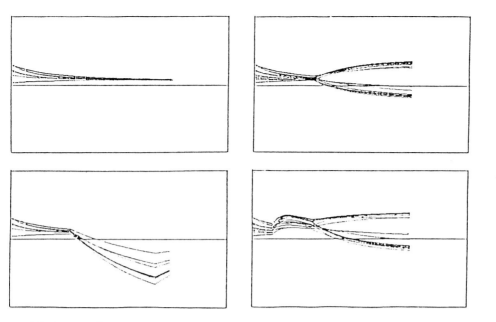

C

FIG. 2-3. *(continued)*

Variable Gains in the Local Feedback Loop

If late-onset myopia develops in some but not all individuals, one must postulate a factor that accounts for this difference. One possible assumption would be that the gains in the feedback loops vary among individuals but are genetically determined constants for each individual. The feedback loop assumption can easily be tested in chicks. A striking feature of deprivation myopia is the enormous variability in refraction after treatment. Because the treatment can be standardized, the variability must be the result of endogenous factors. As described above, deprivation myopia can be induced independently in both eyes because local factors in the eye are responsible for its development. If both eyes are deprived symmetrically, the refractions should remain highly correlated despite the normal variability of deprivation myopia. This situation was, in fact, observed (Fig. 2-4) and supports the hypothesis that the gain in the local mechanism is a genetically determined constant typical for each individual.

"Evidence" for Variable Gains in the Accommodative Feedback Loops

Evidence exists that gains vary among individuals for the central (probably accommodative) feedback loop as well. The results come from human studies, with no data yet available from animal models. There is, however, a gap in the line of arguments because there is no direct experimental proof that accommodation can di-

rectly influence axial eye growth. The results discussed here can describe only accommodation behavior in different refractive groups with no proof that these two factors are causally linked.

Leibowitz and Owens (1975) reported that in the absence of visual stimulation the eye adopts an intermediate resting position somewhere between the far point and the near point. Their finding refutes the commonly held view that the far point is also the resting point of accommodation (Helmholtz, 1855). Because sympathetic as well as parasympathetic innervation of the ciliary muscles have been found (for a review see Gilmartin, 1986), it is assumed that the intermediate resting position of accommodation ("tonic accommodation") is the result of dynamic levels of activity in both systems (McBrien and Millodot, 1987). The observation of Gilmartin et al. (1990) that there are subtle changes in the dynamics of accommodation after pharmacological intervention in the sympathetic pathway supports this interpretation. Two striking features of tonic accommodation are that it varies considerably among individuals (for a review see Owens, 1990), and it is stable over considerable periods (months) (Owens, 1990). Maintaining focus on a near target for some minutes or on a target more distant than the plane of tonic accommodation results in a shift of the dark focus (Ebenholtz, 1991). The shift decays slowly in darkness until the initial level of tonic accommodation is reached. The decay is faster if a distant target was viewed before than for a close target.

With the invention of infrared autorefractors (e.g., the Canon Autoref R-1), small changes in accommo-

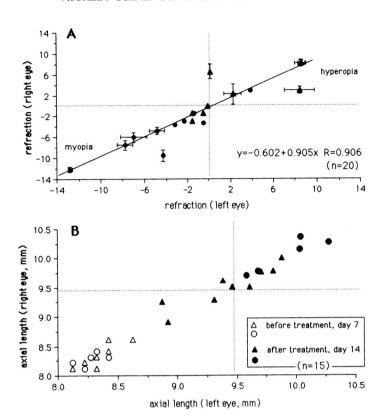

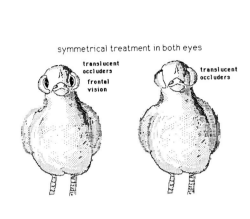

symmetrical treatment in both eyes

translucent occluders
frontal vision

translucent occluders

FIG. 2-4. It was shown previously that deprivation myopia occurs independently in both eyes (see text) with enormous variability among individuals. Here we tested whether the variability is a genetically determined factor that is typical for each individual. Both eyes were deprived symmetrically, and the correlation of refractive errors (A) and axial eye growth (B) were tested. The high correlation and small variability between the two eyes, despite the local control of deprivation myopia, suggests that the variability among individuals results from genetic factors, probably from different gains in the feedback loops. (Redrawn from Schaeffel and Howland, 1991.)

dative tonus (down to less than 0.25 D) can be reliably measured. The opportunity stimulated a number of studies on accommodation behavior in human subjects. It was found that the level of tonic accommodation is somehow related to the refractive state (McBrien and Millodot, 1987), with corrected late-onset myopes having the most distant plane of focus for the resting point of tonic accommodation and hyperopes the closest. Emmetropes have a resting point of accommodation somewhere in between (Fig. 2-5). It was concluded that myopes have a relatively weaker sympathetic innervation of the ciliary muscle than hyperopes or emmetropes. If the sympathetic innervation was responsible for active "negative accommodation for the distance," it could be expected that this process is less effective in the myopic group. Therefore subjects from the different refractive groups were asked to do near work at different distances. It was found that the resting point of tonic accommodation did indeed shift closer to the subjects in the myopic group. There was little change in the emmetropic group, and the hyperopes showed a shift toward a more distant resting position (McBrien

and Millodot, 1987). The shifts in tonic accommodation observed after extensive near work were longlasting, even months (Owens, 1990). In conclusion, there seem to be highly significant differences in accommodative behavior among the different refractive groups (Jones, 1990), and this difference may result in part from different innervation patterns in the ciliary muscles.

The findings on tonic accommodation described above provide an explanation for the differences in refractive development in different individuals. There are two assumptions, however, that have not yet been proved experimentally: (1) the differences in tonic accommodation and plasticity of accommodation behavior are already present before refractive errors develop; and (2) accommodation can influence axial eye growth such that the differences in accommodative behavior would influence the refractive state.

There is then some evidence that the gains in both the local and the accommodative feedback loops are variable among individuals. Because the gain of a feedback loop determines how fast an error is corrected, it could be that people with a fast loop would emme-

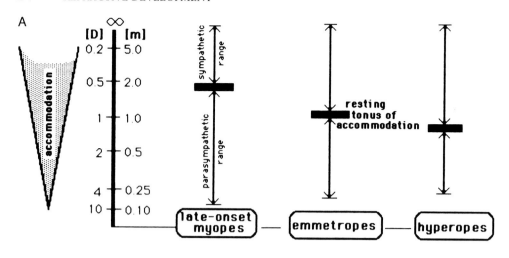

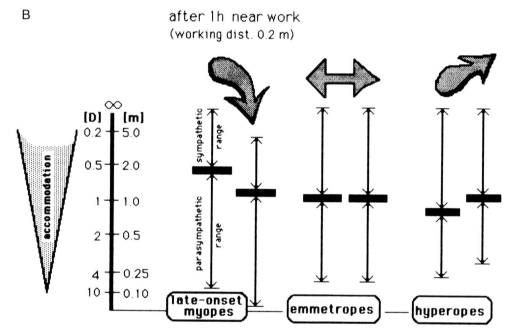

FIG. 2-5. In humans there is evidence that the resting point of tonic accommodation is variable among individuals and is related to the refractive state. (A) Resting points of accommodation in late-onset myopes, emmetropes, and hyperopes. (B) Plasticity of accommodative behavior in the different refractive groups. After a period of extensive near work, the resting point of accommodation shifts closer to the subject, whereas there is little change in emmetropes and even a shift away from the subject in hyperopes. See text for details.

tropize more quickly than others. If true, a person with a fast feedback loop adapts faster to a shorter average viewing distance (e.g., during frequent reading) and becomes myopic, whereas the gain in another person at the time of first reading may already be too low to produce late-onset myopia. Basic to these assumptions is the fact that the emmetropizing mechanism can integrate over the average viewing distances with a long time constant. However, this assumption is already necessary to explain normal refractive development.

TARGETS FOR FUTURE RESEARCH

Avenues for further study point in three directions. First, it is important to find the biochemical pathways that translate the visual signal into a growth response. It has already been determined that the local mechanism in the retina acts directly on the underlying sclera. Second, it is important to know the nature of the visual cues that can change axial eye growth. This question is similar to the question of which stimuli drive accommodation (Kruger and Polla, 1986), although for the local mechanism information from convergence cues and experience are not available. Finally, the role of accommodation during emmetropization is still not clear.

Biochemical Correlates of Deprivation Myopia

Biochemical studies can be divided into two approaches: (1) histological changes and the characterization of changes in tissue properties; and (2) the search for possible changes in retinal transmitters or neuromodulators. Studies are available for both. First, it has been shown that in the chicken axial elongation during deprivation myopia is a real growth process with cell proliferation and increases in cell size, DNA, and protein synthesis (Christensen and Wallman, 1989). These data were collected by autoradiography with ^{3}H-thymidine to measure DNA synthesis and ^{35}S-methionine to measure protein synthesis. In another study, no significant changes in the amount of individual proteins were found by gel electrophoresis (Pickett-Seltner et al., 1988). There are some changes in the histology of the sclera (Rada et al., 1990). Currently, there is enough support for the conclusion that axial elongation is the result of a growth process rather than stretching. Measurements of intraocular pressure changes during deprivation myopia would help to confirm this conclusion but are not available. By contrast, there is some evidence from tree shrew studies that deprivation myopia is the result of stretching of the sclera, which could apparently occur even locally and is augmented by lathyritic agents (McBrien et al., 1989). Because the sclera is also thinning in myopic human subjects, it could be that mammals and birds do indeed differ in this respect.

Stone et al. (1988) found a strong increase of vasointestinal polypeptide (VIP) immunoreactivity in the inner plexiform layer in monkeys during deprivation myopia. The increase was the result of some process prior to an actual growth response because it could also be obtained in adult monkeys where the sensitive period for the induction of deprivation myopia had already passed. The increase in VIP levels seemed to be confined to those eyes that became myopic under conditions of deprivation (Fong et al., 1991). This point is particularly interesting because not all individuals are susceptible to deprivation myopia, probably because the local mechanisms for regulation of axial eye growth have variable gains (see above). VIP can control retinal blood flow and affects smooth musculature (for references see Stone et al., 1988) and could thereby control metabolic activity. Its concentration also seems to be somewhat antagonistic to the dopamine level (Kane et al., 1990), which is particularly interesting with regard to the results described below.

There have been some exciting findings regarding the relation between deprivation myopia and neurotransmitters in the retina. Stone et al. (1989) found that the overall level of retinal dopamine of chickens, as measured by high-pressure liquid chromatography decreases during deprivation myopia. They also showed that by blocking the conversion from dopa to dopamine the synthesis of dopamine was reduced. Furthermore, if the level of dopamine was artificially "raised" by the dopamine agonist apomorphine, deprivation myopia could be reduced or prevented in a dose-dependent fashion. The results must be analyzed with care because they allow the conclusion that the dopamine level is determined not only by the adaptational state of the retina (Iuvone, 1984) and circadian rhythms (fish: Kolbinger et al., 1990; rabbit: Nowak and Zurawska, 1989) but also by the pattern of contrast on the retina. Translucent occluders for the chickens reduced the retinal image brightness little (about 0.5 log units). To produce a reduction in retinal dopamine by an adaptational process of the same magnitude as the one found in deprivation myopia (30–40%), the animal would have to be completely dark-adapted (Brainard and Morgan, 1987). This situation was obviously not the case because the animals were raised under normal light levels. Also another drug that interferes with the normal function of dopaminergic amacrine cells, 6-hydroxydopamine, proved efficient in blocking deprivation myopia without affecting normal axial eye growth and normal vision (Schaeffel and Kohler, personal observation). A role of dopamine during deprivation myopia has also been confirmed in the monkey (Iuvone et al., 1990). Future research must clarify how the local growth-controlling mechanisms can separate the different inputs to the dopamine system (adaptation, circadian, and contrast) to derive an appropriate growth signal.

Excitatory amino acids—quisqualic acid, N-methyl-D,L-aspartate, kainic acid—have also been studied with regard to their effects on eye growth (Barrington et al., 1989). The results are complex because anterior chamber depth, vitreous chamber depth, and eye weight were affected differently for each drug, so a general conclusion cannot yet be drawn. Wildsoet and Pettigrew (1988b) demonstrated that kainic acid could mimic the effects of deprivation myopia to some extent and that the pattern of results was not affected by optic nerve sections.

Finally, because neuroglia cells in the retina (Müller cells) could be responsible for the proliferation of growth factors, their function has been experimentally inhibited by L-α-aminoadipic acid)L-α-AAA) and D-α-AAA (Crewther and Crewther, 1990). D-α-AAA, which causes the Müller cell to swell and reduces the retinal off-response, also caused a marked increase in axial eye growth by a reduction of eye growth under conditions of deprivation. L-α-AAA also causes glial swelling and reduces the on-response, but it acts in opposite ways in normal and deprived eyes. Refractions were not measured. Although the studies described above may provide important information on the general regulation of eye growth, visual function must remain intact during treatment. Otherwise, it is impossible to explore the visual control of eye growth.

Nature of the Visual Information that Triggers Visually Guided Growth

From the results of deprivation myopia, it can be concluded that high contrasts or high spatial frequencies are necessary to inhibit exaggerated axial eye growth that would otherwise occur. To some extent, spatial and temporal contrasts can be exchanged; Gottlieb and Wallman (1987) observed that chickens with occluders do not become myopic if they are raised in stroboscopic light. Here a local detector in the retina is exposed to rapid changes in brightness similar to the condition where a well focused image moves across the retina. The effect may well be mediated by dopamine, as it is has been shown that flickering light results in increased release of dopamine (Kramer, 1971), which could partly compensate for the drop in the overall retinal dopamine content during deprivation myopia (Stone et al., 1989). On the other hand, Cremieux et al. (1989) claimed that cats did become myopic after rearing in stroboscopic light.

It was found that compensatory growth responses can occur in both directions (Schaeffel et al., 1988), thus requiring that the sign of refractive error be detected. Strikingly, the result is similar if no functional accommodation is present (Schaeffel et al., 1990). For a local mechanism in the eye, longitudinal chromatic aberration could provide the information necessary to determine the sign of defocus because color fringes are interchanged if the sign of defocus is reversed (Fincham, 1951). To test the role of chromatic cues, chicks were raised with lenses in monochromatic light. No differences were found between this and a previous experiment in which normally accommodating chicks were raised with lenses in white light (Schaeffel and Howland, 1991). Because accommodation was still possible, it could provide the sign information. The crucial experiment—raising chicks without functional accommodation in monochromatic light with lenses—has not yet been done. One would expect that the sign information is lost and that all eyes become more myopic with no regard to the sign of the lens. However, if the growth response in an eye without accommodation is still appropriate, there is only one explanation left: There must be a detector in the retina that can integrate with a long time constant over the image contrast. If the eye is nearsighted, high contrasts are available only for short viewing distances, but because chicks are mainly concerned about finding food on the ground there is some good contrast most of the time. As a result, axial elongation would be inhibited and the eye would become less myopic. On the other hand, for a hyperopic eye, image contrast is low at all times, resulting in increased axial growth. This way, hyperopia would be rapidly corrected. Further experiments will resolve this question.

One problem the emmetropizing mechanisms have to deal with is longitudinal chromatic aberration. The focal plane for blue light is about 2–3 D in front of the focal plane for red light (Mandelman and Sivak, 1983). One would expect the eye to adopt a refractive state appropriate for green light in the middle of the spectrum where sensitivity is maximal. This question has been studied in the chicken by Rohrer et al. (1992). First, two groups of chicks were raised in monochromatic light from both ends of the spectrum. The light levels were brightness-matched for the chickens by flicker electroretinography. Because of chromatic aberration, if was expected that the two groups would differ in their final refractive states. However, no difference was found. Two explanations were possible: (1) only the mid- and long-wavelength receptors were able to guide emmetropization, with the short-wavelength or ultraviolet receptors having no input to the emmetropizing mechanisms; or (2) the visual acuity of the short-wavelength receptors was too low to detect the defocus provided by the lenses. Therefore chicks were raised with lenses under both light conditions. The result was clear: The lens experiment was successful in deep red light but failed in near-ultraviolet light. A histological analysis showed that, from its sampling interval, the ultraviolet receptor could provide low visual acuity with a depth of focus of 4–6 D, which is too low to detect the weak lenses used (+4 D and −4 D). The result shows that the eye elegantly bypass the problem of chromatic aberration by having low acuity in the blue region where the chromatic change in focal planes is particularly steep. The result also shows that a high acuity system is necessary to guide refractive development.

CONCLUSIONS: WHAT CAN BE LEARNED FROM ANIMAL MODELS REGARDING HUMAN REFRACTIVE DEVELOPMENT?

The results from *animal models* show:

1. There is extensive evidence that visually guided feedback loops control refractive development in the eye.

2. The gains in the loops decrease during development and seem to be proportional to the current growth rate of the eye. There is no evidence that adult eyes ever can become shorter to correct for myopia.

3. There is considerable variability in the gains among individuals.

4. To explain the experimental results, two visually guided loops must be postulated: one acting locally in the eye (matching the photoreceptor plane to the image plane all over the visual field) and one using central pathways (probably involving accommodation). Both mechanisms can detect the amount and sign of defocus.

5. The control of axial eye growth involves the retinal dopamine level.

It can be concluded that for *humans*:

1. The extrapolation of conclusions from animal models to humans is rendered more difficult because it is possible to explain only those physiological types of refractive error that have no additional pathological changes. The animal models had no genetically predetermined defects affecting their refractions, so it can be concluded that their ametropia was a result of experimental manipulations.

2. Visual experience can influence refractive development. Therefore late-onset myopia can be considered an adaptation to the closer average viewing distance.

3. The fact that not all individuals become myopic from near work can be explained from variable gains in the feedback loop that are genetically predetermined.

4. The use of correcting lenses can alter the progression of refractive errors.

5. Once the biochemical pathways that translate visual signals into a growth signal are understood, it may be possible to influence refractive development pharmacologically.

Acknowledgments. The author's work was supported by a grant from the German Research Council (SFB 307-TP A7) and in part by NIH EY-02994 to Howard Howland. The author is grateful to Leilani Peck and Howard C. Howland for carefully reading the manuscript and improving the English.

REFERENCES

AWAYA, S., YASUMA, M., SUGAWARA, M., AND SUZUKI, M. (1979). Studies in visual functions in 50 cases of unilateral congenital ptosis. *Folia Ophthalmol. Jpn.* 30, 195.

BARRINGTON, M., SATTAYASAI, J., ZAPPA, J., AND EHRLICH, E. (1989). Excitatory amino acids interfere with normal eye growth in posthatch chicks. *Curr. Eye Res.* 8, 781–792.

BERCOWITZ, A. B., HARRISON, P. C., AND LEARY, G. A. (1971). Light induced alterations in growth patterns of the avian eye. *Vision Res.* 12, 1253–1259.

BRAINARD, G. C., AND MORGAN, W. W. (1987). Light-induced stimulation of retinal dopamine: a dose-response relationship. *Brain Res.* 424, 199–203.

CALLENDER, M. G., SIVAK, J. G., AND BARRIE, D. L. (1989). Myopia and hyperopia induced in young chicks with convex and concave soft contact lenses. *Invest. Ophthalmol. Vis. Sci.* 31 (suppl.), 253.

CAMPBELL, F. W. (1957). Depth of field in the human eye. *Opt. Acta (Lond.)* 4, 157–164.

CAMPBELL, F. W. (1960). Correlation of accommodation between two eyes. *J. Opt. Soc. Am.* 50, 738–740.

CAMPBELL, F. W., AND GUBISCH, R. W. (1966). The optical quality of the human eye. *J. Physiol. (Lond.)* 186, 558–578.

CHRISTENSEN, A. M., AND WALLMAN, J. (1989). Increased protein synthesis in scleras of eyes with deprivation myopia. *Invest. Ophthalmol. Vis. Sci.* 30 (suppl.), 402.

CREMIEUX, J., ORBAN, G. A., DUYSENS, J., AMBLARD, B., AND KENNEDY, H. (1989). Experimental myopia in cats reared in stroboscopic illumination. *Vision Res.* 29, 1033–1036.

CREWTHER, D. P., AND CREWTHER, S. G. (1990). Pharmacological modification of eye growth in normally rearde and visually deprived chicks. *Curr. Eye Res.* 9, 733–740.

CREWTHER, S. G., NATHAN, J., KIELY, P. M., BRENNAN, N. A., AND CREWTHER, D. P. (1988). The effect of defocussing contact lenses on refraction in cynomolgus monkeys. *Clin. Vis. Sci.* 3, 221–228.

CURTIN, B. J. (1985). *The Myopias: Basic Science and Clinical Management.* Philadelphia: Harper & Row.

EBENHOLTZ, S. M. (1991). Accommodative hysteresis: fundamental asymmetry in decay rate after near and far focussing. *Invest. Ophthalmol. Vis. Sci.* 32, 148–153.

EHRLICH D. (1981). Regional specialization of the chick retina as revealed by size and density of neurons in the ganglion cell layer. *J. Comp. Neurol.* 195, 643–657.

FINCHAM, E. F. (1951). The accommodation reflex and its stimulus. *Br. J. Ophthalmol.* 35, 381–393.

FITZKE, F. W., HAYES, B. P., HODOS, W., HOLDEN, A. L., AND LOW, J. C. (1985a). Refractive sectors in the visual field of the pigeon eye. *J. Physiol. (Lond.)* 369, 33–44.

FITZKE, F. W., SHEEN, F. W., AND HOLDEN, A. L. (1985b). A Maxwellian-view optometer suitable for electrophysiological and psychophysical research. *Vision Res.* 25, 871–875.

FONG, D. S., WIESEL, T. N., RAVIOLA, E., AND REICHLIN, S. (1991). Is lid-fusion myopia caused by an increase in retinal vasoactive intestinal polypeptide (VIP). *Invest. Ophthalmol. Vis. Sci.* 32 (suppl.), 1203.

GILMARTIN, B. (1986). A review of the role of sympathetic innervation of the ciliary muscle in ocular accommodation. *Ophthalmol. Physiol. Opt.* 6, 23–37.

GILMARTIN, B., WINN, B., OWENS, H., AND PUGH, J. R. (1990). The effect of topical beta-adrenergic antagonists on the temporal response characteristics of ocular accommodation in humans. *Proc. Int. Soc. Eye Res.* 6, 96.

GLICKSTEIN, M., AND MILLODOT, M. (1970). Retinoscopy and eye size. *Science* 168, 605–606.

GOLLENDER, M., THORN, F., AND ERICKSON, P. (1979). Development of axial dimensions following eye lid suture in the cat. *Vision Res.* 19, 221–223.

GOTTLIEB, M. D., AND WALLMAN, J. (1987). Retinal activity modulates eye growth. *Soc. Neurosci. Abstr.* 1987, 1297.

GREEN, D. G., POWERS, M. K., AND BANKS, M. S. (1980). Depth of focus, eye size, and visual acuity. *Vision Res.* 20, 827–835.

GREENE, P. R., GUYTON, D. L., PIRO, P., AND SCHOLZ, R. T. (1989). Axial length vs. refraction correlations in the ametropic rhesus monkey eye. *Invest. Ophthalmol. Vis. Sci.* 30 (suppl.), 32.

GUYTON, D. L., GREENE, P. R., AND SCHOLZ, R. T. (1989). Dark-rearing interference with emmetropization in the rhesus monkey. *Invest. Ophthalmol. Vis. Sci.* 30, 761–764.

HAYES, B. P., FITZKE, F. W., HODOS, W., AND HOLDEN, A. L. (1986) A morphological analysis of experimental myopia in young chicks, *Invest. Ophthalmol. Vis. Sci.* 27, 981–991.

HELMHOLTZ, H. (1985). Ueber die Akkommodation des Auges. *Albrecht von Graefes Arch. Ophthalmol.* 1, 1.

HENDRICKSON, P. (1987). *Uber die Entwicklung des Auges.* Zurich: Habilitationsschrift.

HODOS, W., AND ERICHSON, J. T. (1990). Lower-field myopia in birds: an adaptation that keeps the ground in focus. *Vision Res.* 30, 653–659.

HODOS, W., AND KUENZEL, W. J. (1984). Retinal image degradation produces ocular enlargement in chicks. *Invest. Ophthalmol. Vis. Sci.* 25, 652–659.

HOYT, C. S., STONE, R. D., FROMER, C., AND BILLSON, F. A. (1981). Monocular axial myopia associated with eye lid closure in human infants. *Am. J. Ophthalmol.* 91, 197–200.

IUVONE, P. M. (1984). Regulation of retinal dopamine biosynthesis and tyrosine hydroxylase activity in light. *Fed. Proc.* 43, 2709–2713.

IUVONE, P. M., TIGGES, M., STONE, R. A., LAMBERT, S., AND LATIES, A. M. (1990). Apomorphine inhibits development of myopia in visually-deprived infant rhesus monkeys. *Invest. Ophthalmol. Vis Sci.* 31 (suppl.), 254.

JOHNSON, C. A., POST, R. B., CHALUPA, L. M., AND LEE, T. J. (1982). Monocular deprivation in humans: a study of identical twins. *Invest. Ophthalmol. Vis. Sci.* 23, 135–140.

JONES, R. (1990). Accommodative and convergence control system parameters are abnormal in myopia. *Invest. Ophthalmol. Vis. Sci.* 31 (suppl.), 81.

KANE, G. J., KOH, S-W. M., AND RICHARDS, R. D. (1990). Dopamine attenuates the stimulatory effect of VIP on macromolecule secretion at the apical membranes of chick embryonic retinal pigment epithelium. *Invest. Ophthalmol. Vis. Sci.* 31 (suppl.), 370.

KIRBY, A. W., SUTTON, L., AND WEISS, H. (1982). Elongation of cat eyes following neonatal lid suture. *Invest. Ophthalmol. Vis. Sci.* 22, 274–277.

KOLBINGER, W., KOHLER, K., OETTING, H., AND WEILER, R. (1990). Endogenous dopamine and cyclic events in the fish retina. I. HPLC assay of total content, release, and metabolic turnover during light/dark cycles. *Vis. Neurosci.* 5, 143–149.

KRAMER, S. G. (1971). Dopamine: a retinal neurotransmitter. I. Retinal uptake, storage, and light-stimulated release of H³-dopamine in vivo. *Invest. Ophthalmol.* 10, 438–452.

KRUGER, P. B., AND POLLA, J. (1986). Stimuli for accommodation: blur, chromatic aberration and size. *Vision Res.* 26, 957–971.

LAUBER, J. K. (1987). Review: light-induced avian glaucoma as an animal model for human primary glaucoma. *J. Ocular Pharmacol.* 3, 77–99.

LEIBOWITZ, H. W., AND OWENS, D. A. (1975). Anomalous myopias and the intermediate dark focus of accommodation. *Science* 189, 646–648.

MAGUIRE, G. W., SMITH, E. L., III, HARWERTH, R. S., AND CRAWFORD, M. L. (1982). Optically induced anisometropia in kittens. *Invest. Ophthalmol. Vis. Sci.* 23, 253–264.

MANDELMAN, T., AND SIVAK, J. G. (1983). Longitudinal chromatic aberration of the vertebrate eye. *Vision Res.* 23, 1555–1559.

McBRIEN, N. A., AND BARNES, D. A. (1984). A review and evaluation of theories of refractive error development. *Ophthalmic Physiol. Opt.* 4, 201–213.

McBRIEN, N. A., AND MILLODOT, M. (1987). The relation between tonic accommodation and refractive error. *Invest. Ophthalmol. Vis. Sci.* 28, 997–1004.

McBRIEN, N. A., NORTON, T. T., AND McKANNA, J. A. (1989). Scleral and corneal morphometry in lathyritic-enhanced experimental myopia in tree shrew. *Invest. Ophthalmol. Vis. Sci.* 30 (suppl.), 32.

McBRIEN, N. A., MOGHADDAM, H. O., AND REDER, A. P. (1991). Atropine reduces axial elongation and myopia in visually deprived chick eyes. *Invest. Ophthalmol. Vis. Sci.* 32 (suppl.), 1203.

McKANNA, J. A., AND CASAGRANDE, V. A. (1978). Reduced lens development in lid suture myopia. *Exp. Eye Res.* 26, 715–723.

McKANNA, J. A., AND CASAGRANDE, V. A. (1981a). Zonula dysplasia in myopia. In: T. SATO AND R. YANIJ (eds.). *Proceedings of the Second International Conference on Myopia*. Yokohama: Sato Eye Clinic, pp. 21–32.

McKANNA, J. A., AND CASAGRANDE, V. A. (1981b). Atropine affects lid-suture myopia development. *Doc. Ophthalmol. Proc. Ser.* 28, 187–192.

MERRIAM, W. W., ELLIS, F. D., AND HELVESTON, E. M. (1980). Congenital blepharoptosis, anisometropia, and amblyopia. *Am. J. Ophthalmol.* 89, 410.

MILES, F. A. (1972). Centrifugal control of the avian retina. I. Receptive field properties of the retinal ganglion cells. *Brain Res.* 48, 65–92.

MILES, F. A., AND WALLMAN, J. (1990). Local ocular compensation for imposed local refractive error. *Vision Res.* 30, 339–349.

MILLODOT, M. (1981). Effect of ametropia on peripheral refraction. *Am. J. Optom. Physiol. Opt.* 58, 691–695.

MORRIS, V. B. (1987). An afoveate area centralis in the chick retina. *J. Comp. Neurol.* 210, 198–203.

NI, J., AND SMITH, E. L., III. (1989). Effects of chronical optical defocus on the kitten's refractive status. *Vision Res.* 29, 929–938.

NICKLA, D. L., PANOS, S. N., FUGATE-WENTZEK, L. A., GOTTLIEB, M. D., AND WALLMAN, J. (1989). What attributes of visual stimulation determine whether chick eyes develop deprivation myopia? *Invest. Ophthalmol. Vis. Sci.* 30 (suppl.), 31.

NORTON, T. T. (1990). Experimental myopia in tree shrews. In: *Myopia and the Control of Eye Growth*. Ciba Foundation Symposium 155. Chichester: Wiley, pp. 178–199.

NORTON, T. T., ESSINGER, J. A., AND McBRIEN, N. A. (1989). Lid suture myopia in tree shrew despite blockade of ganglion cell action potentials. *Invest. Ophthalmol. Vis. Sci.* 30 (suppl.), 31.

NOWAK, J. Z., AND ZURAWSKA, E. (1989). Dopamine in the rabbit retina and striatum: diurnal rhythm and effect of light stimulation. *J. Neural Transm.* 75, 201–212.

O'LEARY, D. J., AND MILLODOT, M. (1979). Eye lid closure causes myopia in humans. *Experientia* 35, 1478–1479.

OISHI, T., AND LAUBER, J. K. (1988). Chicks blinded with formoguanamine do not develop lid suture myopia. *Curr. Eye Res.* 7, 69–73.

OISHI, T., AND MURAKAMI, N. (1985). Effects of duration and intensity of illumination on several parameters of the chick eye. *Comp. Biochem. Physiol.* 81A, 319–323.

OWENS, D. A. (1990). Near work, accommodative tonus, and myopia. In: T. GROSVENOR AND M. FLOM (eds.). *Researches on Refractive Anomalies: Clinical Applications*. Stoneham, MA: Butterworth-Heinemann.

PICKETT-SELTNER, R. L., SIVAK, J. G., AND PASTERNAK, J. J. (1988). Experimentally induced myopia in chicks: morphometrical and biochemical analysis during the first 14 days after hatching. *Vision Res.* 28, 323–328.

RABIN, J., SLUYTERS, R. C., AND MALACH, R. (1981). Emmetropization: a vision dependent phenomenon. *Invest. Ophthalmol. Vis. Sci.* 23, 561–565.

RADA, J. A., THOFT, R. A., AND HASSELL, J. R. (1990). Extracellular matrix changes in the sclera of chickens with experimental myopia. *Invest. Ophthalmol. Vis. Sci.* 31, 253.

RAVIOLA, E., AND WIESEL, T. N. (1978). Effect of dark rearing on experimental myopia in monkeys. *Invest. Ophthalmol. Vis. Sci.* 17, 485–488.

RAVIOLA, E., AND WIESEL, T. N. (1985). An animal model of myopia. *N. Engl. J. Med.* 312, 1609–1615.

ROHRER, B., SCHAEFFEL, F., AND ZRENNER, E. (1992). Longitudinal chromatic aberration and emmetropization: results from the chicken eye. *J. Physiol.* 449, 363–376.

SCHAEFFEL, F., AND HOWLAND, H. C. (1987). Corneal accommodation in chick and pigeon. *J. Comp. Physiol. [A]* 160, 375–384.

SCHAEFFEL, F., AND HOWLAND, H. C. (1988a). Visual optics in normal and ametropic chickens. *Clin. Vis. Sci.* 3, 83–93.

SCHAEFFEL, F., AND HOWLAND, H. C. (1988b). A mathematical model for emmetropization in the chicken. *J. Opt. Soc. Am. [A]* 5, 2080–2086.

SCHAEFFEL, F., AND HOWLAND, H. C. (1991). Properties of visual feedback loops controlling eye growth and refractive state in the chicken. *Vision Res.* 31, 717–734.

SCHAEFFEL, F., FARKAS, L., AND HOWLAND, H. C. (1987). Infrared photoretinoscope. *Appl. Opt.* 26, 1505–1509.

SCHAEFFEL, F., GLASSER, A., AND HOWLAND, H. C. (1988). Accommodation, refractive error and eye growth in chickens. *Vision Res.* 28, 639–657.

SCHAEFFEL, F., HOWLAND, H. C., AND FARKAS, L. (1986). Natural accommodation in the growing chicken. *Vision Res.* 26, 1977–1993.

SCHAEFFEL, F., TROILO, D., WALLMAN, J., AND HOWLAND, H. C. (1990). Growing eyes that lack accommodation grow to compensate for imposed defocus. *Vis. Neurosci.* 4, 177–183.

SMITH, E. L., III, HARWERTH, R. S., CRAWFORD, M. L. J., AND VON NOORDEN, G. K. (1987). Observations on the effects of form deprivation on the refractive status of the monkey. *Invest. Ophthalmol. Vis. Sci.* 28, 1236–1245.

SORSBY, A. (1967). The nature of spherical refractive errors. In *Report of the Workshop on Refractive Anomalies of the Eye*. NINDB Monograph 5. Washington, DC: U.S. Department of Health, Education and Welfare.

STONE, R. A., LATIES, A. M., RAVIOLA, E., AND WIESEL, T. N. (1988). Increase in retinal vasoactive intestinal polypeptide after eye lid fusion in primates. *Proc. Natl. Acad. Sci. USA* 85, 257–260.

STONE, R. A., LIN, T., LATIES, A. M., AND IUVONE, P. M. (1989). Retinal dopamine and form-deprivation myopia. *Proc. Natl. Acad. Sci. USA* 86, 704–706.

TROILO, D. (1989). The visual control of eye growth in chicks. Doctoral dissertation, City University of New York.

TROILO, D. (1990). Experimental studies of emmetropization in the chick. In *Myopia and the Control of Eye Growth*. Ciba Foundation Symposium 155. Chichester: Wiley, pp. 89–114.

TROILO, D., AND WALLMAN, J. (1987). Changes in corneal curvature during accommodation in chicks. *Vision Res.* 27, 241–247.

TROILO, D., GOTTLIEB, M. D., AND WALLMAN, J. (1987). Visual deprivation causes myopia in chicks with optic nerve section. *Curr. Eye Res.* 6, 993–999.

TROILO, D., JUDGE, S. J., RIDLEY, R., AND BAKER, H. (1990). Myopia induced in a new world primate—the common marmoset (*Callythrix jacchus*). *Invest. Ophthalmol. Vis. Sci.* 31 (suppl.), 254.

VON NOORDEN, G. K., AND LEWIS, R. A. (1987). Ocular axial length in unilateral congenital cataracts and blepharoptosis. *Invest. Ophthalmol. Vis. Sci.* 28, 750–752.

WALLMAN, J., AND ADAMS, J. I. (1987). Development aspects of experimental myopia in chicks. *Vision Res.* 27, 1139–1163.

WALLMAN, J., GOTTLIEB, M. D., RAJARAM, V., AND FUGATE-WENTZEK, L. (1987). Local retinal regions control local eye growth and myopia. *Science* 237, 73–77.

WALLMAN, J., ROSENTHAL, D., ADAMS, J. I., AND ROMAGNANO, L. (1981). Role of accommodation and developmental aspects of experimental myopia in chicks. *Doc. Ophthalmol. Proc.* 28, 197–206.

WALLMAN, J., TURKEL, J., AND TRACHTMAN, J. (1978). Extreme myopia produced by modest changes in early visual experience. *Science* 201, 1249–1251.

WIESEL, T. N., AND RAVIOLA, E. (1977). Myopia and eye enlargement after neonatal lid fusion in monkeys. *Nature* 266, 66–68.

WIESEL, T. N., AND RAVIOLA, E. (1979). Increase in axial length of the macaque monkey eye after corneal opacification. *Invest. Ophthalmol. Vis. Sci.* 18, 1232–1236.

WILDSOET, C. F., AND PETTIGREW, J. D. (1988a). Experimental myopia and anomalous eye growth patterns unaffected by optic nerve section in chickens: evidence for local control of eye growth. *Clin. Vis. Sci.* 3, 99–107.

WILDSOET, C. F., AND PETTIGREW, J. D. (1988b). Kainic acid-induced eye enlargement in chickens: differential effects on anterior and posterior segments. *Invest. Ophthalmol. Vis. Sci.* 29, 311–319.

YINON, U., ROSE, L., AND SHAPIRO, A. (1980). Myopia in the eye of developing chicks following monocular and binocular lid closure. *Vision Res.* 20, 137–141.

3 | Infant accommodation and convergence

RICHARD N. ASLIN

The mature human visual system has evolved the capacity to: (1) select a small portion of the retinal image for close attention; (2) optimize the quality of the retinal image by adjusting its posterior focal distance to match the plane of the retinal receptors; and (3) direct and maintain the two foveas on the object of attention despite changes in object distance. The ability to adjust the optics and binocular alignment of the eyes to match an object's viewing distance affords great efficiency in gathering detailed information about a real-world scene because it reduces the need for fore–aft locomotion. Moreover, because these optical adjustments and binocular eye movements require less than 1 second to complete, detailed information from multiple depth planes can be gathered rapidly.

This chapter summarizes what has been learned since the early 1960s about the accuracy of accommodation and convergence in normal human infants. Not surprisingly, both accommodation and convergence are less accurately controlled in young infants than in normal adults. These empirical findings are discussed in some detail along with the methods of measurement that have enabled researchers to demonstrate developmental improvements in the accuracy of both accommodation and convergence between birth and 6 months of age.

The more interesting question, however, is what mechanisms underlie this rapid postnatal developmental improvement. Four general categories of explanation have been offered to account for the development of improved sensorimotor control (Aslin, 1981). First, young infants may fail to exhibit accurate sensorimotor control because they cannot, or are unmotivated to, direct their attention to the task set forth by the researcher. Second, some fundamental sensory capacity required for guidance of the motor response may be absent or immature. Third, the motor response system itself may be limited by neuromuscular or biomechanical constraints. Fourth, the attentional, sensory, and motor components of a response system may be poorly coordinated, even when these components are each mature. What will become clear from this review is that, despite significant advances in our understanding of infant accommodation and convergence, the past

three decades of research have not revealed a definitive account of the relative contribution of these four possible underlying mechanisms to the normative course of development.

ACCOMMODATION

Accommodation refers to the change in dioptric power of the eye created by alterations in the shape of the crystalline lens. As summarized in Chapter 2, the adult eye has an overall refractive power of approximately 60 diopters (D), and the accommodative system extends that power by approximately 10 D. Thus an emmetropic young adult can maintain optimal retinal image focus on objects ranging in distance from 10 cm to infinity. The presence of significant spherical refractive errors limits this range of accurate focus, either by increasing the near point of focus (in hypermetropia) or by decreasing the far point (myopia). Moreover, the presence of significant astigmatic refractive errors prevents optimal focus of more than one optical meridian at a time.

Accommodative accuracy in human infants has been measured under noncyclopleged conditions using three techniques: retinoscopy, photorefraction, and autorefraction. Haynes and colleagues (1965), Banks (1980), and Brookman (1983) used retinoscopy to assess the accuracy of accommodation in infants under 4 months of age as they fixated a single target at several viewing distances. Haynes et al. (1965) reported that newborns and 1-month-olds showed little or no accommodative response over a 5 D range (Fig. 3-1) but, rather, reverted to a relatively fixed focal distance of 25–20 cm (4–5 D). Both Banks (1980) and Brookman (1983) reported that 2-week-olds and 1-month-olds had considerably better accommodative responsiveness than previously reported by Haynes et al. (1965) (Fig. 3-1). The most important factor associated with this improvement was the use of stimulus targets equated in retinal angle. Haynes et al. (1965) had used a small fixation target whose retinal size declined with increases in viewing distance. Thus at least some of the apparent fixed near-accommodation

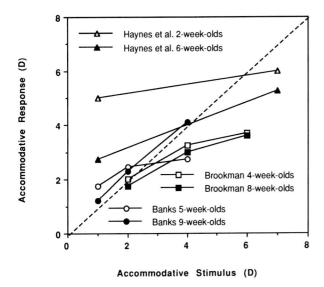

FIG. 3-1. Accommodation stimulus-response functions for 1- to 3-month-olds from studies by Haynes et al. (1965), Banks (1980), and Brookman (1983).

observed by Haynes et al. (1965) was likely the result of an insufficient sensory signal to drive the accommodative response and a tendency to revert to a relatively near focal distance in the absence of a suprathreshold fixation target. Although Banks (1980) and Brookman (1983) reported that infants showed a marked improvement in accommodative accuracy between birth and 5 months of age, errors as large as 1 D were not uncommon even in these older infants. Moreover, if an infant was drowsy or had a significant spherical refractive error, accommodative accuracy was severely reduced.

Several photorefractive techniques, originally developed by Howland and Howland (1974), have been used to assess accommodative accuracy in young infants. The first photorefractive study of infant accommodation (Braddick et al., 1979) used the orthogonal technique in which segmented cylindrical lenses create film images containing features that can be decoded into spherical and cylindrical refractive errors with respect to a fixed camera distance. In agreement with Banks (1980) and Brookman (1983), Braddick et al. (1979) reported that even newborns and 1-month-olds showed reasonably accurate accommodation (±0.6 D) to a target at 75 cm, but these same infants rarely accommodated accurately to a target at 150 cm. Older infants were consistently accurate accommodators to both target distances.

Howland and Sayles (1987) used orthogonal and isotropic photorefraction (which does not utilize cylindrical lenses) to measure accommodative accuracy to a target at 150 cm. They reported that accommodative accuracy was good (mean 0 D error) in a sample of 70 newborn to 6-month-olds. However, the use of a single

target viewing distance did not allow determination of the range of accommodative accuracy. Howland et al. (1987) used this same combination of orthogonal and isotropic photorefraction with an infrared-sensitive television camera to obtain a dynamic estimate of accommodative responses in young infants. They tested 29 infants ranging in postnatal age from 2 to 10 months and reported that the slope of the accommodative stimulus-response function was approximately 0.6, a value that does not differ significantly from the slopes obtained by Banks (1980) and Brookman (1983). They also reported that the accommodative response occurred at a rate of at least 4.6 D/second, a value that is within the adult range. Unfortunately, because of off-axis fixations and vignetting of the photorefraction images, the absolute accuracy of accommodation to the target distances (25, 33, 50, and 100 cm) could not be determined with high confidence. Preliminary results using a similar technique but with eccentric photorefraction has been reported by Atkinson et al. (1988). Riddell and colleagues (1991) have used eccentric photorefraction to obtain estimates of accommodative accuracy in young infants and reported that approximately 50% of the 1-month-olds showed a monotonic accommodative stimulus-response function, but again no data on absolute accommodative accuracy were reported.

The third method that has been used to measure accommodative accuracy in young infants is autorefraction. Autorefractors are commercially available devices that perform rapid retinoscopy while the subject fixates a target. Aslin et al. (1990) succeeded in adapting a particular autorefractor (Canon R-1) for use with young infants and reported that accommodative accuracy was considerably better than that reported by Haynes et al. (1965). However, one puzzling aspect of their data was the presence of significant *over*accommodation in several infants (Fig. 3-2). Whereas most 1- to 3-month-olds showed accommodative stimulus-response slopes that closely matched the slope of 1.0 expected if accommodation were on target, several of the 1-month-olds showed a constant myopic error as large as 2 D.

It is unclear why such myopic accommodative errors have not been observed using other techniques. One possibility is that young infants have a resting position of accommodation that is much nearer than in adults. Aslin and Dobson (1983) reported that the resting position of accommodation, as measured in total darkness, was 1.59 D for a group of four 3-month-olds, whereas adults showed a mean of 1.14 D; and other studies of adults (e.g., Owens and Leibowitz, 1980) have reported means of 1.25 D. Thus there is some limited support for a slightly nearer resting position of accommodation in young infants. However, the consistently high accommodative stimulus-response slopes reported by Aslin et

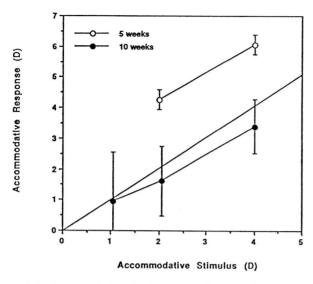

FIG. 3-2. Accommodation stimulus-response functions for 5- and 10-week-olds from a study by Aslin et al. (1990) that used a Canon R-1 autorefractor.

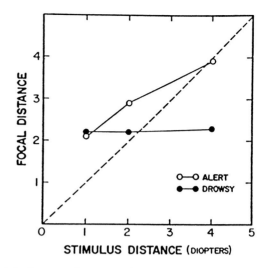

FIG. 3-3. Accommodation stimulus-response functions from a single 5-week-old infant under two conditions of alertness (Reprinted from Banks, 1980 © Society for Research in Child Development.)

al. (1990) for young infants imply that infants of this age are not simply disattending to the near target and reverting to a fixed resting position of accommodation.

Another potential explanation for the myopic accommodation in young infants centers on the near visual-surround that is created by the autorefractor itself. With the Canon R-1 autorefractor, the infant views a target through a beam-splitter and its support frame, which is located less than 10 cm from the infant's face. Rosenfield and Cuiffreda (1991) have shown that knowledge of such a near visual-surround can bias accommodation toward myopia. Although this bias in adults is only approximately 0.5 D, it is possible that young infants, who have a larger depth of focus than adults, may be induced to overaccommodate under these stimulus conditions while maintaining an accommodative state that is within their depth of focus.

The foregoing analysis of findings on infant accommodation suggests that the two primary determinants of accommodative accuracy are attention and detection of the blur signal that drives an accommodative response. Evidence for the role of attentional factors comes from several sources, most notably Banks' (1980) example of a 5-week-old who showed a flat accommodative stimulus-response function when in a drowsy state but a steep slope when alert (Fig. 3-3). Evidence for the role of sensory factors comes from Banks' (1980) and Green et al.'s (1980) analyses of the predicted depth of focus of the infant eye and the relation between measured accommodative accuracy and these predictions. According to Banks' (1980) analysis, accommodative responses typically fall within the predicted depth of

focus, suggesting that detection of the blur signal used in driving accommodation is the primary determinant of accommodative (in)accuracy during early infancy.

A number of studies of acuity and contrast sensitivity support Banks' (1980) model of a primary sensory deficit as the explanation for inaccurate infant accommodation. If infants are incapable of detecting a blur signal to drive accommodation, they should also fail to show deficits in visual sensitivity because of these focusing errors. Fantz et al. (1962), Salapatek et al. (1976), Powers and Dobson (1983), Boltz et al. (1983), and Sokol et al. (1983) have reported that the loss of acuity expected if infants were as sensitive to blur as adults was not observed, either when the acuity targets were presented at viewing distances known to elicit inaccurate accommodation or when lenses were placed in front of the infant's eyes to create a blur signal that was less than the predicted depth of focus. Thus there is now strong support for the role of sensory deficits as a primary reason for accommodative inaccuracies during early infancy.

Although the foregoing analysis suggests that motor factors are relatively unimportant to infant accommodation, there simply is no good information to support or refute such a claim. We know that the accommodative system has at least a 10 D range because accommodation shows spontaneous fluctuations of that magnitude. There may, however, be motor constraints on the amplitude of accommodation in some young infants, either because of limitations in the mechanics of the zonule and ciliary body or because of neuromotor command deficiencies in the signals sent to the ciliary muscles. However, the overaccommodation observed in some infants with the autorefractor suggests that these motor limitations are not widespread.

A final factor that has received little empirical study is the dynamics of the accommodative response in infants. This gap in the literature is entirely the result of technical limitations that may be partially overcome by the use of infrared photorefraction (Howland et al., 1987; Atkinson et al., 1988) or further modifications of autorefractors to enable rapid sequential measurements in real-time (Pugh and Winn, 1988). Although the accommodative system operates under continuous feedback conditions, it is possible that the combination of sluggish dynamics and the ambiguity of an unsigned blur signal may severely limit accommodative accuracy in young infants except for relatively stable target-viewing conditions.

CONVERGENCE

Spatial resolution is highest when the image of an object is projected onto the fovea. The mature visual system has evolved mechanisms to ensure that when attention is directed to an object the eye is rotated to bring that object's image onto the fovea. When both eyes are used for fixation of a target, the eyes must rotate toward or away from each other so the image of the object is projected onto both foveas. These horizontal vergence eye movements—convergence for far-to-near changes in target distance and divergence for near-to-far changes—create the necessary geometrical relations for single or fused percepts of a fixated object. If binocular alignment via vergence eye movements does not lead to projection of a single object's image onto both foveas, the object is either perceived as a double image or the input to one fovea is suppressed to eliminate the confusion associated with the differing apparent directions of the double images. As in the case of accommodation, vergence eye movements allow bifoveal fixation of objects ranging in distance from approximately 10 cm to infinity.

Only one method has been used successfully to measure binocular alignment in young human infants. This method involves photographic or video images of one or both eyes. One variant of this method compares the relative position of the pupil in each eye with the reflection of one or more light sources on the cornea. The other variant simply involves measurement of the distance between the two pupils. Both methods suffer from calibration problems and from a limited sampling rate. Calibration is confounded by the fact that no external feature of the eye (e.g., the center of the pupil) corresponds exactly in all subjects with the line of foveal fixation. Thus all studies of binocular alignment in human infants have relied either on inferences about the absolute alignment of the two eyes during some calibration trials or on the collection of relative changes in

binocular alignment during changes in target viewing distance.

The first systematic study of changes in binocular alignment in young infants was conducted by Ling (1942), who made qualitative judgments of vergence eye movements from movie films as infants viewed a small fixation target moving in distance along the midline. Ling reported that consistent evidence of convergence to near viewing distances did not emerge until 3 months postnatal age. Two subsequent studies (Wickelgren, 1976; Maurer, 1975) gathered quantitative estimates of the alignment of the two eyes using corneal reflection photography. However, both studies assumed that the center of the pupil corresponded with the visual axis connecting the fovea with the object of fixation. Because the pupil center is somewhat temporal of the visual axis these investigators concluded that newborns were exotropic.

Slater and Findlay (1975) overcame these interpretive problems associated with corneal reflection photography in two ways. First, they presented targets at three viewing distances in order to elicit a change in vergence. Second, they used a group calibration procedure to correct for the measurement error associated with the discrepancy between the line of sight and the center of the pupil. They reported that newborns alter their binocular alignment appropriately (within their measurement error of ±2 degrees) to targets at 50 and 25 cm, but that newborns failed to converge any further when the target was placed at 12.5 cm (Fig. 3-4).

Aslin (1977) extended these findings using corneal reflection photography by *moving* the fixation target

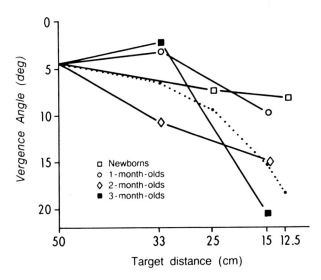

FIG. 3-4. Estimated binocular alignment of newborns (Slater and Findlay, 1975) and 1- to 3-month-olds (Aslin, 1977) to a visual target at various viewing distances. The dashed line represents the vergence angle required to maintain bifoveal fixation. (Reprinted from Aslin, 1988.)

over viewing distances of 10–50 cm and by testing 1- to 3-month-olds. Rather than using a group calibration procedure to interpret these film images, Aslin simply determined whether the relation between pupil center and the corneal reflection created by the target remained constant as the target moved through its range of viewing distances. Although infants as young as 1 month of age altered their binocular alignment in the appropriate direction as the target distance changed, they did not show a sufficient magnitude of change in binocular alignment to support the maintenance of bifoveal fixation until 3 months of age (Fig. 3-4).

As in the case of the accommodative system, there are several basic reasons why young infants may not show appropriate changes in binocular alignment to support bifoveal fixation. Poor attention cannot be ruled out as a significant factor in young infants' poor convergence accuracy, but sensory factors appear to be a more likely explanation. There are two types of sensory signal that trigger convergence in normal adults. The first is the linkage between the accommodative system and the vergence system (see next section), and the second is the misregistration of the two retinal images, which creates retinal disparity. It is important to point out a confusion that pervades the literature on vergence control based on retinal disparity. As cogently summarized by Collewijn and Erkelens (1990), *relative* retinal disparity refers to the difference in separation between two pairs of visual stimuli projected to the two retinas. The use of the term retinal disparity in the literature on binocular depth perception refers to these interocular image differences that support stereopsis. However, for a single target in an otherwise contourless visual field, vergence eye movements can be elicited by *absolute* retinal disparity, that is, the projection of a single target's image onto noncorresponding points in the two retinas. The use of the term retinal disparity in the literature on oculomotor control refers to the presence of noncorrespondence, regardless of whether the stimulus display supports stereopsis. Thus for the control of vergence eye movements based on disparity information, the critical question is whether infants converge or diverge their eyes appropriately to bring the object of attention into interocular retinal correspondence. Because in adults this process results in sensory fusion (the elimination of double images), disparity-driven vergence eye movements are called fusional vergence.

There is qualitative evidence that retinal disparity does not provide as precise a stimulus for fusional vergence in infants as it does in adults. Aslin (1977) placed wedge prisms of various sizes in front of one eye in 3- to 6-month-old infants. The refixation eye movement observed in normal adults to this prism-induced binocular misalignment was not observed in infants until 3–4 months of age (Fig. 3-5). Thus in contrast to the minimally sufficient disparity of less than 1 degree required to elicit binocular realignment in adults, infants appeared to require a disparity of at least 5 degrees for such a refixation response to be elicited. These results may appear to contradict the results of Slater and Findlay (1975) and of Aslin (1977), who showed that newborns and 1-month-olds make vergence eye movements in the appropriate direction but of insufficient magnitude for bifoveation. It is important to note that the total vergence change required in the Slater and Findlay (1975) and Aslin (1977) studies was 13.4 and 10.6 degrees, respectively. Thus if infants have a degraded sensory capacity to detect the disparity signal required to trigger a vergence response, they may make vergence eye movements that fall only within the sensory range of *absolute* disparity detection.

An extension of this sensory-deficit hypothesis is that poor disparity detection may only be a symptom of poor spatial resolution. In adults Kulikowski (1978) and Schor et al. (1984) have shown that low-pass spatially filtered targets increase the extent of the region surrounding the point of binocular fixation within which objects are perceived as single rather than double (Panum's fusion area). Because young infants' contrast sensitivity function is known to be shifted toward lower spatial frequencies than in normal adults, it is possible that the developmental improvement in vergence accuracy is primarily the result of a developmental improvement in contrast sensitivity for medium and high spatial frequencies and not the result of the developmental improvement in *relative* disparity sensitivity required for stereopsis (Held et al., 1980; Birch et al., 1982). For

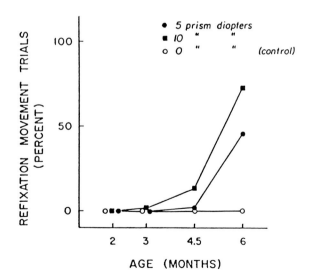

FIG. 3-5. Proportion of trials on which 2- to 6-month-old infants responded appropriately to two magnitudes of prism-induced disparity (Reprinted from Aslin, 1988.)

example, nearly two decades of infant research have revealed that grating acuity improves gradually by a factor of 4–5 between birth and 12 months of age (Dobson and Teller, 1978). A study of the development of acuity and contrast sensitivity by Norcia et al. (1990) using the visual evoked potential (VEP) has replicated this finding by showing that contrast sensitivity for medium to high spatial frequencies improves gradually over the first postnatal year (Fig. 3-6A). Because the detection of interocular image offsets requires medium to high spatial frequency sensitivity, this gradual increase in contrast sensitivity for medium to high spatial frequencies may account for the gradual improvement in vergence accuracy. For example, Schor et al. (1984) reported that the extent of Panum's fusion area in adults is approximately 10 arc minutes for bandpass spatial targets with a center frequency of 5 cycles/degree (cpd). Norcia et al. (1990) reported that infants as young as 9–10 weeks of age have a contrast sensitivity 20 times less than adults at this middle (5 cpd) spatial frequency. If the size of Panum's fusional area in infants is proportional to peak contrast sensitivity (as it is in adults), the extent of Panum's fusion area in 9- to 10-week-olds should be 200 arc minute, a value that is consistent with the prism-induced disparity results from Aslin (1977).

What remains puzzling about this gradual improvement in medium to high spatial-frequency sensitivity and its relation to vergence accuracy is the poor vergence accuracy observed in infants younger than 9–10 weeks of age and the rapid onset of stereopsis at 14 weeks of age. The Norcia et al. (1990) data on contrast

sensitivity may provide a potential explanation of these additional facts. Between birth and 9–10 weeks of age, infants show a rapid improvement in contrast sensitivity even at low spatial frequencies (Fig. 3-6B). Thus there may simply be insufficient contrast sensitivity during early infancy to support all but the coarsest control of vergence. Moreover, if one posits a minimum contrast sensitivity at medium spatial frequencies for the activation of the *relative* retinal disparity (stereopsis) mechanism, this internal threshold could result in the rapid improvement in stereoacuity observed at approximately 14 weeks of age. Held (1993) has raised but rejected a similar threshold account for the rapid onset of stereopsis.

An alternative explanation for the poor vergence accuracy observed in young infants is that their resting position of vergence may be at a far distance, thereby creating an increased motor demand at near viewing distances. However, Aslin (1986) reported that the resting position of vergence, as measured in total darkness, was approximately 25–30 cm in 1- to 4-month-olds, a significantly *nearer* distance than the 100–120 cm resting position in adults. Thus there does not appear to be a motor constraint on near vergence in young infants.

Although attentional and sensory factors appear to offer the best explanation for inaccurate vergence in young infants, it is important to note that, as in the case of the accommodative system, we have no information about the dynamics of the vergence response. Technical limitations, most notably the poor temporal sampling rate of corneal reflection systems, have prevented the collection of real-time vergence responses in young infants. It is possible that sluggish neuromuscular dynam-

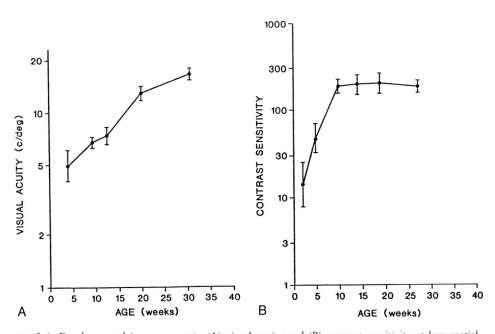

FIG. 3-6. Developmental improvement in (A) visual acuity and (B) contrast sensitivity at low spatial frequencies. (Reprinted from Norcia et al., 1990.)

ics contributes to the inaccurate binocular alignment observed during early infancy.

ACCOMMODATION–CONVERGENCE INTERACTIONS

As outlined above, vergence eye movements receive a trigger signal from the accommodative system as well as from the disparity or fusional system. Similarly, the accommodative system receives a trigger from the vergence system as well as from the detection of blur. These control signals are illustrated in Figure 3-7. The influence of disparity signals on the accommodative system can be revealed only under open-loop conditions, where changes in accommodation have no effect on stimulus blur. Such an experiment requires either a Maxwellian viewing system, with rigid control of head position, or pinhole pupils to increase the depth of focus of the eye. Neither system has yet been used successfully with young infants.

Accommodative-convergence is easier to study than convergence-accommodation because it requires only the measurement of binocular alignment under monocular viewing conditions. Aslin and Jackson (1979) provided the first demonstration of accommodative-convergence in young infants using infrared photography to measure changes in interpupillary distance while the infant fixated a target at far and near viewing distances under monocular conditions. Chromatic filters and a chromatic target constrained the infant's view of the target to a single eye while allowing both eyes to be recorded on infrared-sensitive film. Aslin and Jackson reported that infants as young as 2 months of age showed clear evidence of convergence to a near target (15 cm distance) even under monocular viewing conditions. Thus either the stimulus to accommodation, the actual accommodative response, or some other monocular information for target distance triggered a convergence response. Infants younger than 2 months of age were not tested because the accommodative system was not believed to be reasonably accurate until after 2 months of age. Given more recent evidence that accommodative accuracy is better than originally reported by Haynes et al. (1965), a follow-up study of younger infants seems to be appropriate in the near future.

Two other studies have used a combination of photorefraction and corneal reflection photography to measure the linkage between accommodation and convergence under *binocular* (i.e., closed-loop) viewing conditions. Widdersheim et al. (1990) gathered data from 199 infants and children, but only 5 were under 12 months of age. Unfortunately, the relation between accommodation and convergence was estimated only from group data. Thus the absence of a significant correlation between accommodation and convergence to a binocularly fixated target at 100, 20, and 10 cm viewing distances may have been the result of large individual differences in the accommodative-convergence/accommodation (AC/A) ratios of these subjects. Riddell et al. (1991) also used photorefraction and corneal reflection

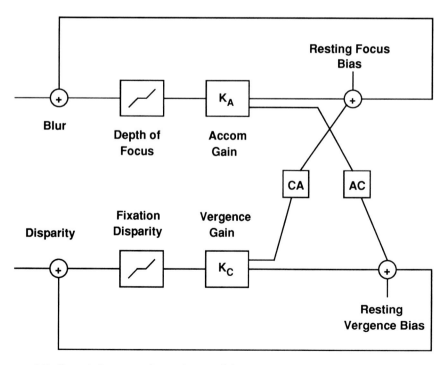

FIG. 3-7. Control elements and organization of the vergence eye movement system.

photography to record accommodation and convergence in 818 infants and young children to targets at 200, 100, 50, 33, and 25 cm viewing distances. Although quantitative estimates of accommodation and convergence accuracy were not reported, nearly half of the youngest infants (1-month-olds) showed monotonic increases in both accommodation and convergence to a decrease in target viewing distance.

Another important aspect of accommodation–convergence interactions is the possibility that some infants have resting positions of accommodation and convergence that are highly discrepant, thereby placing the two systems in conflict when they each receive primary trigger signals (blur for accommodation and disparity for convergence) and secondary trigger signals (accommodative-convergence and convergent-accommodation). Aslin and Dobson (1983) measured the resting positions of accommodation and convergence in total darkness and reported that the consistent positive correlation between accommodation and convergence observed under binocular target viewing conditions was absent in the dark. The resting position of accommodation was stable within the infants, but the resting position of convergence was variable. These results suggest that the set point for vergence effort, reflected in the resting point of vergence, may be significantly different from the resting position of accommodation, thereby requiring a change in the AC/A ratio to maintain accurate binocular fixation under binocular viewing conditions.

Many of these questions concerning the mechanisms underlying vergence control in young infants cannot be answered without some assessment of the dynamics of the vergence response. Unfortunately, to date no binocular eye movement system with sufficient temporal resolution to assess vergence dynamics has been successfully adapted for use with young infants.

SUMMARY AND CONCLUSIONS

From this brief review it is apparent that both the accommodation and convergence systems are inaccurate during the first 3 months of life. Attentional and sensory factors appear to be the primary constraints on both systems, although motor constraints have not been evaluated in detail because of technical limitations that have prevented the assessment of system dynamics. An important characteristic of stimulus displays used to elicit accommodation and convergence in young infants and that is relevant to oculomotor control in natural visual environments has not been manipulated systematically, namely, the presence of multiple targets that compete for the infant's attention. Clearly, there is a need for more detailed, quantitative measures of accommodation and convergence during early infancy and especially their various interactions (e.g., the AC/A ratio). Moreover, the role of maturational versus experiential factors in the development of these oculomotor systems is virtually unknown. Although animal models have been used to characterize the development of spatial vision and refractive errors (Boothe et al., 1985), virtually no animal research has been directed to the oculomotor system, except for studies of the optokinetic response (Hoffmann, 1979; Malach et al., 1981; Sparks et al., 1986). Because of the improvements observed in spatial vision during early infancy and the role of spatial sensitivity in the detection of signals that control oculomotor responses, a program of research aimed at linking these developmental improvements in an animal model appears to be a fruitful avenue for future research.

REFERENCES

ASLIN, R. N. (1977). Development of binocular fixation in human infants. *J. Exp. Child Psychol.* 23, 133–150.
ASLIN, R. N. (1981). Development of smooth pursuit in human infants. In D. F. FISHER, R. A. MONTY, AND J. W. SENDERS (eds.). *Eye Movements: Cognition and Visual Perception.* Hillsdale, NJ: Erlbaum, pp. 31–51.
ASLIN, R. N. (1986). Dark vergence in human infants: implications for the development of binocular vision. *Acta Psychol. (Amst.)* 63, 309–322.
ASLIN, R. N. (1988). Normative oculomotor development in human infants. In G. LENNERSTRAND, G. K. VON NOORDEN, AND E. C. CAMPOS (eds.), *Strabismus and Amblyopia.* London: Macmillan Press, pp. 133–142.
ASLIN, R. N., AND DOBSON, V. (1983). Dark vergence and dark accommodation in human infants. *Vision Res.* 23, 1671–1678.
ASLIN, R. N., AND JACKSON, R. W. (1979). Accommodative-convergence in young infants: development of a synergistic sensory-motor system. *Can. J. Psychol.* 33, 222–231.
ASLIN, R. N., SHEA, S. L., AND METZ, H. S. (1990). Use of the Canon R-1 autorefractor to measure refractive errors and accommodative responses in infants. *Clin. Vision Sci.* 5, 61–70.
ATKINSON, J., BRADDICK, O., WATTAM-BELL, J., ANKER, S., AND NORRIS, V. (1988). Videorefractive screening of accommodation performance in infants. *Invest. Ophthalmol. Vis. Sci.* 29 (suppl.), 60.
BANKS, M. S. (1980). The development of visual accommodation during early infancy. *Child Dev.* 51, 646–666.
BIRCH, E. E., GWIAZDA, J., AND HELD, R. (1982). Stereoacuity development for crossed and uncrossed disparities in human infants. *Vision Res.* 22, 507–513.
BOLTZ, R. L., MANNY, R. E., AND KATZ, B. (1983). The effects of induced blur on infant visual acuity. *Am. J. Optom. Physiol. Opt.* 60, 100–105.
BOOTHE, R. G., DOBSON, V., AND TELLER, D. Y. (1985). Postnatal development of vision in human and nonhuman primates. *Annu. Rev. Neurosci.* 8, 495–546.
BRADDICK, O., ATKINSON, J., FRENCH, J., AND HOWLAND, H. C. (1979). A photorefractive study of infant accommodation. *Vision Res.* 19, 1319–1330.
BROOKMAN, K. E. (1983). Ocular accommodation in human infants. *Am. J. Optom. Physiol. Opt.* 60, 91–99.
DOBSON, V., AND TELLER, D. Y. (1978). Visual acuity in human infants: a review and comparison of behavioral and electrophysiological studies. *Vision Res.* 18, 1469–1483.
COLLEWIJN, H., AND ERKELENS, C. J. (1990). Binocular eye movements and the perception of depth. In E. KOWLER (ed.). *Eye Move-

ments and Their Role in Visual and Cognitive Processes. Amsterdam: Elsevier, pp. 213–261.

FANTZ, R. L., ORDY, J. M., AND UDELF, M. S. (1962). Maturation of pattern vision in infants during the first six months. *J. Comp. Physiol. Psychol.* 55, 907–917.

GREEN, D. G., POWERS, M. K., AND BANKS, M. S. (1980). Depth of focus, eye size, and visual acuity. *Vision Res.* 20, 827–836.

HAYNES, H., WHITE, B. L., AND HELD, R. (1965). Visual accommodation in human infants. *Science* 148, 528–530.

HELD, R. (1993). What can rates of development tell about underlying mechanisms? In C. GRANRUD (ed.). *Carnegie-Mellon Symposium on Cognition: Visual Perception and Cognition in Infancy.* Vol. 23. Hillsdale, NJ: Erlbaum, pp. 75–89.

HELD, R., BIRCH, E., AND GWIAZDA, J. (1980). Stereoacuity of human infants. *Proc. Natl. Acad. Sci. USA* 77, 5572–5574.

HOFFMANN, K-P. (1979). Optokinetic nystagmus and single-cell responses in the nucleus tractus opticus after early monocular deprivation in the cat. In R. D. FREEMAN (ed.). *Developmental Neurobiology of Vision.* New York: Plenum, pp. 63–72.

HOWLAND, H. C., AND HOWLAND, B. (1974). Photorefraction: a technique for study of refractive state at a distance. *J. Opt. Soc. Am.* 64, 240–249.

HOWLAND, H. C., AND SAYLES, N. (1987). A photorefractive characterization of focusing ability of infants and young children. *Invest. Ophthalmol. Vis. Sci.* 28, 1005–1015.

HOWLAND, H. C., DOBSON, V., AND SAYLES, N. (1987). Accommodation in infants as measured by photorefraction. *Vision Res.* 27, 2141–2152.

KULIKOWSKI, J. J. (1978). Limit of single vision in stereopsis depends on contour sharpness. *Nature* 276, 126–127.

LING, B. C. (1942). A genetic study of sustained fixation and associated behavior in the human infant from birth to six months. *J. Genet. Psychol.* 61, 227–277.

MALACH, R., STRONG, N., AND VAN SLUYTERS, R. C. (1981). Analysis of monocular optokinetic nystagmus in normal and visually deprived kittens. *Brain Res.* 210, 367–372.

MAURER, D. (1975). The development of binocular convergence in infants. Doctoral dissertation, University of Minnesota, 1974. *Dissertation Abstr. Intr. B* 35, 6136–B (University Microfilms No. 75–12, 121).

NORCIA, A. M., TYLER, C. W., AND HAMER, R. D. (1990). Development of contrast sensitivity in the human infant. *Vision Res.* 30, 1475–1486.

OWENS, D. A., AND LEIBOWITZ, H. W. (1980). Accommodation, convergence, and distance perception in low illumination. *Am. J. Optom. Physiol. Opt.* 57, 540–550.

POWERS, M. K., AND DOBSON, V. (1982). Effect of focus on visual acuity of human infants. *Vision Res.* 22, 521–528.

PUGH, J. R., AND WINN, R. (1988). Modification of the Canon Auto Ref R1 for use as a continuously recording infra-red optometer. *Ophthalmic Physiol. Opt.* 8, 460–464.

RIDDELL, P. M., GROSE-FIFER, J., HAINLINE, L., AND ABRAMOV, I. (1991). Photorefractive evaluation of infant accommodation and convergence. Topical meeting of the Optical Society of America, Noninvasive assessment of the visual system, Sante Fe, NM, February 6.

ROSENFIELD, M., AND CUIFFREDA, K. J. (1991). Effect of surround propinquity on the open-loop accommodative response. *Invest. Ophthalmol. Visual Sci.* 32, 142–147.

SALAPATEK, P., BECHTOLD, A. G., AND BUSHNELL, E. W. (1976). Infant visual acuity as a function of viewing distance. *Child Dev.* 47, 860–863.

SCHOR, C. M., WOOD, I., AND OGAWA, J. (1984). Binocular sensory fusion is limited by spatial resolution. *Vision Res.* 24, 661–665.

SLATER, A. M., AND FINDLAY, J. M. (1975). Binocular fixation in the newborn baby. *J. Exp. Child Psychol.*, 20, 248–273.

SOKOL, S., MOSKOWITZ, A., AND PAUL, A. (1983). Evoked potential estimates of visual accommodation in infants. *Vision Res.* 23, 851–860.

SPARKS, D. L., MAYS, L. E., GURSKI, M. R., AND HICKEY, T. L. (1986). Long- and short-term monocular deprivation in the rhesus monkey: effects on visual fields and optokinetic nystagmus. *J. Neurosci.* 6, 1771–1780.

WICKELGREN, L. (1967). Convergence in the human newborn. *J. Exp. Child Psychol.* 5, 74–85.

WIDDERSHEIM, K. P., PECK, L. B., AND HOWLAND, H. C. (1990). Studies of accommodation and convergence in infants and young children. *Invest. Ophthalmol. Vis. Sci.* 31 (suppl.), 82.

II. Oculomotor Function
Introduction

CLIFTON M. SCHOR

Virtually no aspect of oculomotor control is fully developed at birth. During development, varying degrees of maturation are found among the oculomotor subsystems. Under these circumstances, one oculomotor system, such as the saccadic, may substitute its function for a less mature system such as the smooth pursuit following response. This particular example of substitution is referred to as "cog wheel" movements, which can be observed in normal neonates (Aslin, 1981). Eventually the smooth pursuit system develops at 2 months, and the infant becomes capable of smooth following movements (Aslin, 1981).

Development of oculomotor control requires maturation of sensory afferent (literally "carried in") processes that transduce the light distribution of the retinal image into neural codes. These codes are interpreted and evoke efferent ("carried out") commands that guide the intra- and extraocular muscles. Precision of these motor responses can be limited by subcomponents in either of these systems. However, much of the limitation during infancy appears at the sensory, or afferent, side of the motor reflex arc. For example, the human fovea is immature in the neonate in comparison to the peripheral retina (see Chapter 17). A major question that remains is to what extent, if any, the immature fovea limits oculomotor performance. The visual cortex is another neural locus that accounts for some of the neonate's sensory defects, as do higher level cognitive factors such as attention, motivation, state level of alertness, distraction, fatigue, and sleepiness. These higher level factors influence even the simplest motor reflexes. For example, the pupil tends to decrease in size during periods of inattention and just before going to sleep (Lowenstein and Loewenfeld 1969), which may produce apparent developmental differences between pupil size at high luminance levels between infants (who sleep or are inattentive much of the time) and adults. Similarly, we have observed in our laboratory that inattentive infants, who effectively sleep with their eyes open, do not exhibit an optokinetic following reflex even though they are totally surrounded by a rotating textured optokinetic drum. In contrast, during an alert state the optokinetic reflex is reliably triggered by the same stimulus. Accordingly, an infant's average oculomotor behavior is not typical of its best performance or potential capability. The lack of cooperation justifies drawing attention to isolated records of unusually good performance as a measure of the potential level of oculomotor development.

There are a variety of classes of oculomotor activity, involving both positioning of the eyes by the extraocular muscles and the intraocular muscles involved in flexing the lens during accommodation.

FIXATIONAL EYE MOVEMENTS

Monocular Fixation

The postnatal changes in morphology of the fovea (see Chapter 17) indicate that approximately the central 5 degrees of the retina is at best partially functional at birth, whereas the parafovea has adult-like structure. Currently, it is unknown if this foveal scotoma influences the characteristics (i.e., stability and accuracy) of monocular fixation. Indeed, infants may utilize extrafoveal sites for monocular and binocular fixation while the fovea develops during the first 3 months of life (Lewis et al., 1978; Bronson 1982). Given the uncertainty of angle kappa (the angle between the pupillary and visual axes) and foveal immaturity, it is impossible at this time to establish if fixation is foveal or has any preferred site during the first 3 months of life. Presumably fixation aligns objects of interest with retinal loci where resolution is highest. Given the reduced visual acuity of the newborn, there is not as specific a site as there is in the adult where a fixation preference would be advantageous.

In adults, fixational movements are composed of irregular slow drugs and fixation saccades that occur at a rate of one to five per second and with a 60-Hz microtremor. The drifts and saccades are both error-producing and error-correcting (Cornsweet, 1956; Steinman et al., 1973). These movements tend to follow the outline of contour in the visual field (St. Cyr and Fender, 1969) and to have idiosyncratic biases that can be responses to imbalances in the vestibuloocular reflex (Schor and Westall, 1986).

Although it is not known what retinal site, if any, is preferred by infants during monocular fixation, infants do stare steadily at objects (Lewis et al., 1978; Hainline, 1985) and infrequently shift their gaze to fixate a new target (Peiper, 1963). The tendency to refixate new objects increases in frequency during the first 3 months of life (Tronick, 1972; Aslin and Salapatek, 1975). It may be due to an increase in the size of the visual field, to the development of a preference for central retinal fixation as opposed to no preference, or to the ability to relinquish fixation and attention of one target in order to capture another. Studies of the dynamics of fixational eye movements in infants ranging in age from 2 weeks to 1 year revealed that infants tend to fixate an object to within 1 degree of some unspecified retinal locus (Hainline et al., 1986). Preschool children and 10-year-olds are reported to have less precise fixation control than that of adults (Kowler and Facchiano, 1982). When the increased range of eye position is caused by large saccades, much of this difference may be attributed to attentional factors (Aslin and Cuiffreda, 1983).

Binocular Fixation

Binocular fixation can be maintained in adults to within a range of 6–10 arc minutes. Static subjective measures of fixation vergence error are referred to as "fixation disparity." These binocular errors rarely exceed 6 arc minutes when heterophoria is corrected with prisms (Ogle, 1964; Schor, 1979). Dynamic objective measures of binocular alignment demonstrated a similar range of variability (Riggs and Neihl, 1960; St. Cyr and Fender, 1969). The components of binocular fixation serve different roles. Yoked saccades (both eyes moving in the same direction) appear to correct fixation errors, whereas drifts tend to be disjunctive (two eyes moving in opposite directions laterally) and to correct overall vergence errors between the two eyes (St. Cyr and Fender, 1969). These errors of binocular alignment do not elicit diplopia, as the retinal image disparities they produce fall within the range of Panum's fusional limits (Schor and Tyler, 1981).

Rudimentary binocular alignment without cosmetically noticeable strabismus is often present at birth but is probably not truly bifoveal until 2–3 months of age, although the exact timing of this onset and its accuracy of alignment are not conclusively established (see Chapters 3, 15, and 22). As noted above, no study has been able to determine which retinal area is used by the infant as the line of sight; and it is possible that while the fovea is immature infants utilize an extrafoveal retinal region during binocular fixation. It is lso unclear to what stimulus the apparent convergence responds. Stimuli could evoke accommodative vergence, disparity vergence, or monocularly driven proximal vergence, none of which requires bifoveal alignment.

VERSIONAL (CONJUGATE) EYE MOVEMENTS

Hering's Law of Yoked Eye Movements

In addition to convergence, which allows the eyes to binocularly fuse objects at various viewing distances, binocular vision also relies on yoked conjugate eye movements to maintain a fixed vergence angle during versional saccadic and pursuit eye movements. Hering's law describes this conjugacy relation as equal movements of the two eyes. Studies by Schor et al. (1990) demonstrated that conjugacy can be recalibrated in adults in response to anisometropic spectacle corrections as well as partial weakening of one or more muscle groups. Their finding suggests a potential for similar response in infants with anisometropia (see Chapter 1).

Ling (1942) observed binocular following (conjugate) eye movements of all types and in all directions in 75 infants during the first 48 hours of their lives. She also reported that the onset of convergence is delayed nearly 2 months in the same infants. There are sparse reports of an apparent lack of conjugacy or independence of eye rotation in the newborn (Guernsey, 1929). These apparent defects may result from an occasional combination of versional and accommodative vergence movements, both of which are present in the neonate.

Saccades

As noted in Chapter 4, rapid shifts of attention from one portion of the visual field to another often evoke a fast, saccadic eye movement that places the image of the new target of regard on the fovea. These movements have short latencies of 180–200 ms and high velocities approaching 1000 degrees/second. Saccadic movements are easily observed in newborns during both wakeful and sleep states. Initially, infants are likely to hold one fixation position, rather than shifting gaze to the periphery. However, the likelihood that a saccade will respond to a peripheral target increases with age and decreases with retinal eccentricity (Aslin and Salapatek, 1975). When a novel stimulus is introduced into the periphery, 1- to 2-month-old infants approach the target with a series of small saccadic steps of equal amplitude that rarely exceed 50% of the target eccentricity, rather than with a single large saccade (Aslin and Salapatek, 1975; Ashmead 1984) (see Chapter 4). By the second week of life the hypometric saccadic sequence reliably directs the line of sight toward a peripheral target. After the second month of life, large single saccades are used to redirect gaze to novel targets. Peripheral targets may be fixated as eccentrically as 30 degrees horizontally and 10 degrees vertically.

Pursuits

Pursuit tracking eye movements are one of the most susceptible oculomotor functions to postnatal development of the fovea and the corresponding development of contrast sensitivity (Kremenitzer et al., 1979). Pursuit responses by the newborn have been reported for simple-ramp or constant-velocity targets of short duration (Kremenitzer et al., 1979; Roucoux et al., 1983; Hainline, 1985) but not in response to sinusoidal varying (pendular) motion (Aslin, 1981; Shea and Aslin, 1984). Pursuit responses in the newborn are brief and intermittent, lasting 300–400 ms per episode. These responses are interrupted by what appears to be catch-up saccades. These early pursuits are evoked by large, 12-degree targets that stimulate parafoveal regions; however, early responses can also be obtained with a small 1.5-degree target if they are made attractive with synchronized music and flashing (Hainline, 1985) or by imaging cartoon characters (Roucoux et al., 1983). Early responses are further enhanced by reducing target velocity (< 10 degrees/second), whereas responses to higher velocities (> 15 degrees/second) can be obtained at 10–12 weeks of age (Roucoux et al., 1983; Hainline, 1985). These upper velocity limitations may result in part from increased latencies for pursuits in neonates, as at high velocities extended latency would result in targets becoming eccentric or even invisible prior to the onset of the pursuit. Perceived contrast is another factor that potentially restricts the upper velocity limit for immature pursuits. Contrast sensitivity improved dramatically during the first 6 months of life (Salapatek and Banks, 1978), and the upper velocity limit for pursuits is clearly restricted by reduced target contrast (Haegerstrom-Portnoy and Brown, 1979; Tychsen and Lisberger, 1986).

REFLEX CONJUGATE EYE MOVEMENTS

Optokinetic Nystagmus

Reflex optokinetic following responses to large, moving patterned fields are more easily evoked in the neonate than pursuit responses to small isolated targets (Dayton et al., 1964; Atkinson and Braddick, 1981). It is due, in part, to the interaction of target size and the immature

fovea. An optokinetic nystagmus (OKN) target that exceeds 5 degrees in diameter stimulates the more developed parafovea, whereas small pursuit targets can easily be restricted to the immature central retina.

Traditionally, OKN has been used to evaluate visual acuity in infants (Gorman et al., 1957; Fantz et al., 1962; Dayton et al., 1964) (see Chapter 26). More recently, it has been used to evaluate the development of binocularity (see Chapter 5). Patients with binocular anomalies of childhood strabismus, monocular cataract, or amblyopia exhibit asymmetry of the optokinetic response. When stimulated monocularly, the slow phase component has a higher velocity in response to nasalward than temporalward field motion, and to downward than to upward field motion (Schor and Levi, 1980). This asymmetry occurs for monocular stimulation of either the preferred or nonpreferred eye and is believed to result from a deficit of cortical binocularity (Hoffman, 1988). Afference from the two eyes converges on the pretectum via binocular cells in the visual cortex. In the absence of binocularity, temporal asynchronies between the two eyes' inputs is believed to result in subcortical suppression of motion signals in the temporalward and, presumably, upward directions (Hoffman, 1988). Latent nystagmus, which is a nasalward slow-phase jerk nystagmus during monocular fixation, is another symptom of this subcortical binocular anomaly (Schor, 1993). Prior to the development of cortical binocularity, infants exhibit a similar horizontal asymmetry of monocular OKN (Atkinson and Braddick, 1981; Naegele and Held, 1982; Hainline et al., 1984a; Schor et al., 1983). After 5 months of age, the infants' OKN becomes symmetrical in the horizontal meridian at about the same time tht stereopsis emerges (Naegel and Held, 1982). OKN remains asymmetrical in adults who had deprived binocularity as a result of cataract (Schor and Levi, 1980; Maurer et al., 1983) or stabismus (Schor and Levi, 1980) prior to 6 years of age. Because symmetrical OKN in normals appears at 3 months of age, the loss of this symmetry at a later time represents deterioration or loss of binocularity rather than arrested development. This loss may persist even though normal visual acuity is restored in monocular cataract (Lewis et al., 1986) (see Chapter 26), amblyopia, and when binocular eye alignment is regained in strabismus (Schor and Levi, 1980). The continued OKN asymmetry suggests that subcortical binocularity may remain disrupted after the recovery of some binocular cortical functions (Schor, 1982).

The slow phase of the optokinetic response increases proportionally with stimulus velocity up to a limit. The upper velocity limit in newborns is approximately 25 degrees/second (Kremenitzer et al., 1979). Improvement in slow phase velocity occurs throughout the first year of life, eventually reaching adult velocity limits of more than 40 degree/second. The gradual improvement in slow following phase parallels the development of contrast sensitivity during the first 5 months of life (Banks and Salapatek, 1978). Reduced target contrast normally reduces the upper velocity limit for smooth following movements in adults (Haegerstrom-Portnoy and Brown, 1979; Tychsen and Lisberger, 1986), suggesting that reduced contrast sensitivity reduces gain of slow phase responses to high stimulus velocities in the infant as well.

Vestibuloocular Reflex

Maintained direction of gaze during body movement is sustained by the optokinetic mechanism at relatively low stimulus velocities and by the vestibuloocular reflex (VOR) during acceleration. The VOR responds to even the smallest head acceleration after a 12-ms latency (Cohen et al., 1981). Like OKN, the VOR to unidirectional acceleration is characterized by slow phase compensatory eye movements interrupted by rapid flicks in the opposite direction. In addition to these dynamic posture responses, there are static gravitational reflexes in which the eyes counter-roll in response to a tilted head posture. The vestibular system is anatomically complete and functional at birth. The endolymphatic and bony labyrinths (Dayal et al., 1973) and the number of myelinated vestibular fibers (Bergstrom, 1973) and vestibular hair cells (Rosenhall, 1972) are mature at birth.

Both the ophthalmostatic and kinetic vestibular responses are present at birth (Peiper, 1963). The VOR is present in term infants but not premature infants, and it is more robust in infants with large than small birth weights (Eviatar et al., 1974). From 1 month of age the VOR evoked by a unidirectional acceleration is of a higher amplitude and velocity than it is later in life. Slow phase amplitude slowly decreases during the first 7 years of life (Orintz et al., 1979). Presumably, higher gains are advantageous to young infants who undergo constant unpredictable passive body motion as a result of adult handling and falling.

NEAR TRIAD AND DISJUNCTIVE EYE MOVEMENTS

Pupillary Reflex

"Near triad" is the term given to the simultaneous response of pupil, accommodation, and vergence to either accommodative or vergence stimuli. The role of pupillary constriction in the triad response is to increase the eye's depth of focus and reduce the demands on the accommodative system, as well as to reduce chromatic

and spherical aberration of the optics of the eye during critical near point inspection tasks.

Pupillary constriction also serves the obvious function of regulating the amount of light entering the eye, particularly during the initial stages of light and dark adaptation. In adults, pupil diameters range from 2 to 8 mm with variation of light level, which results in 16-fold, or 1.2 log unit, change in retinal illumination. The pupillary response has an initial transient or phasic component that is followed by a sustained tonic component. The phasic component has a latency of 300–500 ms and a duration of 1 second (Lowenstein and Lowenfeld, 1969). The tonic or resting state is achieved within several minutes, depending on the time course of light and dark adaptation.

Pupillary responses to light are present at birth in both term and premature infants (Peiper, 1963; Kessen et al., 1972). The pupillary response is also consensual (i.e., both pupils constrict together) at birth. The phasic component of the pupillary response of a 2-month-old infant to step increments in light (.1 .5 log ft.L.) have prolonged latencies (567–467 ms) and smaller amplitudes and are more sluggish than during adulthood. The tonic or resting diameter of the infant's pupil increases during the first 2 months of life (Salapatek and Banks, 1978). The pupil diameter of young infants is highly variable, presumably owing to large variations in level of attention and state of alertness (Banks, 1980a).

Accommodation

At birth, the amplitude of accommodation, extrapolated from Hofstetter's equation (1950), is 18.5 diopters (D). This amplitude is reduced by 1 D every 3 years owing to progressive sclerosis of the lens, which becomes complete at approximately 53 years of age (Hamasaki et al., 1956). Despite their potential capacity, newborns do not fully utilize accommodation because their depth of focus is so large that large changes in target distance do not produce increases in perceived blur; consequently, an accommodative response is unnecessary (see Chapter 3). The accuracy of accommodation agrees closely with the depth of focus. Reduction of depth of focus with maturation in the infant is largely responsible for the improvement in the infant's accommodative response (Banks, 1980b).

Vergence

A variety of sensory functions, including relative depth perception, camouflaged form perception, and perception of motion in depth are enhanced by binocular disparity cues. Our ability to sense or encode these disparities relies heavily on binocular alignment of the eyes to within a fraction of a degree on the object of regard. If this binocular motor alignment is not achieved during early infancy, the binocular sensory functions may not develop adequately to support binocular alignment in the future. In such cases constant strabismus may develop. Subsequent suppression of the deviating eye may deprive it of necessary stimulation during the critical period of development (Movshon and Van Sluyters, 1981), and partial loss of sight (amblyopia) could result.

Vergence eye movements normally respond to both open-loop and closed-loop modes. The open-loop responses do not utilize retinal image disparity feedback and are stimulated by intrinsic innervation (tonic vergence), blue (accommodative vergence), and perceived distance (proximal vergence) (Schor et al., 1992). These responses are refined by a closed-loop response (disparity vergence) that utilizes retinal image disparity as a source of sensory feedback. Currently it is believed that the open-loop vergence responses are present at birth but that the closed-loop disparity vergence develops postnatally.

Tonic Vergence.

Innervation that converges the eyes from the divergent anatomical position of rest to the physiological position of rest is referred to as tonic. The physiological position of rest is usually quantified by the distance phoria test and is normally found to be 1–2 prism diopters exophoric (Morgan, 1964).

Errors of binocular fixation, described for infants earlier in this Introduction, are usually divergent (Wickelgren, 1967; Slater and Findlay, 1975; Aslin, 1977) (see Chapter 22). These errors would represent the physiological position of rest if there were no fusional vergence responses operating prior to 3–4 months of age. One approach to measuring tonic vergence has been to measure binocular eye position during deep sleep (Rethy, 1969). Approximately half of the infants examined by Rethy had 15–35 degrees of divergence during the first few days of life. These observation made by Rethy (1969) suggest that there are marked changes in the tonic vergence during the first few weeks of life. Once in place, however, the changes are long-lasting, as demonstrated by the stability of distance heterophoria throughout life (Hirsch et al., 1948). The process of reducing the distance phoria is referred to as orthophorization (Crone, 1973) and demonstrates the plasticity of tonic vergence innervation. This plasticity is seen with maturity in prism adaptation and in adjustment of heterophoria in response to lenses and prisms worn for short periods (15 seconds) before the eyes (Schor, 1983). Clearly, vergence adaptation would be of benefit to infants during the first 5 years of life when there is rapid growth of the cranium and interpupillary distance.

Accommodative Vergence.

Accommodative vergence is another open-loop response that is believed to be present in the neonate (Aslin, 1987) (see Chapter 3). During the second week of life, monocularly stimulated accommodation results in a reliable convergence of the covered eye (Aslin and Jackson, 1979). As noted in Chapter 3, the magnitude of the AC/A ratio has not been determined in the neonate, principally because of calibration difficulty (Aslin and Jackson, 1979).

Fusional Vergence.

The refinement of binocular alignment is achieved by utilizing feedback from retinal image disparity (Rashbass and Westheimer, 1961). Both the disparity vergence response and binocular sensory functions, such as fusion and stereopsis, rely on the same stimulus (i.e., retinal image disparity). Until the processes that encode and process retinal image disparity develop, there can be no disparity vergence or stereoscopic depth perception. Details of fusional vergence development are reviewed in Chapter 3.

It is clear that the binocular disparity vergence system is the last of the oculomotor functions to develop. Little is known about the dynamics of these responses in immature infants (i.e., latency, velocity, and adaptability), and the age at which the response is fully adult-like is a matter of ongoing discussion (see Chapters 15 and 22). It is remarkable that gross binocular alignment is possible in infants prior to the emergence of disparity vergence, as it is the only vergence component that utilizes retinal disparity feedback to ensure an accurate response (closed loop). It is likely that infants utilize peripheral fusion before binocular vision has developed sufficiently to support stereoscopic depth perception, and that peripheral fusion is too sluggish to be revealed by the loose prism test of asymmetrical vergence (Aslin, 1977) (see Chapter 3).

SUMMARY

This introduction has provided a brief overview of the development of a broad range of oculomotor functions. The two chapters that follow provide an in-depth description of versional reflex and tracking eye movements. Hainline (see Chapter 4) reviews the neural anatomy of saccadic and pursuit eye movements, their behavioral developmental sequence, measurement techniques, and models of infant oculomotor control. Preston and Finocchio (see Chapter 5) review development of the ocular postural reflexes that stabilize retinal image position during movement of the head and body. They describe developmental changes in visual–vestibular interactions as the pursuit system matures. Finally, they review the relation between the development of binocular cortical functions and symmetry of the optokinetic reflex. Related information is also presented by Tychsen in his chapter on the origins of infantile strabismus (see Chapter 22), and Maurer and Lewis in their chapter on visual outcomes in infant cataract (see Chapter 26). These chapters illustrate how postnatal development of the cortex modifies oculomotor functions that are initially controlled at birth by the brainstem.

REFERENCES

ASHMEAD, D. (1984). Parameters of infant saccadic eye movements *Infant Behav. Dev.* 7, 16.

ASLIN, R. N. (1977). Development of binocular fixation in human infants. *J. Exp. Child Psychol.* 23, 133–150.

ASLIN, R. N. (1987). Motor aspects of visual development in infancy. In P. SALAPATEK AND L. COHEN (eds.). *Handbook of Infant Perception. Vol. 1. From Sensation to Perception.* Orlando, FL: Academic Press.

ASLIN, R. N. (1981). Development of smooth pursuit in human infants. In D. F. FISHER, R. A. MONTY, AND J. W. SENDERS (eds.). *Eye Movements: Cognitive and Visual Perception.* Hillsdale, NJ: Erlbaum.

ASLIN, R. N., AND CIUFFREDA, K. (1983). Eye movements of preschool children. *Science* 222, 74–75.

ASLIN, R. N., AND JACKSON, R. W. (1979). Accommodative-convergence in young infants: development of a synergistic sensory-motor system. *Can. J. Psychol.* 33, 222–231.

ASLIN, R. N., AND SALAPATEK, P. (1975). Saccadic localization of visual targets by the very young human infant. *Percept. Psychophys.* 17, 293–302.

ATKINSON, J., AND BRADDICK, O. (1981). Development of optokinetic nystagmus in infants: an indicator of cortical binocularity? In D. F. FISHER, R. A. MONTY, AND J. W. SANDER (eds.). *Eye Movements: Cognition and Visual Perception.* Hillsdale, NJ: Erlbaum.

BANKS, M. S. (1980a). The development of visual accommodation during early infancy. *Child Dev.* 51, 646–666.

BANKS, M. S. (1980b). Infant refraction and accommodation. *Int. Ophthalmol. Clin.* 20, 205–232.

BANKS, M. S., AND SALAPATEK, P. (1978). Acuity and contrast sensitivity in 1-, 2-, 3-month-old human infants. *Invest. Ophthalmol. Vis. Sci.* 17, 361–365.

BERGSTROM 1973

BRONSON, G. W. (1982). *The Scanning Patterns of Human Infants: Implications for Visual Learning.* Norwood, NJ: Ablex.

COHEN, B., HENN, V., RAPHEN, T., AND DENNETT, D. (1981). Velocity storage, nystagmus and visual-vestibular interactions in humans. *Ann. N.Y. Acad. Sci.* 421–433.

CORNSWEET, T. M. (1956). Determination of the stimulus for involuntary drifts and saccadic eye movements. *J. Opt. Soc. Am.* 46, 987–993.

CRONE, R. A. (1973). *Diplopia.* New York: Elsevier.

DAYAL, V. S., FARKASHEDY, J., AND KOKSHANIAN, A. (1973). Embryology of the ear. *Can. J. Otolaryngol.* 2, 136.

DAYTON, G. O., JONES, M. H., RAWSON, R. A., STEELE, B., AND ROSE, M. (1964). Developmental study of coordinated eye movements in the human infant. II. An electroculographic study of the fixation reflex in the newborn. *Arch. Ophthalmol.* 71, 871–875.

EVIATAR, L., EVIATAR, A., AND NARCY, I. (1974). Maturation of neuro-vestibular responses in infants. *Rev. Med. Child Neurol.* 16, 435–446.

FANTZ, R. L., ORDY, L. M., AND UDELF, M. S. (1962). Maturation of pattern vision during the first six months. *J. Comp. Physiol. Psychol.* 55, 907–917.

GORMAN, J. J., COGAN, D. G., AND GELLIS, S. S. (1957). An apparatus for grading the visual acuity of infants on the basis of optokinetic nystagmus. *Pediatrics* 19, 1088–1092.

GUERNSEY, M. (1929). A quantitative study of the eye reflexes in infants. *Psychol. Bull* 26, 160–161.

HAEGERSTROM-PORTNOY, G., AND BROWN, B. (1979). Contrast effects on smooth-pursuit eye movement velocity. *Vision Res.* 19, 169–174.

HAINLINE, L. (1985). Oculomotor control in human infants. In R. GRONER, G. E. KCKONKIE, AND L. MENZ (eds.). *Eye Movements and Human Information Processing.* Amsterdam: Elsevier/North Holland.

HAINLINE, L., LEMERISE, E., ABRAMOV, I., AND TURKEL, J. (1984a). Orientational asymmetries in small-field optokinetic nystagmus in human infants. *Behav. Brain Res.* 13, 217–230.

HAINLINE, L., TURKEL, J., ABRAMOV, I., LEMERISE, E., AND HARRIS, C. M. (1984b). Characteristics of saccades in human infants. *Vision Res.* 24, 1771–1780.

HAMASAKI, D., ONG, J., AND MARG, E. (1956). The amplitude of accommodation in presbyopia. *Am.J. Optom. Arch. Am. Acad. Optom.* 33, 3–14.

HIRSCH, M. J., ALPERN, M., AND SCHULTZ, H. (1948). The variation of phoria with age. *Am. J. Optom. Arch. Am. Acad. Optom.* 25, 535–541.

HOFFMAN, P. K. (1988). Neuronal basis for changes of the optokinetic reflex with strabismus and amblyopia. In G. LENNERSTRAND, G. VON NOORDEN, E. CAMPOS, AND B. BAKER (eds.). *Strabismus and Amblyopia—Experimental Basis for Advances in Clinical Management.* New York: Pergamon.

HOFSTETTER, H. W. (1950). Useful age-amplitude formula. *Opt. World* 38, 42.

KESSEN, W., SALAPATEK, P., AND HAITH, M. M. (1972). The visual response of the human newborn to linear contour. *J. Exp. Child Psychol.* 13, 9–20.

KOWLER, E., AND FACCIANO, D. M. (1982). Kid's poor tracking means habits are lacking. *Invest. Ophthalmol. Vis. Sci. Suppl.* 22, 103.

KREMENITZER, J. P., VAUGHAN, H. G., KURTZBERG, D., AND DAWLING, K. (1979). Smooth-pursuit eye movements in the newborn infant. *Child. Dev.* 50, 442–448.

LEWIS, T. L., MAURER, D., AND BRENT, A. (1986). Effects on perceptual development of visual deprivation during infancy. *Br. J. Ophthalmol.* 70, 214–220.

LEWIS, T. L., MAURER, D., AND KAY, D. (1978). Newborn's central vision: whole or hole? *J Exp. Child Psychol.* 26, 193–203.

LING, B. C. (1942). A genetic study of sustained fixation and associated behavior in the human infant from birth to six months. *J. Genet. Psychol.* 61, 227–277.

LOWENSTEIN, O., AND LOEWENFELD, I. E. (1969). The pupil. In H. DAVSON (ed.). *The Eye,* Vol. 3. Orlando, FL: Academic Press.

MAURER, D., AND SALAPATEK, P. (1976). Developmental changes in the scanning of faces by young infants. *Child Dev.* 47, 523–527.

MAURER, D., LEWIS, T. L., AND BRENT, H. (1983). Peripheral vision and optokinetic nystagmus in children with unilateral congenital cataract. *Behav. Brain Res.* 10, 151–161.

MORGAN, M. W. (1964). The analysis of clinical data. *Optom. Weekly* 65, 27.

MOVSHON, J. A., AND VAN SLUYTERS, R. C. (1981). Visual neural development. *Ann. Rev. Psychol.* 32, 000–000.

NAEGELE, J. R., AND HELD, R. (1982). The postnatal development of monocular optokinetic nystagmus in infants. *Vision Res.* 2, 341–346.

OGLE, K. N. (1964). *Researchers in Binocular Vision.* New York: Hafner.

ORNITZ, E. M., ATWELL, C. W., WATER, D. O., HARTMANN, E. E., AND KAPLAN, A. R. (1979). The maturation of vestibular nystagmus in infancy and childhood. *Acta Otolaryngol. (Stockh.)* 88, 244–256.

PEIPER, A. (1963). *Cerebral Function in Infancy and Childhood.* New York: Consultants Bureau.

RASHBASS, C., AND WESTHEIMER, G. (1961). Disjunctive eye movement. *J. Physiol. (Lond.)* 159, 339–360.

RETHY, I. (1969). Development of simultaneous fixation from the divergent anatomical eye position in the neonate. *J. Pediatr. Ophthalmol.* 6, 92–96.

RIGGS, L. A., AND NEIHL, (1960). Eye movements recorded during convergence and divergence. *J. Opt. Soc. Am.* 50, 913–920.

ROSENHALL, U. (1972). Vestibular macular mapping in man. *Ann. Otol. Rhinol. Laryngol.* 81, 339.

ROUCOUX, A., CULEE, C., AND ROUCOUX, M. (1983). Development of fixation and pursuit eye movements in human infants. *Behav. Brain Res.* 10, 133–139.

SALAPATEK, P., AND BANKS, M. S. (1978). Infant sensory assessment: vision. In F.D. MINIFIE AND L. L. LLOYD (eds.). *Communicative and Cognitive Abilities: Early Behavioral Assessment.* Baltimore: University Park Press.

SCHOR, C. M. (1979). The relationship between fusional vergence eye movements and fixation disparity. *Vision Res.* 19, 1359–1367.

SCHOR, C. M. (1982). Subcortical binocular suppression affects the development of latent and optokinetic nystagmus. *Am.J. Optom. Physiol. Optics* 60, 481–502.

SCHOR, C. M. (1983). Fixation disparity and vergence adaptation. In C. M. SCHOR AND K. CIUFFREDA (eds.). *Vergence Eye Movements: Basic and Clinical Aspects.* Boston: Butterworth.

SCHOR, C. M. (1993). Development of OKN. In F. A. MILES AND J. WALLMAN (eds.). *Reviews of Oculomotor Research. Vol. 5. Visual Motion and Its Role in the Stabilization of Gaze.* Amsterdam: Elsevier, pp. 301–320.

SCHOR, C. M., AND LEVI, D. L. (1980). Disturbances of small-field horizontal and vertical nystagmus in amblyopia. *Invest. Ophthalmol. Vis. Sci.* 19, 683–688.

SCHOR, C., AND TYLER, C. (1981). Spatio-temporal properties of Panum's fusional area. *Vision Res.* 21, 683–692.

SCHOR, C. M., NARAGAN V., AND WESTALL, C. W. (1983). Postnatal development of optokinetic after nystagmus in human infants. *Vision Res.* 23, 1643–1647.

SCHOR, C. M., GLEASON, J., AND HORNER, D. (1990). Selective nonconjugate binocular adaptation of vertical saccades and pursuits. *Vision Res.* 30, 1827–1844.

SCHOR, C. M., ALEXANDER, J., CORMACK, L., AND STEVENSON, S. (1992). Negative feedback control model of proximal convergence and accommodation. *Ophthal. Physiol. Optics.* 12, 307–318.

SHEA, S., AND ASLIN, R. N. (1984). Development of horizontal and vertical pursuits in human infants. *Invest. Ophthalmol. Vis. Sci. Suppl.* 25, 263.

SLATER, A. M., AND FINDLAY, J. M. (1975). Binocular fixation in the newborn baby. *J. Exp. Child Psychol.* 20, 248–273.

ST. CYR, G. S., AND FENDER, D. (1969). The interplay of drifts and flicks in binocular vision. *Vision Res.* 9, 245–265.

STEINMAN, R. M., HADDAD, G. M., SKAVENSKI, A. A., AND WYMAN, D. (1973). Miniature eye movements. *Science* 181, 810–812.

TRONICK, E. (1972). Stimulus control and the growth of the infant's effective visual field. *Percept. Psychophys.* 11, 373–376.

TYCHSEN, L., AND LISBERGER, S. (1986). Visual motion processing for the initiation of smooth-pursuit eye movements. *J. Neurophysiol.* 51, 952–968.

WICKELGREN, C. (1967). Convergence in the human newborn. *J. Exp. Child Psychol.* 5, 74–85.

4 | Conjugate eye movements of infants

LOUISE HAINLINE

Conjugate eye movements are movements of the eyes in the same rather than opposite directions (to distinguish from vergence, for example). The list of eye movements generally described as conjugate includes saccades, pursuit, the vestibuloocular response (VOR), and nystagmic responses, particularly optokinetic nystagmus (OKN). The default case of fixation, no movement of the eyes during intervals of information pickup, also is germane to discussions of oculomotor behavior and its development. This chapter deals with the development of saccades, pursuit, and fixation. Development of the VOR and OKN is discussed in Chapter 5.

There have already been a number of competent reviews of the infant eye movement literature. Comprehensive reviews of the relevant material can be found in Aslin (1985, 1987, 1988), Hainline (1988), and Shupert and Fuchs (1988) among others. I have not attempted another exhaustive review here. Rather than cover the same ground again, my purpose is to deal more with the process and motivation of this body of work from an evaluative perspective.

This chapter first describes these eye movements and some of the most recent information about the organization of the visual system that is responsible for them. I then briefly review the developmental data available on each and describe some of the problems these data pose for infant models that are based on development of the underlying neurophysiology. Because the recording of eye movements requires some degree of technology and their analysis some degree of quantification, I deal next with issues of method and calibration and how they influence the kind of research we can do with infants. This section is followed by an evaluation of shortcomings in how we have been conducting research on these eye movements in infants; it is my belief that it is our extant research "model," rather than technical limitations, that has restricted our ability to understand infant oculomotor development better. To end on a positive note, I offer some suggestions for future research that might advance our understanding of how conjugate eye movements develop in infants.

CLASSES OF CONJUGATE EYE MOVEMENTS

Saccades are among the most rapid movements made by the body. Saccades serve to reorient the visual world on the retina. In humans and other species with spatially inhomogeneous retinas, the primary purpose of saccades is to reorient the area of the retina with the most acute vision, the fovea, to inspect different discrete targets in the world. The presence of a fovea is not deterministic for saccadic movements; saccades also occur in creatures without foveas, although in those cases there is evidence that some parts of the retina (e.g., a visual streak) have higher spatial resolution than others. Evolution of the fovea coincided with the migration of the eyes from the sides of the head to a frontal position, with substantial overlap of the visual fields of the two eyes. In foveate animals, saccades are conjugate movements; the presence of a large degree of frontal visual field overlap increased the requirements for conjugate control of eye movements because having the eyes pointed in different directions is maladaptive in this circumstance. Exact registration of the eyes' two fovea also makes possible fine depth perception from the comparison of the slightly different visual images in the two eyes; the emergence of the fovea in frontal-eyed animals also coincided with the evolution of significant binocular vision and stereopsis, increasing the demand for oculomotor systems that could maintain retinal images on corresponding areas in the two eyes. Clearly, evolution of the fovea in frontal-eyed species exerted considerable selective pressure on the evolution of oculomotor control centers. It is thus remarkable to consider how small a portion ($<0.01\%$) of the total retinal surface is occupied by the fovea. That we are unaware that only one ten-thousandth of the visual field is seen with great clarity is a testament to how well the resulting oculomotor behaviors deal with our nonhomogeneous retinas.

In most cases for afoveate animals, and to a lesser extent in foveate ones, saccades are executed in combination with head movements. The coordination of head and eye movements allows a more flexible and enveloping exploration of the world than eye movements alone permit, although in foveate species smaller saccades (10–15 degrees or less) are often made without accompanying head movements. Some researchers make a distinction between (1) afoveate saccades that anticipate a head movement and occur in species both with and without foveae, and (2) foveate saccades that occur independent of head movement. Another distinction sometimes made is between short-latency "reflexive" saccades and "intentional" saccades, with more variable latencies influenced by conscious, volitional factors, although there is no consensus about some of these distinctions (e.g., Findlay, 1991).

Pursuit, as the term implies, is the movement required to follow a moving target. Pursuit itself can be either saccadic (i.e., a jerky succession of saccades along the path of target movements interspersed with breaks in the following) or smooth (i.e., nonjerky movements of the eye that approximately match the position and velocity of a moving target). Saccadic pursuit is seen in both foveate and afoveate species, but smooth pursuit appears to be a system that evolved with the fovea. As with saccades, in natural circumstances smooth pursuit is often coordinated with head movements. Smooth pursuit is not the only smooth tracking eye movement system. With *optokinetic nystagmus*, slow eye movements that follow the stimulus alternate repetitively with fast eye movements in the direction opposite to stimulus movement. OKN occurs only when large portions of the visual field move; a single target moving against a background does not elicit OKN. The OKN system is also relatively slow to begin tracking, so the movement must continue for at least several seconds before the response begins, but it can continue indefinitely. In the case of the *vestibuloocular response*, smooth eye movements counteract the visual effect of body and head rotation and help to stabilize vision as the organism moves; the VOR is a faster response but adapts quickly to continued stimulation. Both OKN and the VOR are present in afoveate animals.

Once the fovea evolved, it was important to provide a system that would allow interesting objects to be placed on the fovea and kept there even when movement of the observer caused a substantial portion of the environment to be in motion on the retina at the same time. Smooth pursuit tracking is achieved through visual feedback from retinal image slip of the pursuit target on the fovea. At the same time, stabilization of the object's image on the fovea implies that retinal image slip from peripheral contours is substantial, so smooth pursuit must involve a mechanism for suppression of the OKN response to peripheral retinal slip and of the VOR response to the head movements that often accompany following by the eyes. Practiced adults can smoothly pursue objects effectively up to velocities of 30–40 degrees/second and even higher for brief periods of time, but this kind of tracking requires sustained attention. Under normal circumstances adults usually pursue objects with a mixture of smooth pursuit and saccadic tracking.

Fixation in an oculomotor context refers to the act of keeping the eyes immobile for some period of time between other eye movements. In both foveate and afoveate animals, the eyes tend to drift significantly in the dark, even when the subject has been given instructions or is trained to keep the eyes still. In contrast, eye drift is substantially reduced in the light, implying the presence of a mechanism that provides for stable vision even when the head and the environment are not moving. There is some debate about whether the act of fixation is simply a result of the interaction of stabilizing mechanisms (e.g., the VOR and OKN in the face of head and body motion), it is a special case of smooth pursuit, or there is a separate stabilization system for retinal drift during fixation. Whatever the mechanism, during normal fixation the eye is never absolutely still; indeed, if it were, vision would be impossible because absolutely stabilized retinal images rapidly lead to fading of the visual image due to neural adaptation (Troxler fading). There is actually some degree of slow drift (on the order of 1 degree/second) in the normal fixations of adults performing everyday tasks, although highly trained laboratory subjects can reduce drift to fractions of 1 degree/second.

NEURAL MECHANISMS CONTROLLING CONJUGATE EYE MOVEMENTS

Eye movements are made in response to different dimensions of visual and in some cases vestibular stimulation. In order to understand the development of eye movement control, conjugate or otherwise, it is first necessary to consider what is currently known about the structural and functional organization of the visual system. At this point, it is worth addressing the issue of what is meant by the "visual system." There are three aspects that are relevant to eye movements:

1. Sensory aspects. That is, is the stimulus visible? The answer may change with viewing conditions and developmental level.

2. Attentional/motivational aspects. Is the subject alert, attending to the target, and motivated to respond to it?

3. Oculomotor systems directly involved in generating particular classes of eye movements. Are the appropriate neural control centers in place and ultimately connected to the extraocular muscles?

These aspects are conceptually separable but may be difficult to distinguish operationally. Because most oculomotor research has been done on mature subjects, the role of immaturities in sensory and attentional factors has remained relatively unstudied. However, with developing organisms, we cannot ignore the interrelations among these aspects of the visual system—all the more so because it is often difficult to control these factors in order to isolate their relative contributions.

There have been significant advances in the understanding of the functional connectivity in the primate visual system. It is now generally agreed that the visual system consists of a number of parallel visual pathways responsible for coding different aspects of visual stimulation, primary among them color, form, and motion (e.g., Van Essen, 1979; De Yoe and Van Essen, 1988; Livingstone and Hubel, 1988). There are differences among these accounts, for example, in how absolutely segregated the various neural streams or pathways are believed to be, but the substantial agreement about the organization of structures from retina to cortex is striking. One finds the beginning of segregation into parallel streams in both the retina and the lateral geniculate nucleus; and in both structures there is a structural and functional segregation into two types of cells, M and P cells in the retina projecting to magnocellular and parvocellular cells in the lateral geniculate nucleus (LGN). Parvo cells are color-sensitive and have small receptive fields, low contrast sensitivity, and high spatial resolution; they are thought to be responsible for fine visual discriminations of form and color. Magno cells are relatively insensitive to color and have large receptive fields and high contrast sensitivity. Their role is probably much more to support functions relating to movement and stereopsis. Magno cells are also sometimes said to have low spatial resolution. Actually, individual magno cells are often as good as individual parvo cells for detecting spatial patterns. As a system, however, the magno pathway may have lower resolution because these cells are more sparsely distributed and do not spatially sample a stimulus as often as does the parvo system (Kaplan et al., 1990). An earlier belief that parvo cells are associated with the fovea and magno cells with the periphery is now thought to be incorrect; both cell types are found across the retina, and both cover, or "tile," the retinal surface completely (Kaplan et al., 1990).

In the retina, cells that contribute to the parvo pathway project to the dorsal layers of the LGN and then to an identifiable layer (layer 4cβ) in the striate or primary visual cortex (V1). From here, according to De Yoe and Van Essen (1988), they project either to (1) structures labeled "blobs" in layers 2 and 3 of V1, where they show good wavelength sensitivity and low spatial resolution, possibly related to discrimination of hue from spectral and luminance contrast; or (2) structures be-

tween the blobs in layers 2 and 3, where they show selectivity for both wavelength and orientation, implicated in form discrimination deriving from wavelength cues. Both the parvo-blob and parvo-interblob streams project to separate columns subserving color and form in prestriate, secondary visual cortex (V2). From here, the streams project to visual association areas of extrastriate cortex (V3, V4), and the inferior temporal lobes for further, more sophisticated processing.

Cells in the retina that contribute to the magno pathway project through ventral layers of the LGN and then to layer 4Cα in V1. From here they go to level 4B, where their visual fields are especially sensitive to movement. They then connect directly to middle temporal cortex (area MT) or through areas in V2 associated with stereopsis through to MT, which appears to be a region important to the analysis of movement. From here, the magno streams converge on parietal cortex. In De Yoe and Van Essen's account, there is less absolute segregation of function and more interaction among the various pathways than proposed in the original Livingstone and Hubel account, but both models propose that some structures are more responsive than others to the kinds of stimulation necessary for the control of eye movements (Fig. 4-1).

Schiller (1985) has been particularly concerned with the role that these pathways play in eye movement control. Articulating with the magno/parvo segregation, Schiller and colleagues have further posited four pathways for the control of different classes of eye movement (Fig. 4-2). One pathway is responsible for "reflexive," quickly executed saccades to highly discriminable visible targets. This pathway projects from the retina to the superior colliculus and primarily reflects the properties of the broadband (color nonopponent) magno system, i.e., with low spatial frequency resolution, good temporal response, and fast conduction speed. A second broad-band pathway projects to the cortex and is implicated in eye movements (e.g., pursuit, fixation, and the VOR) that require a reaction to retinal image slip. In this pathway, outputs from V1 project directly to the superior colliculus, and indirectly from V1 to area MT, whose outputs also converge eventually on the superior colliculus. A third cortical pathway for oculomotor control links the broad-band and color-opponent pathways to the frontal eye fields (FEFs), with the color-opponent channel providing more extensive inputs. This region appears to be responsible for detailed saccadic analysis of complex visual material, such as is required for visual search. A final pathway for oculomotor control is an inhibitory pathway to the superior colliculus from the substantia nigra. Schiller posited that this pathway allows regulation of the activity in the superior colliculus. All of these channels eventually converge on and receive inputs from structures in the brainstem, primarily for

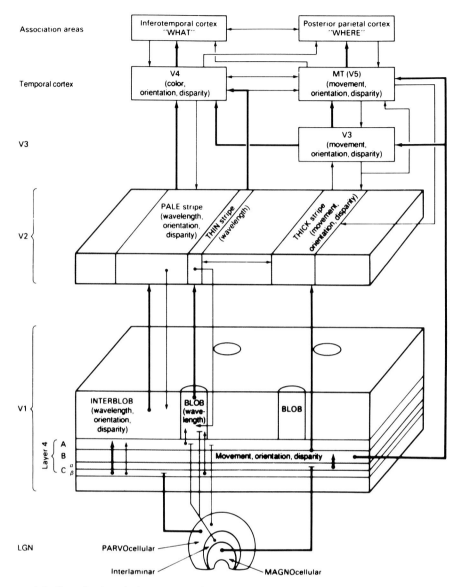

FIG. 4-1. Organization of primate cortex, showing the organization and contributions of the parvocellular system (left) and the magnocellular system (right). (From Levine and Shefner, 1990. By permission.)

fast movements—the pontine parmedian reticular formation (PPRF) for horizontal fast movements and the mesencephalic reticular formation (MRF) for fast vertical movements; and in the cerebellum, primarily for slow movements (the flocculus and the vermis). These lower level oculomotor centers are responsible for innervation of the six extraocular muscles ultimately responsible for executing eye movement.

Superior Colliculus

Because primary interest here is on the control of conjugate movements, it is necessary to discuss in somewhat greater detail the properties of the neural structures thought to be responsible for saccades and pursuit; the information that follows was compiled from a number of sources, including Carpenter (1977), Robinson (1981), Howard (1982), Levine and Shefner (1990), and Richards (1990). Because these eye movements are often accompanied by head movements that stimulate the VOR, interactions with the structures responsible for such coordination are also of interest. The superior colliculus (SC) is heavily involved in visual information processing and particularly in the execution of different types of saccade. The superficial layers of the SC receive visual inputs from the retina, LGN, and V1 (particularly layers 5 and 6), as well as V2, V3, and the FEF. There are also superficial-layer SC projections involved in the control of eye movements to the pulvinar of the thalamus,

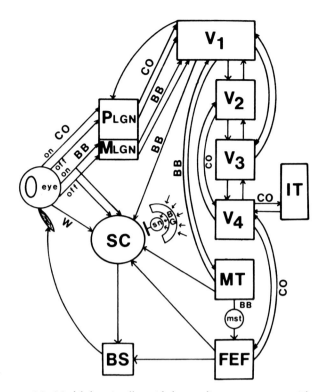

FIG. 4-2. Model for visually guided saccadic eye movements. The color opponent (CO) and broad-band (BB) pathways terminate, respectively, in the parvocellular (P) and magnocellular (M) layers of the lateral geniculate nucleus (LGN) of the thalamus. BB cells also project to the superior colliculus (SC) as do W-like cells. CO and BB axons from LGN terminate in striate cortex (V1), which projects to SC and makes reciprocal connections with V2, V3, and the middle temporal area (MT). V4 connects with V2, inferotemporal cortex (IT), and the frontal eye fields (FEF). MT also sends projections to SC and medial superior temporal area (mst), which itself projects to FEF. The V1–SC connection is driven by the BB system, whereas the V4–FEF connections are primarily CO-driven. The FEF and SC projects to the brainstem (BS) can generate saccadic eye movements independently. The substantia nigra (sn) makes inhibitory connections with the SC. The sn receives its projections from the basal ganglia (BG) which receives inputs from many cortical structures. Saccade generation involves both inhibition (e.g., of sn input to the SC) and excitation (e.g., from the visual cortex to SC). (From Schiller, 1985. By permission.)

from which there are numerous connections throughout the primary visual cortex. The deeper layers of the SC are implicated in saccadic eye movements, attention, and orientation, with some parts of the deep levels responsive to multisensory inputs (e.g., auditory/visual/ somatosensory). The superficial layers are heavily influenced by the broad-band magnocellular channels and may be involved in the analysis of retinal image slip that plays a role in supporting the VOR, smooth pursuit, and fixational mechanisms. No parvocellular retinal structures project to the SC.

Some theorists (e.g., Bronson, 1974) have proposed that a totally subcortical pathway through the SC is

responsible for reflexive-type saccades exhibited during early infancy. However, saccades are controlled by the middle and deep layers of SC, whereas retinal inputs are received in the superficial layers; because there does not appear to be direct connection between the superficial and deeper layers in the SC, visual inputs to the superficial layers that influence the deeper layers in the control of saccades always involve a cortical route. Lesions to primary visual cortex remove responsiveness of the deeper level of SC and eliminate both intentional and reflexive saccades, although spontaneous saccades in the absence of stimulation and quick phases of OKN are preserved. Lesions to the SC result in inaccurate saccades with longer than normal latencies and slower velocities. The SC sends efferents to the thalamus and thence to the FEF and inferior parietal region. Deeper levels also send connections to the motor structures in the brainstem involved in eye and head movements.

One of the most interesting features of the SC is that it appears to be organized according to a spatiocentric topographic map, i.e., according to the position of the organism in space, rather than a retinotopic organization, organized according to the position of a feature on the retina. This map reflects both motor and sensory coding of space. Its existence suggests that the SC plays a role in saccade generation by computing saccades to particular locations in space. The multimodal aspects of the deep layers of the SC are also topographically coded in the same spatial map, suggesting that the SC is also involved in creating a unified spatial map used to localize multimodal stimuli and then coordinating this map with various movements of the eyes, head, and body.

There is also an important inhibitory afferent pathway to the deep and middle layers of the SC from cells in the substantia nigra (SNr). The SNr inhibits firing in the SC in the presence of visual contours or preceding saccades to visual stimuli, but not during spontaneous saccades not elicited by specific visual targets, or anti-saccades, instructed saccades away from visual targets. When inhibiting the SC, the SNr is activated by inputs from cortical areas such as FEF and parietal cortex, acting through nuclei in the basal ganglia. These cortical centers are implicated in the control of voluntary eye movements.

Thus it appears that the SC plays a role in generating short-latency, fast, and accurate reflexive saccades to simple but salient properties of a visual stimulus, and that its activities are modulated by the FEF, which controls saccades that are more attention-directed and voluntary to specific targets, probably taking advantage of the functions controlled by the SC in doing so. At least one function of the FEF appears to be to inhibit reflexive saccades to allow more deliberate inspection of specified targets.

Frontal Eye Fields

The FEFs control voluntary saccades directed to visual targets that attract explicit attention (Bruce and Goldberg, 1984). Cells in the FEF do not fire during reflexive saccades that precede a head movement, spontaneous saccades emitted during free scanning, or smooth pursuit, although they do fire just prior to intentional saccades to specific visual targets. The FEF is well connected to a number of cortical and subcortical areas involved with saccadic eye movements, visual information processing, and attention. The FEFs have a number of direct and indirect connections to the PPRF and MRF in the brainstem, the only cortical area with such direct connections to the brainstem eye movement control centers. The role of FEFs in inhibiting the reflexive saccades controlled by SC by means of the SNr has already been described. There are also numerous connections with parietal area PG, particularly those areas that project to the SC; the PG is part of the inferior parietal lobe, which is an area implicated in various attentional processes. With animals, lesions to the FEF leads to visual neglect but not to major changes to the latency or morphology of saccades. Patients with frontal lobe damage often show at least transient visual neglect. They are reported to show a reduction in exploratory saccades, with difficulty making spontaneous saccades. For these patients, scanning is heavily determined by the physical features of the stimulus; their scanning patterns are unsophisticated and are little influenced by verbal instructions. It thus appears that the FEF serves to free saccades from the specifics of the visual stimulus and allows intentionally directed, flexible, voluntary inspection of visual scenes. Normally, the FEF and the SC work jointly to program morphologically similar saccades that allow a choice between deliberate inspection and grosser scanning of the environment.

Cerebellum

The cerebellum is primarily implicated in the control of slow conjugate movements, with some minor role in saccadic generation controlled by other centers (e.g., Eckmiller, 1987). Damage to the cerebellum leads to disruptions of smooth pursuit and the VOR through saccadic intrusions, reductions in pursuit gain, and increases in latency. The cerebellum is closely connected with the vestibular system; both the flocculus and the vermis have access to information about head and eye movements, but only the vermis receives information about retinal image slip; the pathway is via the pons. Thus the flocculus does not respond to information about retinal slip but can calculate gaze velocity (a sum of the velocities of head and eye). The vermis, with its additional information about retinal slip, can also cal-culate target velocity. Put another way, the vermis can distinguish between changes in the retinal position of an image due to motion of the object in space, in contrast to motion of the eye or head when the object is stationary. The cerebellum plays a role in the coordination of the VOR with smooth pursuit to allow tracking of a single object with or without accompanying head movements.

Smooth pursuit begins with a response to retinal slip at the retina. This information is processed in turn by the SC and movement sensitive cells in V1, which connect to cells with small receptive fields in MT that are selective for direction of movement. The cells in MT that generate pursuit are mostly foveal in origin and are coded according to a retinotopic spatial map. MT also connects to brainstem eye movement structures, one of which may be a brainstem smooth pursuit area. Once smooth pursuit has begun, the cerebellum helps maintain it by providing feedback about target velocity, which is then fed back to the brainstem structures in order to allow accurate foveation of the target to be continued. Maintenance of tracking accompanied by head movements requires active suppression of the VOR, possibly by brainstem regions receiving cerebellar inputs.

Parietal Cortex and Area PG

It is important to remember that most of the eye movement systems in primates are under considerable voluntary control. The FEF's role in voluntary eye movements appears to be mediated by several areas in the parietal cortex (Goldberg and Bruce, 1985; Heilman et al., 1987). One in particular, area PG in the inferior parietal lobe, has a number of connections that appear relevant for eye movement behavior; PG is connected to FEF, the middle temporal (MT) area, the pulvinar, and other regions in the thalamus. Visual inputs to PG are from extrastriate regions (V3 and V4), rather than directly from primary visual cortex. PG appears to play an important role in the analysis of complex target motion and in attention to events occurring in the animal's vicinity, even if a behavioral response is not elicited by these events. Slow pursuit tracking, saccadic eye movements, and fixations on visual targets are associated with PG activity. PG does not appear to generate any eye movement signals; rather, it serves as an attention-mediated modulator of these signals. One of the key properties of PG is that it responds to targets in specific locations, implying that it is important in the organization of spatial attention.

In addition to being involved in spatially coded selective attention, there is evidence that PG and related parts of the inferior parietal region may also be involved in gross modulation of arousal and motivation. There are a number of structures in the reticular formation, including regions in the MRF also involved in eye movements, that appear to exercise global enhancement or diminution of overall attentional processes (Posner and Peterson, 1990). These brainstem structures are interconnected with the limbic system and the parietal lobe. There is direct input from the limbic system (heavily involved with motivational aspects of behavior) into area PG through the cingulate cortex. PG also communicates with the pulvinar in the thalamus and with the SC, which could be a route for influencing eye movements. This type of connectivity suggests that motivational/state-related factors can modulate oculomotor behavior through direct and indirect influence on the PG, which may play an important role in thresholds for detection of significant stimuli and the resulting behaviors that accurately localize these targets with head and eye movements through connections with the FEF and SC.

Selective attentional processes also can be recorded in V4 during attention to form or pattern, but these processes do not appear to be spatially coded. Rather, these centers appear to be more involved in the attentional components of identification or discrimination of an object's configuration. MT, PG, and FEF, in contrast, are involved in spatial aspects of attention to these objects, possibly in parallel with V4−inferior temporal processing. The interconnections of such centers with areas directly involved in the execution of various types of eye movements remind us that it is difficult to decide in the intact, mature organism just where to draw the boundaries during discussions of oculomotor control. Both sensory inputs and motivational/attentional factors influence the way in which eye movements are executed; and when searching for explanations for oculomotor developments, it is important not to forget the breadth of neural involvement in the generation of the various classes of movements. Before dealing with this issue further, let us review some of the data on how infants make conjugate eye movements.

DEVELOPMENTAL DATA ON SACCADES

Morphology of Saccades

Saccadic eye movements, among the most rapid of all muscular responses, serve to point the fovea at targets that must be examined in some detail during a fixation. They are fast presumably to minimize visual "downtime" as the eye moves from fixation to fixation. During the course of a saccade, the eye rapidly accelerates to a peak velocity that is proportional to the amplitude of the saccade and then begins to decelerate as the eye approaches its landing point. Measures of saccadic velocity−amplitude and duration−amplitude relations

("main sequences") (Bahill et al., 1975) have been useful for characterizing the control system for saccades in various populations, as have measures of saccadic accuracy and latency. There is a relatively large clinical literature demonstrating that analysis of precise saccadic parameters is useful diagnostically for a variety of neurological disorders (e.g., Wirtschafter and Weingarden, 1988). From a developmental standpoint, analysis of saccades is interesting because it evaluates the effects of sensory and motor immaturity on these generally rapid, precise visually mediated movements.

There are only two studies on the relation between saccade peak velocity and saccade amplitude during infancy. Hainline et al. (1984) used corneal reflection technology to measure infants' saccades during free examination of different types of visual scene; some were complex, realistic scenes and gradients of contour-rich textures, whereas others were simpler representations of geometric forms. When infants scanned the more complex stimuli, their saccades were as rapid as those of adults for a given saccadic amplitude. However, when infants looked at simpler (more boring?) stimuli, their decreased attention was reflected in significantly lower peak velocity−amplitude functions (Fig. 4-3). Under conditions of reduced arousal, they also observed an increased frequency of poorly formed saccades and saccadic oscillations (back-to-back saccades separated by brief intersaccadic intervals). These observations, true of infants as young as 14 days of age, suggest that the basic structures responsible for the essential morphology of saccades are functional early in life, but that factors relating to attention and arousal and probably a large number of more "cognitive" factors can alter how saccades are executed. Ashmead (1984) using electroculography (EOG) also reported adult-like velocity−amplitude main sequences for individual saccades elicited by targets presented in different locations in the visual field.

Saccadic Accuracy

Ashmead (1984) noted that the form of localization used by infants was markedly different from the pattern normally observed in adults. Saccadic accuracy is usually studied in a demand-saccade situation: Subjects begin by fixating a small, stationary target that then jumps to a new target location. When adults make saccades to such a peripheral target, they usually make an approximately accurate first saccade that may be followed by a small corrective saccade, if needed. Ashmead and other researchers (Aslin and Salapatek, 1975; Salapatek et al., 1980; Roucoux et al., 1983) reported that young infants in particular are considerably less accurate with their initial saccades; when young infants localize small targets presented in isolation, the first saccade grossly

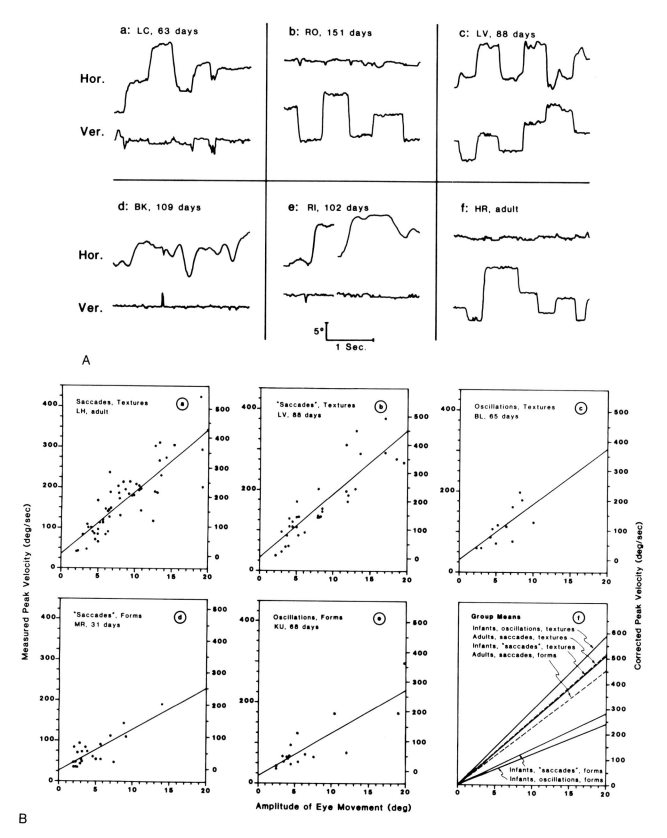

FIG. 4-3. (A) Examples of saccades from infants and adults. Horizontal and vertical eye positions are plotted versus time. Note the saccadic oscillations (D) and the slow saccades (E). (B) Examples of saccadic main sequences, plotting peak velocity versus amplitude of saccade. Main sequences of saccades and saccadic oscillations do not differ. (F) Group regression lines, illustrating the effect on saccadic velocity of stimuli that differ in attentional value for infants. (From Hainline et al., 1984. By permission.)

undershoots the target and is followed by a series of short saccades approaching the target, with each step of the series approximately equal in size (some examples are shown in Figure 4-4). Each step is executed after a normal saccadic interval; and according to Ashmead (1984), each component saccade falls on a main sequence function. The size of the step is related to target eccentricity; steps were longer for more distant targets, shorter for nearer ones. This pattern is reported to diminish over the first few months of life.

Saccadic steps are not commonly observed when infants look at stimuli more visually rich than single points of light on a blank field (Hainline and Abramov, 1985). In fact, even in our own work on demand saccades, we have not observed them with the frequency suggested by earlier studies. Interestingly, they are sometimes observed in adults who are tired or inattentive (Bahill and Stark, 1975), although such saccades are usually not a series of equal-sized steps. Thus it is likely that the steps are not an essential part of the saccadic system itself but a consequence of either or both attentional lapses or problems in localization of the target in space when deprived of other visual landmarks. The most puzzling

thing about the phenomenon of infant saccadic steps is that they are of equal size; in corrective saccade situations, each saccade is usually smaller than the preceding one, as error in retinal position is reduced across successive saccades. This finding would be consistent with each being programmed immediately before execution, based on the current positional error. Unless the whole sequence were programmed in advance with an appropriate step size chosen so the eye successfully lands on target, it seems that such steps would result in cases in which the infant is never able to foveate the target successfully.

Saccadic Latencies

Less attention has been devoted to the issue of saccadic latency in infants. In an adult demand saccade experiment, saccadic latency consists primarily of the time required to plan and execute a saccade; but with free scanning, intersaccadic intervals are more likely to represent the information-processing time associated with selection of a target in addition to the time to plan and execute the next saccade. Current indications are that

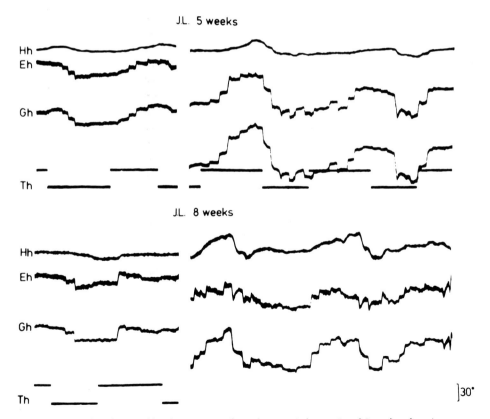

FIG. 4-4. Examples of eye and head movements from the same infant at 5 and 8 weeks of age in response to targets 30 degrees in the periphery. The two left traces show the most common behavior; an alternate behavior is shown in the top right trace. The bottom right trace represents spontaneous scanning in the absence of a stimulus. Note the similarity between saccadic localization and the infant's spontaneous looking behavior. H = head position; E = eye position; G = gaze (head plus eye position); T = target position. Only the horizontal position is indicated. (From Roucoux et al., 1983. By permission.)

in demand saccade paradigms latencies are longer for infants, particularly young infants. Some unpublished data by Regal and Salapatek, reported by Regal et al. (1983), showed that saccadic latencies increased with target eccentricity and decreased with increasing age. One-month-olds were found to have latencies of about 0.5 second for targets presented suddenly 10 degrees peripherally, and almost 1 second for targets presented at 30 degrees. In contrast, for 5-month-olds, latency was about 0.25 second for a 10-degree target and about 0.5 second for the 30-degree target. By comparison, adults' reaction times were about 200 ms for both target eccentricities.

The long latencies seen in infant demand saccade experiments may not mean that infants always take longer to plan and execute the saccades, however. In free scanning situations, we find that infant intersaccadic intervals can be either briefer or longer than those of free-scanning adults depending on stimulus factors, such as the complexity of the stimulus and the density of contours on the retina (Harris et al., 1988). In their work, it was found that for stimuli that filled the retina with visual contours, infants had briefer fixations (200–300 ms on average) than did uninstructed adults viewing the same stimuli, whose fixations were on the order of 400 ms. For stimuli that had fewer contours, infants' fixations (in this case being considered as intersaccadic intervals) were considerably longer, 0.5 second or more. These fixational intervals were modeled as representing both information-processing time and the time needed to program the next saccade (Harris, 1989). Our analysis of the situation is that under these types of test conditions infants' saccades are elicited by the detection of peripheral visual contours in a relatively automatic way. If there is a large number of contours, the next saccade occurs promptly; if there is nothing salient to draw the eye away from the current fixation, it takes longer for a saccade to be triggered.

This point speaks to the difficulty of interpreting "spontaneous" reaction times. It is difficult to think of a manipulation that would make adult and infant saccadic latencies directly comparable. Take answering the telephone as a convenient example; if I am expecting an important call or if I happen to be close to the telephone when it rings, I am apt to answer the phone with a short latency. On the other hand, if I am involved in doing something else, such as an alternative cognitive activity—writing a chapter with my word processor—when the phone rings, I am apt to finish the sentence I am writing and maybe even save the file before I make the motor response to pick up the receiver. If I am daydreaming when the phone rings, there might also be an extended latency before I "come to" enough to organize a response. Such factors would make it difficult to analyze my telephone response latency. Adults

are easily set—explicitly through instructions or implicitly through implied task demands—to ignore all other activities and make rapid saccades to small lights flashing in various parts of the visual field. We cannot, obviously, instruct infants. In fact, it is difficult to imagine what we might do experimentally to ensure that infants will bother to respond quickly to a relatively unimportant target appearing somewhere in space.

Studies investigating the extent of the infants' peripheral field have found that (1) infants are less likely to respond to peripheral targets, and (2) latencies are longer if a central fixation target stays on than if the central target is extinguished as the new target appears in the periphery (Harris and Macfarlane, 1974; Aslin and Salapatek, 1975; Salapatek et al., 1980). This phenomenon is not restricted to infants; adult humans and monkeys have longer saccadic latencies to peripheral targets when a central stimulus is present than when one is absent (Fischer, 1986; Fisher and Breitmeyer, 1987). These results support the supposition that attention to central visual targets normally needs to be disengaged, a process that takes some time, before saccades can be executed to peripheral targets. In the limiting case, the presence of central targets may completely eliminate the peripheral saccade, although the subject may still at some level be aware that a peripheral target has occurred. Finlay and Ivinkis (1982, 1984) coupled the measurement of infants' localization of peripheral targets with change in heart rate and found that 4-month-old infants frequently showed a change in heart rate when a peripheral target appeared, even if no saccade to the new target occurred; this finding indicated that saccadic reactions do not totally reflect what the infant is detecting. It would be interesting to follow this line of research further with methods that would allow heart rate responses to be correlated with more precise measures of saccadic latency.

Possible Interpretations

The above data show that infant and adult saccades differ in various ways. To whom, then, should the infant's behavior be compared? The type of subject usually chosen is the highly practiced, well-motivated adult, whose data are presented in many of the published articles in the eye movement literature. It may not be the best comparison for infant data, however. At first thought, a more appropriate alternative seems to be naive, uninstructed adults; and they *are* probably a more appropriate group than highly practiced adults. In our experience, "off the street," naive adults often perform at much lower levels than the textbooks describe, but perhaps no adult can ever be truly "naive"; such subjects are never totally free of expectations and self-instructions that can influence how they execute various eye movements (e.g., Steinman et al., 1990).

We now have a reasonable understanding of the neural mechanisms responsible for saccades. Can we relate the characteristics of infant saccades to the properties of the underlying mechanisms? When infants are alert, their saccades have normal main sequence properties. In the saccadic centers in the brainstem, several types of neuron are instrumental in the generation of saccades. In order to start the eye in motion, burst neurons begin to fire to excite the nerves connected to the extraocular muscles; at the same time, pause cells (which prevent intrusive saccades and are active all the time except immediately preceding and during a saccade) and tonic cells (which are responsible for keeping the eye steady during and after the saccade is completed) are inhibited. Activity of the burst neurons causes the eye to accelerate from its originally stationary position. After some duration, which is proportional to the amplitude of the saccade, the burst cells stop firing and the eye decelerates to its end position, at which point the pause and tonic neurons resume their firing. Because the duration of the pulse from the burst neurons is directly responsible for the distance that eye moves, burst neurons are the means by which spatial information is converted to neural signals to create appropriate saccades. The existence of the main sequence, the proportional relation between saccadic amplitude and peak velocity, implies that the amplitude of the saccade is "known" to the burst neurons before the saccade is begun (Zee and Robinson, 1979; Robinson, 1981). In the case of an infant's free scanning, where the saccadic target is unknown, it is possible that the signals to the burst neurons represent some random process, so that one sees a random collection of saccadic amplitudes that nevertheless are on the main sequence function. The differences we observe in infants' main sequences across stimuli with different attentional/arousal values might mean only that arousal modulates activity in the burst cells globally. Strictly speaking, then, the existence of main sequence saccades that we reported (Hainline et al., 1984) for free scanning infants does not necessarily tell us that saccades are being made appropriately, although the fact that the amplitude histograms for infants and adults look similar is indirect evidence, in contrast to the hypothesis that random burst cell activity drives infants' free scanning saccades rather than having saccade amplitudes directly determined by salient targets in the visual field (Hainline and Abramov, 1985).

In support of the latter possibility, there are other data that argue for the existence of spatially controlled, topographical mapping during the generation of infant saccades, and they are the step-saccades that have been reported to single targets. As mentioned above, we have some doubts that saccadic steps are a universal property

of saccadic localization of small targets during early infancy, but let us assume for the sake of discussion that they are at least a prevalent property. If, as reported, the steps are equal in size, ultimately reach the target, and are scaled to target eccentricity, and if each component is one the main sequence, it appears necessary to conclude that the duration of the burst neuron activity is not a random process. Rather, these data are consistent with saccades appropriately preplanned to specific locations organized in an appropriate topographic map. On the retina, the image must be a veridical representation of the world, assuming no major optical distortions, but the SC appears to be organized not according to retinal coordinates but in terms of space, as indicated by retinal position and head and eye position (Mays and Sparks, 1980; Sparks, 1986). Thus the existence of more or less correct distance information in the real world implies that at least the SC and its maps are probably in place early, although we still have no explanation for why the steps occur as they do.

Some conclusions about the level of neural control of infant saccades may also be found in an analysis of infant saccadic latencies. The SC saccadic pathway is described as reflexive, quick, and accurate. We observe that latencies in free scanning are either longer or shorter than those of adults, depending on the nature of the stimulus. Fischer and colleagues (Fischer and Boch, 1983; Fischer and Ramsperger, 1984) posited that intentional saccades require the release of attention by centers in the FEF before voluntary saccades can occur. They described a phenomenon of "express" saccades that monkeys and human adults (although possibly not all adults) (Wenban-Smith, 1990) can be trained to make with short latencies, provided a central fixation target is extinguished as a warning that a target step is about to occur. It is possible that some of the brief saccadic intervals observed with infants in free-scanning paradigms are indicative of the fact that under some circumstances FEF influence is minimal. In these cases, as in Harris's (1989) model for saccade generation during free scanning, we may be observing a relatively reflexive SC pathway in control of saccades that are not intentionally directed at particular targets (Fig. 4-5).

This reasoning leaves us, however, with the curious finding that infants' saccadic latencies in demand situations are longer, not shorter, than those of adults. Although it is still possible that it is a property of an immature SC system (monkeys' saccades have longer latencies after collicular lesions) (Wurtz and Goldberg, 1972) or due to higher cortical immaturities (posterior parietal lesions in monkeys also lengthen latencies) (Mountcastle et al., 1981), such explanations are inconsistent with the latency data derived with free-scanning. It is also possible that these longer latencies rep-

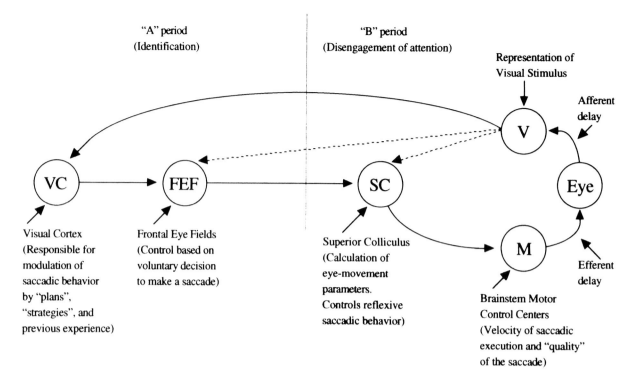

"A" period
(Identification)

"B" period
(Disengagement of attention)

Representation of
Visual Stimulus

Afferent
delay

V

VC

FEF

SC

Eye

Visual Cortex
(Responsible for
modulation of
saccadic behavior
by "plans",
"strategies", and
previous experience)

Frontal Eye Fields
(Control based on
voluntary decision
to make a saccade)

Superior Colliculus
(Calculation of
eye-movement
parameters.
Controls reflexive
saccadic behavior)

M

Efferent
delay

Brainstem Motor
Control Centers
(Velocity of saccadic
execution and "quality"
of the saccade)

FIG. 4-5. Model for the control of saccades by various brain centers. The model states that normally control passes sequentially from the visual cortex (VC) to the frontal eye fields (FEF) to the superior colliculus (SC), and that each level contributes some amount of time to the intersaccadic interval. Dotted lines indicate alternative pathways that control may take with training, pathology, or neurological immaturity. The A and B periods represent two subprocesses that have been established from the analysis of fixation duration distributions (Harris, 1989). Fischer termed these periods "identification" and "disengagement of attention." (After Fischer, 1985, and Harris and Hainline, 1986.)

resent the nascent influence of the centers in the FEF that control intentional saccades, which may take longer to plan for infants or for which the attentional release mechanism in the FEF works more slowly. Such an explanation is consistent with the fact that infants' saccadic latencies are shorter when a central target is extinguished than when it is maintained after a second target appears. This situation illustrates well the problem of determining what causes the behaviors of infants. It is possible that it is simply a sensory effect; latencies to peripheral targets could be longer than in adults because neural activity in the infant peripheral retina is noisier than that in adults, and so a longer integration time or more samples are needed to extract a particular signal. A paradigm in which we have a better certainty that a saccade is intended, rather than simply elicited by the presence of a stimulus, might help to decide among these alternatives. One that comes to mind is an anticipation paradigm, in which one analyzes the properties of latencies and saccades to expected targets. It might be profitable to explore some operant paradigms as well.

There may be insights about the maturity of infants' eye movement control systems that can be derived from clinical observations. In other words, we may be able

to conduct a deconstructionist analysis of what we observe in infant eye movements, informed by what we do *not* observe. There are, of course, some problems with this sort of analysis. For example, there are clinical observations that lesions in V4 cause alexia, but it is not therefore appropriate to conclude that immaturities in V4 are responsible for the fact that infants cannot read. However, clinical data can still provide perspective when direct physiological experimentation is impossible. To cite some examples, pulvinar lesions are associated with a paucity of spontaneous saccades to contralateral visual space. Unilateral frontal lesions are associated with a number of oculomotor problems, including impaired contralateral gaze and problems with visual search. Bilateral frontal lesions are associated with problems initiating saccades and pursuit as well as abnormalities of scanning, including an inability to voluntarily transfer gaze within a structured visual scene. None of these possibilities seems to particularly characterize infant saccadic behavior. At the same time, there are some interesting parallels to certain infant behaviors that are found in Balint syndrome, in which posterior parietal lesions result in an inability to perceive a whole structure from component parts, an inability to coordinate movements of the arms and legs with visual information, and an inability to shift gaze to a novel stimulus that normal adults would immediately attend to; when the patient finally does look at the new target, the eye movements are inaccurate. It is also interesting to note that cerebellar lesions, especially in the vermis, are associated with permanent saccadic dysmetria, possibly because of problems in taking account of mechanical forces of the eye, although these symptoms are not identical to the hypometria that has been reported for infants. Saccadic dysmetria has also been associated with increased postsaccadic drift, a behavior that has not been commonly reported for infants. It is difficult to make a hard case that the absence of these symptoms necessarily points to some level of functioning in appropriate structures for infants, as the order in which different centers begin to function during development may play a critical role in how immaturities are reflected in behavior. Still, such clinical data do support the contention that the infant saccadic system, although not totally adult-like, is not in a "pathological" condition as a result of whatever structures are immature during the early months of life.

DEVELOPMENTAL DATA ON FIXATION

Image Slippage and Motion Detection

Adults are able to keep their eyes still during fixation, especially if they are instructed to do so and are given some amount of practice. The best adult fixational performances include a variety of micro movements (tremors, drifts, and microsaccades, which some consider to be phenomena of the laboratory) (Howard, 1982) that keep the eye steady within minutes of arc. Under normal viewing with an unrestrained head, however, adults do not hold their eyes exceptionally still, yet visual functioning is unimpaired (Skavenski et al., 1979). Adults' detection and identification of many sorts of stimuli are not greatly compromised by drifts of the eye on the order of several degrees per second (Westheimer and McKee, 1975; Murphy, 1978; Kelly, 1979a,b). Thus it appears that whereas steady fixation is within an adult's capability, such behavior is not always demanded by the requirements of many everyday situations, an observation that is an important context for evaluating the stability of infant fixations.

Feedback about drift of a scene's retinal image has been regarded as the visual signal used to maintain stable fixation; systematic drift in one direction can be compensated for by drift or a microsaccade in the other direction to maintain the fixation position. If drift velocity or amplitude becomes too great, the fixation may be terminated as a saccade brings the eye to a different fixation point. Sensitivity to temporal change at the

retina as an image drifts across retinal receptive fields influences how the visual system responds to fixational drift. If the temporal response of retinal cells is sluggish, there might be no feedback to control high drift rates during fixation. Spatial sensitivity also matters. With large receptive fields, the eye might drift a considerable distance or at a high rate before eye position can be corrected. Smaller receptive fields would be needed to detect lower amplitude or slower drifts.

To explore some of these issues developmentally, given what is known about the level of retinal development in infants, we have been examining a number of aspects of infant fixations, including their drift characteristics and durations. It is difficult to separate the issue of drift velocity from the issue of the duration of fixations during infancy. Our data (Hainline and Harris, 1990; Hainline and Abramov, 1991; Harris and Hainline, 1991) suggest that fixational drift is related to fixation duration but in a complex way. As mentioned above, we have been analyzing the duration of fixations from the perspective of a model proposing that fixations are terminated, after a minimum waiting time, by a process with a fixed probability per unit time of fixation that a salient contour in peripheral retina elicits a new saccade (Harris and Hainline, 1986; Harris et al., 1988; Harris, 1989). In general, we find shorter fixation durations for stimuli rich in retinal contours than for those that do not fill the retina with contours and details.

When we look at drift velocity as a function of fixation duration, we again see differences across stimuli for infants (Fig. 4-6). For the more contour-rich stimuli, drift velocity was relatively low, although higher than that observed for adults for equivalent fixation durations, falling to 2.0–2.5 degrees/second for fixations of 300 ms or longer. For briefer fixations with the same stimuli, velocity was often more than 10 degrees/second. In contrast, for simple geometric shapes, spots, and single bars, drift velocity was higher at all fixation durations and never less than 5 degrees/second even for fixations lasting more than 0.5 second. For these stimuli, fixations of 100 ms were associated with drift velocities of as much as 15–18 degrees/second. These data imply that for infants the duration of a fixation is limited by tolerance for slippage of the stimulus' retinal image, which in turn depends on availability of contours to define this slippage. Contour-rich scenes have better controlled fixations, possibly due to the presence of many contours to define drift during an individual fixation. At the same time that they serve to stabilize fixation, these same peripheral contours are likely to elicit a saccade away after some minimal interval. In contrast, stimuli with few visual contours yield longer fixations that are more poorly controlled for retinal slip. Interestingly, we have observed no clear age trends in any of these results over the first year. Nevertheless, the fact

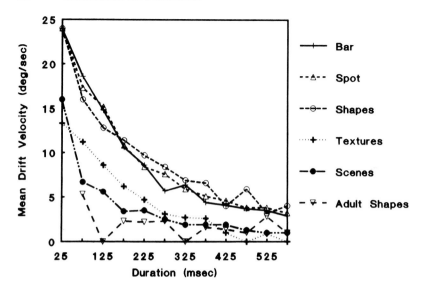

FIG. 4-6. Mean drift velocity observed for fixations of different durations by infants viewing different types of stimuli and an adult group viewing simple geometric shapes. Stimuli seen by infants were a single horizontal or vertical bar, a single small spot, simple geometric shapes, textures such as checkerboards, and complex realistic visual scenes. Note that for infants and to a lesser extent for adults, fixation drift velocity decreases as duration increases; a possible explanation is the presence of a mechanism sensitive to retinal slip that ends a fixation if slip is too great. This effect is moderated in infants by the type of stimulus being viewed; there is less drift for stimuli that fill the retina with more edges. (From Hainline and Abramov, 1991. By permission.)

that we do not observe long infant fixations that also have high drift velocities implies the early existence of a corrective feedback mechanism that is probably visual in origin. That even young infants are sensitive to these factors speaks to the ability of the infant's visual system to communicate information about change in spatial distribution on the retina across time. It would be useful to know more about the ability of the infant's visual system to respond to temporal change in other situations.

Motion Detection

The issue of motion thresholds during infancy is of obvious relevance here (as it is for the issue of the minimal target velocity eliciting pursuit; see below). There is some discrepancy in the motion thresholds that have been reported using forced-choice preferential looking. Some studies report fairly high thresholds for young infants. For example, Aslin and Shea (1990) reported motion thresholds of no better than 9 degrees/second for 6-week-olds and 4 degrees/second for 12-week-olds; and Dannemiller and Freedland (1989) estimated thresholds worse than 6 degrees/second for 8-week-olds and no better than 5 degrees/second for 16-week-olds. Another FPL study by Bradbury et al. (1990), found a threshold sensitivity of 3.5 degrees/second for 12-week-

olds and 1.25 degrees/second for 20-week-olds. In contrast to these high motion detection thresholds, Bushnell (1979) found that 1-month-olds showed reliable evidence of noticing movement of 2.4 degrees/second; and Kaufmann et al. (1985) found a motion threshold of 2.8 degrees/second for the same age group. These lower threshold estimates are more consistent with our smooth pursuit data in which even young infants were found able to begin smooth pursuit of targets moving as slowly as 2.5 degrees/second (see below). The discrepancy raises the possibility that retinal motion detection (which is probably closely related to temporal sensitivity of retinal cells) is more acute than motion-sensitive mechanisms in other sites of the visual system (e.g., in area MT) that may be instrumental in higher order perceptions of motion of real objects. Another issue is which of these motion-sensitive systems influences the voluntary control of behavior; the lower levels, in particular, may not be available for conscious control of behavior. The issue of the temporal sensitivity of vision during early infancy clearly needs much more experimental attention using a variety of methods. Because feedback about retinal and stimulus movement is instrumental to many forms of eye movement control, oculomotor development must be related to the development of the infant's ability to detect and respond to the movement of stimuli.

Accuracy of Refixations

Another aspect of fixation that we have been examining is the ability of the infant to refixate a given target precisely. When a small target is looked at repeatedly, we were interested in how widely scattered infants' fixations would be in the light of their reported foveal immaturities (Hainline et al., 1990). Even highly trained adults refixating the same target show some scatter (with an SD of about 0.1 degree) (de Bie, 1986; Snodderly, 1987). We presented a 1.5-degree target repeatedly in consistent locations in the visual field and measured the coordinates of the infant's fixations each time the same point was viewed. The standard deviations for infants' refixations were roughly constant over the first year and had a mean of about 0.8 degree. The average standard deviation for uninstructed adults was around 0.4 degree (Fig. 4-7). Some of this scatter probably came

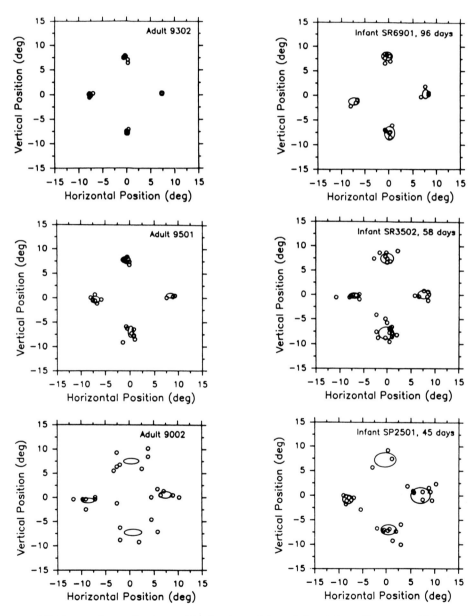

FIG. 4-7. Scatter of mean fixation position for three adults and three infants. No age trend is implied by the choice of infants. Each symbol represents the position of the mean of one fixation when the target was in one of its four terminal locations (7.5 degrees from center, left, right, up, and down). Ellipses represent 1 standard error. Subject 9032 deliberately attempted to fixate a corner of the 1.5 degree square. Note the poor performance of subject 9002, who was not given any specific instructions about how to perform the task. (From Hainline et al., 1990. By permission.)

from the fact that subjects were looking at slightly different portions of the 1.5-degree stimulus across trials. These results are consistent with the hypothesis that even though infants may lack high acuity during the early months, they are able to use some reasonably consistent small retinal area to direct fixations, although it is impossible with present methods to determine what portion of retina this area is.

Possible Interpretations

We interpret the small database currently available on infant fixation to show evidence of an ability to detect retinal slippage of images. The data are consistent with a self-limiting mechanism that keeps retinal slip to some minimum either because the target's image has moved too far on the retina or because it is moving too rapidly; we observe a roughly reciprocal relation between fixation drift velocity and fixation duration, such that the image of the target does not move too far on the retina during a single fixation. When this limit is exceeded, the fixation is terminated by some other eye movement. What we do not know is whether during free scanning this terminating movement is in a corrective direction, that is, to reacquire the target. Here again, we have interpretational difficulties because if the infant fails to show a corrective movement it could also be because another target has become salient. Our informal observation of the data is that this sort of correction does in fact occur, but we need to examine all of the data systematically to discern how common this pattern is. Our data also show that when targets move continuously from one end position to another the coordinates of refixations of a target in a given location are variable, but within small limits that are consistent with attentional rather than oculomotor limitations.

Given the small database on quantitative analysis of infant fixations, some of the things that researchers have not reported about infant fixation may be of interest. There do not appear to be regions in space that infants cannot fixate, as in many clinical disorders, particularly those involving the basal ganglia. Neither do we observe sustained episodes of the several varieties of nystagmus, which is a common neurological symptom with many sorts of damage to oculomotor structures. The occasional episodes of saccadic oscillations (back-to-back saccades without a normal intersaccadic interval) that we observe in young infants when they appear to be a state of reduced arousal (described above) are transient and probably related to small mistimings of the burst and pause neurons (Zee and Robinson, 1979); clinically, this behavior is sometimes referred to as *opsoclonus*. More continuous oscillations, termed *ocular flutter*, are also rarely seen. *Square-wave jerks* are a pattern in which fixations are terminated by inappro-

priate saccades away from a target fixation after a normal intersaccadic interval, again observed in a number of clinical conditions. Frontal lobe lesions have been reported to be associated with impaired fixation due to intrusive saccades. Infants have not been reported to show consistent evidence of square-wave jerks or other major saccadic intrusions in their fixations during scanning. Thus whatever the mechanisms that control fixations, infants do have the ability to keep their eyes relatively still during intersaccadic intervals, almost certainly due to visual feedback from retinal slip.

DEVELOPMENTAL DATA ON PURSUIT

Smooth Pursuit

In studies of smooth pursuit, the principal dependent measure is usually velocity gain, the ratio of the eye's velocity to target velocity. The relation of eye position to stimulus position (phase) is sometimes reported, as are the latency to begin pursuit and the frequency of saccadic intrusions. When a fixated target begins to move, there is some latency before an eye movement is entrained; and if the stimulus movement is rapid, the first movement may be a "catch-up" saccade followed by smooth pursuit or a mixture of smooth and saccadic pursuit. To stabilize a moving target effectively, smooth pursuit gain must to be close to unity.

It has been argued that because smooth pursuit is a foveal function, young infants whose foveae are immature (Abramov et al., 1982; Hendrickson and Yuodelis, 1984; Yuodelis and Hendrickson, 1986) have poorly developed smooth pursuit (e.g., Aslin, 1981, 1988). Some studies have indeed failed to find smooth pursuit in infants younger than about 2–3 months, when targets are reported to be tracked almost exclusively with a series of saccades (Dayton et al., 1964; Aslin, 1981; Atkinson and Braddick, 1981; Shea and Aslin, 1984). Such data are consistent with the notion that smooth pursuit is absent until some critical level of foveal function is achieved, but the absence of pursuit in these studies may be due to other factors. Smooth pursuit may not have been observed either because of the nature of the stimulus movement chosen (i.e., sinusoidal pursuit is poorer than constant velocity pursuit in infants) (Aslin, 1981, versus Shea and Aslin, 1990) or attentional or sensory factors regarding target visibility (large targets still too small to be likely to trigger OKN response are pursued better than smaller targets) (Shea and Aslin, 1984).

Not all the data are consistent with the early absence of smooth pursuit (e.g., Kremenitzer et al., 1979; Roucoux et al., 1983; Hainline, 1985; Shea and Aslin, 1988, 1990; Krinsky et al., 1990) These studies provide data that infants do show episodes of smooth pursuit even early in life, although admittedly only to relatively low target velocities (10 degrees/second or less). Figure 4-8 shows some examples of pursuit from infants and a naive adult. Both Roucoux et al. (1983) and Hainline (1985) found developmental change in the maximum velocity for which smooth pursuit is shown. Other factors that probably make a difference but require more empirical attention are stimulus size (Shea and Aslin, 1984), the profile of target velocity (see above), and the nature of stimulus movement (repetitive target move-

ment yields better pursuit than single excursions) (e.g., Hainline, 1988; Krinsky et al., 1990).

Alternative Forms of Pursuit

A second question is how well infants keep up with a moving target whatever the type of eye movement used. Shea and Aslin (1990) reported some relevant findings for 2-month-olds. They presented infants with small targets moving at fixed velocities of 3–12 degrees/sec-

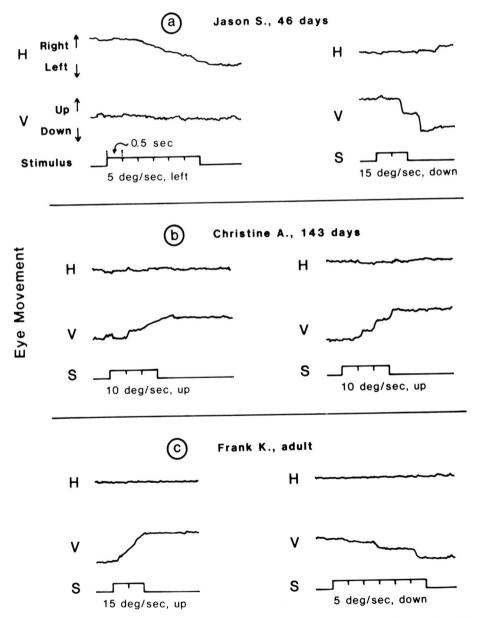

FIG. 4-8. Examples of smooth and saccadic pursuit from two infants and a naive adult. Note that all the subjects show episodes of smooth pursuit but not at all times or under all conditions. (From Hainline, 1988. By permission.)

ond. Eye movement records were processed to remove any saccades that occurred during target movement. They then based an overall measure of pursuit gain on mean eye velocity of the remaining record, that is, with saccades removed. By this measure, infants had pursuit gains considerably less than 1.0, ranging from 0.5 for slow targets to 0.1 for the fastest. The systematic drop in gain was such that average eye velocity was the same for all stimulus velocities. They concluded that moving targets trigger some sort of following response, but one that is not matched to the movement of the stimulus. The problem with this analysis is that filtering out pursuit saccades necessarily reduces pursuit gain and implies that the eye is not "keeping up" with the target, although the effects of such saccades may be to ensure exactly that. Fixations that occurred after the beginning of stimulus movement (representing pursuit latency) or as pauses during following were averaged with the actual smooth pursuit movements, thereby necessarily lowering the calculated gain. In the limiting case with such an analysis, a subject could pursue a target perfectly with a series of saccades interspersed with fixations, and the filtered eye velocity would reflect only the near-zero velocities of the fixations. It is noteworthy that Shea and Aslin reported that most infants showed short episdoes of smooth pursuit with near-unity gains, but because of the form of data analysis employed these episodes could not be evaluated as a separate class of movement.

In our own work on smooth pursuit in infants, we use a different form of initial data analysis that allows the characteristics of smooth pursuit to be investigated as a separate class of any of the eye movements that occur during object tracking. We measured the eye movements of infants 1–7 months old and naive adults as they tracked small targets moving back and forth or up and down several times across a screen at velocities ranging from 2.5 to 15.0 degrees/second; a preliminary analysis was presented by Krinsky et al. (1990). Eye movements were measured with a corneal reflection system, and data were in most cases individually calibrated for eye movement gain and eye position. Eye movement records were individually "parsed" into a succession of component episodes and quantitatively analyzed for each type of movement (i.e., smooth pursuit, fixations, saccades). None of the subjects pursued all targets smoothly and accurately for the entire duration of a trial. For adults, it was presumably because they were uninstructed and did not bother to apply their full pursuit skills to this task; these targets were not particularly difficult for a motivated adult to pursue. Infants spent less time in smooth pursuit than did adults. The incidence of smooth pursuit declined as velocity increased for both infants and adults, as did the average

duration of each "bout" of smooth pursuit. For infants, the proportion of time spent in smooth pursuit ranged from 25% at 2.5 degrees/second to 12% for 15 degrees/second; corresponding values for adults were 57% and 13%, respectively. The duration of each bout of smooth pursuit decreased in both infants and adults as target velocity increased; the mean for both age groups was about 2 seconds for the slowest target, decreasing to around 0.5 second for the fastest velocity. For the episodes when they showed smooth pursuit, both infants and adults stabilized the retinal images rather well; gains for both groups were between 0.9 and 1.0 even at the highest stimulus speeds.

To examine the point at which a moving target elicited pursuit (either smooth pursuit or a catch-up saccade) we measured the latency to the first following movement. Although somewhat longer, infants' latencies compared favorably with those of adults. For both groups, latencies decreased as stimulus velocity increased, suggesting that following movements were elicited when retinal displacement of the stimulus exceeded some criterion value. For smooth pursuit, the latency value ranged from 3 to 5 degrees across velocities (Fig. 4-9). If the response was delayed until the stimulus was displaced even more, the first movement was usually a catch-up saccade. There were few significant age trends, except that the proportion of time spent in smooth pursuit increased with age for the higher velocities. These data suggest that although infants do not pursue moving targets exactly as do naive adults, when they do show smooth pursuit it is similar to the high gain following movements of adults. Even though they are not pursuing smoothly all the time, their total pursuit is a functional mixture of smooth pursuit, saccades, and fixational pauses that maintains the eye on a moving target with acceptable tolerance. At this point, we do not know how to interpret the increase in the frequency of smooth pursuit with age; it may be due to direct improvement in the neural centers responsible for smooth pursuit, but it is also possible that substantial improvement derives from changes in attentional factors and developments in cognitive expectancies about objects and their patterns of movement in the world.

Possible Interpretations

It is important to distinguish logically between the absence of smooth pursuit in species that never evolved foveae and its absence in individual members of a foveate species who might have poorly developed foveae. The fovea is a small region. In many cases, even small targets fall on both foveal and parafoveal regions. Small targets near the threshold of spatial resolution may not be salient enough to capture and hold the infant's at-

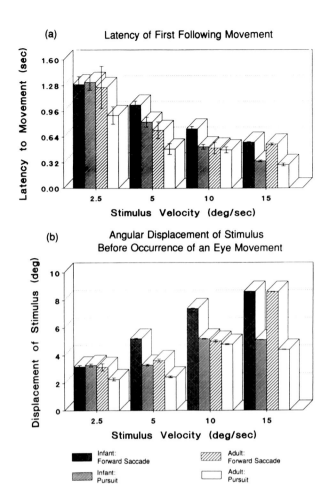

(a) Latency of First Following Movement

(b) Angular Displacement of Stimulus Before Occurrence of an Eye Movement

■ Infant: Forward Saccade
▨ Infant: Pursuit
▨ Adult: Forward Saccade
☐ Adult: Pursuit

FIG. 4-9. Histograms describing some parameters of following eye movements from infants and adults. Small targets were moved at one of four constant velocities several times across the stimulus display. The top graph illustrates the latency of the first movement, whether it was a forward saccade or a smooth pursuit, for the different velocities for infants and adults; the two age groups show a similar pattern of response of latency versus velocity. The bottom graph illustrates how far the stimulus had moved, in degrees, before the first following movement was made. If the stimulus has moved beyond about 5 degrees, the first movement is likely to be a saccade, but it depends on velocity and latency. (From Krinsky et al., 1990. By permission.)

tention for the time required to demonstrate reliable pursuit. If not foveal, it is possible that the pursuit that has been observed in young infants is mediated by a more highly developed parafoveal locus. If such a region has lower spatial resolution, pursuit, though present, may be poorer than that observed at later ages because of the development of sensory abilities. Spatial vision falls off quickly as one moves away from the fovea, but visually normal adults with some practice can pursue objects effectively with peripheral retina (Robinson, 1981).

Further conclusions about the presence or absence of smooth pursuit at a given age during infancy must also deal with the issue of whether smooth pursuit with some retinal region of higher spatial resolution is demanded by the task. We usually follow an object with smooth pursuit in order to inspect its fine details. If such inspection is not necessary, it is less effortful to keep up with the target using saccadic pursuit or a mixture of saccadic and smooth pursuit. Because smooth pursuit is a voluntary response requiring maintained attentional deployment, in uninstructed subjects it is difficult to separate oculomotor from attentional factors. With the exception of the Roucoux et al. (1983) study, which employed a target with facial features, existing studies have used unpatterned spots, circles, or bars as pursuit targets. Such targets have no spatial details that require high resolution vision. Thus there is no compelling reason to follow them using the smooth pursuit system after a brief inspection, assuming the stimulus details are above threshold for a particular infant. My opinion is that there are sufficient data to warrant the conclusion that there is some kind of smooth pursuit system present and functioning even before 2 months, but that it is used only when circumstances require it and then only for lower velocities of stimulus movement unless target movement is sustained for some time. This issue deserves further empirical attention.

A number of clinical conditions are associated with defects or deficits in smooth pursuit. Low-gain pursuit is often associated with drugs such as tranquilizers and anticonvulsants, organic diseases of the cerebellum such as multiple sclerosis, and progressive supranuclear palsy. Unilateral disease in various cortical structures are associated with imbalances in pursuit tone, evidenced by asymmetrical drift and gain. Imbalance in pursuit mechanisms has been associated with some forms of spontaneous nystagmus (Abel et al., 1979). Square-wave jerks are also sometimes seen as intrusions in smooth tracking. If there is any information in the clinical literature relevant to the infant case, it may be to point to cerebellar immaturities as possible reasons for some of the behaviors seen; cerebellar damage is associated with dysmetric saccades (but with normal velocities and latencies), with fixation abnormalities such as ocular flutter, square wave jerks and increased drift, impaired smooth pursuit with the head moving or stationary (i.e., problems with VOR cancellation), many forms of nystagmus, postsaccadic drifts (glissades), increased VOR gain, and vertical misalignment of the visual axes (Zee, 1982). A few of these problems have been associated with infant eye movements, but most have not been observed and probably would have been evident to inspection even if no careful quantitative analyses were done.

DEVELOPMENTAL DATA ON OCULOMOTOR INTERACTIONS

The ability of the visual system to function appropriately depends on the ability of the various oculomotor systems described at the beginning of the chapter to be smoothly coordinated during joint functioning. We are only beginning to understand how these abilities combine developmentally; more complete discussion of the development of the VOR and its role in image stabilization is found in Chapter 5. Most of the work on pursuit, saccades, and fixation in infants has been done with the infant's head and body kept relatively still. Although it is important to understand how these behaviors develop separately, evaluating their development in isolation is highly artificial from the perspective of the evolution of the various eye movement systems and the function they must serve in the everyday life of the infant. There has been some sharp criticism of the tendency to study eye movement systems in isolation, even in adult research where the situation is less complex because all of the systems have reached their final level of organization. Steinman et al. (1990) argued that restricting the study of eye movements to single subsystems evaluated with grossly unnatural stimuli results in a misleading characterization of oculomotor system performance. They proposed that it is the artificial constraints imposed on oculomotor performance in typical laboratory settings that has led to the postulation of numerous separate oculomotor subsystems, and that actually there are only two systems: one responsible for slow movements and another for fast ones. Furthermore, they suggested that performance of the complete oculomotor system acts synergistically with movements of the head and body to yield a well coordinated system for precise orientation of the organism in space. This critique of a prevailing trend in much of the adult eye movement work strikes a resonant chord. It is worth worrying about the possibility that researchers studying the development of eye movement systems in infants may be falling into a similar trap by failing to look at the interactions among the different systems. There are many methodological problems involved in this work, and such analysis is not easy; but more effort should be expended in the direction of studying the coordination of eye movement systems during development.

There have been a few attempts at this sort of program. For example, Roucoux et al. (1983) and Regal et al. (1983) investigated saccades made to small targets when free head movement was allowed. Both studies reported that if head movements were permitted infants often accompanied their saccadic "steps" with coordinated "steps" of the head (Fig. 4-4). It appears to put the phenomenon of saccadic steps in a different light, as these data make it difficult to attribute the phenom-

enon to problems with the saccadic system alone; as before, an immaturity in spatial localization is a parsimonious explanation for both saccadic and head "steps" in this kind of experiment. A study by Daniel and Lee (1990) has investigated developmentally the role that vision plays in stabilizing gaze in the face of head and torso movements. The head and eye coordination of adults and of infants 11–28 weeks of age were recorded as they tracked a moving target when the head and torso were stationary and fixated a stationary target when the torso was turning. In both conditions, infants and adults turned their heads more than their eyes when stabilizing their gaze. Over the developmental interval tested, infants showed improvements in head tracking and in coordinating the head and eye when tracking both types of target. Much of the infant tracking was saccadic, rather than smooth, and head tracking was consistently better than eye tracking. Even by 28 weeks, however, infants were still less skilled than adults in precisely stabilizing their vision under these conditions; of course, we have difficulty excluding motivational/attentional factors as at least partially responsible for the patterns seen in the infants. This sort of work is technically demanding (see below on methods of eye movement recording) but is a valuable contribution to our understanding of how functional vision evolves during the early months. The problem of gaze stabilization in the face of head and body movements must be more difficult for infants than for adults; infants have poor head control and are often passively carried in strange postures that are not under their control. Failure to evaluate the quality of oculomotor behavior in these natural circumstances must necessarily leave us with an incomplete understanding of how infants' vision functions.

Possible Interpretations

Coordination of conjugate eye movements with movements of the head and body is not a primary topic of this chapter, but such issues cannot be ignored if we wish to understand fully how infants are able to execute spatially appropriate and accurate conjugate eye movements. In the review of the material about the neural control of vision and eye movements, it was seen that in both the SC and the cerebellum there is coordination of information about the position of the eye in the head and the position of the head in space. We do not know how early such a spatiocentrically spatial map develops. Infants have been reported, even at young ages, to make directionally appropriate first saccades to targets in various positions in the visual field, which might mean that there is a topologically correct spatiocentric visual map fairly early, but unfortunately all of the current data on early saccadic localization of targets has been done with the head in the equivalent of the upright, straight-ahead position. Under these circumstances, we cannot rule out that correct early localization is due to a retinotopic map, without coordination of information about head position. Interestingly, Kellman et al. (1987) were able to show that, by 4 months, infants could distinguish between the retinal slip caused by moving an object past them and moving them past the object. It would be fascinating to know how early infants are able to demonstrate this ability, presumably mediated by the cerebellum.

DEVELOPMENTAL CONSIDERATIONS IN OCULOMOTOR BEHAVIOR

Models of Infant Oculomotor Control

This brief review of how infants make conjugate eye movements is an interesting but clearly incomplete database from which to draw conclusions about why they act as they do. There have been some attempts to generate models of neural development that systematize data on infant eye movements and attempt to explain their developmental course. Probably best known was an early account by Bronson (1974) suggesting that many forms of visual behavior in infants younger than 2 months, including selective attention and eye movements, could be accounted for by subcortical mechanisms, with behavior being increasingly cortically controlled at later ages. One problem with this model is that it oversimplifies the complex neural connectivities responsible for behaviors such as saccades and pursuit (as well as attentionally mediated behaviors such as habituation). As mentioned above, "reflexive" saccades apparently are mediated by cortical structures and are not exclusively subcortical.

There have been several alternative formulations to explain infant oculomotor development. Aslin (1988) attributed many of the immaturities in infant eye movements to developments on a retinal level, focusing in particular on the problem of spatial calibration on the retina as a result of changes in the organization and connectivity of retinal cells with development. Aslin raised the potentially important point that as the eye increases in size the angular subtense of any small patch of retinal receptors must decrease. In principle, it creates a calibration problem for a growing organism (e.g., how to decide from the position of the image on the retina the eccentricity at which the object is located so a saccade can be programmed). He analyzed the magnitude of the possible problem in all of its ramifications, but it is still unclear that a calibration problem in fact exists. When adults are suddenly challenged by optical distortions induced by lenses, they recalibrate their eye movements quickly, on the order of hours or less. The changes due to growth of the eye in infants, in contrast, are gradual; it is likely that infants would be engaging in a continuous recalibration process as this slow growth occurred. Furthermore, the *data* on infant saccades do not support the existence of such a calibrational problem. Accepting the data on step saccades, they showed that the hypometric saccades that infants make are of equal size, but that the step size increases with target eccentricity. Furthermore, the sum of the amplitudes of the component steps to the target is, on average, equal to the displacement of the target, implying that accurate distance information is available before the series of steps is initiated. Rather than having a calibration problem, infants seem to be using a different strategy to localize, although, as mentioned above, why they do it is far from clear.

Johnson (1990) reviewed much of the recent physiological data on eye movement control, adopting particularly Schiller's suggestion of the four pathways through the SC, MT, FEF, and the inhibitory circuit from the SNr to the FEF. Johnson suggested that many aspects of infant eye movements (particularly smooth pursuit) and attentional processes (e.g., preferential looking, the extent of visual fields, the externality effect, and other features of infant attention) can be accounted for by positing the gradual development of primary visual cortex (V1).

There are probably a number of other scenarios about what is developing that changes how infants make conjugate eye movements. For instance, when preparing this chapter, the data led me to suspect that many of the important changes in oculomotor behavior could also be attributed to developments in the control of attention and arousal from FEF and PG as well as improvements in spatial mapping all through the system. Sensory developments in spatial and temporal aspects of vision, well documented from studies of infants not oriented to oculomotor issues, must also be involved in oculomotor developments; presumably, these sensory changes result from development at a number of levels, from retina to primary visual cortex (V1). Paradoxically, in a chapter on conjugate eye movements, we have almost no good quantitative binocular recordings of eye movements from infants, leaving almost unaddressed the question of the role that binocular aspects of vision play in the control of these types of eye movement.

Although such accounts are intriguing, it is important to evaluate clearly how adequate such treatments are as models of infant development. There are some major difficulties when making connections between the neural structures known to mediate behaviors such as eye movements in the mature organism and the behaviors of infants. First, we know little about the developmental histories of the different pathways or how their developments interact. There is some information available about neural development of the relevant structures, but many of the human data are from old sources (e.g., Conel, 1939–1967). The visual system of the human infant is structurally immature compared to the level of development seen in older children and adults. This immaturity begins at the retina, particularly in the region associated with highest acuity, the fovea (Abramov et al., 1982; Hendrickson and Yuodelis, 1984; Yuodelis and Hendrickson, 1986). At this point we know that these neonatal immaturities have mostly disappeared by the end of the first year, but we still lack detailed information about the time course of many of the changes, especially during the first 2–3 months when visual performance is changing rapidly. The structural immaturity of the fovea is mirrored at successive levels in the visual pathway; there are substantial developments described in the SC, LGN, and V1 (e.g., Hickey, 1977; Huttenlocher, 1979; Garey and De Courten, 1983). At the level of the LGN at least, the magnocellular pathway shows slower and more protracted development (over at least the first year) compared with the parvo system, which undergoes rapid development during the first few months of life (Hickey, 1981).

Other data on visual neural development are from species such as the cat, whose visual system, at least from an oculomotor perspective, is different from that of primates. Unfortunately, we have few relevant physiological data from more relevant species, such as infant monkeys; and even when these data are available, we lack information about how these neural factors map onto behavior at different ages. Our understanding of infant eye movement development would benefit greatly by having more developmental electrophysiological data from young primates. We may simply not have enough information at this point to describe a satisfactory model of the connections between neural development and behavioral change.

A second problem with this type of description is that much of the argument rests on accepting negative findings about the inability of young infants to perform a particular behavior, followed by its emergence at a later developmental stage. Attentional and motivational factors have been demonstrated to play a role in the execution of all eye movements, including all the conjugate ones discussed here. Infants are far more likely to be under the sway of variations in endogenous arousal, controlled by the mechanisms in the brainstem. Exogenous, stimulus-related factors in the environment also clearly influence their attentional processes; preferential looking depends on the infant turning head and eyes to look at one stimulus rather than another, and habituation is based on the same infant's tendency to look away from targets after they have been processed. Until we can figure out a way to give infants explicit instruc-

tions about what we want them to do, the failure of an infant of a particular age to cleanly demonstrate a given class of eye movements should not immediately be taken as evidence that the infant lacks that ability, at least until motivational/attentional factors can be ruled out by testing in a wide variety of settings. An immediately questionable example from the Johnson (1990) report involves smooth pursuit, which Johnson suggested is absent before 2 months because of the immaturity of cortical structures in V1, MT, and their collaterals. The problem, of course, as described above is that there are a number of reports that infants less than 2 months of age do show pursuit under appropriate circumstances, evidence that is not cited by Johnson. What should this information do to Johnson's hypothesis? Does it mean that Johnson is wrong about the maturational state of V1, at least as far as eye movements are concerned? Or should we keep the model and reject the data? Indeed some have suggested that early pursuit is somehow not "real" smooth pursuit but, rather, some form of OKN despite the fact that the eye movements appear much more like pursuit than classical OKN.

Although these various scenarios may (all?) be correct to some degree, the major problem is whether they generate experiments that allow us to decide among them. It seems, on one level, uncharitable to quibble with the masterful job that Johnson, for instance, has done in knitting together the various facts that are emerging about the neural connectivity of the visual system. At the same time, it is important to be explicit about how we would be able to go about verifying that it is correct or, possibly more relevantly, what kinds of data would falsify a given account. In the best case, such treatments can serve as the basis for the positing of specific testable hypotheses that can be empirically addressed using the methods that are available with infants, but many of our predictions may be inherently untestable. Until we know more about neural/behavioral connections in relevant organisms, such generalizations should be regarded as tentative.

Reflexive Versus Volitional Oculomotor Mechanisms

There has been a tendency to assume that behaviors that are present early either in an evolutionary or a developmental time frame are more "reflexive" than behaviors that occur later phylogenetically or ontogenetically. Later emerging behaviors have been regarded as more voluntary, conscious, and controlled. The concept of the reflex is often ill-defined but typically is used to imply that the behavior is present early and apparently occurs without volitional control or the need for learning. In the oculomotor literature, it is common to find behaviors such as OKN and VOR referred to as reflexes, as they occur early in the evolution of the visual system, are seen immediately after birth, and are difficult (though not impossible) to inhibit voluntarily. Pursuit and to a lesser extent saccades are typically seen as more volitional acts, under the organism's conscious control.

However, it has proved difficult to differentiate between "reflexive" behaviors and their more voluntary counterparts. For one thing, it is rare that "reflexive" behaviors are morphologically distinct from similar behaviors under more voluntary or conscious control, diluting the utility of the term, as the distinction then involves an unsubstantiated interpretation of the motivation of a given act. The extensive investigation of the neural control of eye movements has demonstrated how many different neural centers interact in the control of even "reflexive" eye movements. It has thus been difficult, even in direct electrophysiological investigations of oculomotor control centers, to establish which normal eye movements are reflexive, subcortical, and so on, and which are voluntary, cortical, and so on (Richards, 1990). Lacking a good description of the time course and interactions in neural development in eye movement control, it might be possible to follow the process behaviorally if eye movements of a given class generated by different neural pathways are measurably distinct. However, that does not appear to be the case for most of the eye movements that have been studied. Unless there is a good metric or methodology for distinguishing reflexive from volitionally controlled eye movements (or any other neurophysiologically distinct classes) behaviorally, we have no way of knowing what centers are controlling the behaviors we are observing. As tempting as such a dichotomy between reflexive and volitional is, it is more truthful to admit that we have little idea of what structures are in control of an infant's eye movements and at the moment have no methods that are likely to supply such information. Although some imaging techniques such as positron-emission tomography may eventually have developmental application, they have not yet been used for this purpose. Such interpretations of behavior become *ad hoc* and, as such, necessarily circular: What explains the oculomotor behavior of a young infant? Reflexes. How do we know that the behavior is reflexive? Because it is observed in a young infant.

Sensory Factors

The purpose of conjugate eye movement systems is to deal with some of the problems that both foveate and afoveate animals face when maintaining a stable image of objects on the retina as these objects and the animals move about the world. Visual feedback is obviously essential for all of these eye movements. The neural interconnections between sensory and motor areas described above speaks to the impossibility of separating the motor from the sensory aspects of these behaviors. However, most of this work has been done with adult animals whose sensory abilities are stable and well known. If it were always true, focusing oculomotor research on the properties of the eye movements per se, to the exclusion of considerations of the sensory capacity of the organism in question, is probably not a serious problem. However, in the case of human infants, whose functional vision improves markedly during the first year of life, the pressure to understand the mutual influences of sensory and oculomotor factors is particularly acute.

For example, it is well known (as discussed in several chapters in this volume) that infants' spatial vision is relatively poor during early infancy and improves rapidly during the first year. Most of this work, on acuity and to a lesser extent on the full spatial contrast sensitivity function, has been done with stationary stimuli. It has usually been assumed that thresholds obtained with stationary stimuli are representative of vision for stationary retinal images, and it has been common to attribute these improvements in spatial vision to neurally mediated improvements in factors such as photoreceptor packing density, receptive field organization, or narrowing in the bandwidth of spatial frequency channels. Is it likely, however, that improvements in spatial vision are not independent of other developmental processes, particularly oculomotor control. If fixational control itself improves during infancy, oculomotor factors may play as significant a role in improving spatial vision as the other neural factors commonly discussed.

In practice, it is impossible to separate spatial and temporal aspects of vision. Visibility of targets always depends on the joint spatiotemporal sensitivity to a given stimulus (Kelly, 1979a,b). Retinal image motion is an important form of feedback about oculomotor performance. The visual system is more sensitive to temporal change in some spatial frequencies than others. Target visibility is a joint function of sensitivities to the spatial frequencies in the stimulus and the temporal thresholds for each of these frequencies. It is difficult to imagine how an organism could manage adequate visual stabilization without some sensitivity to slippage of images over the retina. Without such feedback, uncontrolled retinal image motion due to poor VOR, pursuit, or other oculomotor stabilization mechanisms is the greatest handicap for clear vision. Thus in order to understand how a given infant controls his or her eye movements, it is necessary not only to understand aspects of spatial vision when retinal images are stationary but also to establish how vision is affected by temporal change on the retina, that is, to study the full spatiotemporal function developmentally. The issue of motion thresholds and their development (see Chapter 10) is also intimately related to how eye movements affect vision in infants.

METHODOLOGICAL CONSIDERATIONS

Research on infant eye movement development is heavily dependent on the development of appropriate methodologies. There are a number of eye movement recording techniques that are inappropriate for use with infants because they involve extreme head restraint or invasive attachments such as contact lenses or heavy glasses; see, for example, Young and Sheena (1975) for a review of general methods for recording eye movements and Aslin (1985) and Maurer (1975) for specific discussions of systems with application to infants. The systems that are available for studying infant eye movements vary considerably in terms of technological sophistication, and each constrains the sort of data that can be obtained. The three methods currently in use with infants are simple observation, the EOG, and television-based corneal reflection methods; these methods have different strengths and weaknesses that are discussed further below. Because, as discussed above, head movements often accompany eye movements, the need to eliminate head movements in order to study eye movements could be, in principle, a hindrance to a full understanding of oculomotor development; one characteristic that differentiates the methods is their tolerance for head movements. All systems, to be maximally useful, require some kind of calibration to relate parameters being measured to eye movement values such as amplitude or direction. There are three general types of calibration that must be considered when measuring eye movements: the amplitude of eye movements (gain calibration), the direction the eye is pointing in space (positional calibration), and how the sampling rate of the recording device changes the characteristics of faster eye movements (bandwidth calibration). The relevant specification for characterizing a system's sensitivity to noise is *resolution* (the minimum eye movement reliably detected by the method) and that for direction of regard is *accuracy* (the error entailed when specifying where the eye is pointing at any observation interval). *Bandwidth* is a measure of the range of frequencies an instrument transmits. These issues are dealt with briefly in the discussion of each method, and then the general issue of calibration of infant eye movements is directly addressed.

Direct Observations

The most inexpensive and simplest method is for an experimenter to observe the infant's eyes directly. The experimenter is often screened from the infant's view and may even view the infant's eyes unobtrusively by means of television equipment. Although such observation is good enough to detect relatively large and slow eye movements, and can specify grossly the direction in which the eyes are pointed, observation alone cannot provide quantitative information about the fine structure of any eye movement. The most frequent use of observation of eye movements is probably in forced-choice preferential looking, where eye movements and direction of gaze are important components of the behaviors an observer uses to specify the location of a stimulus. Another situation in which observation has been used frequently is when specifying the presence or absence of OKN, in which the eye movements are repetitive and often large, so their presence is readily observable. Simple observation is not ideal for small or fast eye movements or for describing how complex sequences of eye movements are linked. For many research applications, it is obviously desirable to be able to obtain more quantitative estimates of eye movements, so the use of observational methods is probably limited to contexts in which eye movements are a robust cue for some other response. I do not want to dismiss observation of eye movements as without merit, however, especially because the other available methods are expensive in terms of time and equipment. For some clinical applications, for example, it may be efficient and appropriate to use simple observation. However, such usage would benefit greatly from validation studies comparing the results from observation and some other, more precise method such as EOG or corneal reflection. At a given observation distance, such a validation would allow us to specify how small or how fast an eye movement must be before it is missed by the observer. Similar validation procedures would also be valuable for training observers by giving them objective feedback about their observations of different eye movements. Although not amenable to calibration in the usual sense, some sort of validation of observation methods is necessary for the most appropriate application of this straightforward means of evaluating eye movements.

Electrooculogram

There is a standing voltage difference between the front and the back of the eye. It is as if the eye contained a battery, oriented from front to rear, that rotates as the eye does. Recording electrodes placed on the face next to each canthus (corner) of the eye can be used to measure eye movements: as the eye rotates, the difference in voltage is recorded by the pair of electrodes. This placement of electrodes allows recording of horizontal movements. At least one more electrode, placed above or below the eye, is needed to record vertical components as well. With enough electrodes and amplifiers, it is possible to simply double this system and record binocularly, although most studies of infants restrict EOG to recording the movements of only one eye.

The EOG procedure is relatively noninvasive and is not difficult to implement. With fast analog-to-digital conversion, it is possible to sample eye position rapidly to allow measurement of fast movements such as saccades, although in practice EOG is used with a wide range of sampling rates. The method does not require that the head be well stabilized, although contractions of the muscles of the face or head generate electrical potentials that can be picked up by the EOG electrodes and mask voltages due to relatively small eye movements. Also, as discussed above, if the subject's head moves, the VOR causes the eyes to compensate by rotating in the opposite direction. Unless there also a way of recording head position, such an eye movement could be misinterpreted as a look away from the stimulus rather than as maintaining fixation. Other problems relate to the source of the voltage that is recorded in the EOG; the absolute magnitude of this potential varies with the eye's state of light or dark adaptation. As adaptation state changes, the signals recorded for movements of the same amplitude change. To avoid such errors, subjects should be preadapted to the average luminance of the stimuli, which should also be controlled to prevent changes in adaptation during a session.

Calibration of the EOG involves relating a particular voltage to a particular direction of regard and a particular change in voltage to an eye movement of a particular amplitude. With adults, it is typically accomplished quickly and usually several times during a recording session to control for drifts in the gain of the signals and adaptation of the visual system by instructing subjects to move their eyes to look at each of a series of locations on the stimulus plane; the separations of these known locations can then be related to the EOG's voltages. With infants, the only recourse is to present calibration targets one at a time and measure responses when the infant appears to be attending to the target. This process is to some extent circular, of course: The device is intended to tell us when the infant is looking at a certain target, but we must know when the infant looks at the target in order to calibrate the device.

Finocchio et al. (1990) have described a clever technique for quickly calibrating infant EOG records that is likely to lead to an increase in infant EOG studies; before this time, there were no satisfactory quick methods for calibrating EOGs with infants; so although the technique was reasonably simple to implement, there was dissatisfaction with the results it yielded. In the Finocchio et al. method, a lighted target is slowly moved to known positions as the infant is observed by a hidden observer, who observes the reflection of this target from the subject's cornea. The observer notes whether the corneal reflections of the target are located symmetrically in the pupils, which indicates central fixation at that particular target position. Using this method, Finocchio and colleagues reported calibration that allows the specification of eye position to an accuracy of ±1 degree over a ±15 degree range. Resolution of minimal eye position change was reported to be about 1 degree. Metz (1984) has suggested an alternative method for calibration of infant EOG and possible other methods for recording eye movements in which a prism is introduced in front of the infant's eye while the infant is looking at an attractive target. With knowledge of the target distance and the value of the prism, if the infant makes a refixation movement to maintain fixation of the target this movement can be calibrated for gain. Finocchio et al. (1990) have tried the method and found that it did not work well because of problems getting reliable fixation and infants' objections to having prisms placed in front of their eyes.

Corneal Reflection Trackers

"Optical" eye trackers focus on some landmarks of the eye and record their changing positions as the eye moves. The landmark that has been most commonly used with infants is the corneal reflection of a fixed, invisible infrared light source (or, sometimes, sources), evaluated with reference to the center of the pupil (e.g., Haith, 1969; Hainline, 1981). As the eye rotates, there are systematic changes in the position of the corneal reflection relative to pupil center (Fig. 4-10). The details of corneal reflection (CR) equipment differ more from laboratory to laboratory than is true for EOG recording, so it is impossible to give a single description of the method's resolution and accuracy; Hainline and Lemerise (1985) included a table that lists the characteristics of a number of such systems. Because the CR systems in use with infants to date have used conventional television technology, the bandwidth of the system is limited by the frame rate of the television raster, 60 Hz in the United States; some applications of CR with infants have used much slower sampling rates because of the use of cinematic rather than television recording. One advantage of this type of technology over EOG is that nothing needs to be attached to the infant; the eye is imaged by a television camera, and this video image is analyzed either manually or automatically to yield information about the point of regard. Unlike EOG, there are no problems with stability of the recording signal across the session. The details of how CR techniques are accomplished vary from system to system. In our laboratory, we collimate the light source used for illumination and to provide the CR, so a significant fraction of the light incident on the retina is reflected

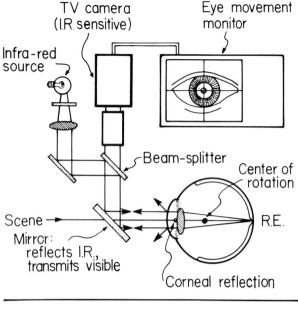

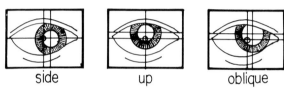

FIG. 4-10. Essential elements of a corneal reflection eye movement recorder used to derive estimates of eye position from the relative positions of the image of an infrared (IR), collimated light source's corneal reflection relative to the subject's pupil. An IR-sensitive television camera images the eye by way of a dichroic beam splitter; the eye has a bright pupil because of light reflected off the fundus from the collimated source. Eye movements, but not head movements, cause differential movement of these landmarks, illustrated at the bottom panel of the figure. (From *Behavioral Research Methods and Instrumentation* 13:21, 1981. © Psychonomic Society. By permission.)

back from the eye into the camera. The result is an image of the eye with a bright pupil that is easier to detect with the automated image detection equipment that specifies point of regard on each sample. Other CR systems use uncollimated light and thus produce images with dark pupils, and they may also have manual rather than automatic scoring of eye position.

The biggest problem for CR systems is movement of the subject's head. The systems work best when the head is kept reasonably still, within the field of view of the camera and at the same distance from the camera at all times. The CR systems currently in use with infants require greater immobilization of the head than is needed with EOG. In our system, for example, the camera imaging the eye is fixed in position, so with the lens we use the head can move only about ±2 cm before the image of the eye is lost; in our laboratory we accomplish this by having a human holding the infant upright, over her shoulder and gently stabilizing the infant's head. In

a system used by Bronson (1990) a tracking mirror allows automatic following of slow head movements over a range of about ±3 cm; in this case, the infant is supine with the head in a cradle. In principle, faster tracking devices or servo mechanisms could follow the eye over a wider range as it moves in a frontoparallel plane, but the speed of such movements is a factor in creating a viable tracking system. Also, such movements of the imaging device can cause optical parallax problems that must be considered (Bronson, 1983). Autofocus lenses in principle could allow some in−out movement but at the cost of variable magnification of movements in the resulting image; such a system would also require dynamic gain adjustments linked to movement of the lens. As yet, no one has devised a scheme to follow the eye adequately with the camera in situations of large head rotations, a serious limitation of the method for some research questions. In the best cases, CR systems can specify change in eye position over a 40 × 40 degree region with reasonably good linearity and with a resolution of 0.5 degree. The accuracy of such a system depends intimately on the characteristics of the system's optics and on the calibration system used.

As with EOG, the CR systems must be calibrated. There are two major parameters that require calibration in any system specifying position of gaze over time: the system's gain (the ratio of measured change to actual change in eye position) and system offset (a measure of where the system says that the eye is pointing on each sample). Gain is related to the differential movement of the two landmarks (most typically, corneal reflection and pupil center), which is determined by the curvature of the cornea, the location of the plane of the pupil as seen through the cornea, and the location of the eye's center of rotation. Infant eyes are smaller than adult eyes, but the maturational growth of the relevant structures is such that a given rotation of the eye produces approximately the same differential motion of the landmarks at all ages (Bronson, 1982; Abramov and Harris, 1984; Hainline et al. 1990). Thus when using a CR system based on corneal reflection and pupil measurements with fixed gain settings, one is able to use a gain calibration appropriate for both the average adult and the average infant. There is some error in gain for any individual who differs markedly from the mean; ideally, estimates of an individual subject's gain can be improved by performing a calibration such as that described above for EOG, namely by having the subject fixate a series of points in succession and obtaining eye position for each target in the set. It is important to note, then, that within some limits uncalibrated CR data from a system referenced to the pupil still allow some valid statements about eye movement changes, both relative and absolute, across subjects of different ages.

This situation would be enhanced by information about the nature of corneal curvature for each subject. We have been working toward obtaining photokeratometric measurements from each infant who serves as an eye movement subject; at this point we are still working on the details of quantitative analysis of the resulting measurements, but ultimately such a system may help to increase the validity of uncalibrated gain measurements without great expenditure of time.

It is not possible to predict the variability of gain measures obtained from uncalibrated EOG systems or from CR systems that reference other landmarks not on the eye itself. There are, for example, some CR systems that measure change in eye position by comparing the position of the corneal reflection relative to the position of an artificial landmark such as a reflective dot placed on the face within the field of view of the camera. Because placement of such a head dot, like placement of the EOG electrodes, is only approximately the same from subject to subject, there is considerable variability in the measurements obtained from different subjects. An average gain is unsatisfactory in these circumstances.

Additional calibrational procedures are required with a CR system to specify point of regard on a particular stimulus. Part of the problem with a pupil-referenced system is that the fovea is not actually on the optic axis of the eye, connecting the center of the pupil through the nodal point to the retina at the back of the globe. When a subject looks at a stimulus, the angle of convergence of the optic axis is less than the angle of convergence of the visual axis, connecting the fovea through the nodal point. The angle between the optic and visual axes in each of the adult's eyes, known as angle α, is about 5 degrees. [Strictly speaking, we do not measure angle α directly but, rather, angle λ, the angle between the line of sight (joining the center of the entrance pupil with the object of regard) and the pupillary axis (joining the center of the entrance pupil to the retina). The differences between these angles is in practice small, and most of the developmental work refers to this angle as α, a practice that is continued here.] Angle α is much larger in young infants, decreasing from about 8–10 degrees to the adult value over the first year (Slater and Findlay, 1972, 1975; London and Wick, 1982; Hainline et al., 1988) (Fig. 4-11). In principle, then, it might be possible to use an average calibration for this fixed offset, as suggested by Salapatek et al. (1972). The problem is that there appears to be substantial variability, in both adults and infants, in the value of angle α (Bronson, 1982, 1990; Hainline et al., 1988), necessitating an individual calibration for the most accurate estimation of spatial points of regard. For most CR systems, another factor that contributes to an unknown extent (unless head position is also measured) is the exact placement of the head with respect to the camera; to the extent that any head movement is allowed, the absolute position of the corneal reflection that corresponds, for example, to viewing the straight-ahead position shifts slightly as the head moves, leading to misestimates of point of regard unless these head movements are calibrated out. This problem is not a large one in systems that allow minimal head movement, but it must contribute to variability in measured eye position both within and across subject sessions. It is possible to set some limits as to how poor uncalibrated positional accuracy is with such systems, but probably it is more conservative simply not to analyze variables related to eye position without some individual positional calibration.

In an early report, Hainline and Lemerise (1982) followed the then prevailing tendency to study infants' scanning of stimuli without individual calibration of CR

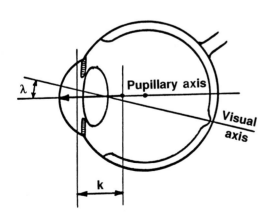

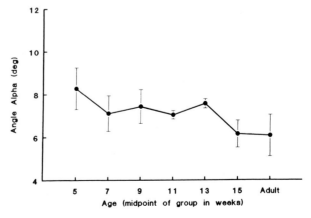

FIG. 4-11. (Left) Angle λ, the angle between the visual axis (joining the center of the entrance pupil with the object of regard) and the pupillary axis (joining the entrance pupil to the retina). This angle is sometimes also called angle α, which is closely related but formed by the intersection of the optic and visual axes. Angle λ is referred to clinically as angle κ. (Right) Note that angle α (or λ) decreases systematically with age during infancy. (From Hainline et al., 1988. By permission.)

data. To compensate for the lack of such data from each infant, they instead allowed wide error margins (± 3–4 degrees) for specifying the position of each fixation on the stimuli. Although the imposition of an error boundary at least took into account the fact of uncertainty when specifying eye position (which had not been done in previous studies), this method has been subject to criticism, which we have addressed specifically elsewhere (Hainline and Lemerise, 1985). With greater reflection on the factors that lead to errors when estimating the location of eye positions spatially with CR systems and more experience with such data, we now believe that it is probably unwise to report positional data without individual calibration; they are more subject to individual variation than are gain values. Our early use of an error boundary when specifying point of regard has also been misunderstood as reflecting the limits of spatial resolution of a CR system with infants (e.g., Shupert and Fuchs, 1988). With the calibration procedures we use now, it is possible to create an infant calibration that allows estimates of infant fixations within ± 1.0 degree of the true position (Hainline et al., 1990).

A final calibration is bandwidth calibration, which is instrument-specific rather than subject-specific, but general for both EOG and CR systems. A system's bandwidth limits how faithfully an instrument alters the characteristics of rapid eye movements; slow sampling rates necessarily distort the measurements of fast eye movements, particularly velocities and durations. CR and EOG systems differ in sampling rate. CR systems' bandwidths are limited by the raster rate of the television camera; although faster scan rates are possible in principle, at this point all the systems in use with infants sample no faster than 60 Hz, as in our system. Bronson (1990), by comparison, uses a 9 Hz sample rate in his CR system. Analog-to-digital conversion for EOG signals can, in principle, be done much faster; but it creates much larger data sets, and practical considerations have led to the selection of slower rates. For example, Finocchio et al. (1990) used a 30 Hz sample rate in their EOG recording. There are some post hoc calibrations that can be done to allow some estimation of how much different velocities of eye movement are underestimated by a given system; Harris et al. (1984) described one such method for the CR system we use.

The implication of much of the foregoing is that it is highly advisable to obtain full calibration from each subject with any method. The problem is that these procedures are not easy to perform on infants; in one review, Shupert and Fuchs (1988) observed that only the brilliant or the foolish undertake studies of infant eye movements. For obvious reasons, I am not going to venture even a tentative classification of the current crop of researchers engaged in this research. Clearly, all involved in the business are interested in getting the best possible data from each infant. The major problem is that to accommodate to the limited periods of alertness and cooperativeness of the average infant researchers are often faced with the Hobson's choice of either gathering (1) a good, clean set of calibration data but no data in the actual experiment, or (2) experimental data with meager calibration data, if any. The EOG calibration devised by the Finocchio group is a step in the direction of fulfilling both of these needs efficiently. There have also been significant improvements in CR methods for calibration. In our earliest paper on CR calibration (Harris et al., 1981), for example, our calibration targets were single flashing lights that were presented one at a time in various positions in the visual field. During the intervening time, we eventually discovered that infants often failed to attend to this discrete jumping of targets from one position to another but would follow if the target moved smoothly from one calibration position to another, resulting in better calibration data over shorter periods of time (e.g., Hainline et al., 1990). This position is essentially the same as the solution reached independently by the Finocchio group.

Such modifications in procedure have been made easier as computers capable of more sophisticated graphics have arrived on the laboratory scene. At this point, the best calibration scheme, in our perspective, is one in which calibration targets are smoothly moved to the desired position, with these calibration trials interspersed throughout the experimental session if it does not compromise the purposes of the experiment. This method gives us a chance to obtain both calibration and experimental data before the infant is lost for that session. It is also highly desirable (see further discussion below) to use targets that are more interesting to infants than simple spots of light. Habituation is a well documented phenomenon in infant research. Calibration targets should be as jazzy as possible and should be changed over the session to maximize the likelihood that infants will look at them, as we desire them to do. There will still be some sessions for which full or even partial calibration data are not available. In some cases, as in gain measurements from CR techniques, the data may still be valid for some types of analysis. In other cases, regardless how difficult it was to obtain the experimental data, it is probably necessary to discard the data until further analyses of uncalibrated adult and infant data allow us to establish better limits for using uncalibrated infant eye movement data from either EOG or CR.

In their review, Shupert and Fuchs (1988) concluded, on the basis of their overview of eye movement methods appropriate for infants, that EOG is probably preferable to CR in most experimental situations involving infants. I have to disagree, as both CR and EOG have problems and advantages. In my judgment, what is more important is to choose the method that best fits the research question. For studies that require some free head movement, EOG is undeniably the method of choice. The importance of understanding the interactions of the various contexts for eye movements is clearly a research question with a high priority. For studies of fixational control, the metrics of saccades, and even some pursuit work, CR has the advantages of being nonintrusive and more stable across a session. With CR, measures such as gain can also be interpreted from the average subject, even without individual calibration. Given the small set of methods we have available, it is counterproductive to impugn one to enhance the status of the other.

CRITIQUE OF INFANT EYE MOVEMENT STUDIES

Dating the beginning is somewhat arbitrary, but it is probably defensible to date the beginning of quantitative study of infant eye movements to the mid-1970s, when the first EOG-based study on step saccades was reported (Aslin and Salapatek, 1975). By some standards, a critical reviewer might be unimpressed about how little we know about the development of infant eye movements as the result of 15 years of research. At the same time, I think it would be a mistake to be too negative about what has been accomplished during this interval. Though possibly neither brilliant nor foolish in the main, the workers in this area have been stubbornly persistent, steadily chipping away at the significant methodological problems of recording, calibrating, and analyzing infant eye movements. Shupert and Fuchs (1988) concluded that we have learned about all we can from qualitative studies of infant eye movements and that it is time to press harder for well-calibrated, quantitative studies; it is difficult to disagree with this proposition, but we must think carefully about what needs to be done to meet this goal.

The special problems when doing infant eye movement research, virtually always discussed in reviews of this topic, are real. Such data are more difficult to collect and analyze than those regarding adult eye movements. Fortunately for us, there has been some significant improvement in the technology available for this effort, and these developments have contributed to our progress. It is likely that the infusion of new technology will continue, and that future research will be the beneficiary. Potential developments that seem on the horizon for CR systems include less expensive high scan rate television cameras, better servo systems for camera tracking of head and eyes, and better, faster algorithms for image analysis that allow improved tracking of landmarks of the eye. As discussed above, we also need improvements in our methods for calibrating and our understanding on how far we can go with the inevitable

data from subjects whose tests could not be calibrated. These problems can be addressed empirically.

To do any kind of quantitative analysis of raw eye movement records from infants is still time-consuming. Early studies were forced to process data with laborious and time-consuming "by hand" scoring of eye position. Advances in image analysis equipment and analog-to-digital converters in laboratory computers have allowed more of the early stages of data analysis to be automated. There are a number of data-processing routines available to facilitate the automated analysis of adult eye movement records, including "parsing" routines. The problem is that most are not robust in the face of noisy data, and infant data are rarely as clean as those of cooperative adults. Our own solution is a semiautomatic "parsing" controlled by an operator, but this process is slower than we would like and limits the rate at which we can quantify data, an obvious prerequisite to more extensive quantitative analysis. The analysis system used by Shea and Aslin (1990) involves less operator interaction, but it also collapses various types of eye movement into one heterogeneous class, which is not advantageous either. Better algorithms for digital signal processing for filtering out noise in eye movement records would be enormously helpful in this regard.

To make better progress in this area, we need to give some thought to what questions we are trying to answer about infant eye movements. Are we attempting to assess the best behavior of which the system is capable at any age—or the typical behavior? The answer to this question, study by study, will allow the informed selection of an appropriate comparison group of adults to provide a context for evaluating the results of a given study. It would be interesting to make more efforts to include age groups other than infants and adults; studies of children's eye movements have their own problems (e.g., Aslin and Cuiffreda, 1983) but can effectively fill in the huge gap in the developmental function between birth and adulthood.

As a seasoned researcher in this area, it is my intuitive opinion that the greatest progress will come from rethinking the way in which we have designed our eye movement studies. Much of the infant research is directly modeled on studies of adult eye movements. A problem with this style of work is that the stimuli have, most of the time, been simple; the prototypical target is a small spot of light generated by a light-emitting diode (LED) or a laser. From the perspective of "pure" research considerations, these targets are desirable because they are small, clearly visible, and easy to control precisely. However, from the perspective of an infant, targets such as this one are not likely to hold attention for long. To elicit maximum performance from infants, we must think about our stimulus choices more carefully. The targets we use must be above sensory threshold for our youngest subjects and should be interesting enough to hold attention for the duration of a recording session. These considerations require more interesting, complex stimuli than we have been using. To avoid specifying stimulus characteristics precisely would be unscientific, but it would also be poor science to fail to accommodate to important characteristics of the subject we are studying. Infants respond best to complex, natural stimuli. To present them only with simple (though easy to specify) stimuli is likely to lead us to underestimate their abilities. Steinman et al. (1990) made the point that the types of experiments and stimuli typically found in adult studies may also be underestimating the oculomotor abilities of adults, so the issue of the "naturalness" of the setting under which eye movements are studied may be a general one, not limited to the case of infants.

The problem of negative evidence, of young infants not exhibiting a particular type of eye movement or showing an immaturity in a given eye movement parameter, is a significant one in this area of work. There has been an unfortunate tendency to accept the null hypothesis in much infant oculomotor research. The infant's failure to move his or her eyes can often plausibly be explained as due to sensory factors (e.g., limitations in spatial vision, temporal or movement thresholds); if infants cannot see the target, they can hardly be expected to make eye movements in response to it. As some of the data on heart rate response to visual targets shows, infants may "detect" a target but not make a movement either because they can see it but not accurately localize it or simply because they are not motivated enough to bother to execute a movement. The lack of motivation can be due to a low state of arousal (e.g., a drowsy behavioral state) or because of environmentally mediated reductions in attention due to habituation. It is, of course, possible that the failure to make an eye movement reflects immaturity in some specifically oculomotor structure, but we cannot automatically assume it to be the case. Better on-going ratings of behavioral state would be of a great help in this regard; the state can be indexed by a standard checklist or supplemental recording of variables such as heart rate. Some eye movement systems, such as our CR system, also give information about changes in pupil diameter that might be of value when evaluating the infant state. Our work on differences in the slope of infants' saccadic main sequence during scanning implies that changes in the microstructure of some eye movements can be sensitive indices of changes in arousal even in infants who appear awake and attentive. The problem of interpreting negative evidence and the type of studies that have traditionally been run in this area of research are also relevant to the process of model building and the task of relating behavioral results to underlying physiological mechanisms.

What should we be doing to improve the yield from our infant eye movement research on conjugate eye movements and other sorts of oculomotor behavior? This review suggests that we give careful attention to how oculomotor behavior is influenced by other characteristics of the infant, particularly to spatiotemporal sensitivities and to the dynamics of attentional processes. It is also important to take advantage of technological advances and improve our algorithms for data analysis. The chronic problem of calibration still requires creative attention. We should rethink the way in which we do experiments and design them from the ground up as experiments appropriate for infant subjects, rather than simply adopting the forms of study that have typified adult work in the field, particularly regarding our choice of stimuli. It would also be beneficial to begin to reach some cooperative agreements across laboratories about common definitions for various eye movements.

Remarkable progress has been made in understanding the neural substrate of eye movement control in the mature organism. At this point the elaboration of an animal model relating the development of oculomotor behavior to the underlying neurological mechanisms would be helpful for understanding what we are observing in the young infant. In addition to the obvious basic science value of this kind of information, such efforts would also extend greatly our ability to use infant eye movement recording as a clinical tool. Quantitative analysis of infant eye movements in clinical contexts offers the potential of new diagnostic insights; in the study of adult eye movements, clinical application has often fed back new insights to the basic researchers that have allowed refinement of our models of oculomotor control. At an eye movement conference during the early 1980s a discussant was asked to comment on whether eye movements could save the earth (Llewllyn-Thomas, 1981); the conclusion was that they could not hurt. We can recast the question here a bit less grandiosely and with a developmental slant by asking whether the studying conjugate infant eye movements can help us to understand infant vision. Infant vision is always operating on a platform formed by two mobile eyes. I believe there are enough potential answers that could flow from consideration of this fact that studies of infant eye movements have a real chance of helping the effort a great deal.

Acknowledgments. The preparation of this chapter, and much of my own research cited, was supported by NIH grant EY03957. In addition, I thank my colleague Israel Abramov for his helpful suggestions and careful reading of the manuscript.

REFERENCES

ABEL, L. A., DAROFF, R., AND DELL'OSSO, L. F. (1979). Horizontal pursuit defect nystagmus. *Ann. Neurol.* 5, 449–452.

ABRAMOV, I., AND HARRIS, C. M. (1984). Artificial eye for assessing corneal-reflection eye trackers. *Behav. Res. Methods Instrum. Comput.* 16, 437–438.

ABRAMOV, I., GORDON, J., HENDRICKSON, A., HAINLINE, L., DOBSON, V., AND LABOSSIERE, E. (1982). The retina of the newborn human infant. *Science* 217, 33–37.

ASHMEAD, D. (1984). Parameters of infant saccadic eye movements. *Infant Behav. Dev.* 7, 16.

ASLIN, R. N. (1981). Development of smooth pursuit in human infants. In D. F. FISHER, R. A. MONTY, AND J. SENDERS (eds.). *Eye Movements: Cognition and Visual Perception.* Hillsdale, NJ: Erlbaum.

ASLIN, R. N. (1985). Oculomotor measures of visual development. In G. GOTTLIEB AND N. A. KRASNEGOR (eds.). *Measurement of Audition and Vision in the First Year of Postnatal Life.* Norwood, NJ: Ablex.

ASLIN, R. N. (1987). Motor aspects of visual development in infancy. In P. SALAPATEK AND L. B. COHEN (eds.). *Handbook of Infant Perception.* Vol. 1. Orlando, FL: Academic Press.

ASLIN, R. N. (1988). Anatomical constraints on oculomotor development: implications for infant perception. In A. YONAS (ed.). *Perceptual Development in Infancy.* Hillsdale, NJ: Erlbaum.

ASLIN, R. N., AND CUIFFREDA, K. J. (1983). Eye movements in preschool children. *Science* 222, 74–75.

ASLIN, R. N., AND SALAPATEK, P. (1975). Saccadic localization of visual targets by the very young human infant. *Percept. Psychophys.* 17, 293–302.

ASLIN, R. N., AND SHEA, S. L. (1990). Velocity thresholds in human infants: implications for the perception of motion. *Dev. Psychol.* 26, 589–598.

ATKINSON, J., AND BRADDICK, O. (1981). Development of optokinetic nystagmus in infants: an indicator of cortical binocularity? In D. F. FISHER, R. A. MONTY, AND J. W. SENDERS (eds.). *Eye Movements: Cognition and Visual Perception.* Hillsdale, NJ: Erlbaum.

BAHILL, A. T., AND STARK, L. (1975). Overlapping saccades and glissades are produced by fatigue in the saccadic eye movement system. *Exp. Neurol.* 48, 95–106.

BAHILL, A. T., CLARK, M. R., AND STARK, L. (1975). The main sequence: a tool for studying human eye movements. *Math. Biosci.* 24, 191–204.

BRADBURY, A., BERTENTHAL, B. I., AND KRAMER, S. J. (1990). Minimum velocity thresholds in 12- and 20-week old infants. *Invest. Ophthalmol. Vis. Sci.* 31 (suppl.), 9.

BRONSON, G. W. (1974). The postnatal growth of visual capacity. *Child Dev.* 45, 873–890.

BRONSON, G. W. (1982). The scanning patterns of human infants: implications for visual learning. *Monographs on Infancy* (Whole No. 2). Norwood, NJ: Ablex.

BRONSON, G. W. (1983). Potential sources of error when applying a corneal reflex eye-monitoring techniques to infant subjects. *Behav. Res. Methods Instrum.* 15, 22–28.

BRONSON, G. W. (1990). The accurate calibration of infants' scanning records. *J. Exp. Child Psychol.* 49, 79–100.

BRUCE, C. J., AND GOLDBERG, M. E. (1984). Physiology of the frontal eye fields. *Trends Neurosci.* 7, 436–441.

BUSHNELL, I. (1979). Modification of the externality effect in young infants. *J. Exp. Child Psychol.* 28, 211–229.

CARPENTER, R. H. S. (1977). *Movements of the Eye.* London: Pion.

CONEL, J. L. (1939–1967). *The Postnatal Development of the Human Cerebral Cortex.* Vols. I–VIII. Cambridge, MA: Harvard University Press.

DANIEL, B. M., AND LEE, D. N. (1990). Development of looking with head and eyes. *J. Exp. Child Psychol.* 50, 200–216.

DANNEMILLER, J. L., AND FREEDLAND, R. L. (1989). The detection of slow stimulus movement in 2- to 5-month-olds. *J. Exp. Child Psychol.* 47, 337–355.

DAYTON, G. O., JONES, M. H., STEELE, B., AND ROSE, M. (1964). Developmental study of coordinated eye movements in the human infant. II. Electrooculographic study of the fixation reflex in the newborn. *Arch. Ophthalmol.* 71, 871–875.

DE BIE, J. (1986). The control properties of small eye movements. Dissertation, Technische Universiteit, Delft, The Netherlands.

DE YOE, E. A., AND VAN ESSEN, D. C. (1988). Concurrent processing streams in monkey visual cortex. *Trends Neurosci.* 5, 219–216.

ECKMILLER, T. (1987). Neural control of pursuit eye movements. *Physiol. Rev.* 67, 797–857.

FINLAY, D., AND IVINKIS, A. (1982). Cardiac and visual responses to stimuli presented both foveally and peripherally as a function of speed of moving stimuli. *Dev. Psychol.* 18, 692–698.

FINLAY, D., AND INVINKIS, A. (1984). Cardiac and visual responses to moving stimuli presented either successively or simultaneously to the central and peripheral visual fields in 4-month-olds. *Dev. Psychol.* 20, 29–36.

FINDLAY, J. (1992). Programming of stimulus elicited saccadic eye movements. In K. RAYNER AND H. A. WHITAKER (eds.). *Eye Movements and Visual Cognition.* New York: Springer-Verlag.

FINOCCHIO, D. V., PRESTON, K. L., AND FUCHS, A. F. (1990). Obtaining a quantitative measure of eye movements in human infants: a method of calibrating the electrooculogram. *Vision Res.* 30, 1119–1128.

FISCHER, B. (1986). The role of attention in the preparation of visually guided eye movements in monkey and man. *Psychol. Res.* 48, 251–257.

FISCHER, B., AND BOCH, R. (1983). Saccadic eye movements after extremely short reaction times in the monkey. *Brain Res.* 260, 21–26.

FISCHER, B., AND BREITMEYER, B. (1987). Mechanisms of visual attention revealed by saccadic eye movements. *Neuropsychology* 25, 73–84.

FISCHER, B., AND RAMSPERGER, E. (1984). Human express saccades: extremely short reaction times of goal-directed eye movements. *Exp. Brain Res.* 57, 191–195.

GAREY, L, AND DE COURTEN, C. (1983). Structural development of the lateral geniculate nucleus and visual cortex in monkey and man. *Behav. Brain Res.* 10, 3–15.

GOLDBERG, M. E., AND BRUCE, C. J. (1985). Cerebral cortical activity associated with the orientation of visual attention in the rhesus monkey. *Vision Res.* 25, 471–481.

HAINLINE, L. (1981). An automated eye movement recording system for use with human infants. *Behav. Res. Methods Instrum.* 13, 20–24.

HAINLINE, L. (1985). Oculomotor control in human infants. In R. GRONER, G. W. MCCONKIE, AND C. MENZ (eds.). *Eye Movements and Human Information Processing.* Amsterdam: Elsevier–North Holland.

HAINLINE, L. (1988). Normal lifespan developmental changes in saccadic and pursuit eye movements. In C. W. JOHNSTON AND F. J. PIROZZOLO (eds.). *Neuropsychology of Eye Movements.* Hillsdale, NJ: Erlbaum.

HAINLINE, L., AND ABRAMOV, I. (1985). Saccades and small-field optokinetic nystagmus in infants. *J. Am. Optom. Assoc.* 56, 620–626.

HAINLINE, L. AND ABRAMOV, I. (1991). Assessing infant visual development: is infant vision good enough? In C. ROVEE-COLLIER

AND L. P. LIPSITT (eds.). *Advances in Infancy Research*. Vol. 7. Norwood, NJ: Ablex.

HAINLINE, L., AND HARRIS, C. M. (1990). The stability of infant fixations. In R. GRONER, G. d'YDEVALLE, AND R. PARHAM (eds.). *From Eye to Mind: Information Acquisition in Perception, Search, and Reading*. Amsterdam: North Holland.

HAINLINE, L., AND LEMERISE, E. (1982). Infants' scanning of geometric forms varying in size. *J. Exp. Child Psychol. 33*, 235–256.

HAINLINE, L., AND LEMERISE, E. (1985). Corneal reflection eye movement recording as a measure of infant pattern perception: what do we really know? *Br. J. Dev. Psychol. 3*, 229–242.

HAINLINE, L., GHEORGHIU, B., AND ABRAMOV, I. (1988). Accommodation and convergence in young infants. *Invest. Ophthalmol. Vis. Sci. 27* (suppl.), 266.

HAINLINE, L., HARRIS, C. M., AND KRINSKY, S. (1990). Variability of refixations in infants. *Infant Behav. Dev. 13*, 321–342.

HAINLINE, L., TURKEL, J., ABRAMOV, I., LEMERISE, E., AND HARRIS, C. (1984). Characteristics of saccades in human infants. *Vision Res. 24*, 1771–1780.

HAITH, M. M. (1969). Infrared television recording and measurement of ocular behavior in the human infant. *Am. Psychologist 24*, 269–282.

HARRIS, C. M. (1989). The ethology of saccades: a non-cognitive model. *Biol. Cybernet. 60*, 401–410.

HARRIS, C. M., AND HAINLINE, L. (1986). Characteristics of fixations in human infants: durations. In J. K. O'REGAN AND A. LEVY-SCHOEN (eds.). *Eye Movements: From Physiology to Cognition*. Amsterdam: North Holland.

HARRIS, C. M., AND HAINLINE, L. (In preparation). A quantitative analysis of eye drift in infant fixations.

HARRIS, C. M., ABRAMOV, I., AND HAINLINE, L. (1984). Instrument considerations in measuring fast eye movements. *Behav. Res. Methods Instrum. Comput. 16*, 341–350.

HARRIS, C. M., HAINLINE, L., AND ABRAMOV, I. (1981). A method for calibrating an eye-monitoring system for use with human infants. *Behav. Res. Methods Instrum. 13*, 11–20.

HARRIS, C. M., HAINLINE, L., ABRAMOV, I., LEMERISE, E., AND CAMENZULI, C. (1988). The distribution of fixation durations in the human infant. *Vision Res. 28*, 419–432.

HARRIS, P., AND MACFARLANE, A. (1974). The growth of the effective visual field from birth to seven weeks. *J. Exp. Child Psychol. 18*, 340–348.

HEILMAN, K. M., WATSON, R. T., VALENSTEIN, E., AND GOLDBERG, M. E. (1987). Attention: behavior and neural mechanisms. In B. MOUNTCASTLE, F. PLUM, AND S. R. GEIGER (eds.). *Handbook of Physiology. Section I. The Nervous System*. Vol. V. Bethesda: American Physiological Society.

HENDRICKSON, A., AND YUODELIS, C. (1984). The morphological development of the human fovea. *Ophthalmologica 91*, 603–612.

HICKEY, T. L. (1977). Postnatal development of the human lateral geniculate nucleus: relationship to a critical period for the visual system. *Science 198*, 836–383.

HICKEY, T. L. (1981). The developing visual system. *Trends Neurosci. 1*, 41–44.

HOWARD, I. P. (1982). *Human Visual Orientation*. New York: Wiley.

HUTTENLOCHER, P. (1979). Synaptic density in human frontal cortex: developmental changes and effects of aging. *Brain Res. 163*, 195–205.

JOHNSON, M. H. (1990). Cortical maturation and the development of visual attention in early infancy. *J. Cogn. Neurosci. 2*, 81–95.

KAPLAN, E., LEE, B. B., AND SHAPLEY, R. M. (1990). New views of primate retinal function. *Prog. Retinal Res. 9*, 273–336.

KAUFMAN, F., STUCKI, M., AND KAUFMANN-HAYOZ, R. (1985). Development of infants' sensitivity for slow and rapid motions. *Infant Behav. Dev. 8*, 89–98.

KELLMAN, P. J., GLEITMAN, J., AND SPELKE, E. (1987). Object and observer motion in the perception of objects by infants. *J. Exp. Psychol. Hum. Percep. Perform. 13*, 586–593.

KELLY, D. H. (1979a). Motion and vision. I. Stabilized images of stationary gratings. *J. Optical Soc. Am. 69*, 1266–1274.

KELLY, D. H. (1979b). Motion and vision. II. Stabilized spatiotemporal threshold surface. *J. Optical Soc. Am. 69*, 1340–1349.

KREMENITZER, J. P., VAUGHAN, H. G., KURTZBERG, D., AND DOWLING, K. (1979). Smooth-pursuit eye movements in the newborn infant. *Child Dev. 50*, 442–448.

KRINSKY, S. J., HAINLINE, L., AND SCANLON, M. (1990). In pursuit of smooth pursuit: a repeated excursion approach. *Infant Behav. Dev. 13*, 462a.

LEVINE, M. W., AND SHEFNER, J. M. (1990). *Fundamentals of Sensation and Perception*. Pacific Grove, CA: Brooks/Cole.

LIVINGSTONE, M., AND HUBEL, D. (1988). Segregation of form, color, movement and depth: anatomy, physiology and perception. *Science 240*, 740–749.

LLWELLYN-THOMAS, E. (1981). Can eye movements save the earth? In D. F. FISHER, R. A. MONTY, AND J. W. SENDERS (eds.). *Eye Movements: Cognition and Visual Perception*. Hillsdale, NJ: Erlbaum.

LONDON, R., AND WICK, B. (1982). Changes in angle lambda during growth: theory and clinical applications. *Am. J. Optom. Physiol. Opt. 59*, 568–572.

MAURER, D. (1975). Infant visual perception: methods of study. In L. B. COHEN AND P. SALAPATEK (eds.). *Infant Perception: From Sensation to Cognition*. Vol. 1. Orlando, FL: Academic Press.

MAYS, L. E., AND SPARKS, D. L. (1980). Saccades are spatially, not retinocentrically, coded. *Science 208*, 1163–1165.

METZ, H. S. (1984). Calibration of saccades in infants. *Invest. Ophthalmol. Vis. Sci. 25*, 1233–1234.

MOUNTCASTLE, V. B., ANDERSON, R. A., AND MOTTA, B. C. (1981). The influence of attentive fixation upon the excitability of the light-sensitive neurons of the posterior parietal cortex. *J. Neurosci. 1*, 1218–1235.

MURPHY, B. J. (1978). Pattern thresholds for moving and stationary gratings during smooth eye movements. *Vision Res. 18*, 521–530.

POSNER, M. I., AND PETERSON, S. E. (1990). The attention system of the human brain. *Annu. Rev. Neurosci. 13*, 25–42.

REGAL, D. M., ASHMEAD, D. H., AND SALAPATEK, P. (1983). The coordination of eye and head movements during early infancy. *Behav. Brain Res. 10*, 125–132.

RICHARDS, J. E. (1990). Neuropsychological basis of eye movements, and the effects of attention on eye movements in the development of infant saccades, smooth pursuit, and visual tracking. Unpublished manuscript.

ROBINSON, D. (1981). Control of eye movements. In V. B. BROOKS (ed.). *Handbook of Physiology: The Nervous System*. Vol. II. Baltimore: Williams & Wilkins.

ROUCOUX, A., CULEE, C., AND ROUCOUX, M. (1983). Development of fixation and pursuit eye movements in human infants. *Behav. Brain Res. 10*, 133–139.

SALAPATEK, P., ASLIN, R. N., SIMONSON, J., AND PULOS, E. (1980). Infant saccadic eye movements to visible and previously visible targets. *Child Dev. 51*, 1090–1094.

SALAPATEK, P., HAITH, M. M., MAURER, D., AND KESSEN, W. (1972). Error in the corneal reflection technique: a note on Slater and Findlay. *J. Exp. Child Psychol. 14*, 493–497.

SCHILLER, P. H. (1985). A model for the generation of visually guided saccadic eye movements. In D. ROSE AND V. G. DOBSON (eds.). *Models of the Visual Cortex*. New York: Wiley.

SHEA, S. L., AND ASLIN, R. N. (1984). Development of horizontal and vertical pursuit in human infants. *Invest. Ophthalmol. Vis. Sci. 25* (suppl.), 263.

SHEA, S. L., AND ASLIN, R. N. (1988). Oculomotor displacement thresholds in young infants. *Infant Behav. Dev. 11*, 287.

SHEA, S. L., AND ASLIN, R. N. (1990). Oculomotor responses to step-ramp targets by young human infants. *Vision Res.* 30, 1077–1092.

SHUPERT, C., AND FUCHS, A. F. (1988). Development of conjugate human eye movements. *Vision Res.* 28, 585–596.

SKAVENSKI, A. A., HANSEN, R. M., STEINMAN, R. M., AND WINTERSON, B. J. (1979). Quality of retinal image stabilization during small natural and artificial body rotations in man. *Vision Res.* 19, 675–683.

SLATER, A. M., AND FINDLAY, J. (1972). The measurement of fixation position in the newborn baby. *J. Exp. Child Psychol.* 20, 248–273.

SLATER, A. M., AND FINDLAY, J. (1975). The corneal reflection technique and the visual preference method: sources of error. *J. Exp. Child Psychol.* 20, 240–247.

SNODDERLY, M. (1987). Effects of light and dark environments on macaque and human fixational movements. *Vision Res.* 27, 401–415.

SPARKS, D. L. (1986). Translation of sensory signals into movements for control of saccadic ocular movements: role of the superior colliculus. *Physiol. Rev.* 66, 118–171.

STEINMAN, R. M., KOWLER, E., AND COLLEWIJN, H. (1990). New directions for oculomotor research. *Vision Res.* 30, 1845–1864.

VAN ESSEN, D. C. (1979). Visual areas of the mammalian cerebral cortex. *Ann. Rev. Neurosci.* 2, 227–263.

WENBAN-SMITH, M. G. (1990). The latency of target elicited saccadic eye movements. MSc thesis, University of Durham.

WESTHEIMER, G., AND MCKEE, S. P. (1975). Visual acuity in the presence of retinal-image slip. *J. Opt. Soc. Am.* 65, 847–850.

WIRTSCHAFTER, J. D., AND WEINGARDEN, A. S. (1988). Neurophysiology and central pathways in oculomotor control: physiology and anatomy of saccadic and pursuit eye movements. In C. W. JOHNSTON AND F. J. PIROZZOLO (eds.). *Neuropsychology of Eye Movements.* Hillsdale, NJ: Erlbaum.

WURTZ, R. M., AND GOLDBERG, M. E. (1972). Activity of superior colliculus in behaving monkey. IV. Effects of lesions on eye movements. *J. Neurophysiol.* 35, 587–596.

YOUNG, L. R., AND SHEENA, D. (1975). Survey of eye movement recording methods. *Behav. Res. Methods Instrum.* 7, 397–429.

YUODELIS, C., AND HENDRICKSON, A. (1986). A qualitative and quantitative analysis of the human fovea during development. *Vision Res.* 26, 847–855.

ZEE, D. S. (1982). Ocular motor abnormalities related to lesions in the vestibulocerebellum in primate. In G. LENNERSTRAND, D. S. ZEE, AND E. L. KELLER (eds.). *The Functional Basis of Ocular Motor Disorders.* Oxford: Pergamon Press.

ZEE, D. S., AND ROBINSON, D. A. (1979). A hypothetical explanation of saccadic oscillations. *Ann. Neurol.* 5, 405–414.

5 | Development of the vestibuloocular and optokinetic reflexes

KAREN L. PRESTON AND DOM V. FINOCCHIO

Vision may be compromised (blurred) whenever the image of the outside world moves across the retina. One function of the oculomotor system is to stabilize gaze by reducing such retinal image motion, or slip, thereby preventing blurred vision from occurring when either the individual or an object of visual interest in the environment moves. The greatest threat to visual acuity occurs during head rotation when the entire visual field appears to move in the opposite direction. The potential for blurred vision caused by head rotation is lessened because compensatory rotational eye movements opposite in direction to those of the head partially stabilize the retinal image. These reflexive eye movements, known as the vestibuloocular reflex (VOR), receive afference from the semicircular canals and provide, in adults, about 60% of the eye velocity needed for complete ocular stabilization. The apparent motion of the visual surround that occurs when the head moves, however, elicits the optokinetic reflex (OKR), which supplements the velocity of the compensatory eye movements generated by the VOR to further reduce retinal image motion. Finally, in primates the slip of images of small objects off the fovea elicits a second, visually guided smooth pursuit (SP) eye movement that further enhances the compensatory eye velocity. Together, the VOR, OK, and SP eye movements provide sufficient compensatory eye velocity to reduce the retinal image motion caused by angular head rotation to a level (<2.5 degrees/second) compatible with clear vision (Westheimer and McKee, 1975).

During early infancy, SP has been shown to be markedly immature, if not absent (Dayton et al., 1964; Barten et al., 1971; Kremenitzer et al., 1979; Aslin, 1981; Shea and Aslin, 1990) and therefore may not contribute significantly to compensatory eye movements until later in development. The VOR and OKR, however, are functional at birth (e.g., Kreminitzer et al., 1979; Wilson and Melvill Jones, 1979) and probably provide most of whatever retinal image stabilization capacity neonates possess. This stabilization is particularly important, as retinal image motion resulting from head ro-

tation could interfere with the development of vision in young infants (Boothe et al., 1985).

Although the VOR and OKR are studied separately in the laboratory, they are inseparable in everyday visual behavior and are closely related to one another. The VOR and OKR generate similar sawtooth or nystagmoid response patterns (vestibular and optokinetic nystagmus, or OKN), which are comprised of a slow phase in the compensatory direction followed by a quick, resetting fast phase. In addition, for both types of compensatory response, the nystagmus continues (after-nystagmus) following cessation of the appropriate stimulus, indicating storage of velocity information during stimulation. It has been suggested that there is a common velocity storage mechanism for both VOR and OKR (Cohen et al., 1977; Raphan et al., 1979; Lisberger et al., 1981). Further evidence for the interrelation of VOR and OKN was reported by Miyoshi et al. (1973), who found that repeated OKN stimulation facilitated VOR habituation. Additionally, Zee and colleagues (1976) reported that patients with labyrinthine disorders showed defects in OKN as well as in the VOR. Recordings from cells in the medial vestibular nucleus (MVN) were found to be modulated by both vestibular and optokinetic inputs (Waespe and Henn, 1977). Finally, Robinson (1981) has reviewed the evidence showing the interdependence of VOR and OKN in relation to the frequency of sinusoidal rotation. At frequencies within the usual physiological range (0.1–3.0 Hz), the VOR gain is stable but drops off dramatically at lower frequencies. The visually driven OKR, however, is most effective at these low frequencies and provides the necessary compensatory eye velocity.

Few quantitative data are available concerning the development and function of the VOR and OKR (Shupert and Fuchs, 1988), for which there are several reasons. The most obvious one is the intractability of infant subjects. Second, the eye movement transducers that make recording in adults relatively simple and precise are generally too intrusive to use with infants. Finally, the inability to convincingly calibrate the usable eye

80

movement monitors in infants has often precluded both precise measurement of the eye movements and quantitative comparison with adults. Therefore most studies of the development of the VOR and OKR are descriptive only and document the presence or absence of the responses at various ages or relative changes in various conditions. Consequently, these studies have led various experimenters to different conclusions regarding the maturational characteristics of eye movements, especially the VOR.

Because only a few studies have examined the concurrent development of the VOR and OKR we review their developmental characteristics separately before returning to a discussion of their cooperative role in the stabilization of retinal images in infants.

DEVELOPMENT OF THE VOR

The VOR is clearly present in neonates (Ornitz et al., 1985; Weissman et al., 1989), and in fact the underlying anatomical structures responsible for the generation of the reflex are remarkably well developed at birth (Rosenhall, 1972; Bergstrom, 1973; Bronson, 1982; Lannou et al., 1983; Ornitz, 1983). Despite this apparent anatomical maturity, the infant VOR differs from that of the adult in several important ways. First, the time constants that describe the decay of the nystagmus when a constant velocity of rotation is maintained are significantly shorter in infants than adults (Ornitz et al., 1979; Weissman et al., 1989), as are the time constants associated with postrotatory-nystagmus (Ornitz et al., 1979). Second, the temporal relation of eye position to head position during sinusoidal rotation (phase shift) shows that neonates manifest a marked phase lead, particularly at low frequencies (Cioni et al., 1984). Third, the gain of the VOR—the ratio of slow phase eye velocity to head velocity—in 1- to 4-month-old infants is 1.0, indicating a perfect compensatory response (Finocchio et al., 1991a). The gain changes slowly throughout childhood until it reaches the adult value of approximately 0.6 (Finocchio et al., in preparation). Finally, visual stimulus modification of the VOR-induced compensatory eye movements is not adult-like until well into childhood.

Time Constants

At a constant velocity of rotation in total darkness, the responsiveness of the labyrinth decreases and the velocity of the slow-phase primary nystagmus (SPEV) decreases exponentially. With continued rotation, the nystagmus reverses direction and becomes anticompensatory (secondary nystagmus) until the VOR is eventually extinguished. The decay of both the primary and secondary nystagmus is characterized by the time constant (time for the SPEV to decay to 37% of its peak value) and total duration. Both increase with age. Weissman et al. (1989) found the time constant of primary nystagmus in newborns (1 to 5 days old) was about 6 seconds and increased slightly to 7.5 seconds in 5-month-old infants (Ornitz et al., 1985). The time constant undergoes further increase during development because it is about 20 seconds in adults (Robinson, 1981; Ornitz et al., 1985). The total duration of primary nystagmus is about 10 seconds in infants (Ornitz et al., 1979; Kaga et al., 1981; Weissman et al., 1989) and about 30 seconds in adults (Ornitz et al., 1985). The time constants of the postrotatory nystagmus following abrupt cessation of the rotatory stimulus also increased with age (Cordero et al., 1983; Clark et al., 1984).

The time constant of infant primary nystagmus is roughly the same as that recorded for the cupula in squirrel monkeys (Fernandez and Goldberg, 1971), and it may therefore be determined primarily by peripheral, mechanical properties of the semicircular canals. Although there have been few anatomical studies, the cupula is not thought to undergo significant growth during development, and therefore it is unlikely that changes in the peripheral apparatus can explain the changes in the time constant with age. The longer VOR time constants of adults are thought to result from the additional activity of central neural processes (putative velocity storage) (Robinson, 1981, 1986). Therefore the increase in the time course of vestibular nystagmus with age likely is due to the maturation of these, as yet incompletely defined, central neural processes.

Phase

In addition to having the correct amplitude and velocity, the VOR must be in the direction opposite to that of the head movement in order to reduce retinal image slip. That is, the eye movements must be 180 degrees out of phase with the head movements. This phase inversion results from a double integration of the head acceleration signal driving the semicircular canals. The first integration occurs in the canals themselves and the second in a neural integrator purportedly located in the nucleus prepositus hypoglossi (Skavenski and Robinson, 1973). Like other characteristics of the VOR, this phase relation is frequency-dependent. In the frequency range of normal adult head movements (0.1–2.0 Hz), however, the phase shift is negligible (Benson, 1970; Skavenski et al., 1979). At higher frequencies (> 5 Hz) there is a phase lag that appears to originate in the mechanics of the orbital tissues. At frequencies below 0.01 Hz, the VOR is dominated by two time constants

(T_A and T_{VOR}) producing a decrease in gain and a phase lead. The phase lead increases further as the frequency of head rotation decreases. Clearly, large phase differences would result in blurred vision. As has been mentioned, however, at low frequencies of head rotation, the visually guided optokinetic response can successfully reduce retinal image motion.

In infants a few days old, eye position exhibits a marked phase lead at frequencies of less than 0.5 Hz; the lead increased to approximately 40 degrees at frequencies between 0.2 and 0.5 Hz (Cioni et al., 1984; Weissman et al., 1989). Moreover, Cioni et al. (1984) reported a phase lead of about 25 degrees at 0.05 Hz in 2-month-old infants and in a control group of children 4–7 years of age. Weissman et al. (1989) discussed several factors that may account for the phase lead observed in young infants. First, they suggested that the VOR depends heavily on visual inputs for "calibration" during early infancy. During the first 2 months of life, the imperfect calibration of the VOR could be due to immaturity of the visual system (Dobson and Teller, 1978; Atkinson, 1984). Second, an increase in T_{VOR} and a delay in onset of the secondary nystagmus following prolonged stimulation occurred in older infants and children in conjunction with a decrement in the phase lead. This finding suggested to these authors that the large phase lead in neonates is partly due to an "adaptation operator" with a much shorter time constant than is observed in older children and adults.

Gain

The efficacy of the VOR in reducing retinal image motion may be assessed by determining the gain of the response, that is, the ratio of the compensatory slow-phase eye velocity to head velocity. Perfect compensation has a gain of 1.0. Whereas determination of the temporal characteristics of the VOR does not require accurate calibration of the eye movement monitor, gain calculation requires conversion of the electrooculography (EOG) voltage into an absolute measure of angular eye position.

Although the lack of an effective calibration procedure has precluded the accurate determination of the VOR gain, several investigators have suggested that the gain in infants is higher than that in adults (Goodkin, 1980; Kaga et al., 1981; Regal et al., 1983; Ornitz et al., 1985; Reisman and Anderson, 1989), whereas others have reported a low gain during infancy, indicating a less efficacious VOR (Cyr et al., 1985; Staller et al., 1986).

Finocchio and colleagues (1990) developed a calibration technique that allows simultaneous measurement of EOG potential and a determination of the sub-

ject's fixation position using corneal light reflection. With this technique, calibration of the infant EOG was accurate to within ±1.0 degree at the most eccentric eye position (±20 degrees) and was used to determine the gain of the VOR during horizontal ramp-and-hold vestibular rotation at velocities between 10 and 40 degrees/second. Our results confirm earlier reports of the VOR gain being higher in infants than in adults. We found that infants 1–4 months old have an average gain of 1.03, compared to that of adult subjects, whose average gain was 0.59 (Finocchio et al., 1991a). Preliminary data for older infants and younger children (Figure 5-1) show that the VOR gain does not begin to drop toward adult levels until 3–5 years of age and is not yet adult-like even in 10- and 15-year-old subjects. We conclude that the infant VOR alone can stabilize retinal image motion due to angular head rotation, at least for velocities between 10 and 40 degrees/second, without assistance from the SP and OK subsystems. On the other hand, adults and (to a lesser extent) children clearly require visual backup systems to achieve retinal image stability, as the VOR gain at these ages is less than 1.0. The higher VOR gain in infants may have evolved to allow improved image quality during visual development when other visual and oculomotor functions are immature.

Visual–Vestibular Interactions

Visual–vestibular interactions occur during head rotation in a visual environment. For example, when adults fixate a stationary target while being rotated, the resultant compensatory gain increases to 1.0 from its value of approximately 0.6 in total darkness (Benson and Barnes, 1978; Collewijn, 1989). The VOR gain of infants, unlike that of adults, remained unchanged when they fixated either a small stationary spot of light (a SP stimulus) (Fig. 5-1) or a stationary full-field gradient of black and white stripes (an optokinetic stimulus) (Finocchio et al., 1991a). Of course, with the VOR gain already near 1.0, visual modification of the VOR is functionally unnecessary in infants. Conversely, when a small target rotates in phase with the head, adults show nearly complete VOR suppression, i.e., a gain approaching zero (Benson and Barnes, 1978; Herman et al., 1982). This cancellation of the VOR is thought to be accomplished by an SP response of equal magnitude in the opposite direction of the VOR. Because young infants have markedly immature SP (Aslin, 1981; Shea and Aslin, 1990), we would expect to see gain near 1.0 in infants. There *was* some suppression of the VOR gain, although less in infants than in adults (Finocchio et al., 1991b). Two-month-old subjects showed a reduction to 85% of normal under these conditions,

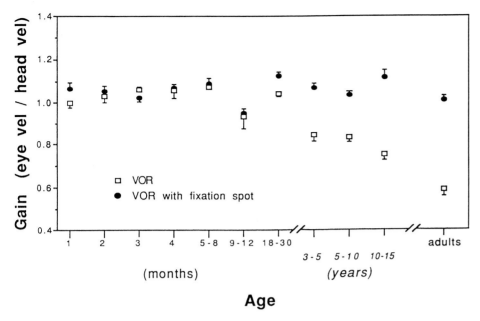

FIG. 5-1. VOR gain (open symbols) and gain of VOR with visual enhancement (closed symbols) as a function of age. One to four month data from Finocchio, Preston, and Fuchs (1991a). Data for older children from Finocchio, Preston, and Fuchs (in preparation).

whereas the adult VOR gain dropped to only 11% of its value in the dark. Three-month-old subjects showed an average gain of 69% of normal, 4-month-olds 65%, 1- to 5-year-olds 51%, and children 6–14 years old 26% of normal. Ornitz and Honrubia (1987) also found poorer VOR gain suppression in infants than adults. Moreover, the ability to suppress the VOR was dependent on rotation velocity, as suppression decreased with increasing head velocity at all ages (Finocchio et al., 1991b).

In summary, infants have shorter time constants, higher gains, and less visual modification of the VOR gain than adults. We may conclude that infants possess a VOR well suited to reflexively compensate for brief periods of head and body rotation. Ornitz et al. (1985) have suggested that the greater VOR gain during infancy is adaptive, as infants undergo frequent passive and active head movement. It may be that the age-related reduction in VOR gain occurs with improvements in gross motor control and volitional, visually guided eye movements as well as maturation of underlying neural processes.

OPTOKINETIC RESPONSE

The OKR occurs during full-field image motion and is thought to have developed early to complement the VOR in retinal image stabilization during head rotation (Robinson, 1981). Because the OKR is a visually guided response it is sometimes difficult to distinguish between the slow eye movements generated by the reflexive OKN and voluntary SP. Honrubia and colleagues (1968) described two distinct types of OKN responses in adult humans referred to as look (implying voluntary tracking of individual features of the optokinetic stimulus) and stare (reflexive) OKN. *Stare-OKN* is thought to be mediated subcortically, whereas *look-OKN* is considered to be, at least in part, a result of cortical, pursuit mechanisms. These two OKN responses may be distinguished on the basis of several features. First, stare-OKN has an upper SPEV limit of approximately 40 degrees/second, whereas the SPEV of look-OKN increases with target velocity to the limits of SP tracking velocity (approximately 50–60 degrees/second). Second, the slow-phase amplitude is greater with fewer fast phases for stare-OKN than for look-OKN. Third, optokinetic afternystagmus follows stare-OKN but not look-OKN. The type of response elicited by an optokinetic stimulus is highly dependent on instructional set for adult subjects. As a result, study of the development of OKN is complicated, as infant subjects cannot be reliably instructed on responses to optokinetic stimuli.

The study of infant OKN is additionally complicated, as its development is dependent on the maturation of other visual functions, e.g., visual acuity, contrast sensitivity, velocity sensitivity, and direction selectivity of target motion as well as the extent of the visual field. It has led various investigators to use optokinetic responses to study these and other aspects of visual capacity (Gorman et al., 1957; Dobson and Teller, 1978; Boothe et al., 1985; Maurer et al., 1989; Roy et al.,

1989; Teller and Lindsay, 1989; Lewis et al., 1990) (see Chapter 9). Unfortunately, it is often difficult to interpret the results of such studies, as the stimulus characteristics sufficient to drive OKN in infants have not been fully explored. The question arises as to whether the absence of OKN is due to a sensory or a motor limitation. Like the VOR, OKN can be elicited in young infants (Enoch and Rabinowicz, 1976; Kremenitzer et al., 1979; Schor, 1981; Roy et al., 1989).

Pursuit Versus Reflexive OKN in Infants

Optokinetic nystagmus may be elicited in an adult monkey at drum velocities up to about 180 degrees/second. The response consists of two components: a rapid rise followed by a gradual rise in slow-phase eye velocity (Cohen et al., 1977). Within about 130 ms after the rotating drum is illuminated, the velocity of the slow phase jumps rapidly (within several hundred milliseconds) to 55–65% of the steady-state velocity. The early, rapid component is thought to be mediated by a "direct," or cortical, pursuit pathway because it shows several features that resemble smooth pursuit. This rapid component is largest in primates, which have excellent pursuit (Lisberger et al., 1981), and is impaired in patients with defective SP (Zee et al., 1976; Baloh et al., 1982). The early phase is followed by a longer, more gradual increase in eye velocity that takes 15–20 seconds to reach full steady-state amplitude. The later phase is thought to be mediated subcortically and is referred to as the "indirect" pathway. If the lights are turned off after a sufficient period of optokinetic stimulation, the OKN persists with first a rapid, then a gradual, decrease in velocity. This persistence is referred to as optokinetic after-nystagmus (OKAN). The rapid drop in eye velocity is thought to reflect the loss of the pursuit component, and the initial eye velocity for OKAN reflects the contribution the indirect pathway was making just before the lights went out (Raphan et al., 1977). It has been suggested that the ensuing OKAN is a gradual release of that OKN velocity accumulated in a velocity storage mechanism in the indirect pathway (Waespe and Henn, 1977; Raphan et al., 1979).

In adult humans, OK responses differ from the monkey in that the SPEV jumps to its steady-state value during the first nystagmic beat (Cohen et al., 1981). The immediate rise in SPEV is thought to reflect the well-developed direct SP pathway. Although there is no apparent gradual buildup of OKN-SPEV, a modest OKAN occurs, indicating that adult humans also have an OKN storage mechanism. The maximum SPEV of human OKAN, however, is low, and its duration short (Cohen et al., 1981; Schor et al., 1983).

These response characteristics in adult monkeys and humans raise interesting questions regarding the development of infant OKN. Because infants do not possess a well-developed SP system, the direct or pursuit optokinetic pathway should show similar immaturities. As a result, the rise in OKN-SPEV in infants may show the slow changing component elicited in monkeys. Unfortunately, few studies characterize the change in velocity toward steady state during the initial phases of optokinetic stimulation. Hainline and Abramov (1985) reported no buildup of slow-phase velocities during *small-field* optokinetic stimulation; however, the 30 × 22 degree stimulus may not have been sufficient to elicit the indirect OK response. Furthermore, infant steady-state velocities were lower than those of the adult, suggesting that only the pursuit pathway was involved in the response to the small-field stimulus.

Although OKAN in adult humans is weak, the infant OKAN is fairly robust in both amplitude and duration (Schor et al., 1983), providing support for the notion that indirect pathways contribute more to the optokinetic response in infants than in adults.

Gain

Little is known about the efficacy of the infant OKR. Data collected during full-field optokinetic stimulation were not calibrated, and therefore only relative velocity information was reported. Experimenters who did attempt calibration either did not test binocularly or used small-field stimuli. In infants 1–3 days old, Kremenitzer et al. (1979) reported an increase in SPEV as the velocity of a full-field stimulus increased from 9 to 25 degrees/second. However, the gain of the response diminished at 32 and 40 degrees/second stimulus velocities, indicating a sensory or motor limit to OKN slow-phase eye movements in neonates. In contrast, adult slow-phase velocities continue to increase with increasing target velocities up to 40 degrees/second. The characteristics of velocity saturation are not known for any stage of early human development, nor is it known when the OKR can match higher stimulus velocities.

Small-field optokinetic targets produce OKN with lower gains in infants up to 1 year of age than in adults (Hainline and Abramov, 1985). As stated above, it may reflect immaturities in the smooth pursuit system rather than the OKR. The data reported by Hainline and Abramov were grouped across ages, so no information is available on developmental trends.

Monocular OKN Asymmetries

Most studies investigating the development of OKN have described the immaturities revealed during monocular stimulation. If an infant views an optokinetic target with either the right eye or the left eye alone, drum movement in a temporal to nasal (T–N) direction elicits qualitatively much stronger OKN than nasal to temporal (N–T) stimulation (for a review see Shupert and Fuchs, 1988). A similar asymmetry has been noted in kittens (Van Hof-van Duin, 1978) and young monkeys (Atkinson, 1979). This asymmetry persists in cats (van Hof-van Duin, 1978; Malach et al., 1981, 1984) and humans with impaired binocular vision (Schor and Levi, 1980; Atkinson and Braddick, 1981; Maurer et al., 1983). The direction-dependent disparity in monocular OKN responses in humans gradually diminishes by about the 20th postnatal week (Naegele and Held, 1982).

Several investigators have noted the concurrent onset of binocularity and a symmetrical OKN. This coincidence, when taken together with evidence for persistent asymmetrical responses in binocularly impaired subjects and the lack of symmetrical responses in nonbinocular animals (Fukuda, 1959; Precht, 1981), has led to the speculation that the developmental changes in monocular OKN are linked to cortical binocular development. Indeed, at least in cats, brainstem structures thought to control OKN, namely the nucleus of the optic tract (Hoffman and Schoppmann, 1981), receive cortical input from binocularly driven cells (Schoppmann, 1981). Schor et al. (1983) have hypothesized that these binocularly driven cortical projections to the optic tract nucleus may also be present in humans and provide the mechanism for development of OKN to temporalward motion. This hypothesis has received support from Hine (1985), who used dichoptic, strobe illumination of optokinetic targets to demonstrate that OKN asymmetry is indeed negatively related to binocular input but is not associated with the same cortical binocular mechanisms that give rise to stereopsis. Rather, subcortical binocular mechanisms appear to be responsible for the production of symmetrical OKN.

A second explanation for poorer OKN to temporalward stimuli has been advanced by several investigators (see Chapter 10). Infant visual evoked responses (VERs) reveal a directional asymmetry in motion processing to monocularly presented gratings undergoing both horizontal and vertical jitter (Norcia et al., 1991). Similar findings have been reported for subjects with early-onset but not late-onset, strabismus (Hamer et al., 1990). Although the test technique does not allow differentiation of the direction of motion producing the weaker VER, poorer motion sensitivity in the temporalward direction would be consistent with asymmetrical OKN such as that found with early development and binocularly deficient subjects. Therefore poor N–T OKN may be, at least in part, the result of delayed development of cortical processing of N–T (temporalward) motion.

In addition to the above hypotheses advanced to explain monocular OKN asymmetry, several other factors have been shown to contribute to the asymmetry. The spatial frequency of the OK stimulus may be a factor (Schor and Narayan, 1981), as high spatial frequencies reveal an asymmetry in older infants (Lewis et al., 1990). Additionally, the development of symmetrical OKN may be dependent, in part, on visual experience, as premature infants showed higher gains for temporalward motion than did the control group matched for gestational age (Roy et al., 1989). Presumably, the premature infant had a longer exposure to visual stimulation.

In summary, although OKN is present at birth, it undergoes several developmental changes, the most notable of which is the development of symmetrical monocular OKN at approximately 4–6 months of age. Whether this change is a result of cortical binocular development, asymmetrical development of direction selective neurons, or some combination of the two awaits further study. Although there has been some suggestion that the gain of the OKR is low in infants, the data are insufficient to determine how effectively and at what velocities the infant OKR reduces retinal image motion.

DISCUSSION

The function of the VOR and OKR is to prevent blurred vision associated with excessive retinal image motion during head rotation. Image stabilization during angular head rotation is particularly important during early infancy, as infants are subjected to frequent passive rotation of the head coupled with the active rotations that occur owing to poor motor control. In addition, the central retina and visually elicited SP eye movements are poorly developed at birth and seem to be dependent, at least in part, on visual experience for maturational improvements. As a result, infants must rely on the VOR and OKR to reduce retinal image motion and facilitate clear vision. Fortunately, the VOR has a gain of about 1.0 in young infants, and it can stabilize retinal images during head movements, at least for velocities of 10–40 degrees/second. There are, as yet, too few quantitative data to determine the head velocities at which OK stimulation elicits eye movements of sufficient velocity to enhance VOR-induced compensatory eye movements.

The infant and adult oculomotor systems do not achieve retinal image stability in the same way. The adult VOR provides only about 60% of the compensatory eye velocity necessary to reduce retinal image motion and must therefore be supplemented by SP and OK eye movements. In addition, adults presumably use an oppositely directed SP response to cancel the VOR (VOR suppression) when it is in conflict with the requirements of vision. If indeed the SP response is the

VOR canceling mechanism, without an adequate SP young infants can only marginally suppress the VOR.

Infant and adult optokinetic responses also differ. Adult OKN is more related to cortical, pursuit pathways, particularly during active attention to elements of the optokinetic stimulus (Honrubia et al., 1968), whereas infant OKN appears to be generated primarily via the indirect pathway. This point is suggested by the slower rise to steady-state eye velocity in infants in contrast to the quick rise seen in adults (Finocchio, Preston, and Fuchs, unpublished observations). Also, infants demonstrate a more robust OKAN than adults, indicating more velocity storage, a feature of indirect OKN.

The adaptability and plasticity of the oculomotor system are seen most dramatically in its ability to deal with the rapid, multiple requirements imposed by the visual system. Often, the visual system places conflicting requirements for image stabilization on the oculomotor system. For example, adults most often track a target moving against a stationary background with a combination of head and eye movements. All of the slow eye movements—VOR, OKR, and SP (and most likely saccades as well)—are joined in stabilizing the retinal image. The head movement elicits the VOR and the moving background the OKR; and both must be suppressed for the SP response to keep the eye on the target. Modulation of the VOR gain is also required when the distance between the individual and the target changes. A larger gain is required for perfect image stabilization at closer distances (Viirre et al., 1986). Again, SP plays a major role in this gain modulation in adults.

If the VOR and OKR consistently fail to reduce retinal image motion, a gradual gain recalibration occurs. In adults this plasticity is facilitated, at least in part, by feedback via the flocculus of the cerebellum from the pursuit system (Robinson, 1975). The default value (about 0.6 in the dark) of the VOR gain in adults may represent a bias toward suppression resulting from the visual situations in which coordinated eye-head tracking occurs, e.g., observing the ball during a tennis match or reading something carried in the hand while walking.

It is clear that the VOR and OKR do not operate independently. The activity of both the VOR and OKR is stored in a velocity-storage integrator (Raphan et al., 1977, 1979; Cohen et al., 1981). Evidence for such storage in adults may be found in the VOR time constant. The cupular time constant is estimated to be approximately 6 seconds, yet vestibular nystagmus is prolonged about threefold in adult humans (for a review see Robinson, 1986). Several investigators (Skavenski and Robinson, 1973; Raphan et al., 1979) have suggested that the cupular time constant is transformed to the VOR time constant by the addition of a signal from a central integrator, which is also part of the OKR. The integrated signal provides a more faithful representation

of head velocity and improves the low-frequency response of the VOR.

As we have described, the presence of OKAN indicates that an optokinetic velocity storage mechanism was charged. There is evidence to suggest that one velocity-storage integrator is common to both the VOR and OKR, and it may be located in the nucleus prepositus hypoglossi (Cannon and Robinson, 1985; Cheron et al., 1987). It is clear from the short VOR time constants in infants that either input to, or activity in, the neural integrator is not fully developed in infants. Infants have a VOR time constant dominated by the cupular activity and not one that represents velocity storage. Conversely, OK velocity storage is more fully developed in infants, as shown by a robust OKAN. Therefore although there may be only one velocity integrator, its input–output relations may be multiple in nature, with different developmental time courses.

In summary, if a stable retinal image is necessary for the development of vision, the infant VOR, with a gain of 1.0, can reduce retinal image motion sufficiently for clear visual processing without the optokinetic and smooth pursuit assistance required during adulthood. Quantitative data regarding the development of the optokinetic and SP systems and their interaction with the VOR are necessary to understand the natural progression of compensatory eye movements and their modulation by visual experience.

REFERENCES

ASLIN, R. M. (1981). Development of smooth pursuit in human infants. In D. F. FISHER, R. A. MONTY, AND J. W. SENDERS (eds.). Eye Movements: Cognition and Visual Perception. Hillsdale, NJ: Erlbaum, pp. 31–51.

ATKINSON, J. (1979). Development of optokinetic nystagmus in the human infant and monkey infant: an analogue to development in kittens. In R. D. FREEMAN (ed.). Developmental Neurobiology of Vision. New York: Plenum Press.

ATKINSON, J. (1984). Human visual development over the first 6 months of life: a review and hypothesis. Hum. Neurobiol. 3, 61–74.

ATKINSON, J., AND BRADDICK, O. (1981). Development of optokinetic nystagmus in infants: an indicator of cortical binocularity? In D. F. FISHER, R. A. MONTY, AND J. W. SENDERS (eds.). Eye Movements: Cognition and Visual Perception. Hillsdale, NJ: Erlbaum, pp. 53–64.

BALOH, R., YEE, R., AND HONRUBIA, V. (1982). Clinical abnormalities of optokinetic nystagmus. In D. LENNERSTRAND, D. ZEE, AND E. KELLER (eds.). Functional Basis of Ocular Motility Disorders. New York: Pergamon Press, pp. 311–320.

BARTEN, S., BIRNS, B., AND RONCH, J. (1971). Individual differences in the visual pursuit behavior of neonates. Child Dev. 42, 313–319.

BENSON, A. J. (1970). Interactions between semicircular canals and gravireceptors. In D. D. BUSBY (ed.). Recent Advances in Aerospace Medicine. Dordrecht, Holland: D. Reidel, pp. 249–261.

BENSON, A. J., AND BARNES, G. (1978). Vision during angular oscillation: the dynamic interaction of visual and vestibular mechanism. Aviat. Space Environ Med. 49, 340–345.

BERGSTROM, B. (1973). Morphology of the vestibular nerve. II. The number of myelinated vestibular nerve fibers in man at various ages. *Acta Otolaryngol. (Stockh.)* 76, 173–179.

BOOTHE, R. G., DOBSON, V., AND TELLER, D. Y. (1985). Postnatal development of vision in human and nonhuman primates. *Annu. Rev. Neurosci.* 8, 495–545.

BRONSON, G. (1982). The scanning patterns of human infants: implications for visual learning. *Monographs on Infancy* (Whole No. 2). Norwood, NJ: Ablex.

CANNON, S. C., AND ROBINSON, D. A. (1985). Neural integrator failure from brainstem lesions in monkey. *Invest. Ophthalmol. Vis. Sci.* 26 (suppl.), 47.

CHERON, G., GODAUX, E., LAUNE, J., AND VANDERKELEN, B. (1987). Disabling of the oculomotor neural integrator by lesions in the region of the propositus and vestibular nuclear complex. *J. Physiol. (Lond.)* 347, 267–290.

CIONI, G., FAVILLA, M., GHELARDUCCI, B., AND LaNOCE, A. (1984). Development of the dynamic characteristics of the horizontal vestibulo-ocular reflex in infancy. *Neuropediatrics* 15, 125–291.

CLARK, D. L., CORDERO, L., AND BATES, J. (1984). Development of postrotatory nystagmus time constants. *Acta Otolaryngol. (Stockh.)* 98, 287–291.

COHEN, B., MATSUO, V., AND RAPHAN, T. (1977). Quantitative analysis of the velocity characteristics of optokinetic nystagmus and optokinetic after-nystagmus. *J. Physiol. (Lond.)* 270, 321–344.

COHEN, B., HENN, V., RAPHAN, T., AND DENETT, D. (1981). Role of velocity storage in visual-vestibular interactions in human. *Ann. N.Y. Acad. Sci* 374, 421–433.

COLLEWIJN, H. (1989). The vestibulo-ocular reflex: is it an independent subsystem? *Rev. Neurol. (Paris)* 145, 502–512.

CORDERO, L., CLARK, D. L., AND URRUTIA, J. G. (1983). Postrotational nystagmus in full term and premature infants. *Int. J. Pediatr. Otorhinolaryngol.* 5, 47–57.

CYR, D., BROOKHAUSER, P., VALENTE, M., AND GROSSMAN, A. (1985). Vestibular evaluation of infants and preschool children. *Otolaryngol. Head Neck Surg.* 93, 463–468.

DAYTON, G. O., JONES, M. H., AIU, P., RAWSON, R. D., STEELE, B., AND ROSE, M. (1964). Developmental study of coordinated eye movements in the human infant. I. Visual acuity in the newborn infant: a study based on induced optokinetic nystagmus by electrooculography. *Arch. Ophthalmol.* 71, 865–870.

DOBSON, V., AND TELLER, D. Y. (1978). Visual acuity in human infants: a review and comparison of behavioral and electrophysiological studies. *Vision Res.* 18, 1468–1483.

ENOCH, J. M., AND RABINOWICZ, I. M. (1976). Early surgery and visual correction of an infant born with unilateral eye lens opacity. *Doc. Ophthalmol.* 41, 371–382.

FERNANDEZ, D., AND GOLDBERG, J. M. (1971). Physiology of peripheral neurons innervating semicircular canals of the squirrel monkey. II. Response to sinusoidal stimulation dynamics of peripheral vestibular system. *J. Neurophysiol* 34, 661–675.

FINOCCHIO, D. V., PRESTON, K. L., AND FUCHS, A. F. (1990). Obtaining a quantitative measure of eye movements in human infants: a method calibrating the electrooculogram. *Vision Res.* 30, 1119–1128.

FINOCCHIO, D. V., PRESTON, K. L., AND FUCHS, A. F. (1991a). Infant eye movements: quantification of the vestibulo-ocular reflex and visual-vestibular interactions. *Vision Res.* 31, 1717–1730.

FINOCCHIO, D. V., PRESTON, K. L., AND FUCHS, A. F. (1991b). A quantitative analysis of the development of VOR suppression in human infants. *Invest. Ophthalmol. Vis. Sci.* 32 (suppl.), 896.

FUKUDA, T. (1959). Unidirectionality of the labyrinthine reflex in relation to the unidirectionality of the optokinetic reflex. *Acta Otolaryngol (Stockh.)* 50, 507–516.

GOODKIN, F. (1980). The development of mature patterns of head-eye coordination in the human infant. *Early Hum. Dev.* 4, 373–386.

GORMAN, J., COGAN, O., AND GILLIS, S. (1957). An apparatus for grading the visual acuity of infants on the basis of optokinetic nystagmus. *Pediatrics* 19, 1088–1092.

HAINLINE, L., AND ABRAMOV, I. (1985). Saccades and small-field optokinetic nystagmus in infants. *J. Am. Opt. Assoc.* 56, 620–626.

HAMER, R. D., NORCIA, A. M., OREL-BIXLER, D., AND HOYT, C. (1990). Cortical responses to nasalward and temporalward motion are asymmetric in early but not late-onset strabismus. *Invest. Ophthalmol. Vis. Sci.* 31, (suppl.), 289.

HERMAN, R., MAULUCCI, R., AND STUYCK, J. (1982). Development and plasticity of visual and vestibular generated eye movements. *Exp. Brain Res.* 47, 69–78.

HINE, T. (1985). The binocular contribution to monocular optokinetic nystagmus and afternystagmus asymmetries. *Vision Res.* 25, 589–598.

HOFFMAN, K. P., AND SCHOPPMANN, A. (1981). A quantitative analysis of the direction-specific response of neurones in the cat's nucleus of the optic tract. *Exp. Brain Res.* 42, 1–12.

HONRUBIA, V., DOWNEY, D. P., MITCHELL, B. A., AND WARD, P. Œ. (1968). Experimental studies on optokinetic nystagmus. *Acta Otolaryngol. (Stockh.)* 65, 441–448.

KAGA, K., SUZUKI, J. I., MARSH, R., AND TANAKA, V. (1981). Influence of labyrinthine hypoactivity on gross motor development of infants. *Ann. N.Y. Acad. Sci.* 374, 412–420.

KREMENITZER, J. P., VAUGHAN, H. G., KURTZBERG, D., AND DOWLING, K. (1979). Smooth pursuit eye movements in the newborn infant. *Child Dev.* 50, 442–448.

LANNOU, J., PRECHT, W., AND CAZIN, L. (1983). Functional development of the central vestibular system. In R. ROMAND (ed.). *Development of Auditory and Vestibular Systems.* Orlando, FL: Academic Press.

LEWIS, T. L., MAURER, D., AND BRENT, H. (1990). The development of visual resolution in infants and toddlers tested monocularly with optokinetic nystagmus. *Clin. Vis. Sci.* 5, 231–242.

LEWIS, T. L., MAURER, D., AND van SCHAIK, C. S. 1990). Monocular OKN acuity is asymmetric in normal 3-month olds. *Invest. Ophthalmol. Vis. Sci.* 31 (suppl.), 7.

LISBERGER, S. G., EVINGER, C., JOHANSON, G. W., AND FUCHS, A. F. (1981). Relationship between eye acceleration and retinal image velocity during foveal smooth pursuit in man and monkey. *J. Neurophysiol.* 46, 229–249.

LISBERGER, S. G., MILES, F. A., OPTICAN, L. M., AND EIGHMY, B. B. (1981). Optokinetic response in monkey: underlying mechanisms and their sensitivity to long term adaptive changes in the vestibulo-ocular reflex. *J. Neurophysiol.* 45, 869–890.

MALACH, R., STRONG, N. P., AND van SLUYTERS, R. S. (1981). Analysis of monocular optokinetic nystagmus in normal and visually deprived kittens. *Brain Res.* 210, 367–372.

MALACH, R., STRONG, N. P., AND VAN SLUYTERS, R. S. (1984). Horizontal OKN in the cat: effect of long term monocular deprivation. *Dev. Brain Res.* 13, 192–205.

MAURER, D., LEWIS, T. L., AND BRENT, H. P. (1983). Peripheral vision and optokinetic nystagmus in children with unilateral congenital cataract. *Behav. Brain Res.* 10, 151–161.

MAURER, D., LEWIS, T., AND BRENT, H. P. (1989). The effect of deprivation on human visual development: studies of children treated for cataracts. In F. J. MORRISON, C. E. LORD, AND D. P. KEATING (eds.). *Applied Developmental Psychology.* Vol. 3. Orlando, FL: Academic Press, pp. 139–227.

MIYOSHI, T., PFALTZ, C. R., AND PIFFKO, P. (1973). Effect of repetitive optokinetic stimulation upon optokinetic an vestibular responses. *Acta Otolaryngol (Stockh.)* 75, 259.

NAEGELE, J. R., AND HELD, R. (1982). The postnatal development of monocular optokinetic nystagmus in infants. *Vision Res.* 22, 341–346.

NORCIA, A. M., GARCIA, H., HUMPHREY, R., HOLMES, R., HAMER,

R. D., AND OREL-BIXLER, D. (1991). Anomalous motion VEPs in infants and in infantile esotropia. *Invest. Ophthalmol. Vis. Sci.* 32, 436–439.

ORNITZ, E. M. (1983). Normal and pathological maturation of vestibular function in the human child. In R. ROMAND (ed.). *Development of Auditory and Vestibular Systems*. Orlando, FL: Academic Press, pp. 479–536.

ORNITZ, E. M., AND HONRUBIA, V. (1987). Developmental modulation of vestibulo-oculomotor function. Presented to the Baranay Society, Bologna, Italy.

ORNITZ, E. M., ATWELL, C. W., WALTER, D. D., HARTMANN, E. E., AND KAPLAN, A. R. (1979). The maturation of vestibular nystagmus in infancy and childhood. *Acta Otolaryngol. (Stockh.)* 88, 244–256.

ORNITZ, E. M., KAPLAN, A. R., AND WESTLAKE, J. R. (1985). Development of the vestibulo-ocular reflex from infancy to adulthood. *Acta Otolaryngol. (Stockh.)* 100, 180–193.

PRECHT, W. (1981). Visual-vestibular interaction in vestibular neurons: functional pathway organization. *Ann. N.Y. Acad. Sci.* 374, 230–248.

RAPHAN, T., COHEN, B., AND MATSUO, V. (1977). A velocity storage mechanism responsible for optokinetic nystagmus (OKN), optokinetic aftr-nystagmus (OKAN) and vestibular nystagmus. In R. BAKER AND A. BERTHOZ (eds.). *Control of Gaze by Brain Stem Neurons: Developments in Neuroscience*. Amsterdam: Elsevier–North Holland, pp. 37–47.

RAPHAN, T., MATSUO, V., AND COHEN, B. (1979). Velocity storage in the vestibulo-ocular reflex arc (VOR). *Exp. Brain Res.* 35, 229–248.

REGAL, D. M., ASHMEAD, D. H., AND SALAPATEK, P. (1983). The coordination of eye and head movements during early infancy: a selective review. *Behav. Brain Res.* 10, 125–132.

REISMAN, J. E., AND ANDERSON, J. H. (1989). Compensatory eye movements during head and body rotation in infants. *Brain Res.* 484, 119–129.

ROBINSON, D. A. (1975). Oculomotor control signals. In G. LENNERSTRAND AND P. BACH-Y-RITA (eds.). *Basic Mechanisms of Ocular Motility and Their Clinical Implications*. New York: Pergamon Press, pp. 337–378.

ROBINSON, D. A. (1981). Control of eye movements. In J. M. BROOKHART, V. B. MOUNTCASTLE, V. B. BROOKS, AND S. R. GEIGER (eds.). *Handbook of Physiology*. Sect. 1, Vol. II, Part 2. Bethesda: American Physiological Society, pp. 1275–1320.

ROBINSON, D. A. (1986). The systems approach to the oculomotor system. *Vision Res.* 26, 91–99.

ROSENHALL, U. (1972). Vestibular macular mapping in man. *Ann. Otorhinolaryngol.* 81, 339–351.

ROY, M. S., LACHAPPELLE, P., AND LEPORE, F. (1989). Maturation of the optokinetic nystagmus as a function of the speed of stimulation in full term and preterm infants. *Clin. Vis. Sci.* 4, 357–366.

SCHOPPMAN, A. (1981), Projections from area 17 and 18 of the visual cortex to the nucleus of the optic tract. *Brain Res.* 22, 1–17.

SCHOR, C. M. (1981). Directional anisotropies of pursuit zztracking and optokinetic nystagmus in abnormal binocular vision. In D. FENDER AND B. COOPER (eds.). *Ocular Motor Symposium*. Pasadena, CA: Cal-Tech Press, pp. 83–104.

SCHOR, C. M., AND LEVI, D. M. (1980). Disturbances of small-field horizontal and vertical optokinetic nystagmus. *Invest. Ophthalmol. Vis. Sci.* 19, 668–683.

SCHOR, C. M., AND NARAYAN, V. (1981). The influence of field size upon the spatial frequency response of optokinetic nystagmus. *Vision Res.* 21, 985–994.

SCHOR, C. M., NARAYAN, V., AND WESTALL, C. (1983). Postnatal development of optokinetic after nystagmus in human infants. *Vision Res.* 23, 1643–1647.

SHEA, S. L., AND ASLIN, R. M. (1990). Oculomotor responses to step-ramp targets by young human infants. *Vision Res.* 31, 1077–1092.

SHUPERT, C., AND FUCHS, A. F. (1988). Development of conjugate human eye movements. *Vision Res.* 28, 585–596.

SKAVENSKI, A. A., AND ROBINSON, D. A. (1973). Role of the abducens neurons in vestibulo-ocular reflex. *J. Neurophysiol.* 36, 724–738.

SKAVENSKI, A. A., HANSON, R., STEINMAN, R., AND WINTERSON, B. (1979). Quality of retinal image stabilization during small natural and artificial body rotations in man. *Vision Res.* 19, 675–683.

STALLER, S. J., GOIN, D. W., AND HILDEBRANDT, M. (1986). Pediatric vestibular evaluation with harmonic acceleration. *Otolaryngol. Head Neck Surg.* 95, 471–476.

TELLER, D. Y., AND LINDSEY, D. T. (1989). Motion nulls for white vs. isochromatic gratings in infants and adults. *J. Opt. Soc. Am.* 86, 1945–1955.

VAN HOF-VAN DUIN, J. (1978). Direction preference of optokinetic responses in monocularly tested normal kittens and light deprived cats. *Arch. Ital. Biol.* 116, 472–477.

VIRRE, E., TWEED, D., MILNER, K., AND VILIS, T. (1986). A reexamination of the gain the vestibulo-ocular reflex. *J. Neurophysiol* 56, 439–450.

WAESPE, W., AND HENN, V. (1977). Vestibular nuclei activity during optokinetic after-nystagmus (OKAN) in the alert monkey. *Exp Brain Res.* 30, 323.

WEISSMAN, B. M., DISCENNA, A. O., AND LEIGH, R. J. (1989). Maturation of the vestibulo-ocular reflex in normal infants during the first 2 months of life. *Neurology* 39, 534–538.

WESTHEIMER, G., AND MCKEE, S. P. (1975). Visual acuity in the presence of retinal-image motion. *J. Opt. Soc. Am.* 65, 847–850.

WILSON, V. J., AND MELVILL JONES, G. (1979). The vestibulo-ocular system. In *Mammalian Vestibular Physiology*. New York: Plenum Press, pp. 249–318.

ZEE, D. S., YEE, R. D., AND ROBINSON, D. A. (1976). Optokinetic responses in Labyrinthine-defective human beings. *Brain Res.* 113, 423–428.

III. Spatial and Chromatic Vision
Introduction

MARTIN S. BANKS

Two events that occurred during the 1970s and 1980s led to the flourishing of experimentation on visual development in human infants. First, animal and human studies showed that the visual experience during infancy had seemingly permanent effects on visual capacity for the remainder of life (Wiesel and Hubel, 1963, 1965; Hubel and Wiesel, 1970; Awaya et al., 1973; Banks et al., 1975; Hohmann and Creutzfeld, 1975). These demonstrations led to our current appreciation of the critical need to assess vision during infancy when preventive treatments have the best chance for success. Second, a number of methodological breakthroughs gave experimentalists tools for the first time to measure visual function rigorously during infancy. The new methodologies were the forced-choice preferential looking paradigm (Teller, 1979), innovative evoked potential techniques (Norcia and Tyler, 1985), and the habituation/dishabituation procedure (Cohen et al., 1971). These two events motivated and made feasible the study of early vision.

Once the interest was established, a large number of experimental investigations were conducted that yielded an excellent and reasonably complete description of the normative development of essentially all important visual capabilities. We learned that visual resolution improves by more than a log unit between birth and adulthood, more so for Vernier than for grating targets (Dobson and Teller, 1978; Norcia and Tyler, 1985; Shimojo and Held, 1987). We learned that contrast sensitivity also improves by at least a log unit during the same period, more so at high spatial frequencies than at low frequencies (Atkinson et al., 1977; Banks and Salapatek, 1978; Norcia et al., 1990). We learned that color vision, as indexed by the ability to make hue discriminations, improves significantly between birth and maturity (Teller and Bornstein, 1987). Studies of light and dark adaptation showed that adaptation mechanisms seem to operate from very early in life, but that infants' sensitivity to light increments at different levels of ambient illumination is poor compared to that of adults

(Hansen and Fulton, 1981, 1991; Dannemiller and Banks, 1983; Dannemiller, 1985; Brown, 1990). We learned that increment sensitivity improves with age in peripheral and central visual fields (Mayer et al., 1988; Maurer and Lewis, 1990). We also learned that "channels" tuned to specific aspects of visual stimulation become more selective during the first months; for example, channels become tuned to narrower bands of spatial frequency (Banks et al., 1985), orientation (Braddick et al., 1986), and directions of motion (Wattam-Bell, 1991). These subjects comprise only a short list of the database on normative development that emerged from two decades of intense study. The chapters in this book provide a reasonably complete review of this database.

For all of the skills listed above, the age-related improvements we observed are dramatic. Having documented these improvements, many investigators of infant vision have now devoted themselves to understanding the mechanisms that underlie the growth of visual capability. The following chapters provide the reader several excellent examples of experimental and theoretical attempts to uncover those mechanisms. The chapters by Banks and Crowell, Wilson, and Brown describe efforts to determine how much of the early deficits in acuity and contrast sensitivity can be explained by immaturities in the eye's optics and the photoreceptors. All three chapters conclude that much, but not all, of the early acuity and contrast sensitivity deficits can be explained by these "front-end" immaturities; Wilson is the most optimistic in this regard and Brown the least. The chapter by Hansen and Fulton reviews what we know about increment sensitivity at different levels of ambient light and comes to a similar conclusion that much, but not all, of the early sensitivity deficits can be understood from the effects of optical and receptoral immaturities. The chapter by Teller and Lindsey describes a neat way to conceptualize the development of chromatic and luminance sensitivity and presents preliminary evidence that chromatic and luminance sensitivity develop at similar rates. Finally, the chapter by

Braddick provides elegant and convincing experimental evidence that the orientation and directional tuning of central visual pathways improves markedly during early development.

These chapters illustrate the current trend to unveil the developmental mechanisms that underlie the visual growth that was documented during the last two decades.

REFERENCES

ATKINSON, J., BRADDICK, O., AND MOAR, K. (1977). Development of contrast sensitivity over the first 3 months of life in the human infant. *Vision Res.* 17, 1037–1044.

AWAYA, S., MIYAKE, Y., AMAIZUMI, Y., SHIOSE, Y., KANDA, T., AND KOMURO, K. (1973). Amblyopia in man suggestive of stimulus deprivation amblyopia. *Jpn. J. Ophthalmol.* 17, 69–82.

BANKS, M. S., AND SALAPATEK, P. (1978). Acuity and contrast sensitivity in 1-, 2-, and 3-month-old human infants. *Invest. Ophthalmol. Vis. Sci.* 17, 361–365.

BANKS, M. S., ASLIN, R. N., AND LETSON, R. D. (1975). Sensitive period for the development of binocular vision. *Science* 190, 675–677.

BANKS, M. S., STEPHENS, B. R., AND HARTMANN, E. E. (1985). The development of basic mechanisms of pattern vision: spatial frequency channels. *J. Exp. Child Psychol.* 40, 501–527.

BRADDICK, O. J., WATTAM-BELL, J., AND ATKINSON, J. (1986). Orientation-specific cortical responses develop in early infancy. *Nature* 320, 617–619.

BROWN, A. M. (1990). Development of visual sensitivity to light and color vision in human infants: a critical review. *Vision Res.* 30, 1159–1188.

COHEN, L. B., GELBER, E. R., AND LAZAR, M. A. (1971). Infant habituation and generalization to differing degrees of stimulus novelty. *J. Exp. Child Psychol.* 11, 379–389.

DANNEMILLER, J. L. (1985). The early phase of dark adaptation in human infants. *Vision Res.* 25, 207–212.

DANNEMILLER, J. L., AND BANKS, M. S. (1983). The development of light adaptation in human infants. *Vision Res.* 23, 599–609.

DOBSON, V., AND TELLER, D. Y. (1978). Visual acuity in human infants: a review and comparison of behavioral and electrophysiological techniques. *Vision Res.* 18, 1469–1483.

HANSEN, R. M., AND FULTON, A. B. (1981). Behavioral measurement of behavioral adaptation in human infants. *Invest. Ophthalmol. Vis. Sci.* 21, 625–629.

HANSEN, R. M., AND FULTON, A. B. (1991). Electroretinographic assessment of background adaptation in 10-week-old human infants. *Vision Res.* 31, 1501–1507.

HOHMANN, A., AND CREUTZFELDT, O. D. (1975). Squint and the development of binocularity in humans. *Nature* 254, 613–614.

HUBEL, D. H., AND WIESEL, T. N. (1970). The period of susceptibility to the physiological efefcts of unilateral eye closure in kittens. *J. Physiol. (Lond.)* 206, 419–436.

MAURER, D., AND LEWIS, T. L. (1990). The development of peripheral vision and its physiological underpinnings. In M. J. WEISS AND P. R. ZELAZO (eds.). *Newborn Attention.* Norwood, NJ: Ablex.

MAYER, D. L., FULTON, A. B., AND CUMMINGS, M. F. (1988). Visual fields of infants assessed with a new perimetric technique. *Invest. Ophthalmol. Vis. Sci.* 29, 452–459.

NORCIA, A. M., AND TYLER, C. W. (1985). Spatial frequency sweep VEP: visual acuity during the first year of life. *Vision Res.* 25, 1399–1408.

NORCIA, A. M., TYLER, C. W., AND HAMER, R. D. (1990). Development of contrast sensitivity in the human infant. *Vision Res.* 30, 1475–1486.

SHIMOJO, S., AND HELD, R. (1987). Vernier acuity is less than grating acuity in 2- and 3-month-olds. *Vision Res.* 27, 77–86.

TELLER, D. Y. (1979). The forced-choice preferential looking procedure: a psychophysical technique for use with human infants. *Infant Behav. Dev.* 2, 135–153.

TELLER, D. Y., AND BORNSTEIN, M. H. (1987). Infant color vision and color perception. In P. SALAPATEK AND L. COHEN (eds.). *Handbook of Infant Perception.* Orlando, FL: Academic Press.

WATTAM-BELL, J. (1991). Development of motion-specific cortical responses in infancy. *Vision Res.* 31, 287–297.

WIESEL, T. N., AND HUBEL, D. H. (1963). Effects of visual deprivation on morphology and physiology of cells in the cat's lateral geniculate body. *J. Neurophysiol* 26, 978–993.

WIESEL, T. N., AND HUBEL, D. H. (1965). Comparison of the effects of unilateral and bilateral eye closure on cortical unit responses in kittens. *J. Neurophysiol.* 28, 1029–1040.

6 | Front-end limitations to infant spatial vision: Examination of two analyses

MARTIN S. BANKS AND JAMES A. CROWELL

After more than a decade of intense research, it is now widely recognized that visual sensitivity early in life is rather poor (Dobson and Teller, 1978; Banks and Salapatek, 1983; Brown, 1990). For example, contrast sensitivity and grating acuity during the first month of life are at least an order of magnitude worse than during adulthood. From birth to maturity the eye undergoes significant growth (Larsen, 1971), and the morphology of the photoreceptors, particularly the foveal cones, changes strikingly. Because these changes are extensive, it is natural to wonder to what extent optical and receptoral maturation causes the observed changes in visual sensitivity. The answer to this question is controversial; and, interestingly, the controversy stems primarily from differing assumptions about how age-related anatomical changes in the eye and retina ought to affect visual sensitivity rather than from disagreements about what those anatomical changes are. Specifically, Banks and Bennett (1988) and Wilson (1988) (see also Chapter 32) have used the same quantitative data on the growth of the eye and the photoreceptors to reach essentially opposite conclusions. Banks and Bennett concluded that age-related changes in eye size and foveal cone properties were not sufficient to account for the observed disparities between neonatal and adult contrast sensitivity and acuity, and Wilson concluded that they were nearly sufficient.

Obviously, the issue under debate is important to our understanding of visual development. If Wilson is right, the sometimes dramatic postnatal changes in retinal circuitry, lateral geniculate cell size and circuitry, and arborization of visual cortex have little measurable effect on our standard measures of visual sensitivity. In this chapter we examined the developmental analyses of Banks and Bennett and of Wilson more carefully and concluded that they actually lead to similar conclusions: In both cases, the authors showed that changes in eye size and foveal cone properties can account for much of the observed improvement in contrast sensitivity and grating acuity but are insufficient to explain all of it.

The chapter is organized as follows. First we describe the independent and combined effects of filtering and sampling that occurs in the front-end of the visual system; the experienced reader may wish to skim this section. Then we describe the Banks and Bennett (1988) analysis of the extent to which optical and receptoral immaturities limit early sensitivity. We next describe Wilson's (1988) (see also Chapter 32) developmental model, followed by a discussion and evaluation of the differences between the two analyses. We then modify Wilson's model by making more reasonable assumptions for some of the modeling parameters and examine the predictions of that model. Finally, we compare the predictions of the two approaches and discuss implications.

FILTERING AND SAMPLING BY THE OPTICS, RECEPTORS, AND NEURAL TRANSFER FUNCTION

Our analysis is based on the spatial contrast sensitivity function (CSF), which relates the inverse of the contrast required to detect a target to the target's spatial frequency; later we discuss the models' predictions of acuity. Signals entering the visual system are affected by the optics, the properties of the receptor lattice, the properties of individual receptors, and the postreceptoral processes. The models under consideration here assume that all these factors can be represented by linear filtering and sampling stages, so we can represent their effects in the following way:

$$g(x,y) = P^2 \cdot T \cdot E \cdot \{[i(x,y) * o(x,y) * r(x,y)] \cdot s(x,y)\} * n(x,y) \qquad (1)$$

where $\cdot$ and $*$ = multiplication and convolution, respectively; i = the stimulus (specifically, its luminance function); g = the output of the sequence of processing stages; P = the numerical aperture of the eye (the pupil

91

diameter divided by the focal length)[1]; T = the transmittance of the ocular media (the proportion of incident photons that reach the retina); E = the efficiency of individual receptors in converting incident photons into isomerizations (specifically, the proportion of photons incident to the outer segments that are absorbed by the photopigment); $o(x, y)$ = the optical quality of the eye (i.e., the optical point-spread function); $r(x, y)$ = the aperture of individual receptors; $s(x, y)$ = the sampling function specifying the positions of receptors in the lattice; and $n(x, y)$ = the postreceptor transfer function. This equation can also be written in the spatial frequency domain as:

$$G(u, v) = P^2 \cdot T \cdot E \cdot \{[I(u, v) \cdot O(u, v)$$
$$\cdot R(u, v)] * S(u, v)\} \cdot N(u, v) \quad (2)$$

where G, I, O, R, S, and N = the Fourier transforms of the functions represented by lower-case letters in Eq. (1); and u and v = horizontal and vertical spatial frequencies, respectively.

Before considering the Banks and Bennett and Wilson analyses, we examine the influence of each of these factors on contrast sensitivity in a manner that is mostly model-independent. Using optical, anatomical, densitometric, and psychophysical data in the literature, we can provide suitably accurate estimates of the transmission of the signal through the ocular media and formation into the retinal image and of the sampling and isomerizing properties of the receptor mosaic. We use these estimates to derive CSFs for two different assumptions about the shape of the neural transfer function (NTF), represented by $N(u, v)$. These two assumptions represent two simple models of the variation in receptive field size as a function of preferred spatial frequency.

Figure 6-1 represents the approach. Two stimuli—a grating (α) and a uniform field (β)—are presented and processed through the stages shown. Finally, a decision strategy is used to judge whether the grating or uniform field was presented on a given trial. The decision strategy used here is an ideal decision rule, that is, an optimal rule for discriminating α from β given the constraints imposed by the processing stages. We employ an ideal decision rule because it is the only rule that preserves all the discrimination information available (Geisler, 1984; Watson, 1985); in this way, we can examine the

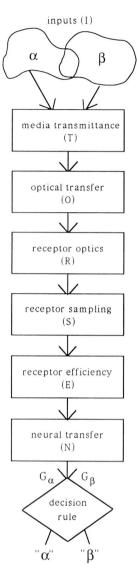

FIG. 6-1. Sequential ideal-observer analysis approach (Geisler, 1984). Two stimuli—a grating (α) and a uniform field (β)—are passed through the various processing stages shown here. At the end of the sequence, an ideal decision rule is used to determine the discriminability of the processed stimuli. We can determine the effect of the various stages on contrast sensitivity by making all stages but one perfect (or fixing them at some reasonable value) and varying the parameters of the stage of interest.

information losses that occur during the processing stages under consideration rather than during the decision process itself.

PUPIL, MEDIA TRANSMITTANCE, AND RECEPTOR EFFICIENCY

Three of the factors—the numerical aperture (P), the transmittance of the ocular media (T), and the efficiency of the photopigment-laden part of the receptors (E)—

1. Variations in pupil diameter have two effects on retinal image formation. First, it affects the proportion of photons incident to the eye that pass into the retinal image. This effect is represented by our value P. Second, the optical quality of the eye is affected by the diameter of the pupil too (Campbell and Gubisch, 1966); larger pupils are generally associated with poorer optical quality. This second effect is represented by $o(x, y)$, or in the frequency domain by $O(u, v)$, which represents the optical transfer function of the eye.

affect only the proportion of photons approaching the eye that are actually caught and produce signals; these effects are independent of the spatial frequency of the stimulus. Obviously, a change in the space-average luminance of the input stimuli has the same effect. Both approaches under consideration here—those of Banks and Bennett (1988) and of Wilson (1988) (see also Chapter 32)—assume that changes in photon catch affect contrast sensitivity according to square-root law (Rose, 1952; Barlow, 1958). Specifically, a K-fold increase in photon catch leads to a square root of K-fold increase in contrast sensitivity. Square-root law is a consequence of the Poisson probability distribution that describes the statistical properties of light. Incorporating this assumption in the models examined later is equivalent to assuming that contrast sensitivity is limited by quantal fluctuations in the stimulus. To show the effects of changes in P, T, E, or the space-average luminance of the stimulus, we have computed the contrast sensitivity of a system with perfect optics $[O(u, v)]$, that is, optics that pass all spatial frequencies with equal fidelity, perfect receptor optics $[R(u, v)]$ (all frequencies passed with equal fidelity through the receptors), and a flat neural transfer function $[N(u, v)]$ (meaning that all frequencies are passed with equal strength through the postreceptoral circuits). In mathematical terms, we set the functions $O(u, v)$, $R(u, v)$, and $N(u, v)$ to constants so their effects on contrast sensitivity do not vary with spatial frequency. An ideal decision rule was used to compute the contrast sensitivity of such a system; the ideal decision rule, derived by Geisler (1984), consists in responding based on the value of the following decision variable (C):

$$C = \sum_{i=1}^{n} Z_i \ln(\alpha_i/\beta_i)$$

where Z_i = the observed photon catch at the ith receptor; and α_i and β_i = the expected catches at the ith receptor if either stimulus α or β was present. The ideal decision rule consists in constructing a weighting function $\ln(\alpha_i/\beta_i)$, which in the tasks we consider here is nearly equivalent to constructing a template of the expected grating target. In this chapter, we consider two-alternative, forced-choice experiments: The value of C is computed for each alternative, and the one with the higher value of C is assumed to have contained stimulus α. Other details of this system are provided in Table 6-1. Figure 6-2 shows the resulting CSFs. The parameter of the functions is the number of photons presented to the receptors per unit area per second. The upper function shows ideal contrast sensitivity when space-average luminance is 50 candelas per square meter (cd/m^2) and pupil diameter is 6 mm (retinal illuminance, the product of external luminance and pupil area, is 1413 trolands).

TABLE 6-1. *Values Used for Modeling*

Factor	Neonate	15 Month-old	Adult
Media transmittance (555 nm)	0.54	0.54	0.54
Pupil diameter (mm)	2.2	2.7	3.3
Posterior nodal distance (mm)	11.7	14.4	16.7
Receptor aperture (min)	0.35	0.67	0.48
Receptor spacing (min)	2.30	1.27	0.58
Outer segment length (μm)	3.1	22.5	50.0
Isomerization rate (555 nm)	0.05	0.28	0.50

The media was assumed to transmit 54% of the light (at 555 nm) incident on the cornea to the retina, and the photopigment was assumed to absorb 50% of the photons at 555 nm incident on receptors and other amounts at different wavelengths in correspondence with the L- and M-cone pigment sensitivities. The two lower functions show sensitivity when the retinal illuminance is reduced by 1 or 2 log units, which could be achieved (all other factors remaining constant) by reducing the external luminance by these values, reducing media transmittance by these values, or reducing the numerical aperture of the eye by the square root of these values. For each log unit of reduction in the number of incident photons, sensitivity falls by 0.5 log unit, thus obeying square-root law. Changes in receptor efficiency have the same effect.

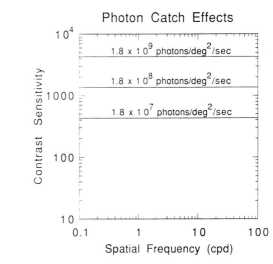

FIG. 6-2. Effect of photon catch on ideal contrast sensitivity. The three curves are ideal CSFs; the parameter of the functions is the number of photons presented to the receptors per unit area per second. The upper function shows ideal contrast sensitivity when retinal illuminance equals 1413 td, target duration is 250 ms, and large grating patches are presented. The two lower functions show sensitivity when either the retinal illuminance is reduced by 1 or 2 log units or the media transmittance is lowered by the same amounts. For each log unit of reduction in the number of incident photons, sensitivity falls by 0.5 log unit, thus obeying square-root law. Changes in receptor efficiency have the same effect.

OPTICS

Next we examine the influence of the optical quality of the eye. We do so by constructing a system in which the media transmittance and receptor efficiency are those of the mature fovea, and the receptor apertures and receptor spacing are set to small values so they do not affect the calculated sensitivities. The optical transfer functions (OTFs) used in this analysis are from Campbell and Gubisch (1966), who measured OTFs at different pupil diameters using the double-pass technique.[2] Again, an ideal decision rule is used to discriminate α and β based on the information available in G_α and G_β. Figure 6-3 shows the normalized contrast sensitivity of such a system limited by the optics. Optical transfer is poorer at larger pupil diameters. Note, for example, the spatial frequency at which transfer falls to 1% at different pupil diameters: 57, 50, 40, and 30 cycles per degree (cpd) at 2, 3, 3.8, and 5.8 mm, respectively.

RECEPTOR APERTURE

To consider the influence of receptor optics on contrast sensitivity we again assume perfect optics and a flat neural transfer function and then vary the diameter of the receptor apertures. Other details of this system are given in Table 6-1. The receptor apertures are represented by cylinder functions of various diameters. Figure 6-4 plots the contrast sensitivities of this observer for different aperture diameters; the sensitivity of the system with an aperture of 0.48 minute has been set to 1 and the others plotted relative to that value. The plots are equivalent to the Fourier transforms of cylinder functions; that is, they are sombrero functions whose first zeroes occur at 1.22 times the reciprocals of the aperture diameters (Gaskill, 1978). The functions have small bumps at higher spatial frequencies, but in the interest of clarity they were suppressed in this figure.

Two effects are evident: (1) At small diameters, the CSF extends to high spatial frequencies, which makes intuitive sense: Receptors integrate light across their apertures, so large receptors are less able to signal fine detail in the image. (2) The low-frequency end of the CSF is higher for large receptor diameters. This finding also makes sense because an array of large receptors ought to collect more light than an array of small receptors with the same spacing. Banks and Bennett (1988) referred to the second effect as *retinal coverage*, arguing that the percentage of the retinal area covered by receptor apertures determines the proportion of incident photons that can be delivered to the photopigment.

2. Measuring the quality of an image reflected off the retina; the image passes through the optics twice.

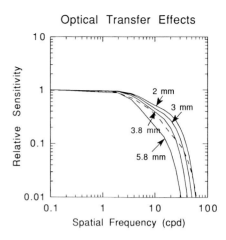

FIG. 6-3. OTFs for different pupil diameters. The solid curves are data from Campbell and Gubisch (1966) for pupil diameters of 2.0, 3.0, 3.8, and 5.8 mm; the dashed curve is M.S.B.'s OTF for a 4-mm pupil. Considering only the solid curves, it is clear that increasing pupil diameter has no effect at low frequencies but leads to greater and greater attenuation at high frequencies. This figure also demonstrates that M.S.B.'s optics are exceptionally good at high frequencies.

RECEPTOR SPACING

To examine the influence of receptor spacing on contrast sensitivity we construct a system with perfect optics, a flat neural transfer function, and receptor apertures of 0.48 minute, the value assumed for the mature fovea. Again an ideal decision rule is employed. Other details are given in Table 6-1. Figure 6-5 displays CSFs for such a system with receptor spacing varying from

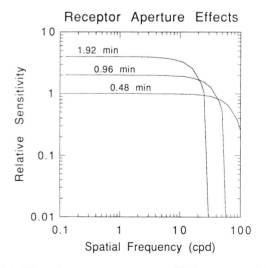

FIG. 6-4. Effect of receptor aperture size on ideal contrast sensitivity. The curves here are normalized CSFs for an ideal observer with perfect optics and a flat NTF and receptor apertures represented by cylinder functions of various sizes. Note that as the aperture size increases: (1) low-frequency sensitivity increases because the receptors are catching more photons; and (2) high-frequency sensitivity decreases because individual receptors are integrating over larger areas.

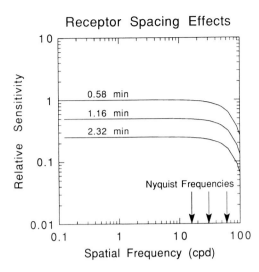

FIG. 6-5. Effect of receptor spacing on ideal contrast sensitivity. The ideal observer used to make this figure had perfect optics, a flat neural transfer function, and receptor apertures of 0.48 minute (Table 6-1). Receptors were arranged hexagonally. Note that (1) as receptor spacing increases from 0.58 to 2.32 minutes, sensitivity decreases; (2) this drop in sensitivity is independent of spatial frequency and in particular bears no relation to the Nyquist frequency. From left to right, the three arrows indicate the Nyquist frequencies for 2.32-, 1.16-, and 0.58-minute spacings, respectively.

etry.[3] The fact that discrimination performance in a contrast sensitivity experiment is not necessarily limited by the Nyquist sampling frequency of the receptor lattice is significant because all too often researchers assume that the Nyquist frequency imposes a hard limit on high-frequency vision (e.g., Jacobs and Blakemore, 1988). Spatially aliased gratings could well attract infants' fixations in forced-choice preferential looking (FPL) experiments and drive visual evoked potentials (VEPs), so there is no reason to believe that the Nyquist frequency of the receptor lattice can predict or limit infants' performance in these tasks. The more likely culprits are the processes that limit intensity discrimination (e.g., photon noise, internal noise, sampling efficiency) and processes that affect signal strength at high spatial frequencies (e.g., optical quality, receptor aperture). This point is bolstered by the observation that adults' and infants' grating acuity varies greatly with luminance (Shlaer, 1937; Brown et al., 1987; Allen et al., 1992; Coletta and Ethirajan, 1991); the Nyquist frequency of the adult foveal cone lattice is always about 60 cpd, but the highest resolvable spatial frequency drops with decreasing luminance to about 10 cpd at low photopic levels.

NEURAL TRANSFER FUNCTION

Obviously, postreceptoral information processing affects contrast sensitivity as well. Here we consider two of the possible neural transfer functions one could assume and describe their influence on contrast sensitivity. The detection of targets of various spatial frequencies is best modeled by assuming that the visual system possesses bandpass detection mechanisms (e.g., Campbell and Robson, 1968; Blakemore and Campbell, 1969). Let us assume for the moment that these mechanisms differ only in the manner in which they combine information from different receptors, that is, that the levels of noise produced within the circuits serving these mechanisms are identical, that the temporal summation properties of the mechanisms are identical, and so on. Now consider two assumptions about the manner in which the sizes of these mechanisms vary with preferred spatial frequency: (1) the mechanisms might have a con-

0.58 minute (the value assumed for the mature fovea) to 2.32 minutes. There are two important points here. First, increases in receptor spacing lead to poorer contrast sensitivity, which makes sense because with receptors of fixed aperture size a lattice of widely spaced receptors catches fewer photons than one with finely spaced receptors. For every doubling of receptor spacing, the number of photons incident on receptor apertures decreases by a factor of 4; therefore, following square-root law, sensitivity decreases by a factor of 2. Second, the contrast sensitivity of the model system does not dip in the region of the Nyquist frequency, the highest spatial frequency a lattice can signal without distortion due to aliasing. The Nyquist frequencies are indicated by the arrows; the leftmost arrow is associated with a spacing of 2.32 minutes and the rightmost with a spacing of 0.58 minutes. The fact that contrast sensitivity does not dip near or above the Nyquist frequency might seem surprising at first, but recall that an ideal decision rule uses all of the information available to discriminate one stimulus from another. If the information from the grating is aliased to a lower spatial frequency, the ideal decision rule simply constructs a weighting function to detect the alias. This result is consistent with Williams' (1985a,b) observation that the adult foveal CSF extends smoothly beyond the Nyquist frequency of 60 cpd to nearly 180 cpd once the optics of the eye are bypassed by laser interferom-

3. Williams' result and the one shown in Figure 6-5 would not be observed if all three of the following conditions obtained: (1) if the lattice geometry were perfectly regular; (2) if the grating's orientation was 30 degrees from vertical such that its bars lined up with the smallest spaced columns of receptors; (3) if the grating was presented in sine phase so that, at the Nyquist limit, it would present zero-crossings to each column of receptors. These conditions are not generally met because the lattice is not perfectly regular and the eye moves continually, so a grating is seldom in sine phase with respect to the sensing lattice for the duration of a stimulus presentation.

stant size in degrees; or (2) the mechanisms might have a constant bandwidth in log cycles per degree. The spatial receptive fields of these two mechanisms are shown in Figure 6-6A,B. The dashed line in each figure represents a mechanism tuned to a spatial frequency of F cpd; the solid line represents a mechanism tuned to 2F cpd, twice the frequency of the first. The spatial frequency tuning functions of these mechanisms, obtained by Fourier transformation, are displayed in Figures 6-6C,D. The mechanisms of constant size have different bandwidths (the widths of the tuning curves in Figure 6-6C) but the same peak sensitivity (the heights of the tuning curves). Mechanisms of constant bandwidth have different peak sensitivities. The difference in the peak sensitivities is a consequence of the assumption of square-root law (discussed above): The diameters of mechanisms of constant bandwidth are inversely proportional to preferred spatial frequency, so the areas are inversely proportional to the square of the preferred frequency. According to square-root law, therefore, the peak sensitivity of constant bandwidth mechanisms is inversely proportional to the square-root of the square of preferred frequency; that is, it is inversely proportional to preferred frequency.

Receptive Field Profiles

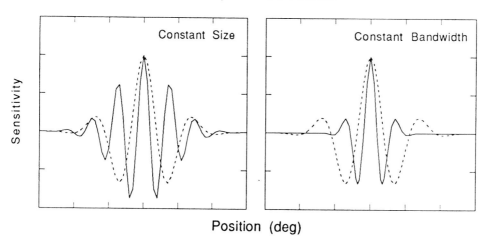

Spatial Frequency Tuning Functions

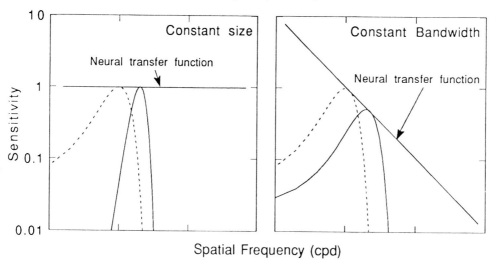

FIG. 6-6. Spatial receptive field profiles and spatial frequency tuning functions for mechanisms of constant size (in degrees) or constant bandwidth (in log spatial frequency). The two upper graphs are the receptive field profiles, and the lower two are the tuning functions. The two graphs on the left are for constant-size mechanisms, and the two on the right are for constant-bandwidth mechanisms. The dashed curves are for a mechanism with a preferred frequency of F, the solid curves for a mechanism with a preferred frequency of 2F. Note that constant-size mechanisms lead to a flat NTF and constant-bandwidth mechanisms to an NTF with a slope of −1.

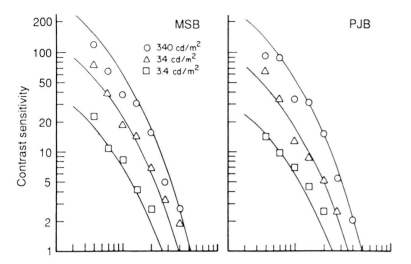

FIG. 6-7. Ideal observer (solid curves) and human (symbols) CSFs for two observers at three luminances from the data of Banks et al. (1987). The data were collected at luminances of 3.4, 34.0, and 340.0 cd/m²; the ideal observer CSFs are for the same luminances. The ideal CSFs have been shifted down by a single scale factor for each observer. The fact that the curves have the same shape indicates that variation in human performance with spatial frequency can be explained by the factors built into the ideal observer; the fact that human and ideal observers show similar variation in sensitivity with luminance indicates that human observers follow square-root law over this range of spatial frequencies and luminances.

The CSF of a system limited by the neural transfer function only is shown in Figure 6-6 for constant size and constant bandwidth mechanisms. Note again that under the constant size assumption the contrast sensitivity of the system is independent of spatial frequency, and under the constant bandwidth assumption the sensitivity of the system is inversely proportional to spatial frequency.

PREDICTING ADULT DATA

Before turning to development, it is important to consider how the factors shown in Figure 6-1 affect contrast sensitivity in mature visual systems. Banks et al. (1987) used an ideal decision rule applied in the fashion suggested by Figure 6-1 to calculate the best possible contrast sensitivity the human adult fovea could have given the constraints of the processing stages shown. The values they used for each of the factors discussed above are given in Table 6-1. In a sense, Banks et al. (1987) assumed a constant bandwidth NTF because they restricted the ideal observer to detection of gratings with a fixed number of cycles. Therefore the ideal observer used weighting functions such as those of Figure 6-6A to make detection judgments.

Banks and colleagues also measured contrast sensitivity psychophysically in two adult observers under the same conditions presented to the ideal observer. Figure 6-7 displays the ideal and human adult CSFs. The data points are contrast sensitivities from 5 to 40 cpd col-

lected at 3.4, 34, and 340 cd/m². As expected, contrast sensitivity declines monotonically from medium to high spatial frequencies, and sensitivity is greater for high than for low luminances. The solid lines are the ideal CSFs for the same stimulus conditions, shifted downward as a unit (by 1.33 log units for observer M.S.B. and 1.43 log units for P.J.B.) to fit the data. The similarity of shapes demonstrates that the high-frequency rolloff of the adult foveal CSF can be explained by consideration of information losses among the factors discussed above, assuming a constant-bandwidth NTF.[4] This observation implies in turn that efficiency beyond the last stage shown in Figure 6-1 is constant from 5 to 40 cpd for adult foveal vision. The fact that real and ideal CSFs are affected similarly by changes in luminance implies that square-root law holds under these conditions and that efficiency beyond the last stage shown in Figure 6-1 is constant across this range of photopic luminances. It is important to note that the similarity in shapes between the human and ideal CSFs breaks down at low spatial frequencies where lateral interactions not incorporated in the ideal observer affect contrast sensitivity (Crowell and Banks, in preparation). We return to the modeling of low-frequency sensitivity later.

---

4. For gratings of fixed size (in degrees), the high-frequency slope of the ideal CSF is shallower than the observed slope because the ideal weighting function incorporates information from all available grating cycles, but human adults do not appear to summate information across all cycles.

Tracking information losses through the front-end stages shown in Figure 6-1 by using an ideal observer analysis allows one to predict the high-frequency rolloff of the adult CSF. Having shown the independent effects on contrast sensitivity of all the front-end processing stages, we now turn to development and the models of Banks and Bennett (1988) and Wilson (1988) (see also Chapter 32). We develop three models: the Banks and Bennett model in the framework of the above discussion, the Wilson model, and a modified version of the Wilson model incorporating more realistic assumptions.

BANKS AND BENNETT ANALYSIS OF DEVELOPMENT

Developmental Changes in Optics, Pupil, and Media Transmittance

Banks and Bennett (1988) examined the influence of eye growth and receptor maturation on the development of acuity and contrast sensitivity. They first examined the four optical properties that are important to the transmission of signals into the retinal image: eye size (specifically, posterior nodal distance), numerical aperture (pupil diameter divided by focal length), ocular media transmittance, and the OTF. The newborn's eye is significantly smaller than that of the adult. Because image magnification is proportional to the posterior nodal distance of an eye (the distance between the "center point" of the optics and the retina), an object of a given size projects to a smaller area on the retina (expressed in millimeters) in the newborn than in the adult. Banks and Bennett (1988) reported the posterior nodal distances of the newborn and adult eyes as 11.7 and 16.7 mm, respectively, a ratio of 1.43 (the adult/15-month-old ratio is about 1.16). Thus the retinal image of a small object is 1.43 times greater in the adult eye than in the newborn eye (when the image size is expressed in millimeters), a fact that should favor fine detail vision in the adult. In terms of the equations described above, in which all factors are expressed in degrees, it has the effect of enlarging the newborn's receptor aperture $[r(x, y)]$ and spacing $[s(x, y)]$.

Two factors affect the proportion of photons incident on the cornea that make it to the retina: the numerical aperture of the eye (P), and the transmittance of the ocular media (T). Retinal illuminance is proportional to the eye's numerical aperture. The newborn pupil is smaller than that of the adult: According to Salapatek and Banks (1978), 1-month-old and adult diameters at 66 cd/m² are 2.4 and 3.9 mm, respectively. However, the numerical apertures of the two eyes are similar because the age-related increase in pupil diameter is offset by the increase in posterior nodal distance (Dannemiller and Banks, 1983; Brown et al., 1987). Consequently,

we assumed that the retinal illuminance associated with a given target luminance does not change with age. Two elements affecting ocular media transmittance are known to change with development: the crystalline lens and macular pigments. In both cases transmittance is probably higher in the young eye (Bach and Seefelder, 1914; Werner, 1982; Bone et al., 1988), but the differences are small at all but short wavelengths. Banks and Bennett (1988) built differences in media transmittance into their calculations mostly because they examined some hue discriminations involving short wavelengths; here we assume the media transmittance is constant with age because we are concerned with spatial vision and broadband lights only. Thus we assume that the retinal illuminance associated with a given target luminance is the same in newborns and adults (i.e., P and T are the same).

No measurements of OTF $[O(u, v)]$ of the human newborn have been reported, but it is likely that the optical quality of the newborn eye greatly exceeds the resolution performance of the visual system as a whole. Banks and Bennett (1988) assumed therefore that the OTF is adult-like at birth, and we follow that assumption here by using adult OTFs from Campbell and Gubisch (1966) for all ages.

Retinal Development

Banks and Bennett (1988) also considered the effects of receptor maturation. Several investigators have reported that the retina is immature at birth, particularly in and around the fovea (Bach and Seefelder, 1914; Abramov et al., 1982; Hendrickson and Yuodelis, 1984; Yuodelis and Hendrickson, 1986). For instance, the diameter of the rod-free area of the retina decreases from about 5.4 degrees at birth to 2.3 degrees at maturity, a developmental change that is apparently the consequence of postnatal migration of foveal cones toward the center of the retina. Figure 6-8 shows tangential sections of the retina near the center of the fovea at birth, 15 months, and adulthood. An individual cone is outlined for clarity in each photograph. As one can see, the foveal cones of the newborn human are strikingly immature: Neonatal inner segments are much broader and shorter than their mature counterparts, and neonatal outer segments are much shorter than the adult versions. The cones of the retinal periphery are also immature at birth (see Chapter 17), but the differences between young and old versions are not as distinct as in the fovea.

In the adult, the inner segment of a foveal cone acts as a funnel, gathering light and guiding it to the outer segment where it isomerizes the photopigment. Banks and Bennett (1988) calculated the ability of the new-

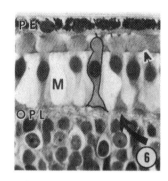

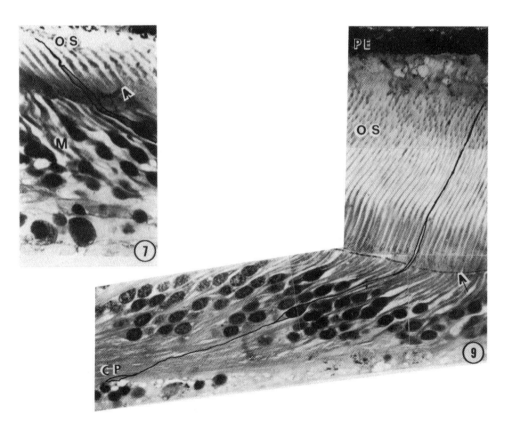

FIG. 6-8. Tangential sections of the retina near the center of the fovea at birth, 15 months, and adulthood. The magnification is the same in each panel. An individual cone is outlined for clarity in each photograph. The outer segments of the receptors are labeled OS, and the inner segments are just below the outer segments. See text for further discussion.

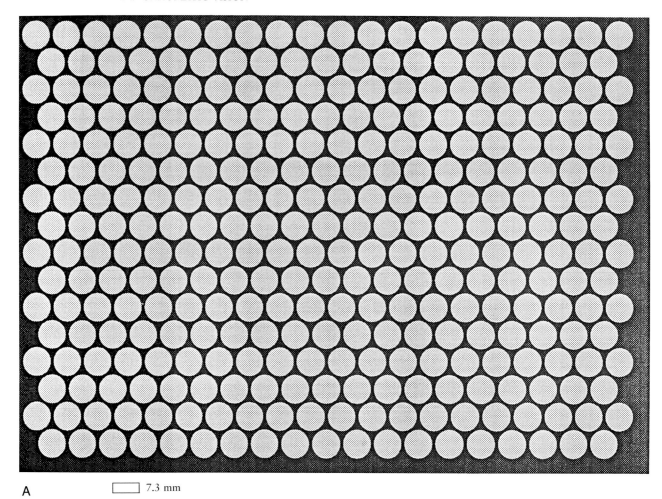

A   □ 7.3 mm

FIG. 6-9. Foveal cone lattices for (a) an adult and (b) a newborn. The white bars represent 0.5 minute. The gray areas represent the effective light collecting areas, that is, the receptor apertures. See text for further discussion.

born's foveal cone inner segments to perform this function. They concluded that the funneling or waveguide property of the immature inner segment cannot work properly; any photons that are not aimed directly at an outer segment are not absorbed. In other words, the effective aperture of newborn foveal cones appears to be the outer segment itself, a conclusion also reached by Brown et al. (1987) and Wilson (1988; see Chapter 32). Taking the smaller size of the newborn's eye into account, the angular diameter of the effective aperture—the outer segment—is approximately 0.35 minute. The effective aperture of adult foveal cones is, of course, the inner segment and is about 0.48 minute (Miller and Bernard, 1983; MacLeod et al., 1992). The effective aperture at 15 months is probably the inner segment, and its diameter is about 0.67 minute.

Banks and Bennett (1988) also calculated the average spacing between foveal cones, assuming a regular hexagonal arrangement. Based on the anatomical data of Yuodelis and Hendrickson (1986), they reported values

of 2.3, 1.27, and 0.58 minutes in the newborn, 15-month, and adult central foveae, respectively. The spacing changes are a consequence of receptor migration and increasing eye size. The Nyquist frequencies associated with such lattices are given by $1/\sqrt{3} * d)$ (Snyder and Miller, 1977) and are 15.1, 27.2, and 59.7 cpd for newborns, 15-month-olds, and adults, respectively.

These intercone distances and effective aperture diameters were used to construct the receptor lattices shown in Figure 6-9. The white bars represent 0.5 minute. The gray areas represent the effective light-collecting areas, that is, the receptor apertures. The effective collecting areas cover 2% of the fovea in newborns, 25% in 15-months-olds, and 62% in adults. Clearly, most incident photons are not collected within newborn cone apertures.

The efficiency of the outer segment (E)—that is, the proportion of photons striking the outer segment that are absorbed—also varies between neonates and adults. As shown in Figure 6-8, the lengths of newborn and

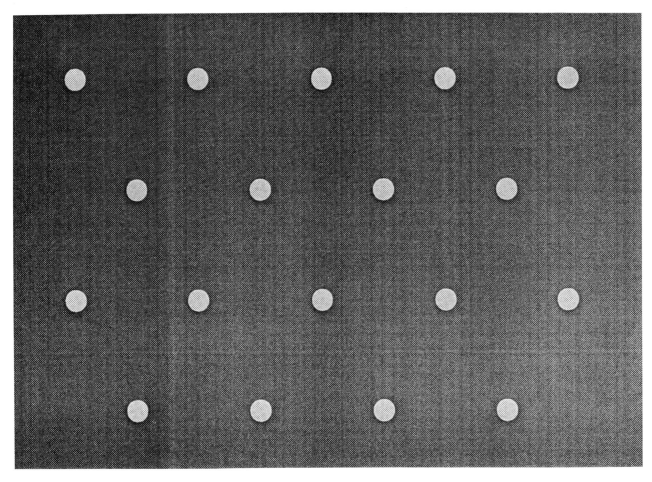

B   ⬚ 7.3 mm

FIG. 6-9. (continued)

adult outer segments differ substantially. In the cental fovea, the adult/newborn lengths ratio is about 16:1 and adult/15-month lengths ratio is about 2.2:1. Banks and Bennett assumed that the newborn and adult outer segments differ only in their widths and lengths (i.e., the photopigment concentrations and extinction coefficients are the same). They used Beer's law[5] to estimate the proportions of incident photons that produce isomerizations (Wyszecki and Stiles, 1982). By their calculations, the 16:1 and 2.2:1 path length ratios produce 10:1 and 1.8:1 ratios of the number of isomerizations for a given number of incident photons.

Taking into account the age-related changes in the factors discussed above and listed in Table 6-1, Banks and Bennett (1988) estimated that the adult central foveal cone lattice absorbs 350 times more photons than does the newborn lattice and four times more photons than the 15-month-old lattice. Stated another way, if identical patches of light are presented to newborn and adult eyes, roughly 350 photons are effectively absorbed in adult foveal cones for every photon absorbed in newborn cones. Because an ideal decision rule is used, the modeling of Banks and Bennett follows square-root law. Thus the 350-fold loss in newborns' photon catch should produce a roughly $\sqrt{350}$ (18.7-fold) drop in contrast sensitivity, and the fourfold loss in the 15-month catch should produce a twofold drop.

To summarize, Banks and Bennett (1988) assumed that four front-end properties of the visual system change with increasing age. (1) Image magnification increases with eye growth. (2) The effective receptor aperture $[r(x, y)]$ increases in size as the inner segment begins to act as a funnel. (3) The receptor spacing $[s(x, y)]$ decreases as cones migrate toward the fovea. (4) The efficiency of the outer segment (E) increases as it grows longer. As stated above, the consequence of increased image magnification is to decrease the aperture size and spacing of the receptors expressed in angular units.

_____

5. The number of absorptions is equal to $k * (1 - 10^{-c \cdot e \cdot l})$, where c = pigment concentration, e = extinction coefficient, l = segment length, and k = a constant.

Therefore the effects of these four developmental factors on Eqs. 1 and 2 are to: (1) make the newborn receptor aperture slightly smaller, decreasing its diameter from the adult value of 0.48 minute (Miller and Bernard, 1983) to about 0.35 minute; (2) increase the spacing between newborn cones from 0.58 minute to 2.3 minutes; and (3) decrease the newborn outer segment efficiency by a factor of 10. The 15-month aperture at 0.67 minute is actually larger than that in the adult; the 15-month values for the other factors fall between the neonatal and adult values but are closer to those of the adult.

In the next sections, we isolate these three effects and show, step by step, how they affect contrast sensitivity. As above, we do it by placing an ideal decision rule at the output of the schematic visual system in Figure 6-1 and varying the parameter under consideration while holding other parameters fixed.

Consequences of Age Changes in Outer Segment Efficiency

The effect of age-related changes in the outer segment efficiency (E) is shown in Figure 6-10. As in Figure 6-2, we assumed experimental conditions similar to those under which infant CSFs have been measured. Space-average luminance was 50 cd/m², large grating patches were used, and the pupil was natural with a diameter of 6 mm. The target duration was 250 ms, and threshold was the contrast required to achieve 71% correct, in a two-interval, forced-choice procedure. For construction of Figure 6-10, the OTF [$O(u, v)$] and NTF [$N(u, v)$] were flat, and receptor spacing [$s(x, y)$] and aperture diameter [$r(x, y)$] were set to 0.58 and 0.48 minute,

respectively, the values in the adult fovea. Media transmittance (T) and numerical aperture (P) were set to adult values for the fovea (Table 6-1). The curves show the contrast sensitivity of a system with an ideal decision rule when the adult, 15-month, and neonate outer segment efficiencies are those reported by Banks and Bennett (1988) and reproduced in Table 6-1.

Consequences of Age Changes in Receptor Spacing and Aperture

Figure 6-11 illustrates the effect of changes in receptor spacing and the diameter of the receptor aperture. Here peak sensitivity is normalized to 1 for the adult system, and the neonate and 15-month sensitivities are plotted relative to those values. When constructing this figure, the media transmittance and numerical aperture were set to adult values, the OTF and NTF were flat, and the outer segment efficiency was set to adult values. The figure shows that coarse receptor spacing and small receptor apertures in the neonate lead to reduced sensitivity for an otherwise ideal system. The 15-month sensitivity falls between that of the adult and the neonate.

Combined Effects

Figure 6-12 shows the CSFs once all the factors are included. At all ages, we assumed adult values for media transmittance, numerical aperture, and optical transfer [3.8 mm data of Campbell and Gubisch (1966)]. We also assumed a constant-bandwidth NTF. We then plugged in the age-appropriate values for receptor spacing, receptor aperture, and outer segment efficiency once the effect of image magnification had been incorpo-

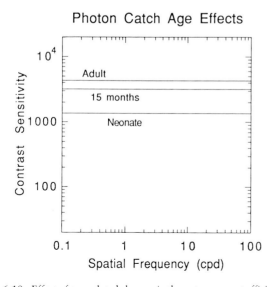

FIG. 6-10. Effect of age-related changes in the outer segment efficiency (E) on contrast sensitivity. See text for explanation.

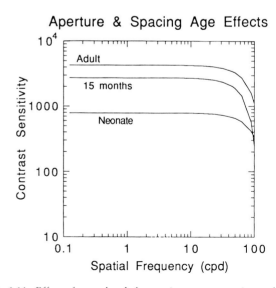

FIG. 6-11. Effect of age-related changes in receptor spacing and the diameter of the receptor aperture. See text for explanation.

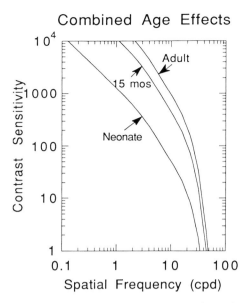

FIG. 6-12. CSFs once all factors are included. See text for explanation.

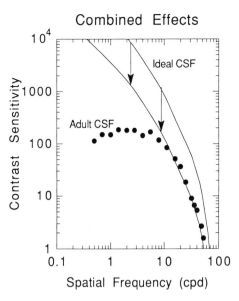

FIG. 6-13. Human adult and ideal CSFs. The data points represent the contrast sensitivity of observer M.S.B., which was measured at 50 cd/m², with large grating patches, 250 ms target duration, natural pupil of 6 mm, and 21FC procedure. The ideal CSF is for the same conditions, assuming mechanisms of constant bandwidth. The ideal CSF, once shifted downward by 1.4 log units (indicated by arrows), fits the data reasonably well from 6 to 60 cpd.

rated. The resulting CSFs are those of ideal observers, limited by the factors incorporated, for the assumed experimental conditions. There are clear developmental differences in the resulting CSFs; the neonatal CSF is essentially the same as the adult CSF shifted down by a factor of 18.7 ($\sqrt{350}$). The 15-month CSF falls between those of the neonate and the adult; it is nearly equivalent to an adult CSF shifted down by a factor of 2.

The differences among these functions represent the presumed consequences of information losses due to lower image magnification and the reduced photon catch that stems from greater receptor spacing, smaller receptor apertures, and lower outer segment efficiency. The differences are large, but are they large enough to account for the observed differences between real neonates and adults? To answer this question, let us evaluate a specific hypothesis.

Developmental hypothesis: Spatial contrast information losses are the same in neonatal and adult visual systems except for the losses caused by reduced image size and reduced photon catch resulting from receptor immaturities.

To evaluate this hypothesis, we conducted an experiment in which we measured the CSF of an experienced adult observer under conditions such as those used to measure CSFs in infants. The conditions were the same as those assumed for the construction of the ideal CSFs of Figures 6-2 through 6-5: two-interval, forced-choice procedure, large grating patches, luminance of 50 cd/m², duration of 250 ms, and natural pupil diameter of 6 mm. The resulting CSF is shown in Figure 6-13.

Figure 6-13 also shows the ideal CSF for the same conditions. Note that the ideal CSF is about 0.7 log

units higher than the empirical one across a broad range of spatial frequencies. However, when the ideal CSF is shifted downward, as shown by the arrows, it fits the empirical function well from 5 to 60 cpd, a result consistent with the earlier observations of Banks et al. (1987). Thus we can fit the observed contrast sensitivity data across a broad range of spatial frequencies if we assume that the processes not included in our analysis simply cause a uniform 0.7 log unit loss of contrast sensitivity.

If the developmental hypothesis stated above is correct—that information losses in the neonatal and adult visual systems are the same except for losses due to the immaturities incorporated in the model—we should be able to fit the neonate's empirical CSF by shifting the age-appropriate ideal CSF downward by the same 1.4 log units required to fit the adult data. We have done so in Figure 6-14. We have also plotted the behavioral data of Banks and Salapatek (1978) and the electrophysiological data of Norcia et al. (1990). The functions of Norcia et al. were collected at 220 cd/m², so we have shifted them downward according to square-root law to make them comparable. It is clear that the shifted ideal CSFs do not fit the observed data; much larger shifts than predicted by the Banks and Bennett (1988) analysis would be required to fit the data. We conclude, as did Banks and Bennett, that information losses among the front-end mechanisms they modeled are insufficient to account for the observed sensitivity deficits. The de-

Banks & Bennett Predictions (Neonate)

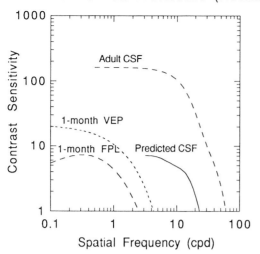

Wilson Adult Channels

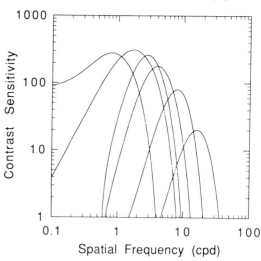

FIG. 6-14. Banks and Bennett neonate prediction and observed infant CSFs. The upper curve is the adult CSF used as a starting point for the modeling. The curve is the neonate prediction under the assumption that square-root law holds. As in Banks and Bennett (1988), the predictions have not been extended to low spatial frequencies, where square-root law does not hold in adults. The dotted curve represents 1-month VEP data from Norcia et al. (1990) and the dashed curve 1-month FPL data from Banks and Salapatek (1978). The preretinal, age-related changes considered by Banks and Bennett clearly do not account for the low contrast sensitivity observed in neonates.

FIG. 6-15. The six spatial-frequency-tuned channels of Wilson's model of adult spatial vision. The bandwidths of the channels were determined using a masking technique (Wilson et al., 1983); their vertical positions have been shifted to fit the adult VEP CSF of Norcia et al. (1990). Wilson's model of human visual development (Wilson 1988, see Chapter 32) consists of a set of transformations that are applied to these six functions.

velopmental hypothesis we entertained earlier is therefore false. Immaturities must exist at other stages of visual processing that are significant enough to limit performance more in neonates than those stages do in adults. Thus the earlier hypothesis must be replaced by one that states that postreceptoral immaturities also contribute significantly to the contrast sensitivity deficits observed early in life.

WILSON MODEL OF DEVELOPMENT

Description of the Model

Wilson's (1988; see Chapter 32) analysis has both similarities and dissimilarities to the Banks and Bennett (1988) analysis. His analysis is based on a model of adult contrast sensitivity and on two simple assumptions about human ocular and retinal development. The model of adult sensitivity incorporates the six spatial-frequency-tuned channels shown in Figure 6-15. The adult CSF is the envelope of the sensitivities of these six channels. The sensitivities have been shifted vertically to fit the adult VEP contrast sensitivity data of Norcia et al. (1990).

In his developmental model, Wilson transformed the channels of the adult model according to his assumptions about the developmental factors that have im-

portant effects on spatial visual tasks. Wilson assumed that only two significant developmental changes occur: (1) the photoreceptor outer segments become longer and hence absorb more of the incident photons; and (2) the photoreceptors move closer together allowing the adult visual system to signal higher spatial frequencies more accurately.

To incorporate the first factor, Wilson simply assumed that both the adult and infant visual systems follow square-root law at all spatial frequencies. He calculated that the adult's outer segment captures 7.2 times more photons than does that of the neonate; thus the effect of outer segment growth is to increase adult sensitivity by a factor of $\sqrt{7.2}$, or 2.7 relative to the neonate, independent of spatial frequency.

The implementation of the second factor is more complicated. Wilson made the following assumptions: (1) neonate foveal cones are 4.6 times farther apart than adult foveal cones; (2) the connections between cones and higher-order neurons do not change over the course of development, so a given higher-order neuron takes inputs from the same number of photoreceptors with the same weightings in neonates and adults; and (3) the size of the photoreceptor aperture (in degrees) does not change with age. These three assumptions have the following consequence: For a grating imaged on the retina, the neonate should have a 2.7 times lower sensitivity to a given spatial frequency as has the adult for a grating of a frequency 4.6 times higher. Figure 6-16A represents

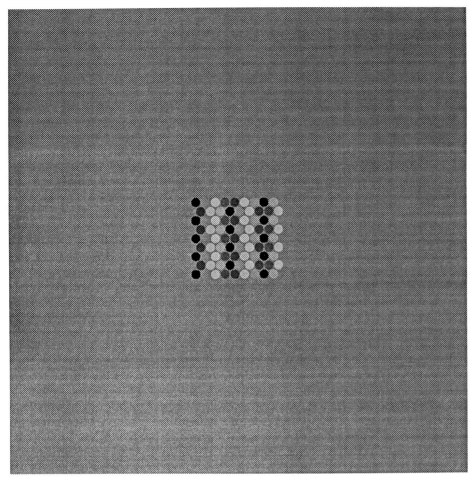

A

FIG. 6-16. Principle behind Wilson's horizontal shift. Circles represent individual receptor apertures, the gray value of each circle corresponding to the photon catch when a grating is presented. (A) Pattern of photon catches for an adult lattice (spacing equals 0.58 minute) when stimulated by a 30 cpd grating. (B) Photon catches when a neonatal lattice (spacing equals 0.58 × 4.6, or 2.67 minutes) is stimulated by a 6.5 cpd grating.

a photoreceptor lattice, with the receptors lined up with the peaks and troughs of a sinewave. The circles represent individual cones, with the intensities representing their photon catches. Figure 6-16B represents a lattice in which the receptors are 4.6 times farther apart; the photoreceptors line up with the peaks and troughs of a grating with a frequency 4.6 times higher than the grating in Figure 6-16A. When constructing the figure, we assumed that the eye's optics passed the two gratings equally well. Clearly, the spatial patterns of photoreceptor responses are identical in the two cases. If the photoreceptors catch the same number of photons (i.e., if they have the same aperture size), the total number of photons available to detect the sine wave is the same, and sensitivity should be equal in the two cases. This shift of sensitivity to lower spatial frequencies in the neonate is represented in Wilson's original model (Wilson, 1988) by a rigid 4.6-fold shift on the log-frequency axis of the adult channels to the left.

There is a complicating factor, however: Not all spatial frequencies are transmitted to the retina with equal fidelity. As described earlier in the chapter, the optics of the eye and the receptor aperture act as low-pass filters, severely attenuating the contrasts of high-frequency targets. These effects must be taken into account before the horizontal shift is applied. Wilson's original model did not take them into account, so the predicted acuities and contrast sensitivities were erroneous. In his revised model (see Chapter 32), the effects were taken into account as we describe here. To represent the attenuating effect of the optics, Wilson assumed a simplified version of an OTF $[O(u, v)]$ described by Geisler (1984) for a pupil diameter of 2 mm. He discussed the receptor aperture and its low-pass filtering

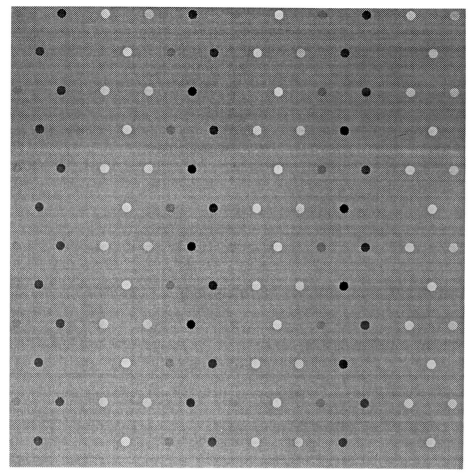

B

FIG. 6-16. (*continued*)

effects but chose to ignore it because the effects are small at the spatial frequencies of interest here. To determine the sensitivity of his adult model to retinal image contrast, Wilson divided the channel sensitivities by the OTF. This operation is illustrated in Figure 6-17. The dashed curves are the channel sensitivities from Figure 6-15, and the solid lines are the sensitivities after division by the OTF. They represent the channel sensitivities to retinal image contrasts rather than to external stimulus contrasts. The effect is to raise sensitivity to high frequencies.

To represent the consequence of cone migration, Wilson then applied a rigid shift to the left. The effect is illustrated in Figure 6-18; again the dashed curves represent the positions of the channels from the previous figure. He next put the optics back in. Wilson assumed that infant and adult OTFs are identical, so it involved multiplying the channels obtained from the prior steps by the same OTF. The 2-mm OTF is nearly flat with a value of about 1 from 1–10 cpd; hence this operation has little effect. In other words, by this set of assump-

tions, the shape of the neonate's CSF is determined almost entirely by the shape of the NTF.

Finally, to account for the neonate's shorter outer segments, Wilson divided the channel sensitivities by 2.7, as shown in Figure 6-19. The envelope of the resulting curves represents Wilson's prediction for the neonate's CSF. A similar sequence of operations with different parameters led to his predicted CSF for 15-month-olds.

Figure 6-20 shows Wilson's predicted CSF along with the infant CSF data of Norcia et al. (1990) and Banks and Salapatek (1978). The prediction matched the Norcia data at 2 months rather well but did not match Norcia's 1-month data or Banks and Salapatek's 1- or 2-month data; the younger infants' sensitivity was simply lower than predicted. Thus Wilson's model with parameters from neonatal anatomy does not fit neonatal data.

Figure 6-21 shows Wilson's predicted CSF for 15-month-olds along with the 8-month data from Norcia et al. (1990). The predicted and observed functions are

Dividing Out the Optics

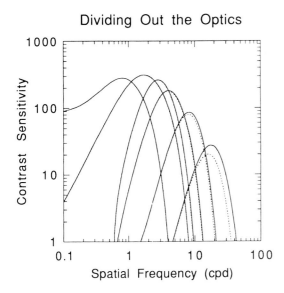

Neonate Prediction

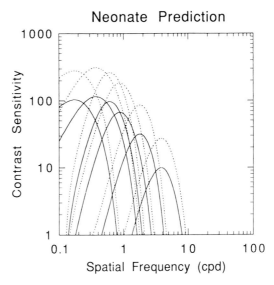

FIG. 6-17. First transformation of Wilson's (see Chapter 32) model: dividing out the OTF. Dotted and solid curves represent the positions of the channels before and after the transformation; the dotted curves are largely obscured because the transformation has no effect at low spatial frequencies. The envelope of the solid curves corresponds to the adult NTF; note that the cutoff point of the NTF implies that there is a neural limit that makes adults incapable of detecting frequencies higher than 42 cpd (at luminances around 220 cd/m²), contradicting the results of Williams (1985b) (see text).

FIG. 6-19. Third and fourth transformations of Wilson's model (see Chapter 32): multiplying by the neonate OTF and incorporating the effect of reduced outer segment length. The neonate OTF is assumed to be identical to that of the adult, which Wilson assumed is flat with a value of about 1.0 to around 10.0 cpd; multiplying by this OTF therefore has little effect. The effect of reduced outer segment length is a rigid downward shift by a factor of 2.7. Again, the dotted and solid curves represent the positions of the channels before and after the transformation. The envelope of the solid curves here corresponds to the predicted neonate CSF.

Horizontal Shift (Cone Migration)

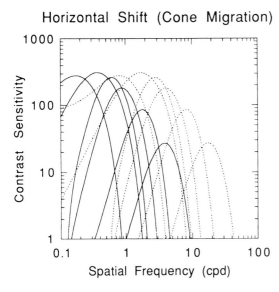

Wilson '91 Prediction (Neonate)

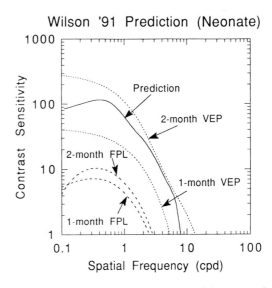

FIG. 6-18. Second transformation of Wilson's model (see Chapter 32): a rigid leftward shift by a factor of 4.6, reflecting the effect of photoreceptor migration. As in Figure 6-17, the dotted and solid curves represent the positions of the channels before and after the transformation. The envelope of the solid curves here corresponds to the neonate NTF.

FIG. 6-20. Wilson's prediction for neonates (solid curve) and some observed CSFs (see Chapter 32). The dotted curves are functions fit to data of Norcia et al. (1990); the data were collected at 1 and 2 months using a sweep-VEP technique. The dashed curves are functions fit to FPL data collected by Banks and Salapatek (1978) at 1 and 2 months. Although the VEP and FPL data were collected at different luminances, they have not been shifted in this figure (unlike in Figure 6-14). The Wilson prediction is close to the 2-month VEP CSF, but this comparison is not appropriate because the model prediction should be compared only to the 1-month data. Even before modifying Wilson's assumptions, the model does not fit the data.

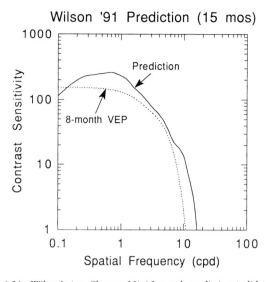

FIG. 6-21. Wilson's (see Chapter 32) 15-month prediction (solid curve) and an observed CSF. The dotted curve is a function fit to the data of Norcia et al. (1990); the data were collected at 8 months using a sweep-VEP technique. The fit is good before we modify Wilson's assumptions.

reasonably similar, but again the match occurs at different ages for the model and data. Wilson (see Chapter 32) also derived grating acuity predictions from his predicted contrast sensitivities and claimed that they matched the observations of Norcia et al. (Norcia and Tyler, 1985; Norcia et al., 1989) reasonably well near the end of the first year and moderately well during the first month. He concluded, therefore, that the major contribution to poor contrast sensitivity early in life is immaturities among front-end mechanisms.

Evaluation of the Wilson Model

When developing his model, Wilson made some assumptions that strike us as questionable: (1) the choice of data to which the adult model was fit (Norcia et al. 1990) to establish the starting point for the modeling; (2) that square-root law holds at all spatial frequencies at the illuminances at which the studies were run; (3) that the eye's optics in those studies are well represented by the OTF for a 2 mm pupil (Fig. 6-3); and (4) that the size of the photoreceptor aperture (in degrees) does not change with age. In this section, we discuss the problems with these assumptions. Later, we develop a version of Wilson's model incorporating assumptions that we think are more plausible.

Choice of Data Sets. The choice of data sets to represent adult and infant contrast sensitivities is important. The experimental conditions under which adults and infants were tested should be as similar as possible and should

be consistent with as many modeling parameters as possible.

When making the decision, one must consider the response measure. One could use behavioral techniques, such as the forced-choice preferential looking method (FPL) (Teller, 1979), or electrophysiological techniques, such as the sweep VEP (Norcia and Tyler, 1985). In the case of behavioral techniques, one must worry about differing effects of attention span in the adult and infant and other task variables that might affect performance (such as whether the method of adjustment or a two-alternative, forced-choice procedure was used in the adult). In the case of electrophysiological techniques, one must consider several effects that might change with age, such as signal conductance through the skull and sensitivity to different temporal frequencies.

Wilson (1988; see Chapter 32) used VEP estimates of adult and infant CSFs, according to Norcia et al. (1990), as the data to be modeled. Their choice may be the best one because the method used to determine sensitivity is identical in infants and adults; it does bring with it a problem, however. In infants sweep VEP estimates of sensitivity are generally higher than behaviorally estimated sensitivities, but in adults sweep VEP estimates are generally *lower* than behavioral estimates (Norcia and Tyler, 1985; Norcia et al., 1990; Allen et al., 1992). Some of this age-related difference between the two techniques is almost certainly due to reduced motivation on the infant's part, which presumably affects behavioral measurements more than VEP measurements. Of course, motivational variations are difficult to model quantitatively, which argues for using VEP data. On the other hand, signal conductance through the skull is an important determinant of VEP signal strength; and because adults have thicker skulls than infants, the VEP signal may be more attenuated in mature observers. In our opinion, this conductance effect may well lower adult sensitivity relative to the infant, an effect that should be explicitly included in any model of the development of VEP sensitivity. The omission of this factor makes Wilson's model fit the data better than it should given the factors he considered.

Also when choosing the data set to model, one must consider the stimulus conditions: the luminance, size, duration, and flicker rate of the stimulus, the observer's pupil diameter, the threshold criterion, and more. We discuss this issue in the next two sections.

Assumption of Square-Root Law. The most important of the four questionable assumptions is the one concerning the relation between sensitivity and the number of caught photons. Both Wilson (1988, 1993) and Banks and Bennett (1988) assumed square-root law when calculating the effects of reduced numbers of captured photons on contrast sensitivity. Banks and Bennett restricted their prediction to spatial frequencies above 3 cpd, but Wilson made predictions for frequencies as low as 0.15 cpd. The problem is that square-root law does not hold at all spatial frequencies and luminances. As van Nes and Bouman (1967), Kelly (1977), and Koenderink and van Doorn (1978) have shown, for every spatial frequency there is a retinal illuminance above which sensitivity ceases to rise with increasing illumination. In other words, the visual system follows Weber's rather than square-root law at sufficiently high illuminances, and the illuminance at which this transition occurs is lower for lower spatial frequencies. Assuming (as Banks and Bennett did) that infants and adults are affected similarly by reductions in the number of available photons, it means that the effect of reduced photon catch due to shorter outer segments and more widely spaced photoreceptors is probably smaller than predicted by Wilson, particularly at low spatial frequencies. We discuss this point in greater depth later for both the Wilson and the Banks and Bennett analyses.

Optics. The third problem concerns the OTF [$O(u, v)$] Wilson used to represent the effects of the human optics in the Norcia et al. (1990) experiment. This OTF is a simplified version of an equation fit by Geisler (1984) to modulation transfer measurements made by Campbell and Gubisch (1966) for a 2-mm artificial pupil. Geisler's full 2-mm OTF is shown in Figure 6-3; the equation Geisler used is the difference of two gaussians. Wilson argued that because he was primarily interested in predicting acuity, he only needed to use one of the two gaussians: the one extending to higher spatial frequencies. This assumption allowed him to derive a simple analytical expression for his infant acuity prediction, but the assumption is questionable because his infant acuity prediction is down in the region affected by the second, lower-frequency gaussian and because he later went on to predict the entire neonate CSF, the shape of which is certainly affected by the second gaussian. These errors are not significant, however, because they are quantitatively small.

A more serious problem is Wilson's implicit assumption that the pupil diameters of the observers in the experiments of Norcia et al. (1990) were 2 mm. Those experiments were run at a luminance of 220 cd/m² with natural pupils. At that luminance, adult pupil diameters are 2.4–4.3 mm, with a mean of about 3.5 mm (Spring and Stiles, 1948). Campbell and Gubisch's (1966) OTF for a 3.8-mm pupil is shown as the solid curve in Figure 6-3. The attenuation of high frequencies is obviously more severe at 3.8 than at 2.0 mm. Consequently, the use of a 3.8-mm OTF, which is more realistic for the experimental conditions under consideration here, has a significant effect on the infant predictions, particularly on the predictions of acuity and high-frequency contrast sensitivity. We show this later.

Receptor Aperture. Wilson assumed that the angular diameter of the receptor aperture is about 0.5 minute and does not change with development, which follows from his assumption that the outer segment is the effective aperture of foveal cones (see discussion of Figure 32-1). The problem is that the effective receptor aperture in the adult fovea is the inner segment, not the outer segment (Miller and Bernard, 1983; MacLeod et al., 1992), and the diameter of the mature inner segment is larger than that of the outer segment. Banks and Bennett assumed that the effective cone apertures are the inner segment in adults and outer segments in neonates; the corresponding diameters are 0.48 and 0.35 minute in adults and neonates, respectively. At 15 months, the receptor aperture is probably the inner segment which, at 0.67 minute, is considerably larger.

The size of the receptor aperture affects the proportion of incident photons that are captured by the receptors and, owing to the low-pass filtering of the aperture [$R(u, v)$], it affects the high-frequency slope of the CSF. The effects are small, but we include them in the reanalysis of Wilson's model anyway.

DIFFERENCES BETWEEN THE APPROACHES

We now turn to the differences between the Wilson and the Banks and Bennett analyses. Wilson (see Chapter 32) argued that the key difference is the way in which the effects of cone migration are incorporated. Wilson assumed that all connections between photoreceptors and higher neurons are maintained in development, so a neuron responding to a range of low frequencies at birth responds to a higher range at maturity because the receptors that feed it have moved closer together. Thus the effect of tighter receptor spacing with increasing age is a horizontal shift on the log spatial frequency axis. As pointed out by Wilson (see Chapter 32), Banks and Bennett incorporated the spacing effect as a vertical shift. Wilson claimed that it requires that the connections change with age. This statement is false. In fact, given square-root law and the NTFs [$N(u, v)$] assumed by Banks and Bennett for the adult and the infant, these two methods of implementing the effects of cone migration are exactly equivalent.

To understand, consider a developing visual system in which the only change from birth to maturity is a fourfold decrease in receptor spacing. This shrinking of the photoreceptor lattice would be represented in Wilson's model by shifting the NTF to the right by a factor of 4; in the Banks and Bennett analysis, this lattice would capture a higher proportion of the incident pho-

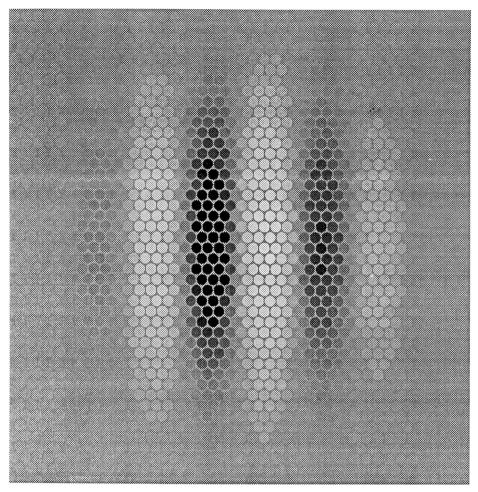

A

FIG. 6-22. Adult and infant receptive fields from Banks and Bennett (1988). Circles represent individual photoreceptors, with the gray value of each circle corresponding to the weight applied to the output of that photoreceptor. (A) Adult receptive field tuned to 10 cpd. (B) Adult receptive field tuned to 40 cpd. (C) Neonate receptive field tuned to 10 cpd; it is identical to the receptive field in (B) except that the photoreceptors are four times farther apart, making the point that the Banks and Bennett model can be thought of as a horizontal-shift model (provided it is restricted to regions of the spatial-frequency axis where square-root law holds and a linear NTF with a slope of − 1 is a good approximation).

tons (by a factor of 4²); so if square-root law holds, the NTF should be shifted upward by a factor of 4. Recall, however, that Banks and Bennett assumed at intermediate and high spatial frequencies (the only range over which they made a prediction) that the NTF is a line with slope − 1 on a log-log plot. Obviously, for this NTF a horizontal shift by a factor of 4 is equivalent to a vertical shift by the same amount. This point is made another way in Figure 6-22, which shows three sample ideal weighting functions (the model's equivalent of receptive fields) from the Banks and Bennett analysis. Figure 6-22A shows the adult weighting function when the stimulus to be detected is a Gabor patch of 10 cpd. Each circle represents an individual cone, the size representing the diameter of the aperture, and the intensity

representing the weight assigned to the output. Figure 6-22B shows the adult function for detecting 40 cpd and Figure 6-22C the infant function for detecting 10 cpd. Note that the infant weighting function for detecting 10 cpd is just a stretched version of the adult function for detecting 40 cpd. Thus given an implicit NTF of the sort assumed by Banks and Bennett and square-root law, the vertical-shift method of Banks and Bennett is perfectly compatible with connections being maintained between photoreceptors and higher neurons. Therefore the Wilson and Banks and Bennett analyses are equivalent on this point.

Earlier, we discussed some assumptions in Wilson's model, which to us seem questionable: the choice of data to represent the adult, the OTF, that square-root

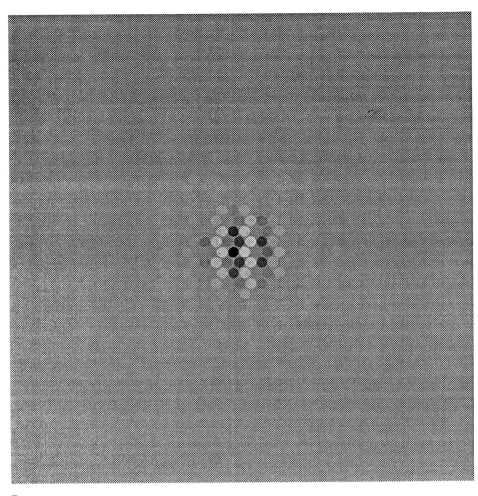

B

FIG. 6-22. (*continued*)

law holds everywhere, and the omission of the effects of changing receptor aperture. We have changed these assumptions to more reasonable ones in the next section in which we modify the Wilson model. The most significant of the assumptions is the manner in which square-root law was applied, and the difference on this point between the two analyses probably represents a difference in philosophy: Wilson's approach is simply bolder than that of Banks and Bennett. Wilson used a model of adult spatial vision as his starting point and applied the presumed effect of reduced photon catch everywhere. Banks and Bennett attempted to keep the number of assumptions to a minimum by starting with an ideal observer and tracing information losses due to immature optics and photoreceptors. They made only developmental predictions on the portion of the CSF for which square-root law holds in adults and for which the ideal observer analysis of Banks et al. (1987) predicted the shape of the adult CSF. Hence Wilson applied square-root law at all spatial frequencies, whereas Banks and Bennett applied it only to frequencies above 3 cpd.

Assumptions about the domain over which square-root law applies are crucial to modeling the factors of interest here. We know in adults that contrast sensitivity tends to follow square-root law at low to moderate photopic illuminances and medium to high spatial frequencies; and that sensitivity tends to follow Weber's law at high illuminances and low spatial frequencies (van Nes and Bouman, 1967; Kelly, 1977; Koenderink and van Doorn, 1978). Unfortunately, we do not know the range of spatial frequencies and illuminances in which square-root law holds in infants; that is, we do not know the relation between infant photopic contrast sensitivity and light level (Dannemiller and Banks, 1983; Brown et al., 1987; Fiorentini et al., 1990; Allen et al., 1992). Until such data are available, the best one can do is consider the relation in adults and assume that it is similar in infants. We have done so when creating modified versions of Wilson's model: Specifically, we assumed both square-root law and the law implied by van Nes and Bouman's data with the expectation that the correct assumption is contained within these extremes.

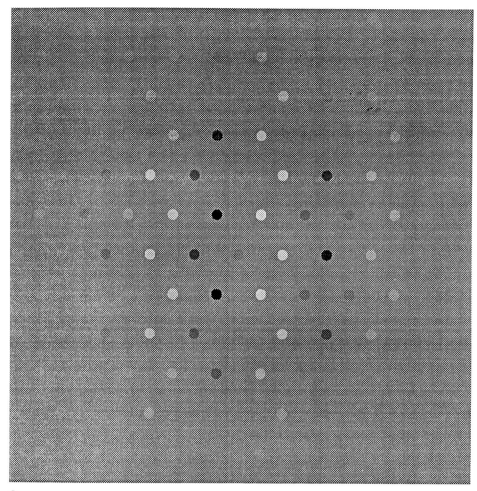

C

FIG. 6-22. (continued)

MODIFIED VERSION OF WILSON'S MODEL

The central concept of Wilson's model—that cone migration causes a horizontal shift of the NTF toward higher spatial frequencies with maturation—is interesting and plausible, but we questioned some of his assumptions about modeling parameters and data sets. Thus we modified his model by incorporating more plausible parameters and more representative data sets while retaining the underlying principle.

First, because we think that considering only VEP data artificially decreases the adult–neonate gap that has to be explained, we used a psychophysical CSF to represent the adult. The CSF data were collected by M.S.B., who has measured his own OTF using the technique of Santamaria et al. (1987); this consideration is important because there is considerable variation in optical quality among individuals (Howland and Howland, 1976; Artal et al., 1988). For most spatial fre-

quencies the stimuli were sine wave gratings, but at the highest frequencies we used square waves, a maneuver that allowed us to measure more of the high-frequency limb of the CSF. Space-average luminance was 50 cd/ m². Under these conditions, M.S.B.'s (natural) pupil diameter is 6 mm, resulting in a retinal illuminance of approximately 1400 td. Stimulus duration was 250 ms. At every spatial frequency, at least 10 grating cycles were presented. Thresholds were estimated using a 2IFC procedure and a two-down, one-up staircase. The choices of luminance, duration, and size of the stimulus reflect compromises in our attempt to make the data comparable to the conditions under which infant CSF's have been measured.

The function fit to these data is shown in Figure 6-13. This adult CSF is different in shape from the envelope of the six mechanisms in Wilson's adult model, probably reflecting the fact that M.S.B.'s optics are unusually sharp. Therefore, instead of fitting the mechanisms of Wilson's adult model to these data, we applied the transformations of Wilson's developmental model directly to the adult CSF.

We used the measured OTF of the adult observer. Unfortunately, the largest pupil diameter for which we have his OTF was 4 mm, and his pupil diameter in the psychophysical experiment was 6 mm. This OTF is shown by the dashed curve in Figure 6-3 and was used to divide the adult data before executing the horizontal shift. To estimate the OTFs of the infants in the Banks and Salapatek (1978) and Norcia et al (1990) studies, we needed some idea of their pupil diameters; we used the average observer of Spring and Stiles (1948), who at Banks and Salapatek's luminance of 55 cd/m² had a pupil diameter of about 4.5 mm and at Norcia's luminance of 220 cd/m² a diameter of about 3.5 mm. Neonatal pupil diameters appear to be smaller than those of adults, but the numerical apertures are similar. Because the numerical aperture, rather than the pupil diameter per se, is the best predictor of optical quality (Gaskill, 1978), we used Campbell and Gubisch's 3.8-mm OTF to represent the infant optics for these conditions (3.8 being the closest measured value to 3.5–4.5 mm). Specifically, the 3.8-mm OTF was used to multiply the NTF after the horizontal shift. The effects due to age-related changes in the aperture transfer function [$R(u, v)$] were also incorporated, but these effects are small.

As stated above, we modeled the effect of the reduced photon catch due to the shorter outer segment (E) assuming both square-root law and the law implied by van Nes and Bouman's (1967) data. The adult-to-neonate drop in contrast sensitivity implied by square-root law is a rigid vertical shift by a factor of 3.4 (we used the number supplied by Banks and Bennett instead of that given by Wilson to simplify the comparison of the models). The change from adulthood to 15 months is smaller, a factor of 1.3. To implement the changes implied by van Nes and Bouman's data, we assumed that the effect of changes in illuminance on contrast sensitivity are similar in adults and neonates except for a fourfold shift in the frequency at which the effects occur (and a twofold shift for 15-month-olds). The changes implied by van Nes and Bouman's data are smaller than those implied by square-root law at lower spatial frequencies. Indeed, below 2 cpd there is no effect of reduced photon catch.

We also modified Wilson's assumptions about age-related changes in the receptor aperture. Wilson's representation of the effects of photoreceptor migration by a rigid horizontal shift on a log-frequency axis involves the implicit assumption that the aperture diameter does not change with age (see Chapter 32). As discussed above, the aperture width changes from 0.35 minute in the neonate to 0.67 minute at 15 months to 0.48 minute in the adult. In order to model the effect of changing

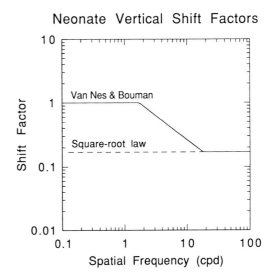

FIG. 6-23. Neonate vertical shift factors for our modification of Wilson's model (see Chapter 32) under two assumptions about how reduced photon catch affects contrast sensitivity. These figures show the combined effects of reduced outer segment length and changing photoreceptor aperture diameter. Dashed line is the shift factor assuming square-root law holds at all spatial frequencies; it is a rigid downward shift by a factor of 5.9. Solid line is the shift factor using the data of van Nes and Bouman (1967); it is smaller than the square-root law shift, and there is no shift below 2 cpd.

aperture size on photon catch, we divided the number of photons caught by the adult receptor lattice by the ratio of the adult aperture area to the infant aperture area. Again, we used the same two assumptions (square-root law and the van Nes and Bouman data) to calculate the effect of reduced quantum catch on sensitivity. Figure 6-23 shows the vertical shift factor, combining the outer segment length effect and the receptor aperture effect for the neonate under these two assumptions. The dashed lines represent square-root law and the solid lines the van Nes and Bouman data. The shift factor for 15-month-olds is much smaller than that for neonates: Assuming square-root law, it is a factor of only 1.3.

The results of all these changes on the neonate and 15-month predictions are shown in Figure 6-24. The solid curves represent the two predictions, based on the square-root law and on van Nes and Bouman's data[6]; the dotted curves represent infant VEP data, and the dashed curves are infant FPL data. In all cases, the discrepancy between predictions and data is considerable; the predicted infant sensitivities across a broad range of medium and high spatial frequencies are a log unit or more higher than the observations. We could not generate an acuity prediction because the curves

---

6. The predictions shown are for the Banks and Salapatek data (1978). The predictions for the Norcia et al. (1990) data are slightly higher but so similar that we did not plot them separately.

Modified Wilson Prediction (Neonate)

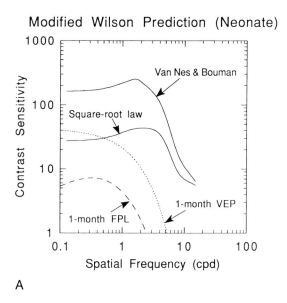

A

Modified Wilson Prediction (15 mos.)

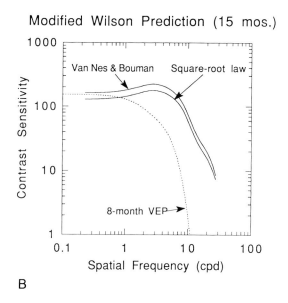

B

FIG. 6-24. Modified Wilson neonate (A) and 15-month (B) predictions. Solid curves are the model predictions under both square-root law and van Nes and Bouman (1967) assumptions; dotted curves represent VEP data from Norcia et al. (1990); and dashed curves represent FPL data from Banks and Salapatek (1978). The predictions approach the data only at low spatial frequencies.

never approach the horizontal axis; in order to make such a prediction, we would need adult data at sensitivities much less than 1.

Thus once more reasonable assumptions about some of the modeling parameters are employed, Wilson's model still does not account for the low contrast sensitivity of the human neonate; indeed, the prediction is farther off than before. The predictions of the original model at

15 months were similar to 8-month data, which is not the case with the modified model: predicted medium- and high-frequency sensitivities at 15 months are 0.5– 1.5 log units higher than the observations at 8 months. Presumably, contrast sensitivity improves between those two ages, so perhaps data collected at 15 months will ultimately confirm the predictions.

We have applied the same assumptions about square-

Same NTF Prediction (Neonate)

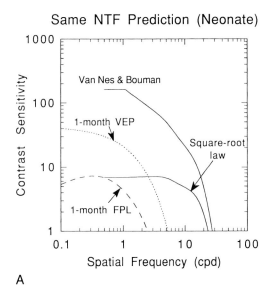

A

Same NTF Prediction (15 mos.)

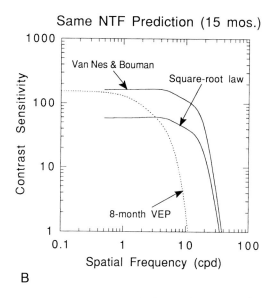

B

FIG. 6-25. Neonate (A) and 15-month (B) predictions under the assumption that the infant NTF is identical to that of the adult at all spatial frequencies, in contrast to laterally shifted, as in Wilson's model, or identical only at high spatial frequencies, as in the Banks and Bennett model. Unlike these two models, the neural implementation of this assumption would require that connections between

receptors and higher neurons be broken and reestablished over the course of development. At each age, all receptive fields would have the same spatial profiles; adult cortical neurons would have to take inputs from many more photoreceptors. None of these assumptions comes close to explaining the observed CSFs.

root law and van Nes and Bouman's data to the Banks and Bennett model. The results are shown in Figure 6-25.

Having taken the liberty of modifying Wilson's model to include modeling parameters more similar to those used in the Banks and Bennett analysis, we should delineate any remaining differences between the two approaches. The approaches are similar in regard to how they treat changes in outer segment efficiency and eye size; so once we included the OTF and receptor apertures used by Banks and Bennett at different ages and inserted the same adult CSF as the starting point for modeling, what differences if any remain? There are three: (1) The effects of cone migration: Banks and Bennett assumed that the only direct consequence of cone migration is to change the photon catch and that that produces a vertical shift in predicted contrast sensitivity; Wilson assumed that the consequence of migration is a change in the preferred frequencies of his six channels and that that produces a horizontal shift of the NTF. (2) The shape of the NTF: Banks and Bennett implicitly assumed a constant-bandwidth NTF, whereas Wilson implicitly assumed an NTF of a different shape (at low and intermediate frequencies anyway) that was required to account for his adult CSF data. (3) The assumed domains over which square-root law applies: Banks and Bennett restricted their analyses to spatial frequencies for which that assumption has been shown to be valid in adults, and Wilson applied square-root law everywhere. Interestingly, the differing assumptions concerning cone migration have no effect on the predictions because, for the NTF implied by Banks and Bennett's analysis, their vertical shifts due to changes in cone spacing are exactly equivalent to Wilson's horizontal shifts. So the only differences are in the shapes of the NTFs and the domain over which square-root law is assumed to apply. It is important to note that on the high-frequency limb of the CSF the assumptions in regard to NTFs and square-root law are similar.

CONCLUSION

Yuodelis and Hendrickson's (1986) description of the development of foveal cones in human infants stimulated two analyses of the factors limiting spatial vision early in life. Although the analyses used essentially the same values for the factors under examination, they came to nearly opposite conclusions. Banks and Bennett (1988) concluded that these factors imposed important constraints but by themselves were insufficient to explain the poor contrast sensitivity and acuity of human neonates; they argued that immaturities among postreceptoral processes must also limit early spatial vision.

Wilson (1988) (see also Chapter 32), on the other hand, concluded that these factors were nearly sufficient and, by inference, that postreceptoral processes are not a major limit to early vision.

This chapter reviewed the two analyses and showed that neither model as originally stated actually fits the observed data, although Wilson's predictions come closer. However, some of the assumptions in Wilson's model are questionable. To see the effects of these assumptions, we modified his model while retaining its main principles. We found that these modifications led to a poorer fit, particularly at intermediate to high spatial frequencies where the modified Wilson model falls a log unit short of fitting the observed data. Consequently, both sorts of analysis lead to the conclusion that optical and photoreceptor immaturities alone are insufficient to explain the low contrast sensitivity and acuity of the human infant.

A useful result of these analyses would be a quantification of the unexplained gap between infant and adult sensitivity (the sensitivity loss that cannot be explained by age-related changes in optics and receptors). This is, unfortunately, impossible at this time because we simply do not know enough about how infants' performance is affected by the level of illumination in the tasks considered here: As we showed, differing assumptions about the effect of illumination lead to widely disparate predictions. Until we know more about this subject, further progress in understanding the effects of front-end immaturities will be difficult to achieve.

Acknowledgments. The authors thank Kirk Swenson for assistance in producing the cone lattice schematics and Stanley Klein for comments on an earlier version. This research was supported by NIH grant HD-19927 to M.S.B.

REFERENCES

ABRAMOV, I., GORDON, J., HENDRICKSON, A., HAINLINE, L., DOBSON, V., AND LABOSSIERE, E. (1982). The retina of the newborn human infant. *Science* 217, 265–267.

ALLEN, D., BENNETT, P. J., AND BANKS, M. S. (1992). The effects of luminance on FPL and VEP acuity in human infants. *Vision Res.* 32, 2005–2012.

ARTAL, P., SANTAMARIA, J., AND BESCOS, J. (1988). Phase-transfer function of the human eye and its influence on point-spread function and wave aberration. *J. Opt. Soc. Am.* [A] 5, 1791–1795.

BACH, L., AND SEEFELDER, R. (1914). *Atlas zur Entwicklungsgeschichte des Menschlichen Auges.* Berlin: Verlag von Wilhelm Engelmann.

BANKS, M. S., AND BENNETT, P. J. (1988). Optical and photoreceptor immaturities limit the spatial and chromatic vision of human neonates. *J. Opt. Soc. Am.* [A] 5, 2059–2079.

BANKS, M. S., AND SALAPATEK, P. (1978). Acuity and contrast sensitivity in 1-, 2-, and 3-month-old human infants. *Invest. Ophthalmol. Vis. Sci.* 17, 361–365.

BANKS, M. S., AND SALAPATEK, P. (1983). Infant visual perception.

In M. Haith and J. Campos (eds.). *Biology and Infancy*. New York: Wiley, pp. 435–471.

Banks, M. S., Geisler, W. S., and Bennett, P. J. (1987). The physical limits of grating visibility. *Vision Res.* 27, 1915–1924.

Barlow, H. B. (1958). Temporal and spatial summation in human vision at different background intensities. *J. Physiol. (Lond.)* 141, 337–350.

Blakemore, C., and Campbell, F. W. (1969). On the existence of neurons in the human visual system selectively sensitive to the orientation and size of retinal images. *J. Physiol. (Lond.)* 203, 237–260.

Bone, R. A., Landrum, J. T., Fernandez, L., and Tarsis, S. L. (1988). Analysis of macular pigment by HPLC: retinal distribution and age study. *Invest. Ophthalmol. Vis. Sci.* 29, 843–849.

Brown, A. M. (1990). Development of visual sensitivity to light and color vision in human infants: a critical review. *Vision Res.* 30, 1159–1188.

Brown, A. M., Dobson, V., and Maier, J. (1987). Visual acuity of human infants at scotopic, mesopic, and photopic luminances. *Vision Res.* 27, 1845–1858.

Campbell, F. W., and Gubisch, R. W. (1966). Optical quality of the human eye. *J. Physiol. (Lond.)* 186, 558–578.

Campbell, F. W., and Robson, J. G. (1968). Application of Fourier analysis to the visibility of gratings. *J. Physiol. (Lond.)* 197, 551–556.

Coletta, N. J., and Ethirajan, K. (1991). Interference fringe acuity as a function of light level. *Invest. Ophthalmol. Vis. Sci.* 32 (suppl.), 699.

Dannemiller, J. L., and Banks, M. S. (1983). The development of light adaptation in human infants. *Vision Res.* 23, 599–609.

Dobson, V., and Teller, D. Y. (1978). Visual acuity in human infants: a review and comparison of behavioral and electrophysiological techniques. *Vision Res.* 18, 1469–1483.

Fiorentini, A., Pirchio, M., and Spinelli, D. (1990). Scotopic contrast sensitivity in infants evaluated by evoked potentials. *Invest. Ophthalmol. Vis. Sci.* 19, 950–955.

Gaskill, J. D. (1978). *Linear Systems, Fourier Transforms, and Optics*. New York: Wiley.

Geisler, W. S. (1984). Physical limits of acuity and hyperacuity. *J. Opt. Soc. Am. [A]* 1, 775–782.

Hendrickson, A., and Yuodelis, C. (1984). The morphological development of the human fovea. *Ophthalmology* 91, 603–612.

Howland, B., and Howland, H. C. (1976). Subjective measurement of high-order aberations of the eye. *Science* 193, 580–582.

Jacobs, D. S., and Blakemore, C. (1988). Factors limiting the postnatal development of visual acuity in the monkey. *Vision Res.* 28, 947–958.

Kelly, D. H. (1977). Visual contrast sensitivity. *Opt. Acta (Lond.)* 24, 107–129.

Koenderink, J. J., and van Doorn, A. J. (1978). Visual detection of spatial contrast; influence of location in the visual field, target extent and illuminance level. *Biol. Cybern.* 30, 157–167.

Larsen, J. S. (1971). The sagittal growth of the eye. IV. Ultrasonic measurement of the axial length of the eye from birth to puberty. *Acta Ophthalmol. (Copenh.)* 49, 873–886.

MacLeod, D. I. A., Williams, D. R., and Makous, W. (1992). A visual nonlinearity fed by single cones. *Vision Res.* 32, 347–363.

Miller, W. H., and Bernard, G. D. (1983). Averaging over the foveal receptor aperture curtails aliasing. *Vision Res.* 23, 1365–1370.

Norcia, A. M., and Tyler, C. W. (1985). Spatial frequency sweep VEP: visual acuity during the first year of life. *Vision Res.* 25, 1399–1408.

Norcia, A. M., Tyler, C. W., and Hamer, R. D. (1990). Development of contrast sensitivity in the human infant. *Vision Res.* 30, 1475–1486.

Rose, A. (1942). The relative sensitivities of television pick-up tubes, photographic film, and the human eye. *Proc. IRE* 30, 293–300.

Salapatek, P., and Banks, M. S. (1978). Infant sensory assessment: vision. In F. D. Minifie and L. L. Lloyd (eds.). *Communicative and Cognitive Abilities: Early Behavioral Assessment*. Baltimore: University Park Press.

Santamaria, J., Artal, P., and Bescos, J. (1987). Determination of the point-spread function of human eyes using a hybrid optical-digital method. *J. Opt. Soc. Am. [A]* 4, 1109–1114.

Shlaer, S. (1937). The relation between visual acuity and illumination. *J. Gen. Physiol.* 21, 165–187.

Snyder, A. W., and Miller, W. H. (1977). Photoreceptor diameter and spacing for highest resolving power. *J. Opt. Soc. Am* 67, 696–698.

Spring, K. H., and Stiles, W. S. (1948). Variation of pupil size with change in the angle at which the light stimulus strikes the retina. *Br. J. Ophthalmol* 32, 340–346.

Teller, D. Y. (1979). The forced-choice preferential looking procedure: a psychophysical technique for use with human infants. *Infant Behav. Dev.* 2, 135–153.

Van Nes, F. L., and Bouman, M. A. (1967). Spatial modulation transfer in the human eye. *J. Opt. Soc. Am.* 57, 401.

Watson, A. (1985). The ideal observer concept as a modeling tool. In *Frontiers of Visual Science: Proceedings of the 1985 Symposium*. Washington, DC: National Academy of Sciences, pp. 32–37.

Werner, J. S. (1982). Development of scotopic sensitivity and the absorption spectrum of the human ocular media. *J. Opt. Soc. Am.* 72, 247–258.

Williams, D. R. (1985a). Aliasing in human foveal vision. *Vision Res.* 25, 195–205.

Williams, D. R. (1985b). Visibility of interference fringes near the resolution limit. *J. Opt. Soc. Am. [A]* 2, 1087–1093.

Wilson, H. R. (1988). Development of spatiotemporal mechanisms in infant vision. *Vision Res.* 28, 611–628.

Wilson, H. R., McFarlane, D. K., and Phillips, G. C. (1983). Spatial frequency tuning of orientation selective units estimated by oblique masking. *Vision Res.* 23, 873–882.

Wyszecki, G., and Stiles, W. S. (1982). *Color Science: Concepts and Methods, Quantitative Data and Formulae*. New York: Wiley.

Yuodelis, C., and Hendrickson, A. (1986). A qualitative and quantitative analysis of the human fovea during development. *Vision Res.* 26, 847–855.

7 | Development of the human visual field

D. LUISA MAYER AND ANNE B. FULTON

Why study the visual field of infants? First, the gradient of sensitivity from central to peripheral retinal loci, which in adults has been ascribed to cortical scaling (e.g., Virsu and Rovamo, 1979) or to ganglion cell density (e.g., Frisen and Frisen, 1976; Drasdo, 1977; Perry and Cowey, 1985; Wassle et al., 1989; Banks et al., 1991), remains to be described for the developing visual system. Second, study specifically of peripheral vision, contrasted with central vision, delineates the contribution of central versus peripheral retinal stimulation on photopic visual functions. Much research on infant photopic vision has been intended and assumed to study central visual field (i.e., foveal capacities); examples include acuity and contrast sensitivity, spectral sensitivity, and color vision. However, peripheral visual function may contribute to the presumed measurement of foveal function using preferential looking (PL) methods because with PL infants detect eccentrically located stimuli. The final reason is that clinical needs compel the development of perimetric methods for the assessment of young patients.

The visual field of adults is measured using kinetic or static methods. In both, a peripheral light is presented while the adult subject constantly fixates a stimulus in the center of a perimeter (most often a hemisphere). The adult signals when the light is seen, usually with a buzzer press. For kinetic testing, the light spot is moved along a radius or meridian from a nonseeing portion of the visual field to a seeing portion. The eccentric position at which the adult first detects the light on a number of meridia plots the circumference of the field for that light. This circumference is called the *isopter* for that target. In static perimetry, spots of light are presented briefly at discrete peripheral locations. The adult's threshold (or a measure related to threshold) for detecting the light spot is derived from responses to different light intensities.

Visual fields of infants have been tested using both kinetic and static behavioral perimetry. With either method, an adult observer determines when the infant is fixating centrally and then initiates presentation of a peripheral stimulus. The index of stimulus detection is the infant's eye movement away from central fixation in the direction of the stimulus. The observer reports

the direction of the infant's eye movement usually toward one of a known set of coordinates (e.g., horizontally, right or left). A match between the observer's directional judgment and the meridian of the peripheral target is evidence that the infant detected the target at the tested location. Of course, this conclusion relies on various procedural and statistical controls, including ensuring that the infant's eye position prior to peripheral stimulus detection is central, the observer is unaware of peripheral target position, and the target stimulus is presented on sufficient trials to achieve statistical significance.

Three infant perimetry procedures in current use that have provided normal data are described. Problems with testing when using these procedures that may affect interpreting infant's visual fields are discussed. A section on clinical applications of infant perimetry methods is provided. Psychophysiological and electrophysiological methods that have the potential to assess visual fields of infants are mentioned. We are aware of only one electrophysiological study of infants' visual fields; it differentiates peripheral and central visual field sensitivity using swept visually evoked potentials and has been reported in abstract form only (Allen et al., 1989). Maturation of binocular and monocular visual field extent estimated by behavioral perimetry techniques are presented, and monocular field extent of infants is discussed in terms of adult visual field extent.

METHODS TO ASSESS VISUAL FIELDS OF INFANTS

Three behavioral infant perimetry methods have been described (Mohn and van Hof-van Duin, 1986; Mayer et al., 1988; Maurer and Lewis, 1991; Lewis and Maurer, 1992) and clinical applications reported for two of the methods.

Kinetic Perimetry

Mohn and van Hof-van Duin (1986) developed a method of kinetic perimetry in which an examiner moves a white

117

styrofoam sphere [6 degrees diameter, 0.2 log candelas per square meter (cd/m^2)] on the end of a thin black wire along the surface of one of four black arcs (luminance, -0.2 log cd/m^2). A second adult elicits the infant's central fixation with an identical white sphere presented at the intersection of the arcs. From a central viewing position, this examiner judges the infant's eye movements away from fixation. A third adult holds the infant at a fixed distance from the center of the arcs. Figure 7-1 illustrates this technique.

The peripheral extent at which the observer judges the direction of eye movement correctly is scored, and the median of several trials provides the infant's visual field extent on that meridian. Data from infants with a large number of non-stimulus-directed eye movements are excluded from analysis. This method has been used to obtain normative data on binocular and monocular visual field extent between birth and 10 years of age (Mohn and van Hof-van Duin, 1986; Schwartz et al., 1987; Heersema, 1989; Wilson et al., 1991; Quinn et al., in press); as well as to test visual fields of young patients (van Hof-van Duin and Mohn, 1986, 1987; Groenendaal et al., 1989; Luna et al., 1989, in press; Scher et al., 1989; Van Hof-van Duin et al., 1989).

The white sphere kinetic method requires only simple materials and, in principle, is easy to administer. It can be used to test individual patients, from the newborn period throughout infancy and early childhood. A potential limitation of the technique for clinical applica-

tion is high variability in measured extents. Standard deviations of binocular and monocular hemifield extents for different age groups of normal infants ranges from $\pm$ 5 to $\pm$ 12 degrees (Mohn and van Hof-van Duin, 1986). Dobson and colleagues (Luna et al., 1992) reported 95% limits of binocular field extent for healthy preterm infants that are consistent with the variability from normal infants, ranging from $\pm$ 24 degrees at age 4 months (corrected for preterm birth) to $\pm$ 10 degrees at age 24 months.

Such high variability may be due to aspects of kinetic perimetry procedures that interact with infants' attentional limitations. The presence of a central stimulus, necessary in the white sphere procedure, results in increased latency and variability of infants' eye movements toward peripheral targets (Aslin and Salapatek, 1975). The probability of making a correct eye movement toward a peripheral target is also reduced in the presence of a central target (Aslin and Salapatek, 1975; MacFarlane et al., 1976; Hood and Atkinson, 1990; Maurer and Lewis, 1991). The initiation or latency of eye movements may be inhibited by the infant's sucking on a pacifier during testing (MacFarlane et al., 1976) and by holding the infant's chin during testing (Fig. 7-1), probably because infants' eye movements are yoked with head movements (Roucoux et al., 1981, 1983). Infants also make spontaneous, non-stimulus-related eye movements that may be expected to increase variability.

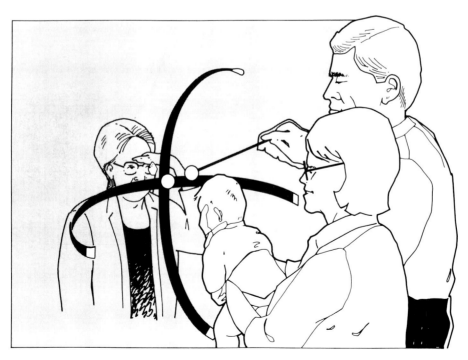

FIG. 7-1. White sphere kinetic arc perimetry method developed by Mohn and van Hof-van Duin (1986). (From Schwartz et al. 1987. By permission.)

Static Perimetry

Lewis and Maurer (1992; Maurer and Lewis, 1991) developed a method of static perimetry in which a 3- or 6-degree diameter light (luminance 2.2 log cd/m², flashed at 3 Hz) is presented at fixed locations with 15-degree intervals on the horizontal meridian in a black hemicylinder (luminance −0.3 log cd/m²). Central fixation is elicited by flashing lights that are extinguished when the centrally located observer judges the infant's fixation to be central. A peripheral stimulus on the right or left is illuminated when the central stimulus is extinguished and remains on until the observer first detects an eye movement away from central fixation. The directions of first eye movements on stimulus trials are compared to those on control trials in which no stimulus occurs. The most eccentric stimulus locus to which the infants' eye movements are statistically significantly greater than on control trials provides the maximum extent for that age group. This method was used to obtain monocular field extent in groups of normal infants between birth and 6 months.

The advantages of this technique are that a central fixation stimulus is not present when the peripheral target is presented, and the peripheral target is not extinguished until the infant makes an eye movement. Both factors act to maximize the probability that an infant will make an eye movement away from the central target. Non-stimulus, control trials are mandatory in this technique to control for chance responses. The major disadvantage of this procedure is that data cannot be derived from individual infants because of infants' limited tolerance for the large number of test trials required for statistical significance and because of infants' position biases (T. Lewis, personal communication).

Hybrid Static-Kinetic Perimetry

Futenma (1977) reported a method to assess visual fields of handicapped children who could not cooperate for standard perimetry. A single 180-degree arc perimeter is rotated to test various meridia; the arc contains 0.9-degree lights at 5-degree intervals and a 2.3-degree central fixation light. The peripheral lights are illuminated for 0.5 second starting at a far peripheral position and stepped in toward more central positions until the child makes an eye movement response. This method can be considered a hybrid of static and kinetic perimetry, as the stimuli are presented in one position for an interval and then moved to a more central position.

We developed a similar perimetry procedure for infants and young children (Cummings et al., 1988; Mayer et al., 1988). Stimuli are 0.7-degree light-emitting diodes (LEDs) (luminance 1.2 log cd/m²) embedded in a hemisphere (background luminance −0.2 log cd/m²) at 7-degree intervals on 24 meridia. Central fixation is elicited by four LEDs, 2.5 degrees from a central observation hole, that flash in synchrony with auditory tones. The tone pattern continues after the central LEDs are extinguished to aid in maintaining central fixation during peripheral stimulus presentation. The observer, viewing the infant through the central hole in the hemisphere or in a video image transmitted by a camera behind the central hole, determines when the infant is fixating centrally and signals a second adult to begin peripheral stimulus presentation. The peripheral LEDs are illuminated for 3 seconds at successive 7-degree positions starting at a far peripheral position. The observer makes a four-alternative forced-choice judgment of stimulus direction in one of four quadrants. Using this method, binocular and monocular visual field extents of 6- to 7-month-old infants were estimated on each of eight meridia (Mayer et al., 1988). The same method was used to test field extent in 2- to 5-year-old children and young patients with field defects (Cummings et al., 1988).

Visual fields of 6- to 7-month-old infants using the LED hybrid kinetic-static method are shown in Figure 7-2 (Mayer et al., 1988). An adult-like ovoid shape of the infants' binocular field, representing the relative construction of superior and inferior fields compared to temporal fields, is shown. This adult shape is also found using the white sphere kinetic method in all ages (Mohn and van Hof-van Duin, 1986), including newborns (Schwartz et al., 1987). For the LED method, the infants' binocular field extents are the same as those of adults on most meridia (Fig. 7-2). Monocular fields in the same age infants show near-adult extents in the temporal field but constriction of the nasal field relative to that in adults (Fig. 7-2).

The advantages of the LED hybrid technique are the following: (1) The presence of a central fixation stimulus during peripheral stimulation is not necessary; (2) the visual field of an individual infant can be assessed, making the technique clinically applicable; (3) the technique provides a field circumference (isopter) that has a known relation to standard Goldmann isopters in patients with field defects (Cummings et al., 1988); and (4) variability is less than with the white sphere kinetic method although still relatively high. The range of variation in monocular field extent is between 0 and 28 degrees for a group of 6- to 7-month-old infants, depending on the meridia (Mayer et al., 1988).

Disadvantages of this technique are the same as for the kinetic white sphere method. Maintaining the infant's central fixation during peripheral stimulus presentation is the primary difficulty. Infants often make spontaneous eye movements, not elicited by peripheral stimuli, apparently due to procedural factors causing restlessness or distress, for example, wariness, or dis-

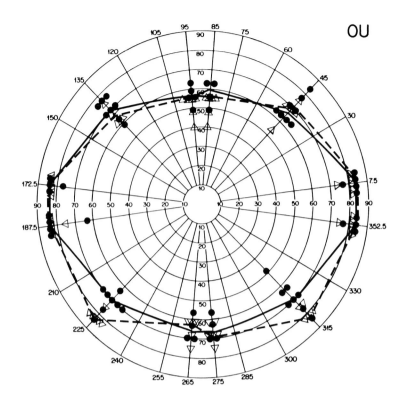

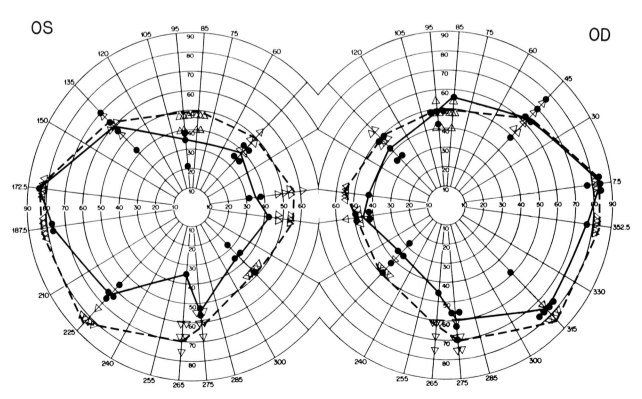

FIG. 7-2. Visual fields of infants and adults using the hybrid kinetic-static perimetry method (0.7 degree, flashing light). OU = binocular; OD = monocular right; OS = monocular left. Infants' mean age: binocular 6.4 months; monocular 7.4 months. Points are medians of three to five trials per subject. ● infant data; △ adult data. The solid line connects the median infant fields and the dashed line the median adult fields. (From Mayer et al., 1988. By permission.)

comfort wearing the adhesive eye patch. Infants are easily distracted by external noises, which cause orienting eye movements. Older infants may look to previously detected peripheral target locations. These non-stimulus-related behaviors may be expected to increase false positives and variability. False positives may cause overestimation of field extent if control trials, scoring corrections, or strict statistical criteria are not used. In infants with field defects, kinetic scans may have long durations, leading to an increased probability of non-stimulus-related eye movements. Experience of this type when testing young patients with the LED hybrid kinetic method led us to use static testing at fixed positions instead of the kinetic presentation (see below).

Peripheral Field Sensitivity

Peripheral visual field sensitivity of adults is tested by measuring luminance thresholds for spots of light at various positions in the visual field. Peripheral visual field sensitivity can also be tested using patterned targets to measure acuity or contrast sensitivity. Data from studies of the peripheral contrast sensitivity and acuity of mature primates have produced models of the spatial scale of retinal ganglion and cortical cell distributions versus eccentricity (e.g., Virsu and Rovamo, 1979; Perry and Cowey, 1985). The few studies of photopic field sensitivity of infants focus on age-dependent increases in relative sensitivity of central versus peripheral loci or between peripheral loci.

Light Sensitivity. Although considerable research on scotopic sensitivity, representing peripheral retinal function under rod-mediated conditions, has been reported (see Chapter 8), to our knowledge only a single, unpublished study of photopic peripheral light sensitivity in human infants exists. In a doctoral study, Guez (1978) tested binocular peripheral light thresholds in 13 infants, ages 8 to 21 weeks, using a procedure similar to that of Lewis and Maurer (see above). Stimuli were 1 degree diameter lights flashed at 3 Hz for 3 seconds against a 0.6 log cd/m² background at 15 and 40 degrees eccentric to fixation. Adults showed little variation in thresholds between 15 and 40 degrees, which is not surprising given that field sensitivity varies little with eccentricity using a large target (1 degree) (Aulhorn and Harms, 1972; Johnson, 1987). The infants' thresholds were on average 4 log units higher than adult thresholds at the same loci.

Peripheral Acuity and Contrast Sensitivity. Sireteanu and colleagues reported binocular and monocular peripheral grating acuities of 2- to 12-month-old infants obtained using first fixation responses in a preferential looking (PL) paradigm (Sireteanu et al., 1984a,b; Sire-

teanu and Fronius, 1987). Stimuli were 12 degree diameter, luminous gratings presented to the right or left of center in a dark surround and paired with a blank, equiluminant stimulus at the same eccentricity. The inner grating edge was 4 degrees or 12.5 degrees from the central peephole. Peripheral acuity increased with age, in parallel with grating acuity assessed during free-viewing PL. At 4 degrees eccentricity, peripheral monocular acuity (hemifield unspecified) was 1.0 log unit less than that of adults at 3.5 months and 0.4 log unit less at 10 months.

The difference between peripheral and free-viewing PL in the Sireteanu studies was slight, 0.1–0.2 log cycles per degree (cpd), at all ages tested. Adults, tested with the same stimuli, showed a larger difference between peripheral and central acuities—0.4–0.6 log unit difference between foveal and 10–20 degrees eccentric loci—in agreement with other studies (e.g., Kerr, 1971; Wertheim, 1980). However, the conditions of testing peripheral and free-viewing PL acuity in infants are probably not adequate to differentiate between peripheral and "central" or foveal acuity. With PL, infants are stimulated to fixate centrally prior to presentation of the grating stimulus, which often appears abruptly. The typical response and one that gives the observer the strongest cue to grating position is a saccade or series of saccades to the right or left position immediately upon stimulus presentation. Therefore it is possible that the "central," or free-viewing, PL grating acuities reported in the Sireteanu studies are based, at least in part and at some ages, on the infant's detection of gratings at peripheral loci. This point would explain the small differences between infant's peripheral and free-viewing grating acuities.

Clinical Applications of Infant Perimetry Methods

Kinetic Perimetry: White Sphere Method. To date, detailed clinical studies using the white sphere kinetic technique (see above) have been limited to binocular visual field assessment. With this method, preterm infants at risk of neurological impairment due to perinatal hypoxia or periventricular echolucencies or echodensities have shown constricted binocular visual fields during early infancy (van Hof-van Duin et al., 1986, 1987, 1989; Groenendaal et al., 1989; Scher et al., 1989), and normal binocular field extent is reported for preterm, low risk infants (van Hof-van Duin et al., 1992) and infants with bronchopulmonary dysplasia and no neurological or ocular disorders (Luna et al., 1992). Field constriction may resolve for some high-risk infants (Groenendaal et al., 1989); but in other, more severely impaired infants visual field defects persist (Scher et al., 1989).

Binocular visual fields have been reported in infants with structural ocular damage due to retinopathy of prematurity (ROP) (Luna et al., 1989). Visual field constriction was seen only in infants who had experienced active ROP in the nasal retina and not in those with temporal retinal involvement or no active ROP. Constriction in the binocular temporal field is consistent with abnormal peripheral nasal retina.

These studies provide evidence for the feasibility and utility of the white sphere kinetic technique for binocular visual field assessment in infants at risk of visual field defects. However, assessment of monocular fields is needed to interpret field defects in relation to the site and extent of visual pathway abnormalities. The clinical value of this technique could be improved further by using smaller targets after the age range in which kinetic field extent for the 6-degree target is asymptotic, or 12–24 months (Heersema, 1989; Luna et al., 1992).

Hybrid Kinetic Perimetry and Visual Field Defect Screening.

We have assessed visual fields in young patients using the hybrid static-kinetic method and a static modification (Mayer et al., 1987, 1988; Mayer and Fulton, 1989). The hybrid method appears sensitive and specific to major field defects secondary to chiasmal and postchiasmal lesions, such as bitemporal or hemifield defects in older pediatric patients (Cummings et al., 1988). However, because infants with neurological disorders are difficult to test reliably with kinetic perimetry due to eye movement disorders and attentional difficulties (Mayer et al., 1987), we developed a clinical test protocol using the LED perimeter and the same four-alternative forced-choice procedure but with static presentation of the stimuli (Mayer and Fulton, 1989). Peripheral stimulus locations were based on the most eccentric position that at least 90% of normal infants detected in kinetic presentation (Mayer et al., 1988). Eight meridia were tested in each eye at 35–70 degrees eccentricity, depending on the quadrant. Homonymous defects were inferred from abnormal responses on the same meridia in each eye. This strategy has high specificity: None of the 20 normal infants ages 6–9 months showed a homonymous quadrantanopsia (Mayer and Fulton, 1989). Results from young patients with intracranial tumors, head trauma, severe hydrocephalus, or neonatal asphyxia suggest that the method is sensitive to homonymous hemifield and quadrantic defects (D. Mayer, in preparation). Constricted fields or relative defects are inferred based on testing at more central loci than normal screening positions.

Infant perimetry methods attempted to date and their clinical utility will become evident through application to well-defined patient groups. Despite limitations, these methods represent an advance over qualitative, confrontation techniques and provide quantitative measures of peripheral vision that can be used to follow patients over time. More research is required to determine if subtle defects can be reliably detected and followed.

Psychophysiological and Electrophysiological Methods

Psychophysiological and electrophysiological measures have been used to assess peripheral vision in adults—in particular to investigate visual pathway abnormalities; however, there have been few reports of these techniques being used in pediatric patients. A heart-rate index of orienting was used to study peripheral vision of 4-month-old infants (Finlay and Ivinkis, 1982, 1984). Evidence for covert orienting based on heart rate changes was obtained to peripheral stimuli that did not elicit overt orienting.

Other promising techniques for infants include (1) pupillometric responses, shown to detect a hemifield defect due to an optic tract lesion in an adult patient (Barbur and Forsyth, 1986; Kardon et al., 1991); (2) binocular optokinetic nystagmus (OKN) asymmetry, which can provide localizing information of the site of a hemispheric lesion causing a hemifield defect; and (3) the electroretinogram (ERG) to spatially localized stimulation, reported in normal adults (Sutter, 1985; Marx and Zrenner, 1990).

Visually evoked potential (VEP) methods have also shown promise for assessing visual fields of infants. VEP methods can reveal asymmetrical responses from right and left hemispheres in patients with unilateral visual pathway abnormalities (e.g., Howe, 1977) that, however, are lateralized differently depending on the stimulus field, pattern element size, and recording electrode placement (e.g., Blumhardt et al., 1977; Holder, 1985). A report of two cases described laterally asymmetrical binocular flash and pattern VEPs consistent with isolated occipital lobe abnormalities in a 9-month-old infant and a 4-year-old child (Lambert et al., 1990).

In a single study of infants (published as an abstract: Allen et al., 1989), the relatively new, swept VEP method (Norcia and Tyler, 1985) (see Chapter 30) was used to differentiate between central and peripheral acuity and contrast sensitivity. Responses were obtained using sine-wave gratings presented simultaneously to the central field (4 degrees diameter) and to a peripheral locus (8–16 degrees) in infants age 10–39 weeks. Gratings were phase-alternated at a different temporal frequency (6 or 8 Hz) at the central and peripheral loci. Central grating acuity was higher than peripheral acuity by about 0.5 log unit at all ages, similar to the behaviorally obtained difference between central and 10-degree presentation reported for adults (Kerr, 1971; Wertheim, 1980). Contrast sensitivity for low spatial frequency gratings at either central or peripheral loci did not vary with age after age 5 months.

MATURATION OF THE INFANT VISUAL FIELD

Binocular Field Extent

Many more studies of binocular than monocular visual fields of infants have been reported, undoubtedly because testing any infant visual function is easier if done binocularly. Figure 7-3 illustrates average data from all studies of the binocular horizontal extent of the photopic visual field of infants from which field extent could be estimated.

Newborn to Age 2 Months. The horizontal extent of the binocular hemifield does not vary markedly during the first two postnatal months, as illustrated in Figure 7-3. The mean extent of the hemifield obtained in these studies ranges between 17 and 34 degrees during the neonatal period and between 29 and 38 degrees at age 2 months. Test conditions expected to influence field size in adults (e.g., background luminance, stimulus size, and contrast) as well as temporal variations in stimuli and procedural factors differ among studies. Therefore some of the variation among extents obtained in different studies at similar ages may be due to these factors.

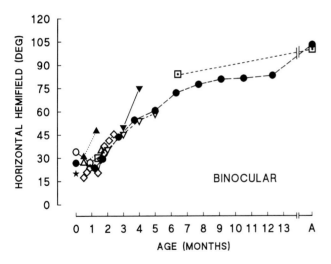

FIG. 7-3. Binocular hemifield extent on the horizontal meridian as a function of the age of the infants (newborn to about 1 year); adult data are from the same stimulus and apparatus indicated as A on the age axis. Mean or median extents were taken from the best estimates for each study. Newborn: ★ 0.55 × 19.3 degrees line (static) (Lewis et al., 1978); newborn to 8 weeks: ○ 6-degree white sphere (kinetic) (Schwartz et al., 1987); 5–53 weeks: ● 6-degree white sphere (kinetic) (Mohn and van Hof-van Duin, 1986); 2–10 weeks: ◇ 6 × 5 × 2 degrees rectangle (kinetic) (Tronick, 1972); 2 and 7 weeks: △ 3 degrees light with 1.5 degrees square inset (flashing) (Harris and MacFarlane, 1974); 2.0 and 5.5 weeks: ▲ 3 degrees light with 1.5 degrees square inset (flashing) (MacFarlane et al., 1976); 1 and 2 months: □ 3.1 degree annular light (static) (Aslin and Salapatek, 1975); 2–5 months: ▽ 8 degree colored ball (moving) (DeSchonen et al., 1978); 3 and 4 months: ▼ 4 × 13 degree stripes (moving) (Finlay et al., 1982); 6.4 months (mean): ⊡ 0.7-degree light (flashing) (Mayer et al., 1988).

For example, the most extensive hemifield during this early period, 47.5 degrees at age 1 month, is obtained under conditions expected to maximize peripheral field extent in infants: a temporally modulated peripheral stimulus, no central stimulus during peripheral stimulus presentation, and no use of a pacifier (MacFarlane et al., 1976).

Some studies, in particular those using kinetic perimetry and a constantly present central stimulus, have found a reduction in field extent between the newborn period and age 4–5 weeks (Mohn and van Hof-van Duin, 1986; Schwartz et al., 1987) that cannot be explained by differences in stimulus conditions. This phenomenon can be described as an inability to disengage orienting to one visual stimulus to attend to another (Stechler and Latz, 1966; Slater, 1988; Johnson, 1990), which is hypothesized because of the onset of corticocollicular inhibition (via the substantia nigra and basal ganglia) at age 1 month (Johnson et al., 1991).

Infants Older Than 2 Months. The mean horizontal extent of the binocular hemifield increases monotonically between ages 2 and 12 months (Fig. 7-3), although relatively few data are reported from infants older than age 5 months. Mean extent of the binocular hemifield ranges between 40 and 50 degrees at about age 3 months (Tronick, 1972; DeSchonen et al., 1978; Finlay et al., 1982; Mohn and van Hof-van Duin, 1986) and between 70 and 84 degrees at about age 6 months (Mohn and van Hof-van Duin, 1986; Mayer et al., 1988). Adult-like hemifield extent of 90–100 degrees is not achieved at the oldest ages tested, 6–12 months. Heersema (1989) reported that children's binocular and monocular horizontal field extents are asymptotic and adult-like for most meridia by about age 2 years with the white sphere kinetic technique. An asymptote in binocular field extent with the white sphere kinetic technique was also shown in a study of healthy preterm infants age 12–24 months using age corrected for preterm birth (Luna et al., 1992).

Agreement between studies that have used three-dimensional stimulus objects (i.e., 6- to 8-degree spheres or rectangles), rather than lights, is excellent in the age range 2–5 months (Fig. 7-3) (Tronick, 1972; DeSchonen et al., 1978; Mohn and van Hof-van Duin, 1986). Studies using luminous stimuli to assess infants older than 2 months (Finlay et al., 1982; Mayer et al., 1988) have shown more extensive horizontal hemifields than studies using nonluminous stimuli. Only one study reported variation in background intensity: Van Hof-van Duin and Mohn (1987) reported that kinetic field extent is reduced when 6-degree white spheres are moved against gray (luminance not specified) rather than black arc meridia.

In summary, the binocular horizontal hemifield increases monotonically after age 2 months up to age 12–24 months, at which time, using 6-degree targets, extent is asymptotic and adult-like (Heersema, 1989; Luna et al., in press). Children's mean extents are similar to those of adults for nasal and temporal quadrants, though not for inferior quadrants (Heersema, 1989). Quinn and colleagues (1991), using the same white sphere kinetic technique to test monocular fields of older children, reported continued, albeit slight, expansion of the visual field from age 4 years to adulthood.

Monocular Visual Field Extent

Monocular field extent of infants has been reported using the perimetry techniques discussed earlier in the chapter (Mohn and van Hof-van Duin, 1986; Mayer et al., 1988; Maurer and Lewis, 1991; Lewis and Maurer, 1992). Figure 7-2 illustrates the shape and extent of monocular fields of 6- to 7-month-old infants tested with the hybrid static-kinetic method.

Field extent on the horizon obtained with the three infant perimetry techniques (Mohn and van Hof-van Duin, 1986; Mayer et al., 1988; Lewis and Maurer, 1992) is represented separately for the temporal (Fig. 7-4A) and nasal (Fig. 7-4B) hemifields. Infants between term and 6 months were tested with the static method and between 2 and 10 months with the kinetic method. Temporal and nasal hemifield extents increase monotonically for both kinetic and static techniques and with both static stimuli. Extent at age 7–8 months (Mayer et al., 1988) tested with the LED hybrid static-kinetic technique agrees well with that tested using the white sphere kinetic technique (Mohn and van Hof-van Duin, 1986) for both nasal and temporal hemifields.

Fields were more extensive to the static 6-degree target compared to the 3-degree static or 6-degree kinetic stimuli at most ages. Marked differences between data obtained with the two static stimuli are seen between term and age 2–3 months. For example, infants at every age up to 3 months, including neonates, detected the 6-degree light at 30 degrees in the nasal field, whereas the 3-degree light was not detected at 15 degrees in the nasal field until age 3 months. These differences are likely due to the greater total luminance of the 6-degree target than either the 3-degree static or 6-degree kinetic stimuli. Kinetic targets produce more extensive rather than less extensive fields than static targets of the same size and luminance (Riddoch, 1917; Safran and Glaser, 1980; Casson et al., 1991).

Larger differences in absolute extent between techniques are shown for the temporal hemifield (Fig. 7-4A) than for the nasal field (Fig. 7-4B) at various ages. Better agreement between stimuli in the nasal field

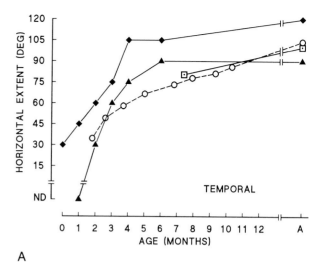

A

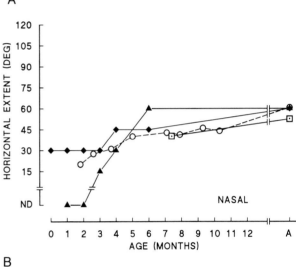

B

FIG. 7-4. Monocular temporal (A) and nasal (B) field extent on the horizontal meridian for infants (newborn to about 10 months) obtained using three perimetry techniques. Adult data (A on age axes) were obtained using the same techniques and stimuli. Data are best estimates of group thresholds for field extent. Newborn to 6 months: ◆ 6-degree light (flashing) (Maurer and Lewis, 1991) (statistical criterion $p < 0.01$); ▲ 3-degree light (flashing) (Lewis and Maurer, 1992) (statistical criterion: $p < 0.01$); 8–44 weeks: ○ 6-degree white sphere (kinetic) (Mohn and van Hof-van Duin, 1986); 7.4 months (mean): ☐ 0.7-degree light (flashing, kinetic) (Mayer et al., 1988).

may be due to the steeper gradient of nasal field sensitivity resulting in relative constriction of the nasal field for all stimuli compared to the temporal field (Aulhorn and Harms, 1977).

In the temporal field, beginning at age 2 months, agreement between techniques and stimuli is more consistent, and the maturation curves are approximately parallel. In the nasal field, extent to the 6-degree static stimulus is greater than to the 3-degree static stimulus except at age 6 months, when this trend reverses. The latter may be attributed to statistical or sampling error.

Because only stimulus area differed between the 6- and 3-degree stimulus conditions, the generally greater extent for the 6-degree than the 3-degree stimulus is undoubtedly due to differences in total stimulus intensity (area × luminance). The larger differences between data obtained with the 6- and 3-degree stimuli during the early postnatal months compared to the later postnatal months suggests that spatial summation in the peripheral visual field may differ across these ages, and consequently that these two stimulus areas may not be psychophysically equivalent across the first 6 postnatal months.

To evaluate maturation of temporal and nasal monocular fields with each technique in the same relative terms, the data from Figure 7-4 are plotted in Figures 7-5 and 7-6 separately for each technique as the percent of adult extent for the same stimuli. Figure 7-5 shows that for the white sphere kinetic technique the maturation of nasal and temporal fields has a common course. Both the white sphere and LED hybrid kinetic techniques show temporal and nasal field extents at age 7–8 months that are 75–80% of the adult value. Thus with kinetic stimulus presentation, maturation of the nasal field appears to follow a course similar to that of the temporal field.

The data obtained with the static technique describe a different picture (Fig. 7-6A,B). The course of maturation is more rapid for both temporal and nasal hemifields tested using the static method and either stimulus than by the kinetic method. In addition, maturation of

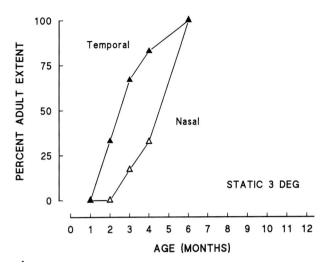

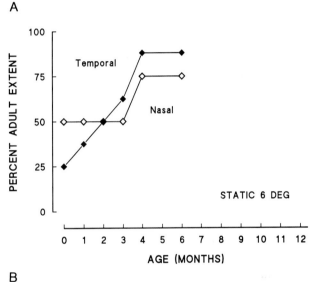

B

FIG. 7-6. Percent adult extent on the horizontal meridian of infants tested with the static method (Maurer and Lewis, 1991; Lewis and Maurer, 1992). Adults were tested using the same technique and stimuli. (A) Data obtained with the static 3-degree stimulus. (B) Data obtained with the static 6-degree stimulus. Temporal field data are indicated by solid symbols and nasal field data by open symbols.

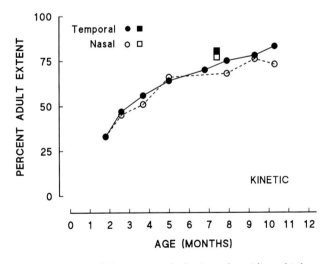

FIG. 7-5. Percent adult extent on the horizontal meridian of infants tested with the kinetic white sphere technique (Mohn and van Hof-van Duin, 1986) and LED hybrid static-kinetic technique (Mayer et al., 1988). Adults were tested using the same technique and stimulus. Data obtained with the white sphere kinetic method are indicated by circles and those obtained by the LED kinetic method by squares. Temporal field data are indicated by solid symbols and nasal field data by open symbols.

the nasal field lags behind that of the temporal field for static stimuli. This delayed maturation is most clearly seen in the 3-degree static data (Fig. 7-6A). The data for the 6-degree static stimulus (Fig. 7-6B) are difficult to interpret as the temporal and nasal curves cross and neither reaches 100% of adult extent, although 100% of adult extent is reached by age 6 months for the smaller, 3-degree stimulus (Fig. 7-6A). This discrepancy between the 6-degree and 3-degree static stimulus data may be due to scattered light in the 6-degree light as adults detected this large, bright (2.2 log cd/m²) light at 120 degrees in the temporal field (Lewis and Maurer, 1992), a physically unlikely eccentricity.

SUMMARY OF MATURATION OF INFANT VISUAL FIELDS AND IMPLICATIONS

The studies discussed above reported a monotonic increase in monocular field extent with age. Internal consistency for each technique was illustrated for the static method by the generally greater extent to the 6-degree stimuli than to the 3-degree stimuli; and for the white sphere kinetic technique, nearly identical maturation of the temporal horizontal hemifield as the binocular horizontal hemifield (compare Figures 7-3 and 7-4A) (Mohn and van Hof-van Duin, 1986). Differences between data obtained with the kinetic and static techniques and between the two static stimuli are attributed to differences in stimulus luminance. However, when the infant data are plotted relative to adult field extents for the same stimuli, differences in the course of maturation of temporal and nasal field between techniques are evident. The kinetic techniques show a common course of nasal and temporal field maturation, and the static method shows a lag in nasal maturation.

Is there evidence for maturation of anatomical structures consistent with the above behavioral data on visual fields of human infants? The growth of the infant eye may be sufficient to explain an increase in kinetic field extent with age. For example, at postnatal age 6 months, the human infant retinal area is about 70% that of the adult (Robb, 1982) and the sagittal length of the eye is about 72% that of the adult (Larsen, 1971). These values are in good agreement with the 75–80% of adult horizontal hemifield extent estimated for infants at ages 7–8 months tested with kinetic techniques (Fig. 7-5).

The common course of nasal and temporal hemifield extent based on kinetic perimetry (Fig. 7-5) might be attributed to growth of temporal and nasal hemiretinae. As estimated from cone density versus eccentricity distributions in rhesus macaque retinae (Packer et al., 1990, data from their Figure 7), the extent of nasal retina (corresponding to the temporal field) is about 60% that of the adult at postnatal age 3 weeks and 70% at age 6 weeks. Figure 7-7 illustrates these data from Packer et al. (1990). Using the conversion factor of 1 week macaque age to 1 month human infant age, by which time grating acuity development in the two species coincides (Teller, 1981), the macaque values are close to the values for the kinetic perimetry data in Figure 7-5 at comparable human ages. The overall course of growth of the infant macaque temporal and nasal retina is similar, and the maximum difference between temporal and nasal retinal extents is no greater than 6% up to age 13 weeks. Cone densities in nasal and temporal retina of macaque infants also show a parallel change (decrease) with age. Moreover, cone density is greater in nasal than temporal retinal loci at all ages after E152

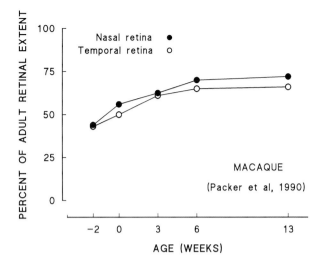

FIG. 7-7. Infant macaque retinal extent (nasal retina ●; temporal retina ○) in terms of percent of adult macaque retina (based on Figure 7 in Packer et al., 1990). Data from animals between embryonic day 152 (−2 weeks on age axis) and 13 weeks postnatal age are shown. Embryonic day 165 is approximately term and is denoted as zero on the age axis.

(E152 = −2 weeks), with cone density differences of the same relative magnitude as in adult macaque hemiretinae (Figure 7 in Packer et al., 1990). Thus the age-related growth and redistribution of cones in temporal and nasal hemiretinae in macaque infants is qualitatively similar to the maturation of human infant visual field extent as seen using behavioral kinetic methods.

To explain a lag in nasal field maturation using static stimuli (Fig. 7-6) at the retinal level requires larger qualitative or quantitative relative differences between temporal and nasal retinal cells or between ganglion cell projections in infant primates than in adult primates. As mentioned, developmental anatomical studies show comparable nasotemporal asymmetries in cone and ganglion cell anatomy and distributions. Moreover, the nasotemporal division between contralaterally and ipsilaterally projecting retinal ganglion cells is distinct as early as 50 days prior to birth in the fetal rhesus macaque (Chalupa and Lia, 1991). However, it has been proposed by Guillery (1988) that different ganglion cell types, which have different birth dates in the nasal and temporal retinae in the cat (Walsh and Polley, 1985), may also differ in terms of the growth rate of their geniculate projections. Specifically, the uncrossed, contralateral projection (from temporal retinal ganglion cells) may be delayed in its growth relative to the crossed, ipsilateral projection (nasal retinal ganglion cells).

Lewis and Maurer (1992) have suggested an alternative, but possibly related, explanation for nasal versus temporal field maturation differences in their study: relatively later maturation of projections from cortex to the nucleus of the optic tract, which govern nasally directed eye movements. Earlier maturation of direct collicular input would be associated with more mature temporally directed eye movements. This explanation does not reconcile the lack of nasal–temporal differences in maturation for kinetic perimetry, as the same infant eye movements are relied on when using the static perimetry method. Only a complicated hypothesis regarding differential maturation of different retinal ganglion cell types in nasal and temporal retinae seem to reconcile these data adequately.

In fact, the methods and data obtained by these techniques cannot address the most interesting and relevant questions regarding the infant peripheral field: What is the sensitivity gradient of the infant's visual field, and how does it mature? To answer this question requires direct measurement of photopic peripheral sensitivity during infancy. A working hypothesis to guide such study is that maturation of the human visual field can be modeled as a constant shift with age from lower to higher sensitivity of the adult central-to-peripheral sensitivity gradient. Alternatively, the infant's peripheral field may have a steeper sensitivity gradient than the adult field. This idea appears to be an implicit assumption of several researchers in this area, possibly due to studying the extent of the visual field. One implication arising from this notion is that the peripheral field matures later than the central visual field. We suggest that the increasing peripheral extent of the visual field could be a consequence of increasing sensitivity of the visual field. To test these hypotheses requires measuring static thresholds for several stimulus areas at several eccentric loci in temporal and nasal fields and in different age groups.

A quantitative model of the gradient of adult human peripheral spatial vision has been reported by Banks and colleagues (1991) using cone/ganglion cell ratios derived from anatomical measurements in adult human retinas (Curcio and Allen, 1990). Peripheral cone morphological development has not been studied as extensively as has foveal cone development (Drucker and Hendrickson, 1989) (see Chapter 17), nor has cone to ganglion cell convergence been reported for infant primate retinae. However, Packer et al. (1990) suggested that differential growth of the primate retina outside the posterior pole likely accounts for the development of the ganglion cell density gradient just as it does for cone density changes. Consistent with our hypothesis of a constant shift with age in the gradient of peripheral field sensitivity is a conjecture based on the suggestion of Packer et al. (1990) that the same relative convergence of cones on ganglion cells with eccentricity persists as the eye grows and as cell soma size and dendritic fields increase.

We conclude that the field of infant perimetry is in its beginning stages. Behavioral methodologies have been developed and each has strengths and weaknesses, most due to the nature of the infant subject and the dependence on infant eye movements. The swept VEP technique has the potential to surmount inferential difficulties when interpreting data on peripheral visual function that rely on eye movements. Two of the behavioral techniques have clinical potential and represent an advance over confrontation methods with pediatric patients in that stimuli and field extent can be quantitated. These techniques provide a means to assess infants at risk of field defects and to increase knowledge regarding the age-related effects of visual pathway insults on peripheral vision.

The available data on normal maturation of the photopic visual field are limited to estimates of field extent. The early phase of maturation of visual field extent appears similar to that of visual acuity development with rapid improvement during the first 6 months. Study of the continuing maturation of the visual field requires use of smaller or dimmer stimuli, as field extent appears to asymptote for the large and bright stimuli used to date between age 6 and 12 months. Studies to elucidate maturation of visual field sensitivity are needed.

REFERENCES

ALLEN, D., TYLER, C. W., AND NORCIA, A. M. (1989). Development of grating acuity and contrast sensitivity in the central and peripheral visual field of the human infant. *Invest. Ophthalmol. Vis. Sci.* 30 (suppl.), 311.

ASLIN, R. N., AND SALAPATEK, P. (1975). Saccadic localization of visual targets by the very young human infant. *Percept. Psychophys.* 17, 293–302.

AULHORN, E., AND HARMS, H. (1972). Visual perimetry. In *Handbook of Sensory Physiology*. Vol. VII/4. Berlin: Springer-Verlag.

BANKS, M. S., SEKULER, A. B., AND ANDERSON, S. J. (1991). Peripheral spatial vision: limits imposed by optics, photoreceptors, and receptor pooling. *J. Opt. Soc. Am. [A]* 8, 1775–1787.

BARBUR, J. L., AND FORSYTH, P. M. (1986). Can the pupil response be used as a measure of visual input to the geniculostriate system? *Clin. Vision Sci.* 1, 107–111.

BLUMHARDT, L. D., BARRETT, G., AND HALLIDAY, A. M. (1977). The asymmetrical visual evoked potential to pattern reversal in one half field and its significance for the analysis of visual field defects. *Br. J. Ophthalmol.* 61, 454–461.

CASSON, E. J., OSAKO, M., JOHNSON, C. A., AND HWANG, P. (1991). Temporal and spatial properties of optic neuritis patients manifesting statokinetic dissociation. *Appl. Opt.* 30, 2136–2142.

CHALUPA, L. M., AND LIA, B. (1991). The nasotemporal division of retinal ganglion cells with crossed and uncrossed projections in the fetal rhesus monkey. *J. Neurosci.* 11, 191–202.

CUMMINGS, M. L., VAN HOF-VAN DUIN, J., MAYER, D. L., HANSEN, R. M., AND FULTON, A. B. (1988). Visual fields of young children. *Behav. Brain Res.* 29, 7–16.

CURCIO, C. A., AND ALLEN, K. A. (1990). Topography of ganglion cells in human retina. *J. Comp. Neurol.* 300, 5–25.

DE SCHONEN, S., MCKENZIE, B., MAURY, L., AND BRESSON, F. (1978). Central and peripheral object distances as determinants of the effective visual field in early infancy. *Perception* 7, 499–506.

DRASDO, N. (1977). The neural representation of visual space. *Nature* 266, 554–556.

DRUCKER, D. N., AND HENDRICKSON, A. E. (1989). The morphological development of extrafoveal human retina. *Invest. Ophthalmol. Vis. Sci.* 30 (suppl.), 226.

FINLAY, D., AND IVINKIS, A. (1982). Cardiac and visual responses to stimuli presented both foveally and peripherally as a function of speed of moving stimuli. *Dev. Psychol.* 18, 692–698.

FINLAY, D., AND IVINKIS, A. (1984). Cardiac and visual responses to moving stimuli presented either successively or simultaneously to the central and peripheral visual fields in 4-month-old infants. *Dev. Psychol.* 20, 29–36.

FINLAY, D., QUINN, K., AND IVINKIS, A. (1982). Detection of moving stimuli in the binocular and nasal visual fields by infants three and four months old. *Perception* 11, 685–690.

FRISEN, L., AND FRISEN, M. (1976). A simple relationship between the probability distribution of visual acuity and the density of retinal output channels. *Acta Ophthalmol. (Copenh.)* 54, 437–444.

FUTENMA, M. (1977). Perimeter for children or mentally handicapped. *J. Jpn. Ophthalmol. Soc. [Nichigenkai Shi]* 81, 19–28 [in Japanese].

GROENENDAAL, F., VAN HOF-VAN DUIN, J., BAERTS, W., AND FETTER, W. P. F. (1989). Effects of perinatal hypoxia on visual development during the first year of (corrected) age. *Early Hum. Dev.* 20, 267–279.

GUEZ, J. R. (1978). Peripheral visual sensitivity in infants: a methodological study. Doctoral dissertation, Pennsylvania State University.

GUILLERY, R. W. (1988). Retinal representations in prethalamic visual pathways. In C. Kennard and F. C. Rose (eds.). *Physiological Aspects of Clinical Neuro-Ophthalmology.* Chicago: Year Book Medical Publishers.

HARRIS, P., AND MACFARLANE, A. The growth of the effective visual field from birth to seven weeks. *J. Exp. Child Psychol.* 18, 340–348.

HEERSEMA, T. (1989). Development of the visual field of human infants and young children. Doctoral dissertation, Department of Physiology I, Erasmus University, Rotterdam, The Netherlands.

HOLDER, G. E. (1985). Pattern visual evoked potential in patients with posteriorly situated space-occupying lesions. *Doc. Ophthalmol.* 59, 121–128.

HOOD, B., AND ATKINSON, J. (1990). Sensory visual loss and cognitive deficits in the selective attentional system of normal infants and neurologically impaired children. *Dev. Med. Child Neurol.* 32:1067–1077.

HOWE, J. W. (1977). The causes and assessment of visual field defects in young children. *Br. Orthop. J.* 34, 46–53.

JOHNSON, C. A. (1987). Peripheral visual function at various adaptation levels. In *Night Vision, Current Research and Future Directions.* Washington, DC: National Academy Press.

JOHNSON, M. H. (1990). Cortical maturation and the development of visual attention in early infancy. *J. Cogn. Neurosci.* 2, 81–85.

JOHNSON, M. H., POSNER, M. I., AND ROTHBART, M. K. (1991). Components of visual orienting in early infancy: contingency learning, anticipatory looking, and disengaging. *J. Cogn. Neurosci.* 3, 335–344.

KARDON, R. H., KIRKALI, P. A., AND THOMPSON, H. S. (1991). Automated pupil perimetry. *Ophthalmol.* 98, 485–496.

KERR, J. L. (1971). Visual resolution in the periphery. *Percept. Psychophysics* 9, 375–378.

LAMBERT, S. R., KRISS, A., AND TAYLOR, D. (1990). Detection of isolated occipital lobe anomalies during early childhood. *Dev. Med. Child Neurol.* 32, 451–455.

LARSEN, J. S. (1971). The sagittal growth of the eye. IV. Ultrasonic measurement of the axial length of the eye from birth to puberty. *Acta Ophthalmol.* 49, 873–886.

LEVENTHAL, A. G., AULT, S. J., VITGEK, D. J., AND SHOU, T. (1989). Extrinsic determinants of retinal ganglion cell development in primates. *J. Comp. Neurol.* 286, 170–189.

LEWIS, T. L., AND MAURER, D. (1992). The development of the temporal and nasal visual fields during infancy. *Vision Res.* 32, 903–911.

LEWIS, T. L., MAURER, D., AND KAY, D. (1978). Newborns' central vision: whole or hole? *J. Exp. Child Psychol.* 26, 193–203.

LUNA, B., DOBSON, V., CARPENTER, N. A., AND BIGLAN, A. W. (1989). Visual fields development in infants with stage 3 retinopathy of prematurity. *Invest. Ophthalmol. Vis. Sci.* 30, 580–582.

LUNA, B., DOBSON, V., AND GUTHRIE, R. D. (1992). Grating acuity and visual field development in infants with bronchopulmonary dysplasia. *Dev. Med. Child Neurol.* 34, 813–821

MACFARLANE, A., HARRIS, P., AND BARNES, I. (1976). Central and peripheral vision in early infancy. *J. Exp. Child Psychol.* 21, 532–538.

MARX, R., AND ZRENNER, E. (1990). Sensitivity distribution in the central and midperipheral visual field determined by pattern electroretinography and harmonic analysis. *Doc. Ophthalmol.* 73, 347–357.

MAURER, D., AND LEWIS, T. L. (1991). The development of peripheral vision and its physiological underpinnings. In M. J. Weiss and P. R. Zelazo (eds.). *Newborn Attention.* Norwood, NY: Ablex.

MAYER, D. L., AND FULTON, A. B. (1989). Efficient method to screen visual fields of pediatric patients. *Invest. Ophthalmol. Vis. Sci.* 30 (suppl.), 242.

MAYER, D. L., FULTON, A. B., AND CUMMINGS, M. C. (1987). The LED perimeter. II. Fields of young patients. *Invest. Ophthalmol. Vis. Sci.* 28 (suppl.), 302.

MAYER, D. L., FULTON, A. B., AND CUMMINGS, M. F. (1988). Visual fields of infants assessed with a new perimetric technique. *Invest. Ophthalmol. Vis. Sci.* 29, 452–459.

MOHN, G., AND VAN HOF-VAN DUIN, J. (1986). Development of the binocular and monocular visual fields of human infants during the first year of life. *Clin. Vis. Sci.* 1, 51–64.

MOHN, G., AND VAN HOF-VAN DUIN, J. (1990). Development of spatial vision. In D. M. Regan (ed.). *Vision and Visual Dysfunction.* London: Macmillan.

NORCIA, A. M., AND TYLER, C. W. (1985). Spatial frequency sweep VEP:visual acuity during the first year of life. *Vision Res.* 25, 1399–1408.

PACKER, O., HENDRICKSON, A. E., AND CURCIO, C. A. (1990). Developmental redistribution of photoreceptors across the *Macaca nemestrina* (pigtail macaque) retina. *J. Comp. Neurol.* 298, 472–493.

PERRY, V. H., AND COWEY, A. (1985). The ganglion cell and cone distributions in the monkey's retina: implications for central magnification factors. *Vision Res.* 25, 1795–1810.

QUINN, G. E., FEA, A. M., AND MINGUINI, N. (1991). Visual fields in 4 to 10 year old children using Goldmann and double arc perimeters. *J. Pediatr. Ophthalmol. Strabismus* 28, 314–319.

RIDDOCH, G. (1917). Dissociation of visual perception due to occipital injuries, with especial reference to appreciation of movement. *Brain* 40, 15–57.

ROBB, R. M. (1982). Increase in retinal surface area during infancy and childhood. *J. Pediatr. Ophthalmol. Strabismus* 19, 16–20.

ROUCOUX, A., CROMMELINCK, M., GUERIT, J. M., AND MEULDERS, M. (1981). Two modes of eye-head coordination and the role of the vestibulo-ocular reflex in these two strategies. *Dev. Neurosci.* 12, 309–315.

ROUCOUX, A., CULEE, C., AND ROUCOUX, M. (1983). Development of fixation and pursuit eye movements in human infants. *Behav. Brain Res.* 10, 133–139.

SAFRAN, A. B., AND GLASER, J. S. (1980). Statokinetic dissociation in lesions of the anterior visual pathway. *Arch. Ophthalmol.* 98, 291–295.

SCHER, M. S., DOBSON, V., CARPENTER, N. A., AND GUTHRIE, R. D. (1989). Visual and neurological outcome of infants with periventricular leukomalacia. *Dev. Med. Child Neurol.* 31, 353–365.

SCHWARTZ, T. L., DOBSON, V., SANDSTROM, D. J., AND VAN HOF-VAN DUIN, J. (1987). Kinetic perimetry assessment of binocular visual field shape and size in young infants. *Vision Res.* 27, 2163–2175.

SIRETEANU, R., AND FRONIUS, M. (1987). The development of peripheral acuity in human infants. In H. Kaufman (ed.). *Transactions of 16th Meeting European Strabismological Association.* Giessen: pp. 221–227.

SIRETEANU, R., KELLERER, R., AND BOERGEN, K-P. (1984a). The development of peripheral visual acuity in human infants: a preliminary study. *Hum. Neurobiol.* 3, 81–85.

SIRETEANU, R., RENTSCHLER, I., KELLERER, R., AND BOERGEN, K. P. (1984b). Entwicklung der peripheren Sehscharfe beim Saugling. *Fortschr. Ophthalmol.* 81, 483–486.

SLATER, A. (1988). Habituation and visual fixation in infants: information processing, reinforcement and what else? *Eur. Bull. Cogn. Psychol.* 8, 517–523.

STECHLER, G., AND LATZ, E. (1966). Some observations of attention and arousal in the human infant. *J. Am. Acad. Child Psychiatry* 5, 517–525.

SUTTER, E. E. (1985). Multi-input VER and ERG analysis for objective perimetry. In: *Proceedings: IEEE Engineering in Medicine and Biology Society*, pp. 414–419.

TELLER, D. Y. (1981). The development of visual acuity in human and monkey infants. *Trends Neurosci.* 4, 21–24.

TRONICK, E. (1972). Stimulus control and the growth of the infant's effective visual field. *Percept. Psychophysics* 11, 373–376.

VAN HOF-VAN DUIN, J., AND MOHN, G. (1986). Visual field measurements, optokinetic nystagmus and the visual threatening response: normal and abnormal development. *Doc Ophthalmol. Proc. Ser.* 45, 305–317.

VAN HOF-VAN DUIN, J., AND MOHN, G. (1987). Early detection of visual impairments. In H. Galjaard, H. F. R. Prechtl, and V. Velickovic (eds.). *Early Detection and Management of Cerebral Palsy.* Dordrecht: Martinus Nijhoff.

VAN HOF-VAN DUIN, J., EVENHUIS-VAN LEUNEN, A., MOHN, G., BAERTS, W., AND FETTER, W. P. F. (1989). Effects of very low birth weight (VLBW) on visual development in the first year after term. *Early Hum. Dev.* 20, 255–266.

VAN HOF-VAN DUIN, J., HEERSEMA, D. J., GROENENDAAL, F., BAERTS, W., AND FETTER, W. P. F. (1992). Visual field and grating acuity development in low-risk preterm infants during the first 2½ years after term. *Behav. Brain Res.* 49, 115–122.

VIRSU, V., AND ROVAMO, J. (1979). Visual resolution, contrast sensitivity, and the cortical magnification factor. *Exp. Brain Res.* 37, 475–494.

WALSH, C., AND POLLEY, E. H. (1985). The topography of ganglion cell production in the cat's retina. *J. Neurosci.* 5, 741–750.

WASSLE, H., GRUNERT, U., ROHRENBECK, J., AND BOYCOTT, B. B. (1989). Cortical magnification factor and the ganglion cell density of the primate retina. *Nature* 341, 643–646.

WERTHEIM, T. (translated by I. L. Dunsky) (1980). Peripheral visual acuity. *Am. J. Optom. Physiol. Opt.* 57, 915–924.

WILSON, M., QUINN, G., DOBSON, V., LUNA, B., AND BRETON, M. (1991). Normative values for visual fields in 4 and 5 year old children using kinetic perimetry. *J. Pediatr. Ophthalmol. Strabismus* 28, 151–154.

8 | Development of scotopic retinal sensitivity

RONALD M. HANSEN AND ANNE B. FULTON

Infant and adult scotopic functions differ significantly. This chapter considers psychophysical and electroretinographic (ERG) studies of scotopic sensitivity, including spectral sensitivity, spatial and temporal summation, background, and bleaching adaptation, that have demonstrated immaturities of infants' scotopic function. Explanations of these immaturities involve modern concepts of retinal sensitivity and gain control (e.g., Shapley and Enroth-Cugell, 1984; Hood, 1988; MacLeod et al., 1989; Hood and Greenstein, 1990; Walraven et al., 1990).

SPECIFICATION OF RETINAL ILLUMINANCE FOR INFANT EYES

To specify the retinal illuminance produced by a stimulus, pupillary diameter and the focal length of the eye, as well as losses in the ocular media, must be considered. The average diameter of the dark-adapted pupil is 5.2 mm (SD 0.15) in 10-week-old infants and 7 mm (SD 0.15) in adults (Fig. 8-1A). The axial length of the eye (Fig. 8-1B) increases from about 16.5 mm at term to 20 mm at age 1 year; it is about 24 mm in adults (Larsen, 1971; Hirano et al., 1979; Sampaolesi and Caruso, 1982; Gordon and Donzis, 1985). Retinal illuminance varies directly with pupillary area and inversely with the square of the posterior nodal distance.

For the dark-adapted condition, the pupillary area/posterior nodal distance ratio is about the same for 8- to 10-week-old infants and adults. Thus corneal irradiances near absolute threshold produce about equal retinal illuminances for infants and adults (Fulton et al., 1986; Brown et al., 1987; Brown, 1990). All results in this chapter are in units of retinal illuminance (log scotopic Troland, or log scot Td) appropriate for age.

Steady scotopic backgrounds (Fig. 8-2) with intensities less than about +1 log scot Td have little effect on pupillary diameter of infants or adults (Spring and Stiles, 1948; Alpern and Ohba, 1972; Birch and Birch, 1987). Brighter backgrounds cause significant constrictions of both infants' and adults' pupils, which must be taken into account to specify retinal illuminance.

LIGHT LOSSES IN THE OCULAR MEDIA

Preretinal absorption by the ocular media is less for infants than for adults (Werner, 1982; Hansen and Fulton, 1989). Light losses in the eye are mainly due to absorption of light by the lens with only negligible absorption by the cornea, vitreous, and neural retina (Wyszecki and Stiles, 1982). To estimate losses in infants' eye, Hansen and Fulton (1989) compared psychophysical thresholds of 10-week-old infants at 400 and 560 nm. Rhodopsin absorbs equally at these wavelengths (Bowmaker and Dartnall, 1980). However, at one wavelength (400 nm) the lens absorbs light strongly, whereas at the other (560 nm) absorption by the lens is negligible. Thus any difference in threshold is due to losses in the preretinal ocular media. The median estimated ocular media density at 400 nm is 0.75 log unit for 10-week-old infants compared to 1.46 log units for young adults (Hansen and Fulton, 1989). These results (Fig. 8-3) along with other psychophysical data (Powers et al., 1981) and visual evoked potential data (Werner, 1982) show that media density increases throughout life, and that there is a large amount of normal intersubject variability (Norren and Vos, 1974; Wyszecki and Stiles, 1982; Pokorny et al., 1987).

MEASUREMENTS OF DARK-ADAPTED SENSITIVITY

Psychophysics

Psychophysical procedures used to estimate infants' absolute thresholds are modifications of the two-alternative forced-choice preferential looking method (Teller, 1979). The dark-adapted infant is shown large, brief (usually <1000 ms) stimuli presented eccentrically. An adult observer reports stimulus position (forced choice) based on the infant's head and eye movements.

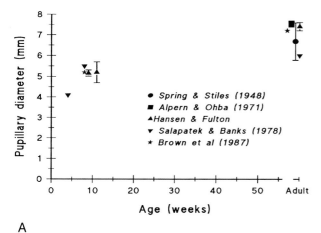

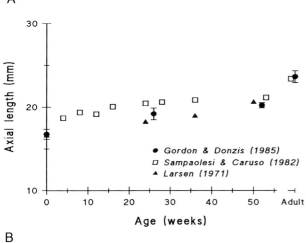

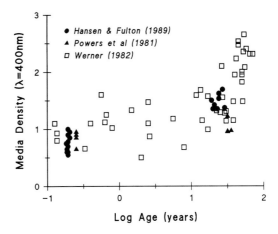

FIG. 8-3. Media density at 400 nm as a function of age for infants and adults. Psychophysical (Powers et al., 1981; Hansen and Fulton, 1989) and visual evoked potential (VEP) results (Werner, 1982) are shown.

FIG. 8-1. (A) Dark-adapted pupillary diameter as a function of age. The sources of the data are indicated in the key. (B) Axial length of the eye determined using ultrasonography as a function of age.

Thresholds have been estimated with the method of constant stimuli and staircase methods (e.g., Wetherill and Levitt, 1965).

The course of scotopic sensitivity increase during infancy, derived from cross-sectional dark-adapted threshold data, is shown in Figure 8-4 (Hansen and Fulton, 1981; Powers et al., 1981; Hamer and Schneck, 1984; Schneck et al., 1984; Brown, 1986, 1988; Hansen et al., 1986). There is reasonable agreement among threshold estimates across laboratories. Infants' dark-adapted thresholds average 1.40 log units higher than adults' at age 4 weeks, 1.10 log units higher at age 10 weeks, and 0.65 log unit higher at age 18 weeks.

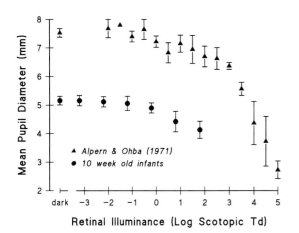

FIG. 8-2. Mean pupillary diameter (±1 SD) as a function of background intensity for 10-week-old infants and adults. (From Alpern and Ohba, 1972. By permission.)

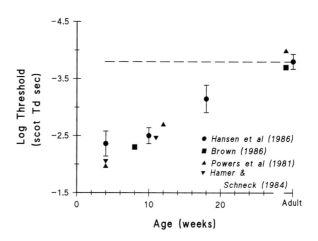

FIG. 8-4. Dark-adapted psychophysical threshold as a function of age for infants and adults. Thresholds were measured using the two-alternative forced-choice preferential looking method. Error bars show ±1 SD. The dashed line represents the average threshold for adults.

ERG b-Wave Results

Dark-adapted infant and adult sensitivities have also been estimated with the b-wave of the electroretinogram (ERG). The b-wave is taken to be an indicator of on bipolar cell activity (Stockton and Slaughter, 1989), and thus it samples activity of cells at a more distal retinal level than psychophysical measures. To estimate b-wave sensitivity, dark-adapted infants are shown a range of stimulus intensities, and the b-wave responses are recorded (Fig. 8-5).

The relation between the peak to trough amplitude of the b-wave and stimulus intensity is

$$V/V_{max} = I^n/(I^n + \sigma^n) \qquad (1)$$

where V = the b-wave amplitude produced by a flash of intensity I; V_{max} = the maximum b-wave response; n = unity. A measure of sensitivity derived from b-wave data is log σ, the flash intensity required to produce a half-maximum (semisaturated) response (Fulton and Rushton, 1978; Arden et al., 1983; Massof et al., 1984; Birch and Fish, 1986; Fulton and Hansen, 1988). The shape of the b-wave stimulus response function, indexed by the exponent n, does not change with development (Fulton and Hansen, 1985, 1990; Birch et al., 1990; Fulton et al., 1991b; Hansen and Fulton, 1991).

The saturated response, V_{max}, increases from about 75 μV at 4 weeks to about 375 μV for adults (Fulton and Hansen, 1982, 1985, 1989). Developmental increases in V_{max} could result from (1) changes in the number of functioning rods, (2) improved synaptic transmission from receptors to second-order neurons, or (3) an increase in the size of responses of postreceptoral neurons. Changes in eye size alone are unlikely to account for increases in V_{max} (Chen et al., 1992).

The b-wave data confirm the psychophysical result that infants are less sensitive than adults (Fig. 8-6). The development of b-wave sensitivity (log σ) roughly parallels psychophysical sensitivity development, although the change in b-wave sensitivity (<1 log unit) is less than the change in psychophysical sensitivity (>1 log unit). At age 4 weeks b-wave sensitivity averages 0.94 log unit less than that of adults, and at 10 weeks sensitivity averages 0.39 log unit lower (Fulton and Hansen, 1982, 1985, 1987, 1989; Fulton et al., 1991b; Hansen and Fulton, 1991). Results from a study (Birch et al., 1990) that included preterm infants are consistent with these data. Infant b-wave sensitivity becomes adultlike by about age 6 months (Fulton and Hansen, 1982, 1985).

For both infants and adults, b-wave sensitivity (log σ) is about 1.8 log units above b-wave threshold, defined as the flash intensity required to produce a small (10–20 μV) response (Fulton and Rushton, 1978). The average b-wave threshold for a 10 μV criterion response

DARK ADAPTED

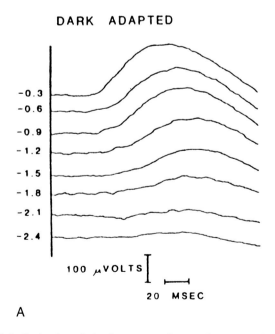

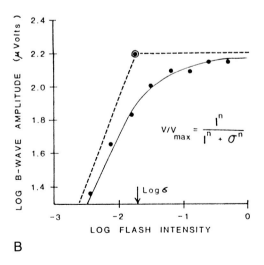

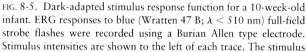

A

B

FIG. 8-5. Dark-adapted stimulus response function for a 10-week-old infant. ERG responses to blue (Wratten 47 B; λ < 510 nm) full-field strobe flashes were recorded using a Burian Allen type electrode. Stimulus intensities are shown to the left of each trace. The stimulus occurred at the start of each trace. Trough-to-peak b-wave amplitudes were measured and plotted as a function of log flash intensity. The smooth curve represents Eq. 1. The intersection of the horizontal and oblique asymptotes have coordinates log σ and log V_{max}.

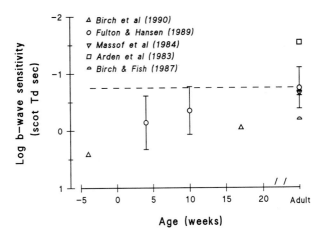

FIG. 8-6. Log b-wave sensitivity as a function of age. Average infant results are from Fulton and Hansen (1989). Error bars represent ±1 SD.

is −2.17 (SD 0.11) log scot Td second for adults and −1.42 (SD 0.44) log scot Td second for 10-week-old infants (Fulton and Hansen, 1989). For adults, b-wave threshold is still nearly 2 log units above psychophysical threshold (Finkelstein et al., 1968; Fulton and Rushton, 1978; Sieving and Nino, 1988).

MECHANISMS OF INCREASED SENSITIVITY: CHANGES IN QUANTAL CATCH

Scotopic sensitivity improvement during infancy could be caused by increased quantal catch, resulting, for example, from increased rhodopsin content. Decreases in quantum catch can be simulated by placing a neutral density filter in front of the eye (Massof et al., 1984; Hood, 1988; MacLeod et al., 1989). For dark-adapted adults, the filter causes b-wave sensitivity (log σ) to decrease, but there is no change in V_{max}.

The distribution of V_{max} and log σ for infants and adults is shown in Figure 8-7A. The infants' b-wave data are not simply shifted horizontally relative to the adult distribution as predicted by reduced quantal catch. Between age 4 weeks and adulthood there are systematic changes in *both* log σ and log V_{max}. Infant V_{max} values increase from about 70 μV to 150 μV between ages 4 and 10 weeks. During this period, log σ changes 0.4 log unit. Thus changes in quantal catch alone do not explain developmental increases in b-wave sensitivity. A more complex model that includes both receptoral and postreceptoral factors is needed (Hood, 1988, see Chapter 29).

Steady scotopic backgrounds also reduce b-wave sensitivity, but until the backgrounds are fairly intense they do not change log V_{max} appreciably. A similar relation between background intensity and V_{max} holds for 10-

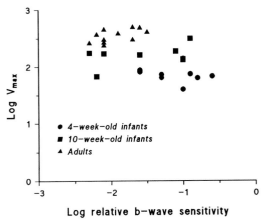

A

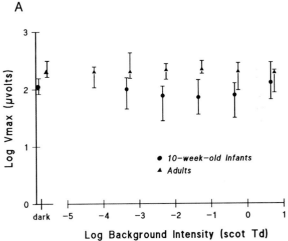

B

FIG. 8-7. (A) Log maximum b-wave amplitude (V_{max}) as a function of b-wave log σ. Data from 4- and 10-week-old infants and young adults are shown (Fulton and Hansen, 1989). (B) Log V_{max} as a function of background intensity for 10-week-old infants and adults (Hansen and Fulton, 1991). Error bars represent the range.

week-old infants (Fig. 8-7B). Scotopic backgrounds that reduce b-wave sensitivity by up to 2.8 log units have little effect on log V_{max} for either infants or adults. For adults, other data show that V_{max} decreases significantly for backgrounds brighter than about +2 log scot Td (Fulton and Rushton, 1978).

AXIAL DENSITY OF RHODOPSIN IN ROD OUTER SEGMENTS

Increases in the axial density of rhodopsin in the rod outer segment could lead to increased quantum catch and improved sensitivity. The b-wave data do not exclude the hypothesis that the axial density of rhodopsin in infant rod outer segments is less than that of adults. The absorbance of rhodopsin in rod outer segments is proportional to the path length of light through the pigment and the concentration of rhodopsin in the rod (Goldstein and Williams, 1966). By the Beer-Lambert relation, increases in rhodopsin density broaden the absorption spectrum. This "concentration broadening" effect changes the shape of psychophysically determined spectral sensitivity functions. For adults, the relation between the rod spectral sensitivity function and the absorption spectrum of rhodopsin is fairly well established (Bowmaker and Dartnall, 1980; Alpern, 1987).

The spectral sensitivity functions of infants as young as 1 month old derived from cross-sectional data have a shape similar to that of the adult scotopic luminous efficiency function (V'_λ), with a peak at about 500 nm (Dobson, 1976; Powers et al., 1981; Werner, 1982; Clavadetscher et al., 1988). To examine these functions in detail, spectral sensitivity functions of individual infants were measured using the preferential looking method and 440–640 nm stimuli (Fig. 8-8A). When sensitivity was expressed as a percent of the maximum sensitivity, the points for 10-week-old infants consistently fell below those of adults (Fig. 8-8B), suggesting that the adult spectral sensitivity functions were wider as predicted by concentration broadening.

Thresholds of infants and adults corrected for losses in the ocular media (Hansen and Fulton, 1989) were compared quantitatively to the absorption spectrum of human rhodopsin (Bowmaker and Dartnall, 1980) to estimate the peak axial density of rhodopsin in the rod outer segment (D_{max}) and the wavelength of peak absorbance (λ_{max}). The curve fitting procedure was based on the method used by Alpern (1987).

The wavelength of peak absorption did not vary systematically with age and averaged about 494 nm (range 489–504 nm) for both infants and adults. The average value of D_{max} inferred from functions fit to individual subject's data was 0.10 (SEM 0.046) for 10-week-old infants and 0.291 (SEM 0.095) for adults. This result is consistent with the notion that rhodopsin densities are low at the time sensitivity is low.

Assuming that dark-adapted sensitivity is proportional to rhodopsin content, threshold elevations for infants relative to adults can be predicted from:

$$\theta_{infant}/\theta_{adult} = 1 - 10^{D(infant)}/1 - 10^{D(adult)} \qquad (2)$$

Using the values of D_{max} obtained in this analysis, an average 0.46 log unit threshold elevation for 10-week-old infants relative to the adult value is predicted. It differs from the observed psychophysical threshold elevations of 1.1 log unit or more (Fig. 8-4) but agrees with the average difference in b-wave sensitivities (0.39 log unit) (Fig. 8-6).

Is this estimated value of D_{max} for 10-week-old infants plausible? Histological measures of rod outer segment length (Drucker and Hendrickson, 1989) (see Chapter 17) at retinal sites near those tested in psychophysical studies found that the length increases about threefold. Assuming that rhodopsin concentration in the outer segment remains constant, as it does in the developing rat retina (Rapp et al., 1990), a threefold increase in D_{max} is expected from the histological results. In addition, measurement of the total rhodopsin content of infant eyes found a median rhodopsin content (2.52 nmol) of about one-third the adult median (6.77 nmol). These measurements predict that infant sensitivity should be 0.5 log unit lower than adult sensitivity (Fulton et al., 1991a).

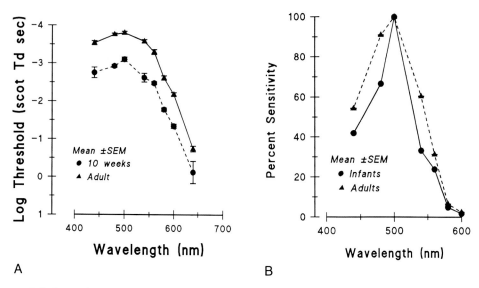

FIG. 8-8. Spectral sensitivity results. (A) Average threshold (± 1 SEM) is plotted as a function of wavelength for 10-week-old infants and adults. (B) Threshold expressed as a percent of the maximum sensitivity (500 nm) is plotted as a function of wavelength for infants and adults.

Thus three lines of evidence—measurement of extracted rhodopsin, measurement of rod outer segment length, and the value of D_{max} inferred from dark-adapted spectral sensitivity functions—are consistent with a receptoral origin for at least for part of the reduced scotopic sensitivity of infants. Although rhodopsin content appears an important controller of b-wave sensitivity for dark-adapted infants, it cannot be the sole determinant of psychophysical threshold.

TEMPORAL SUMMATION FUNCTIONS

Increasing stimulus duration leads to increased sensitivity for detection of brief stimuli up to a critical duration of about 100 ms; further increases in stimulus duration have little effect on sensitivity. Infant and adult b-wave log σ values vary with stimulus duration in similar ways (Fulton et al., 1991b). There is complete temporal summation for stimuli of less than 100 ms and little change in sensitivity with longer durations (Fig. 8-9). These results are consistent with previously reported adult b-wave data (Alpern and Farris, 1956). Estimated critical duration for dark-adapted 10-week-old infants, derived from b-wave log σ, is similar to that of adults (Fulton et al., 1991b).

Other temporal characteristics of infants' b-waves, such as their rise time, fall time, and integration time, differ from those of adults, suggesting that some duration-dependent information is signaled differently by infants' b-waves (Fulton et al., 1991b). For example, integration time (Baylor and Hodgkin, 1973; Baylor et al., 1984), a measure of the width of the b-wave at the baseline

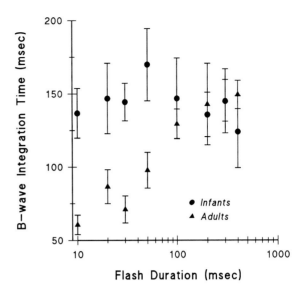

FIG. 8-10. Integration times for b-wave responses to stimuli $< \log \sigma$ are shown as a function of log flash duration.

normalized by its peak amplitude, is nearly constant for infants over a range of 10- to 400-ms flash durations (Fig. 8-10). Adult integration times, however, increase with flash duration up to the critical duration (about 100 ms) and then remain nearly constant (Fulton et al., 1991b).

Infant psychophysical temporal summation functions differ markedly from those of adults (Fig. 8-11). The temporal summation function of individual infants is a line with slope -0.5, suggesting stimulus detection in noise with square-root law improvement in sensitivity based on probability summation over time. Adults tested with the same range of stimulus durations show complete summation for durations up to about 100 ms and

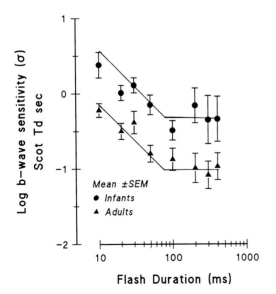

FIG. 8-9. Temporal summation. Log b-wave (σ) sensitivity is plotted as a function of log stimulus duration for infants and adults tested by Fulton et al. (1991b).

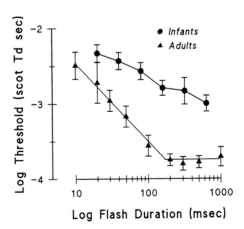

FIG. 8-11. Psychophysical temporal summation functions of infants and adults. Thresholds for detecting 10 degrees diameter, blue ($\lambda <$ 510 nm) flashes presented 20 degrees from fixation (Fulton et al., 1991) were determined using the forced choice preferential looking method.

almost no decrease in threshold at longer durations. Fulton et al. (1991b) concluded that these psychophysical immaturities are primarily a consequence of rod immaturities.

POSTRECEPTORAL POOLING: SPATIAL PROCESSING

Age-dependent changes in convergence of photoreceptors onto second-order neurons are a potential source of sensitivity increase at a postreceptoral level. In adults the critical area for complete spatial summation is thought to reflect receptive field size. Psychophysical studies with

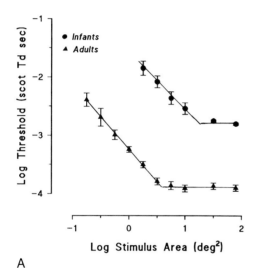

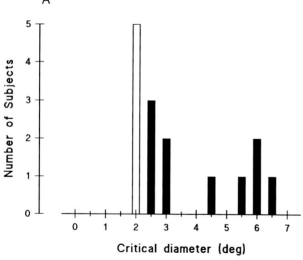

A

B

FIG. 8-12 Spatial summation. (A) The average value of log threshold is plotted as a function of log stimulus area for infants and adults. Error bars represent standard errors. Estimated critical areas are determined from the intersection of a line with slope −1 through the thresholds for small stimuli and a line with slope 0 through the threshold for 10 degrees diameter stimulus. (B) Distribution of critical areas of dark-adapted infants and adults (Hansen et al., 1992). Infant results are represented by filled bars and adult results by the open bar.

dark-adapted infants have shown that the critical area of 4- to 11-week-old infants is larger than that of adults (Hamer and Schneck, 1984; Schneck et al., 1984; Hansen et al., 1992). Critical areas of individual dark-adapted 10-week-old infants were derived from thresholds for a range of stimulus sizes (Fig. 8-12A) by Hansen et al. (1992). Data from individual infants showed that the critical area of each of the infants tested was larger than the critical area of any of the adults tested, although some infants had critical areas only slightly larger than those of adults (Fig. 8-12B). There was a broad overlap between the data of Hansen et al. (1992) and previously reported cross-sectional infant data (Hamer and Schneck, 1984; Schneck et al., 1984).

Because infants' psychometric functions are shallower than those of adults (Hamer and Schneck, 1984; Schneck et al., 1984; Hansen et al., 1986; Brown, 1988; Fulton et al., 1991b) the effects of spatial probability summation (Watson, 1979; Gorea and Tyler, 1985) must be considered to estimate infant critical areas accurately. In both adult and infant subjects, the second branch of the spatial summation function, where threshold changes must be due to the effect of spatial probability summation, had slopes that were not significantly different from zero. This finding suggested that spatial probability summation has similar effects on infant and adult thresholds. Thus it is unlikely that spatial probability summation alone accounts for the large critical areas of infants. Hansen et al. (1992) concluded, rather, that decreases in receptive field size may account for developmental decreases in critical area.

BACKGROUND ADAPTATION IN INFANTS

Psychophysics

Rod increment threshold functions of infants have a similar shape to those of adults (Hansen and Fulton, 1981; Dannemiller and Banks, 1983; Brown, 1986; Hansen et al., 1986). The effects of steady, dim backgrounds on the thresholds of 4-, 10-, and 18-week-old infants (Fig. 8-13) were studied by Hansen et al. (1986). Subjects were tested in the dark-adapted condition and while adapted to a range of scotopic backgrounds (−3 to +1 log scot Td).

The slope of the linear portion of the increment threshold function was about 0.5 for 4- to 6-week-old infants (Hansen and Fulton, 1981; Dannemiller and Banks, 1983; Hansen et al., 1986) and 0.83 for 10-week-olds compared to the value of about 1.0 found for adults. Based on increment thresholds from an achromat and increment thresholds on backgrounds of differing colors, it has been argued that the slope of 1.0 obtained for blue stimuli on red backgrounds results

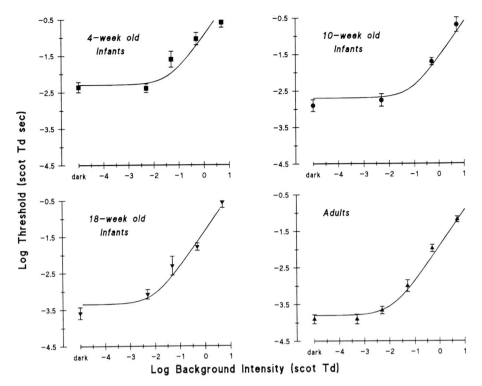

FIG. 8-13. Average psychophysical increment threshold functions of 4-, 10-, and 18-week-old infants and adults. Stimuli were 10 degrees diameter, 1000 ms blue ($\lambda < 510$ nm) flashes presented 20 degrees from fixation. Each point is the mean of five thresholds in that adaptation condition. Error bars are ±1 SD. The smooth curve represents Eq. 3 fit to these threshold data.

from rod–cone interactions (Sharpe et al., 1989). Thus the shallow increment thresholds of young infants may reflect the absence of rod–cone interactions.

Models of Light Adaptation

In the mammalian retina, scotopic adaptation to backgrounds has been documented to occur in the rods (Matthews, 1991; Nakatani et al., 1991), and there is substantial evidence that postreceptoral cells are involved in sensitivity control and background adaptation (Penn and Hagins, 1972; Baylor et al., 1984; MacLeod et al., 1989). Two-stage models of sensitivity control during light adaptation with adults have been proposed (e.g., Hood, 1988; MacLeod et al., 1989; Hood and Greenstein, 1990). In these models, the first site has the properties of rod photoreceptors, and the second stage combines postreceptoral mechanisms of gain control (Shapley and Enroth-Cugell, 1988; Walraven et al., 1990). These models provide explicit predictions that can be compared to infants' increment threshold data.

For example, Brown (1986) concluded that immaturities in scotopic background adaptation are sited proximal to the photoreceptor (i.e., at the second stage) because backgrounds elevated thresholds of 8-week-old infants and adults by equal amounts. The data of Han-

sen et al. (1986) showed that although backgrounds produced similar threshold elevations for infants and adults, threshold elevations were smaller for 4- and 10-week-old infants than for adults. By age 18 weeks, infant and adult threshold elevation were nearly identical (Fig. 8-14).

The psychophysical increment threshold functions of individual infants and adults (Hansen et al., 1986) were fit to:

$$S = S_{DA} + \log [(I + A_o)/A_o] \qquad (3)$$

where S = the threshold at background intensity I; S_{DA} = the dark-adapted (no background) threshold; and A_o = the *eigengrau*, defined as the background intensity that elevates threshold 0.3 log units above the dark-adapted level (Barlow, 1972; Hood, 1988). The distribution of S_{DA} and A_o is shown in Figure 8-15. The predictions of the two-stage model are shown as dashed lines. The horizontal line shows the locus expected if there were *only* postadaptation site immaturity. Dark-adapted thresholds differ between infants and adults, but the *eigengrau* remains constant. Receptoral, or pre-adaptation, site immaturity causes both threshold and *eigengrau* to be affected equally. The data would fall along the diagonal line. The lines are positioned to meet at the average adult values of dark-adapted threshold

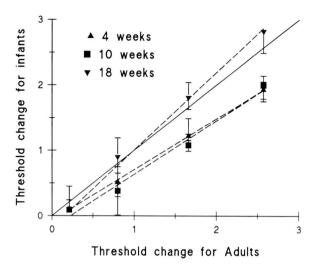

FIG. 8-14. The average threshold elevation produced by each background for 4-, 10-, and 18-week-old infants as a function of the average threshold elevation produced by the same background for adults. The solid line has a slope of 1.0.

and *eigengrau*. Although there is an increase in *eigengrau* with threshold, the slope of the best fitting line through these points is 0.66, not the slope of 1.0 predicted by receptoral immaturity. Thus the psychophysical data are consistent with receptoral immaturity but do not rule out postreceptoral immaturities.

Background Adaptation Assessed Using the b-Wave

To further investigate scotopic background adaptation, Hansen and Fulton (1991) examined ERG b-wave background adaptation functions of 10-week-old infants and adults. The b-wave stimulus response relation was recorded in the dark-adapted condition and then in the presence of steady full-field -3.5 to $+1.0$ log scot Td backgrounds (Fig. 8-16). The b-wave data show that the infant Weber-Fechner functions are of similar shape but are shifted vertically; that is, dark-adapted sensitivity is less than that in adults. The horizontal shift of the background adaptation function, manifested by an increase in *eigengrau*, is less definite.

When Eq. 3 was fit to individual background adaptation functions, the average dark-adapted b-wave sensitivity of infants (-0.30 log scot Td) was significantly lower than that in adults (-0.72 log scot Td). The *eigengrau* values of 10-week-old infants and adults overlapped. The average *eigengrau* of infants was -1.35 (SD 0.23) log scot Td compared to an average -1.53 (SD 0.17) log scot Td for adults. The distribution of dark-adapted sensitivities and *eigengrau* values are compared to the predictions of a two-stage model of adaptation in Figure 8-17. For comparison, the psychophysical results (Hansen et al., 1986) are also plotted on this graph. For both psychophysical and b-wave data sets, infant results depart from the diagonal line predicted by receptoral immaturities.

The *eigengrau* is thought to reflect intrinsic retinal noise (Barlow, 1972; Baylor, 1987). Previously, results have shown that psychophysical and b-wave *eigengraus* are similar for adults (Biersdorf et al., 1965; Fulton and

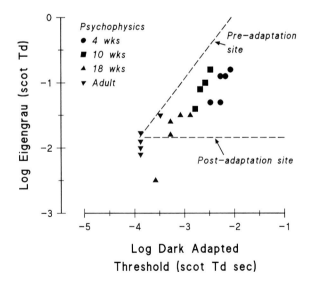

FIG. 8-15. Log *eigengrau* (A_0) is plotted as a function of log dark-adapted threshold (S_{DA}). Eq. 3 was fit to the increment threshold data of individual infants tested at age 4 weeks (circles), 10 weeks (squares), and 18 weeks (triangles). Predictions derived from a two-stage model of adaptation are shown as dashed lines positioned to pass through the average adult results (inverted triangles). The oblique line (slope = 1) is the locus predicted by a first site immaturity and the horizontal line (slope = 0) the prediction of a second site immaturity.

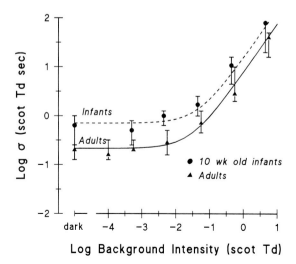

FIG. 8-16. Average b-wave background adaptation functions of 10-week-old infants and adults. Stimuli were 50 ms, full field blue ($\lambda < 510$ nm). The steady full-field backgrounds were red ($\lambda > 610$ nm) and produced retinal illuminances of -3.5 to $+1.0$ log scot Td. The smooth curves represent Eq. 3.

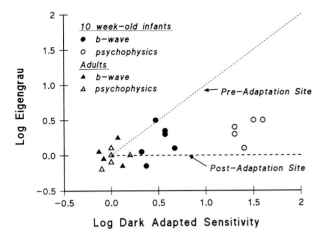

FIG. 8-17. *Eigengrau* (A_0) derived from b-wave background adaptation data (Fig. 8-12). is plotted as a function of the dark-adapted sensitivity (S_{DA}) for individual infants and adults. The dashed oblique line has a slope of 1 and represents the predicted distributions of S_{DA} and A_0 resulting from a receptoral immaturity and the horizontal dashed line (slope = 0) the distribution resulting from postreceptoral immaturity. The open circles are values of S_{DA} and A_0 for previously reported psychophysical increment threshold functions for 10-week-old infants. Adult psychophysical results are represented by open triangles.

Rushton, 1978). A similar result has been found for 10-week-old infants (Hansen et al., 1986; Hansen and Fulton, 1991). Thus we have no evidence that intrinsic retinal noise imposes limitations on the scotopic vision of infants different from those in adults.

In the context of a two-stage adaptation model, available psychophysical and ERG b-wave data do not rule out immaturities at either stage but are consistent with developmental changes at both stages. Small changes in the *eigengrau* suggest that part of the reduced sensitivity of infants has a receptoral origin. The b-wave results suggest that this effect may be as small as 0.23 log unit (Hansen and Fulton, 1991) or, from the psychophysical data (Hansen et al., 1986), as large as 0.4 log unit. However, psychophysical threshold elevations exceed the shifts in the *eigengrau*, and equal backgrounds produce about equal sensitivity reductions for adults and infants. Thus an immaturity at or beyond the second stage must also be present.

DYNAMICS OF BLEACHING ADAPTATION

Following exposure to stimuli that bleach a large proportion of rhodopsin, the slow recovery of sensitivity (governed by photochemical factors) and rhodopsin content in adults follow parallel exponential courses with time constants of about 400 seconds (Rushton, 1961; Alpern, 1971). Not even abbreviated preferential looking methods are quick enough to follow these sen-

sitivity changes because of the time required to estimate each threshold (Fulton and Hansen, 1987; Brown, 1990). However, changes in b-wave log σ and in pupillary diameter provide two measures that can be used to monitor the time course of adaptation with infants.

For adults, pupillary dilation in the dark following a large full-field bleach has the same time course as rhodopsin regeneration measured using reflection retinal densitometry (Alpern and Ohba, 1972; Hansen and Fulton, 1986). A modification of Alpern and Ohba's (1972) method was used to follow pupillary recovery of 10-week-old infants (Hansen and Fulton, 1986). Pupillary diameter was measured for 30 minutes in the dark after exposure for 2 minutes to a 5.4 log scot Td bleach. For adults, this light bleaches more than 90% of the rhodopsin present.

Pupillary diameter increased exponentially for both infants and adults (Fig. 8-18A). The time constant of the best fitting exponential function through each subject's data averaged 399 seconds (SD 31) for infants and 401 seconds (SD 42) for adults (Hansen and Fulton, 1986). Thus rhodopsin regeneration kinetics of 10-week-old infants are the same as those of adults. These data also provide evidence that by age 10 weeks the human visual pathways from the retina to the tectum and the contralateral pupil are functionally equivalent to those of adults.

After the same bleaching exposure, recovery of b-wave sensitivity was followed for 10-week-old infants and adults (Fulton and Hansen, 1987). Four or five b-wave stimulus response functions were measured during 30 minutes in the dark following exposure to the adapting light. Log σ increased with time in the dark (Fig. 8-18B). Although b-wave sensitivity increased less in infants (0.8 log unit) than in adults (1.5 log units), the time constant of exponential functions fit to the b-wave data were nearly identical (average 404 seconds for infants and 407 seconds for adults).

During rod dark adaptation small increases in the amount of rhodopsin present are associated with large changes in sensitivity (Dowling, 1960; Rushton, 1961). Specifically, *log* threshold is proportional the amount of rhodopsin present. When the changes in pupillary diameter, indicating rhodopsin content, and b-wave sensitivities are compared, similar sensitivity–rhodopsin relations are found (Fig. 8-19) for infants and adults (Fulton and Hansen, 1987). Thus the complex mechanisms that govern the log-linear relation are in place as early as age 10 weeks.

SUMMARY

The infant psychophysical and b-wave data presented provide a demonstration of immaturities of scotopic

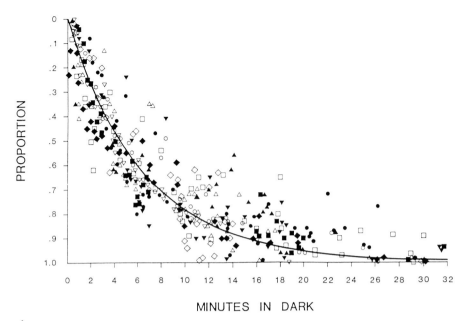

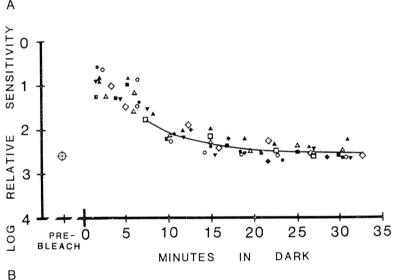

FIG. 8-18. (A) Pupillary recovery of infants. Pupil diameter is plotted as a function of time after a 2-minute, 5.4 log scot Td adapting exposure. The smooth curve is an exponential function, with 399 seconds time constant representing the average time course of changes in infant pupil diameter. (B) Recovery of infant b-wave sensitivity as a function of time. The curve is an exponential function with time constant of 404 seconds. Each subject is represented by a different symbol.

function during the early postnatal period. The data suggest that both receptoral and postreceptoral immaturities are present. Rod immaturities are deduced from developmental shifts in the *eigengrau* of increment threshold functions, psychophysical spectral sensitivity functions, increases in rhodopsin content, and immaturities of psychophysical temporal summation functions. The a-wave, which provides a measure of photoreceptor function (Hood and Birch, 1990a,b,c,) has not been investigated systematically for human infants.

It should be noted that infants' b-wave implicit times are prolonged relative to those in adults (Fulton and Hansen, 1985); it may result from a receptoral immaturity (see Chapter 29). The evidence for postreceptoral or postadaptation site immaturities results from the large spatial summation areas of infants and the fact that equal background intensities produce approximately equal changes in sensitivity for both infants and adults. Thus although the data provide evidence of immaturities at both stages of the model, they do not allow us

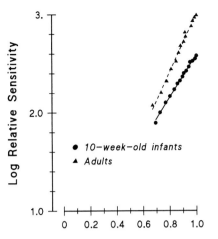

Proportion of Rhodopsin Present

FIG. 8-19. Log relative sensitivity as a function of rhodopsin present. The points were derived from the mean b-wave and pupillary data in Figure 8-18. The slopes of the lines are 2.94 for adults and 2.19 for infants.

to specify the "critical immaturity" (Brown, 1990) that limits scotopic performance of infants.

Acknowledgments. We thank Christine Canniariato, Joanne Daly, and Linda Medwar for their assistance. This project was supported by NIH grant EY-05325.

REFERENCES

ALPERN, M. (1971). Rhodopsin kinetics in the human eye. *J. Phys. (Lond.)* 217, 447–471.

ALPERN, M. (1987). A note on the action spectrum of human rod vision. *Vision Res.* 27, 1471–1480.

ALPERN, M., AND FARIS, J. J. (1956). Luminance duration relationship in the electrical response of the human retina. *J. Opt. Soc. Am.* 46, 845–850.

ALPERN, M., AND OHBA, N. (1972). The effects of bleaching and backgrounds on pupil size. *Vision Res.* 12, 943–951.

ARDEN, G. B., CARTER, R. M., HOGG, C. R., POWELL, D. J., ERNST, W. J. K., CLOVER, G. M., AND QUINLAN, M. P. (1983). A modified ERG technique and the results obtained in X-linked retinitis pigmentosa. *Br. J. Ophthalmol.* 67, 419–430.

BARLOW, H. (1972). Dark and light adaptation. In L. M. HURVICH AND D. JAMESON (eds.). *Handbook of Sensory Physiology. Vol. VII/4. Visual Psychophysics.* Berlin: Springer, pp. 1–28.

BAYLOR, D. A. (1987). Photoreceptors and vision. *Invest. Ophthalmol. Vis. Sci.* 28, 34–49.

BAYLOR, D. A., AND HODGKIN, L. A. (1973). Detection and resolution of visual stimuli by turtle photoreceptors. *J. Physiol. (Lond.)* 234, 163–198.

BAYLOR, D. A., NUNN, B. J., AND SCHNAPF, J. L. (1984). The photocurrent, noise and spectral sensitivity of rods of the monkey *Macaca fasicularis. J. Physiol. (Lond.)* 357, 575–607.

BIERSDORF, W. R., GRANDA, A. M., AND LAWSON, H. F. (1965). Electrical measurement of incremental thresholds in the human eye. *J. Opt. Soc. Am.* 55, 454–455.

BIRCH, D. G., AND FISH, G. E. (1986). Rod ERG's in children with hereditary retinal degeneration. *J. Pediatr. Ophthalmol. Strabismus* 23, 227–232.

BIRCH, E. E., AND BIRCH, D. G. (1987). Pupillometric measures of retinal sensitivity in infants and adults with retinitis pigmentosa. *Vision Res.* 27, 499–505.

BIRCH, E. E., BIRCH, D. G., PETRIG, B., AND UAUY, R. (1990). Retinal and cortical function in very low birthweight infants at 36 and 57 weeks post conception. *Clin. Vis. Sci.* 5, 363–373.

BOWMAKER, J. K., AND DARTNALL, H. J. A. (1980). Visual pigments of rods and cones of a human retina. *J. Physiol. (Lond.)* 298, 501–511.

BROWN, A. M. (1986). Scotopic sensitivity of the two-month-old human infant. *Vision Res.* 26, 707–711.

BROWN, A. M. (1988). Saturation of rod initiated signals in 2-month-old human infants. *J. Opt. Soc. Am. [A]* 5, 2145–2158.

BROWN, A. M. (1990). Development of visual sensitivity to light and color in human infants: a critical review. *Vision Res.* 30, 1159–1188.

BROWN, A. M., DOBSON, V., AND MAIER, J. (1987). Visual acuity of infants at scotopic, mesopic and photopic luminances. *Vision Res.* 27, 1845–1858.

CLAVADETSCHER, J. E., BROWN, A. M., ANKRUM, C., AND TELLER, D. Y. (1988). Spectral sensitivity and chromatic discriminations in 3- and 7-week-old human infants. *J. Opt. Soc. Am. [A]* 5, 2093–2105.

CHEN, J.-F., EISNER, A. E., BURNS, S. A., HANSEN, R. M., LOU, P. L., KWONG, K. K., AND FULTON, A. B. (1992). The effect of eye shape on retinal responses. *Clin. Vis. Sci.* (in press).

DANNEMILLER, J. L., AND BANKS, M. S. (1983). The development of light adaptation in human infants. *Vision Res.* 23, 599–609.

DOBSON, V. (1976). Spectral sensitivity of the 2-month-old infant as measured by the visually evoked potential. *Vision Res.* 16, 367–374.

DOWLING, J. E. (1960). Chemistry of visual adaptation in the rat. *Nature* 188, 114–118.

DRUCKER, D. N., AND HENDRICKSON, A. E. (1989). The morphological development of extrafoveal human retina. *Invest. Ophthalmol. Vis. Sci.* 30 (suppl.), 226.

FINKELSTEIN, D., GOURAS, P., AND HOFF, M. (1968). Human electroretinogram near the absolute threshold of vision. *Invest. Ophthalmol.* 7, 214–218.

FULTON, A. B., AND HANSEN, R. M. (1982). Background adaptation in human infants: analysis of b-wave results. *Doc. Ophthalmol. Proc. Ser.* 31, 191–197.

FULTON, A. B., AND HANSEN, R. M. (1985). Electroretinography: application to clinical studies with infants. *J. Pediatr. Ophthalmol. Strabismus* 22, 251–257.

FULTON, A. B., AND HANSEN, R. M. (1987). The relationship of retinal sensitivity and rhodopsin in human infants. *Vision Res.* 27, 697–704.

FULTON, A. B., AND HANSEN, R. M. (1988). Scotopic stimulus/response relations of the b-wave of the electroretinogram. *Doc. Ophthalmol.* 68, 293–304.

FULTON, A. B., AND HANSEN, R. M. (1989). Development of scotopic OP's in human infants. *Invest. Ophthalmol. Vis. Sci.* 30 (suppl.), 314.

FULTON, A. B., AND RUSHTON, W. A. H. (1978). The human rod ERG: correlation with psychophysical responses in light and dark adaptation. *Vision Res.* 18, 793–800.

FULTON, A. B., ABRAMOV, I., ALLEN, J., GWIAZDA, J., HAINLINE, L., O'NEILL, J., RAYMOND, P., AND VARNER, D. (1986). In M. WAXLER AND V. M. HITCHINS (eds.). *Optical Radiation and Visual Health.* Boca Raton, FL: CRC Press, p. 138.

FULTON, A. B., DODGE, J., HANSEN, R. M., SCHREMSER, J-L., AND WILLIAMS, T. P. (1991a). The quantity of rhodopsin in young human eyes. *Curr. Eye Res.* 10, 977–982.

FULTON, A. B., HANSEN, R. M., YEH, Y-L., AND TYLER, C. W.

(1991b). Temporal summation of dark adapted 10-week-old infants. *Vision Res.* 31, 1259–1269.

GOLDSTEIN, E. B., AND WILLIAMS, T. P. (1966). Calculated effects of "screening pigments." *Vision Res.* 6, 39–50.

GORDON, R. A., AND DONZIS, P. B. (1985). Refractive development of the human eye. *Arch. Ophthalmol.* 103, 785–789.

GOREA, A., AND TYLER, C. W. (1985). A new look at Bloch's law for contrast. *J. Opt. Soc. Am.* [A] 3, 52–61.

HAMER, R. D., AND SCHNECK, M. E. (1984). Spatial summation in dark adapted human infants. *Vision Res.* 24, 77–85.

HANSEN, R. M., AND FULTON, A. B. (1981). Behavioral measurement of background adaptation in human infants. *Invest. Ophthalmol. Vis. Sci.* 21, 625–629.

HANSEN, R. M., AND FULTON, A. B. (1986). Pupillary changes during dark adaptation in human infants. *Invest. Ophthalmol. Vis. Sci.* 27, 1726–1729.

HANSEN, R. M., AND FULTON, A. B. (1987). Scotopic spectral sensitivity of human infants. *Invest. Ophthalmol. Vis. Sci.* 28 (suppl.), 4.

HANSEN, R. M., AND FULTON, A. B. (1989). Psychophysical estimates of ocular media density of human infants. *Vision Res.* 29, 687–690.

HANSEN, R. M., AND FULTON, A. B. (1991). Electroretinographic assessment of background adaptation in 10-week-old human infants. *Vision Res.* 31, 1501–1507.

HANSEN, R. M., FULTON, A. B., AND HARRIS, S. J. (1986). Background adaptation in human infants. *Vision Res.* 26, 771–779.

HANSEN, R. M., HAMER, R. M., AND FULTON, A. B. (1992). The effect of light adaptation on scotopic spatial summation in 10-week-old infants. *Vision Res.* 32, 387–392.

HIRANO, S., YAMAMOTO, Y., TAKAYAMA, H., SUGATA, Y., AND MATSUO, K. (1979). Ultrasonic observations of eyes in premature babies. Part 6. Growth curves of ocular axial length and its components. *Acta Soc. Ophthalmol. Jpn.* 83, 1697–1693.

HOOD, D. C. (1988). Testing hypotheses about development with electroretinographic and increment threshold data. *J. Opt. Soc. Am.* [A] 5, 2159–2165.

HOOD, D. C., AND BIRCH, D. G. (1990a). The a-wave of the human electroretinogram and rod receptor function. *Invest. Ophthalmol. Vis. Sci.* 31, 2070–2081.

HOOD, D. C., AND BIRCH, D. G. (1990b). A quantitative measure of the electrical activity of human rod photoreceptors using electroretinography. *Vis. Neurosci.* 5, 379–387.

HOOD, D. C., AND BIRCH, D. G. (1990c). The relationship between models of receptor activity and the a-wave of the ERG. *Clin. Vision Sci.* 5, 293–297.

HOOD, D. C., AND GREENSTEIN, V. C. (1990). Models of the normal and abnormal rod system. *Vision Res.* 30, 51–68.

LARSEN, J. S. (1971). The sagittal growth of the eye. IV. Ultrasonic measurements of the axial length of the eye from birth to puberty. *Acta Ophthalmol.* (Copenh.) 49, 873–886.

MACLEOD, D. I. A., CHEN, B., AND CROGNALE, M. (1989). Spatial organization of sensitivity regulation in rod vision. *Vision Res.* 29, 965–978.

MASSOF, R. W., WU, L., FINKELSTEIN, D., PERRY, C., STARR, S. J., AND JOHNSON, M. A. (1984). Properties of electroretinographic intensity-response functions in retinitis pigmentosa. *Doc. Ophthalmol.* 57, 279–296.

MATTHEWS, H. R. (1991). Incorporation of chelator into guinea pig rods shows that calcium mediates mammalian photoreceptor light adaptation. *J. Physiol.* (Lond.) 432, 93–105.

NAKATANI, K., TAMURA, T., AND YAU, K-L. (1991). Light adaptation in retinal rods of the rabbit and two other non-primate mammals. *J. Gen. Physiol.* 97, 413–435.

NORREN, D. VAN, AND VOS, J. J. (1974). Spectral transmission of the human ocular media. *Vision Res.* 14, 1237–1244.

PENN, R. D., AND HAGINS, W. A. (1972). Kinetics of the photocurrent of retinal rods. *Biophys. J.* 12, 1073–1094.

POKORNY, J., SMITH, V. C., AND LUTZ, M. (1987). Aging of the human lens. *Appl. Opt.* 26, 1437–1440.

POWERS, M. K., SCHNECK, M. S., AND TELLER, D. Y. (1981). Spectral sensitivity of human infants at absolute visual threshold. *Vision Res.* 21, 1005–1016.

RAPP, L. M., TOLMAN, B. L., KONTZ, C. A., AND THUM, L. A. (1990). Predisposing factors to light induced photoreceptor cell damage: retinal changes in maturing rats. *Exp. Eye Res.* 51, 177–184.

RUSHTON, W. A. H. (1961). Dark adaptation and the regeneration of rhodopsin. *J. Physiol.* [Lond.] 156, 166–178.

SALAPATEK, P., AND BANKS, M. S. (1978). Infant sensory assessment: Vision. In F. D. MINIFIE AND L. L. LOYD (eds.). *Communicative and Cognitive Abilities: Early Behavioral Assessment.* Baltimore: University Park Press, pp. 61–106.

SAMPAOLESI, R., AND CARUSO, R. (1982). Ocular echometry in the diagnosis of congenital glaucoma. *Arch. Ophthalmol.* 100, 574–577.

SCHNECK, M. E., HAMER, R. D., PACKER, O. S., AND TELLER, D. Y. (1984). Area threshold relations at controlled retinal locations in 1-month-old human infants. *Vision Res.* 24, 1753–1763.

SHAPLEY, R., AND ENROTH-CUGELL, C. (1984). Visual adaptation and retinal gain control. *Prog. Retinal Res.* 3, 263–346.

SHARPE, L. T., FACH, C., NORDBY, K., AND STOCKMAN, A. (1989). The incremental threshold of the rod visual system and Weber's law. *Science* 244, 354–356.

SIEVING, P. A., AND NINO, C. (1988). Scotopic threshold response (STR) of the human electroretinogram. *Invest. Ophthalmol. Vis. Sci.* 29, 1608–1614.

SPRING, K. H., AND STILES, W. S. (1948). Variation of pupil size with change in the angle at which the light stimulus strikes the retina. *Br. J. Ophthalmol.* 32, 340–346.

STOCKTON, R., AND SLAUGHTER, M. M. (1989). B-wave activity of the electroretinogram: a reflection of on-bipolar cell activity. *J. Gen. Physiol.* 93, 101–122.

TELLER, D. Y. (1979). The forced choice preferential looking method: a psychophysical technique for use with human infants. *Infant Behav. Dev.* 2, 135–153.

WALRAVEN, J., ENROTH-CUGELL, C., HOOD, D. C., MACLEOD, D. I. A., AND SCHNAPF, J. L. (1990). The control of visual sensitivity. In L. SPILLMAN AND J. S. WERNER (eds.). *Visual Perception: The Neurophysiological Foundations.* San Diego: Academic Press, pp. 53–101.

WATSON, A. B. (1979). Probability summation over time. *Vision Res.* 19, 515–522.

WERNER, J. S. (1982). Development of scotopic sensitivity and the absorption spectrum of the human ocular media. *J. Opt. Soc. Am.* 72, 247–258.

WETHERILL, G. B., AND LEVITT, H. (1965). Sequential estimation of points on a psychometric function. *Br. J. Math. Stat. Psychol.* 18, 1–10.

WYSZECKI, G., AND STILES, W. S. (1982). *Color Science: Concepts and Methods, Quantitative Data and Formulas.* New York: Wiley.

9 | Infant color vision: OKN techniques and null plane analysis

DAVIDA Y. TELLER AND DELWIN T. LINDSEY

Much has been learned about the development of color vision during early infancy, but much remains unknown. Extensive reviews have been published by Teller and Bornstein (1987), Brown (1990), and Banks and Bennett (1988), so a general literature review is not attempted here.

As a rough characterization of the behavioral literature on chromatic discriminations, it is fair to say that color vision—the capacity of an infant to respond to purely chromatic stimulus differences—emerges rapidly during early infancy. One-month-olds generally fail to demonstrate chromatic discriminations and therefore must be missing some of the processing elements required for the task. Many 2-month-olds, in contrast, clearly succeed in making chromatic discriminations, especially when large stimuli and large color differences are used. Thus the neural machinery, including photoreceptors and postreceptoral neural processing, sufficient for at least minimal chromatic discrimination is already functional at 2 months. The time course of the change from this rudimentary color vision system to adult-like sensitivity to color differences is almost completely unknown.

Two interesting hypotheses to account for the immaturity of infant color vision have been offered. The first hypothesis, developed most explicitly by Brown (Clavadetscher et al., 1988; Brown, 1990), is that under at least some circumstances infant vision may be more *rod-dominated* (dominated by signals initiated by rod rather than cone photoreceptors) than is that of adults. The second, developed most explicitly by Banks and his collaborators (Banks and Bennett, 1988; Banks and Shannon, 1993; c.f. Teller and Lindsey, 1988; Brown, 1990), is that infants may simply suffer from a *uniform loss* of sensitivity to both luminance and chromatic differences, and that there may be no need to postulate the existence of any immaturity specific to chromatic processing per se.

During the past few years, we have been working in three related areas of research on color vision: (1) the use of three-dimensional spaces and three-dimensional geometry as a means of representing theories of color vision; (2) the psychophysics of adult color vision, especially the perception of motion at isoluminance; and (3) the use of moving stimuli and optokinetic nystagmus (OKN) in tests of color vision and related functions in human infants.

In this chapter, we attempt to unite these topics. First, we present a brief introductory sketch of the approach to color theory through the use of three-dimensional color spaces. This approach has provided us with a consistent, provocative, geometrically based framework for thinking about both infant and adult color vision. To our knowledge, no other integrated introduction to this material is available (for a simpler treatment, see Teller and Lindsey, 1993; for a broader treatment, see Teller, 1991), and we hope to provide the non-specialist with at least an intuitive sense of the value of this kind of geometrical modeling. Some of the earlier data on infant color vision, as well as the *rod dominance hypothesis* proposed by Brown and the *uniform loss* hypothesis proposed by Banks, are translated into this framework.

Second, we review and describe the use of moving stimuli and OKN-based techniques, as they potentially apply to infant color vision testing. Our particular variant of OKN color testing is described, and our first two experiments are presented and interpreted in the context of three-dimensional color spaces. These experiments, though preliminary, provide some new data and approaches that bear on the rod dominance and uniform loss hypotheses.

Three disclaimers are in order at the outset. The first concerns the definition of OKN. In the eye movement literature this term is sometimes reserved to refer to specific stimulus conditions or specific response characteristics, and distinctions between at least two forms of OKN are made (e.g., Schor and Narayan, 1981). In the present context, we are using the term more loosely, to refer to the whole set of directional, OKN-like eye movement patterns that an adult can see by watching the response of the infant's eyes to gratings moving across a video screen.

The second disclaimer concerns the legitimacy of OKN-based techniques for the assessment of infant color vision. Adult color vision is usually studied with small, precisely localized, stationary stimuli and voluntary verbal responses, and not with large moving fields and OKN-like eye movements. Unfortunately, precise, sustained fixation and verbal responses are not part of the infant's behavioral repertoire, whereas OKN-like eye movements in response to large moving fields are. In a way, the present research effort reminds one of the man who dropped his keys in the middle of the block but looked for them under the lamp post at the corner because the light was better there. Our plan is to study both infant and adult color vision with OKN-based techniques and mend our fences with classical color science as we go along.

The third disclaimer is that the theoretical work and the infancy work are just now converging, and the infancy work is only just getting started. Thus the stimuli we have used with infants to date are not perfectly chosen with respect to the color space we have come to use in our adult work, and the data are not yet extensive. Nonetheless, experiments performed to date suggest that the territory under the lamp post will turn out to be interesting.

THREE-DIMENSIONAL COLOR SPACES

Null Plane Analysis

To begin at the beginning: Three kinds of photoreceptors—L (long-), M (mid-), and S (short-wavelength-sensitive) cones—are found in the human fovea. The fourth kind of photoreceptor, the rods, are added to the three cone types in the extrafoveal retina. The probability that a quantum of light will be absorbed by a photoreceptor depends on the wavelength of the quantum. The *spectral sensitivity curves* of the four photoreceptor types are shown in Figure 9-1.

A fundamental property of the process of quantal absorption is that its effect on a photoreceptor is independent of the wavelength of the quantum. Remarkably, each individual photoreceptor discards wavelength information, and the only effect that light of any given wavelength composition can have on the visual system is to produce a particular quantum catch rate in each of the photoreceptor types. Thus the existence of only three kinds of cone places a profound and irreversible limitation on our foveal color and brightness vision and leads directly to the trichromacy of color vision (Cornsweet, 1970).

Cone Excitation Space. Because human foveal color/brightness vision is limited to three degrees of freedom, color theorists have often used three-dimensional geometry to represent the coding and recoding of color/brightness information. For example, the initial encoding stage can be represented as a three-dimensional *cone excitation space*, with the quantum catches of the three cone types used to define the cardinal axes of the space, as shown in Figure 9-2. Any given visual stimulus can produce a set of three quantum catch rates: L, M, and S. Visual stimuli can be represented as points in this space, in terms of their effects on the visual system.

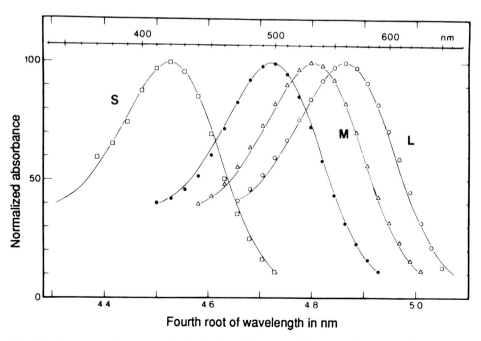

FIG. 9-1. Spectral sensitivity curves for the L, M, and S cones and the rods. (After Dartnall et al., 1983.)

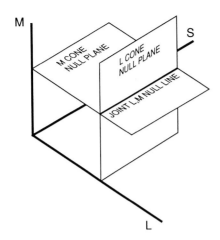

FIG. 9-2. Three-dimensional photoreceptor space. Quantum catches of the L, M, and S cones are represented on the three axes. Planes perpendicular to the L and M axes represent L and M cone null planes, respectively. Their intersection represents a joint null line for both L and M cones.

Metamers—stimuli of different wavelength composition that yield identical responses in each of the three cone types, respectively, and are thus indiscriminable—plot to the same point in cone excitation space.

Three-dimensional color spaces are also useful for allowing easy representation of the existence of silent substitution sets, or *null planes*, for the individual cone types. That is, a plane perpendicular to the L cone axis represents a set of stimuli that yield identical quantum catches in the L cones. A spatial pattern (e.g., a set of stripes) composed of stimuli chosen to lie in such a null plane would produce no special variation across the matrix of L cones; therefore, where the picture presented by the L cone matrix is concerned, the field might as well be spatially homogeneous. Planes perpendicular to the M or S axes similarly represent null planes for M and S cones, respectively. Spatial patterns composed of stimuli selected from a null plane for one cone type allow us to reduce the *cone contrast* to zero for that cone type and thereby explore the properties of vision when the spatial variations in the stimulus are confined to the remaining two cone matrices.

Furthermore, the intersection of two such null planes, such as the null planes for L and M, represents a joint silent substitution set, or a *joint null line*, for two cone types simultaneously. Along this line, the cone contrasts are zero for both of these two cone types. Spatial patterns made from stimuli selected from a joint null line can be used to explore the properties of vision when the spatial variation in the input pattern is confined to a single cone type. Figure 9-2 shows a joint null line along which L-cone contrast and M-cone contrast are both zero; the contrast in a spatial pattern made from stimuli represented along this line would be confined to the S-cone matrix.

Postreceptoral Channels Space. The particular neural code originated by the photoreceptors is short-lived. Signals from the three cone types are recombined, probably several times at different levels of serial processing, to form recoded signals in (at least) three postreceptoral neural channels. The question of which cone types contribute to which neural channels has been a matter of debate among color theorists; a summary of the various theories has been represented by Boynton (1979, p. 248).

A particularly simple and useful model of an early postreceptoral processing stage in human vision was first proposed by Ingling and Tsou (1977) and popularized by Boynton (1979). This scheme has received support from both psychophysical and physiological experiments (e.g., Krauskopf et al., 1982; Derrington et al., 1984; Lennie et al., 1990) and is adopted here. This model suggests that at some stage of neural processing there are three particular channels concerned with color/brightness vision: a *luminance* channel and two *chromatic channels*, which we call the r/g and *tritan* channels, respectively. The signal in each channel is formed by a linear combination of inputs from two or three cone types. L and M signals are summed to produce the signal in the luminance channel (L + M) and differenced to produce the signal in the r/g channel (L − M). The signal in the tritan channel is produced by differencing the S cone signal with the sum of L and M [S − (L + M)].

Like the signals in the three cone types, the signals in the three putative postreceptoral channels can be represented on the axes of a three-dimensional space. Figure 9-3 shows a simplified version of the *postreceptoral channels space* developed by Derrington et al. (1984) to display the characteristics of this model of color vision. The origin of this space is at a (somewhat arbitrary) "white" point. The vertical axis represents activity in the putative luminance channel. The plane perpendicular to the luminance axis is a null plane for the luminance channel, in short, an *isoluminant plane*. More specifically, it here represents a set of lights of different chromaticities, matched in luminance by an internationally recognized standard photopic spectral sensitivity curve [Judd's (1951) modified V_λ] and here called the V_λ *isoluminant plane*. The two lines in the isoluminant plane are the putative chromatic axes: the r/g axis at the 0- to 180-degree azimuth, and the tritan axis at the 90- to 270-degree azimuth. These axes represent the activity levels in the r/g and tritan channels, respectively. For further discussion and alternate choices of the luminance (or achromatic) axis, see Flanagan et al., 1990, and Lindsey, in preparation.

As described above, the signals in each of the putative postreceptoral channels are composed of linear sums or differences between photoreceptor signals. It follows that the cone excitation space of Figure 9-2 can be

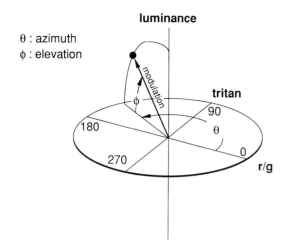

FIG. 9-3. Three-dimensional channels space. The model of postreceptoral processing described by Boynton (1979) and others is incorporated into this spatial representation. Vertical axis represents the signal in the luminance channel, which sums input from L and M cones. The plane perpendicular to the luminance axis and spanned by the r/g and tritan axes represents a V_λ-defined isoluminant plane through the origin. The horizontal axis at azimuth 0–180 degrees represents the signal in the r/g channel, which differences inputs from the L and M cones. The horizontal axis at azimuth 90–270 degrees represents the signal in the tritan channel, which differences the S cones from the sum of L and M cones. By convention, stimuli that appear reddish plot near 0 degrees, and the color circle proceeds counterclockwise from this point. Stimuli represented at 90 degrees appear greenish yellow, those at 180 degrees, greenish, and those at 270 degrees, violet. (After Derrington et al., 1984.)

transformed into the postreceptoral channels space of Figure 9-3 by means of an origin shift, axis rotations, and axis scaling. The same piece of three-dimensional space is still being represented, distorted but otherwise intact; in particular, planes (e.g., L, M, and S cone null planes) defined in one space remain planes in the other.

With the information we already have and a little work, it is possible to locate the L, M, and S cone null planes defined in Figure 9-2 in the new coordinate system of Figure 9-3. Because by hypothesis the S cones make no contribution to the r/g signal, the S cone null plane intersects the isoluminant plane along the r/g axis. The L and M cone null planes similarly intersect the isoluminant plane along the tritan axis (Derrington et al., 1984). More technically, with our particular choice of axis scaling (Palmer et al., 1993) the S cone null plane tilts above the tritan axis at an elevation of 45 degrees. The M and L cone null planes fall just above and just below the r/g axis, at +2.4 degrees and −1.3 degrees, respectively.

A useful two-dimensional format for representing tilts of other planes with respect to the V_λ plane is shown in Figure 9-4. Figure 9-4A,B shows locations of the L, M, and S cone null planes in postreceptoral channels space. On the azimuth at which a particular null plane

(either a cone null plane or an empirical isoluminant plane) intersects the V_λ plane, the elevation is zero; and where it deviates most, the elevation is maximal. The geometry of the situation is such that elevation varies approximately sinusoidally with azimuth between these two points, as shown in Figure 9-4C,D. Furthermore, the amplitude and phase of this sinusoidal variation provide a useful characterization of the tilt of a particular null plane.

Tilt of the Isoluminant Plane. The term *photometry* refers to methods for matching two lights of different wavelength composition in luminous efficiency, or *luminance*. The two most established photometric methods are heterochromatic flicker photometry (HFP) and minimally distinct border matches (MDBs). With both of these methods, lights of a series of different wavelengths can be matched against a standard white. In other words, photometry can now be conceptualized as the operation of selecting a white light (ideally coinciding with the white light represented at the origin of the space) and determining the chromatic lights that fall in the isoluminant plane passing through that white light.

In the postreceptoral channels model described above, the isoluminant plane is exactly the V_λ plane. However, empirical photometric matches vary somewhat with stimulus parameters, retinal eccentricity, and photometric technique; and individual differences in HFP and MDB judgments are well known. The V_λ isoluminant plane therefore certainly is not precisely accurate for most observers under most conditions. In fact, empirically determined isoluminant planes typically are tilted with respect to the V_λ plane, and this tilt can be specified by the methods already presented in Figure 9-4. As is discussed below, a great deal of information concerning the visual substrate can be gleaned from analysis of the tilt of an individual subject's isoluminant plane with respect to the V_λ plane.

Lindsey (1990a, in preparation) has augmented the postreceptoral channels model by developing a quantitative model of possible causes of variations in the tilt of an empirical isoluminant plane with respect to the V_λ isoluminant plane. In his analysis, there are five—and only five—factors that can cause such variations in tilt. They are variations in the relative proportions of L versus M cones, the density of lens pigmentation, the density of macular pigmentation, inputs from S cones, and inputs from rods. None appears explicitly in the postreceptoral channels model as presented up to this point, and we here digress to discuss these complicating factors.

Of the five factors, it turns out that only one factor yields a tilt at azimuth zero, or cosine phase (Fig. 9-4C). That factor is the L/M ratio, or the relative weighting of L and M cone inputs used to model the luminance

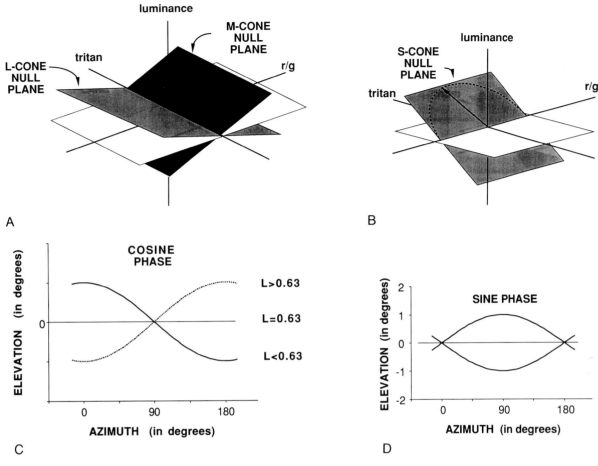

A

B

C

D

FIG. 9-4. (A,B) Representation of the L and M cone null planes (A) and the S cone null plane (B) in channels space. The L and M cone null planes intersect the isoluminant plane along the tritan axis, with maximum elevations of −1.3 and 2.4 degrees, respectively (not to scale). The S cone null plane intersects the isoluminant plane along the r/g axis, with a maximum elevation of 45 degrees (not to scale.)

(C,D) Representation of tilts of other planes with respect to the V_λ isoluminant plane in two-dimensional plots of elevation against azimuth. Planes that intersect the isoluminant plane along the tritan axis produce a cosine-phase variation of elevation with azimuth (C), whereas those that intersect along the r/g axis produce a sine-phase variation (D).

signal (L + M). Various weightings of L and M cone inputs yield a family of planes that all intersect on the tritan axis, bounded by the M and L cone null planes at +2.4 degrees and −1.3 degrees (Fig. 9-4A). The original V_λ isoluminant plane is obtained by weighting the L and M cones in the proportion 0.63:0.37.

In contrast to the relatively simple situation for tilts in cosine phase, it turns out that the other four factors—macular pigment, lens pigment, S cones, and rods—potentially contribute tilts at or near 90 degrees azimuth in sine phase.

The first two factors are the densities of two intraocular pigments: the macular pigment and the pigment in the lens. As it happens, population average values for the densities of both of these pigments are already incorporated into V_λ; that is, the V_λ standard observer looks out through average values of lens and macular pigment. There are substantial individual differences in the concentrations of these intraocular pigments, how-

ever, and any deviation from the population average values means that an individual's isoluminant plane is tilted with respect to the V_λ plane.

Figure 9-5A shows the effect of variations in macular pigment density on the elevation of the isoluminant plane. The density already incorporated into Judd's modified V_λ, 0.65, yields an elevation of zero, and lower and higher pigment densities yield positive and negative tilts, respectively. A similar array of curves describes the effects of variations in lens pigmentation (not shown). Figure 9-5B shows calculations for a wide range of combinations of lens and macular pigment densities; all yield tilts that are nearly (although not exactly) in sine phase.

The final two factors are contributions from S cones and rods, respectively. According to the assumptions of the original channels model, described above, the luminance signal is composed of summed signals from L and M cones, and neither S cones nor rods should con-

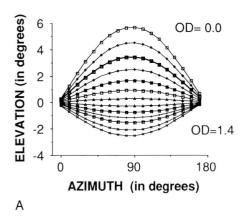

A

FIG. 9-5. (A) Influence of various concentrations of macular pigment on the tilt of the isoluminant plane with respect to the V_λ plane. From top to bottom the peak optical densities are 0, 0.1, . . . , 1.0, 1.2, and 1.4. A macular pigment density of 0.65 is assumed for the standard observer and is automatically incorporated into V_λ; thus this concentration yields a tilt of zero. (B) Influence of various combinations of lens and macular pigment densities on the tilt of the isoluminant plane. Lens densities at 400 nm: △ 2.0; ▲ 1.6; □ 1.0. For each lens density, macular pigment densities range from 0 (topmost symbol) to 1.4 (lowest symbol). All reasonable combinations of lens and macular pigment densities yield tilts in nearly sine phase, particularly when the overall tilt is positive and greater than 2 degrees.

tribute. If an S cone input were to occur, however, it would contribute a component of tilt toward the S cone null plane, exactly in sine phase. In the extreme, if the luminance channel were controlled exclusively by the S cones, the isoluminant plane would coincide with the S cone null plane and have an elevation of 45 degrees above the tritan axis (Fig. 9-4B).

Finally, we consider the consequences of complicating the model of Figure 9-3 by assuming that rod photoreceptors provide an input to the luminance channel. Rod photoreceptors occur in abundance outside the foveal region, and their luminous efficiency curve has been presented in Figure 9-1. In fact, there is general agreement that rod-initiated signals do not have a separate neural channel, and therefore a rod contribution to the luminance channel is likely outside the fovea. If large stimuli are to be used, the postreceptoral channels model must be modified to accommodate such a contribution. (There is no universal agreement on the question of whether rod-initiated signals also share the chromatic channels; this possibility is ignored for the present purposes.)

It can be shown that sets of stimuli that produce equal rod quantum catches also occupy planes—*rod null planes*—in three-dimensional spaces initially defined in terms of cones. However, the exact location of the rod null plane in spaces such as those in Figures 9-2 and 9-3 depends on the exact primaries used to generate the stimuli (D'Zmura and Lennie, 1986; Young and Teller, 1991). With the primaries we use, the rod null plane cuts the isoluminant plane at azimuth 168 degrees, and its maximum deviation from the V_λ plane is 18 degrees at azimuth 78 degrees. Thus a rod contribution to the luminance channel would introduce a component of tilt

in this direction of a magnitude that would depend on the relative weights of rod with respect to L and M cone inputs. If the luminance channel were controlled exclusively by rod inputs, the new isoluminant plane would coincide with the rod null plane.

In sum, Lindsey's analysis identifies and quantifies five factors that influence the tilt of the empirical isoluminant plane. It would, of course, be useful to be able to reverse the process and use the tilt of the empirical isoluminant plane to sort out individual differences in the factors that influence the tilt of the plane. However, there is a problem: Tilt is specified by only 2 degrees of freedom: azimuth and elevation (or the amplitude and phase of the best-fitting sinusoid as illustrated in Figure 9-4). Auxiliary information or assumptions are needed to reduce the number of degrees of freedom, especially in the case of sine phase components.

Infant Null Planes. Only a few studies of infant spectral sensitivity are available to date (for reviews see Teller and Bornstein, 1987; Brown, 1990). In general, infant spectral sensitivity has been found to be similar to that of adults tested with similar techniques under similar stimulus conditions. However, some of these studies show an apparent increase in the influence of rod-initiated signals for infants compared to adults, and these results form a major basis for Brown's (1990) hypothesis of increased rod dominance in infant vision.

Unfortunately, with one exception (Maurer et al., 1989; also see below), none of the published studies has been carried out with techniques that approximate classically accepted photometry (i.e., with flicker photometry or minimally distinct border judgments). Moreover, because both HFP and MDB require the psychophysical subject to make rather sophisticated perceptual judgments, neither technique seems readily adaptable for use with infants (Teller et al., 1992). Thus virtually no direct estimates of infant null planes are available.

The analysis of infant null planes would provide an interesting contribution to developmental studies of color vision. If infant isoluminant planes could be established photometrically and the degrees of freedom problem bypassed, tilt differences might be used to assess developmental changes in the various factors that contribute to the tilt of the isoluminant plane. For example, one could address the maturation of infant L and M cones and the maturity of their weightings in the infant luminance channel (Brown and Teller, 1989; Maurer et al., 1989). One could also determine if Brown's rod dominance hypothesis, derived from studies in which nonstandard techniques have been employed, would receive support from more classical photometry.

Discrimination Ellipsoids

We turn now to the question of just detectable changes of luminance and chromaticity. Starting at a point such as the "white" origin of the postreceptoral channels space shown in Figure 9-3, one can ask how large a change of luminance or chromaticity (or both) is required for a psychophysically detectable change to occur. Historically, *detection* or *discrimination thresholds* have been measured in many directions from the chosen origin and the thresholds in the two opposite directions from the origin averaged (e.g., Brown and MacAdam, 1949). More recently, *modulation thresholds* (Teller and Lindsey, 1993) have been measured for many vectors *through* the origin (e.g., Noorlander and Koenderink, 1983).

In either case, for the color-normal trichromatic observer, the resulting data tend to form ellipses in two dimensions, or ellipsoids in three dimensions, around the chosen origin. Theoretically, thresholds measured along the luminance, tritan, and r/g axes reveal the sensitivity of the observer to signals in each of these channels in isolation, and thresholds measured at intermediate azimuths and elevations reveal the sensitivity of the observer to combinations of signals in two or all three channels. [The exact shapes of the ellipsoids depend on the summation rules for signals in the three channels (Wyszecki and Stiles, 1982; Graham, 1989; Poirson and Wandell, 1990) and are beyond the scope of this chapter.]

Russian Dolls Model. Discrimination ellipsoids tested under any two conditions may or may not be identical in size and shape. In general, luminance thresholds and chromatic thresholds change with stimulus parameters, such as spatial and temporal frequency, with light and dark

adaptation, and with the psychophysical task; and these changes need not be identical on all three axes.

Equal changes of sensitivity on all three axes would yield a pair of nested, identically shaped discrimination ellipsoids, scaled to each other by equal multiplicative factors. Such a picture reminds us of a set of Russian dolls, nested and identical, with each doll scaled up in size exactly in proportion to the one that fits inside it. For this reason, we refer to this class of models as the *Russian dolls model*. A Russian dolls model, then, does not deal with the shape of any one ellipsoid. Rather, it states that a specific *relation* holds between two discrimination ellipsoids; that is, they are identical in three-dimensional shape and orientation, differing only by a single multiplicative scaling factor.

These ideas are illustrated in Figure 9-6. Parts A, B,

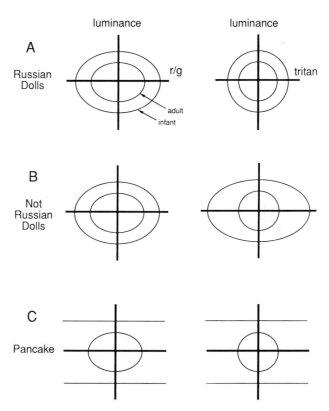

FIG. 9-6. Discrimination ellipsoids. Each pair of figures represents two vertical cuts through the same ellipsoid, one in the r/g-luminance plane (left) and one in the tritan-luminance plane (right). The inner contour represents the discrimination surface for adults and the outer contour that for infants. (A) Outer ellipsoid differs from the inner one by a single scaling factor. Differences between infants and adults conform to a Russian dolls model. (B) Luminance and r/g sensitivities scale equally, but the infants show a greater loss on the tritan axis. Differences between infants and adults depart from a Russian dolls model along the tritan axis. (C) Chromatic discriminations are impossible for infants, and their discrimination contour takes the form of two parallel planes (a "pancake") above and below the isoluminant plane. Differences between infants and adults depart strongly from a Russian dolls model.

and C of Figure 9-6 each represent two cuts through the origin of postreceptoral channels space, with cuts along the r/g and tritan axes represented on the left and right, respectively. Figure 9-6A shows a pair of discrimination ellipsoids that differ by a constant scaling factor; these ellipsoids illustrate a Russian dolls model. Figure 9-6B shows a pair of ellipsoids with equal scaling factors on the luminance and r/g axes but a much larger difference on the tritan axis; in this situation, a Russian dolls model can be rejected.

Russian dolls models are interesting as a class for two reasons. First, because the thresholds for two tasks are tied together by a constant scaling factor on all axes, a Russian dolls model in one coordinate system remains a Russian dolls model in any linear transformation of that coordinate system. For example, a Russian dolls model in cone excitation space (Fig. 9-2) remains a Russian dolls model in postreceptoral channels space (Fig. 9-3). Second, any spatiotemporal noise that is uncorrelated with the stimulus does not upset the Russian dolls relation.

Russian dolls models can be proposed for changes in sensitivity with stimulus parameters or task variables in adults (Lindsey, 1990b). More importantly in the present context, they can also be proposed as descriptions of development. We return to this point below.

Pancakes and Cigars. Elliptical discrimination contours are not, however, expected under all conditions, as shown in Figure 9-6C. Suppose that an initial task is used that yields the inner discrimination contour in Figure 9-6C. If a second psychophysical task is used that the subject can perform on the basis of luminance signals but not on the basis of chromatic signals, the discrimination surface degenerates to two parallel planes (a "pancake") separated from the isoluminant plane by plus or minus the luminance modulation threshold (Teller and Lindsey, 1990, 1993). Moreover, if the subject can perform the second task on the basis of luminance signals and the signals in one chromatic channel but not the other, the discrimination surface resembles a tube (or "cigar") with the long axis oriented along the disabled chromatic axis. Both of these situations are, of course, serious departures from the Russian dolls model.

Infant Discrimination Thresholds. The infant chromatic discrimination paradigm first employed by Peeples and Teller (1975) and used in several subsequent experiments on infant chromatic discrimination (Teller et al., 1978; Hamer et al., 1982; Packer et al., 1984; Varner et al., 1985; Clavadetscher et al., 1988) can now be translated into the context of postreceptoral channels space. In the Peeples and Teller paradigm, two kinds of measurement are used. First, infant luminance discrimination thresholds are measured by testing the in-

fant with a series of luminances of a white test field in a white surround. Second, the infants are tested with a chromatic target, presented at each of a series of relative luminances in the same white surround.

The translation is as follows. The stimuli used in the luminance discrimination task probe a series of points along the luminance axis. The infant's performance at each point, above or below 75%, locates that point, respectively, outside or inside the discrimination contour as it crosses the luminance axis; and the threshold (75% correct) provides a measurement of the width of the discrimination ellipsoid on the luminance axis.

Similarly, the chromatic discrimination function provides an exploration of a series of points falling on a vertical line parallel to the luminance axis but displaced outward from it to a high chromatic value. Again, the infant's performance at each point, above or below 75% correct, locates that point, respectively, outside or inside the discrimination contour in that region of space.

If all points, including the infant's isoluminance point, fall outside the contour, the contour is bounded on that particular chromatic axis, and the infant is said to have made a purely chromatic discrimination. This outcome occurs with some chromatic stimuli, such as red versus white, as shown in Figure 9-7A. If one or more points fall inside the contour, the contour may be unbounded on that chromatic axis, and the infant has failed to make a chromatic discrimination. In the extreme, identical luminance and chromatic discrimination functions are seen, as shown in Figure 9-7B. Such data are consistent with the infant's having a pancake- or cigar-shaped discrimination contour, rather than a discrimination ellipsoid.

The literature to date on infant chromatic discriminations may be summarized in the language of postreceptoral channels space by saying that the discrimination contour of 1-month-olds may well be a pancake, or nearly so, whereas the discrimination contour of 2-month-olds is bounded on at least some chromatic axes. However, compared to adults, even 2-month-olds are remarkably insensitive to chromatic differences, in the sense that they require large test fields and large chromatic differences in order to demonstrate chromatic discrimination (Teller et al., 1978; Packer et al., 1984).

Russian Dolls Model and Infant Color Vision. The Russian dolls analysis provides an interesting heuristic for thinking about several proposed models that bear on the topic of infant color vision. This first is the *uniform loss* model, discussed early in the chapter. The question is, given that young infants are remarkably insensitive to isoluminant chromatic stimuli, why is it true? In comparison to adults, do infants suffer from a differential loss of chromatic with respect to luminance sensitivity or, as Banks and others have suggested, simply

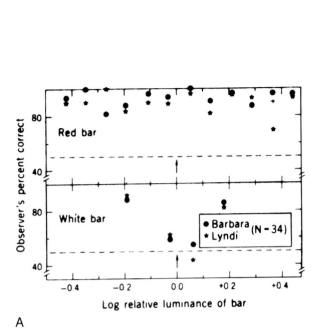

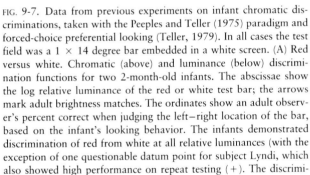

A

B

FIG. 9-7. Data from previous experiments on infant chromatic discriminations, taken with the Peeples and Teller (1975) paradigm and forced-choice preferential looking (Teller, 1979). In all cases the test field was a 1 × 14 degree bar embedded in a white screen. (A) Red versus white. Chromatic (above) and luminance (below) discrimination functions for two 2-month-old infants. The abscissae show the log relative luminance of the red or white test bar; the arrows mark adult brightness matches. The ordinates show an adult observer's percent correct when judging the left–right location of the bar, based on the infant's looking behavior. The infants demonstrated discrimination of red from white at all relative luminances (with the exception of one questionable datum point for subject Lyndi, which also showed high performance on repeat testing (+). The discrimi-

nation functions for red versus white (above) clearly differ from the luminance discrimination functions for the same two subjects (below). These data support the conclusion that (for these stimuli) the infant discrimination contour is bounded near the 0 degrees end of the r/g axis. (From Peeples and Teller. By permission.) (B) Yellow-green versus white. Chromatic (○) and luminance (■) discrimination functions for three infant subjects. The U-shaped chromatic discrimination function for yellow-green versus white closely resembles the luminance discrimination function. These data support the possibility that (for these stimuli) the infant discrimination contour may be unbounded near the 90-degree end of the tritan axis. (From Teller et al., 1978. By permission.)

from a uniform loss of sensitivity to both chromatic and luminance differences? In the present context, this question becomes: Do infants suffer the same losses of sensitivity on all axes of color space? Does a Russian dolls model hold for the relation between infant and adult discrimination contours?

In fact, we would argue that the ideal observer analysis of infant color vision presented by Banks and his associates (Banks and Bennett, 1988; Banks and Shannon, 1993), although apparently complex, reduces precisely a Russian dolls model. With an ideal observer analysis applied to adults, both luminance and chromatic thresholds are predicted on the basis of the combination of L, M, and S cone contrasts (Mullen, 1985; Geisler, 1989). The infant ideal observer analysis centers on the immaturities of the infant's foveal photoreceptors (Yuodelis and Hendrickson, 1986). All three

photoreceptor types are assumed to be equally immature, and nothing about the analysis upsets the fundamental dependence of predicted thresholds on cone contrasts. For this reason, a constant infant/adult threshold ratio is predicted for all axes in color space, which is precisely the defining characteristic of the Russian dolls models.

As it turns out, infants' chromatic discrimination performance is correctly predicted by the infant ideal observer for some chromatic discriminations but not others. In particular, infants are less sensitive than predicted along the tritan axis. To model this deficiency, Banks and Bennett abandoned their initial assumption of equal immaturity of all classes of photoreceptor in favor of a second model that eliminates S cone inputs entirely from the model of the infant retina. The second model thus departs from being a Russian dolls model and produces a discrimination contour corresponding to a cigar along the tritan axis. (Alternatively, infants' relative tritan deficiency can be equally well be modeled by continuing to assume equal immaturities of all three photoreceptor types but a differential loss of tritan sensitivity introduced at the postreceptoral channels level.)

As a second example of a Russian dolls model, we consider noise models (see Chapter 11). Any model of development in which developmental trends are attributed solely to an increased noise level in infants, and in which such noise is assumed to affect luminance and chromatic channels equally, would conform to the Russian dolls prediction.

As a final example, we consider a class of models in which development is modeled in whole or in part by a shift of the spatial contrast sensitivity function (CSF) along the spatial frequency axis (Wilson, 1988). In adults, spatial CSFs are band-pass for luminance-modulated gratings, and more nearly low-pass for isoluminant gratings (e.g., Mullen, 1985), as shown in Figure 9-8. For a stimulus fixed in spatial frequency at, for example, 1 c/d, the luminance/chromatic sensitivity ratio shifts as the luminance and chromatic CSFs shift together along the spatial frequency scale. Thus this model would violate a Russian dolls prediction and predict a gain of chromatic with respect to luminance sensitivity during development.

This final example is important because it illustrates the fact that the interpretation of departures from Rus-

sian dolls behavior is not necessarily simple. The finding of larger losses on chromatic axes than on the luminance axis during development might initially suggest that the chromatic channels are delayed with respect to the luminance channel during development. In this case, however, the differential loss would be attributed most fundamentally to development of *spatial*, rather than chromatic, mechanisms.

Summary. We have tried to describe the unique advantages of using three-dimensional spaces as a means of representing the information available in a three-channel color/brightness system and the changes of coding of this information from one processing level to the next. The concept of null planes and their locations—particularly the question of the tilt of the isoluminant plane—provides a useful conceptual framework for asking questions about developmental changes in spectral sensitivity and its underlying chromatic mechanisms. Discrimination contours in three-dimensional space provide a means for asking questions about developmental changes in chromatic discrimination. In particular, Russian dolls models provide a means of asking whether infants suffer a differential loss of chromatic (with respect to luminance) sensitivity during development. We argue that these themes serve to unite a variety of theories of visual development within a single, fundamentally simple context; and we believe that in the future the development of color vision can be profitably studied in this context.

One final note: The data on infant discrimination ellipsoids, cited above, are the fruit of some 15 years of infant color testing. Yet it obviously remains incomplete. To measure thresholds in all directions in color space is a major task, perhaps prohibitively large in infants. If progress is to be made before the sands have run entirely through the glass, an alternative, more efficient approach to infant color testing is needed. It is to one possible alternative approach that we now turn.

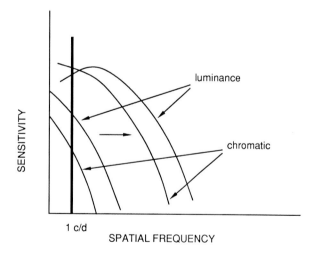

FIG. 9-8. Model of visual development based solely on a shift of spatial scale. The two rightward curves show spatial contrast sensitivity functions for adults. The luminance CSF is band-pass, and the chromatic CSF is low-pass; the two curves approach each other in the vicinity of a spatial frequency of 1 cpd (vertical line). The two leftmost curves show (hypothetical) infant luminance and chromatic CSFs generated by a leftward shift of the adult functions together. Chromatic contrast sensitivity now falls well below luminance contrast sensitivity at 1 cpd. The outcome departs from a Russian dolls model, although the fundamental developmental change is confined to the spatial domain.

MOVING STIMULI AND OPTOKINETIC NYSTAGMUS

We now consider the twin topics of visual motion and optokinetic nystagmus. At the practical level, moving stimuli are uniquely important to the study of visual development because they evoke a special response or set of responses—optokinetic nystagmus (OKN)—that are not available for use with other kinds of visual stimuli. OKN-like eye movements have long been known to occur from early infancy onward; historically, moving stimuli in combination with OKN responses provided the first paradigm ever used for quantitative estimation of the visual acuity of infants (Gorman et al., 1957).

In this section, by way of background, we introduce the uses of moving stimuli as they are currently being incorporated into studies of adult color vision. We begin with the concept of visual losses at isoluminance and the importance of these losses in defining photometric systems. We then describe some current work in adults, in which motion perception and motion nulling are being developed as photometric techniques. Finally, we discuss the use of moving stimuli—motion photometry and motion nulling—in combination with OKN responses as an approach to studying infant color vision and related topics.

Motion Photometry

Visual Losses at Isoluminance. A major theme of visual psychophysics has been the exploration of the striking perceptual losses that occur when isoluminant patterns are used as visual stimuli. That is, in adult subjects, many visual functions, including accommodation, border perception, stereopsis, flicker perception, hyperacuities, and the perception of motion, are poorly sustained when spatial or temporal patterns are made up of sets of stimuli selected to lie within a common isoluminant plane (for references to the isoluminance literature see Lindsey and Teller, 1990).

Although there is general agreement that these losses of perceptual function occur, there is less agreement as to their cause(s). Much of the most recent literature supports the notion that many, if not all, of the visual losses at isoluminance should be attributed to the diminished cone contrasts produced by isoluminant stimuli. It is argued that when luminance-modulated and chromatically modulated stimuli are equated in terms of cone contrasts they are found to have nearly equivalent detection thresholds (Mullen, 1985). Moreover, thresholds for other visual functions, such as vernier acuity (Krauskopf and Farell, 1991), and orientation and spatial frequency discrimination (Webster et al., 1990) are similar for both luminance-modulated and chromatically modulated stimuli when evaluated in comparison to detection thresholds for the same stimuli. It was a variant of this latter point—the question of whether discrimination/detection ratios are the same for luminance-modulated as for chromatically modulated stimuli—that led us to the original articulation of the "Russian dolls conjecture" for adult color vision (Lindsey, 1990b).

At present the question of whether there are important losses of visual function at isoluminance, not attributable to losses of cone contrast, remains unresolved. An apparent exception to this rule—a special loss of perception at isoluminance not attributable solely to cone contrasts—occurs for the perception of motion in small grating patches (Lindsey and Teller, 1990). A second exception apparently occurs for visual accommodation (Switkes et al., 1990).

Photometry. As discussed above, photometry is the enterprise of equating stimuli of different chromaticities in luminance. Whatever their causes, we believe that various specific perceptual losses at isoluminance form the basis for the various classical photometric methods. Flicker photometry is a feasible psychophysical task because flicker—temporal resolution—passes through a distinctive perceptual minimum at isoluminance, and the minimally distinct border technique works because borders also go through a distinctive perceptual minimum at the isoluminance point. To return to the present context, neither of these techniques is feasible for use with infants.

Motion Photometry. Moreland (1982, 1987) suggested that the distinctive motion minimum seen at isoluminance might make motion-based photometry feasible. To explore this possibility, we have investigated the reliability and other properties of adult minimum motion settings. Subjects viewed small patches of moving gratings and adjusted the elevation of modulation to find those elevations at which the perception of motion ceased. We found that subjects could set the upper and lower boundaries of motion perception near isoluminance with high reliability, and that, at least for one subject, these boundaries traced out perfect pancakes over the entire color gamut of the video system used to generate the stimuli (Teller and Lindsey, 1993).

Motion Nulling

In an important related paradigm called motion nulling, the subject views two stimulus components, such as sine or square-wave gratings, superimposed on each other and moving in opposite directions. When adult subjects view such stimuli, they report seeing motion in the direction of the component with the higher luminance or, if average luminances are equated, in the direction of the component with the higher contrast. However, as the relative luminances or contrasts are varied, a point is found at which neither direction of motion predominates; this point is the motion null point.

Motion nulling techniques have been developed and applied to studies of color vision, most notably by Anstis and Cavanagh (1983). These authors used motion nulling to define the isoluminance points of luminance-modulated stimuli of different chromaticities and began the development of motion nulling as a form of motion photometry. The effects of spatial and temporal frequency on motion nulls have been explored (Cavanagh et al., 1987), as has the additivity of luminance matches made with motion nulls (Kaiser et al., 1989).

Nulling Metric. Motion nulling can also be used to address the question of relative sensitivities to luminance modulated versus chromatically modulated stimuli (Cavanagh and Anstis, 1986, 1991). That is, suppose a luminance-modulated grating of a fixed contrast were moved in one direction and a chromatic grating of variable chromatic contrast in the other direction. The value of the chromatic contrast, required to null the fixed luminance contrast, could provide a metric for the relative efficacies of the two stimuli in producing the perception of motion. By this metric, equal nulling values at two ages would imply equal relative efficiencies of the two stimuli at the two ages, and departures from equal nulling values would be taken as evidence of differential losses of sensitivity to one of the two stimuli.

Motion Thresholds and Motion Nulling in Infant Subjects. The importance of motion thresholds and motion nulling techniques in the context of this chapter is that these techniques might provide the much-needed alternative approach to the evaluation of infant color vision. In particular, motion nulls of various chromatic gratings against a standard white might be a particularly sensitive metric for studying the question of tilts of the infant isoluminant plane. Furthermore, motion nulls in which luminance and chromatically modulated stimuli are pitted against each other, allows one to address the question of differential loss of sensitivity to different stimuli during development. Under these conditions, the identity of null values for infants and adults would provide support for a Russian dolls model. In contrast, if infants require extra chromatic contrast to null a fixed luminance contrast, evidence for a differential loss of chromatic sensitivity would be provided.

A major advantage of motion nulling techniques is that they may be expected to have a minimal measurement error. Behavioral measurements of infant visual function necessarily come with large error bars attached; and if two thresholds have to be measured in order to evaluate the relative efficiency of two stimuli, the measurement errors compound. In the case of nulling techniques, the signals initiated by the two stimuli are processed simultaneously within the same infant subject and nulled against each other before the introduction of measurement error.

OKN and OKN Nulling Techniques

What about testing infants? As mentioned above, the use of large, moving visual fields as stimuli and the observation of OKN-like eye movements as responses has a venerable history in studies of visual development (Dobson and Teller, 1978). These techniques have been used most recently in studies of infant visual acuity by Lewis and colleagues (1990) and in studies of contrast sensitivity in adults (Hainline et al., 1986; Leguire et al., 1991) and infants (Hainline et al., 1986).

In addition, Maurer et al. (1989) have used the motion nulling technique developed by Anstis and Cavanagh (1983) to assess the relative efficiency of broad-band red, yellow, green, and blue stimuli in infant subjects. A group of 1- to 3-month-old infants were tested along with their mothers. For both red versus green and yellow versus blue gratings, the group average null values for mothers and infants were virtually identical. In addition, a deuteranomalous mother and her infant son showed motion nulls shifted in the direction appropriate to deuteranomaly. The work of Maurer et al. suggested immediately to us that the infant and adult null planes have similar tilts. Their successes encouraged us to attempt further development of infant OKN and OKN nulling techniques for use with infant subjects.

In summary, the literature suggests that two variants of OKN experiments can be used effectively with infant subjects. In a classical OKN experiment (Fig. 9-9A) the stimulus consists of a single grating moving across the screen in one of two possible directions (e.g., leftward or rightward). Such stimuli can be used to find contrast thresholds for both luminance-modulated and chromatically modulated gratings. Alternatively, in an OKN *nulling* experiment (Fig. 9-9B), the stimulus consists of two superimposed grating components moving across the screen in opposite directions. If both stimuli are modulated in luminance, the nulling paradigm can be used to carry out motion photometry; and if the two stimuli are modulated along luminance versus chromatic axes, the paradigm can be used to test the relative sensitivity of infant (or adult) subjects to modulation on the two dimensions.

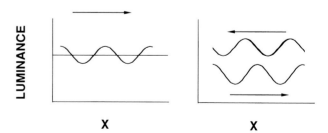

FIG. 9-9. Stimuli used in motion (left) and motion nulling (right) paradigms. In the motion paradigm, a single grating stimulus moves either leftward or rightward (shown) across the video screen. In the motion nulling paradigm, two grating stimuli are superimposed on the screen and move in opposite directions.

EXPERIMENTS WITH INFANT SUBJECTS

General Techniques

In our variant of OKN techniques, stimuli are produced on a color video system. The stimuli fill the entire video display screen and subtend about 50 × 50 degrees. We have used low spatial frequency sinusoidal gratings (0.2–0.5 cycles per degree, or cpd) moving at velocities of 15 to 25 degrees/second (Schor and Narayan, 1981; Roy et al., 1989).

Video cameras above or to the side of the display allow observation of the infant's face and eye movements. An adult observer watches the infant's eye movements on a remote video and judges the presence or absence and the direction of OKN-like eye movements on a trial-by-trial basis.

Two methodological comments are in order. The first is that we are still experimenting with the details of our observational technique somewhat, and we are not always using a strict, two-alternative forced-choice paradigm (Hainline et al., 1986, 1987; Lewis et al., 1990). For example, we have sometimes allowed the observer three categories of response: "OKN leftward," "OKN rightward," or "no OKN." The reason is that forced-choice techniques, although elegant, are known to be inefficient; and for infant testing efficiency is critical. In the service of higher efficiency, we hope to develop an observational coding scheme for judging the infants' eye movements. Ideally, for a fixed stimulus, a couple of trials on which several clear, directionally appropriate OKN-like beats are judged to occur should be sufficient to establish that that stimulus elicits OKN. Of course, measures of interobserver reliability are critical for validating such a method.

The second comment is that it is of course possible to record the infant's eye movements and evaluate them quantitatively, with either electrooculography (EOG) or video technology. Such techniques are clearly proper when the quantitative characteristics of the eye movements are under study (e.g., Naegele and Held, 1982; Finocchio et al., 1990). We also hope to undertake a comparative study to determine if eye movement recording would provide additional power and efficiency in eye-movement-based tests of infant vision.

Experiment I: Tilts of the Isoluminant Plane

Methods. In our first experiment using OKN-like responses to investigate infant color vision (Teller and Lindsey, 1989), an OKN nulling technique was employed. Informally, the stimuli can be described as consisting of two components superimposed on the video screen and moving simultaneously across the screen in opposite directions.

The *standard* component was a 0.3 cpd vertical white/black grating moving across the screen at a speed of 25 degrees/second (7.5 Hz). Its contrast was fixed at 50% with respect to its space-average luminance of 1.3 candelas (cd)/m^2.

The *test* component consisted of an isochromatic, luminance-modulated red/black, green/black, or blue/black grating of the same space-average luminance, spatial frequency, and orientation moving at the same speed in the opposite direction. The contrast of the test grating varied from trial to trial, and the goal of the experiment was to find the contrast of the isochromatic test grating needed to null the fixed 50% contrast of the white standard grating.

Results. Individual psychometric functions for five infants and five adults are shown in Figure 9-10 and the group average functions in Figure 9-11. The psychometric functions for the adults are steep and regular, and individual differences are small. Remarkably, the same is true for the infants. Furthermore, infant and adult null values are remarkably alike; the small difference in means for the red grating is not statistically significant.

Beyond the similarity of infant and adult data, the absolute values of the null points are also of interest. The contrast of the standard grating was 50%, and all three test gratings were matched to the standard in space-average luminance. Hence if equal contrasts are always required for a null, 50% contrast (log contrast 1.7) would be required to null the standard grating in each case. This prediction is true for the red and green gratings but not for the blue grating, for which the null occurs at a log contrast of about 1.4. Why should it be?

Analysis. To address this question, we return to the analysis of the isoluminant plane in postreceptoral channels space (Lindsey, 1990a, in preparation). As discussed above, there is only one factor, the L/M ratio, that imparts a tilt to the r/g axis (i.e., in sine phase). However, there are four factors that impart tilts to the tritan axis (cosine phase) either exactly or nearly: (1) variations in S-cone input; (2) variations in rod input; (3) macular pigment concentration; and (4) lens pigment concentration.

The standard V_λ isoluminant plane derives from measurements obtained from adults with small, foveally fixated fields. The present data, however, are obtained from large fields, so that one expects peripheral as well as foveal retina to contribute to the isoluminant points determined with large fields. In particular, one expects decreased concentration of macular pigment and potentially increased contribution of rod-initiated signals.

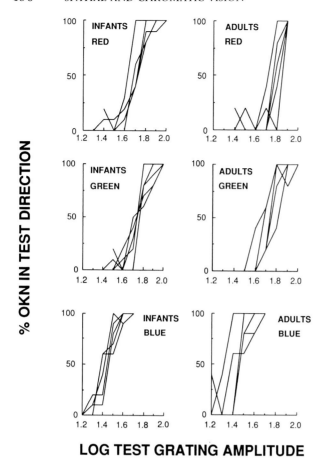

LOG TEST GRATING AMPLITUDE

FIG. 9-10. Results for individual subjects from experiment I, in which luminance-modulated red, green, and blue test gratings were nulled against a white standard grating of 50% contrast (1.7 log contrast). The abscissae show the contrast of the test gratings. Psychometric measurements from five infants and five adults are shown for red (top), green (middle), and blue (bottom) video phosphors. The functions are regular; individual differences are small; and infant and adult contrast thresholds are similar. (After Teller and Lindsey, 1989.)

To analyze the data from our infant experiment, a large-field standard photopic observer was devised. For the tilt component at 0 degrees, we assume standard L and M cone weights of 0.63 and 0.37, respectively. For the tilt components at or near 90 degrees we make three simplifying assumptions. The first is a return to one of the original assumptions of the channels model described above: that S cones do not provide an input to the luminance channel, so the S cone weight for the luminance channel is zero. The second is that for large fields the foveal contribution to the mechanism that drives OKN is negligible, so the effective macular pigment concentration is assumed to be zero. The third is to assume an average lens density of 0.75 for infants (Hansen and Fulton, 1989) and 1.60 for adults (Smith and Pokorny, 1975).

Calculations show that under these assumptions the isoluminant plane should have a tilt whose cosine component should lie close to the 90-degree axis, with an elevation of +5.6 degrees for adults and +4.2 degrees for infants. These tilts come about largely because of the removal of macular pigment from the large-field standard observer. In contrast, a *rods-alone* hypothesis—that rod inputs alone control the infants' OKN responses in this experiment—would predict a tilt of +18 degrees elevation shifted to an azimuth of 78 degrees.

The results of the analysis are shown in Figure 9-12. The data are from five infants and ten adults, and the curves are the predictions of the corrected null plane for the large-field standard observer with no rod input. The data appear to be consistent with those for the large-field standard observer, without the need to invoke rod inputs. It can be seen by inspection that a shift of the predicted curve to the left and an increase in peak

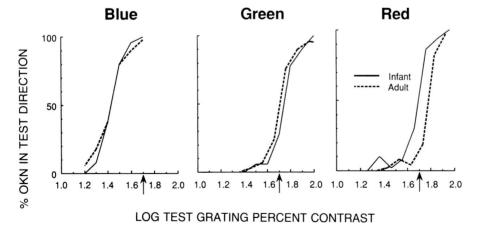

LOG TEST GRATING PERCENT CONTRAST

FIG. 9-11. Group average psychometric functions from experiment I. The slopes of infant and adult functions are similar, as are the threshold values. The arrows on the abscissae show the predicted contrast thresholds if equal contrasts (log contrast 1.7) are required for the motion null for all three test gratings. The contrast threshold for the blue test stimuli depart from the predicted value in the direction that less contrast is required than was predicted. (After Teller and Lindsey, 1989.)

INFANTS

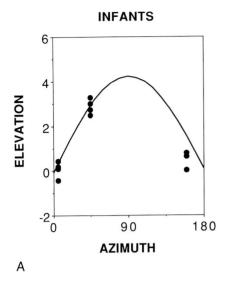

ADULTS

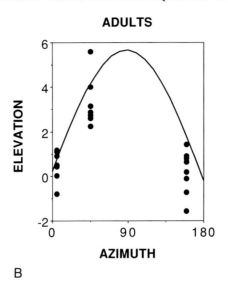

A   B

FIG. 9-12. Solid line represents the prediction of tilt of infant and adult null planes based on a model incorporating V_λ, lens pigmentation, and macular pigmentation (see text). Data points are the results of experiment I for individual subjects. The fit of the model to the data is reasonable, suggesting that inputs from S cones or rods to the luminance channel are not required.

amplitude, which would be consistent with an excitatory rod input, would make the fit worse. With the limited data available, the possibility of minor contributions from rods certainly cannot be rejected. However, the possibility that rod-initiated signals solely or largely control the infants' OKN responses can obviously be rejected. This outcome is of some interest, particularly in view of the low luminances and large fields used in the experiment.

Furthermore, because infants and adults show highly similar data, the experiment lends no support to the rod dominance hypothesis discussed earlier in the chapter. Perhaps this difference in outcome occurs because the peripheral retina is dominating the OKN responses of both adults and infants under the present conditions, whereas the smaller test fields used in earlier experiments are somehow more affected by the well-known immaturity of the infant foveal region (Yuodelis and Hendrickson, 1986).

Experiment 2: Discrimination Ellipsoids and Motion Nulls

We turn now to a second line of experimentation on infant color vision using OKN techniques. This line, which is still in its preliminary stages, is aimed at the question of whether infants suffer from a differential loss of sensitivity for chromatically-modulated, in contrast to luminance-modulated, stimuli. Both 1- and 2-month-old infants have been tested but so far with only a limited range of stimuli (Teller and Lindsey, 1988).

Methods. The experiment has three parts. In part 1, yellow/black luminance-modulated gratings are used alone, and OKN contrast thresholds are measured for these luminance-modulated stimuli. In part 2, high-chromatic-contrast red/green chromatic gratings are used alone. Because the isoluminant values of the red and green phosphors is not known in advance for infant subjects, the "R/G ratio"—the *luminance* contrast between the red and green components of the grating—is varied from trial to trial. In part 3, the nulling paradigm is used: Luminance-modulated gratings and red/green gratings are nulled against each other. For part 3, the contrast of the luminance-modulated grating was set to 15%, as this value proved to provide a good range of response values in adult subjects. The R/G ratio of the chromatic grating was also varied from trial to trial in part 3 of the experiment.

Results. The results of Part 1, with luminance-modulated gratings, are shown in Figure 9-13. The various symbols show the percents of trials in which OKN in the appropriate direction, OKN in the wrong direction, and no OKN were judged to occur. As before, the pattern of results is consistent and encouraging: For the infant subjects, direction-appropriate OKN increases, and the other two response categories decrease, as stimulus contrast increases.

For adult subjects, a 2% luminance modulation (the lowest modulation available in the apparatus) was sufficient to drive OKN on virtually all trials, and luminance-modulation thresholds could not be measured. For

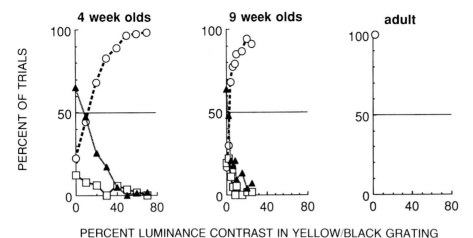

FIG. 9-13. Experiment II. Group-average results for part 1, yellow/black gratings alone. The abscissa shows the contrast for the yellow/black grating, and the ordinate shows the percent of trials on which OKN was judged to occur in the direction appropriate to the motion of the yellow/black grating (○), the red/green grating (□), or on which no OKN was judged to occur (▲). Infants, especially 4-week-olds, showed lowered contrast sensitivity with respect to adults.

9-week-olds, gratings of about 3% contrast were sufficient to drive directionally appropriate OKN. For 4-week-olds, gratings of about 12% contrast were required. These results confirm the general finding of reduced contrast sensitivity in infant subjects, although the response of 9-week-olds to 3% contrast gratings reveals an unusually high level of absolute sensitivity.

The results of part 2, with red/green gratings, are shown in Figure 9-14. In this instance, the abscissa shows the *luminance* contrast in the red/green grating. Zero on the abscissa indicates the adult isoluminance point (i.e., the point at which the luminances of the red and green are equated for adult subjects).

For adults and 9-week-olds, the red/green gratings were sufficient to drive directionally appropriate OKN at all relative luminances, including by inference the individual subject's isoluminance point. For these subjects, the chromatic contrast used is above the modulation threshold, even at isoluminance. The performance of 4-week-olds, on the other hand, falls apart near the (adult) isoluminance value; only half of the trials produce directionally appropriate OKN. Note, however, that OKN is consistently judged to be in the right direction more often than in the wrong direction, so even the 4-week-olds demonstrate a marginal OKN response to isoluminant red/green gratings of high chro-

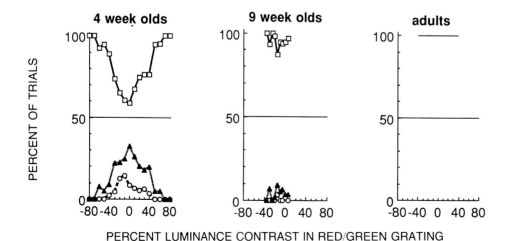

FIG. 9-14. Experiment II. Group average results from part 2, red/green gratings along. The abscissa shows the luminance contrast in the red/green grating. Ordinate and symbols are as in Figure 9-13. Both adults and 9-week-olds show directionally appropriate OKN to all relative luminances of the red/green grating. Four-week-olds show lowered sensitivity to the red/green grating near the adult isoluminance point.

matic contrast. These results confirm findings in the earlier infant color vision literature: Infants about 2 months of age can make chromatic discriminations when chromatic differences are large, and 1-month-olds demonstrate only marginal discrimination capabilities (Teller and Bornstein, 1987; Clavadetscher et al., 1988).

Obviously, these modulation threshold data are incomplete, in that threshold values have not yet been measured for all age groups on all combinations of luminance and chromatic contrast. Hence we do not yet know the shapes of the discrimination ellipsoids for the different age groups, and we cannot yet use these data to defend or reject a Russian dolls model.

The results of part 3—red/green nulled against luminance-modulated gratings—are shown in Figure 9-15. Again, the various symbols show the percents of trials in which OKN was judged to occur in the direction appropriate to the red/green grating or appropriate to the luminance modulated grating, or no OKN was reported. For chromatic gratings that are far from (adult) isoluminance, OKN is driven in the direction of the red/green grating.

For a range of values near the adult isoluminance point, for all age groups the response in the red/green direction is reduced by the presence of the luminance-modulated grating. For 9-week-olds and adults, the response reverses, and OKN is driven in the direction of the luminance-modulated grating during most trials. Of all age groups, the performance of 4-week-olds is least changed by the 15% luminance-modulated nulling grating.

Why might this be? The widths of the minima found in part 3 of this experiment are obviously related to the luminance modulation thresholds found in part 1. As luminance modulation is added to the chromatic modulation, the adult function rises most steeply, the 9-week-olds' function rises less steeply, and the 4-week-olds' functions are the shallowest. In fact, for 4-week-olds the 15% contrast luminance-modulated grating used to null the chromatic grating in part 3 is only barely above threshold in part 1, and it is therefore not surprising that it leads to only minimal interference with the chromatic grating. Perhaps it is for this reason that the 4-week-olds, if anything, show a more robust response to the red/green grating than do the other two age groups.

In any case, the differences between groups are small, and the experiment would have to be replicated with other values of stimulus parameters—particularly with higher contrasts of the luminance-modulated grating used to null the red/green grating—before any claim of meaningful group differences could be supported.

Analysis. We have argued above that comparative null values in infants and adults provide a novel but useful metric of differential losses of sensitivity to different stimuli. Equal nulls across age groups provide evidence of uniform losses of sensitivity in both the luminance and the red/green channel in the infant compared to the adult.

Although they are preliminary, the present results are thus difficult to reconcile with any specific losses of r/g chromatic sensitivity and are consistent with the idea of a generalized loss of sensitivity that applies equally to both luminance and r/g channels. They are thus consistent with earlier data from our laboratory, as reanalyzed by Banks and Bennett (1988), and with a Russian dolls model for r/g versus luminance axes.

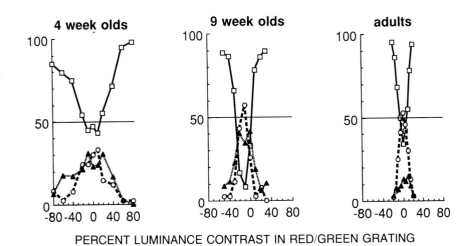

FIG. 9-15. Experiment II. Group average results from part 3, nulling of yellow/black against red/green gratings. Axes and symbols are as in Figures 9-13 and 9-14. The yellow/black nulling grating was set to 15% contrast. For all age groups, the red/green grating shows a minimum in its control over the direction of OKN near the adult isoluminance point. The percents correct at the minimum fall in the range between 10% and 50% for all three age groups. The data thus conform, at least approximately, to a Russian dolls model.

No nulling data are yet available for the tritan axis, nor for any noncardinal axes of color space. A full test of the Russian dolls model in the nulling paradigm thus awaits further experimentation. Exploration of the tritan axis will be particularly interesting in view of Banks and Bennett's ideal detector analysis and their prediction that the Russian dolls model will fail for tritan stimuli.

One final point: In the earlier series of infant chromatic discrimination experiments from our laboratory and in the second of the three experiments described above, a discrimination failure (such as that shown by 4-week-olds in Figure 9-13) provides an estimate of the infants' isoluminance point. However, a discrimination success (such as that shown by 9-week-olds in Figure 9-13) yields no estimate of the isoluminance point. When a nulling paradigm is used, however, it is always possible to increase the contrast of the luminance-modulated nulling grating and find a response minimum. Thus nulling experiments also provide estimates of infants' isoluminance values.

To date, all of the minima we have observed with motion nulling have been close to adult isoluminance values. Thus the results of experiments I and II are consistent on this point, and all are consistent with the conclusion that rod-initiated signals do not provide a major input to the OKN-generating signal under the range of conditions we have tested.

SUMMARY AND CONCLUSIONS

We are in the process of developing quantitative OKN and OKN nulling techniques for studying luminance and chromatic processing in human infants. We are working in the context of a three-dimensional geometrical model of the postreceptoral channels that underlie chromatic and achromatic vision.

This model puts the classic questions of infant color vision in a geometrical context. The question of spectral sensitivity, and the influence of different receptor inputs and preretinal pigment densities on spectral sensitivity becomes the question of the tilt of the isoluminant plane; the question of chromatic discrimination becomes the question of chromatic modulation thresholds within the isoluminant plane; and the question of differential losses in luminance versus chromatic channels becomes the question of the relative robustness of luminance-modulated versus chromatically modulated stimuli in the OKN nulling paradigm.

To date, these OKN and OKN nulling techniques appear to have an important potential for increasing the efficiency of infant testing. First, in nulling experiments the expected psychometric functions span the full range from 0% to 100%, with consequent increases in

statistical efficiency (McKee et al., 1985). Second, the psychometric functions we have seen so far are remarkably steep and regular, and individual differences are remarkably small. Third, rating scales, behavioral coding, and eye movement recording can potentially be applied in a search for further increases in efficiency. Finally, a single measurement, rather than two, is required to test the relative efficacy of two stimuli within the infant subject; and the nulling takes place inside the subject, before the introduction of measurement error.

None of these advantages can undo the disadvantages mentioned early in the chapter: the need for large fields, the limitation to moving stimuli, and the unorthodoxy of using OKN-like eye movements in color vision experiments. Nonetheless, the regularity of the initial data encourages us to continue studies of infant color vision using these paradigms.

REFERENCES

ANSTIS, S. M., AND CAVANAGH, P. (1983). A minimum motion technique for judging equiluminance. In: *Color Vision: Physiology and Psychophysics.* London: Academic Press.

BANKS, M. S., AND BENNETT, P. J. (1988). Optical and photoreceptor immaturities limit the spatial and chromatic vision of human neonates. *J. Opt. Soc. Am.* [A] 5, 2059–2079.

BANKS, M. S., AND SHANNON, E. (1993). How optical and receptor immaturities limit the vision of human neonates. In C. GRANRUD (ed.). *Visual Perception and Cognition in Infancy.* Hillsdale, NJ: Erlbaum.

BOYNTON, R. (1979). *Human Color Vision.* New York: Holt, Rinehart, & Winston.

BROWN, A. M. (1990). Development of visual sensitivity to light and color vision in human infants: a critical review. *Vision Res.* 30, 1159–1188.

BROWN, A. M., AND TELLER, D. Y. (1989). Chromatic opponency in 3-month-old human infants. *Vision Res.* 29, 37–46.

BROWN, W. R. J., AND MACADAM, D. L. (1949). Visual sensitivities to combined chromaticity and luminance differences. *J. Opt. Soc. Am.* 39, 808–834.

CAVANAGH, P., AND ANSTIS, S. M. (1986). Do opponent-color channels contribute to motion? *Invest. Ophthalmol. Vis. Sci.* 27 (suppl.), 291.

CAVANAGH, P., AND ANSTIS, S. M. (1991). The contribution of color to motion in normal and color deficient observers. *Vision Res.* 31, 2109–2148.

CAVANAGH, P., MACLEOD, D. I. A., AND ANSTIS, S. M. (1987). Equiluminance: spatial and temporal factors and the contribution of blue-sensitive cones. *J. Opt. Soc. Am.* [A] 4, 1428–1438.

CLAVADETSCHER, J. E., BROWN, A. M., ANKRUM, C., AND TELLER, D. Y. (1988). Spectral sensitivity and chromatic discriminations in 3- and 7-week-old human infants. *J. Opt. Soc. Am.* [A] 5, 2093–2105.

CORNSWEET, T. N. (1970). *Visual Perception.* Orlando, FL: Academic Press.

DARTNALL, BOWMAKER, AND MOLLON (1983). Microspectrophotometry of human photoreceptors. In J. D. MOLLON AND L. D. SHARPE (eds.). *Color Vision: Physiology and Psychophysics.* New York: Academic Press.

DERRINGTON, A. M., KRAUSKOPF, J., AND LENNIE, P. (1984). Chromatic mechanisms in lateral geniculate nucleus of macaque. *J. Physiol. (Lond.)* 357, 241–265.

DOBSON, V., AND TELLER, D. Y. (1978). Visual acuity in human infants: a review and comparison of behavioral and electrophysiological studies. *Vision Res.* 18, 1469–1483.

D'ZMURA, M., AND LENNIE, P. (1986). Shared pathways for rod and cone vision. *Vision Res.* 26, 1273–1280.

FINOCCHIO, D. V., PRESTON, K. L., AND FUCHS, A. F. (1990). Obtaining a quantitative measure of eye movements in human infants: a method of calibrating the electrooculogram. *Vision Res.* 30, 1119–1128.

FLANAGAN, P., CAVANAGH, P., AND FAUREAU, O. E. (1990). Independent orientation-selective mechanisms for the cardinal directions of colour space. *Vision Res.* 30, 769–778.

GEISLER, W. S. (1989). Sequential ideal-observer analysis of visual discriminations. *Psychol. Rev.* 96, 267–314.

GORMAN, J. J., COGAN, D. G., AND GELLIS, S. S. (1957). An apparatus for grading the visual acuity on the basis of optokinetic nystagmus. *Pediatrics* 19, 1088–1092.

GRAHAM, N. (1989). *Visual Pattern Analyzers.* New York: Oxford University Press.

HAINLINE, L., CAMENZULI, C., ABRAMOV, I., RAWLICK, L., AND LEMERISE, E. (1986). A forced-choice method for deriving infant spatial contrast sensitivity functions from optokinetic nystagmus. *Invest. Ophthalmol. Vis. Sci.* 27 (suppl.), 266.

HAINLINE, L., DE BIE, J., ABRAMOV, I., AND CAMENZULI, C. (1987). Eye movement voting: a new technique for deriving spatial contrast sensitivity. *Clin. Vision Sci.* 2, 33–44.

HAMER, R. D., ALEXANDER, K. R., AND TELLER, D. Y. (1982). Rayleigh discriminations in young human infants. *Vision Res.* 22, 575–587.

HANSEN, R., AND FULTON, A. B. (1989). Psychophysical estimation of ocular media density of human infants. *Vision Res.* 29, 687–690.

INGLING, C. R., AND TSOU, B. H. (1977). Orthogonal combinations of three visual channels. *Vision Res.* 17, 523–529.

JUDD, D. B. (1951). *Report of U.S. Secretariat Committee on Colorimetry and Artificial Daylight.* Paris: Bureau Central CIE.

KAISER, P. K., VIMAL, R. L. P., COWAN, W. B., AND HIBINO, H. (1989). Nulling of apparent motion as a method for assessing sensation luminance: an additivity test. *Color Res. Appl.* 14, 187–191.

KRAUSKOPF, J., AND FARELL, B. (1991). Vernier acuity: effects of chromatic content, blur and contrast. *Vision Res.* 31, 735–749.

KRAUSKOPF, J., WILLIAMS, D. R., AND HEELEY, D. W. (1982). Cardinal directions in color space. *Vision Res.* 22, 1123–1131.

LEGUIRE, L. E., ZAFF, B. S., FREEMAN, S., ROGERS, G. I., BREMER, D. L., AND WALT, N. (1991). Contrast sensitivity of optokinetic nystagmus. *Vision Res.* 31, 89–97.

LENNIE, P., KRAUSKOPF, J., AND SCLAR, G. (1990). Chromatic mechanisms in striate cortex of macaque. *J. Neurosci.* 10, 649–669.

LEWIS, T. L., MAURER, D., AND BRENT, H. P. (1990). The development of visual resolution in infants and toddlers tested monocularly with optokinetic nystagmus. *Clin. Vis. Sci.* 5, 231–241.

LINDSEY, D. T. (1990a). Linear analysis of eccentricity-dependent changes in the null-based isoluminant plane. Presented at the Optical Society of America Annual Meeting, Boston. *OSA Techn. Dig.* 15, 166.

LINDSEY, D. T. (1990b). Are there fundamental losses of visual function at isoluminance? Presented at the Optical Society of America Annual Meeting, Boston. *OSA Techn. Dig.* 15, 135.

LINDSEY, D. T. (in preparation). Linear analysis of eccentricity-dependent changes in the null-based isoluminant plane.

LINDSEY, D. T., AND TELLER, D. Y. (1990). Motion at isoluminance: discrimination/detection ratios for moving isoluminant gratings. *Vision Res.* 30, 1751–1761.

MAURER, D., LEWIS, T., CAVANAGH, P., AND ANSTIS, S. (1989). A new test of luminous efficiency for babies. *Invest. Ophthalmol. Vis. Sci.* 30, 297–303.

MCKEE, S. P., KLEIN, S. A., AND TELLER, D. Y. (1985). Statistical properties of forced-choice psychometric functions: implications of probit analysis. *Percept. Psychophys.* 37, 286–298.

MORELAND, J. D. (1982). Spectral sensitivity measured by motion photometry. In V.G. VERRIEST (ed.). *Docum. Ophthalmol. Proc. Series 33.* The Hague: Dr. W. Junk, pp. 61–66.

MORELAND, J. D., AND TODD, D. T. (1987). Motion photometry and the spectral sensitivity of colour defectives. In MARRÉ, TOST, AND ZENKER (eds.). *Normal and Pathologic Colour Vision.* Halle, Germany: Martin Luther Universität, pp. 39–42.

MULLEN, K. T. (1985). The contrast sensitivity of human colour vision to red-green and blue-yellow chromatic gratings. *J. Physiol. (Lond.)* 359, 381–400.

NAEGELE, J. R., AND HELD, R. (1982). The postnatal development of monocular optokinetic nystagmus in infants. *Vision Res.* 22, 341–346.

NOORLANDER, C., AND KOENDERINK, J. J. (1983). Spatial and temporal discrimination ellipsoids in color space. *J. Opt. Soc. Am.* 73, 1533–1543.

PACKER, O., HARTMANN, E. E., AND TELLER, D. Y. (1984). Infant color vision: the effect of test field size on Rayleigh discriminations. *Vision Res.* 24, 1247–1260.

PALMER, J., MOBLEY, L. A., AND TELLER, D. Y. (1993). Motion at isoluminance: discrimination/detection ratios and the summation of luminance and chromatic signls. *J. Opt. Soc. Amer.* [A] 10 (in press).

PEEPLES, D. R., AND TELLER, D. Y. (1975). Color vision and brightness discrimination in two-month-old human infants. *Science* 189, 1102–1103.

POIRSON, A. B., AND WANDELL, B. A. (1990). The ellipsoidal representation of spectral sensitivity. *Vision Res.* 30, 647–652.

ROY, M. S., LACHAPELLE, P., AND LEPORE, F. (1989). Maturation of the optokinetic nystagmus as a function of the speed of stimulation in fullterm and preterm infants. *Clin. Vis. Sci.* 4, 357–366.

SCHOR, C., AND NARAYAN, V. (1981). The influence of field size upon the spatial frequency response of optokinetic nystagmus. *Vision Res.* 21, 985–994.

SMITH, V. C., AND POKORNY, J. (1975). Spectral sensitivity of the foveal cone photopigments between 400 and 500 nm. *Vision Res.* 15, 161–171.

SWITKES, E., BRADLEY, A., AND SCHOR, C. (1990). Readily visible changes in color contrast are insufficient to stimulate accommodation. *Vision Res.* 30, 1367–1376.

TELLER, D. Y. (1979). The forced-choice preferential looking procedure: a psychophysical technique for use with human infants. *Infant Behav. Dev.* 2, 135–153.

TELLER, D. Y. (1991). Color vision. In: *Encyclopedia of Human Biology.* Orlando, FL: Academic Press.

TELLER, D. Y., AND BORNSTEIN, M. (1987). Infant color vision and color perception. In P. SALAPATAK AND L. COHEN (eds.). *Handbook of Infant Perception, Vol. I. From Sensation to Perception.* Orlando, FL: Academic Press.

TELLER, D. Y., AND LINDSEY, D. T. (1988). OKN isoluminance points and equivalent achromatic contrasts in infants and color-normal and color-deficient adults. Presented at the Optical Society of America Annual Meeting, Santa Clara, CA. *OSA Techn. Dig.* 11, 64.

TELLER, D. Y., AND LINDSEY, D. T. (1989). Motion nulls for white vs. isochromatic gratings in infants and adults. *J. Opt. Soc. Amer.* [A] 6, 1945–1954.

TELLER, D. Y., AND LINDSEY, D. T. (1990). Motion photometry: additivity and the isoluminant plane. Presented at the Optical Society of America Annual Meeting, Boston. *OSA Techn. Dig.* 15, 166.

TELLER, D. Y., AND LINDSEY, D. T. (1993). OKN nulling techniques and infant color vision. In C. GRANRUD (ed.). *Visual Perception and Cognition in Infancy.* Hillsdale, NJ: Erlbaum.

TELLER, D. Y., AND LINDSEY, D. T. (1993). Motion at isoluminance: motion dead zones in three-dimensional color space. *J. Opt. Soc. Amer. [A]* 10 (in press).

TELLER, D. Y., LINDSEY, D. T., MAR, C. M., SUCCOP, A., AND MAHAL (1992). Infant temporal contrast sensitivity at low temporal frequencies. *Vision Res.* 32, 1157–1162.

TELLER, D. Y., PEEPLES, D. R., AND SEKEL, M. (1978). Discrimination of chromatic from white light by two-month-old human infants. *Vision Res.* 18, 41–48.

VARNER, D., COOK, J. E., SCHNECK, M. E., McDONALD, M., ET AL. (1985). Tritan discriminations by 1- and 2-month-old human infants. *Vision Res.* 25, 821–831.

WEBSTER, M. A., DeVALOIS, K. K., AND SWITKES, E. (1990). Orientation and spatial-frequency discrimination for luminance and chromatic gratings. *J. Opt. Soc. Am. [A]* 7, 1034–1049.

WILSON, H. R. (1988). Development of spatiotemporal mechanisms in infant vision. *Vision Res.* 28, 611–628.

WYSZECKI AND STILES (1982). Color Science: Concepts and Methods, Quantitative Data and Formulae (2nd ed.). New York: Wiley.

YOUNG, R. S. L., AND TELLER, D. Y. (1991). The determination of lights that are isoluminant for both scotopic and photopic vision. *J. Opt. Soc. Am. [A]* 8, 2048–2052.

YUODELIS, C., AND HENDRICKSON, A. (1986). A qualitative and quantitative analysis of the human fovea during development. *Vision Res.* 26, 847–855.

10 | Orientation- and motion-selective mechanisms in infants

OLIVER BRADDICK

If we lacked the ability to analyze the orientation of edges or the direction of visual motion, the usefulness of vision would be devastatingly reduced. Physiological (Hubel and Wiesel, 1962, 1977) and psychophysical (Braddick et al., 1978; De Valois and De Valois, 1988) studies show orientation selectivity to be pervasive during early visual processing, so pervasive as to virtually compel the idea that scene analysis and object recognition depend on initial representations in terms of oriented primitives. Orientation is also one of the most important properties in determining the perception of visual textures (Beck, 1966; Olson and Attneave, 1970; Nothdurft, 1990). Visual motion serves as a basis for perceptual functions as diverse as hand-eye control, event recognition, object segmentation, three-dimensional structure perception, and monitoring and control of self-motion (Nakayama, 1985; Braddick, in press). It is clear, then, that knowledge of how orientation and motion processing develop is critical for understanding the basis of the infant's developing perceptual competences.

There is another reason why orientation and motion selectivity are scientifically significant for our understanding of visual development. Along with binocularity, they are the best-defined operations known to be performed by the primary visual cortex. Specificity for orientation or motion direction is not found in the pathway leading to the cortex in primates and other higher mammals. The development of these two functions therefore provides a test for the maturity of specifically cortical function in the vision of human infants, a question that has been central to the discussion of the neural basis of visual development (Bronson, 1974; Atkinson, 1984). Evidence about this development comes from two complementary techniques: visual evoked potentials (VEPs) and behavioral indicators of discrimination, primarily habituation-recovery methods and forced-choice preferential looking.

DEVELOPMENT OF ORIENTATION SELECTIVITY

Orientation-Specific VEPs

Visual evoked potentials are electrical brain signals recorded from the scalp that can be identified by their consistent temporal relation to a stimulus event. Any orientation-selective neuron should, by definition, generate a signal where there is a suitable change of stimulus orientation. However, such a change (e.g., switching between gratings oriented 45 degrees either side of vertical) also involves local luminance and contrast changes that will elicit signals from neurons with nonoriented receptive fields as well. It is conceivable that the orientation-specific and nonspecific VEP responses could be distinguished by their topography, latency, or waveform; but the history of attempts to reach an agreed and unambiguous classification of VEP components and their origins is not an encouraging one. Instead, our alternative approach is to create a "designer stimulus" that can isolate any orientation-specific response. Figure 10-1 illustrates the stimulus sequence, in which the abrupt changes in orientation are embedded in a series of pattern displacements (random phase shifts of the grating) (Braddick et al., 1986). For a neuron with a nonoriented (i.e., circularly symmetrical) field, the orientation reversal illustrated between frames 3 and 4 may produce a phase shift of the grating relative to the receptive field center (depending on the exact location of the receptive field), but it is indistinguishable from the effects of the displacement, or jitter, between the other frames. Only an orientation-selective neuron can generate a response to the orientation changes that is distinctive from the responses to the intervening jitter.

This special response component associated with the orientation reversals is identified by recording "steady-state" VEPs in which the periodic components at dif-

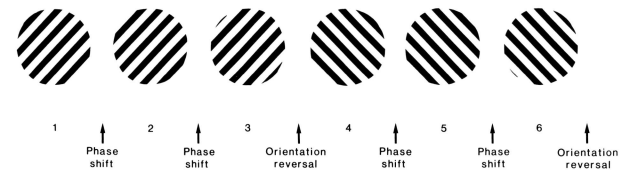

FIG. 10-1. Stimulus sequence for eliciting the orientation-reversal VEP.

ferent temporal frequencies can be analyzed. A component at the frequency of the jitter is likely to be present but is of little interest. A statistically reliable response (Wattam-Bell, 1985) at the frequency of the orientation reversals (or at harmonics of this frequency lower than the jitter frequency) is evidence for a contribution from orientation selective mechanisms.

In early work (Braddick et al., 1986), the displacements occurred at a rate of 25 per second, accompanied by orientation reversals on every third frame as shown in Figure 10-1 (i.e., 8.33 reversals per second, referred to henceforth as 8 reversals/second). This stimulus was found to generate a clear orientation reversal VEP (OR-VEP) in adults and infants around 2 months of age, but we could find no evidence for OR-VEPs in a group of newborns. These same newborn infants showed reliable VEPs for a pattern-appearance control stimulus, in which frames 4, 5, and 6 of the sequence in Figure 10-1 were replaced by a uniform field of mean luminance equal to the grating. This control indicated that the spatial frequency of the grating (0.2 cycle per degree, or cpd) and the temporal frequency of the jitter were within the range that could effectively activate the newborn's visual system. Furthermore, although the strongest VEP component in this case occurs at the first harmonic of the pattern appearance frequency (4 Hz in this case), a number of the newborns also showed a significant second-harmonic response (i.e., at the same 8 Hz response frequency that would be expected for the OR-VEP). It was concluded that neither the spatiotemporal properties of the stimulus nor the temporal characteristics of the required response were outside the range of the newborn system; rather, newborns appeared to lack the cortical machinery necessary to respond specifically to the orientation changes in the stimulus. Longitudinal study of a group of infants born at term showed that the first age at which the OR-VEP could be detected was, on average, around 6 weeks.

Does this finding mean that, before 6 weeks, the infant's visual system is "orientation-blind"? More recent work strengthens the case that the development of the OR-VEP does indeed reflect maturation of a specific cortical mechanism but shows that the course of this maturation is more complex than a simple onset of orientation sensitivity.

Temporal and Spatial Determinants of the OR-VEP

Braddick et al. (1989) performed a second longitudinal study similar to that outlined above, but with each infant tested at two rates of orientation reversal: 8 reversals/second, as before, and 3 reversals/second (embedded in random jitter at 25 per second in each case). To ensure comparability, the two temporal frequencies were tested in interleaved blocks. The median onset of the OR-VEP response for 8 reversals/second occurred at 5–6 weeks, similar to that found in the earlier study. For the 3 reversals/second stimulus, however, the OR-VEP could be first detected, on average, at 3 weeks of age. The infants in this study were also tested with phase-reversal (PH) stimuli; that is, gratings of constant orientation in which the black and white stripes are periodically interchanged, at the same two frequencies. This PH-VEP response does not imply any orientation selectivity; and, like the pattern-appearance response, it can readily be recorded at birth. Figure 10-2 shows a striking example in which the 3 reversals/second OR-VEP emerges between 2 and 3 weeks, whereas the phase-reversal VEP is present throughout.

It is clear in Figure 10-2 that the measured amplitude of the OR-VEP is considerably smaller than that of the phase-reversal response at both ages, which raises the question: Does the appearance of the OR-VEP indicate the specific development of an orientation-selective mechanism, or does it simply reflect a general increase of VEP amplitudes with age during this period, allowing the weak OR-VEP response to emerge from noise? The example of Figure 10-2 does not support such an effect of a general increase, as the accompanying PH-VEP responses show little amplitude change between 2 and 3 weeks. This finding was confirmed by the study as a whole. For each individual, over the interval when the

Recordings taken from the same infant one week apart.

Age 2 weeks, 1 day..

A strong phase-reversal
signal occurs at 3 reversals/sec:

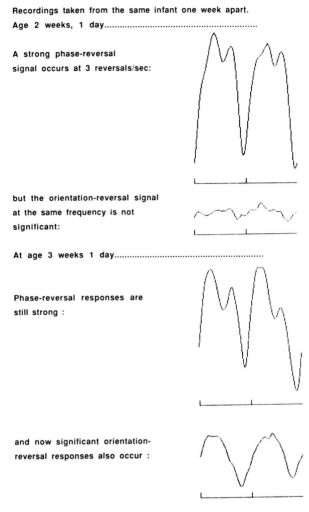

but the orientation-reversal signal
at the same frequency is not
significant:

At age 3 weeks 1 day.......................................

Phase-reversal responses are
still strong :

and now significant orientation-
reversal responses also occur :

FIG. 10-2. Orientation- and phase-reversal VEP waveforms recorded from the same infant in two runs 1 week apart. Stimulus trace below each record (duration 0.67 second) indicates timing of two reversals at a rate of 3 reversals/second.

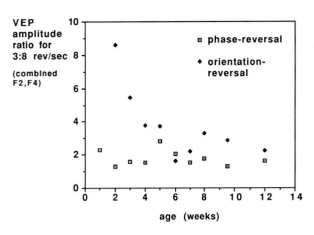

FIG. 10-3. Mean ratio (VEP amplitude for 3 reversals/second stimulus/)(VEP amplitude for 8 reversals/second stimulus) as a function of age for a group of 22 longitudinally tested infants (individual infants contributed between one and eight points). Amplitude measure is $\sqrt{(F2^2 + F4^2)}$ where $F2$ and $F4$ = amplitudes of components at reversal frequency and double the reversal frequency, respectively. Recording blocks at the two frequencies were interleaved in a single run.

OR-VEP became significant, the amplitude ratio of OR-VEP/PH-VEP consistently increased. Thus the increase in the OR-VEP was more than proportional to any increase in the non-orientation-specific response and must at least in part reflect a specific developmental process in the underlying orientation-sensitive mechanism.

Similarly, we can ask whether the difference in the age of onset for the OR response to 3 and 8 reversals/second reflects specific properties of the orientation mechanism or simply a more general improvement in the high-frequency response of the visual system with age. There undoubtedly is such an improvement (e.g., Moskowitz and Sokol, 1980), but it is inadequate to explain the orientation effect. For the phase-reversal stimulus we used, the ratio of response amplitudes for 3 and 8 reversals/second shows little change from 2 to 12 weeks (Fig. 10-3). The figure also shows the corresponding ratios for the OR stimulus, which drop steeply

between 2 and 6 weeks as the 8 reversals/second response emerges. This sharp relative improvement in the high frequency response is specific to the orientation mechanism. Even after the 8 reversals/second OR response has become established, the ratio plotted is consistently higher for OR than for PH responses. That is, the two responses show different temporal frequency characteristics.

A similar contrast between the two responses can be found in their spatial frequency selectivity. Figure 10-4 shows how in 11- to 16-week-old infants the optimal gratings for eliciting the OR-VEP have a higher spatial frequency than for the PH-VEP (Atkinson et al., 1990). The optimal spatial frequency for the OR-VEP, around 1 cpd in the group plotted in Figure 10-4, has increased by about one octave from that found in 8-week-olds.

All this evidence supports the view that the OR-VEP is generated by a distinctive, rapidly developing mechanism different from that responsible for the conventional phase-reversal VEP. The two processes are distinguished by a relatively strong high spatial-frequency response and relatively weak high temporal-frequency response in the oriented mechanism, and by the difference in their developmental course over the first 2–3 months.

In particular, the orientation-selective response is first seen with low temporal frequency stimulation. The 3-week-old onset for 3 reversals/second does not necessarily represent the earliest possible orientation response, but lower temporal frequencies would lengthen the recording runs needed to average weak VEP signals, leading to severe practical difficulties when gathering

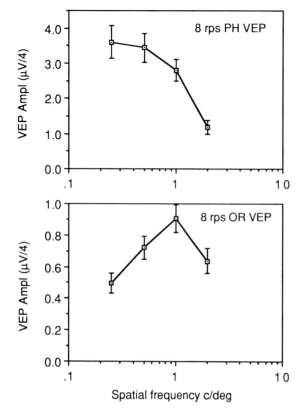

FIG. 10-4. Variation of mean VEP amplitude with spatial frequency for phase-reversal (above) and orientation-reversal (below) stimuli. Subjects: 24 infants aged 11–16 weeks. Temporal frequency: 8 reversals/second. Recording blocks at the four spatial frequencies were interleaved in a single run. See legend to Figure 10-3 for an explanation of amplitude measure.

data from young infants. Behavioral experiments, discussed below, may provide a better way to explore the low temporal-frequency range.

OR Response in Infants Born Preterm

There is ample evidence from animal studies that the development of cortical function is strongly influenced by visual input. How far is the development of orientation selectivity in human infants a determinate process of maturation, and how far is it a response to visual stimulation? We have tested OR-VEP responses at two reversal frequencies in a group of very-low-birth weight infants, born at 24–32 weeks' gestation; the tests were done at ages 5 and 12 weeks postterm. No systematic difference was apparent in the proportion of infants showing positive responses in comparison with a control group born at term (Fig. 10-5) (Atkinson et al., 1990; Visual Development Unit, 1990). There is no evidence, then, that this aspect of cortical development has gained from the additional weeks of postnatal visual exposure in the premature group (or that these infants, who were healthy at the time of testing, have suffered

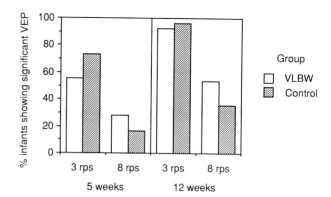

FIG. 10-5. Percentage of infants in very low birth weight and control groups who showed a statistically reliable orientation-reversal VEP response at ages 5 and 12 weeks postterm, for stimulus frequencies of 3 and 8 reversals/second. (Statistical test: phase consistency across blocks by "circular variance" (Wattam-Bell, 1985).) The relatively low proportion of both groups showing a response to 8 reversals/second at age 12 weeks can be attributed to the use of a spatial frequency of 0.25 cpd, which proved to be suboptimal for this age group (see data of Figure 10-4).

delays from their initially at-risk condition). Although it is likely that the detailed course of development can be biased in important ways by experience, and deprivation of normal experience may disrupt or retard it, the initiation of cortical orientation selectivity seems to reflect a timetabled unfolding of neural capacities that are apparently unable or unready to be accelerated by visual input at prenatal stages.

Anisotropy of the OR-VEP

All the work on the OR-VEP described so far has used an alternation between oblique orientations 90 degrees apart (or close to this value in the original report by Braddick et al., 1986). This protocol has been extended in two ways: (1) by looking for any special properties of horizontal and vertical orientations; and (2) by measuring the response to smaller orientation changes as a test for the degree of orientation selectivity of the underlying mechanism.

The original studies used oblique rather than horizontal-vertical (H-V) orientations to exclude any artifactual responses due to H-V anisotropy, introduced by either the raster structure of the display or astigmatism in the subject's eye. However, the developmental course of H-V OR responses is an interesting question, given suggestions that cells responding to these "primary" orientations may develop first and serve as a basis for developing a more complete set of cortical orientation detectors. The problems of potential artifacts can be excluded by photorefractive screening of subjects for astigmatism and by maintaining symmetrical oblique orientations on the monitor screen but physically rotating the monitor through 45 degrees to achieve the H-V display. A longitudinal group of infants tested with both H-V and ± 45 degree orientation reversals at 8 reversals/second showed a closely similar age function for the onset of the OR-VEP to each pair of orientations (Fig. 10-6) (Wattam-Bell et al., 1987). There is no evidence, then, that the horizontal and vertical meridians have any special status in the initial development of the mechanism underlying the OR-VEP. This does not mean, however, that all orientations are equivalent for the mechanism. In the OR display, each cycle of the sequence includes two orientation changes. There is no reason why the two transitions, from +45 to −45 degrees and from −45 to +45 degrees, should be anything other than symmetrical, so they would be expected to make equivalent contributions to the VEP. We therefore look for a response at the reversal rate (i.e., the second harmonic of the fundamental frequency), which was 8 Hz in the experiment under discussion.

In most cases a first-harmonic response (4 Hz in this case), which would imply an asymmetry between the two orientations, was not found for alternating obliques in either infant or adult subjects. However, most adults do show a marked first-harmonic response (as well as a second harmonic) to H-V alternation, indicating that horizontal and vertical orientations do *not* play an equivalent role in the orientation-selective mechanism. This first harmonic component was not present when the response to H-V alternation first became visible at around 6 weeks of age, but we have detected it in most infants aged 12 weeks and over (Fig. 10-6). Thus the organization of the orientation-selective mechanism undergoes important development beyond its initial emergence. It is possible that this development could reflect asymmetries in the visual environment. Another possibility is that, because binocular disparities are predominantly horizontal, vertical and horizontal contours may play different parts in stereoscopic processing. This idea gains some support from the close coincidence between the age at which the OR-VEP anisotropy becomes apparent and that at which the stereo system begins to function (Birch et al., 1982; Braddick and Atkinson, 1983) (see Chapters 12 and 13).

Orientation Tuning of the OR Response

If we take the alternation between gratings at ± 45 degrees and reduce the angle on either side of the vertical, the amplitude of the OR-VEP declines, presumably reflecting the extent to which orientation-sensitive neurons respond differently to the two orientations used. Hence it can be taken as a measure of the orientation tuning of the mechanism. The data presented in Figure 10-7 (Atkinson et al., 1990) show that for 10- to 16-week-old infants, the amplitude of response drops to

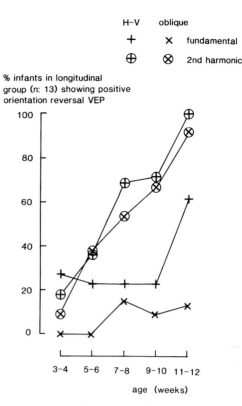

FIG. 10-6. Percentage of infants in a longitudinal group (*n* = 13) showing statistically reliable orientation-reversal VEP responses, as a function of age, for gratings alternating between 0 and 90 degrees (H-V) and ± 45 degrees (oblique). Symbols in circles refer to responses at the reversal frequency (2nd harmonic), plain symbols to responses at half this frequency (fundamental); the latter imply a response anisotropy between the two orientations. (See legend to Figure 10-5 for statistical criterion.)

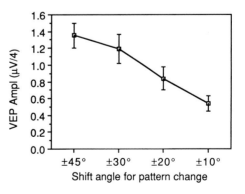

FIG. 10-7. Amplitude of the orientation reversal VEP as a function of the size of orientation change, in a group of infants aged 9–16 weeks. In each run, recording blocks with orientations of ± 45 degrees were interleaved with blocks of one other orientation pair, and amplitudes have been normalized with respect to the amplitude obtained for ± 45 degrees in the same run. At least 20 infants contributed to each point. Orientations were always symmetrical around vertical.

half its maximum height for orientations of ±15 degrees. (We recognize the limitations of this simple measure of tuning; in particular, the likelihood that the VEP amplitude saturates when the mechanism is strongly driven means that it cannot be taken as reliably indicating the shape of a *sensitivity* function).

In adults, OR-VEPs can be measured for orientation changes between +5 and −5 degrees or even smaller angles, implying considerably sharper tuning than in infants. However, the interpretation of the adult function is not straightforward; a *minimum* in response amplitude is often found in the range ±10 to ±20 degrees, suggesting that distinct processes may be involved in the generation of VEPs, yielding two peaks at large and small orientation differences. Manny and Fern (1990) have taken the width of the small-angle peak as a measure of orientation tuning, but it is not clear what model of the underlying process would justify this measure.

We can also look for evidence of the early development of orientation tuning. Testing of a longitudinal group (Atkinson et al., 1990) showed little change between 10 and 15 weeks. The function appeared flatter for 5-week-olds; however, this flattening principally reflected the weaker responses in this young group, which meant that at ±20 degrees and below the responses were dominated by noise. Although responses to small orientation changes become easier to detect with age, we have no positive evidence for a sharpening of the orientation tuning curve between 5 and 15 weeks. It remains a challenge to devise a method that can adequately characterize the orientation selectivity of mechanisms that can only just be detected near the first emergence of any selective response; until we can make this characterization, it is difficult to know whether the mechanisms become more selective or simply more responsive during early development.

Behavioral Measures of Orientation Discrimination

From the point of view of visual function, we are interested not only in whether orientation-selective mechanisms are present in the visual system but also in whether the information they potentially provide plays any part in the infant's perception and visually controlled behavior. It is also possible that behavioral discriminations may provide a more sensitive test than VEPs of what operations the infant visual system can perform. It is essential, then, to complement VEP studies of orientation with behavioral tests.

A number of studies have seemed to imply orientation-based discriminations in newborns. However, it is not always possible to be confident that orientation was the only basis for the observed performance. For example, Fantz et al. (1975) reported that, in a range of displays, newborns showed a fixation preference for a pattern composed of curved lines over a straight-line version matched in contour length. It is attractive to interpret this finding as a preference for the figure containing a greater range of contour orientations, perhaps because a larger number of cortical detectors is activated (Haith, 1978). However, patterns with different radii of curvature at corners would differentially activate circularly symmetrical receptive fields of various sizes, and this pattern of activation might be the basis of a preference. Another case is the work of Slater and Sykes (1977), which showed discrimination in a habituation-recovery test between vertical and horizontal gratings. One possible artifact here could be contrast differences introduced by the common astigmatism of infancy (Howland et al., 1978; Mohindra et al., 1978), whose axis is most commonly close to horizontal or vertical. Another is the predominance of horizontal eye movements that would generate more temporal modulation from vertically oriented than from horizontally oriented contours. Some habituation studies have presented the test grating stimulus in a fixed phase, which leaves open the possibility that infants habituate to the presence of a dark (or light) patch at a particular location.

A procedure that avoids these criticisms tests the recovery of looking time to one oblique grating after habituation to the symmetrically opposite oblique, with the phase of the grating randomized on each trial to avoid any positional cues. Using this method Maurer and Martello (1980) showed that 6-week-olds could discriminate opposite obliques. For younger infants in our laboratory (Atkinson et al., 1988) we first used a different approach, designed to be as comparable as possible to our VEP technique. The infant was habituated to a grating undergoing 25 Hz phase jitter, as in frames 1–3 of Figure 10-1 but with a constant orientation. When a habituation criterion was reached, orientation changes between ±45 degrees, at 8 reversals/second, were introduced into the stimulus. Infant groups aged 5–6 weeks and older showed recovery of looking time when the orientation reversals were introduced, but newborns and 2- to 4-week-olds did not, in agreement with the age of onset of the OR-VEP for 8 reversals/second. The behavioral method, unlike VEPs, is possible with static stimuli: Our initial testing of newborns habituated to one static oblique grating (but no consistent phase) and tested with the opposite oblique showed no evidence of discrimination.

Slater and colleagues (1988), however, modified the habituation method so that the test phase involved preferential looking at the novel and habituated orientations presented side by side. Using this method they found evidence of orientation discrimination by newborns, a finding successfully replicated by Atkinson et al. (1988).

Clearly, results from newborns are sensitive to the test procedure, although the apparent dependence of orientation performance on temporal frequency is not simply a consequence of the test procedure used. Hood et al. (1992) used the paired-comparison procedure that was successful with newborns viewing static gratings to test discrimination between (1) a grating of constant orientation undergoing phase jitter at 25 Hz and (2) a grating in which orientation reversals were embedded in the jitter. A group of 1-month-olds showed significant preference for the reversing orientation in the test phase at 3 reversals/second but none at 8 reversals/second. This finding is consistent with the presence of an OR-VEP at the lower frequency but not at the higher one, which would be expected in this age group.

Thus there are at least two aspects of development relevant to the behavioral results: (1) an increase in the temporal resolution of orientation-sensitive mechanisms, which although present at birth must be sluggish; and (2) an inability of newborns, perhaps due to limitations of the visual information represented in memory, to perform relatively difficult discriminations unless both stimuli are present simultaneously.

A different behavioral approach does not rely on orientation discrimination as such. Held et al. (1989; Yoshida et al., 1990) used preferential looking to test infants' detection of a vertical grating on one screen against a background grating that appears on both screens and examined the orientation specificity of the masking effect of the background. One-month-olds showed no variation in masked threshold for masking orientations ranging from 10 to 90 degrees, implying that the mechanism responsible for detection is initially orientation nonselective. A gradual increase in selectivity occurs from 2 months to 8 months. When interpreting these results it should be realized that a selective mechanism may be present and might contribute to orientation discrimination performance at a given age, but it may not be the most sensitive mechanism for the infant's detection of contrast.

Mechanisms of Orientation Selectivity

When temporal frequency is taken into account, the results of behavioral and VEP studies seem to be in good accord. Of course, this agreement does not prove that they demonstrate the same underlying processes. Potential nonoriented cues have hopefully been excluded from the behavioral discrimination displays, but it is conceivable that infants could respond to positional relations that imply orientation without using neurons that are in any sense specialized for orientation-selective responses. It is also possible that infants could perform a discrimination based on the response of a small number of selective neurons, too small to yield a measurable VEP with current techniques.

Conversely, the orientation-selective neurons giving rise to the OR-VEP might be only a subset of those that can control orientation discrimination behavior. All pattern VEP responses imply some kind of nonlinearity (otherwise, equal and opposite transitions stimulating different populations of linear neurons would cancel out). In the case of the OR-VEP, a cell with an oriented receptive field showing simple linear spatial summation would yield a response that varied randomly at the orientation reversal, depending on the spatial phase in which the new orientation appeared. (Consider the cases where a bright bar, a dark bar, or a bright-dark edge is centered on the parallel receptive field.) The population of such responses over space and time would not be distinct from those to the jitter displacements among which the orientation change is embedded. Cortical complex cells, on the other hand, show spatial nonlinearities that enable them to respond in the same way to a grating in their preferred orientation regardless of its spatial phase. Although it is unlikely that any cortical cell is truly linear, it is possible that the OR-VEP has a disproportionate contribution from complex cells. Simple cells might then be relatively invisible in the VEP but contribute strongly to behavioral discrimination, especially at low temporal frequencies.

Although the orientation selectivity of cortical neurons has been known for nearly 30 years, there is still no definitive account of the neural connectivity that determines this property. The original model of Hubel and Wiesel (1962), in which an oriented receptive field is built up from the spatial arrangement of on- and off-center lateral geniculate nucleus (LGN) afferents, almost certainly describes just one of several relevant types of connection. There is much evidence that intracortical inhibition exists between cells tuned to different orientations (e.g., Orban, 1984, Ch. 12; Ramoa et al., 1986) and plays an important part in determining their selectivity (von der Malsburg, 1973; Sillito, 1975). If it is true that there are several types of synaptic organization that contribute to the orientation properties of cortical cells, it would not be surprising if they appeared at different stages of development. Indeed, connectionist models involving synapses that are modified by the correlation of pre- and postsynaptic activity would lead us to expect that one type of connection (e.g., anisotropic input to a particular cortical cell from LGN afferents) might be needed to guide the organization of others, e.g., cross-orientation inhibition (Linsker, 1986), progressively sharpening the overall tuning. Morrone and Burr (1986) measured how phase-reversal VEP amplitude depended on grating contrast in the presence and absence of an orthogonal "masking" grating that did not directly affect the VEP recording because of its different temporal frequency. They argued that a change in slope of the contrast-response function was evidence for the action of cross-orientation inhibition and found this effect in adults; in infants it first appeared between the ages of 6 and 8 months. Wilson (1988) has speculated more generally that the onset of inhibitory mechanisms may play an important part in the development of visual function during the first 8 months of life.

If cross-orientation inhibition is present, it may play a complex part in determining the OR-VEP or behavioral response to dynamic stimuli. First, an adequate model would have to reckon with not only the inhibitory interactions between neurons simultaneously activated by a given stimulus but also with inhibitory effects that might persist from the previous orientation in the sequence. Second, the effects of inhibition would be in part mutual and recurrent, and they might be expected to have rather different dynamics from the effects of a direct input. The study of how the temporal frequency response of the OR-VEP develops may yet provide important clues as to how inhibitory processes act at different stages.

For detailed understanding of the OR-VEP, one must also consider its relation to the phase-reversal response. Because orientation selectivity is a specifically cortical process, we have suggested that the emergence and development of the OR-VEP is an indicator of the more general maturation of visual cortical function. It is generally assumed, however, that pattern-reversal VEPs, which we have seen to have a different developmental course, originate in cortical activity. The basis for this assumption is not strong, and in some cases (e.g., auditory brainstem responses) subcortical activity can yield measurable evoked potentials at the scalp. If the pattern-reversal VEP does originate in the region of the visual cortex, however, there are several ways in which it could be reconciled with the developmental course of the OR-VEP.

1. VEPs do not necessarily represent the action potentials of cortical neurons. [In fact, it has been argued that action potentials are too short-lasting to produce the large, relatively slow mass activity measured in the VEP; see the discussion in Regan (1972, Ch. 1).] PH-VEPs could originate in the topographical area of primary visual cortex but primarily from postsynaptic potentials, which reflect the nonoriented properties of the input to the cortex as much as the organization of the cortical responses themselves. Ad hoc assumptions would be required, however, to explain the difference in the temporal and spatial sensitivity of the two responses.

2. It is possible that the OR-VEP and PH-VEP arise at the same site but reflect responses to different patterns of input. So, for example, the cross-orientation inhibition discussed above might impose different spatial and temporal properties on the OR-VEP response to orientation changes than on the PH-VEP response, which is independent of orientation.

3. Phase-reversal responses may be detectable from a population of cortical neurons that do not contribute to the OR response. A number of possibilities can be suggested. The possible absence of a simple-cell contribution to the OR-VEP has already been discussed; such cells, regardless of whether they are oriented at any particular stage of development, would be expected to play a large part in the phase-reversal response. In the adult primate, there are a large number of cells in layer 4C that have nonoriented receptive fields (Poggio et al., 1975; Bullier and Henry, 1980) and so should not contribute to the OR-VEP but would be activated by the phase-reversal stimulus. Again, it is not obvious how these proposals would account for the higher spatial-frequency response and lower temporal-frequency response of the OR-VEP compared to the PH-VEP. These properties are suggestive of the differences between cell properties in the magno- and parvocellular pathways (Derrington and Lennie, 1984). Thus it is possible that the OR-VEP reflects specifically the development of orientation selectivity in cortical cells forming part of the "parvo stream," consistent with the role often proposed for that pathway in the transmission of information for spatial pattern processing (Atkinson, in press).

MOTION-SELECTIVE MECHANISMS

When evaluating the development of visual responses to motion, it is important to realize that a response to a moving stimulus, even a response that requires a moving stimulus, does not necessarily provide evidence for a true motion mechanism. It is well established that young infants show a visual preference for moving over static patterns (e.g., Volkmann and Dobson, 1976). The moving pattern produces temporal modulation, however, and it is also known that infants show a preference for full-field flicker, i.e., temporal modulation without motion, to remarkably high rates (Regal, 1981). Any genuine use of visual motion requires information about the direction of motion, and the usual physiological or psychophysical criterion for motion sensitivity in the visual pathway is a difference in response to opposite directions of motion (i.e., directional selectivity).

There is a close logical and actual association between selectivity for motion direction and that for orientation. The preferred contour orientation of a visual neuron defines a preferred motion axis at right angles; in many cases the "aperture problem" (Adelson and Movshon, 1982) means that its responses can be informative only about the component of motion along this axis. To allow the dissociation of orientation selectivity and directional selectivity in visual responses, it is common to use two-dimensional random-dot patterns, which can have a particular direction of motion without any dominant orientation component.

Directional VEP Responses

Wattam-Bell, in our laboratory, has used a random-dot-based VEP technique, analogous to the OR-VEP, to investigate the development of directional responses during infancy (Wattam-Bell, 1988, 1991). The random-dot pattern oscillates vertically, its direction of motion reversing four times per second. If the dot pattern was constant, it would be in identical positions at equal times before and after each reversal, and this periodicity could generate signals at the reversal rate even in mechanisms that were insensitive to motion direction. To avoid this problem, the random-dot pattern is replaced by an uncorrelated pattern (a "jump") at each reversal of direction. These jumps, however, could themselves elicit a VEP response even if there was no response to the intervening motion. The reversals are therefore embedded in a sequence of eight jumps per second, in which alternate jumps are not accompanied by any change in direction. Because the motion is in fact generated by a discrete step every video frame (50 Hz) the overall sequence is:

... 5 steps up → jump → 5 steps up → jump(R) →

5 steps down → jump → 5 steps down →

jump(R) → 5 steps up ... etc.

where (R) = a jump accompanied by a motion reversal. The steady-state VEP can be analyzed for components at the jump frequency (8 Hz) and at the reversal frequency (4 Hz); the latter component can arise only from mechanisms that respond differentially to the two directions of motion. Figure 10-8 illustrates VEP records from an infant subject tested with two velocities at ages 8 and 14 weeks. The higher-frequency "jump" response is clear at both ages with the slower velocity stimulus, but at 8 weeks there is no detectable response to the reversals of direction. By 14 weeks the directional response (four cycles across the trace) is visible at both velocities.

The spatiotemporal stimulation of the visual system depends not only on the display but also on any optokinetic or pursuit eye movements it elicits. To check whether the directional VEP was an artifactual result of eye movements, Wattam-Bell (1991) recorded EOGs simultaneously with VEPs in some infants. The amplitudes of the eye movements were generally small and showed no systematic variation with the presence of a significant directional VEP. The latter seems genuinely to reflect sensory mechanisms responding to the direction of motion.

A group of infants studied longitudinally showed the first statistically significant VEP to motion reversals at

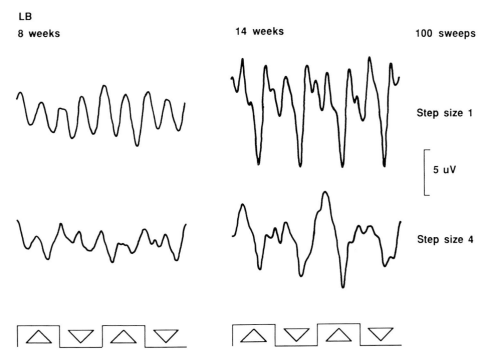

FIG. 10-8. Motion VEP records from the same infant at ages 8 weeks (left) and 14 weeks (right). Trace at the bottom indicates the four reversals of direction during the 0.96 second averaging sweep. At 8 weeks, only a response at twice the reversal frequency is detectable; it can be attributed to the interleaved incoherent "jumps" in the stimulus sequence (see text). At 14 weeks this component is still visible but accompanied by a strong response at the frequency of direction reversals (four cycles across the record), seen at both stimulus velocities. (From Wattam-Bell, 1991. By permission.)

a median age of 74 days when tested with a stimulus velocity of 5 degrees/second (Wattam-Bell, 1991). On the same occasions, they were also tested at 20 degrees/second; for this higher velocity, the median age of onset was significantly later (89 days). There are two striking features of these results: (1) that these motion-specific responses develop at least 4 weeks later than orientation-specific responses measured by a closely analogous technique and at a similar reversal frequency; and (2) that the motion responses are seen earlier at the lower velocity.

In adults, the response was found to have a greater amplitude for 20 degrees/second stimuli than for 5 degrees/second. The developmental difference between these velocities, then, does not simply reflect a uniform increase in the strength of the motion-specific VEP. Rather, there appears to be a slow-to-fast progression in the development of responses to different velocities. It must be borne in mind that the velocity sensitivity of a motion mechanism is determined by its spatial and temporal properties; in particular, when (as here) the appearance of motion is generated by a sequence of discontinuous displacements, the size of the displacements rather than the velocity per se may be the relevant limiting factor (see Baker and Braddick, 1985). Some progress in distinguishing spatial from temporal or velocity limits on performance comes from behavioral studies reported below.

The slow-to-fast sequence suggests that testing with velocities lower than 5 degrees/second might reveal directional responses at an earlier age than 10 weeks. Both logic and behavioral evidence, however, suggest that there must also be a *lower* limit of discriminable velocity, and it would be surprising if performance at this end of the velocity spectrum did not also improve with age. With this constraint, it seems unlikely that directionally specific VEP responses would be observed at or before the ages of 3–6 weeks, where we have seen orientation-specific responses emerging. However, there are obviously a number of parameters to be explored before we can present a full picture of the development of directional responses. They include, notably, the reversal rate, which has such a clear effect on the OR-VEP, and the spatial frequency content of the pattern.

Behavioral Discrimination of Differential Motion

As with orientation discrimination and other visual functions, behavioral and VEP methods can test the infant's capabilities for processing motion information. The two approaches are complementary, and conclusions based on information from both are much more secure than from either one alone. As argued above, a reversing-motion random-dot pattern can isolate the presence of directional selectivity in the infant's visual system, and Wattam-Bell (1990) has used this stimulus for behavioral as well as VEP testing.

In the behavioral version, a 10-degree strip of the random-dot pattern, which appears 5 degrees either left or right of the display midline, moves at the same speed as the rest of the pattern and reverses direction at the same moments; but it is always moving down when the background moves up, and vice versa. For an observer who can detect the direction of motion, this strip appears as a sharply defined object oscillating against a homogeneous background. The infant's detection of the strip is tested by forced-choice preferential looking. Wattam-Bell (1990) used a staircase procedure that adjusted the velocity from trial to trial to determine the maximum velocity (V_{max}) at which an infant discriminated the target strip. With this display, adults showed a V_{max} of around 120 degrees/second. The infant limit, as would be expected from the VEP results, was a function of age: for an 8- to 9-week-old group the median limit was 12 degrees/second, and it rose steadily to 33 degrees/second for 14- to 15-week-old infants. Among the 8- to 9-week-olds, about 40% of the infants showed no evidence of discrimination at 8 degrees/second, the lowest velocity tested. Presumably if these infants were capable of directional discrimination at all, their V_{max} was lower than 8 degrees/second.

Many models of directional motion detectors involve the comparison of spatially separated locations across a temporal delay. V_{max} is determined by both the maximum spatial range and the minimum time interval with which such detectors operate. These factors can be dissociated, as motion on the video display is in fact temporally sampled. Normally this sampling is at the video frame rate (20 ms interval), but Wattam-Bell (1990) tested infants also with a display that was displaced only on every second frame (i.e., at 40 ms intervals). For adults, it drastically reduced V_{max} but by a factor that meant that the maximum spatial displacement between frames (D_{max}) was constant, a result consistent with the findings of others, such as Baker and Braddick (1985). A similar relation was found in a group of 12- to 15-week-old infants, who showed a mean D_{max} of 0.7 degree compared with an adult value of 2.6 degrees for this display. Thus a change in the spatial range is the limiting factor that determines the increase of V_{max} between 12 weeks and adulthood. The developing spatial characteristics are presumably also responsible for at least part of the slow-to-fast progression up to age 12 weeks, although work currently in progress suggests that temporal characteristics also play a role in determining velocity sensitivity in younger infants.

It is worth noting that the implied spatial development is in the direction of small to large scale within the range of the spatial interactions required. It is the opposite of the coarse-to-fine development familiar from studies of infant spatial vision. In adults, D_{max} is increased by removing high spatial frequencies from the image (Chang and Julesz, 1983; Cleary and Braddick, 1990), and so it might have been expected that as the developing infant becomes sensitive to higher spatial frequencies D_{max} would decline. Such a result has indeed been reported from a preferential looking study of 12- and 20-week-olds by Kramer and Bertenthal (1989). In this study, however, the positive stimulus was a random-dot kinematogram consisting of strips moving coherently against an incoherent dynamic background. Low-pass temporal filtering of such a display produces an apparent spatial difference between the regions (a "smearing" of the coherently moving dots along the direction of motion), which does not depend on the stimulation of directional mechanisms. Thus it is possible that the apparent decrease in D_{max} represented the effects of improved temporal resolution with age, rather than the properties of a true motion mechanism. The counterphase motion of target and surround in Wattam-Bell's (1990) experiments requires directional discrimination and concurs with the VEP results in showing an increase of D_{max} in development.

Other behavioral studies of infants have concentrated on the lower rather than on the upper velocity threshold for motion detection. Experiments with moving line or spot targets (Kaufmann et al., 1985; Dannemillar and Freedland, 1989, 1991; Aslin and Shea, 1990) and with random-dot kinematograms (Kramer and Bertenthal, 1989; Bradbury et al., 1990) have all found that the lowest detectable velocity (V_{min}) or the corresponding minimum discrete displacement (D_{min}) decreases between ages 8 and 20 weeks. In most of these experiments, the task required discrimination between moving and stationary targets, which does not necessarily imply directional information, and the limit may be set simply by the improving spatial and temporal resolution of the infant's visual system. For example, Freedland and Dannemillar (1987) tested 5-month-olds' preference for an oscillating over a stationary random-dot pattern. They argued that their results imply mechanisms similar to those of adults in terms of temporal characteristics but of poorer spatial resolution. This argument is plausible, but the experiment cannot demonstrate with confidence that these mechanisms yielded a directional signal. Aslin and Shea (1990) found thresholds of 9 degrees/second in 6-week-olds and 3–4 degrees/second in 12-week-olds that were determined by velocity, not temporal frequency. This finding implies spatiotemporal interaction rather than simply detection of temporal modulation; although it still does not prove directionality, there is a strong case that such an interaction is associated with motion processing. Bradbury et al. (1990) tested preferential looking for a velocity-modulated dot pattern against a pattern moving uniformly at the same speed,

a task that *does* require directional discrimination. They reported a value of V_{min} of 3 degrees/second at age 12 weeks and 1 degree/second at 20 weeks.

The overall picture, then, is that the upper and lower thresholds for directional responses diverge with age. We do not yet know the detailed form of these functions. However, it seems likely that as younger infants are tested the two thresholds will come together, and below this age motion discrimination is not possible anywhere in the velocity range. No behavioral studies have yet provided any evidence of motion detection in infants before 6 weeks, and the earliest demonstration of directional discrimination so far is at 8 weeks. The data make it clear that, to find the true onset of directional motion processing, test stimuli must be correctly located in a rather critical velocity range between the immature lower and upper thresholds for motion. Given the success of suitably chosen habituation-recovery methods in demonstrating young infants' capabilities for pattern discrimination, it is also important to add this approach to VEP and FPL studies of motion sensitivity.

MOTION SELECTIVITY: DISCUSSION

Motion selectivity is vital for many visual functions, and it has been found as a prominent feature of information processing in every visual system where it has been sought, from insects through amphibia and birds to rabbits, cats, and primates. Given this evolutionary and functional importance, one might expect to find it as one of the earliest forms of visual processing in the developing human infant. On the contrary, it appears to lag behind the development of pattern processing as reflected in the OR-VEP and in a variety of behavioral discriminations.

Directionality and OKN

One of the phylogenetically primitive functions of motion information is to stabilize the orientation of the organism. In species with movable eyes, including humans, it is the eyes that are stabilized; and this mechanism is reflected in the optokinetic response to large-field movement. Optokinetic nystagmus (OKN) is present at birth (Dayton et al., 1964; Kreminitzer et al., 1979), which strongly suggests that somewhere in the newborn's visual system there must be directionally selective neurons that can detect the retinal slip signal needed to control OKN. However, it is likely that this site is subcortical. In infants under 2–3 months of age, OKN with monocular stimulation shows a directional asymmetry; stimuli in temporal-to-nasal motion are effective, whereas those in the reverse direction are not (Atkinson, 1979; Atkinson and Braddick, 1981). In cats this asymmetry is known to be a property of the distribution of directional selectivity between the pretectal nuclei of the optic tract on each side. A symmetrical monocular OKN response depends on a descending pathway from the cortex to these nuclei. This dependence is consistent with the idea that the appearance of nasal-to-temporal OKN in 8- to 12-week-old infants depends on the development of cortical motion selectivity, a timetable that fits well with the VEP and behavioral data outlined above. Mohn's (1989) finding that the asymmetry persists to later ages for high stimulus velocities fits with the finding of a slow-to-fast developmental progression. This view implies that the subcortical pathway controlling neonatal OKN does not make a measurable contribution to the VEP. (It should be noted that in Wattam-Bell's experiments the motion was vertical; this motion elicits OKN less well than horizontal directions, which was one of the reasons for selecting it.) Smooth pursuit for a discrete target is believed to require cortical mechanisms and is developmentally distinct from OKN (Atkinson and Braddick, 1981). Pursuit is not reliably seen before 6–8 weeks and, like other indicators of cortical motion processing, operates for progressively increasing stimulus velocities with age (Aslin, 1987; Shea and Aslin, 1988).

Although this picture is consistent, there are indications that it is incomplete. Norcia et al. (1989, 1990) recorded infants' VEPs for oscillatory displacements of monocularly viewed gratings. They found that young infants showed a first harmonic response, that is, an asymmetry between leftward and rightward displacements. The phase of this component reversed between stimulation of the two eyes, implying that it depends on a nasotemporal asymmetry. These findings are in good accord with the findings of an OKN asymmetry, as is the longer persistence of the VEP asymmetry at higher velocities (Norcia et al., 1989, 1990). However, they imply that either (1) this VEP response to horizontal grating displacements, unlike that to vertical reversals of random-dot motion, can be generated by subcortical mechanisms; or (2) that the asymmetry in the VEP, and presumably at least part of that in monocular OKN, reflects asymmetries in cortical as well as subcortical motion processing. The latter view tends to be supported by findings of asymmetries in pursuit responses (Atkinson and Braddick, 1981; Tychsen and Lisberger, 1986). It is possible that this motion-related VEP can be recorded from cortical structures at a younger age than Wattam-Bell's response to random-dot reversals, although most of the data of Norcia et al. have been gathered from infants aged 10 weeks and older.

Motion-Dependent Perceptual Capabilities

It is interesting to compare the evidence for the relatively late development of directional responses with evidence that infants can perform some complex perceptual tasks that appear to depend on motion information. An example of the latter is the ability of 4-month-olds to discriminate between three-dimensional forms distinguished only (and subtly) by "structure-from-motion" in random-dot patterns (Arterberry and Yonas, 1988). The nature of this display makes it unlikely that the discrimination could be based on processing it as a static sequence of positional or configurational information. There can be less confidence on this point for displays that contain more static form information. Nonetheless, the ability to integrate local velocity information for global object and event perception is strongly suggested by the experiments of Gibson and her coworkers (Gibson et al., 1979; Walker et al., 1980), which showed that infants are sensitive to the distinction between rigid motions and nonrigid deformations, and by the finding of Kellman and Spelke (1983) that infants can group spatially separated parts of a partially occluded object that share a common motion. All these experiments have been carried out with infant subjects aged 3–5 months, and so there is no direct conflict with data on the onset of directional responses. Nonetheless, there is a striking implication that within rather few weeks of the basic motion information first becoming available in the visual system the infant can use this information in complex and sophisticated ways.

It is worth noting that a number of the behavioral tests of infants' motion detection (including those from our laboratory) depend on infants' attention to a region of the display containing relative motion. It is possible that this attention is associated with the use of relative motion for segmenting surfaces in depth. This view gains some support from the finding of Dannemillar and Freedland (1991) that 8- to 20-week-olds showed a preference for a region moving faster than the background or in the opposite direction, but not for a region moving slower than the background. Thus when we are attempting to analyze elementary motion detection in infants, at least some of our methods may depend on processes that use motion information for segmentation, perception of three-dimensional structure, and other "higher" perceptual functions.

Another, possibly simpler task that uses motion information is the recognition that an object is "looming," or approaching on a collision path. Yonas (1981) provided a detailed review of work on infants' responses to looming, from which it is clear that reports of such stimuli eliciting avoidance responses in newborns are open to other interpretations. The presence of a head-retraction response specific to the looming configuration has not been proved earlier than age 4 months. An increase in blink rate caused by looming can be found in 1-month-olds (Yonas et al., 1979), although the probability of its occurrence is low and is still increasing at 10 weeks (Pettersen et al., 1980). Sensitivity to motion-in-depth appears to depend on specific mechanisms (Beverly and Regan, 1973), and it is possible that these mechanisms, at least in controlling specific responses, can develop independently of more general-purpose mechanisms of directional selectivity.

Overall, these perceptual experiments raise the possibility that tasks selected for the ecological relevance of their global stimuli may reveal infant abilities that are surprising in the light of formally simpler tests designed to isolate relatively low-level visual mechanisms. We must, however, also be careful not to make unwarranted assumptions about what stimulus information the infants are using for the more complex perceptual tasks. Experiments that defined the critical stimulus properties for these tasks (e.g., the range of image velocities required) would be valuable.

Relation Between Motion and Other Visual Selectivities

Most cells in visual cortex, outside layer $4C\beta$, are orientationally selective; and their preferred direction of motion is normally, if not always, orthogonal to their preferred orientation. Thus the organization of directional selectivity cannot develop independently of orientation selectivity. In the cat and monkey cortex, there is a rich topographical organization of "orientation columns" in an orderly sequence (Hubel and Wiesel, 1974, 1977; Albus, 1985; Blasdel and Salama, 1986; Swindale et al., 1987). It is widely believed that this spatial ordering reflects the developmental processes by which orientation selectivity is established and refined (Swindale, 1982; von der Malsburg and Cowan, 1982). The topographical organization of directionality has not been the subject of as much study. However, cells in a column with preferred orientation 30 degrees, for example, may have a preferred direction of either 120 or −60 degrees. It appears that these opposed directions are not promiscuously mixed (Swindale et al., 1987). If the ordering of motion directions was established before that of contour orientation, there should be sequences of columns going through the full 360-degree cycle of directions; a subsequent development of orientation selectivity consistent with the preferred direction for each cell would lead to two cycles of orientation within each cycle of direction, as contours at 0 and 180 degrees are equivalent. If 180-degree cycles of orientation were established first, however, it would be difficult if not impossible for the developing system to superimpose 360-degree cycles. What is in fact found in cat cortex (Swindale et al., 1987) is that 180-degree orientation cycles exist, often circling around "singularities" in the cortical map; this arrangement necessarily implies that there must be places where there are discontinuous 180-degree jumps of direction between neighboring cortical locations, and this situation is what is found. This evidence is thus consistent with a developmental sequence in which the ordering of orientation columns is established first (even if sketchily), and direction selectivity must be added to the plan at a later stage, the sequence that our VEP results suggest for human development. It is not clear, however, whether there is any intrinsic reason why this sequence of events is more biologically or geometrically feasible than the reverse sequence.

This discussion has treated directional and orientational selectivity as two properties of a single population of cortical neurons. There is much evidence (Maunsell and Newsome, 1987; DeYoe and Van Essen, 1988; Livingstone and Hubel, 1988), however, that motion information is carried by a specific subsection of the visual pathway, the "magno stream" originating in alpha retinal ganglion cells and transmitted through the magnocellular layers of the LGN, layers $4C\alpha$ and 4B of area V1, and the thick stripes of V2 to area MT of extrastriate cortex in primates. It is possible, then, that the directional responses we have studied depend on the development of selectivity in this pathway; the possibility that the OR-VEP may depend on activity in the parvo pathway has already been tentatively suggested. In this context it is interesting to note that the processing of binocular disparity also develops relatively late (onset at around 12–16 weeks) (Birch et al., 1982; Braddick and Atkinson, 1983; Smith et al., in press) compared to orientation selectivity; disparity selectivity is a property that has been reported predominantly within the magno pathway (DeYoe and Van Essen, 1988). Hopefully, further work will help us understand whether the developmental dissociation between motion and orientation reflects a sequence in the development of different structures in the visual pathway or of different properties within a common system of neurons.

Acknowledgments. The contribution to this work of John Wattam-Bell and Janette Atkinson goes far beyond the cited references. It has also depended on the work and support of other past and present members of the Visual Development Unit including Shirley Anker, Carol Evans, Nicola Gardner, Bruce Hood, Sarah Rae, Hilary Stobart, Jo Tricklebank, and Frank Weeks. The Unit is supported by grants from the Medical Research Council of Great Britain.

REFERENCES

ADELSON, E. H., AND MOVSHON, J. A. (1982). Phenomenal coherence of moving visual patterns. *Nature* 300, 523–525.

ALBUS, K. (1985). A microelectrode study of the spatial arrangement of isoorientation bands in the cat's striate cortex. In D. ROSE AND V. G. DOBSON (eds.). *Models of the Visual Cortex*. Chichester: Wiley.

ARTERBERRY, M. E., AND YONAS, A. (1988). Infants' sensitivity to kinetic information for three-dimensional object shape. *Percept. Psychophys.* 44, 1–6.

ASLIN, R. (1987). Motor aspects of visual development in infancy. In P. SALAPATEK AND L. B. COHEN (eds.). *Handbook of Infant Perception*. Orlando, FL: Academic Press.

ASLIN, R. N., AND SHEA, S. L. (1990). Velocity thresholds in human infants: implications for the perception of motion. *Dev. Psychol.* 26, 589–598.

ATKINSON, J. (1979). Development of optokinetic nystagmus in the human infant and monkey infant: an analogue to development in kittens. In R. D. FREEMAN (ed.). *Developmental Neurobiology of Vision*. NATO Advanced Study Institute Series. New York: Plenum Press.

ATKINSON, J. (1984). Human visual development over the first six months of life: a review and a hypothesis. *Hum. Neurobiol.* 3, 61–74.

ATKINSON, J. (in press). Infant eyes and infant brain. In R. L. GREGORY, J. HARRIS, AND P. HEARD (eds.). *The Artful Brain*. Oxford: Oxford University Press.

ATKINSON, J., AND BRADDICK, O. J. (1981). Development of optokinetic nystagmus in infants: an indicator of cortical binocularity? In D. F. FISHER, R. A. MONTY, AND J. W. SENDERS (eds.). *Eye Movements; Cognition and Visual Perception*. Hillsdale, NJ: Erlbaum.

ATKINSON, J., BRADDICK, O. J., WEEKS, F., AND HOOD, B. (1990). Spatial and temporal tuning of infants' orientation-specific responses. *Perception* 19, 371.

ATKINSON, J., HOOD, B., WATTAM-BELL, J., ANKER, S., AND TRICK-LEBANK, J. (1988). Development of orientation discrimination in infancy. *Perception* 17, 587–595.

BAKER, C. L., AND BRADDICK, O. J. (1985). Temporal properties of the short range process in apparent motion. *Perception* 14, 181–192.

BECK, J. (1966). Effect of orientation and shape similarity on perceptual grouping. *Percept. Psychophys.* 1, 300–302.

BEVERLY, K. I., AND REGAN, D. (1973). Evidence for the existence of neural mechanisms selectively sensitive to the direction of motion in space. *J. Physiol. (Lond.)* 235, 17–29.

BIRCH, E. E., GWIAZDA, J., AND HELD, R. (1982). Stereoacuity development for crossed and uncrossed disparities in human infants. *Vision Res.* 22, 507–513.

BLASDEL, G. G., AND SALAMA, G. (1986). Voltage-sensitive dyes reveal a modular organization in monkey striate cortex. *Nature* 321, 579–585.

BRADBURY, A., BERTENTHAL, B. I., AND KRAMER, S. J. (1990). Minimum velocity thresholds in 12- and 20-week infants. *Invest. Ophthalmol. Vis. Sci.* 31 (suppl.), 9.

BRADDICK, O. J. (in press). The many faces of motion perception. In R. L. GREGORY, J. HARRIS, AND P. HEARD (eds.) *The Artful Brain*. Oxford: Oxford University Press.

BRADDICK, O. J., AND ATKINSON, J. (1983). Some recent findings on the development of human binocularity: a review. *Behav. Brain Res.* 10, 141–150.

BRADDICK, O. J., ATKINSON, J., AND CAMPBELL, F. W. (1978). Channels in vision: basic aspects. In R. HELD, H. LEIBOWITZ, AND H. L. TEUBER (eds.). *Handbook of Sensory Physiology. Vol. VIII. Perception*. Heidelberg: Springer-Verlag.

BRADDICK, O., ATKINSON, J., WATTAM-BELL, J., AND HOOD, B. (1989). Characteristics of orientation-selective mechanisms in early infancy. *Invest. Ophthalmol. Vis. Sci.* 30 (suppl.), 313.

BRADDICK, O. J., WATTAM-BELL, J., AND ATKINSON, J. (1986). Orientation-specific cortical responses develop in early infancy. *Nature* 320, 617–619.

BRONSON, G. W. (1974). The postnatal growth of visual capacity. *Child Dev.* 45, 873–890.

BULLIER, J., AND HENRY, G. H. (1980). Ordinal position and afferent input of neurons in monkey striate cortex. *J. Neurophysiol.* 193, 913–935.

CHANG, J. J., AND JULESZ, B. (1983). Displacement limit for spatial frequency filtered random-dot cinematograms in apparent motion. *Vision Res.* 23, 1379–1385.

CLEARY, R., AND BRADDICK, O. J. (1990). Masking of low fre-

quency information in short-range apparent motion. *Vision Res.* 30, 317–327.

DANNEMILLAR, J. L., AND FREEDLAND, R. L. (1989). The detection of slow stimulus movement in 2- to 5-month-olds. *J. Exp. Child Psychol.* 47, 337–355.

DANNEMILLAR, J. L., AND FREEDLAND, R. L. (1991). Detection of relative motion by human infants. *Dev. Psychol.* 27, 67–78.

DAYTON, G. O., JONES, M. H., AIU, P., RAWSON, R. A., STEELE, B., AND ROSE, M. (1964). Developmental study of co-ordinated eye movements in the human infant. I. *Arch. Ophthalmol.* 71, 865–870.

DERRINGTON, A. M., AND LENNIE, P. (1984). Spatial and temporal contrast sensitivities of neurones in lateral geniculate nucleus of macaque. *J. Physiol. (Lond.)* 357, 219–240.

DE VALOIS, R. L., AND DE VALOIS, K. K. (1988). *Spatial Vision*. Oxford: Oxford University Press.

DEYOE, E. A., AND VAN ESSEN, D. C. (1988). Concurrent processing streams in monkey visual cortex. *Trends Neurosci.* 11, 219–226.

FANTZ, R. L., FAGAN, J. F., AND MIRANDA, S. B. (1975). Early visual selectivity. In L. B. COHEN AND P. SALAPATEK (eds.). *Infant Perception: From Sensation to Cognition*. Vol. 1. New York: Academic Press.

FREEDLAND, R. L., AND DANNEMILLAR, J. L. (1987). Detection of stimulus motion in 5-month-old infants. *J. Exp. Psychol. Hum. Percept. Perform.* 13, 566–576.

GIBSON, E. J., OWSLEY, C. J., WALKER, A., AND MEGAW-NICE, J. (1979). Development of the perception of invariants: substance and shape. *Perception* 8, 609–619.

HAITH, M. M. (1978). Visual competence in early infancy. In R. HELD, H. LEIBOWITZ, AND H. L. TEUBER (eds.). *Handbook of Sensory Physiology. Vol. VIII. Perception*. Berlin: Springer-Verlag.

HELD, R., YOSHIDA, H., GWIAZDA, J., AND BAUER, J. (1989). Development of orientation selectivity measured by a masking procedure. *Invest. Ophthalmol. Vis. Sci.* 30 (suppl.), 312.

HOOD, B., ATKINSON, J., BRADDICK, O. J., AND WATTAM-BELL, J. (1992). Orientation selectivity in infancy: behavioral evidence for temporal sensitivity. *Perception* 21, 351–354.

HOWLAND, H. C., ATKINSON, J., BRADDICK, O. J., AND FRENCH, J. (1978). Infant astigmatism measured by photorefraction. *Science* 202, 331–333.

HUBEL, D. H., AND WIESEL, T. N. (1962). Receptive fields, binocular interaction, and functional architecture, in the cat's striate cortex. *J. Physiol. (Lond.)* 160, 106–154.

HUBEL, D. H., AND WIESEL, T. N. (1974). Sequence regularity and geometry of orientation columns in the monkey striate cortex. *J. Comp. Neurol.* 158, 267–294.

HUBEL, D. H., AND WIESEL, T. N. (1977). Functional architecture of macaque monkey visual cortex. *Proc. R. Soc. Lond. B.* 198, 1–59.

KAUFMANN, F., STUCKI, M., AND KAUFMANN-HAYOZ, R. (1985). Development of infants' sensitivity for slow and rapid motions. *Infant Behav. Dev.* 8, 89–95.

KELLMAN, P. J., AND SPELKE, E. S. (1983). Perception of partly occluded objects in infancy. *Cog. Psychol.* 15, 483–524.

KRAMER, S. J., AND BERTENTHAL, B. I. (1989). Infants' sensitivity to motion in random-dot kinematograms. *Invest. Ophthalmol. Vis. Sci.* 30 (suppl.), 312.

KREMINITZER, J. P., VAUGHN, H. G., KURTZBERG, D., AND DOWLING, K. (1979). Smooth-pursuit eye movements in the newborn infant. *Child Dev.* 50, 442–448.

LINSKER, R. (1986). From basic network principles to neural architecture. *Proc. Nat. Acad. Sci. USA* 83, 8778–8783.

LIVINGSTONE, M., AND HUBEL, D. (1988). Segregation of form, color, movement, and depth: anatomy, physiology, and perception. *Science* 240, 740–749.

MANNY, R. E., AND FERN, K. D. (1990). The orientation-response function in infants and adults. *Invest. Ophthalmol. Vis. Sci.* 31 (suppl.), 8.

MAUNSELL, J. H. R., AND NEWSOME, W. T. (1987). Visual processing in monkey extrastriate cortex. *Annu. Rev. Neurosci.* 10, 363–401.

MAURER, D., AND MARTELLO, M. (1980). The discrimination of orientation by young infants. *Vision Res.* 20, 201–204.

MOHINDRA, I., HELD, R., GWIAZDA, J., AND BRILL, S. (1978). Astigmatism in infants. *Science* 202, 329–331.

MOHN, G. (1989). The development of binocular and monocular optokinetic nystagmus in human infants. *Invest. Ophthalmol. Vis. Sci.* 30 (suppl.), 49.

MORRONE, M. C., AND BURR, D. C. (1986). Evidence for the existence and development of visual inhibition in humans. *Nature* 321, 235–237.

MOSKOWITZ, A., AND SOKOL, S. (1980). Spatial and temporal interaction of pattern-evoked potentials in human infants. *Vision Res.* 20, 699–708.

NAKAYAMA, K. (1985). Biological image motion processing: a review. *Vision Res.* 25, 625–660.

NORCIA, A. M., HUMPHRY, R., GARCIA, H., AND HOLMES, A. (1989). Anomalous VEPs in infants and in infantile esotropia. *Invest. Ophthalmol. Vis. Sci.* 30 (suppl.), 327.

NORCIA, A. M., HAMER, R. D., AND OREL-BIXLER, D. (1990). Temporal tuning of the motion VEP in infants. *Invest. Ophthalmol. Vis. Sci.* 31 (suppl.), 10.

NOTHDURFT, H. C. (1990). Texton segregation by associated differences in global and local luminance distribution. *Proc. R. Soc. Lond. B.* 239, 295–320.

OLSON, R., AND ATTNEAVE, F. (1970). What variables produce similarity grouping? *Am. J. Psychol.* 83, 1–21.

ORBAN, G. A. (1984). *Neuronal Operations in the Visual Cortex.* Berlin: Springer-Verlag.

PETTERSEN, L., YONAS, A., AND FISCH, R. O. (1980). The development of blinking in response to impending collision in preterm, full-term, and post-term infants. *Infant Behav. Dev.* 3, 155–165.

POGGIO, G. F., BAKER, F. H., MANSFIELD, R. J. W., SILLITO, A., AND GRIGG, P. (1975). Spatial and chromatic properties of neurons subserving foveal and parafoveal vision in rhesus monkey. *Brain Res.* 100, 25–59.

RAMOA, A. S., SHADLEN, M., SKOTTUN, B. C., AND FREEMAN, R. D. (1986). A comparison of inhibition in orientation and spatial frequency selectivity of cat visual cortex. *Nature* 321, 237–239.

REGAL, D. (1981). Development of critical flicker frequency in human infants. *Vision Res.* 21, 549–555.

REGAN, D. (1972). *Evoked Potentials in Psychology, Sensory Physiology, and Clinical Medicine.* London: Chapman & Hall.

SHEA, S., AND ASLIN, R. (1988). Oculomotor responses to step-ramp targets by young human infants. *Invest. Ophthalmol. Vis. Sci.* 29 (suppl.), 165.

SILLITO, A. M. (1975). The contribution of inhibitory mechanisms to the receptive field properties of neurones in the striate cortex of the cat. *J. Physiol.* (*Lond.*) 250, 305–329.

SLATER, A. M., AND SYKES, M. (1977). Newborn infants' responses to square-wave gratings. *Child Dev.* 48, 545–553.

SLATER, A. M., MORISON, V., AND SOMERS, M. (1988). Orientation discrimination and cortical function in the human newborn. *Perception* 17, 597–602.

SMITH, J. C., ATKINSON, J., AND WATTAM-BELL, J. (1993). The development of sensitivity to binocular correlation and disparity in infants, and its relationship to optokinetic nystagmus. *Vision Res.* (in press).

SWINDALE, N. V. (1982). A model for the formation of orientation columns. *Proc. R. Soc. Lond. B.* 215, 211–230.

SWINDALE, N. V., MATSUBARA, J. A., AND CYNADER, M. S. (1987). Surface organization of orientation and direction selectivity in cat area 18. *J. Neurosci.* 7, 1414–1427.

TYCHSEN, L., AND LISBERGER, S. (1986). Maldevelopment of visual motion processing in humans who had strabismus with onset in infancy. *J. Neurosci.* 6, 2495–2508.

VISUAL DEVELOPMENT UNIT (1990). Visual development in the very-low-birthweight infant. Poster presented at the 4th European Conference on Developmental Psychology, Stirling.

VOLKMANN, F. C., AND DOBSON, M. V. (1976). Infant responses of ocular fixation to moving visual stimuli. *J. Exp. Child Psychol.* 22, 86–99.

VON DER MALSBURG, C. (1973). Self-organization of orientation-selective cells in the striate cortex. *Kybernetik* 14, 85–100.

VON DER MALSBURG, C., AND COWAN, J. D. (1982). Outline of a theory for the ontogenesis of iso-orientation domains in visual cortex. *Biol. Cybernet.* 45, 49–56.

WALKER, A., OWSLEY, C. J., MEGAW-NICE, J., GIBSON, E. J., AND BAHRICK, L. E. (1980). Detection of elasticity as an invariant property of objects by young infants. *Perception* 9, 713–718.

WATTAM-BELL, J. (1985). Analysis of infant visual evoked potentials (VEPs) by a phase-sensitive statistic. *Perception* 14, A33.

WATTAM-BELL, J. (1988). The development of motion-specific cortical responses in infants. *Invest. Ophthalmol. Vis. Sci.* 29 (suppl.), 24.

WATTAM-BELL, J. (1990). The development of maximum velocity limits for direction discrimination in infancy. *Perception* 19, 369.

WATTAM-BELL, J. (1991). Development of motion-specific cortical responses in infancy. *Vision Res.* 31, 287–297.

WATTAM-BELL, J., BRADDICK, O. J., MARSHALL, G., AND ATKINSON, J. (1987). Development and anisotropy of the orientation-specific VEP. *Invest. Ophthalmol. Vis. Sci.* 28 (suppl.), 5.

WILSON, H. R. (1988). Development of spatiotemporal mechanisms in infant vision. *Vision Res.* 28, 611–628.

YONAS, A. (1981). Infants' responses to optical information for collision. In R. N. ASLIN, J. R. ALBERTS, AND M. R. PETERSEN (eds.). *The Development of Perception: Psychobiological Perspectives.* Orlando, FL: Academic Press.

YONAS, A., PETTERSEN, L., AND LOCKMAN, J. J. (1979). Sensitivity in 3- and 4-week-old infants to optical information for collision. *Can. J. Psychol.* 33, 268–276.

YOSHIDA, H., GWIAZDA, J., BAUER, J., AND HELD, R. (1990). Orientation selectivity is present in the first month and subsequently sharpens. *Invest. Ophthalmol. Vis. Sci.* 31 (suppl.), 8.

11 | Intrinsic noise and infant visual performance

A N G E L A M . B R O W N

One of the recurring themes of this book is how noise may affect the visual sensitivity of infants to a variety of stimuli. This chapter is organized around the theme of noise, a term I use in the context of three phenomena.

1. *Photon noise.* It is impossible to deliver exactly a given number of photons to the retina in any particular spatiotemporally, spectrally defined stimulus. Rather, it is possible to deliver a stimulus only with an average of that number of photons. Photons are quantal (all-or-none), random, independent events; therefore the number of photons in a given stimulus is Poisson distributed. Hence for more than about 30 photons, the expected value and the variance of the number of photons delivered in a particular stimulus are equal, and the probability density function is close to a Gaussian "normal" distribution.

2. *Intrinsic noise.* The physiological activity at most stages of the visual system is almost never nil, even in the absence of any visual stimulus or of any change in stimulation. Rather, at each stage there is activity that is unrelated to the onset or offset of a stimulus and to stimulus magnitude when a stimulus is present. Whatever the average value of this resting activity, it is assumed to vary randomly over time. Following the doctrine of specific nerve energies, that variation is assumed to be indistinguishable from the variation in activity induced by a dim or low-contrast stimulus. The application of the Theory of Signal Detectability to the detection of stimuli is based on this assumption. This stimulus-independent physiological activity is known as the intrinsic noise of the visual system.

a. The visual pigment in the outer segments of the photoreceptors initiate visual signals by isomerizing and causing physiological changes in the electrical conductance of the outer segment cell membrane. The isomerization of a molecule of visual pigment may be caused in two ways: It may be due to absorption of a photon of light (photoisomerization), or it may occur spontaneously as a result of the heat of the body. These thermal isomerizations occur randomly even in the absence of light and are commonly considered to be one of the main sources of intrinsic noise in the retina (Barlow, 1957).

b. Every neuron in the body has a baseline level of activity. For some cells (e.g., ganglion cells), the baseline is the rate of occurrence of spontaneous action potentials. These events are random (presumably Poisson); inasmuch as their rate varies randomly, and variation in their rate also occurs in response to a stimulus, spontaneous variation in baseline response rate may be mistaken for a stimulus-initiated response. A similar argument applies to cells that do not fire action potentials, although in that case the domain of interest is the graded membrane potential rather than the firing rate.

3. *Response variability.* When the stimulus is well above its detection threshold, the response it generates is large compared to the intrinsic noise. Nevertheless, responses are variable even for a given "constant" stimulus. As a minimum, the standard deviation of the response must increase at least as fast as the square root of the stimulus magnitude because the photons in the stimulus are Poisson processes, so the variance of the number of photons in the stimulus is equal to the mean number of photons. The action potentials generated at many stages of the visual system may also be Poisson processes, at least for responses well short of saturation.

The standard deviation of the response to a given stimulus determines the stimulus increment required to achieve some predetermined performance criterion (e.g., for the increment to be correctly identified on 75% of trials in a forced-choice experiment). If Poisson processes were the only cause of response variability, the increment threshold function (across all stimulus domains) would be 0.5 on log-log coordinates (Barlow, 1957). For large, long-duration stimuli, this "ideal" square-root behavior is not generally observed. Most adult increment threshold functions have slopes somewhere between 0.5 and 1.0. One explanation is that the variability in response increases faster than the mean response. For example, a slope of 1.0 is attained and Weber's law is obeyed when the standard deviation

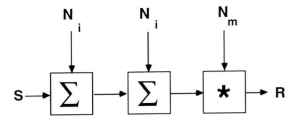

FIG. 11-1. Sources of noise in the visual system. S = the stimulus. It is a random variable because of the Poisson statistics of light. N_i = intrinsic noise from several sources, which are combined with the visual response to S. Some combination rules are linear, some may be nonlinear. N_m = a source of contrast-dependent noise that affects the standard deviation of the response to a given stimulus. R = the subject's response

(rather than the variance) is proportional to the mean stimulus magnitude.

These various noise sources are shown in Figure 11-1. The stimulus is variable because of photon noise. Furthermore, intrinsic noise is combined with the visual signal at several stages of the visual system, where summation is indicated by a sigma; some of those combination rules may not be linear addition. The resulting signal is then transmitted via a neural channel with contrast-dependent noise.[1]

This simple model includes variables that allow it to be applied to a variety of visual phenomena. However, the physiological substrates of the free parameters are different, depending on which phenomenon is being considered. For example, in the case of measuring the absolute threshold for a flashed test light, the intrinsic noise is likely to be primarily the thermal isomerization of the visual pigment (item 2a, above), which is likely to be linearly added to the primary response to the test flash. On the other hand, when the contrast detection and discrimination thresholds are measured, the luminances are typically high enough that the thermal isomerization rate is negligible compared to the rate of photoisomerization. Other sources of intrinsic noise (see item 2b, above) predominate. Those sources of intrinsic noise may be combined nonlinearly with the visual signal (this subject is discussed in greater detail below, in the section on my experiments). Wherever it occurs, such a nonlinearity is important because it can divide the sources of noise into those that must be distal to it (e.g., photon noise) and those that must be proximal to it (e.g., contrast-dependent noise in the transmission line). It is important to remember, though, that psychophysical experiments alone probably cannot establish the site of the nonlinearity.

In the rest of this chapter, these sources of noise are discussed in four contexts. First, the sensitivity of the

infant visual system to stimulation of the rods and the contribution of Hansen and Fulton are discussed. That section leads to a discussion of the Weber fraction of infant rods, which is mathematically equivalent to their contrast threshold, and the inverse of their contrast sensitivity (Graham, 1989, pp. 530–535). Next, the contrast sensitivity (or the inverse of the Weber fraction) of infant cones is related to infant color vision in a discussion of Chapter 9. Next, the "ideal observer" described in Chapter 6 is discussed. Finally, an experiment of mine is presented that is used to evaluate the relative amounts of intrinsic noise and response variability in infants' and adults' perception of contrast.

INFANT ROD VISION AND THE CONTRIBUTION OF HANSEN AND FULTON

Infant rods are suspected to have shorter photopigment-bearing outer segments (ROS) than adult rods. This finding suggests that the optical density of infants' rods should be lower than that of adults by a factor determined by the difference in ROS length:

$$D_\lambda = C \cdot 1 \cdot e_\lambda$$

where: D_λ = the optical density of rhodopsin at a given wavelength in common log units; c = molar concentration of rhodopsin within the ROS; l = ROS length; and e_λ = extinction coefficient at a given wavelength.

The optical density measured by Hansen and Fulton in 10-week-olds is 0.46 log units lower than in adults (see Chapter 8). Given the uncertainties inherent in calculations of this nature,[2] this estimate is not far from 0.19 log units' difference, which is the predicted difference derived from three assumptions: (1) that the rods of the adult have an optical density of 0.35 (Alpern and Pugh, 1974); (2) that the length of the ROS of newborn infants is 45% of that of adults (derived from Fig. 17-3); and (3) that the concentration of infant rhodopsin, the packing density of the rods, and the cross-sectional area of the ROS that contains them do not differ from the adult. It can be shown that violations of the third assumption do not importantly affect the conclusions to be drawn here (Brown, Fulton, and Hansen, in preparation).

Three consequences of reduced optical density (due to reduced ROS length) suggest themselves to the psychophysical community.

---

1. This general model is similar to that described by Pelli (1990).

2. The growth in ROS length is still somewhat uncertain because of the small number of retinas examined to date and the considerable variability in morphology among individuals. However, ROS length appears to grow slowly enough that only a small error should be introduced by comparing the morphology data from a 1-week-old retina and the psychophysical data on 10-week-olds.

1. The actual proportion of photons absorbed from a given light should be lower during infancy than during adulthood by an amount determined by the Beer-Lambert relation:

$$A_\lambda = 1 - 10^{-D_\lambda}$$

where A_λ = proportion of incident photons absorbed by rhodopsin.

2. The spectral sensitivity of infant rod vision (its action spectrum) should be narrower than the spectral sensitivity of adult rod vision. The action spectrum is also predicted by the Beer-Lambert relation, taking the wavelength dependence of the extinction spectrum into account (Dartnall, 1957). This effect is also known as differential "self-screening" at different wavelengths (Brindley, 1970).

3. The number of spontaneous thermal isomerizations per second should be lower in infants than in adults. If a certain proportion of the available rhodopsin molecules are isomerized per second (on average) because of the heat of the body, a subject who has fewer rhodopsin molecules (e.g., an infant) should have a smaller absolute number of spontaneous (thermal) isomerizations per second.

Hansen and Fulton measured the action spectrum of infant and adult night vision at detection threshold and indeed found that the action spectra of 10-week-old infants and adults differ in a way that is consistent with the hypothesis that the rods have lower optical density during infancy than during adulthood. This inference is based on item 2 above. These authors go on to suggest that the reduced optical density is largely responsible for the higher infant absolute test detection threshold of infants. This inference is based on item 1, above. However, items 1 and 3 must be considered together when predicting the effects on test threshold. Shorter outer segment length predicts fewer photoisomerizations from the test light (because of item 1) but also less intrinsic noise (due to item 3). Conversely, longer outer segment length predicts more photoisomerizations but also more intrinsic noise. In either case, the result would be little net change in absolute test threshold.

Absolute and increment test threshold may be assumed to depend on the square root of the number of quantal events in the region of the test stimulus, at least at absolute threshold, when there is no adapting field. This point may also apply when the intensity of the adapting field is low (Barlow, 1965). These quantal events may come from both spontaneous isomerizations and the photoisomerizations from the adapting field:

$$\text{Crit} = \frac{P_T}{\sqrt{P_B + N}}$$

where Crit = the critical value of the signal-to-noise

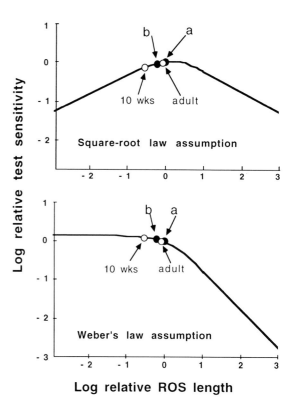

FIG. 11-2. Log test sensitivity measured under full dark adaptation. Sensitivity is in log units relative to the adult value predicted for an optical density of 0.35. **a** = adult value for optical density = 0.35; **b** = infant value, assuming a rod outer segment (ROS) length that is 45% of the adult value (see Chapter 17). ○ = values for adults and infants, based on optical density values from Hansen and Fulton (see Chapter 8). (Top) Predictions under a square-root law assumption. (Bottom) Predictions under a Weber's law assumption (see text for further explanation).

ratio[3]; P_T = number of photons absorbed from the test flash; P_B = number of photons absorbed from the adapting background (equal to zero when absolute threshold is measured); and N = number of spontaneous thermal isomerizations that occur over the spatiotemporal region of the stimulus (intrinsic noise).

The relation between test sensitivity in the dark and the length of the ROS, under the square-root assumption, is shown in the upper panel of Figure 11-2. Both axes have been normalized to the adult values, assuming an adult optical density of 0.35 (a in Fig. 11-2). The function shows a maximum value near the adult ROS length. Below that maximum, the function has a positive slope of about $+1/2$, because the numerator (P_T) increases approximately linearly with ROS length (and optical density), whereas the denominator increases only as the square root of the length and therefore of the

---

3. The stimulus is assumed to be "seen" if the response value (Crit) is exceeded and "not seen" otherwise.

optical density. As ROS length increases, the function approaches a negative slope of $-1/2$, because the numerator shows little further increase with increased ROS length, whereas the denominator continues to increase as the square root of length. The open data points are placed at the optical density values measured by Hansen and Fulton for 10-week-old infants.[4]

Alternatively, increment threshold data may be assumed to obey Weber's law. In that case, Crit is assumed to be proportional to the number of quantal events:

$$\text{Crit} = \frac{P_T}{P_B + N}$$

When this function is evaluated at absolute threshold, i.e., when $P_B = 0$, Crit is nearly constant for short ROS. This is because the rate of photoabsorption increases nearly linearly with increases in length for short ROS (i.e., at low values of optical density, where "self-screening" is negligible). The amount of intrinsic noise (N) also increases linearly over this range. The increases in P_T and N, being nearly linear and proportionate, cancel from their ratio. For long ROS, P_T approaches a constant value, whereas N continues to increase linearly, yielding a near-linear falloff in predicted absolute threshold. The transition between the near-constant part of the function to the near-linear falloff occurs at just about the length of the adult ROS. This point is illustrated in the bottom panel of Figure 11-2.

No matter which model one prefers, the linear model (which predicts Weber's law for the rising part of the increment threshold function) or the square root model (which predicts a square root law), little change in the absolute threshold is predicted from the optical density values estimated by Hansen and Fulton for 10-week-olds and adults. The empirical data on infant absolute threshold, however, are incompatible with that conclusion. The absolute threshold in infants is much higher in infants than in adults: the infant threshold at age 10 weeks is $1.2-1.4$ log units higher than that of adults when psychophysical measurements are made. Whatever the uncertainty about the length of infant ROS, predicted rod thresholds for infants are much lower than those observed empirically.

In addition to the much higher absolute threshold during infancy than during adulthood, there is a much higher increment threshold. The absolute and increment thresholds are related to the amount of intrinsic noise in the retina by means of the "equivalent *eigengrau*." Intrinsic noise cannot be measured directly in a psychophysical experiment. Rather, the "equivalent *eigengrau*" may be estimated as the amount of light that

should have the same visual effect as the intrinsic noise itself. Intrinsic noise is considered to have the same effect as some adapting background made up of real light, as it is a constant signal that is present in all conditions. Increasing the amount of intrinsic noise therefore makes the test threshold increase, as though an adapting background of real light were being added. Equivalent *eigengrau* may therefore be measured by estimating the luminance of the background that is just intense enough to elevate test threshold above its dark-adapted value by a factor of 2.[5]

A maturational change in the length of the ROS would not be expected to produce any major change with age in test increment threshold for intense adapting backgrounds. The equivalent noise becomes negligible compared to the response to the background at high background intensities. The change in the rate of photoisomerization with ROS growth is multiplicative and simply disappears from the expression of Weber's law:

$$\frac{kT}{kB} = \frac{T}{B} = \text{constant}$$

To a first approximation, the adult data obey Weber's law, so no maturational change in the Weber fraction (or test increment threshold) is predicted. Contrary to this prediction, there is a large difference between infants and adults in the increment threshold value, and the predicted increment threshold based exclusively on reduced ROS length does not agree with the infant data at all. This relation is shown in Figure 11-3.

The absolute and increment thresholds of infants and adults are related in such a way that a small difference with age in the amount of equivalent *eigengrau* may be measured in some experiments (see Figs. 8-15 and 8-17). A measurable equivalent *eigengrau* change cannot be due to the different length of the ROS, as argued above. Rather, it must be due to separate effects on the ability of the rods to generate signals and on the actual amount of intrinsic noise. Tradition aside, the intrinsic noise need not be due entirely to thermal isomerizations of the visual pigment: Every neuron in the visual system has a variable baseline activity in the absence of a stimulus, and this activity cannot be distinguished from light-induced responses. Therefore it is not unreasonable to suppose that the amount of intrinsic noise and the magnitude of visual signals might develop independently, causing developmental changes in the amount of equivalent *eigengrau*.

---

4. I am grateful to P. E. King-Smith for discussion of this point.

5. Under the standard descriptive model of the increment threshold function, where Weber's law is assumed, equivalent *eigengrau* may be estimated by fitting a line to the log-log increment threshold function and extrapolating that line to find where it crosses the absolute threshold value on the y-axis.

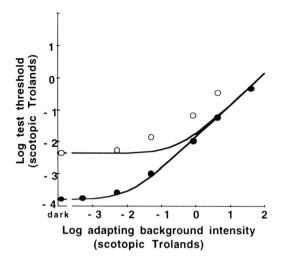

FIG. 11-3. Increment threshold data for infants (○) and adults (●) obtained by Hansen and Fulton (see Chapter 8). The solid lines are the predicted increment threshold functions assuming that Weber's law is obeyed and that infants and adults differ in sensitivity only because of reduced photoabsorption (the dark glasses hypothesis of MacLeod, 1978).

In any case, the observed changes in the equivalent eigengrau are minor compared to the large differences in absolute test detection threshold, however it is measured. The effects on test increment threshold are also comparatively large. What is responsible for this discrepancy? As I and others (Brown, 1986; Hood, 1988) have argued before, it is most parsimonious to assume that much of the discrepancy between infant and adult data is due to critical immaturities that are in the test detection pathway, but not the adaptation pathway, and are therefore proximal to the site of light adaptation. To the extent that absolute and increment test threshold values are elevated by different amounts during infancy, distal immaturities may also be involved. Unfortunately, it is not easy to identify these immaturities or measure their magnitudes because the temporal and spatial pooling of signals in infant vision are known to be greater during infancy than during adulthood, as Hansen and Fulton reported (see Chapter 8). Other things being equal, increased pooling should produce increased sensitivity (or lower thresholds). Thus the extensive pooling in infant vision should counteract the critical immaturities that are responsible for poor infant sensitivity (Brown, 1988); and the exact amount of sensitivity reduction on a per-unit-area basis is difficult to estimate (Brown, 1990).

The conclusion of Hansen and Fulton that infant optical density is reduced relative to that of adults is consistent with the morphological data. It is not, however, a major determinant of the absolute threshold of the

infant's night vision, at least starting at age 10 weeks, because the reduction in photoabsorption is almost perfectly counteracted by the reduction in *eigengrau* intrinsic noise. A second type of noise is required to account for the overall insensitivity of the infant rod increment threshold function. As discussed earlier in the chapter, this second type of noise depends on stimulus luminance.

INFANT COLOR VISION AND THE CONTRIBUTION OF TELLER AND LINDSEY

The contribution of Teller and Lindsey (see Chapter 9) elaborates on the prediction based on line element theory that subjects who have reduced luminance contrast sensitivity of one or more chromatic mechanisms also have reduced sensitivity to changes in color. That is, large Weber fractions must also produce "MacAdam ellipses" (which are actually ellipsoids) that are enlarged in one or more directions in color space. The direction(s) in three-dimensional color space in which the ellipsoids are enlarged depends on the level of visual processing at which the impaired sensitivity occurs. The classical example from color vision is subjects with reduced contrast sensitivity in one of the cone mechanisms, whose ellipses are enlarged in the CIE diagram along the protan, deutan, or tritan lines, according to which mechanism is impaired. Teller and Lindsey point out that reduced cone contrast sensitivity is not the only kind of contrast impairment a subject (e.g., an infant) could have. For example, a subject with selectively impaired chromatic discrimination would have enlarged ellipses within the equiluminant plane but no enlargement in the luminance direction. The particular dimensionalization of color space can be chosen to emphasize the level of color processing at which the impairment occurs: for example, selective impairment of the short-wavelength sensitive cones (S cones) or their pathways can be well illustrated by ellipses elongated along the tritan dimension of the MacLeod and Boynton (1979) and Krauskopf et al. (1982) color spaces. In those spaces, selective impairment of the red/green color dimension is also clearly revealed and has an appearance that is clearly distinctive from separate impairment of either of the long-wavelength (L) or middle-wavelength (M) cones.

The particular case of interest here, though, is the case in which the MacAdam ellipsoid is simply allometrically enlarged proportionately in all three directions. Teller and Lindsey call this case the "Russian dolls" situation (see Fig. 9-6). For example, suppose that infants and adults differ from each other only because all three infant cone types have proportionately larger Weber fractions, or if infant red/green, tritan, and luminance channels have proportionately reduced contrast sensitivity. In either case, infants' MacAdam ellipsoids in three-dimensional color space would be geometrically similar to those of adults, only allometrically enlarged, and would nest perfectly outside the adult ellipsoids, just as the nesting Russian dolls enclose one another. Teller and Lindsey emphasize that the important feature of the "Russian dolls" case is that whenever the ellipsoids are geometrically similar in one dimensionalization they are geometrically similar in all other dimensionalizations as well. In other words, in the case of "Russian dolls" similarity between infant and adult data, chromatic and luminance discrimination thresholds give no clues as to the level of visual processing where the critical immaturity occurs. In fact, equal impairment of all three color channels (at whatever level of processing) is not even required: Under most models, reduced infant sensitivity of the "detector," or the "homunculus" that mediates behavior on the basis of color signals, could also produce an allometric relation between infant and adult discrimination ellipsoids in color space.

It was for this reason that I have been exploring the problem of contrast sensitivity in infants. There is abundant evidence that infants have impaired contrast discrimination along every direction in color space in which they have been tested (for reviews see Teller and Bornstein, 1987; Brown, 1990). Whether or not the discrimination ellipses of infants and adults turn out to be related by a perfectly allometric transformation, it is certainly possible that a more central impairment at the detector level could co-occur with possible selective impairment in the chromatic channels at one or more levels of color vision processing. My goal, then, is to partition the reduced contrast sensitivity of infants into a part that is due to critical immaturities in the more distal parts of the visual system, which could be responsible for violations of the Russian dolls relation (if they occur) and to critical immaturities that might occur more centrally, which could affect all dimensions of color space equally, introducing a "Russian dolls" component to the relation between infant and adult ellipsoids.

This point is illustrated in Figure 11-4, where adults' and infants' color discrimination ellipses are not related by an allometric transformation, but distal insensitivity in the distal color vision channels and proximal insensitivity to contrast co-occur. In the top diagram the proximal immaturity predominates and contributes a large allometric component to the difference between adult and infant ellipses; in the bottom diagram the proximal immaturity is smaller, and immaturities in both luminance and red/green color channels predominate.

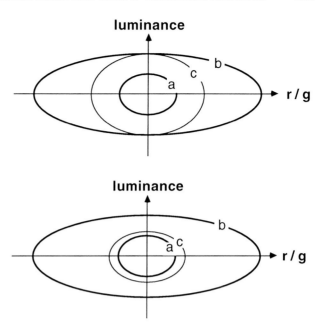

FIG. 11-4. "MacAdam" discrimination ellipses in a color space defined by luminance and red/green chromatic axes. a = adults; b = infants; c = the adult ellipse scaled allometrically to a larger size, representing a critical immaturity of the central visual nervous system, proximal to the sites where luminance and chromatic information are represented in independent channels. (Top) Proximal immaturity predominates, with a secondary immaturity in the chromatic channel. (Bottom) Critical immaturities within the chromatic and luminance channels predominate over proximal immaturities.

IDEAL OBSERVER THEORY AND THE CONTRIBUTION OF BANKS AND CROWELL

An ideal observer is a model of a hypothetical subject who is limited by the Poisson statistics of light (also known as photon noise), which must limit the performance of any device that processes the information contained in light images. Banks' and Crowell's version of the ideal observer (see Chapter 6) includes the optics of the eye and the foveal cones, which are important for predicting the physical limits on the performance of such a device. Unlike a real observer, the ideal observer has no other sources of noise and makes optimum use of all the information available. For example, the ideal observer has perfect knowledge of the physical parameters and location of the stimulus to be detected. The purpose of working through an ideal observer model is to distinguish between those aspects of human performance that are inherent in the stimulus, the optics of the eye, and the morphology of the cones, and those that are due to the physiological nature of the visual system.

Banks and Crowell (see Chapter 6) extend the ideal observer model to the visual performance of infants. The idea here is that infant visual performance must be worse than adult performance because of immaturities in the optics of the eye and the morphology of the retina. The ideal detector model predicts how much worse infant performance should be based on these factors alone and allows one to estimate what aspects of the empirically observed visual capabilities of infants are further limited by critical immaturities of a physiological nature.

Ideal Observer

Because the ideal observer possesses no intrinsic noise, the fundamental limit on the performance of the ideal observer is the statistical nature of light. The performance of the ideal observer is calculated for a two-alternative forced choice stimulus situation. That is, the ideal observer is confronted with two stimulus locations (or intervals)—one that contains stimulus α (a gabor spatial frequency grating pattern) and one of that contains stimulus β (a matched uniform field)—and decides, on the basis of the pattern of photon absorptions in the foveal cones, which stimulus location or interval contains stimulus α. The ideal observer makes this decision by calculating, for each location or interval, the likelihood ratio between the probabilities of the observed response given that α is present or β is present. The ideal observer chooses the location for which this likelihood ratio is greater. The threshold for the grating is attained when this strategy yields a d' of 0.96 (for a full description of this analysis see Geisler, 1984).

To apply this analysis to the problem of the human visual system, one must predict the pattern of photon absorptions in the foveal cones on the basis of the illuminance pattern on the retina. The predicted pattern of absorption is based on the Poisson nature of light, the optical properties of the eye, the distribution of the cones, the physical dimensions of the individual cones, and the optical density of the photopigment they contain. In this way, the ideal detector model is similar to the model I considered for rod vision earlier in the chapter.

If the human eye were truly an ideal detector (i.e., if there were no optical part of the eye or cone morphology to consider), its sensitivity would be independent of the spatial frequency of the stimulus.[6] All the rest of the properties of the eye are low-pass filters and have decreasing modulation transfer at high spatial frequencies. The details of how they do it are spelled out by Banks and Crowell in Chapter 6 and do not need further elaboration here. When all the components of the model are taken into account, the resulting predicted contrast sensitivity function falls off continuously over the spa-

tial frequency range above 5 cycles/degree (cpd). The predicted overall level of the contrast sensitivity is high.

Ideal Versus Human Visual Performance

A large part of Banks and Crowell's Chapter 6 is devoted to evaluating the correspondence between the empirical contrast threshold data obtained on infants and adults and the predicted thresholds of the ideal observer. The first point to be made here is that the overall level of performance of the human falls far short of ideal. The ideal adult observer should be able to detect a 5-cpd sine-wave grating at 50 cd/m² when it has a contrast of only 0.0004, whereas a human adult actually detects that same grating at a contrast of about 0.005, a discrepancy of a factor of 12.5 (1.1 log units) (see Fig. 6-13). The second point is that the human and ideal contrast sensitivity functions (CSFs) for stimuli above about 10 cpd are similar in shape over a range of luminances, and their absolute levels depend similarly on luminance. Thus the real and ideal CSFs agree well once the overall discrepancy of 0.8–1.4 log units, depending on the size and fixation of the stimulus (see Figs. 6-7 and 6-13), has been taken into account. This fact suggests that no physiological explanation for the shape of the CSF is required for that spatial frequency range. Indeed, one may argue that any physiological model that predicts different physiological sensitivity at different spatial frequencies above 10 cpd or that has different physiological gains at different luminances can be ruled out by this correspondence between ideal and observed CSFs.

The neonatal ideal observer prediction is even farther from human infant performance than in the case of the adult. The ideal neonate should be able to detect a 2-cpd stimulus at a contrast of 0.002 (see Fig. 6-12); a human neonate cannot even detect stimuli at that spatial frequency, according to psychophysical data, as their psychophysical visual acuity is in the neighborhood of 1 cpd (Brown and Yamamoto, 1986; Dobson et al., 1987). For 2-month-olds, the behavioral visual acuity is about 2 cpd, measured at about 85% contrast (Dobson and Teller, 1978). The contrast threshold of a 2-month-old is about 5.6% at 2 cpd, as measured using visual evoked potentials (VEPs) (interpolated from Fig. 8 in Norcia et al., 1990). These discrepancies in contrast sensitivity measured at 2 cpd are factors of about 588 (2.77 log units) for psychophysical data and 28 (1.45 log units) for VEP data. Because the ideal observer predictions are based on the morphology of the newborn eye, whereas the real observer data are from 2-month-old infants, these discrepancies are underestimations of the true ratios between real and ideal thresholds for infants.

---

6. It is under the assumption that the area of the stimulus, in square cycles, is constant with spatial frequency. Therefore if the spatial frequency in cycles per degree is doubled, the area must be divided by 4.

Banks and Crowell stress that the discrepancies between real and ideal performance are a substantive topic for developmental research. For example, suppose that the discrepancies were not developmental in nature, and that the only differences between real and ideal performance were common to all visual systems. If that were the case, the real/ideal ratios would be identical for infants and adults. The numbers cited in the previous paragraph clearly refute such an interpretation. Banks and Crowell further consider this possibility by predicting the infant contrast threshold as the empirical adult log contrast sensitivity less a factor at each spatial frequency for the ratio between infant and adult ideal performance. They convincingly reject the hypothesis, as there is a huge difference, in both the performance level and the shape of the contrast sensitivity function, between the infant contrast sensitivity predicted in this manner and the empirical data. For example, at 2 cpd the prediction is in error by a factor of 7.4 (0.9 log units) for the VEP and a factor of 27 (1.44 log units) for psychophysics. The discrepancy between ideal and human neonatal observers is much greater at high spatial frequencies than at low spatial frequencies. This point can be seen in Figure 6-14. It means that there must be spatial-frequency-dependent maturation in the physiological modulation transfer function.

Applying the Ideal Observer to Infant Vision

The main problem when applying the ideal observer to predicting infant visual function is that the ideal observer is currently implemented using data obtained from the infant fovea. Banks and Bennett (1988) and Dobson and I (Brown et al., 1987) were working on the problem of the receptor mosaic at about the same time, and our quantitative results generally agreed. We reached different conclusions, however. Banks and Bennett concluded that the right thing to do next is to explain the discrepancy between the prediction of the foveal neonatal ideal observer and the data. Dobson and I concluded that the infants were in all likelihood relying primarily on their extrafoveal retinas for the visual signals mediating visual performance in most experiments.

In many adult experiments, the fovea is the region of the retina that generates the best visual signals. The foveal cones have no interspersed rods and therefore capture quanta over a larger fraction of the retinal surface than do extrafoveal cones. Foveal cones have higher optical density than peripheral cones because their outer segments are longer. Furthermore, the foveal "cortical magnification factor" is much larger than in the periphery; that is, more of the visual cortex and other parts of the brain are devoted to processing signals originating in the foveal retina. Thus even when the stimulus falls on both the fovea and the extrafoveal retina, adult visual performance is limited by the morphology of the foveal cones.

The same need not be true of infants. For one thing, stimuli generally do fall on the extrafoveal retina in most infant experiments—because grating stimuli are generally larger than the 5.6 degrees subtended by the neonatal fovea, and infant fixation is at best crudely controlled. Furthermore, the extrafoveal retinal mosaic is much more adult-like than the foveal receptor mosaic, suggesting that the stimuli not only fall on extrafoveal as well as foveal cones but that more photons per square degree per second are absorbed from any given stimulus by extrafoveal cones than from foveal cones.

To test this idea, I compared the proportion of incident photons absorbed by the cones in the fovea to the proportion absorbed in the "rod ring," a region of the retina at an eccentricity of 4–5 mm from the fovea, in the neighborhood of the optic disc (Fig. 11-5). Morphological parameters were obtained from two sources: Hendrickson (see Chapter 17, which contains data on human infants) and Packer et al. (1990), whose report contains data on macaque infants. The two species appear to be fairly similar in their retinal development, except for the fovea, which is less mature in human neonates than in macaque neonates. I have repeated the calculations from Appendix C of Brown et al. (1987). These calculations required three parameters for each retinal region as a function of age. The first parameter is the length of the cone outer segment; the second is the diameter of the optical aperture of the cones; and the third is the packing density of the cones on the retina. The cone outer segment length was taken from Figures 17-1 and 17-3. The second and third parameters together determine the fraction of the retinal surface that collects light. The second and third parameters for the fovea also came from Hendrickson's data, but the cone packing density in the rod ring does not appear there. As shown in Figure 11-5C, the packing density of the macaque changes little with age, and the adult human and macaque packing densities are similar (Packer et al., 1990). The receptor inner segment diameter, which is an estimate of the optical aperture of the cones at this retinal eccentricity, is also similar for macaque and human at comparable ages (birth, puberty, and adulthood) and is approximately constant with age. Because both the diameter and packing density are approximately constant with age, the fraction of the retinal surface that absorbs light also shows little change between birth and adulthood. Therefore for lack of human data, the macaque parameters for receptor aperture and packing density were used.

The result of that exercise is as follows: For adults, there are about 6.5 times as many photons per square degree per second absorbed by foveal cones as by cones located in the rod ring at a given level of retinal illu-

FOVEA   ROD-RING   COMPARISON

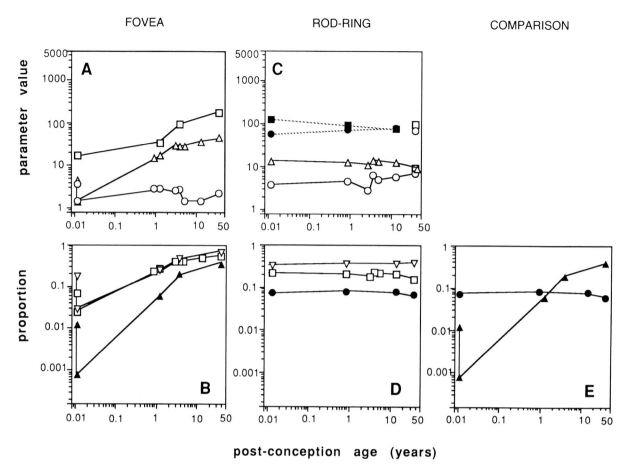

post-conception age (years)

FIG. 11-5. Parameters used to calculate the proportion of photons incident at the retina that are absorbed by the cones located in the fovea (A,B) or in the "rod ring" (C,D). (A,C) Anatomical parameters: □ (human) and ■(macaque) cone packing density, in thousands of cones per square mm; ○ (human) and ● (macaque) optical aperture for a typical individual cone, in microns; △ human cone outer segment length in microns. (B,D) Quantities derived from A and C. ▽ = proportion of retinal surface within the optical aperture of the cones; □ = proportion of photons entering the cone inner segment that are absorbed in the outer segment, calculated from the outer segment length using the Beer-Lambert law. Filled symbols (fovea ▲, rod-ring ●) = the net proportion of photons incident on the retina that are absorbed by the cones. (C,D) Parameters for the cones located in the rod-ring. Infant data from the macaque are separated from adult human data by an interrupted line. Note that the pediatric rod-ring depend on parameters from the macaque (see text) and are separated from the adult rod-ring data, which depend only on human parameters. (E) Proportion of photons incident on the retina that are absorbed by the cone photopigment for the fovea and the rod-ring as a function of age.

minance. On the other hand, for infants there are about 23.4 times as many photons per square degree per second absorbed by cones located in the rod ring of the infant as in the infant's fovea (the two data points near birth were averaged for these estimates[7]). Looking at it another way, there are about 0.8% as many photons absorbed by the neonatal fovea as by the adult fovea; but in the rod ring there are about the same number of incident photons per square degree per second absorbed by the infant's cones as by the adult cones.

It is thus unlikely that the performance of the new-born infant is importantly limited by the photoreceptor mosaic of the fovea. Assuming ideal square-root behavior, contrast threshold should be 4.84 times higher (0.68 log unit) in the infant fovea than in the periphery, in contrast to 2.55 times lower (0.41 log unit) in the adult fovea than in the periphery. The theoretical contrast sensitivity functions (CSFs) for the retinal periphery may be estimated by translating the CSF for the fovea vertically by that amount. When the ideal adult CSFs are translated thus (see Fig. 6-12), ideal infant and adult contrast sensitivity functions nearly coincide. Visual acuity goes from their foveal estimates of 34 and 66 cpd, respectively, to a nearly equal peripheral estimate of about 40 cpd. When empirical adult CSF is used (see Fig. 6-14), predicted infant visual acuity goes from 24.0 cpd to 34.8 cpd. These differences in pre-

---

7. The data at ages 1 and 7 days are different, as can be seen from Figure 17-3. All the developmental data are open for revision as more individual retinas are examined.

dicted visual acuity are modest because the CSF falls off precipitously at high spatial frequencies.

It may be a different matter for infants beyond the first week of life. The problem here is that all the calculations for early infancy, in this exercise and in Chapter 6, are based on data from infants aged 1 week or less, whereas the functional data (VEPs and behavior) are typically from infants 6–12 weeks of age. The low rate of photon absorption in the neonatal fovea is mostly due to the unusual shape of the foveal cones at birth. The cones may change shape quickly, possibly allowing the inner segments to act as waveguides within the first few months of life. Some reconciling hypothesis of this nature may be necessary to reconcile these calculations with the results of Allen and colleagues (1989) (see also Fig. 30-10), who reported that the visual acuity of infants as young as 10 weeks was better and contrast sensitivity higher in the central than in the peripheral visual field. As of this writing, the anatomical data are not available to resolve the important issue of the time course of foveal development.

What Determines Infant Visual Performance?

If, as I contend, the infant is using the extrafoveal retina in visual experiments, the "ideal" infant observer has an overall contrast sensitivity near that of the adult ideal observer, in contrast to the prediction of Banks and Crowell. Of course, this idea makes the agreement between the ideal and human infant data even worse (see footnote 7, above). What critical immaturities are responsible for this huge discrepancy? As discussed earlier in the chapter, one possible explanation is intrinsic noise within the visual nervous system that is added to the sensory signal. Another possibility is the unreliability of the sensory response itself. In the next section, I discuss an experiment designed to estimate these sources of noise and evaluate their importance for determining infant visual sensitivity.

CONTRAST DISCRIMINATION EXPERIMENT

In this section, I discuss data I have been collecting on contrast discrimination in infants. I performed this experiment because of my interest in infant color vision: I wanted to be able to divide the causes for poor contrast sensitivity during infancy into a proximal ("late") part, which seemed likely to affect all directions in color space equally, and a distal ("early") part, which might affect different color channels differently, as discussed above in the section on Teller and Lindsey's contribution. This experiment has led me to a better understanding of the role of noise in infant visual perception.

Methods

Contrast discrimination data on adults and infants were collected using the slow eye movement, or (OKN) "optokinetic nystagmus nulling," method that was described in Chapter 9. I used two stimulus types. In one data set the standard stimulus, which had a contrast of C, was a 20-degree patch of 0.5 cpd green grating at about 13 cd/m² average luminance, and it drifted to the left or to the right at 15 degrees/second. The experimental stimulus was superimposed on the standard stimulus. It had the same size, spatial frequency, color, and speed; but it drifted in the opposite direction. Its contrast was C + ΔC. In the second data set, all conditions were identical, except that the stimulus was 45 degrees across, had a luminance of 65 cd/m², and was white.

I have measured the probability that the experimental stimulus dominates the direction of motion as a function of the contrast of the experimental stimulus, C + ΔC. For both the 7-week-old infants and the adults, it was done by judging the direction of the smooth components of their OKN eye movements. In a separate series of experiments, adult subjects made direct psychophysical judgments of the direction of stimulus motion.

Data Analysis

When *detection threshold* is measured, the standard grating has a contrast (C) of zero. For detection threshold, the contrast increment (ΔC) is never negative, so the psychometric function ranges from $p = 0.5$ to $p = 1.0$, where p is the probability that the experimental stimulus, whose contrast is C + ΔC, dominates the direction of perceived motion or OKN. When *discrimination threshold* is measured, the standard grating has a nonzero contrast (C > 0), and the psychometric function ranges between $0 < p < 0.5$ to $p = 1.0$. When the standard grating is well above threshold (and clearly visible on all trials), the discrimination psychometric function ranges between $p = 0$ and $p = 1$ because when ΔC is negative the standard stimulus has higher contrast than the experimental stimulus (C > C + ΔC), and the experimental stimulus dominates the direction of motion only rarely. All psychometric functions for discrimination pass through the ordinate value of $p = 0.5$ when C = C + ΔC, as the standard and experimental gratings are identical except for moving in the opposite directions. The result is a stationary, contrast-reversing grating, i.e., a "standing wave." To an adult observer, it may look stationary, or it may seem to move in either direction with equal probability.

These psychometric functions were used to create contrast increment threshold functions by calculating

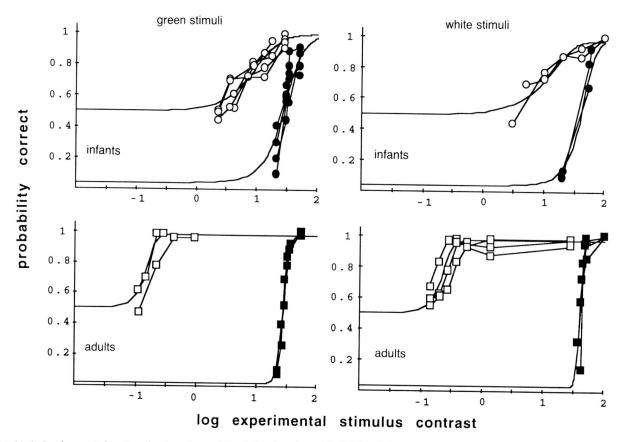

FIG. 11-6. Psychometric functions for detection and discrimination of gratings. Individual data are shown for adults and infants in the experiment using green stimuli (left two graphs) and for adults in the experiment using white stimuli (lower right graph); the upper right hand graph shows averages for four or five infants per data point. The left-hand data set (open symbols) in each graph are for standard stimuli of zero contrast (the detection condition); the right-hand data sets (filled symbols) are for standard stimulus of 40% contrast (a discrimination condition). The curves are the psychometric functions predicted by the model described in the text.

ΔC from the difference between $C + \Delta C$ (the contrast of the experimental stimulus that produces 75% performance) and C (the contrast of the standard stimulus). The 75% point on the psychometric function was estimated by fitting a Weibull function using a maximum likelihood method.[8]

Results

The basic data are shown in Figures 11-6 and 11-7. Figure 11-6 shows the psychometric functions and Figure 11-7 the contrast increment threshold functions.

When $C = 0$, the adult psychometric functions were steep (Fig. 11-6, white squares), whereas the infant psychometric functions were much more gradual (Fig. 11-6, white circles). Furthermore, the contrast detection threshold for adults was about 0.2%, and that for in-

fants was about 10%. This difference can be seen in both the psychometric functions (the infant contrast detection data shown by white circles in Figure 11-6 are far to the right of the adult contrast detection data shown by white squares) and the contrast increment threshold functions (the infant thresholds for $C = 0$, shown by the white circles near the y-axis in Figure 11-7, are far above the adult thresholds, shown by black circles). On the other hand, the differences between the psychometric functions at high contrast were smaller. There, psychometric functions for infants were only somewhat shallower than for adults (compare the black circles to the black squares in Figure 11-6). Adults and infants differed in ΔC sensitivity only by a factor of 3 (Fig. 11-7), which is larger than that reported in experiment I in the Teller and Lindsey contribution but is certainly far less than the factor of 50 difference in infant and adult grating detection threshold.

Finally, the adult contrast increment threshold data (Fig. 11-7, filled symbols) show a large and characteristic improvement in contrast increment threshold, with increasing contrast up to about the point where the

---

8. I am grateful to Dr. William Swanson for providing the computer program.

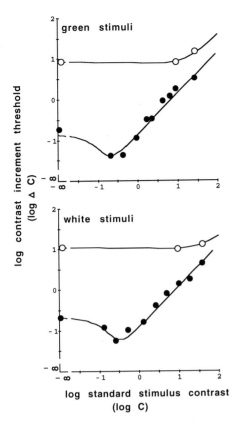

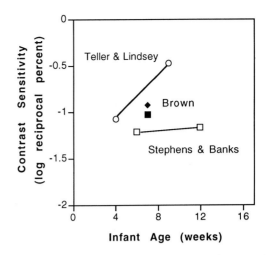

FIG. 11-8. Infant contrast detection thresholds as a function of postnatal age. Open circles: Data from Teller and Lindsey (see Chapter 9) measured with the OKN technique and heterochromatic stimuli. Filled symbols: results of the present experiment, measured with OKN and green stimuli (♦) or white stimuli (■). Open squares: Data from Stephens and Banks (1987), measured using preferential looking and white stimuli.

FIG. 11-7. Contrast increment threshold functions for infants (○) and adults (●). The curves are from the model described in the text.

standard stimulus becomes visible. This phenomenon is the "dipper function" discussed below.

It is interesting to compare the contrast sensitivity (the inverse of contrast detection threshold) obtained in the present experiment with those obtained by other authors (Fig. 11-8). The contrast threshold here is intermediate between those reported by Teller and Lindsey (1989), also obtained using OKN, and that obtained by Stephens and Banks (1987), which were obtained using preferential looking.

Discussion

I have fitted these data with a version of the standard model of contrast discrimination (Foley and Legge, 1981). To apply the standard model to these data, I divide the visual system into two stages (Sperling, 1989).

The first stage of the model is the sensory part (Fig. 11-9; Table 11-1), similar to that illustrated in Figure 11-1: A sensory response is computed that is a combination of the response to the stimulus (S) and a separate source of intrinsic contrast noise (N_i). This intrinsic noise is different from the *eigengrau* that was discussed in the earlier section on luminance increment threshold functions. It is different because, unlike *ei-*

gengrau, it depends on stimulus luminance, and the probability that the observer will mistake it for the test stimulus depends on the test stimulus spatial frequency. It is the noise source that is responsible for the fact that the luminance increment threshold function approximately obeys Weber's law. It is independent of stimulus contrast, however, and therefore remains fixed throughout conditions of the present experiment.

The second stage of the model introduces "postsensory" noise in Sperling's (1989) model. That noise is random trial-to-trial variation in the value of the response (R). It determines the critical value that the response R + ΔR to experimental stimulus of contrast C + ΔC must attain in order for contrasts C and C + ΔC to be discriminable. The second-stage noise (N_m) is multiplicative in the sense that it is proportional to the sensory response. It is responsible for the fact that a Weber/Fechner law is approximately obeyed for contrast discrimination at high contrast values. In this particular version of the model, this point is realized by making the standard deviation of the response at that stage proportional to its input.

TABLE 11-1. *Formulas for Figure 11–9.*

Location in diagram	Expected value	Variance
A	$(S_i^E + N_i^E)^{1/E}$	$(S_i^E + N_i^E)^{1/2E}$
B	$(S_i^E + N_i^E)^{1/E}$	$(S_i^E + N_i^E)^{1/E}$
C	$R_l - R_r$	$(N_m R_l + R_r)$

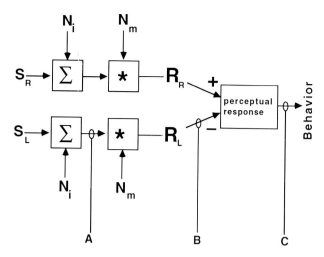

FIG. 11-9. Model from Figure 11-1, elaborated for the OKN contrast discrimination experiment. S_R, S_L = stimuli moving to the right and left, respectively; N_i = intrinsic noise; N_m = contrast-dependent noise; R_R, R_L = responses to right and leftward moving stimuli, respectively. Formulas for the expected value and standard error of the visual signal at the points indicated by A, B, and C are shown in Table 11-1.

If the intrinsic contrast noise (N_i) were simply added to the sensory signal in the first stage, that is, if the sensory stage were linear, the contrast increment threshold function would be monotonically increasing, as is the luminance increment threshold function (Fig. 11-3). However, the contrast increment threshold function is *not* monotonically increasing (Fig. 11-7), so a linear model cannot work. The contrast transducer function is assumed to be an accelerating nonlinearity, which produces a nonmonotonic contrast increment threshold function because of subthreshold summation. Such an assumption is at the heart of both the standard (Foley and Legge, 1981) and stimulus uncertainty (Pelli, 1985) models of contrast discrimination (Graham, 1989, p. 290). An explanation for the decrease of the contrast increment threshold (ΔC) with increasing values of standard stimulus contrast (C) is presented in the Appendix.

The model has three free parameters (Fig. 11-10). First is the amount of *intrinsic contrast noise* (N_i). It controls the minimum value of the response because the intrinsic noise is present even when there is no stimulus. The intrinsic noise is expressed in units of equivalent contrast. Its main effects on the contrast increment threshold function occur at low contrast values, where C is small compared to the amount of intrinsic noise. The less the intrinsic sensory noise, the lower the sensory signal in the absence of a stimulus, the lower the absolute contrast detection threshold, and the further down and to the left on the contrast increment threshold function the dipper function occurs (Fig. 11-10A,D).

The second parameter, E, controls the shape of the transducer function. This nonlinear function describes the way in which the intrinsic sensory noise and the linear sensory response are combined. I model it with a Minkowski metric of variable *exponent*, E (Fig. 11-10B):

$$R = (N_i^E + S^E)^{1/E}$$

For large E, the transition in the transducer function is sharp between the constant region (where the sensory response is small compared to the intrinsic sensory noise) to the function with unit slope (where the sensory response is large compared to the intrinsic sensory noise); for small values of E, the transition is gradual (Fig. 11-5B). The Minkowski function is shown by one of the sigmas in Figure 11-1 and both sigmas in Figure 11-9. The value of E is determined by the β parameter for the slope of the Weibull psychometric function for grating detection (Pelli, 1987). The value of E also determines the depth of the dip in the contrast increment threshold function (Fig. 11-10E): Once E has been fitted to the psychometric function for contrast detection, no additional free parameter is allowed for the depth of the dip.

The third free parameter of the model determines the amount of *contrast-dependent noise* during the second stage and therefore controls the psychophysical criterion for discrimination between the contrasts C and C + ΔC. This parameter (N_m) is controlled by the constant of proportionality between the expected value of the response amplitude and the standard deviation of the response amplitude (Fig. 11-5C). The amount of contrast-dependent noise governs the vertical position of the whole log contrast increment threshold function and determines the Weber/Fechner fraction for contrast (Fig. 11-10F).

The last stage of the model is the perceptual response stage, illustrated in Figure 11-11. The expected value of the response is the difference between the expected values of the responses to the rightward and leftward moving stimuli (R_r and R_l in Fig. 11-9). This differencing operation is standard for modeling luminance increment threshold functions (Hood and Finkelstein, 1986). The variance of the response is the sum of the variances of R_r and R_l. The psychometric function of the probability that the net motion of the grating pair is, for example, to the left is explicitly predicted by this model. It is the probability that the sensory response to the leftward moving grating is greater than the sensory response to the rightward moving grating. It may be determined by finding the area under the response curve for signal differences greater than zero (i.e., that falls to the right of the vertical line at zero in Figure 11-11).

Table 11-2 shows the optimum model parameters obtained by least-squares fits to the contrast increment

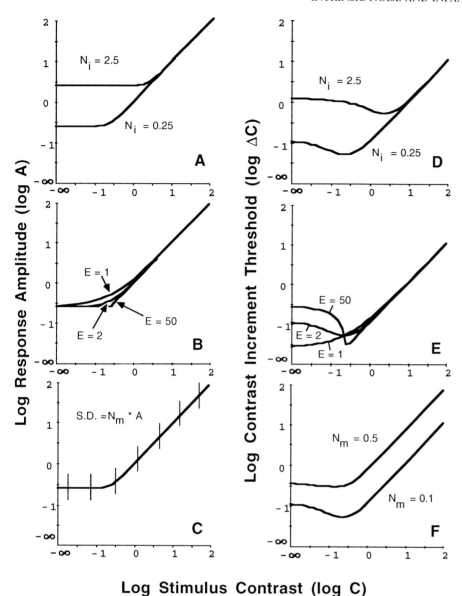

FIG. 11-10. (Left) Transducer functions. (Right) Contrast increment threshold functions. The graphs illustrate the three parameters of the model. (A,D) Effects of changing intrinsic noise. (B,E) Effects of changing the Minkowski exponent. (C) Variability of the sensory response is assumed proportional to the response amplitude. (F) Effects of changing N_m.

threshold data on infants and adults. The three free parameters were fitted to each data set by the following method: The value of the *exponent* E was determined by averaging the values of β from maximum likelihood fits of the Weibull to the individual subjects' psychometric functions for grating detection (the C = condition). The *intrinsic sensory noise*, N_i (which controls contrast detection threshold), and the *contrast-dependent noise*, N_m (which controls the overall level of the contrast increment threshold function), were estimated by a least-squares fit to the threshold data.

The amount of intrinsic noise was 88 times as great for infants as for adults for the green stimulus and 182

times as great for the white stimulus. The shallow slope of the infant psychometric function for C = 0 requires a low value for the Minkowski exponent E (open circles in Figure 11-6). The average values of E for infants were 1.30 for green stimuli and 1.15 for white stimuli. The average values for adults were 3.47 for green stimuli and 3.25 for white stimuli. The infant contrast discrimination data dip slightly below the contrast detection threshold, as predicted by the fact that E is not quite unity. The amount of contrast-dependent noise differs between infants and adults by a factor of about 2.3 for the green stimuli and 1.2 for the white stimuli. The differences between the parameters fit to the two

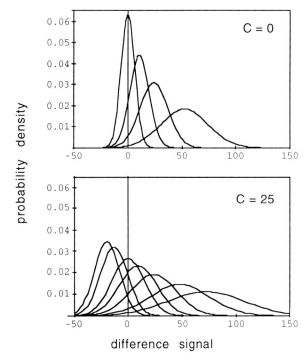

FIG. 11-11. Distributions of difference signals (i.e., the response at point C in Figure 11-8) for standard stimulus contrasts of zero (top panel) and 25% (bottom panel). The different distributions are the predicted difference signals elicited by different comparison stimuli $(C + \Delta C)$. When the comparison stimulus produces a greater signal than the standard stimulus, the difference signal is positive. The probability that a subject will perceive the standard stimulus as having the greater contrast (and therefore dominating the direction of motion) is the area under the appropriate curve falling to the right of the upright line at zero on the abscissa.

data sets may look large, but they are not statistically significant and are based on nonsystematic differences between the data sets on the order of 0.1 log units (Fig. 11-7). These data sets suggest that there is much more intrinsic contrast noise in infant vision than in adult vision, and the contrast-dependent noise in the second stage is a much less important determinant of infant performance.

TABLE 11-2. *Fitted parameter values.*

Subjects	$N_i{}^a$(%)	E^b	$N_m{}^c$
Infants			
White stimuli	51	1.207	0.14
Green stimuli	14	1.312	0.32
Adults			
White stimuli	0.28	3.25	0.12
Green stimuli	0.17	3.47	0.14
Infant/adult ratio			
White stimuli	182	0.371	1.167
Green stimuli	82	0.378	2.285

[a]Equivalent intrinsic contrast noise.
[b]Exponent of the Minkowski threshold nonlinearity.
[c]Standard deviation of the response.

CONCLUSIONS

This discussion of noise in the infant's visual system concludes by relating the sources of noise revealed by the contrast discrimination experiment back to the three studies being reviewed.

As discussed above (Fig. 11-5), adult foveal cones absorb about 2.0 log units more photons from a given stimulus than do infant foveal cones. However, consideration of photon noise predicts that adult foveal contrast detection thresholds should be only about 1.0 log(10) unit higher than infant foveal contrast detection thresholds. Because the difference in rate of photo-absorption in the visual periphery is probably negligibly different for infants and adults, contrast threshold in the visual periphery should also be negligibly different. Thus photon noise alone cannot explain the nearly 2.0 log unit difference in contrast threshold between infants and adults.

Two types of intrinsic sensory noise have been discussed. One is the *eigengrau* of the rod increment threshold experiment, which is classically attributed to the thermal isomerization of molecules in the rod outer segment. The amount of *eigengrau* intrinsic noise for rods is not significantly different between infants and adults; the amounts of infant and adult *eigengrau* intrinsic noise for cones have never been compared, but the timely emergence of infant color vision suggests that they are similar. The other type of sensory noise is intrinsic contrast noise. The amount of intrinsic contrast noise is much greater in infants than in adults. We know this fact because contrast detection thresholds are mich higher for infants than for adults. The two experiments reported in this chapter have estimated intrinsic contrast noise to be 80–180 times as great in 7-week-olds as in adults.

The nonlinearity in the contrast discrimination model occurs at the point where the intrinsic contrast noise is combined with the sensory signal. After that nonlinearity, contrast-dependent noise controls the standard deviation of the response, which in turn controls the critical value of incremental response required to signal the difference between two stimuli. Infants' and adults' response standard deviations differ little by comparison to the difference between them in the amount of intrinsic contrast noise.

What effect would these critical immaturities have on infant color discrimination? The immaturities that are due to increased response standard deviation (i.e., greater contrast-dependent noise) are modest and would likely produce only modest distortions in color space. Being late in processing, at "postsensory" levels where the psychophysical criterion is determined and presumably all color channels are processed together, they would likely produce allometric distortions in color space.

On the other hand, the large differences between infants and adults in intrinsic contrast noise, because they are at an earlier stage of visual processing, could conceivably affect the various dimensions of color space differently, depending on the level of color vision processing at which they occur. Such critical immaturities could therefore produce large nonallometric distortions of infant color space. Of course, the amount of intrinsic contrast noise added to each of the three dimensions (at each level of color vision processing) may also happen to be equal for infants at each age. This point would be predicted, for example, if the critical immaturity were some general property of the infant visual nervous system.

These results, taken together, suggest that the most important critical immaturities are in the amount of intrinsic contrast noise that occurs after the site of ordinary light and dark adaptation but before the site where the psychophysical performance criterion is established. These immaturities have important effects on infant contrast detection threshold and color vision but have little effect on sensitivity at the retinal level and little effect on the contrast discrimination threshold.

Acknowledgments. I am grateful to Drs. D. T. Lindsey and P. E. King-Smith for helpful comments on earlier drafts of this chapter, and to Drs. A. B. Fulton and R. M. Hansen for discussion about rods. I am also grateful to Dr. D. Pelli for turning my attention to *eigengrau*. I wish to acknowledge Ms. E. McSweeney and Ms. S. Taylor for their technical assistance in running the experiments reported here. Supported by NIH EY08083 and a grant from the Ohio Lions Eye Research Foundation.

REFERENCES

ALLEN, D., TYLER, C. W., AND NORCIA, A. M. (1989). Development of grating acuity and contrast sensitivity in the central and peripheral visual field of the human infant. *Invest. Ophthalmol. Vis. Sci.* 30 (suppl.), 311.

ALPERN, M., AND PUGH, E. N., JR. (1974). The density and photosensitivity of human rhodopsin in the living retina. *J. Physiol. (Lond.)* 237, 341–370.

BANKS, M. S., AND BENNETT, P. J. (1988). Optical and photoreceptor immaturities limit the spatial and chromatic vision of human neonates. *J. Opt. Soc. Am. [A]* 5, 2059–2079.

BARLOW, H. B. (1957). Increment thresholds at low intensities considered as signal/noise discriminations. *J. Physiol. (Lond.)* 136, 469–499.

BARLOW, H. B. (1965). Optic nerve impulses and Weber's law. *Cold Spring Harbor Symp. Quant. Biol.* 30, 539–546.

BRINDLEY, G. (1970). *Physiology of the Retina and Visual Pathway*. London: Camelot Press, p. 221.

BROWN, A. M. (1986). Scotoptic sensitivity of the 2-month-old human infant. *Vision Res.* 26, 707–710.

BROWN, A. M. (1988). Saturation of rod-initiated signals in 2-month-old human infants. *J. Opt. Soc. Am. [A]* 5, 2145–2158.

BROWN, A. M. (1990). Development of visual sensitivity to light and color vision in human infants: a critical review. *Vision Res.* 30, 1159–1188.

BROWN, A. M., AND YAMAMOTO, M. (1986). Visual acuity in new-born and preterm infants measured with grating acuity cards. *Am. J. Ophthalmol.* 102, 245–253.

BROWN, A. M., DOBSON, V., AND MAIER, L. (1987). Visual acuity of infants at scotopic, mesopic, and photopic luminances. *Vision Res.* 27, 1845–1858.

DARTNALL, H. J. A. (1957). *The Visual Pigments*. London: Methuan; New York: Wiley.

DOBSON, V., AND TELLER, D. Y. (1978). Visual acuity in human infants: a review and comparison of behavioral and electrophysiological studies. *Vision Res.* 18, 1469–1483.

DOBSON, V., SCHWARTZ, T. L., SANDSTROM, D. J., AND MICHEL, L. (1987). Binocular visual acuity in neonates: the acuity card procedure. *Dev. Med. Child Neurol.* 29, 199–206.

FOLEY, J. M., AND LEGGE, G. E. (1981). Contrast detection and near-threshold discrimination in human vision. *Vision Res.* 21, 1041–1503.

GEISLER, W. S. (1984). Physical limits of acuity and hyperacuity. *J. Opt. Soc. Am. [A]* 1, 775–782.

GRAHAM, N. V. (1989). *Visual Pattern Analyzers*. Oxford: Oxford University Press.

HOOD, D. C. (1988). Testing hypotheses about development with electroretinographic and incremental-threshold data. *J. Opt. Soc. Am. [A]* 5, 2159–2165.

HOOD, D. C., AND FINKELSTEIN, M. A. (1986). Sensitivity to light. In K. R. BOFF, L. KAUFMAN, AND J. P. THOMAS (eds.). *Handbook of Perception and Human Performance*. New York: Wiley.

KRAUSKOPF, J., WILLIAMS, D. R., AND HEELEY, D. W. (1982). Cardinal directions of color space. *Vision Res.* 22, 1123–1131.

MacLEOD, D. I. A. (1978). Visual sensitivity. *Annu. Rev. Psychol.* 29, 613–645.

MacLEOD, D. I. A., AND BOYNTON, R. M. (1979). Chromaticity showing cone excitation by stimuli of equal luminance. *J. Opt. Soc. Am.* 69, 1183–3386.

NORCIA, A. M., TYLER, C. W., AND HAMER, R. D. (1990). Development of contrast sensitivity in the human infant. *Vision Res.* 30, 1475–1486.

PACKER, O., HENDRICKSON, A. E., AND CURCIO, C. A. (1990). Developmental redistribution of photoreceptors across the *Macaca nemestrina* (pigtail macaque) retina. *J. Comp. Neurol.* 298, 472–293.

PELLI, D. G. (1985). Uncertainty explains many aspects of visual contrast detection and discrimination. *J. Opt. Soc. Am. [A]* 2, 1508–1531.

PELLI, D. G. (1987). On the relation between summation and facilitation. *Vision Res.* 27, 119–123.

PELLI, D. G. (1990). The quantum efficiency of vision. In C. BLAKEMORE (ed.). *Coding and Efficiency*. Cambridge: Cambridge University Press, pp. 3–24.

SPERLING, G. (1989). Three stages and two systems of visual processing. *Spatial Vision* 4, 183–207.

STEPHENS, B. R., AND BANKS, M. S. (1987). Contrast discrimination in human infants. *J. Exp. Psychol. [Hum. Percept.]* 13, 558–565.

TELLER, D. Y., AND BORNSTEIN, M. H. (1987). Infant color vision and color perception. In *Handbook of Infant Perception*. Vol. 1. Orlando, FL: Academic Press, pp. 185–236.

TELLER, D. Y., AND LINDSEY, D. T. (1989). OKN motion nulls for white vs. isochromatic gratings in infants and adults. *J. Opt. Soc. Am. [A]* 6, 1945–1954.

APPENDIX

To understand why a threshold nonlinearity predicts a dip in the contrast discrimination threshold, we need two assumptions. One is the shape of the nonlinear transducer function. Let us begin by assuming that the response (R) is constant at low contrast values and then increases linearly with contrast thereafter (shown by the bold line in Figure 11-12A). The other assumption needed is the criterion according to which threshold is determined. Two stimuli of differing contrast are assumed discriminable if the response R + ΔR to the higher contrast stimulus (whose contrast is C + ΔC) exceeds the response (R) to the lower contrast (C) stimulus by an amount sufficient to make R + ΔR > R on 75% of trials. The average response increment ΔR sufficient to meet this criterion depends on the standard deviation of R. Without loss of generality, I assume that the standard deviation of R is proportional to R; the existence of the dip is unaffected by the particular assumption made, so long as the standard deviation N_m (in linear units) does not decrease with R. The critical value of R + ΔR is shown as a function of contrast by the light line in Figure 11-12.

To determine the value of C + ΔC for discrimination between the standard and experimental stimuli, consult Figure 11-12A. C is the value of the standard stimulus; R is the response to that value; and R + ΔR is the criterial response for discrimination. C + ΔC is the contrast of the stimulus that produces the response R + ΔR. Thus ΔC is the contrast discrimination thresh-

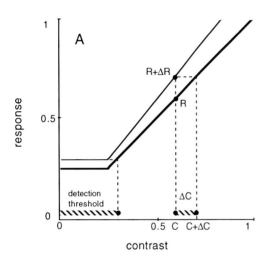

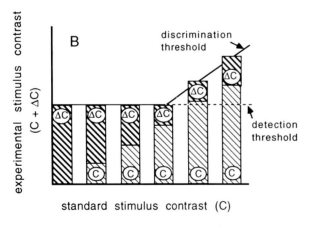

FIG. 11-12. (A) Contrast transducer function for a discontinuous threshold nonlinearity. See appendix for details. (B) Histogram showing how the standard contrast (C) and the contrast increment (ΔC) combine to attain contrast discrimination threshold for a range of standard stimulus contrasts near the contrast detection threshold. The four left-hand bars of the histogram show the contributions of subthreshold values of C and ΔC to the experimental stimulus composition at contrast detection and discrimination threshold; the two right-hand bars show the contributions for barely detectable values of C.

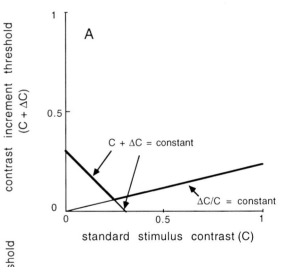

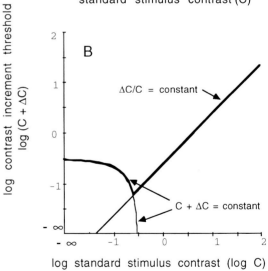

FIG. 11-13. (A) Contrast increment threshold function, in linear units, for the transducer function shown in Figure 11-13A. The constraint lines are discussed in the Appendix text. (B) Same graph as in (A), only in logarithmic coordinates.

old, shown by the hatched bars in the figure. ΔC is indicated for C = 0, which is the contrast detection threshold, and a higher value of C on the rising part of the transducer function.

It can be seen that under these assumptions the critical value of R + ΔR is constant over a range of subthreshold values of C. Let us consider a range of standard stimulus contrasts (C) that are below the contrast detection threshold (the first four bars of the histogram in Figure 11-12B). For each subthreshold value of C, the contrast increment (ΔC) is increased until the experimental and standard stimuli can just be discriminated, that is, until the contrast C + ΔC just attains the discrimination threshold (indicated by the continuous line). Because the detection and discrimination thresholds are equal over this range, the task of dis-

criminating between the standard and experimental stimuli reduces to the problem of simply detecting the experimental stimulus: Whenever the experimental stimulus is not above threshold, the subject cannot see either stimulus and fails at the task. For increasing values of the standard stimulus C, the detection threshold for the composite C + ΔC remains constant. At the same time, the amount of contrast contributed to the constant threshold contrast by C (the standard stimulus contrast) increases and the contrast contributed by ΔC (the contrast of the increment) diminishes. This segment of the contrast increment threshold function can be described by the equation C + ΔC = constant (Fig. 11-13A) where the value of the constant is the contrast detection threshold indicated in Figure 11-12A. In logarithmic coordinates (Fig. 11-13B) the decrease in

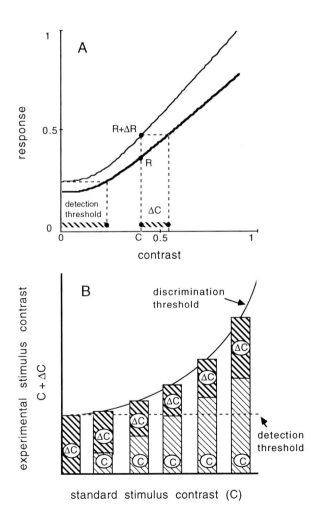

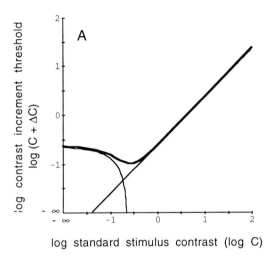

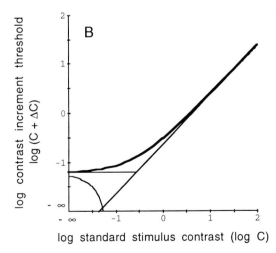

FIG. 11-14. (A) Contrast transducer function for a nonlinearity of the form: R = $(S^E + N_i^E)^{1/E}$, where R, S, N_i, and E are defined in the chapter text, and E = 3. (B) Histogram similar to that in Figure 11-13B, only for the contrast transducer function shown in (A).

FIG. 11-15. Contrast increment threshold functions relative to logarithmic coordinates for the continuous transducer functions shown in Figure 11-15A (A) and Figure 11-16A (B). The constraint lines are discussed in the Appendix text.

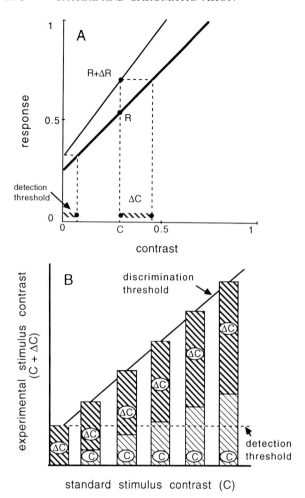

FIG. 11-16. (A) Linear contrast transducer function. (B) Histogram, similar to that in Figure 11-13B, only for a linear contrast transducer function.

threshold and the constraint line curve downward in a "dipper"-shaped function.

When the transducer function begins to rise on its linear part (the last two bars of the histogram in Figure 11-12B), the contrast increment threshold function begins to obey Weber's law because the standard deviation of R is proportional to R. The increase in threshold is indicated by the increasing parts of Figures 11-12B and 11-13.

The decrease in contrast increment threshold with increasing values of the standard stimulus depends on the fact that the transducer function is an accelerating "threshold" nonlinearity. It does not, however, depend on the exact shape of the nonlinearity, as illustrated in Figures 11-14 and 11-15A. Continuous versions of the nonlinearity in Figures 11-12 and 11-13 may be generated by using finite values of E (the Minkowski exponent: see the text for discussion); and so long as $E > 1$ the dipper-shaped contrast increment threshold function is predicted. For example, the series in Figures 11-14 and 11-15A were generated using $E = 3$. The constraint lines in Figure 11-15A are the same equations as in Figure 11-13B.

Finally, when $E = 1$ and the transducer function is the linear sum of signal (S) and intrinsic noise (N_i), the contrast increment threshold function is monotonically increasing. This increase can be seen in Figures 11-15B and 11-16. In that case, the critical value of R + ΔR increases faster than the standard stimulus contrast. Accordingly, ΔC (the contrast increment threshold) increases monotonically with C. The constraint lines calculated as in Figure 11-13B are shown, together with a horizontal line at contrast detection threshold.

IV. Binocular Vision
Introduction

E I L E E N E . B I R C H

The formal study of binocular vision has a long history, dating from at least the 1600s. It includes contributions from the fields of mathematics, physics, anatomy, ophthalmology, neurophysiology, psychology, and philosophy. The long and complex evolution of our understanding of binocular vision has fascinated and stimulated a small group of scientists and physicians to pursue research in this field, which may be daunting to those who do not work with the concepts of binocular vision on a regular basis. A colleague who works in the area of color vision recently expressed this common viewpoint succinctly by stating: "Thinking about binocular vision makes my brain hurt." Hopefully, the next three paragraphs will provide a brief and not too painful summary of the basics for those who are unfamiliar with the terminology of *single binocular vision*.

The two eyes look in the same direction and largely overlap in their visual fields—the first fundamental fact about single binocular vision; that is, both eyes must be capable of seeing and must be capable of simultaneously fixating the same point in space. If one eye has poor or absent vision or if the ability to coordinate the positions of the two eyes is compromised in any way (e.g., due to strabismus), normal binocular vision is not possible.

The visual direction of gaze can be represented by a line drawn from the object of regard to the foveola, and all other directions in visual space can be judged relative to this visual axis. Binocularly corresponding points, then, are retinal points that, when stimulated separately, are associated with the same visual direction. This is the second basic fact about normal binocular vision; that is, it is not possible to see double with corresponding retinal points, as they share a common relative visual direction. If the images falling on corresponding retinal points are similar, they fuse into a single percept. On the other hand, if the images falling on corresponding points are dissimilar, either rivalry (alternation of the two images in space and time) or suppression (only one of the two images perceived) occurs. Given a fixation

point, the set of all other points in space that fall on corresponding retinal points is called the *horopter*.

Because the two eyes are separated by the interpupillary distance, the two images formed in the eyes differ slightly in the positions of some image components on the retina. The binocular disparity in retinal position for some components of the image forms the basis for stereoscopic depth perception, the third basic fact about normal binocular vision—information about relative depth can be recovered from binocular disparity. Initially, the concept of single binocular vision at the horopter appears to be incompatible with binocular disparity. However, stimuli do not need to fall on exactly corresponding retinal points in the two eyes to give rise to single vision. Each retinal point in one eye is associated with a small area in the other eye (rather than a single point), which is called Panum's area. Any pair of similar stimuli that fall within Panum's area are perceived as a single object. Disparity between the positions of these stimuli gives rise to the percept of depth relative to the point of fixation. The perception of depth based on the cue of retinal disparity is called *stereopsis*. Objects located in front of the fixation point have crossed binocular disparity (both images fall on temporal retinal points), and objects located behind the fixation point have uncrossed binocular disparity (both images fall on nasal retinal points). At least within Panum's area, the amount of binocular disparity is monotonically related to the amount of depth perceived relative to the fixation point. Stereopsis is a unique sensation, much as is color vision, in that it is difficult to describe to a person who lacks this visual capacity. Although there are many other cues to depth perception, the precision of stereopsis for judgments about relative depth is at least an order of magnitude better than judgments based on other cues.

The development of single binocular vision in infants remains an area of active research. In essence, many of the studies of the normal development of binocular vision address one or both of the following questions: (1) What does the infant perceive at birth? (2) When does the infant achieve single binocular vision and stereopsis? The answers depend on information regarding the maturation of eye and head size, of accommodation and vergence, and of the physiological substrate for stereoptic vision (including the retinal mosaic and the central nervous system). Although there are still many questions to be answered about the development of binocular vision, there is general agreement that infants do not show any evidence of stereopsis at birth; instead, in most normal infants there is an abrupt onset of stereopsis at about 4 months of age. After the age of onset, stereoacuity improved rapidly. Prior to the onset of stereopsis, most of the evidence suggests that young infants have simultaneous perception with the two eyes and may have a primitive form of fusion that resembles superimposition of the two monocular images.

The general agreement regarding the onset of stereopsis among various laboratories using numerous psychophysical and electrophysiological techniques is unusual in the field of infant vision. This agreement has fostered a multidisciplinary approach to research that has led to rapid progress in our understanding of this aspect of visual function. Since the initial psychophysical and electrophysiological reports regarding the onset of stereopsis in the human infant were published in 1980, the field has moved on to studies of stereoacuity development, fusion and rivalry, binocular summation, and possible relations among stereopsis, fusion, hyperacuity, and acuity development. Data from these studies, in conjunction with anatomical, neurophysiological, and psychophysical data from animal models, have formed the basis for the construction of detailed models of binocular development. Furthermore, the rapid pace of research on the normal developmental course has provided a firm basis for clinical research into the factors that lead to disruption of single binocular vision in congenital and early-onset eye disorders.

Despite the consensus on basic data about normal development, there remain many issues that are still under active investigation and issues about which questions concerning the interpretation of data continue to promote active dialogue. To gently initiate the reader who may be unfamiliar with the field of binocular visual development (or visual development in general), three cautions are offered here.

First, there are many examples in the literature of papers that give particular emphasis to whether one technique is "better" than another. That is, is one technique capable of demonstrating a visual capacity earlier than other techniques, or does one technique measure a more rapid rate of visual development than other techniques? Whereas this approach may motivate optimization of infant vision testing protocols, it also can obscure the benefits of a multifaceted approach to the study of visual development. Discrepancies among findings obtained with different measurement protocols have been casually attributed to "problems" with one of the protocols rather than recognizing that each protocol may tap a different aspect of visual function.

As an example, take the finding of significant interocular differences in acuity during early development, which has been documented in several psychophysical studies but which is not found in visual evoked potential studies. One possible interpretation of this discrepancy is that the interocular differences found psychophysically are an artifact due to larger variability of psychophysical threshold estimates than are visual evoked potential estimates. Although this hypothesis seems reasonable and is an easy way to dismiss the discrepancy, it simply is not tenable. Psychophysical studies do show higher variability in acuity estimates, and interocular acuity difference scores show even more variability than acuity. However, the interocular differences found psychophysically in young infants have been shown to exceed test-retest differences for the same eye in several psychophysical studies; that is, the interocular differences are statistically significant and cannot be regarded as an artifact of the test protocol. An alternative hypothesis is that the discrepancy occurs because psychophysical and visual evoked potential protocols tap different aspects of visual function. For example, psychophysical protocols generally allow free viewing and require not only that the visual system is capable of resolving the stimulus but also that the infant see the stimulus and generate an appropriate gaze response. Visual evoked potential protocols, on the other hand, are biased toward evaluation of the central 10 degrees of visual field (due to cortical topography) and assess electrical activity that occurs at the site of entrance to the striate cortex; the electrical activity at this site may be unrelated to the child's ability to see or produce visually guided behavior. Despite the important implications for understanding the development of single binocular vision, the factors responsible for the discrepancy between psychophysical and electrophysiological estimates of interocular differences have not been identified.

Second, there are many examples in the literature where a test protocol is described as a technique capable of evaluating "binocular function," or "binocularity." The terms binocular function and binocularity are broad, and their use has led to some confusion. For example, "normal binocularity" has been used to describe both simultaneous perception (absence of suppression) and adult-level stereoacuity. This vague terminology has led to misunderstandings in the literature. A new test protocol from one laboratory may be described as a valid measure of binocularity, whereas another laboratory argues that the protocol is not valid because results correlate poorly with stereopsis test results. This argument against test validity is not useful because "binocularity" and "stereopsis" are not synonymous.

Third, a prevalent misconception in the clinical research literature is that a technique showing a higher level of visual function at a given age, a more rapid rate of development, or lower intersubject variability among normal infants is necessarily more sensitive to abnormal vision in infants with congenital or early-onset eye disorders. Although a large separation between normal and abnormal scores and high score reliability are important factors, this protocol-oriented approach overlooks a crucial factor; that is, to be sensitive to visual abnormality, the test must measure an aspect of visual function affected by the particular disease process. This statement means that the sensitivity of protocols to abnormality must be evaluated empirically for each of the many congenital and early-onset eye disorders.

With these cautions in hand, it seems worthwhile to reiterate a point made earlier. There is a general consensus across protocols on the basic timetable for the development of normal single binocular vision. Moreover, the weight of evidence suggests that the limiting factor in the normal development of stereopsis is maturation of the brain, which is not to disregard the sensitivity of the developmental process to disruption by binocular imbalance, such as misalignment of the visual axes or abnormal acuity. This sensitivity forms the basis for clinical research on the development of binocular function in infantile esotropia, unilateral cataract, and other congenital and early-onset eye disorders. In the absence of any infantile eye disorder, however, studies of the development of binocular function may provide insights into the development of the central nervous system. This fact has led to several examples in the literature of the use of stereopsis as an index of the rate of cortical maturation, including studies of the influence of perinatal nutrition on, and the hormonal regulation of, central nervous system development.

The five chapters in this section summarize our current state of knowledge about infant binocular vision.

The chapter by Shinsuke Shimojo reviews data on the development of fusion within the context of developmental constraints on emerging binocular function. Special emphasis is placed on the crucial role of eye-of-origin information in the development of mature binocular vision. A review of the evidence for the sudden onset and rapid development of stereopsis in normal infants is provided in Eileen Birch's chapter, which also addresses the etiology of binocular sensory deficits in infantile eye disorders and the finding that at least some esotropic infants have the sensory capacity for stereopsis during the first year of life.

Changes in axial length, interpupillary distance, and retinal mosaic during infancy require adaptations in binocular function to maintain precision and accuracy in sensory and motor function. Clifton Schor discusses details of these growth parameters and their influence on the horopter and motor control of binocular eye alignment. A two-stage model of human binocular development is proposed by Richard Held. His model includes an immature stage, characterized by simple summation of signals from corresponding retinal loci, and a mature stage, characterized by preservation of eye-of-origin information, disparity selectivity, and interocular inhibition. This model is consistent with a remarkable variety of data, including anatomical, electrophysiological, and psychophysical, from animal models and human infants. Especially provocative is the suggestion that the transition between immature and mature stages may represent a window of risk for the onset of strabismus. In the final chapter, Christopher Tyler discusses several aspects of binocular function that have only recently been examined empirically, including interocular acuity differences, dichoptic summation, and occlusion depth. Although fusion and stereopsis are the most compelling aspects of binocular function and have the most direct relevance to clinical research, basic research in these areas should provide new insights into the normal process of visual development.

12 | Development of interocular vision in infants

SHINSUKE SHIMOJO

Three issues are addressed in this chapter. First, I review studies related to the onset of binocular functions and offer a hypothesis about critical developmental constraints together with supporting evidence. In the second part I review some recent findings in adult psychophysics that have implications regarding the development of binocular functions. Toward the end of this chapter, I briefly describe a theoretical framework to integrate these two sets of findings into a more comprehensive understanding of adaptability and plasticity of binocular functions. *Interocular*, not just binocular, processes based on the eye-of-origin information are the key to these discussions.

ONSET OF BINOCULAR FUNCTIONS

Fusion, Stereopsis, and Rivalry

Fusion, stereopsis, and rivalry are the binocular functions with which we deal in this chapter. *Fusion* is the visual system's capability of integrating the corresponding points and similar visual images in the two eyes into a single vision when the difference between the two retinal images is within a certain limit (Panum's fusible area). *Stereopsis* is the visual system's capability of recovering information about relative depth in the physical world from disparities between the two retinal images. Unlike these cases, *binocular rivalry*, or vigorous alternations of patches between the two visual images, occurs when the visual inputs are drastically different. Particularly strong interocular suppression occurs when one eye sees horizontal stripes and the other eye sees vertical stripes. It may be worth noting here that rivalry is not just a default value of fusion, and that fusion is not just a default value of rivalry. Rather, these two components seem to be different processes with different spatiotemporal characteristics (Kaufman, 1974; Wolfe, 1983, 1986).

Onset of Stereopsis and Improvement of Stereoacuity

The onset age of stereopsis has been assessed by various techniques, such as the preferential looking (PL) method

(Held et al., 1980; Birch et al., 1982), a variation of it utilizing the infant's pursuit eye movements to a cyclopean target (Fox et al., 1980), and the visually evoked potentials (VEP) method (Atkinson and Braddick 1976; Petrig et al., 1981). It has been reported unanimously that there is no evidence of stereopsis in very young infants, with the onset age of it being 2–6 months of age for more than 90% of infants (mean age 3–4 months). What follows it is rapid improvement in stereoacuity—rapid relative to the improvement of grating acuity (Held et al., 1980; Birch et al., 1982).

Onset of Fusion/Rivalry Discrimination

Rivalrous stimuli are known to be aversive to older infants, who show a clear preference to a fusible stimulus over a rivalrous stimulus. This finding provides convincing evidence for discrimination (Birch et al., 1985). The results of several studies employing the VEP technique (Braddick et al., 1980; Petrig et al., 1981; Atkinson et al., 1991) have agreed with those from the PL study (Birch et al., 1985) in that the mean onset age of fusion/rivalry discrimination is roughly the same as that of stereopsis: 3–4 months on average (though some of these VEP studies failed to distinguish response to disparity from that to interocular correlation). Could it be just a coincidence, or does it indicate that there is a common underlying neurological constraint? High correlations between the onset ages of these two kinds of binocularity in both group and individual data (Birch et al., 1985) indicate the latter.

Processing of Binocular Inputs During the Prestereoptic Period

It has been well known ever since Fantz' remarkable report in 1963 that the newborn can discriminate a patterned stimuli from a homogeneous visual field. Fantz and his colleagues argued that this finding should be taken as evidence that some, even if minimal, cortical functions exist at birth because a major lesion of the cortex disabled pattern discrimination in a wide range of mammalian species (Fantz et al., 1962). Thus pattern vision is a product of visual processing before the onset age of stereopsis. (We call this interval the *prestereoptic period*). On the other hand, we know from the above-mentioned literature that the way inputs from the two eyes are integrated in the prestereoptic visual system should be significantly different from that in the stereoptic visual system. Thus there seems to be a "missing link" between our understanding of monocular development and that of binocular development.

PRESTEREOPTIC VISUAL SYSTEM

Hypothesis of Nonselective Convergence

The high correlation of onset age that was observed between coarse stereopsis and fusion-rivalry discrimination suggests that there is a common developmental change in the cortical structure underlying the acquisition of these binocular functions (Held, 1985). What, then, could be the prestereoptic mode of interaction between the two eyes? One intuitively obvious possibility would be "superposition" as if the two monocular images were simply added point for point. The visual system during the prestereoptic period may simply combine inputs from corresponding loci on the two retinas nonselectively into a common binocular representation without calculating disparity or fusing two identical images or causing interocular suppression between them. To be more specific, the following set of hypotheses may be postulated about binocular interaction in the prestereoptic visual system (Shimojo et al., 1986):

1. The "prestereoptic" system has only a common representation in which inputs from the two eyes are nonselectively combined ("superposition" hypothesis).
2. The information about the eye of origin (from which eye the input comes) is therefore lost at a relatively early cortical stage in the "prestereoptic" visual processing.
3. It is the loss of monocular representations and labels of eye of origin that precludes stereopsis and fusion-rivalry discrimination, which requires selective combination of inputs from each eye.

Could these propositions possibly be consistent with what has been known about anatomy of the visual pathways during this period? In fact, they are well predicted by Held's (1985) anatomical model of binocularity development. He speculated that when an adult-like ocular dominance segregation is attained in visual cortex there is a transition from a binocular-unit-based system to a monocular-unit-based system in layer IV of area V1, enabling the system to maintain separate monocular representations of visual inputs together with the eye-of-origin information, thus serving as a basis for disparity computation and interocular suppression. (This model is illustrated in Figure 12-9 and is discussed later in the chapter.) We have tested specific behavioral predictions deriving from these hypotheses, and the next two sections summarize the results.

Supporting Evidence: Interocularly Combined Grids

Healthy infants who were aged 1–8 months, orthotropic, and within the normal range of refractive error participated in this experiment. They wore goggles with orthogonally polarized filters, and each was held on the parent's lap. The viewing distance was 70 cm from two black rear-projection screens (17 × 27 degrees) that were located side by side. The infant subjects were tested once a week by the two-alternative, forced-choice preferential looking (FPL) paradigm. The observer, who was blind to the stimulus, judged in each trial to which side the infant preferred to gaze. Fifteen trials were performed for each of the three kinds of stimuli. (For more detailed descriptions of the subjects, apparatus, and procedures, see Shimojo et al., 1986.)

Figure 12-1 shows the stereograms that were used as stimuli. The spatial frequency of the stripes (0.4 cycle per degree, or cpd) and the duty cycle (0.37) were the same for these three pairs of stimuli. Examine Figure 12-1C first. For the control stimulus (stimulus pair C), grids were presented on one screen (left in this example, though the position was randomized across trials in the experiment), and stripes were presented on the other screen (right); all these patterns were identical for the two eyes; that is, they were interocularly identical and therefore fusible. Virtually all the infant subjects, regardless of their ages, consistently showed a preference for the grid side over the stripe side. This finding presumably reflected the infant's preference for the intersecting stripes in the grids, which is a special case of the general tendency of preference for a more complicated pattern (Karmel, 1969a,b). Thus this preference is a form of pattern detection that is independent of binocular interaction.

Let us now see the experimental stimulus illustrated in the upper half of Figure 12-1A (stimulus pair A). Here vertical stripes were presented to one eye and horizontal stripes to the other eye on one screen (left, in this example), whereas the other screen (right) contained interocularly identical, fusible stripes. Adult observers who had normal stereopsis perceived not intersections but segmented and constantly altering patches of vertical and horizontal stripes (binocular rivalry), as illustrated in the second-from-bottom figure in Figure 12-1A. Intersections between the dichoptically presented stripes were perceived only when interocular

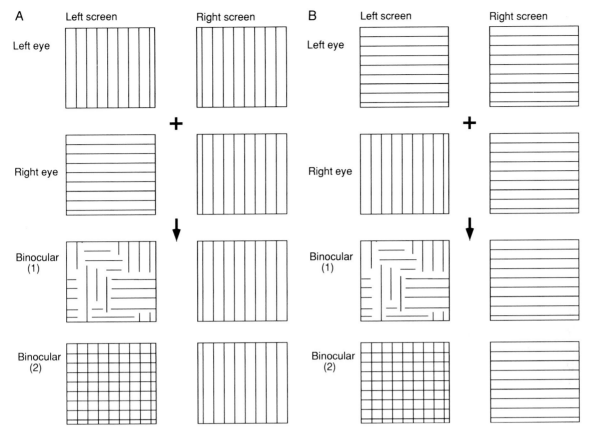

FIG. 12-1. Stimulus pairs. The image presented to the left eye, the image presented to the right eye, binocular perception when interocular suppression exists (Binocular 1), binocular perception when interocular suppression is lacking (Binocular 2) are shown in each figure. (A) Stimulus pair A (experimental condition). Interocularly orthogonal stripes were presented on one screen (left screen, in this example), whereas interocularly identical stripes were presented on the other (right) screen. (B) Stimulus pair B (control condition 1). It was similar to stimulus pair A except that interocularly identical stripes were horizontal. (C) Stimulus pair C (control condition 2). Interocularly identical grids were presented on one screen (left screen, in this example), and interocularly identical stripes were presented on the other (right screen). (From Shimojo et al., 1986. By permission.) *Figure continued*

suppression was avoided by such means as flickering stimuli ("abnormal fusion") (Wolfe, 1983). Our reasoning was as follows: If our hypothesis of nonselective convergence is correct, the binocular representation of the visual inputs in the presstereoptic visual system would be similar to the bottom-most figure in Figure 12-1A, and the infants may be expected to prefer the interocularly orthogonal stripes over the interocularly identical stripes because of the interocularly emergent grids. The same preferential response would be expected for the other stimulus, illustrated in Figure 12-1B (stimulus pair B) because the only difference between the two stereograms was the orientation of interocularly identical stripes. Most infants older than 4 months, however, would prefer the fusible (interocularly identical) pattern over the rivalrous (interocularly orthogonal) one in these stimulus stereograms, as expected from our previous study (Birch et al., 1985). Thus our prediction

was peculiar: Tested longitudinally, an infant should show a dramatic shift of preference exactly at the time when the "eye labeling" process allows selective combination of inputs in binocular processing.

The longitudinal data were highly consistent with this prediction as shown in Figure 12-2, where frequency of preference for the interocularly identical stripes (right side of Figure 12-1A) is plotted as a function of age for each infant. Horizontal lines in the graphs indicate the statistically significant levels of preference ($p = 0.036$ in the two-tailed test). Thus almost all the infants tested showed the predicted shift of preference from the interocularly orthogonal stripes to the interocularly identical stripes, though some (4 of the 25) infants showed an oscillation of preference before they eventually showed a consistent preference for the interocularly identical stripes (see the right bottom graph in Figure 12-2, for example). The mean age of this shift was 14.2 weeks.

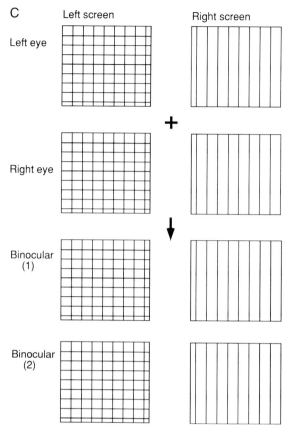

C

Left screen   Right screen

Left eye

+

Right eye

↓

Binocular
(1)

Binocular
(2)

FIG. 12-1. *(continued)*

The longitudinal data obtained with the stimulus pair B (Figure 12-1B) were also plotted on the same graphs in Figure 12-2 as asterisks. The results were in good agreement. Cross-sectional data shown in Figure 12-3 were consistent with the longitudinal data. Here the proportion of infants who reached a preference criterion for the interocularly identical stripes is plotted as a function of age. Two other functions obtained with the checkerboard and random-dot stereograms, and another function obtained with line stereograms were drawn from the previous studies (Birch et al., 1985) and plotted on the same graph. These four functions have been obtained from independent groups of subjects, and yet they show excellent agreement.

Other Evidence

The hypothesis of nonselective convergence was further tested for other aspects of visual perception, such as: (1) number of items; (2) contrast; (3) spatial frequency; and (4) color. A new group of infant subjects was tested with the "interocular grid" stimulus (Figure 12-1A) on a weekly basis. Only those who had been shown to be in the prestereoptic period (32 infants) participated in these experiments. They were tested only once during this period and once again during the "stereoptic pe-

riod," defined as before and after the preferential shift in the "interocular grid" test. Otherwise, the general method was similar to that of the previous experiment (for more details see Shimojo, 1985).

Number of Items. See Figure 12-4A for an example of the stimulus pairs (stimulus pair D). Monocularly, just one horizontal bar was presented on each screen, but on one screen (right in this example) there was a vertical offset between the two eyes, so nonselective binocular convergence would result in totally different configurations between the two screens: a single bar on one side (left in this example) and two bars on the other. Thus the infants during the prestereoptic period should show a clear preference for the side of the interocularly doubled stripes because it contains more contour, though this preference should disappear when the stimulus is viewed monocularly. These predictions were confirmed by the results, as shown in Figure 12-4B, where percentage of preference was plotted for binocular and monocular viewing conditions for each infant. The lines in the graphs indicate within-subject comparisons of the conditions.

As a control experiment, another type of stimulus pair was employed (stimulus pair E, Fig. 12-4C). In this stereogram, both sides were interocularly identical and fusible; but one side contains one stripe, whereas the other contains two. If the infant's preference for the interocularly doubled stripes in the previous stereogram was in fact due to nonselective convergence, within-subject correlations between that and this fusible control should be high. This prediction was also supported, as shown in Figure 12-4D.

Contrast. See Figure 12-5A for an example of the stimulus pairs (stimulus pair F). Horizontal stripes were presented to each eye on each screen, but they were interocularly out-phased (0.25 cycle) on one screen (left in this example) and interocularly counter-phased on the other (right). Nonselective interocular summation would lead to a highly complicated pattern on the out-phased side, as indicated at the bottom left of Figure 12-5A, whereas pretty much homogeneous gray field appeared on the counter-phased side as indicated at bottom right. During the prestereoptic period the infants should show a preference for the out-phased side, though this preference should disappear when the stimulus was viewed monocularly. These predictions were supported by the results, as shown in Figure 12-5B. The preference should also disappear even under binocular viewing during the stereoptic period because *both* screens would now cause vigorous rivalry. This prediction was consistent with the results, as shown in Figure 12-5C.

The interpretation of the infant's preference for the interocularly out-phased pattern would still be ambiguous because not only did the interocularly mixed contrast vary more, so did the amount of contour between

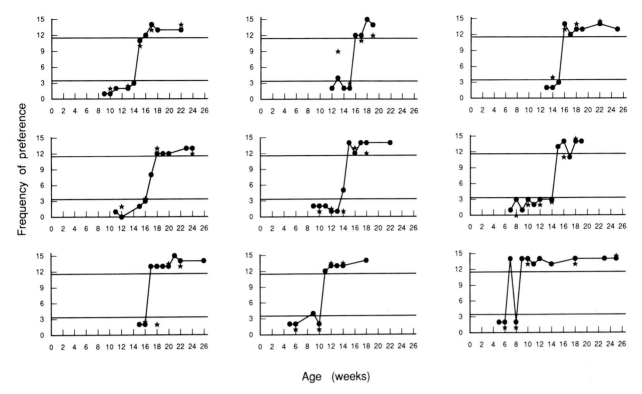

FIG. 12-2. Examples of longitudinal data (obtained with the stimulus pair A). Data of nine infants are shown here. Frequency of preference for the interocularly identical stripes (the right side of Figure 12-1A) is plotted as a function of age for each infant. Frequency of preference for the interocularly identical stripes in the control stimulus B (Fig. 12-1B) is also plotted (*). Horizontal lines in the graphs show the statistically significant levels of preference ($p = 0.036$). (From Shimojo et al., 1986. By permission.)

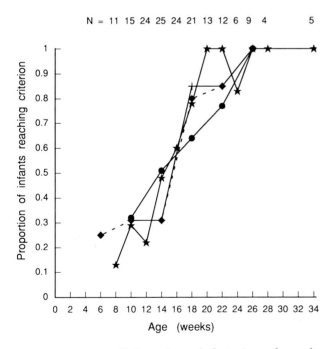

FIG. 12-3. Percentage of infants who reached criterion preference for the interocularly identical pattern in the current study (★) and in a previous study (Birch et al., 1985). ● = checkerboard correlograms; + = random-dot correlograms. The percentage of infants who reached criterion preference for stereoscopic depth (45 minutes) is also obtained from the same study and plotted (♦). (From Shimojo et al., 1986. By permission.)

the two screens in the hypothetical binocular representation. To distinguish these two possible cues to preference, another kind of stimulus pair was employed (stimulus pair G, Figure 12-5D). This pair is similar to the previous pair except that stripes were same-phased instead of 0.25 cycle out-phased on one screen (left in this example). Unlike the previous stimulus, the amount of contour would be the same between the two screens, whereas contrast would be clearly higher on one screen in the nonselective binocular representation, as shown at the bottom of Figure 12-5D. If during the prestereoptic period the infant still showed a preference for the same-phased side, it might be taken as evidence for interocular mixture of contrast. If a preference were found in stimulus pair F (Fig. 12-5A) but not in pair G (Fig. 12-5D), the preference should be mainly on amount of interocularly summed contour. The results clearly support the amount of contour as the main preferential cue, though there might have been some additional effect of contrast (Fig. 12-5E). During the stereoptic period, however, the preference for the same-phased stripes in the stimulus pair G reached the statistically significant level (Fig. 12-5F). This result was expected because one screen was fusible, whereas the other was rivalrous in the stimulus pair G, unlike stimulus pair F, which was rivalrous on both screens. Thus the preferential shift from the prestereoptic to the stereoptic periods in

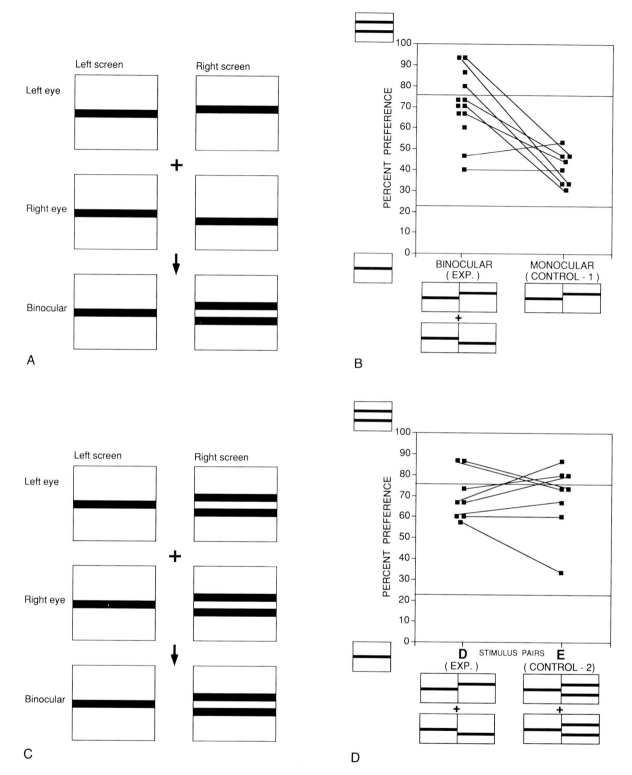

FIG. 12-4. Stimuli and results of the "number of items" experiment. (A) Experimental stimulus pair D. The bottom pair of figures (BINOCULAR) show the binocular representation that is expected under nonselective convergence of inputs from two eyes. (B) Percent preference for interocularly displaced bars in binocular and monocular viewing conditions. Zero percent on the ordinate indicates 100% preference for the other side (the interocularly same-positioned bar, in this case). Each point on the graph represents each infant in each condition. Lines connect data obtained from the same individual infants. All tests were done during the prestereoptic period. (C) Control stimulus pair E. Unlike the experimental stimulus (D), both left and right screens are interocularly identical. (D) Percent preference for two bars over one bar in experimental stimulus pair D and control stimulus pair E. All tests were done during the prestereoptic period. (From Shimojo, 1985. By permission.)

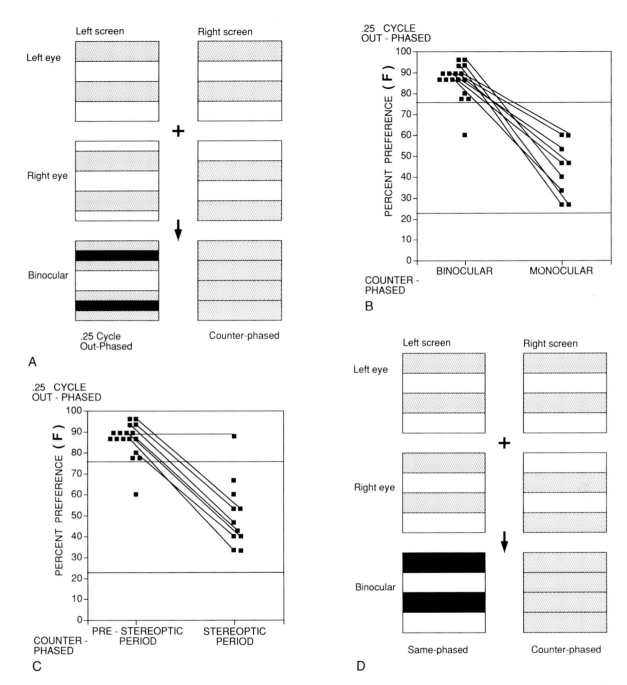

FIG. 12-5. Stimuli and results of the "contrast" experiment. (A) Experimental stimulus pair F. The bottom pair of figures (BINOCULAR) show the binocular representation that is expected under nonselective convergence of inputs from two eyes with linear summation of contrast between eyes. (B) Percent preference for out-phased stripes in stimulus pair F in binocular and monocular viewing conditions during the prestereoptic period. Each point on the graph represents each infant in each condition. Lines connect data obtained from the same individual infants. (C) Percent preference for out-phased stripes in stimulus pair F in binocular viewing during prestereoptic and stereoptic periods. (D) Stimulus pair G. It was similar to stimulus pair F except that interocularly same-phased stripes, instead of 0.25 cycle out-phased stripes, were used on one screen (left screen, in this example). (E) Percent preference for out-phased stripes in stimulus pair F and for the same-phased stripes in stimulus pair G during the prestereoptic period. (F) Percent preference for the same-phased stripes in stimulus pair G during the prestereoptic and stereoptic periods. (G) Individual results. The same sets of data as in the previous figures are replotted individually for each of four infants. The ages when each infant was tested are indicated under the abscissa for each graph. (From Shimojo, 1985. By permission.) *Figure continued*

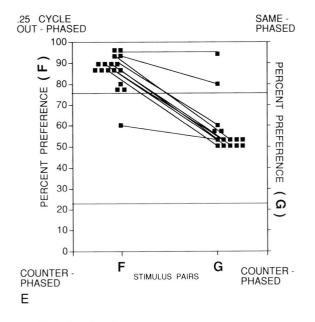

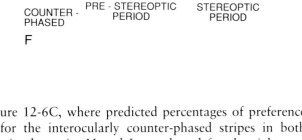

FIG. 12-5. *(continued)*

stimulus pair G was in a direction opposite to that for stimulus pair F, individual examples of which are shown in Figure 12-5G.

To summarize, the infant's preference for the out-phased stripes may be explained most plausibly by the nonselective combination of contour.

Spatial Frequency. See Figure 12-6A for an example of the stimuli (stimulus pair H), where one screen is just a homogeneous white field in both eyes, and the other screen contains horizontal stripes in each eye. The stripes are identical between eyes (0.75 cpd, 0.28 duty cycle) except that they are counter-phased. Nonselective convergence of inputs from two retinas may result in twice as high (1.5 cpd) spatial frequency, as shown at the bottom of the figure. If the infant's grating acuity, which can be measured independently using the conventional method, is between 0.75 and 1.50 cpd, the infant would not show any preference in binocular viewing because the summated spatial frequency is beyond its resolution. With monocular viewing, on the other hand, it should show a preference for the 0.75 cpd stripes over the homogeneous white field. Four infants had been selected from the 11 infants who had participated in this experiment, based on the above-mentioned grating acuity criterion of 0.75–1.50 cpd. Stimulus pair I (Fig. 12-6B) is similar to stimulus pair H except that instead of the homogeneous white field the same stripes with the same phase between eyes are given on the other screen (see the right half of Fig. 12-6B). In this case, the same infant would show a preference for the same-phased stripes only in binocular viewing if nonselective convergence occurs. These predictions are illustrated in Fig-

ure 12-6C, where predicted percentages of preference for the interocularly counter-phased stripes in both stimulus pairs H and I are plotted for the right eye, binocularly, and the left eye viewing conditions.

These double V-shaped predictions were consistent with the results obtained from the four infants, as shown in Figure 12-6D, suggesting that interocular summation of spatial frequency may in fact occur at the central level of visual processing.

Color. When opponent colors such as red and green are presented to the two eyes dichoptically, most normal adult observers perceive rivalry of colors. When the hue difference between two stimuli is less—red in one eye and yellow in the other, for example—interocular color mixture sometimes occurs and an intermediate color (orange in the example) may be perceived. This phenomenon has been called cortical color mixture (for a review see DeWeert and Levelt, 1976) because color channels in monocular pathways first converge at the cortical level. If the prestereoptic system indeed loses the eye-of-origin information at an early stage and therefore lacks the ability of interocular suppression, color channels would be nonselectively pooled at this level. Consequently, the same kind of interocular color mixture should occur even in the opponent color (red/green) case. Something like yellowish white would be seen, which is less saturated than the monocular originals.

Figure 12-7A shows stimulus pair J, used in the experiment. One screen (left in this example) contained an interocularly identical color (red or green), whereas the other screen (right in this example) contained in-

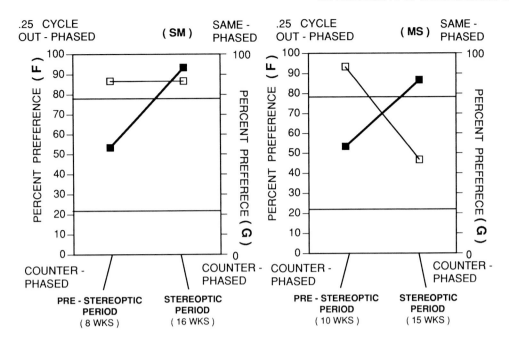

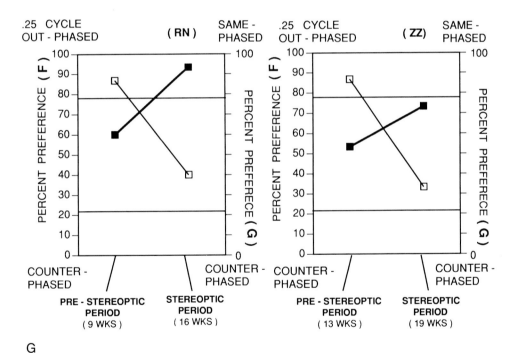

G

FIG. 12-5. (continued)

terocularly opponent colors (red/green). Because infants are known to prefer a colored stimulus over a noncolored or a less-colored stimulus even at 2 months of age (Peeples and Teller, 1975; for a review see Teller and Bornstein, 1982), a preference for the interocularly identical color would be predicted during the prestereoptic period. During the stereoptic period, on the other hand, it is likely that the preference would shift to the interocularly opponent colors because rivalry causes alternation of colors on this side. Even though infants avoid monochromatic rivalry (Birch et al., 1985), they show a preference for a flickering or moving colored stimulus over a stationary one (Volkmann and Dobson, 1976). As expected, most of the 10 infants who participated in the experiment showed a preference for the interocularly identical color over the interocularly op-

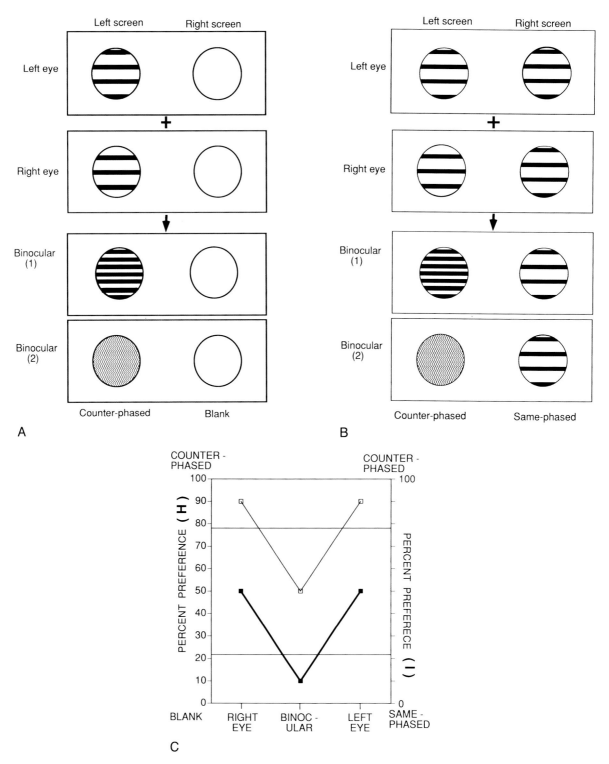

FIG. 12-6. Stimuli and results of the "spatial frequency" experiment. (A) Stimulus pair H. The two bottom pairs of figures (BINOCULAR) show the binocular representations that are expected under nonselective convergence of inputs from two eyes. BINOCULAR (1) = when the spatial frequency of interocularly converging stripes is lower than grating acuity of the infant. BINOCULAR (2) = when the spatial frequency of interocularly converging stripes is beyond grating acuity of the infant. (B) Stimulus pair I. It was similar to stimulus pair F except that interocularly same-phased stripes, instead of a blank field, were used on the other screen (right, in this example). (C) Theoretical predictions of preference during the prestereoptic period. Percent preference expected for the counter-phased stripes in the stimulus pair H (□) and pair I (■) are plotted for right eye, binocular, and left eye viewing conditions, respectively. (D) Individual data. Data obtained from four infants were plotted individually in the same way as the previous prediction graph. Grating acuity of each infant that had been measured independently is indicated at the top of each graph. (From Shimojo, 1985. By permission.) *Figure continued*

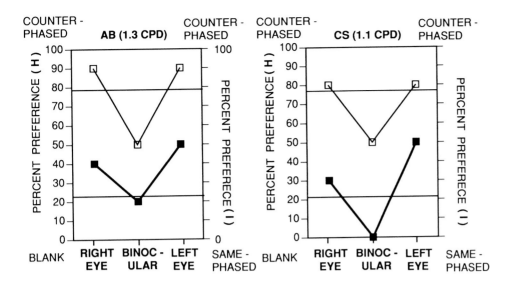

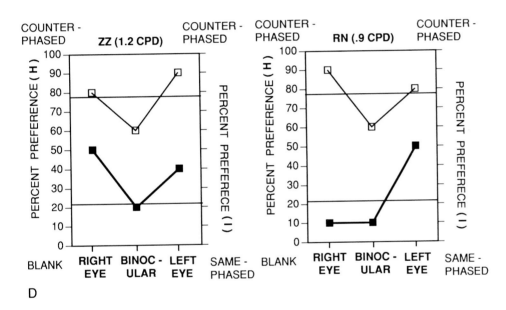

D

FIG. 12-6. *(continued)*

ponent colors during the presterooptic period, whereas they shifted their preference to the interocularly opponent colors during the stereoptic period (Fig. 12-7B).

A control experiment showed that no preference for one color (red) or the other (green) was found during either period when both screens contain interocularly identical colors. Thus the preferential responses observed during both periods cannot be attributed to a simple preference for monocular color per se. In another control experiment, a color was given on one screen in interocularly identical fashion, whereas the other screen was kept white; a consistent preference for the color side was found during both presterooptic and stereoptic periods. This result suggests that color mixture of red

and green may have in fact occurred and been the cause for the preference during the presterooptic period.

Thus overall the data are consistent with the hypothesis of nonselective convergence during the prestereoptic period.

Underlying Neuronal Mechanisms

As thus far described, the data suggest that the neonatal visual system seems to be nonselective to the eye of origin and selective to spatial location for various aspects of visual information, such as orientation of edges, number of items, contrast, spatial frequency, and color. What can be the underlying neuronal mechanisms? What

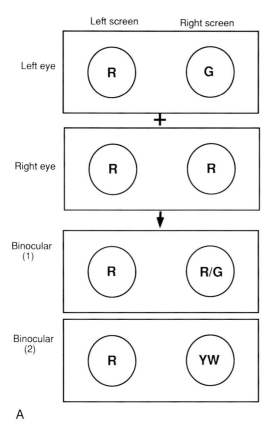

A

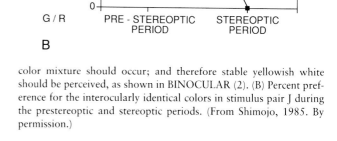

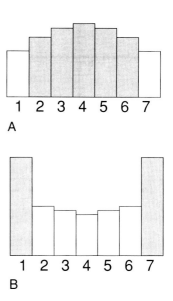

B

FIG. 12-7. Stimuli and results of the "color" experiment. (A) Stimulus pair J. When there is interocular suppression, altering mutual suppression between red and green should occur (on the right screen, in this example), as shown in BINOCULAR (1). When color channels in two eyes are nonselectively pooled without interocular suppression, color mixture should occur; and therefore stable yellowish white should be perceived, as shown in BINOCULAR (2). (B) Percent preference for the interocularly identical colors in stimulus pair J during the prestereoptic and stereoptic periods. (From Shimojo, 1985. By permission.)

is the critical difference between the prestereoptic visual system and the stereoptic visual system that determines the onset age of stereopsis and fusion/rivalry functions?

Figure 12-8 shows hypothetical ocular dominance distributions of neurons in layer IV in neonatal (prestereoptic) and adult (stereoptic) visual systems. We propose that most neurons are nonselectively binocular during the prestereoptic period, whereas most are monocular or selective during the stereoptic period. Even though there is no electrophysiological or anatomical evidence directly supporting these assumptions in the human, there has been some indirect evidence reported in the kitten (LeVay et al., 1978) and the newborn monkey (Rakic, 1976; Hubel et al., 1977; LeVay et al., 1980). If most units are in fact nonselectively binocular in the neonatal system, it would be reasonable to assume that these binocular units play a major role in visual processing by the neonate. In the mature system, on the other hand, monocular units play a major role. Figure 12-9 (Held, 1985) shows hypothetical neuronal pathways in layer IV of the neonatal and mature systems. In the neonatal system (Fig. 12-9A) most neurons re-

FIG. 12-8. Hypothetical ocular dominance histograms during the prestereoptic (A) and stereoptic (B) periods. As indicated by shading, "binocular" neurons are originally dominant during the prestereoptic period, and monocular neurons become dominant later during the stereoptic period. (From Shimojo, 1985. By permission.)

NEONATE

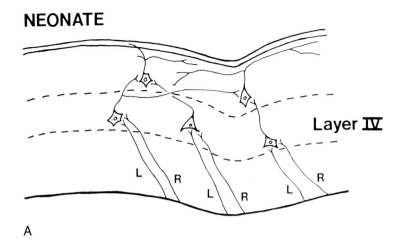

Layer IV

A

MATURE

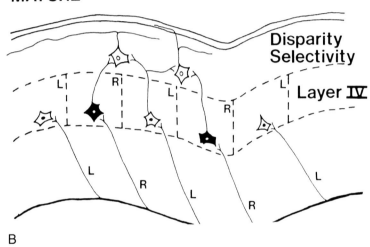

Disparity
Selectivity

Layer IV

B

FIG. 12-9. Hypothetical physiological structures of the prestereoptic (A) and stereoptic (B) visual systems. (A) Geniculostriate afferents from both eyes synapse on the same neurons in layer IV, thereby losing information about the eye of origin. (B) Geniculostriate afferents are segregated on the basis of eye of origin, and consequently recipient neurons in layer IV may send their axons to neurons outside that layer to synapse on neurons that may be disparity selective. (From Held, 1985; Shimojo, 1985. By permission.)

ceive inputs from two eyes and are usually balanced between eyes. As a consequence, visual inputs from the eye should be pooled and processed nonselectively. As soon as the structural segregation of eyes is established (Fig. 12-9B), most of the neurons receive input only from one eye; and therefore monocular representations of visual inputs with the *labeling of eye* (which eye the input comes from) are available at a higher level for binocular functions, such as disparity detection. In fact, existence of disparity-tuned detectors in area 17 and 18 has been established in the kitten (Pettigrew, 1974), the adult cat (Barlow et al., 1967) and the monkey (Poggio and Fischer, 1977; Poggio and Talbot, 1981).

Physiology researchers have pointed out, however, that some of monocular neurons (categories 1 or 7 in the ocular dominance histogram) are in fact binocular and disparity-tuned in the sense that one eye input is excitatory and the other inhibitory (Gardner and Raiten, 1986; Freeman and Ohzawa, 1990). Based on these data, some have pointed to the possibilities that: (1) ocular dominance segregation is established by maturation of inhibitory networks and thus by variations of excitatory/inhibitory balance between the eyes at each neuron level; and (2) it is these "monocular" neurons that play a critical role in disparity detection. This viewpoint is not inconsistent with ours because even in this account the labeling of eye should be established for stereopsis, and it explains how the system can change from an eye-non-selective to an eye-selective one.

In short, we hypothesize that a transition from an ocularly nonselective to an ocularly selective system occurs as a consequence of, or at least contingently with, columnar segregation of ocular dominance. The advantages of this hypothesis are as follows.

1. It explains why predictions of the hypothesis of "nonselective convergence" are supported in a variety of visual properties such as edge orientation, number of items, contrast, spatial frequency, and color.

2. It explains why a preferential shift occurs in some of our experiments (the "grids" and the color experiment), that is, why the same infant shows opposite preferences before and after a certain age.

3. There are some other lines of evidence, such as "binocular beat" (Baitch and Srebo, 1990) and lack of probability summation (see Chapter 13), that indicate the nonselective nature of prestereoptic binocular interaction (see Chapter 15).

4. It explains why coarse stereopsis and fusion/rivalry functions have roughly the same ages of onset.

5. It explains why the onset of stereopsis is highly correlated with the age of substantial completion of ocular dominance segregation in various species.

The last point may require explanation. A survey of the literature (Held, 1985) suggests that stereopsis is found behaviorally at about the age when substantial ocular dominance segregation is achieved. It is so in the kitten (LeVay et al., 1978; Timney, 1981), in the monkey (LeVay et al., 1980; O'Dell et al., 1991), and probably in the human (Held, 1985). It may not be self-evident why it should be so because ocular dominance segregation simply means structural grouping of two kinds of monocularly driven neurons. We hypothesize that the synaptic changes responsible for ocular dominance segregation are also responsible for increasing the population of monocular (eye-selective) neurons, and that the mechanism of disparity detection is based on these eye-labeled units. This interpretation seems to be consistent with current knowledge about ocular dominance segregation, as mentioned above. There is yet another line of evidence in favor of this notion. Evidence has been found for amblyopia caused by esotropia at and after an average age of 4 months, but not in subjects younger than that (Mohindra et al., 1979; Jacobson et al., 1981, 1982; also see Chapter 13). The coincidence of onset ages among stereopsis, fusion/rivalry functions, and strabismic amblyopia may be explained by the attainment of ocular dominance segregation and the eye-specific representations of visual input at that age. [It may also be related to the reason why the presence or absence of stereopsis at 3–5 months of age is

directly related to the magnitude of interocular acuity differences (Birch, 1985)].

We admit that this interpretation of the findings is not the only one. Another obvious alternative is to assume that most units in layer IV are ocular-selective even during the prestereoptic period, and that nonselective convergence occurs only at higher levels. This interpretation is possible but not plausible, considering the above-mentioned physiological and anatomical findings about ocular dominance segregation. For higher-level convergence to occur, there should be monocular representations found at a higher level than layer IV. At any rate, the point is that regardless of the validity of anatomical specification of the locus, the only simple and consistent interpretation of the data so far is the nonselective convergence of the inputs from corresponding retinal loci.

As for the issue of how the visual system can change from ocular nonselectivity to selectivity, there are several possibilities: (1) rewiring of the neuronal connections, as suggested by LeVay et al. (1978) and Shatz and Kirkwood (1984); (2) activation and degeneration of synaptic connections (the possibility that the stereoptic pathways and units do exist even during the prestereoptic period, and that they simply have to be activated to overcome the prestereoptic subsystem); and (3) development of inhibitory networks, as suggested by Gardner and colleagues (1985); Gardner and Raiten, 1986). The question as to which of these hypotheses is correct may be answered only by anatomical and electrophysiological studies. It should be enough here to say that any of these possibilities would be consistent with the hypothesis of nonselective convergence.

INTEROCULAR VISION AND OCCLUSION CONSTRAINTS

After the hypothetical completion of the eye-selective cortical representations, highly intelligent binocular computations become possible at higher levels. In fact, it is only recently that psychophysical researchers started realizing how cleverly the mature binocular system utilizes the eye-of-origin information to accomplish various visual tasks. Before we consider the issues concerning acquisition of binocularity, it would be helpful to take a look at these findings.

"Slit-Motion" Effects

Imagine a situation where an observer is binocularly viewing a vertical bar moving laterally behind a vertically elongated slit (Fig. 12-10) (Shimojo et al., 1988). As illustrated in the figure, there is a time lag between the stimuli to the two eyes, and the amount of lag is

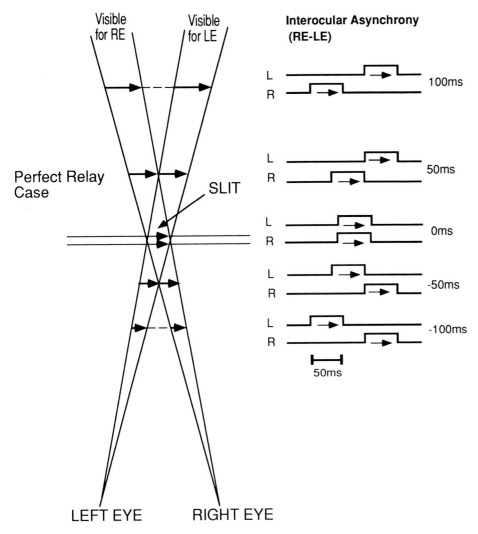

FIG. 12-10. Relation between real-world situations of slit view (left) and our simulated motions (right), where an identical target motion is presented within a slit for various degrees of interocular asynchrony (IOA). Note that positive IOAs (right eye followed by left eye when the motion is rightward), including those with no temporal overlap (IOAs greater than the perfect relay case as shown at the top), are compatible with the constraints imposed by occlusion. In contrast, negative IOAs (left eye followed by right eye) are *not* compatible with real-world situations because targets moving in front of the occluder should always be seen binocularly. RE = right eye; LE = left eye. (From Shimojo et al., 1988. By permission.)

positively correlated with the depth from the slit (occluding surface) to the target. At one particular depth, the offset of the stimulus to one eye coincides with the onset of the stimulus to the other eye (the "perfect relay case") (Fig. 12-11A). The direction of motion of the bar constrains the sequential order of the monocular stimuli to the eyes: Rightward motion is visible to the right eye first and then to the left eye. On the other hand, leftward motion is visible to the left eye first and then to the right eye. They are the only possible real-world combinations if the bar is single and moving laterally behind the slit. Seemingly possible combina-

tions such as "leftward motion—left eye first" are impossible in reality (because if the moving bar is in front of the surface it should be visible from both eyes at the same time; see P2 in Figure 12-11B). Note that these constraints that govern the way distal stimuli determine retinal stimuli are purely optical. This regularity in *ecological optics*, however, instantly raises an intriguing possibility for *inverse ecological optics* because information about a single object at certain depth could be correctly recovered from two asynchronized motion inputs to the eyes, the visual system knowing these optical constraints either explicitly or implicitly. Thus, theo-

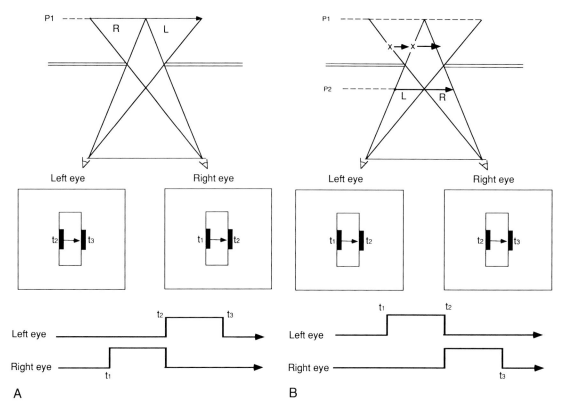

FIG. 12-11. Vertical bar moving behind a vertical slit. The physical structure seen from above (top of figure), the simulated stimulus presented to each eye (middle), and the temporal relation of monocular stimuli (bottom) are shown. (A) Perfect relay case where the target appears in the left eye just as the target in the right eye disappears from view. (B) Case of reversed ocular order. Smooth motion of a single target at a depth behind the slit was observed in the perfect relay case, whereas two targets moving side by side right behind the slit were observed in the reversed case. In our experiment, these two kinds of stimulus were presented in the top and the bottom halves of the slit. The center-to-center separation between the two stimuli was 1.7 degrees, the size of the bar target was 32×32 minutes, and the slit width was 20 minutes at the observation distance of 80 cm. (From Shimojo et al., 1988. By permission.)

retically, depth can be recovered without simultaneous spatial disparity, given direction of motion, the interocular order, and asynchrony.

To see if the human visual system actually uses these real-world constraints to determine depth, we simulated the "perfect relay case" on a cathode-ray tube stereo display. Note that, apart from the interocular asynchrony (IOA), each eye receives exactly the same motion trajectory on corresponding retinal points (Shimojo et al., 1988). Our observations revealed that a seamless motion of a single target is in fact perceived as lying at a depth behind the slit (P1 in Fig. 12-11A). The visual system thus interprets the stimuli that are given sequentially to the two eyes as resulting from one object under smooth motion, rather than from two objects at arbitrary depths. Reversing the sequence of stimuli to the eyes without changing the direction of motion, however, causes a completely different perception (Fig. 12-11B). Instead of a single target, the observer sees two bars moving side by side that appear just behind the

slit ($X \rightarrow X \rightarrow$ at the top of Fig. 12-11B). This perceptual interpretation is perfectly reasonable, considering the fact that the reversed stimulus display violates the above-mentioned "slit motion" constraints.

These observations were confirmed in naive subjects. Moreover, by manipulating the interocular asynchrony and asking the subject to judge the depth, we found that perceived depth kept increasing as a function of IOA even beyond the "perfect relay" limit (for IOAs up to 100 ms). In other words, even when there was a time gap between the inputs to the two eyes, perceived depth could be larger than the "perfect relay case," as inverse ecological optics would indicate (Fig. 12-10). (For more detailed description of the method and the results, see Shimojo et al., 1988.) These findings are significantly different from the stereoscopic depth effect that accompanies the interocular delay of a stroboscopically shifting target without temporal overlap of the stimuli to the two eyes (Lee, 1970; Morgan, 1975; Burr and Ross, 1979). The reasons are because there is major asymmetry between the valid and the invalid cases, and because depth keeps growing when IOA becomes larger beyond the perfect relay timing. Needless to say, the ocular order information, which is based on the eye-of-origin of moving stimuli, is indispensable for this kind of perceptual problem solving. The findings suggest that the occlusion-related optogeometric rules are in fact implemented at early cortical levels of visual information processing where the eye-of-origin information is available. In this regard, the stereoscopic depth mechanism presumably based on the interocular asynchrony in the visual cortex (Gardner et al., 1985) may be relevant.

Occlusion Constraints and "DaVinci Stereopsis"

For another example of how the visual system utilizes the eye-of-origin information, see Figure 12-12. When a surface partly occludes another surface and there are discontinuity edges between them, there are always parts of back surfaces that are interocularly unpaired or visible only from one eye, as indicated by shadows in Figure 12-12A. To be more specific, a region next to the left occluding edge is seen only from the left eye, whereas a region next to the right occluding edge is seen only from the right eye. Other combinations, such as "left region seen from right eye" or "right region seen from left eye," are totally impossible ecologically (Fig. 12-12B).

These constraints, which are stationary counterparts of the "slit motion" constraints, would provide a surprising amount of information to the visual system if they were implemented. Theoretically, the following two directions of inference would be possible about the three-dimensional layout of surfaces and objects.

1. If an unpaired target is presented next to an interocularly paired surface, it should be in back of this fusible surface. However, it is true only if the spatial relation between the unpaired and the fusible surface is valid in terms of the above-mentioned occlusion constraints (Fig. 12-12).

2. If a stimulus is unpaired and shown to only one eye (e.g., the left eye) it would be a strong indicator that there should be an occluding surface and edge right next to the unpaired stimuli (right side of the unpaired stimuli in this case).

Nakayama and Shimojo (1990) psychophysically demonstrated that the human visual system behaves as though it implements these two kinds of inference in a bottom-up fashion. First, see Figure 12-13A, where occlusion geometry defines a specific constraint zone (the shadowed region in the figure), in which only the monocularly viewed object can exist. Note that the leading edge of the zone recedes as a function of the target's

distance to the edge of surface. Interestingly, the perceived depth of the unpaired stimulus actually behaved that way in a disparity matching experiment (Fig. 12-13B,C), up to 30 arc minutes distance from the edge at least (filled circles, Fig. 12-13D). It is so, however, only when the relation between the eye of the unpaired stimulus and the occluding edge was ecologically valid (Figure 12-13B). When it was invalid, the depth function was flat near zero (open circles, Fig. 12-13D). These findings correspond to the above-mentioned inference 1. Second, just by presenting several fusible dots and a few unpaired dots, an observer could experience an illusory occluding surface and edge. An example of the effects is illustrated in Figure 12-14. Illusory occluding edges are perceived with "knife cut" sharpness: one to the right of left-eye-only dots, and the other to the left of right-eye-only dots. More important to note here is that this fragmentary figure of a triangle is seen as an occluding surface that is clearly in front of the surrounding field of dots, even though there is no crossed disparity explicitly available anywhere. This formation of illusory occluding edges and surface by unpaired dots corresponds to the above-mentioned inference 2. (For more detailed descriptions of the method and the results see Nakayama and Shimojo, 1990.)

These findings, together with the "slit motion" effects suggest that the eye-of-origin information is utilized for depth and other aspects of visual perception.

Escape from Rivalry

Perhaps more relevant to the implications from the infant studies is the "escape from rivalry" effect, first reported by Shimojo and Nakayama (1990). Examine Figure 12-12A,B once again as it raises another intriguing question about binocularity, though it is about rivalry this time. According to classical textbooks and reviews, stereopsis and rivalry mechanisms are relatively independent of each other (e.g., Kaufman, 1974; Wolfe, 1983, 1986); and whenever there is a region on one retina where the visual stimulus is not similar to the counterpart at a corresponding locus on the other retina, this region undergoes vigorous suppression. It would, however, have a peculiar consequence in our daily visual experience. As well illustrated in Figure 12-12, whenever a surface partly occludes another surface with discontinuity edges between them, there should always be parts of the back surfaces that are interocularly unpaired regions. Does this fact, then, imply that we should find all regions surrounding boundary contours of objects rivalrous or suppressed? Our daily experience obviously indicates otherwise. Perhaps the textbooks and reviews were overly simplistic. Would it not be the case that the conclusion of independence has been made because most psychophysical experiments

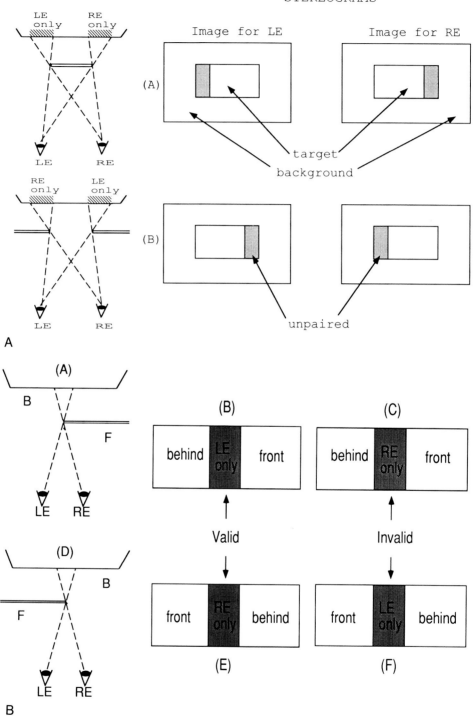

FIG. 12-12. Occlusion constraints and monocularly viewed (interocularly unpaired) zones. (A) Top views of surface occlusion (at left) with corresponding random-dot stereograms (at right). Monocularly viewed (interocularly unpaired) zones are indicated by shading. LE = left eye; RE = right eye. A. Case of occluding surface in the middle. B. Case of a "hole" in the middle. (B) Analysis of occlusion constraints. A. Top view of the case where a front surface is on the right side. B. Valid eye-of-origin of unpaired stimulus between the two surfaces in the case illustrated in A. C. Invalid eye-of-origin in case A. D. Top view of the case where a front surface is on the left side. E. Valid eye-of-origin in case D. F. Invalid eye-of-origin in case D. (From Shimojo and Nakayama, 1990; and Nakayama and Shimojo, 1990. By permission.)

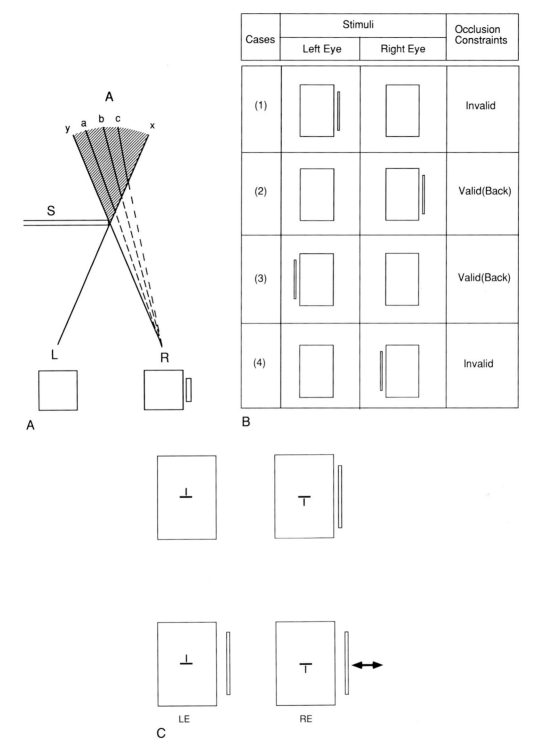

FIG. 12-13. Depth perception by interocularly unpaired stimulus. (A) Occlusion geometry. At the bottom are binocular images for right-eye-only stimulus in relation to fused binocular square. At the top is a top view of occlusion configuration with visibility lines for each eye (Lx and Ry), which delineate the regions of visibility of each eye occasioned by the presence of the binocularly viewed occluder (S). Depth ambiguity line segments for the right eye (a,b,c) define a depth constraint zone (shaded region). (B) Occlusion constraint table, showing valid and invalid combinations of unpaired monocular line-segments in relation to fused image regions. (C) Example of the stimulus used in the depth matching experiment. The observer sees one of the vertical bars binocularly (at the bottom) and sets its disparity to match the perceived depth of the unpaired bar at the top. (D) Disparity matching results. Matched disparity to unpaired points is plotted as a function of horizontal distance from the left or the right edges of the binocularly fused occluder. The leading edge of depth constraint zone illustrated as Lx in (A) is shown as dotted oblique lines. Open circles represent valid monocular stimulus, and solid circles represent invalid monocular stimulus. (From Nakayama and Shimojo 1990. By permission.) *Figure continued*

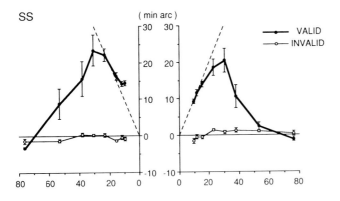

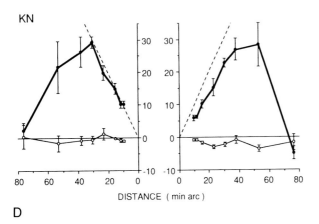

D

FIG. 12-13. *(continued)*

had been conducted with unpaired stimuli being ecologically invalid? Would it not be that the unpaired region escapes from rivalry when it is ecologically valid in relation to neighboring disparity defined surfaces? If so, it would make more sense biologically because these unpaired regions carry real information about the back surface, whereas invalid unpaired regions may be just noise.

Shimojo and Nakayama (1990) tested these possibilities. Figure 12-15A illustrates an example of the

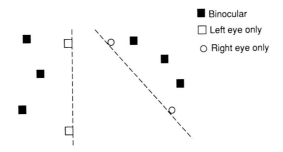

FIG. 12-14. Illusory occluding surface and edges. Dashed lines denote the location of the subjective edges, which partially delineate the triangular surface. (From Nakayama and Shimojo, 1990. By permission.)

stimuli. Region Al in the figure is a valid unpaired region that is naturally caused by disparity of the front surface, whereas Cl is an invalid unpaired region that is created artificially by replacing the original random-dot texture within this region and another totally uncorrelated dot texture. A vertical disparity case (Fig. 12-15B) was added as a control. The subject was asked to decide which had been suppressed more frequently after comparing these two regions in a stereogram. Figure 12-15C shows the results: The "competitive" regions, or the invalid

(A) Horizontal Disparity

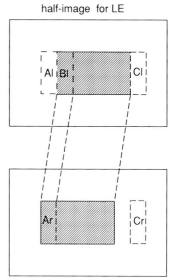

(B) Vertical Disparity

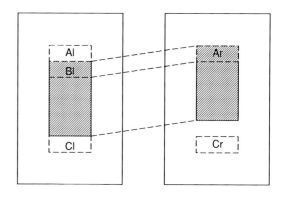

FIG. 12-15. Escape from rivalry in valid unpaired zone. Stimulus stereograms used in the experiment. Retinally corresponding regions are denoted by A, B, and C. Eye is specified by l and r. Dotted lines indicate correspondence with a disparity. (A) Horizontal disparity condition. (B) Vertical disparity condition. (C) Results. Mean rates of suppression for the "competitive" side (or ecologically invalid side in the case of horizontal disparity) are shown for the crossed, uncrossed, and vertical disparity conditions. (From Shimojo and Nakayama, 1990. By permission.) *Figure continued*

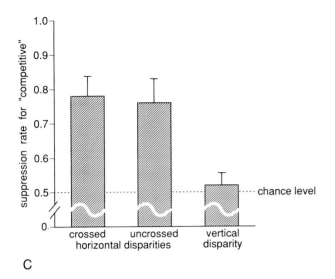

C

FIG. 12-15. *(continued)*

regions in the horizontal cases, were judged to be clearly more rivalrous. The chance-level result in the control condition with vertical disparity suggests that the escape-from-rivalry effect is outcome of depth process, not just of fusion process.

The results suggest that the occlusion-related constraints, as illustrated in Figure 12-12, are internalized by the visual system. Even though this statement solely concerns the human's visual system and potentially that of animals, it has a critical implication for computational vision as well because possible implementation of these constraints would enable artificial systems to do a faster global search not only for the best match between the eyes but also for the best candidates for discontinuity edges.

I have discussed three sets of psychophysical findings on binocularity in normal adults. Implications could be summarized in the following three points.

1. There are specific rules in ecological optics that are closely related to surface occlusion.
2. These rules are based on the explicit eye-of-origin information.
3. There is converging evidence for efficient implementation of these constraints in the human visual system.

CONCERNING ACQUISITION OF INTEROCULAR VISUAL FUNCTIONS

Broader Concept of Stereopsis

Traditionally, stereopsis has been regarded as depth perception based on disparities between the images appearing *simultaneously* on the retinas; that is, simul-taneous spatial disparity has been considered the primitive for stereopsis. The "slit motion" finding, together with DaVinci stereopsis and the "escape from rivalry" findings, makes this "simultaneous disparity" view of stereopsis dubious. This view assumes interocularly paired inputs as the only useful cues for depth perception, whereas the above-mentioned stereo effects are based on unpaired cues. Thus interocularly unpaired stimuli seem to be far more important than just "noise" in various aspects of binocular perception. For the visual system to utilize both the unpaired stimuli and the paired stimuli, eye-of-origin information is indispensable. In fact, without this information, it would be impossible to discriminate a valid unpaired stimulus from an invalid stimulus, the kind of discrimination necessary for any of the above-mentioned effects to occur. Neither would it be possible to discriminate a crossed disparity from the same amount of uncrossed disparity because the only difference between these two disparities is the sign of disparity, which is determined by the eye-of-origin labeling. Meanwhile, the infant studies suggest that completion of monocular representation or the eye-of-origin labeling be the basis of the onset of binocular functions, such as stereopsis and fusion/rivalry discrimination.

Based on all these facts and speculations, let us consider a new concept of stereopsis that neither requires simultaneous stimulation of the two eyes nor limits its input to interocularly pairable stimuli. This broader concept of *binocularity* may be defined as depth perception and any other visual functions that are based on the eye-of-origin labeling in the visual pathways. It is certainly broader as a concept because it includes both the classical stereopsis based on interocularly paired stimuli (let us call this "Wheatstone stereopsis") and DaVinci stereopsis based on interocularly unpaired stimuli. Moreover, the list of included visual functions extends to fusion/rivalry discrimination, depth perception of interocularly unpaired target either moving ("slit-motion") or stationary (DaVinci stereopsis), formation of illusory occluding edges and surfaces (DaVinci stereopsis), and escape from rivalry.

In summary, then, the eye-of-origin labeling, rather than spatial disparity per se, should be considered as the primary requirement for binocularity because:

1. It seems to be the common basis for onset of both stereopsis and fusion/rivalry discrimination earlier in infants.
2. It is represented at earlier cortical levels than are disparities in the visual pathway.
3. It explains a broader range of visual perception, particularly when there are limited paired stimuli and yet the visual system offers an interpretation that is highly adaptive to the external world.

Adaptiveness and Learnability of Binocular Processes

An intriguing question concerns acquisition of the occlusion constraints in relation to the onset age of stereopsis. Let us take the example of valid unpaired regions escaping from rivalry. When and how does the infant acquire this visual capability of utilizing these constraints? Would a considerable learning period be required after the onset of stereopsis in individual infants? Or would these constraints be acquired side by side with stereopsis? The latter seems more likely considering the vigorous reorganization of neural connections during the critical period (Huttenlocher et al., 1982), though the former would be possible, too. This purely empirical question could possibly be answered by an infant experiment utilizing the infant's tendency to avoid a rivalrous stimulus and to prefer a fusible stimulus. For example, a stimulus pair such as is illustrated in Figure 12-15A may be presented to the infant subject; and its preference between the valid unpaired region (Al in the figure) and the invalid unpaired region (Cl) may be judged by an observer. Because the valid region would escape from rivalry in the visual system that has already implemented the occlusion constraints, a significant preference for this side over the invalid side would be expected. Thus comparing the onset age of a significant preference in this experiment with the onset age of stereopsis for each infant would clearly answer the question.

In a more general theoretical framework, the findings related to the eye-of-origin labeling and the ecological analysis of occlusion constraints suggest a possibility that these apparently intelligent interocular functions are learned by experience during the time course of binocular development. To illustrate this point, reconsider the ecologically valid cases of "slit-motion" (Fig. 12-11A), DaVinci stereopsis (Fig. 12-13A), and "escape from rivalry" (Fig. 12-15A). These cases are the combinations of relevant visual information, such as direction of motion, eye of origin/ocular order, and disparity of neighbors, which are encountered by the visual system regularly in daily life. On the other hand, the ecologically invalid combinations are rarely encountered, except in highly abnormal situations. The point here is two-fold; First, binocular visual sampling is systematic and constrained enough so there are numerous opportunities for the visual system to internalize these external rules of optics by simple, contingency-based learning rules such as the Hebbian rule. Second, starting from the neural labeling of eye-of-origin and applying this kind of learning rule, we could possibly understand the suspiciously coincidental onset of various binocular functions on one hand and the highly adaptive behavior of the adult interocular (not just binocular) visual system on the other. In this regard, neurophysiological and computational studies that emphasize the importance of synchrony or contingency of neuronal activities for development and plasticity of cortical visual processes are encouraging (Stent, 1973; Miller et al., 1989), although we may still have to understand the effects of visual experience and of spontaneous neuronal activities differently in the same Hebbian-type framework (Chapman et al., 1986; Jacobson et al., 1986; Linsker 1986a,b; Reiter et al., 1986; Stryker and Harris, 1986; for reviews see Brown et al., 1990; Constantine-Paton et al., 1990; Linsker, 1990).

Acknowledgments. This chapter is based on the author's collaboration with Richard Held, Eileen E. Birch, Joseph Bauer Jr., Kathleen M. O'Connel, Ken Nakayama, and Gerald H. Silverman. They also gave helpful comments on an early draft. I thank these colleagues. I also thank Yasuto Tanaka and Michiteru Kitazaki for preparation of the figures.

REFERENCES

Atkinson, J., and Braddick, O. (1976). Stereoscopic discrimination in infants. *Perception* 5, 29–38.

Atkinson, J., Smith, J., Anker, S., Wattam-Bell, J., Braddick, O., and Moore, T. (1991). Binocularity and amblyopia before and after early strabismus surgery. *Invest. Ophthalmol. Vis. Sci.* 32, 820.

Baitch, L., and Srebro, R. (1990). Binocular interactions in sleeping and awake human infants. *Invest. Ophthalmol. Vis. Sci.* 31, 251.

Barlow, H. B., Blakemore, C., and Pettigrew, J. D. (1967). The neural mechanisms of binocular depth discrimination. *J. Physiol. (Lond.)* 193, 327–342.

Birch, E. E. (1985). Infant interocular acuity differences and binocular vision. *Vision Res.* 25, 571–576.

Birch, E. E., Gwiazda, J., and Held, R. (1982). Stereoacuity development for crossed and uncrossed disparities in human infants. *Vision Res.* 22, 507–513.

Birch, E. E., Shimojo, S., and Held, R. (1985). Preferential-looking assessment of fusion and stereopsis in infants aged 1–6 months. *Invest. Ophthalmol. Vis. Sci.* 26, 366–370.

Braddick, O., Atkinson, J., Julesz, B., Kropfl, W., Bodis-Woller, I., and Roab, E. (1980). Cortical binocularity in infants. *Nature* 288, 363–365.

Brown, T. H., Kairiss, E. W., and Keenan, C. L. (1990). Hebbian synapses: biophysical mechanisms and algorithms. *Annu. Rev. Neurosci.* 13, 475–511.

Burr, D. C., and Ross, J. (1979). How does binocular delay give information about depth? *Vision Res.* 19, 523–532.

Chapman, B., Jacobson, M. D., Reiter, H. O., and Stryker, M. P. (1986). Ocular dominance shift in kitten visual-cortex caused by imbalance in retinal electrical-activity. *Nature* 324, 154–156.

Constantine-Paton, M., Cline, H. T., and Debski, E. (1990). Patterned activity, synaptic convergence, and the NMDA receptor in developing visual pathways. *Annu. Rev. Neurosci.* 13, 129–154.

DeWeert, Ch. M. M., and Levelt, W. J. M. (1976). Comparison of normal and dichoptic colour mixing. *Vision Res.* 16, 59–70.

Fantz, R. L. (1963). The origin of form perception. *Sci. Am.* 204, 66–72.

Fantz, R. L., Ordy, J. M., and Udelf, M. S. (1962). Maturation of pattern vision in infants during the first six months. *J. Comp. Physiol. Psychol.* 55, 907–917.

Fox, R., Aslin, R. N., Shea, S. L., and Dumais, S. T. (1980). Stereopsis in human infants. *Science* 207, 323–324.

FREEMAN, R. D., AND OHZAWA, I. (1990). On the neurophysiological organization of binocular vision. *Vision Res.* 30, 1661–1676.

GARDNER, J. C., AND RAITEN, E. J. (1986). Ocular dominance and disparity-sensitivity—why there are cells in the visual cortex driven unequally by the 2 eyes. *Exp. Brain Res.* 64, 505–514.

GARDNER, J. C., DOUGLAS, R. M., AND CYNADER, M. S. (1985). A time-based stereoscopic depth mechanism in the visual cortex. *Brain Res.* 328, 154–157.

HELD, R. (1985). Binocular vision—behavioral and neural development. In V. MEHLER AND R. FOX (eds.). *Neonate Cognition: Beyond the Blooming, Buzzing Confusion.* Hillsdale, NJ: Erlbaum, pp. 37–44.

HELD, R., BIRCH, E. E., AND GWIAZDA, J. (1980). Stereoacuity of human infants. *Proc. Natl. Acad. Sci. USA* 77, 5572–5574.

HUBEL, D. H., WIESEL, T. N., AND LEVAY, S. (1977). Plasticity of ocular dominance columns in monkey striate cortex. *Philos. Trans. R. Soc. Lond.* [Biol.] 278, 377–409.

HUTTENLOCHER, P. R., DECOURTEN, C., GAREY, L. G., AND VAN DER LOOS, H. (1982). Synaptogenesis in human visual cortex—evidence for synaptic elimination during normal development. *Neurosci. Lett.* 33, 247–252.

JACOBSON, S. G., MOHINDRA, I., AND HELD, R. (1981). Age of onset of amblyopia in infants with esotropia. *Doc. Ophthalmol.* 30, 210–216.

JACOBSON, S. G., MOHINDRA, I., AND HELD, R. (1982). Visual acuity of infants with ocular diseases. *Am. J. Ophthalmol.* 93, 198–209.

JACOBSON, M. D., REITER, H. O., AND STRYKER, M. P. (1986). Ocular dominance shift in kitten visual-cortex caused by imbalance in retinal electrical-activity. *Nature* 324, 154–156.

KARMEL, B. Z. (1969a). Complexity, amount of contour, and visually dependent behavior in hooded rats, domestic chicks, and human infants. *J. Comp. Physiol. Psychol.* 69, 649–657.

KARMEL, B. Z. (1969b). The effect of age, complexity, and amount of contour on pattern preferences in human infants. *J. Exp. Child Psychol.* 7, 339–354.

KAUFMAN, L. (1974). *Sight and Mind—An Introduction to Perception.* New York: Oxford University Press.

LEE, D. N. (1970). Spatio-temporal integration in binocular-kinetic space perception. *Vision Res.* 10, 65–78.

LEVAY, S., STRYKER, M. P., AND SHATZ, C. J. (1978). Ocular dominance columns and their development in layer IV of the cat's visual cortex: a quantitative study. *J. Comp. Neurol.* 179, 223–244.

LEVAY, S., WIESEL, T. N., AND HUBEL, D. H. (1980). The development of ocular dominance columns in normal and visually deprived monkeys. *J. Comp. Neurol.* 191, 1–51.

LINSKER, R. (1986a). From basic network principles to neural architecture: emergence of spatial-opponent cells. *Proc. Natl. Acad. Sci. USA* 83, 7508–7512.

LINSKER, R. (1986b). From basic network principles to neural architecture: emergence of spatial-opponent cells. *Proc. Natl. Acad. Sci. USA* 83, 8390–8394.

LINSKER, R. (1990). Perceptual neural organization: some approaches based on network models and information theory. *Annu. Rev. Neurosci.* 13, 257–281.

MILLER, K. D., KELLER, J. B., AND STRYKER, M. P. (1989). Ocular dominance column development: analysis and simulation. *Science* 245, 605–615.

MOHINDRA, I., JACOBSON, S. G., THOMAS, J., AND HELD, R. (1979). Development of amblyopia in infants. *Trans. Ophthalmol. Soc. UK* 99, 344–346.

MORGAN, M. J. (1975). Mechanisms of interpolation in human spatial vision. *Nature* 256, 639–640.

NAKAYAMA, K., AND SHIMOJO, S. (1990). DaVinci stereopsis: depth and subjective occluding contours from unpaired image points. *Vision Res.* 30, 1811–1825.

O'DELL, C. D., QUICK, M. W., AND BOOTHE, R. G. (1991). The development of stereoacuity in infant rhesus monkeys. *Invest. Ophthalmol. Vis. Sci.* 32, 1044.

PEEPLES, D., AND TELLER, D. Y. (1975). Color vision and brightness discrimination in two-months-old infants. *Science* 189, 1102–1103.

PETRIG, B., JULESZ, B., KROPFL, W., BAUMGARTNER, G., AND ANLIKER, M. (1981). Development of stereopsis and cortical binocularity in human infants: electro-physiological evidence. *Science* 213, 1402–1404.

PETTIGREW, J. D. (1974). The effect of visual experience on the development of stimulus specificity by kitten cortical neurons. *J. Physiol.* 237, 49–74.

POGGIO, G. F., AND FISCHER, B. (1977). Binocular interaction and depth sensitivity of striate and prestriate cortical neurons of the behaving rhesus monkey. *J. Neurophysiol.* 40, 1392–1405.

POGGIO, G. F., AND TALBOT, W. H. (1981). Mechanisms of static and dynamic stereopsis in foveal cortex of the rhesus monkey. *J. Physiol. (Lond.)* 315, 469–492.

RAKIC, P. (1976). Prenatal genesis of connections subserving ocular dominance in the rhesus monkey. *Nature* 261, 467–471.

REITER, H. O., WAITZMAN, D. M., AND STRYKER, M. P. (1986). Cortical activity blockade prevents ocular dominance plasticity in the kitten visual-cortex. *Exp. Brain Res.* 65, 182–188.

SHATZ, C. L., AND KIRKWOOD, P. A. (1984). Prenatal development of functional connections in the cat's retinogeniculate pathway. *J. Neurosci.* 4, 1378–1397.

SHIMOJO, S. (1985). Pre-stereoptic binocular vision in infants. PhD thesis, Department of Psychology, Massachusetts Institute of Technology.

SHIMOJO, S., AND NAKAYAMA, K. (1990). Real world occlusion constraints and binocular rivalry. *Vision Res.* 30, 69–80.

SHIMOJO, S., BAUER, J., O'CONNELL, K. M., AND HELD, R. (1986). Pre-stereoptic binocular vision in infants. *Vision Res.* 26, 501–510.

SHIMOJO, S., SILVERMAN, G. H., AND NAKAYAMA, K. (1988). An occlusion-related mechanism of depth perception based on motion and interocular sequence. *Nature* 333, 265–268.

STENT, G. S. (1973). A physiological mechanism for Hebb's postulate of learning. *Proc. Natl. Acad. Sci. USA* 70, 997–1001.

STRYKER, M. P., AND HARRIS, W. A. (1986). Binocular impulse blockade prevents the formation of ocular dominance columns in cat visual-cortex. *J. Neurosci.* 6, 2117–2133.

TELLER, D. Y., AND BORNSTEIN, M. H. (1982). Infant color vision and color perception. In S. SALAPATEK AND L. B. COHEN (eds.). *Handbook of Infant Perception.* Orlando, FL: Academic Press.

TIMNEY, B. N. (1981). The effect of early and late monocular deprivation on binocular depth perception in cats. *Dev. Brain Res.* 14, 1433–1439.

VOLKMANN, F. C., AND DOBSON, M. V. (1976). Infant responses of ocular fixation to moving visual stimuli. *J. Exp. Child Psychol.* 22, 86–99.

WOLFE, J. M. (1983). Influence of spatial frequency, luminance, and duration on binocular rivalry and abnormal fusion of briefly present, dichoptic stimuli. *Perception* 12, 447–456.

WOLFE, J. M. (1986). Stereopsis and binocular rivalry. *Psychol. Rev.* 93, 269–282.

13 | Stereopsis in infants and its developmental relation to visual acuity

EILEEN E. BIRCH

The capacity to extract information about a three-dimensional world from a pair of two-dimensional retinal images has been the subject of scientific study for centuries. In the modern era, the complex stimulus cues and computations that contribute to veridical depth perception have been elaborated. Appreciation of the complexity of this perceptual function has led to a new line of scientific inquiry: Is depth perception innate or learned? Early studies of infants' responses to depth used paradigms involving the visual cliff (Walk and Gibson, 1961; Campos et al., 1970; Scarr and Salapatek, 1970; Walters and Walk, 1974), impending collision (Bower et al., 1971), size and shape constancy (Bower, 1964, 1965, 1966a,b; Caron et al., 1978), and reaching (Cruickshank, 1941; Fantz, 1961, 1966; Bower, 1972). In general, these early studies of infants' locomotor, postural, and affective responses to depth were unable to assess the degree to which postnatal improvement in response to depth may be attributable to developmental changes in perception, response, or both. In addition, because the infants' responses to depth were the focus of much of this research, many of the early studies used naturalistic test situations that contained multiple cues to depth, both monocular and binocular.

More recently, studies on the development of stereoscopic depth perception have attempted to limit available stimulus cues to binocular disparity and to rigorously measure disparity detection or discrimination. The motivation for this shift in approach to the study of depth perception has been, in part, to forge a close link with the vast amounts of neurophysiological and neuroanatomical data on visual development that became available during the 1960s and 1970s. During the same time span, pediatric ophthalmology began to shift toward an emphasis on early diagnosis and treatment. This shift produced an urgent need for more quantitative methods for assessing infant vision. The focus of this chapter is on the information that has emerged since 1980, including procedures used to assess stereopsis in infants, normal development of stereopsis and stereoacuity, the relation between stereopsis and visual acuity in normal development, and current models of binoc-

ular neural development. In addition, preliminary clinical applications aimed toward improved screening, diagnosis, and research capabilities for infantile eye disorders are reviewed.

PARADIGMS FOR ASSESSMENT OF STEREOPSIS IN HUMAN INFANTS

Since 1980, two classes of stimuli have been used to study the onset age for stereopsis in the human infant: line stereograms and random dot stereograms. Line stereograms are based on the presentation of similar monocular contours to the two retinas, but some of the contours contain a relative disparity in position for the two eyes. Because each of the monocular images provides form information and because the relative disparity between the images can be computed on a point-by-point basis, line stereograms are said to test "local stereopsis." Line stereograms used in studies of infant stereopsis usually have been static slide-projected images (Held et al., 1980; Birch et al., 1982; Granrud, 1986). Line stereogram studies have relied on forced-choice preferential looking (FPL) responses for data acquisition. In the FPL paradigms, the infant is shown a pair of matched stereograms side by side. One stereogram contains binocular disparity, and one has zero binocular disparity. If the infant is able to discriminate the disparate from the nondisparate stereogram, the infant gazes at the disparate stereogram consistently over a number of trials. An observer, unaware of the randomly assigned position of the disparate stimulus, watches the infant and documents the gaze preference. If the infant prefers to gaze at the disparate stimulus over a sufficient number of trials to meet a criterion for statistical significance, the infant can be said to demonstrate stereopsis.

Random dot stereogram studies have included slide-projected stimuli (Atkinson and Braddick, 1976; Birch and Hale, 1989) and video stimuli (Fox et al. 1980; Shea et al., 1980; Petrig et al., 1981; Leguire et al., 1983; Archer et al., 1986). Random dot stereograms are composed ideally of two monocular images that provide no monocular form information; only when the images are viewed stereoscopically does a form emerge from the random arrays of dots. In theory, no monocular form information is available, and the form is detected only when a global structure emerges in the binocular view; this paradigm has been termed "global stereopsis." In fact, static random dot stereograms are rarely ideal, and it may be possible for the viewer to detect binocular disparity by comparing shifting contours in alternating monocular views. Video presentation allows for the use of dynamic random dot stereograms in which the two monocular dot patterns are changed continuously while the binocular disparity is held constant. Because each changing monocular pattern appears as "snow," monocular cues are virtually eliminated. Data acquisition for random dot stimuli has been varied, including FPL (Atkinson and Braddick, 1976; Birch and Hale, 1989), electrooculography (Leguire et al., 1983; Archer et al., 1986); and visual evoked responses (Petrig et al., 1981). FPL methods with random dot stereograms are similar to those described above for use with line stereograms (Atkinson and Braddick, 1976; Birch and Hale, 1989). A variant of FPL with random dot patterns has been used to show a single stereogram with movement of the stereoscopic form toward the left or to the right of the video screen (Fox et al., 1980; Shea et al., 1980; Dobson and Sebris, 1989). The observer's task is then modified to deciding whether the infant is tracking the form to the left or to the right. This moving stereoscopic form has also been used as a stimulus for electrooculographic (EOG) recordings of saccadic (Archer et al., 1986) or pursuit (Leguire et al., 1983) responses. In the EOG test paradigm, the infant's ability to generate the appropriate eye movements is verified initially by recording saccades or pursuit of a monocularly visible form similar in shape and size to the stereoscopic form. Given the presence of measurable, even if immature, eye movement responses in this monocular control condition, similar responses to the stereoscopic form can be interpreted as evidence for stereopsis. Visual evoked response tests of stereopsis utilize random dot stimuli that change in depth over time, usually a slow square-wave or sine-wave alternation between nondisparate and disparate states (Petrig et al., 1981). In adults with stereopsis, a voltage change can be recorded from the scalp over the occipital cortex as the disparity state is alternated. Infants who show similar voltage changes are considered to demonstrate stereopsis.

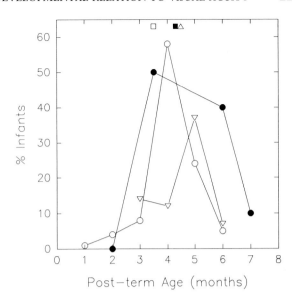

FIG. 13-1. Distribution of onset ages for stereopsis obtained with line stereograms and forced-choice preferential looking (FPL) (○) (Birch et al., 1983), dynamic random dot stereograms and FPL (▽) (Fox et al., 1980), and dynamic random dot stereograms and visual evoked potentials (●) (Petrig et al., 1981). Also shown are mean onset ages from studies with insufficient information to specify distributions (Archer et al., 1986: △; Reuss, 1981: ■; Shea et al., 1980: □).

to a stimulus with coarse binocular disparity and to a stimulus with no binocular disparity. Most studies concerned with the onset age have used coarse binocular disparities ranging from 30 to 60 minutes. Despite the diversity of stimulus generation and data acquisition techniques, remarkably good agreement exists among the various studies on the average age for onset of stereopsis in the human infant. Onset ages from several studies are shown in Figure 13-1; although a small percentage of infants demonstrate stereopsis by 2 months of age, most normal infants show an abrupt onset of stereopsis at 3–5 months of age. Longitudinal studies have shown that the typical infant shows no consistent response to binocular disparity during the first 8–10 weeks of life, first discriminates binocularly disparate from nondisparate stimuli sometime during weeks 11–20, and then continues to show reliable discrimination during follow-up tests conducted weeks or months later (Held et al., 1980; Birch et al., 1982). A sex difference in onset age has been reported, with females demonstrating stereopsis slightly earlier than males (Gwiazda et al., 1989).

ONSET OF STEREOPSIS IN THE HUMAN INFANT

The onset of stereopsis has been defined as the youngest age at which an infant is able to respond differentially

FACTORS THAT MAY DETERMINE AGE OF ONSET

Several factors that may account for the abrupt onset of stereopsis have been considered.

1. It may require maturation of the macula sufficient to support a minimum level of monocular resolution (Aslin and Dumais, 1980).

2. It may require the attainment of accurate vergence control (Aslin and Dumais, 1980; Braddick and Atkinson, 1983).

3. It may require cortical maturation sufficient to preserve eye of origin information and sufficient to support disparity coding (Birch et al., 1982; Atkinson, 1984; Held, 1988; Wilson, 1988).

Retinal Maturation

The immature macula of the neonate is characterized by large interphotoreceptor spacing, which is consistent with the poor acuity measured during the first 2 months of life (Hendrickson and Youdelis, 1984; Youdelis and Hendrickson, 1986; Wilson, 1988). Most studies of infant stereopsis have taken the poor spatial resolution of the young infant into account when designing stimuli for the investigation of stereopsis by using patterns well within the acuity limit of the newborn infant; typical stimuli range from 45 to 120 minutes wide. This approach appears to be reasonable for minimizing the potentially confounding influence of acuity development on the measurement of stereopsis development because adults blurred with cycloplegia and lenses continue to demonstrate stereopsis until their acuity is so degraded they can no longer perceive the monocular patterns that comprise the stereogram (Levy and Glick, 1974; Donzis et al., 1983). Therefore spatial resolution, though poor during the first 2 months of life, should be sufficient to support detection of coarse binocular disparities.

Retinal immaturity is unlikely to be the sole limiting factor when determining the onset age for stereopsis for two additional reasons. First, no abrupt change in acuity has been found to accompany the onset of stereopsis. In fact, the time span over which stereopsis emerges is typically characterized by minimal or no change in grating acuity. Figure 13-2 shows the mean developmental curve for grating acuity during the time span of the onset of stereopsis. Although acuity shows considerable postnatal improvement, no sudden change in acuity occurs at the onset for stereopsis. The inset to Figure 13-2 shows typical results from a single infant who participated in a longitudinal study of stereopsis and grating acuity development. The figure illustrates that, like the group means, individuals show little or no change in acuity during the onset of stereopsis.

Second, several investigators have reported that discrimination of crossed disparities has an earlier age of onset than discrimination of uncrossed disparities (Held et al., 1980; Reuss, 1981; Birch et al., 1982). Figure 13-3 shows the percentage of infants in various age

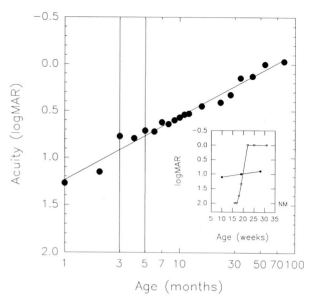

FIG. 13-2. Visual acuity development during as measured by FPL (Birch and Hale, 1988). The age range between the solid vertical lines encompasses the ages of onset for most human infants. (*Inset.*) Visual acuity and stereoacuity development in an infant. NM = not measurable.

groups who demonstrated stereopsis when tested with crossed disparity line stereograms or with uncrossed disparity line stereograms. These cross-sectional data provide clear evidence for the earlier onset of sensitivity to crossed disparity. Similar results have been reported for individual infants tested longitudinally with both crossed and uncrossed disparities (Birch et al., 1982). There is no simple way to fit this difference in onset ages by a model that accounts for the abrupt onset of stereopsis by retinal maturation alone (Birch et al., 1982).

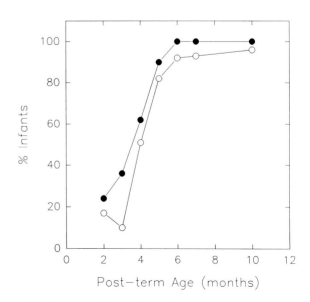

FIG. 13-3. Percent of infants who reached criterion for stereopsis when tested with crossed (●) or uncrossed (○) disparity. (Birch et al., 1982.)

Vergence

It is known that newborns are capable of bifoveal fixation in some experimental paradigms (Slater and Findlay, 1975), but it is also known that the control of vergence undergoes considerable postnatal maturation (Aslin and Dumais, 1980). This point raises the possibility that the neural mechanisms of stereopsis are mature at birth, but that stereopsis may become apparent only when the control of vergence is accurate and stable enough to maintain near-zero absolute disparity (bifoveal fixation). Whether neonatal or infantile vergence is accurate and reliable in the settings under which stereopsis tests have been conducted has not been studied directly. However, two lines of evidence argue against the maturation of vergence control as being the sole factor in determining onset age. First, as discussed above, for many infants the ability to discriminate crossed disparities appears earlier in development than the ability to discriminate uncrossed disparities (Held et al., 1980; Reuss, 1981; Birch et al., 1982). It is difficult to see how immature vergence control might differentially affect the ability to make these two classes of stereo discrimination. Second, Birch et al. (1983) described a periodic stereoscopic stimulus specifically designed to be insensitive to small vergence errors. These stereograms were composed of seven black bars spaced approximately 1.4 degrees apart; in the disparate stimulus, alternate bars were displaced laterally. Periodic line stereograms allow for multiple fusion loci determined by the periodicity of the bars so that, with an approximate upper limit of 25 prism diopters of misalignment of the visual axes, fusion of at least two bars may provide a basis for stereoscopic depth perception. Despite the greater tolerance for vergence error in this paradigm, infants showed the same average onset age for stereopsis as other infants who had been tested with stimuli requiring precise eye alignment.

Cortical Maturation

Although the anatomical substrate for stereopsis remains an area of active study (Ohzawa et al., 1980; Hubel and Livingstone, 1987; Yeshurun and Schwartz, 1987; LeVay and Voight, 1988), anatomical segregation of inputs from the two eyes to the visual cortex is a prerequisite for preserving eye of origin information and therefore stereopsis. The segregated ocular dominance columns that characterize the mature monkey and human primary visual cortex are at best immature and possibly absent in monkeys and humans at birth (LeVay et al., 1978, 1980; Hickey and Peduzzi, 1987). Studies of the anatomical development of the monkey primary visual cortex suggest that ocular dominance column segregation begins 3 weeks prenatally (Rakic,

1976) but is not completed until at least 6 weeks after birth (LeVay et al., 1980). That the onset of stereopsis in the human infant may reflect maturation of visual cortex has been suggested by several authors (Birch et al., 1982; Held, 1988; Wilson, 1988). This hypothesis is consistent with the finding that synaptogenesis continues postnatally in the striate cortex of the human infant, reaching a peak between 2 and 8 months (Huttonlocher et al., 1982). If the onset of stereopsis does represent the achievement of a milestone of visual cortical development, it is probably not a unique consequence of cortical maturation. Other qualitative changes in visual function appear at approximately 2–3 months, including spatial frequency tuning, contrast constancy, and phase discrimination; these qualitative improvements have been linked to cortical maturation (Bronson, 1974; Atkinson, 1984; Dubowitz et al., 1986; Mohn and van Hof-van Duin, 1986).

WHAT ARE INFANTS DISCRIMINATING?

Normal infants aged 5 months or older typically discriminate stimuli containing horizontal binocular disparity from stimuli that are not disparate. Whether this discrimination is accompanied by the percept of depth, which is the hallmark of stereopsis, is not known. Two lines of evidence are available from which we can infer that the infant discriminates the disparity and that the disparity gives rise to the percept of depth.

Binocular vertical disparities and large binocular horizontal disparities provide two cases in which stimuli may be constructed to be similar in all respects to those used for stereo tests, with the exception that the stimuli do not give rise to the percept of depth. In adults such stimuli are seen as rivalrous. These two classes of stimuli can match or exaggerate all of the stimulus parameters of the stereoscopic stimulus, including disparity between the monocular images, degree of correlation between the monocular images, and general characteristics of the monocular images (e.g., line figure or random dot pattern, contrast, mean luminance). If the infant is responding on the basis of binocular disparity alone, we would expect the infant to show similar responses to binocular vertical disparity, large binocular horizontal disparity, and moderate binocular horizontal disparity because the infant is not able to distinguish the class of binocular disparity that gives rise to the percept of depth from other classes of binocular disparity. On the other hand, if the infant is responding to the percept of depth associated with moderate binocular horizontal disparity, we would expect the infant to respond differently when presented with moderate binocular horizontal disparity than when presented with vertical or large horizontal disparity. In fact, infants who consistently prefer to look at stimuli with moderate binocular horizontal disparity over stimuli with zero disparity show either no preference or avoidance of the disparate stimulus when the disparity is vertical or large (Fox et al., 1980; Birch et al., 1982). These results suggest that the infant is responding to the percept of depth and not simply to binocular disparity; that is, the infant is likely demonstrating true stereopsis.

A more direct approach to determining whether the infant sees disparate stimuli in depth involves the use of reaching responses (Granrud, 1986). Under binocular viewing conditions, infants who demonstrate the ability to discriminate disparate from nondisparate line stereograms reach more consistently for the nearer of two objects than infants who show no evidence of disparity discrimination. Under monocular viewing conditions, the two groups of infants showed comparable reaching behavior, suggesting that the groups did not differ in their ability to produce the appropriate response. Furthermore, infants who demonstrate the ability to discriminate disparate from nondisparate stimuli show evidence of size constancy, whereas infants who show no evidence of disparity discrimination do not. These data provide clear evidence that the onset of disparity discrimination signals a significant change in the infant's ability to perceive objects' sizes and distances.

STEREOACUITY DEVELOPMENT DURING INFANCY

Several studies of human infants have documented improvements in stereoacuity (the smallest binocular horizontal disparity discriminable from zero disparity). To date, all studies of stereoacuity development have used line stereograms (Held et al., 1980; Birch et al., 1982). The use of line stereograms simplifies presentation of disparities that are smaller than the pattern element size; therefore large pattern elements that are within the acuity limits of young infants can be used to present very small binocular disparities. After the abrupt onset of stereopsis at 3–5 months of age, the average infant attains a stereoacuity of 60 seconds or better by 6 months of age (Birch et al., 1982). The averaging of ages obscures what is a remarkably rapid improvement in stereoacuity; that is, the developmental curve for stereoacuity is steeper for individual infants than for the sample as a whole. Examples of individual infants' developmental stereoacuity functions are shown in Figure 13-4. Individual infants' stereoacuities improved from 60 minute arc to 60 second arc over a time span of 5–6 weeks.

In clinical evaluation of esotropic patients, comparisons among standardized stereo tests, base out prism tests, the Worth four dot test, and amblyoscopic tests have led to a better understanding of different grades of stereoacuity. Stereoacuity of 400 seconds or more

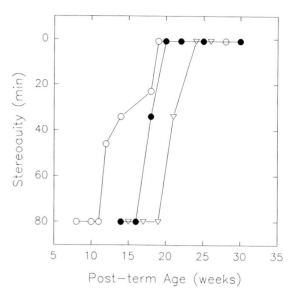

FIG. 13-4. Representative individual developmental stereoacuity curves. (Birch et al., 1982.)

may be considered evidence of peripheral binocularity, stereoacuity of 80–200 seconds may be considered evidence of macular binocularity, and stereoacuity of 60 seconds or less may be considered evidence of foveal binocularity (Parks, 1968, 1969; Okuda et al., 1977). Looking at the stereoacuity data available during infant development within this context suggests that peripheral binocular function may develop at 3–4 months of age, followed by a rapid developmental progression toward the macula; finally, bifoveal fusion is achieved at 6–8 months of age. Alternatively, it may be that some aspects of infant foveal vision at 3 months of age resemble adult peripheral vision but rapidly mature by 6–8 months.

No studies of infant random dot stereoacuity development have been published, but one study of infant rhesus monkey random dot stereoacuity has suggested that a similar developmental course occurs (O'Dell et al., 1991). Infant rhesus monkeys had a mean age of onset of 4 weeks and had attained stereoacuity of 88 seconds by a mean age of 8 weeks. The time courses for the development of several visual functions in the infant rhesus monkey have been related to human development by adjusting the age scales by a factor of 4 (i.e., substitute "months" for "weeks"). When this adjustment is made for the stereoacuity data, the agreement between human infant line stereogram results and rhesus infant random dot stereogram results is excellent.

HYPERACUITY

Hyperacuities comprise a group of visual functions in which the minimum detectable visual angle is less than the resolution acuity (Snellen or grating acuity). In adults, stereoacuity and vernier acuity are both hyperacuities, as the minimum detectable angle is as much as 1.0 log unit smaller than resolution acuity (Westheimer, 1975). Although the anatomical substrates of hyperacuities remain ill-defined, it is generally accepted that hyperacuities depend on cortical function. Hyperacuities exhibit several properties consistent with the use of positional cues from a pool of receptors, including insensitivity to modest motion or blur, degradation by feature separation, and degradation by competing features located nearby. In addition, the cortical basis of vernier acuity is supported by the findings that visually evoked potentials can be recorded in response to vernier offset, that cats without striate cortex retain normal visual acuity but have reduced vernier acuity, and that single neurons in the visual cortex show hyperacuity for vernier offsets (Swindale and Cynader, 1986; Zak and Berkley, 1986).

During development, vernier acuity follows a time course similar to that of stereoacuity in that vernier acuity is not hyperacute until an average age of 4 months. Prior to 4 months, vernier acuity is poorer than grating acuity and has been called "hypoacute" (Shimojo and Held, 1987). The concordance in emergence of hyperacuities suggests that a common mechanism for spatial localization may underlie both visual functions (Held, 1988). The finding that vernier acuity, like stereoacuity, has a more rapid developmental rate of improvement than visual acuity has led to the hypothesis that vernier acuity may provide another index of cortical maturation (Shimojo et al., 1984). However, rapid improvement of vernier acuity during the first 6 months of life also is consistent with developmental changes in the aperture, spacing, and efficiency of foveal cones (Banks and Bennett, 1988). Therefore although it is clear that cortical function is necessary for optimal vernier acuity, the limiting factors in the development of vernier acuity remain to be determined.

SIMULTANEOUS PERCEPTION, FUSION, AND STEREOPSIS

Simultaneous perception of two monocular images, fusion of two monocular images, and stereopsis are three distinct and essential aspects of normal binocular vision (Parks, 1975). Worth (1903) considered these three components to be hierarchically organized, a view consistent with a large body of clinical data. However, it is clear that stereopsis is possible without fusion, and that fusion does not imply stereopsis (Burian, 1936); therefore simultaneous perception, fusion, and stereopsis are regarded as independent features of binocular single vision (Parks, 1975; von Noorden, 1980).

Simultaneous perception appears to be present from

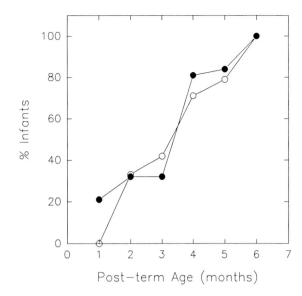

FIG. 13-5. Percent of infants who reached criterion for fusion (○) and for stereopsis (●). (From Birch et al., 1985. By permission.)

birth in the human infant. Shimojo et al. (1986) showed that prior to the onset of stereopsis (before 3.5 months) infants do not alternately suppress each eye but, instead, superimpose dichoptically presented images even when they are sufficiently different as to induce rivalry in adults. Fusion and stereopsis appear to emerge nearly simultaneously in development (Petrig et al., 1981; Birch et al., 1985; Gwiazda et al., 1989), as illustrated in Figure 13-5.

ACUITY AND STEREOPSIS

Acuity development is summarized in another chapter and is discussed here only in the context of its relation to the development of stereopsis. Acuity development has been studied extensively, and many experimental techniques have been employed, including FPL, visual evoked potential, optokinetic nystagmus, and pattern electroretinography. To date, the only paradigm within which both acuity and stereopsis data have been gathered for the same infants is the FPL technique. Therefore the acuity data discussed here are limited for the most part to results using this procedure.

Interocular Acuity Differences

The magnitude of interocular differences in acuity varies with age during the first year of life. As shown in Figure 13-6, interocular acuity differences average slightly under 1.0 octave in infants aged 5 months and younger and decrease to approximately 0.5 octave by 6 months of age. Interocular acuity differences of 1.0 octave or more found in about 40% of infants under 2 months of age

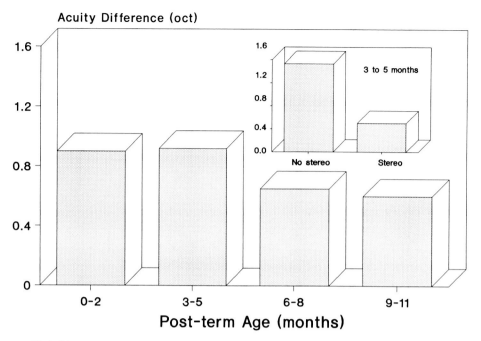

FIG. 13-6. Mean interocular acuity differences (absolute value of right eye acuity minus left eye acuity in octaves) as a function of age. (*Inset*) Mean interocular acuity differences for two subgroups of 3- to 5-month-old infants: those who failed to reach criterion for stereopsis and those who reached criterion for stereopsis. (Birch, 1985.)

and in few infants aged 6 months or older (Atkinson et al., 1982; Dobson, 1983; Birch, 1985; Birch and Hale, 1988; Thompson and Drasdo, 1988). As shown in the Figure 13-6 inset, 3- to 5-month-old infants demonstrating stereopsis have, on average, smaller interocular acuity differences than do 3- to 5-month-old infants who fail to demonstrate stereopsis (Birch, 1985). These data suggest a possible relation between the development of monocular acuity and of stereopsis; that is, the third to fifth months of life may be a period of binocular competition that culminates in small interocular differences and the onset of binocular single vision (Birch et al., 1985; Birch and Hale, 1988).

Monocular Versus Binocular Acuity

Binocular acuity and monocular acuity are comparable during the first 4–6 months of life; thereafter, binocular acuity is superior to monocular acuity (Atkinson et al., 1982; Dobson, 1983; Birch, 1985; Birch and Hale, 1988; Thompson and Drasdo, 1988). Although at first glance the onset of superiority of binocular acuity over monocular acuity appears to be consistent with the emergence of stereopsis at 4–6 months of age, it is in fact difficult to reconcile with predictions of probability summation for two eyes. Probability summation predicts an acuity advantage for two eyes over one when two assumptions are met: (1) the two eyes must have

similar acuities; and (2) the two eyes must function as independent detectors (Green and Swets, 1966). One or both of these assumptions must be incorrect for early human development. That is, the two eyes must have sufficiently different acuities, or the two eyes must not function independently before 4–6 months of age. As discussed above, significant interocular differences in acuity have been documented in some infants during the first few months of life, so probability summation may not predict a significant binocular advantage in this age range. In addition, both anatomical data and psychophysical data suggest that the two eyes may not function independently in young infants (Held, 1985; Shimojo et al., 1986).

One study (Birch and Swanson, 1992) explicitly examined the predictions of probability summation and the adequacy probability summation when describing monocular and binocular acuity development. As shown in Figure 13-7, probability summation predicts a binocular acuity advantage beginning at birth and persisting throughout infancy and early childhood. This result suggests that the interocular differences in acuity present in some infants during the first several months of life are not so great as to preclude a binocular acuity advantage.

The absence of probability summation during the early months of life is consistent with the hypothesis that the two eyes do not function independently. Prior to the

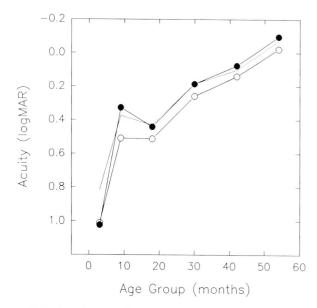

FIG. 13-7. Actual monocular (○) and binocular acuities (●) and binocular acuities (dotted line) predicted by probability summation.

onset of fusion and stereopsis, the human may have a primitive form of binocularity in which the visual system superimposes the inputs from the two retinas regardless of image content (Shimojo et al., 1986). Consistent with this concept, anatomical data from the monkey and human suggest that the immature primary visual cortex lacks segregation into ocular dominance columns so that both retinas provide inputs to common cells (LeVay et al., 1980; Held, 1985; Hickey and Peduzzi, 1987). This convergence of monocular inputs onto common cells cannot support a binocular advantage due to probability summation if both signal and noise are summed linearly. As visual development proceeds, segregation of ocular dominance columns provides for separate left and right eye "channels" (Poggio and Fischer, 1977; LeVay et al., 1980) and for the preservation of eye of origin information required for stereopsis. Independent right eye and left eye channels following ocular dominance column segregation also may provide the anatomical basis for the nonlinear combination of signal and noise that characterizes probability summation.

Clinically, the finding of probability summation of acuity beyond 4 months of age suggests mature cortical organization (e.g., segregation into ocular dominance columns) but does not necessarily imply the capability for stereopsis. Failure to find probability summation for acuity in an infant over 6 months of age suggests immature cortical organization (e.g., lack of segregation into separate right and left eye channels) or that one of the monocular channels is so weak that its contribution to probability summation does not result in a binocular acuity advantage.

NEURAL MECHANISMS OF BINOCULAR DEVELOPMENT

The cortical basis of binocular development has been studied extensively in the cat and monkey (reviewed by Blakemore, 1978; Hubel, 1982; Wiesel, 1982). Early on, afferents from each eye are intermixed throughout layer IV of the striate cortex, with terminal arbors distributed over a much larger area of cortex than in the mature animal (LeVay and Stryker, 1979). Segregation of axons from the two eyes begins prenatally but proceeds postnatally, resulting in the development of ocular dominance columns. In the cat, stereopsis is first measurable behaviorally at the same age that ocular dominance segregation becomes mature anatomically (Pettigrew, 1974; LeVay et al., 1978; Timney, 1988). The segregation is most likely achieved through an active process of competition for common postsynaptic targets (von Noorden and Middleditch, 1975; von Noorden et al., 1976; Hubel et al., 1977; Rakic, 1981). In the human there are few data on anatomical development, but available evidence suggests that ocular dominance column segregation occurs during the first several postnatal months (Hickey and Peduzzi, 1987). Extensive synaptic proliferation occurs in the human infant during the second through eighth months of life followed by a decline in synaptic density to reach adult levels at about 10 years of age (Takashima et al., 1980; Huttenlocher et al., 1982; Garey and deCourten, 1983). Wilson (1988) has proposed that the synaptic proliferation in the striate cortex represents the development of inhibitory processes crucial to mature visual function, including stereopsis.

The period of rapid anatomical development coincides with a period of vulnerability to disruption by environmental events. The concept of a "sensitive period" in visual development has become well accepted. The sensitive period is characterized by rapid anatomical and physiological change, emergence and tuning of visual function, and dependence of the progress of these changes on the visual environment (von Noorden and Crawford, 1970; Hubel, 1982; Wiesel, 1982). Amblyopia is the most studied effect of early abnormal visual experience, particularly the amblyopia that results in poor acuity in one eye and reduced binocular function associated with monocular patterns deprivation or strabismus.

Monocular pattern deprivation due to unilateral ptosis, occlusion, or aphakia during the first weeks or months of life leads to permanent visual impairment, including acuity, contrast sensitivity, and binocular deficits in humans (Awaya et al., 1973, 1979, 1980; von Noorden, 1981; Birch and Stager, 1985; Birch et al., 1986; Tytla et al., 1988) and monkeys (von Noorden et al., 1970; von Noorden, 1973; Harwerth et al., 1981, 1983). In

the monkey, monocular pattern deprivation is known to result in anatomical and physiological cortical changes. Ocular dominance columns driven by the deprived eye are narrower than normal, whereas those driven by the nondeprived eye are wider than normal (Hubel et al., 1977; Blakemore et al., 1978; LeVay et al., 1980). Few binocularly responsive cortical cells are found following deprivation (Hubel et al., 1977; Blakemore et al., 1978; von Noorden and Crawford, 1981). These changes most likely result from competition between the two eyes because they do not occur if a lesion in the lateral geniculate nucleus prevents signals from the nondeprived eye from reaching the cortex (von Noorden, 1976) and because the effect is found only in cortical areas that receive input from both eyes (Hubel et al., 1977).

Strabismus results in diplopia owing to misalignment of the visual axes and subsequently to suppression of one image (von Noorden, 1980). This suppression is a kind of visual deprivation, particularly if a strong fixation preference develops so that one eye is suppressed constantly. Habitual suppression of the nonfixing eye results in reduced acuity, contrast sensitivity, and binocular function (Parks, 1975; von Noorden, 1980). Even when a strong fixation preference does not develop, alternating suppression precludes simultaneous visual experience and leads to permanent impairment of binocular function. In the monkey visual cortex, surgically induced or prism-induced strabismus results in a paucity of binocular cells and, when a fixation preference exists, a shift in the distribution of ocular dominance columns toward the preferred eye (Crawford and von Noorden, 1979, 1980; Crawford et al., 1983).

The need for normal sensory experience during development means that binocular function must develop during the first 6−8 months of life or it will never develop normally (Banks et al., 1975; Vaegan and Taylor, 1979). It has been suggested that the vulnerability of binocular function during development is a necessary feature because of growth of the face and increase in interpupillary distance during the early months of life; a plastic system allows for recalibration. Consistent with this hypothesis is the finding that, in the kitten, sensitivity to monocular pattern deprivation begins to decline as the rate of growth of the interpupillary distance begins to slow (Timney, 1990).

STEREOPSIS AND ACUITY IN INFANTILE ESOTROPIA

What was once termed "congenital esotropia" has been renamed "infantile esotropia" because of the observation that the esotropia is seldom present at birth (Costenbader, 1958; Nixon et al., 1985). The term "congenital esotropia" is consistent with the hypothesis of Worth (1903) that infants with esotropia have a "congenital defect in fusion faculty"; that is, the optimum outcome of treatment would be a cosmetic realignment of the eyes. The new term, infantile esotropia, is consistent with the hypothesis advanced by Chavasse (1939) that all infants have an innate capacity for fusion but this capacity can be disrupted by postnatal influences such as esotropia. This approach suggests that esotropia may be curable; that is, normal binocular vision may be restored. Although suggestive of normal sensory capacity, the fact that the esotropia does not become manifest until some months after birth does not unequivocally imply that the pathways for bifoveal fusion are innately present. A more direct approach to this question has been to evaluate prospectively the development of binocular function in infants with esotropia or at risk for developing esotropia.

Studies of emerging binocular function in young esotropic infants are hampered by several factors. First, the ideal age for the evaluation of innate capacity for stereopsis in infantile esotropes is 3−5 months, as this age corresponds to the onset of stereopsis in normal infants. However, only a small proportion of infantile esotropes have been diagnosed and referred for evaluation and treatment by 5 months. Second, the misalignment of the visual axes present in infantile esotropia precludes stereopsis because images are not presented within Panum's area and cannot be fused even if the sensory capacity for fusion is intact. Third, if amblyopia is present in association with the esotropia, stereopsis may be precluded because one eye is unable to resolve the monocular pattern. Each of these issues has been addressed in a pair of studies that recruited a large number of infantile esotropes and tested them prior to any treatment (including 31 infants aged 3−5 months), compensated for the misalignment of visual axes (by using prisms and stereograms designed to be insensitive to small residual deviations), and measured acuity of each eye to ensure that it was capable of resolving the monocular patterns that comprised the stereogram (Birch and Stager, 1985; Stager and Birch, 1986). The percentages of normal and esotropic infants who demonstrated stereopsis are shown as a function of age in Figure 13-8. Approximately equal percentages demonstrated stereopsis during months 3 and 4. However, during months 5−14 most normal infants demonstrated stereopsis, whereas few esotropic infants did. These results suggest that stereoscopic pathways are present and functional in many 3- and 4-month-old esotropic infants corrected with prisms. Although most older esotropic infants failed to demonstrate stereopsis even with compensatory prisms, clinical studies have shown that they have the capacity to recover some stereopsis when surgically straightened by age 2 years (Taylor, 1974; Ing, 1981). A similar developmental course has been reported for a single esotropic infant tested longitudi-

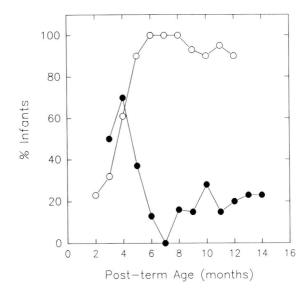

FIG. 13-8. Percent of normal and esotropic infants who reached criterion for stereopsis. All esotropic infants were diagnosed by age 6 months, had no known neurological or neuromuscular disorders, and were tested at the initial visit prior to any treatment. (Stager and Birch, 1986.)

nally with shadow-casted stimuli (Bechtoldt and Hutz, 1979).

The seemingly normal onset of stereopsis in young infantile esotropes raises the possibility that, under ideal conditions, infants with esotropia may be capable of achieving normal binocular single vision. This view is supported by advocates of early surgical intervention (Chevasse, 1939; Parks, 1968, 1969, 1975, 1977; Taylor, 1974; Ing, 1981; Ing et al., 1981). With current early screening and treatment protocols, including occlusion therapy, optical correction, and surgery when indicated, the best outcome to be anticipated is what has been termed *monofixation syndrome* (Parks, 1969). Monofixation syndrome is defined as a small residual deviation (8 prism diopters or less), peripheral fusion with normal vergence amplitudes, normal or near-normal acuity in both eyes, and a small foveal suppression scotoma that precludes bifoveal fixation. In fact, despite the recent popularity of early surgery, not a single case of normal stereoacuity in a child with a history of infantile esotropia has been reported, regardless of the age at surgery (von Noorden, 1980). Stereoacuity in monofixation syndrome may range between 60 and 3000 seconds; stereoacuity of more than 60 seconds is considered to be a marker for monofixation. The achievement of bifoveal fusion requires postoperative alignment within Panum's area, 6–10 minute arc. Although this level of accuracy is a rare surgical achievement, a procedure that results in an incomitant correction at an early age might allow the infant to develop a head turn to refine the deviation to within

Panum's area and utilize the inherent capability for bifoveal fusion (Stager and Birch, 1986). Similar head turns have been noted in Duane's retraction syndrome (resulting in bifoveal fusion) and in some infants immediately after injection with botulinum toxin (Oculinum) (Magoon, 1989).

Although it is generally accepted that early surgical treatment of infantile esotropia is associated with a high success rate of establishing adequate alignment, the possible benefits of early surgery for the development of fusion and stereopsis are less clear. Large-scale retrospective reviews of clinical data have reported that fusion and stereopsis are more commonly found in children whose eyes were initially aligned by age 24 months than in those whose eyes were initially aligned after 24 months (Taylor, 1974; Ing, 1981). Prospective studies of the development of stereopsis in children with a history of infantile esotropia showed that, after early successful surgery, approximately 35% of them had stereopsis, demonstrated by random dot stereograms by 3–5 years of age (Birch et al., 1990). Figure 13-9 summarizes outcomes following surgery in several studies. Note the general agreement among studies in that not all children are able to achieve stereopsis, even when postsurgical alignment is excellent. Discrepancies among the studies may be related to differences in stimuli used (line stereogram versus random dot) and differences in treatment, including postsurgical care. The percent of children demonstrating stereopsis continues to increase

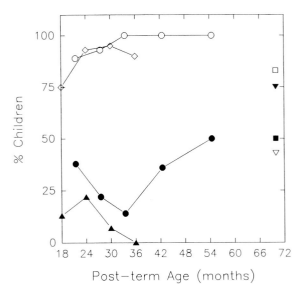

FIG. 13-9. Percent of esotropic infants who reached criterion for stereopsis following surgery in prospective studies (Birch et al., 1990: (●); Dobson and Sebris, 1989: ▲) and retrospective studies (Taylor, 1974: □; Ing, 1981: ▼; Robb and Rodier, 1987: ■; Pratt-Johnson and Tillson, 1983: ▽). Also shown are the percentages of normal children who reached criterion in two studies of preschool children (Birch et al., 1990: ○; Dobson and Sebris, 1989: ◇).

slightly well into early childhood. Some of this increase may result from "fine tuning" of alignment as the child participates in ongoing treatment. It has also been suggested that stereopsis may show a slower rate of maturation or delay in development in children with a history of infantile esotropia (Birch et al., 1990).

SUMMARY AND CONCLUSIONS

Studies of stereopsis have provided a wealth of information about the development and maintenance of single binocular vision in the human infant. A wide variety of stimuli and responses have been refined to utilize the infants' limited response capabilities and attention span to obtain reliable, quantitative, and objective information about developing binocular function. Despite the diversity of methodologies, a consensus on six basic findings has emerged.

1. Response to stereoscopic stimuli is absent at birth.
2. Stereopsis has a sudden onset at about 3–5 months of age.
3. The onset of response to crossed disparities often precedes the onset of response to uncrossed disparities.
4. Following the onset of stereopsis, there is a period of rapid improvement in stereoacuity over the next several weeks.
5. The infants' responses to moderate and small binocular horizontal disparities most likely represent responses to perceived depth.
6. The most likely candidate for the limiting factor in the onset of stereopsis is cortical development.

The interdisciplinary nature of research on the development of stereopsis has included psychophysical, electrophysiological, and anatomical studies of healthy human infants, clinical studies of humans with infantile eye disorders, and neurophysiological and neuroanatomical data from neonatal animals. The convergence of information from these various disciplines has led to significant advances in our understanding of the developing structure and function of the visual areas of the brain and of abnormal development due to infantile visual deprivation.

REFERENCES

ARCHER, S. M., HELVESTON, E. M., MILLER, K. K., AND ELLIS, F. D. (1986). Stereopsis in normal infants and infants with congenital esotropia. *Am. J. Ophthalmol.* 101, 591–596.

ASLIN, R. N., AND DUMAIS, Y. (1980). Binocular vision in infants: a review and a theoretical framework. *Adv. Child Dev. Behav.* 15, 53–94.

ATKINSON, J. (1984). Human visual development over the first 6 months of life—a review and hypothesis. *Hum. Neurobiol.* 3, 61–74.

ATKINSON, J., AND BRADDICK, O. (1976). Stereoscopic discrimination in infants. *Perception* 5, 29–38.

ATKINSON, J., BRADDICK, O., AND PIMM-SMITH, E. (1982). 'Preferential looking' for monocular and binocular testing of infants. *Br. J. Ophthalmol.* 66, 264–268.

AWAYA, S., MIYAKE, Y., IMAIZUMA, Y., SHIOSE, Y., KANDA, T., AND KOMURO, K. (1973). Amblyopia in man, suggestive of stimulus deprivation amblyopia. *Jpn. J. Ophthalmol.* 17, 69–82.

AWAYA, S., SUGAWARA, M., AND MIYAKE, S. (1979). Observations in patients with occlusion amblyopia. *Trans. Ophthalmol. Soc. UK* 99, 447–454.

AWAYA, S., SUGAWARA, M., MIYAKE, S., AND ISOMURA, Y. (1980). Form deprivation amblyopia and the results of its treatment—with special reference to the critical period. *Jpn. J. Ophthalmol.* 24, 241–250.

BANKS, M. S., AND BENNETT, P. J. (1988). Optical and photoreceptor immaturities limit the spatial and chromatic vision of human neonates. *J. Opt. Soc. Am. [A]* 5, 2059–2079.

BANKS, M. S., ASLIN, R. N., AND LETSON, R. D. (1975). Sensitive period for the development of human binocular vision. *Science* 190, 675–677.

BECHTOLDT, H. P., AND HUTZ, C. S. (1979). Stereopsis in young infants and stereopsis in an infant with congenital esotropia. *J. Pediatr. Ophthalmol. Strabismus* 16, 49–54.

BIRCH, E. E. (1985). Infant interocular acuity differences and binocular vision. *Vision Res.* 25, 571–576.

BIRCH, E. E., AND HALE, L. A. (1988). Criteria for monocular acuity deficit in infancy and early childhood. *Invest. Ophthalmol. Vis. Sci.* 29, 636–643.

BIRCH, E. E., AND HALE, L. A. (1989). Operant assessment of stereoacuity. *Clin. Vis. Sci.* 4, 295–300.

BIRCH, E. E., AND STAGER, D. R. (1985). Monocular acuity and stereopsis in infantile esotropia. *Invest. Ophthalmol. Vis. Sci.* 26, 1624–1630.

BIRCH, E. E., AND SWANSON, W. H. (1992). Probability summation of grating acuity in the human infant. *Vision Res.* 10, 1999–2003.

BIRCH, E. E., GWIAZDA, J., AND HELD, R. (1982). Stereoacuity development for crossed and uncrossed disparities in human infants. *Vision Res.* 22, 507–513.

BIRCH, E. E., GWIAZDA, J., AND HELD, R. (1983). The development of vergence does not account for the onset of stereopsis. *Perception* 12, 331–336.

BIRCH, E. E., SHIMOJO, S., AND HELD, R. (1985). Preferential-looking assessment of fusion and stereopsis in infants aged 1–6 months. *Invest. Ophthalmol. Vis. Sci.* 26, 366–370.

BIRCH, E. E., STAGER, D. R., AND WRIGHT, W. W. (1986). Grating acuity development following early surgery for congenital unilateral cataract. *Arch. Ophthalmol.* 104, 1783–1787.

BIRCH, E. E., STAGER, D. R., BERRY, P., AND EVERETT, M. E. (1990). Prospective assessment of acuity and stereopsis in amblyopic infantile esotropes following early surgery. *Invest. Ophthalmol. Vis. Sci.* 31, 758–765.

BLAKEMORE, C. (1978). Maturation and modification in the developing visual pathway. In R. HELD, H. W. LEIBOWITZ, AND H. L. TEUBER (eds.). *Handbook of Sensory Physiology. Vol. VIII. Perception.* Berlin: Springer-Verlag.

BLAKEMORE, C., GAREY, L. J., AND VITAL-DURAND, F. (1978). The physiological effects of monocular deprivation and their reversal in the monkey's visual cortex. *J. Physiol. (Lond.)* 283, 223–262.

BOWER, T. G. R. (1964). Discrimination of depth in premotor infants. *Psychonom. Sci.* 1, 368.

BOWER, T. G. R. (1965). Stimulus variables determining space perception in infants. *Science* 149, 88–89.

BOWER, T. G. R. (1966a). The visual world of infants. *Sci. Am.* 215, 80–92.

BOWER, T. G. R. (1966b). Perception and shape constancy in infants. *Science* 151, 832–834.

BOWER, T. G. R. (1972). Object perception in infants. *Perception* 1, 15–30.

BOWER, T. G. R., BROUGHTON, J. M., AND MOORE, M. K. (1971). The development of the object concept as manifested by changes in the tracking behavior of infants between 7 and 20 weeks of age. *J. Exp. Child. Psychol.* 11, 182–193.

BRADDICK, O., AND ATKINSON, J. (1983). Some recent findings on the development of human binocularity: a review. *Behav. Brain Res.* 10, 141–150.

BRONSON, G. B. (1974). The postnatal growth of visual capacity. *Child Dev.* 45, 873–890.

BURIAN, H. M. (1936). Studien uber zweiaugiges Tiefensehen bei ortlicher Abblendung. *Grafes Arch. Ophthalmol.* 136, 172.

CAMPOS, J. J., LANGER, A., AND KROWITZ, A. (1970). Cardiac responses on the visual cliff in prelocomotor human infants. *Science* 170, 196–197.

CARON, A. J., CARON, R. F., AND CARLSON, V. R. (1978). Infant perception of the invariant shape of objects varying in slant. *Child. Dev.* 50, 716–721.

CHAVASSE, F. B. (1939). *Worth's Squint*. Philadelphia: Blakiston, pp. 519–521.

COSTENBADER, F. D. (1958). Clinical course and management of esotropia. In J. H. ALLEN (ed.). *Strabismus Ophthalmic Symposium II.* Vol. 1. St. Louis: Mosby, pp. 325–353.

CRAWFORD, M. L. J., AND VON NOORDEN, G. K. (1979). The effects of short-term experimental strabismus on the visual system in *Macaca* mulatta. *Invest. Ophthalmol. Vis. Sci.* 18, 496–505.

CRAWFORD, M. L. J., AND VON NOORDEN, G. K. (1980). Optically induced concomitant strabismus in monkeys. *Invest. Ophthalmol. Vis. Sci.*, 19, 1105–1109.

CRAWFORD, M. L. J., VON NOORDEN, G. K., MEHARG, L. S., RHODES, J. W., HARWERTH, R. S., SMITH, E. L., AND MILLER, D. D. (1983). Binocular neurons and binocular function in monkeys and children. *Invest. Ophthalmol. Vis. Sci.* 24, 491–495.

CRUICKSHANK, R. M. (1941). The development of visual size constancy in early infancy. *J. Gen. Psychol.* 58, 327–351.

DOBSON, V. (1983). Clinical applications of preferential looking measures of visual acuity. *Behav. Brain Res.* 10, 25–38.

DOBSON, V., AND SEBRIS, S. L. (1989). Longitudinal study of acuity and stereopsis in infants with or at risk for esotropia. *Invest. Ophthalmol. Vis. Sci.* 30, 1146–1157.

DONZIS, P. B., RAPPAZZO, J. A., BURDE, R. M., AND GORDON, M. (1983). Effect of binocular variations of Snellen's visual acuity on Titmus stereoacuity. *Arch. Ophthalmol.* 101, 930–932.

DUBOWITZ, L. M. S., MUSHIN, J., DE VRIES, L., AND ARDER, G. N. (1986). Visual function in the newborn infant: is it cortically mediated? *Lancet* May 17, 1139–1144.

FANTZ, R. L. (1961). The origin of form perception. *Sci. Am.* 204, 66–72.

FANTZ, R. L. (1966). Pattern discrimination and selective attention as determinants of perceptual development from birth. In A. H. KIDD AND J. L. RIVOIRE (eds.). *Perceptual Development in Children.* New York: International Universities Press, pp. 143–173.

FOX, R., ASLIN, R. N., SHEA, S. L., AND DUMAIS, S. T. (1980). Stereopsis in human infants. *Science* 207, 323–324.

GAREY, L. J., AND deCOURTEN, C. (1983). Structural development of the lateral geniculate nucleus and visual cortex in monkey and in man. *Behav. Brain Res.* 10, 3–13.

GRANRUD, C. E. (1986). Binocular vision and spatial perception in 4- and 5-month-old infants. *J. Exp. Psychol. [Hum. Percept.]* 12, 36–49.

GREEN, D. M., AND SWETS, J. A. (1966). *Signal Detection Theory and Psychophysics.* New York: Krieger, pp. 37–44.

GWIAZDA, J., BAUER, J. A., JR., AND HELD, R. (1989). Binocular function in human infants: correlation of stereoptic and fusion-rivalry discriminations. *J. Pediatr. Ophthalmol. Strabismus* 26, 128–132.

HARWERTH, R. S., CRAWFORD, M. L. J., SMITH, E. L., AND BOLTZ, R. L. (1981). Behavioral studies of stimulus deprivation amblyopia in monkeys. *Vision Res.* 21, 779–789.

HARWERTH, R. S., SMITH, E. L., BOLTZ, R. L., CRAWFORD, M. L. J., AND VON NOORDEN, G. K. (1983). Behavioral studies on the effects of abnormal early visual experience in monkeys: spatial modulation sensitivity. *Vision Res.* 23, 1501–1510.

HELD, R. (1985). Binocular vision—behavioral and neural development. In V. MEHER AND R. FOX (eds.). *Neonate Cognition: Beyond the Blooming, Buzzing Confusion.* Hillsdale, NJ: Erlbaum, pp. 37–44.

HELD, R. (1988). Development of cortically mediated visual processes in human infants. In C. VON EULER, H. FORSSBERG, AND H. LAGERCRANTZ (eds.). *Neurobiology of Early Infant Behavior.* Stockholm: Stockton Press, pp. 155–164.

HELD, R., BIRCH, E. E., AND GWIAZDA, J. (1980). Stereoacuity of human infants. *Proc. Natl. Acad. Sci. USA* 77, 5572–5574.

HENDRICKSON, A. E., AND YOUDELIS, C. (1984). The morphological development of the human fovea. *Ophthalmology* 91, 603–612.

HICKEY, J. L., AND PEDUZZI, J. D. (1987). Structure and development of the visual system. In P. SALAPATEK AND L. COHEN (eds.). *Handbook of Infant Perception.* Orlando, FL: Academic Press, pp. 1–42.

HUBEL, D. H. (1982). Exploration of the primary visual cortex. *Nature* 299, 515–524.

HUBEL, D. H., AND LIVINGSTON, M. S. (1987). Segregation of form, color, and stereopsis in primate area 18. *J. Neurosci.* 7, 3378–3415.

HUBEL, D. H., WIESEL, T. N., AND LeVAY, S. (1977). Plasticity of ocular dominance columns in monkey striate cortex. *Philos. Trans R. Soc. Lond. [Biol.]* 278, 377–409.

HUTTENLOCHER, P. R., deCOURTEN, C., GAREY, L. J., AND VAN DER LOOS, H. (1982). Synaptogenesis in human visual cortex—evidence for synapse elimination during normal development. *Neurosci. Lett.* 33, 247–252.

ING, M. R. (1981). Early surgical alignment for congenital esotropia. *Trans. Am. Ophthalmol. Soc.* 79, 625–663.

ING, M. R., COSTENBADER, F. D., PARKS, M. M., AND ALBERT, D. M. (1981). Early surgical alignment for congenital esotropia. *Am. J. Ophthalmol.* 61, 1419–1427.

LEGUIRE, L. E., ROGERS, G. L., AND FELLOWS, R. R. (1983). Toward a clinical test of stereopsis in human infants. *Invest. Ophthalmol. Vis. Sci.* 24 (suppl.), 34.

LeVAY, S., AND STRYKER, M. P. (1979). The development of ocular dominance columns in the cat. *Soc. Neurosci. Symp.* 4, 83–89.

LeVAY, S., AND VOIGHT, T. (1988). Ocular dominance and disparity coding in cat visual cortex. *Vis. Neurosci.* 1, 395–414.

LeVAY, S., STRYKER, M. P., AND SHATZ, C. J. (1978). Ocular dominance columns and their development in layer IV of the cat's visual cortex: a quantitative study. *J. Comp. Neurol.* 179, 223–244.

LeVAY, S., WIESEL, T. N., AND HUBEL, D. H. (1980). The development of ocular dominance columns in normal and visually deprived monkeys. *J. Comp. Neurol.* 161, 1–51.

LEVY, N. S., AND GLICK, E. B. (1974). Stereoscopic perception and Snellen visual acuity. *Am. J. Ophthalmol.* 78, 722–724.

MAGOON, E. H. (1989). Botulin therapy in pediatric ophthalmology. *Int. Ophthalmol. Clin.* 29, 30–32.

MOHN, G., AND VAN HOF-VAN DUIN, J. (1986). Development of the binocular and monocular fields of human infants during the first year of life. *Clin. Vis. Sci.* 1, 51–64.

NIXON, R. B., HELVESTON, E. M., MILLER, K., ARCHER, S. M., AND ELLIS, D. (1985). Incidence of strabismus in neonates. *Am J. Ophthalmol.* 100, 798–801.

O'DELL, C. D., QUICK, M. W., AND BOOTHE, R. G. (1991). The development of stereoacuity in infant rhesus monkeys. *Invest. Ophthalmol. Vis. Sci.* 32, 1044.

OHZAWA, I., DEANGELIS, G. C., AND FREEMAN, R. D. (1990). Stereoscopic depth discrimination in the visual cortex: neurons ideally suited as disparity detectors. *Science* 249, 1037–1041.

OKUDA, F., APT, L., AND WATNER, B. (1977). Evaluation of the TNO random-dot stereogram test. *Am. Orthoptic J.* 27, 124.

PARKS, M. M. (1968). Summary and conclusion; symposium: infantile esotropia. *Am. Orthoptic J.* 18, 19–22.

PARKS, M. M. (1969). The monofixation syndrome. *Trans. Am. Ophthalmol. Soc.* 67, 609–657.

PARKS, M. M. (1975). *Ocular Motility and Strabismus.* New York: Harper & Row.

PARKS, M. M. (1977). Operate early for congenital strabismus. In R. J. BROCKHURST, S. A. BORUCHOFF, B. T. HUTCHINSON, AND S. LESSELL (eds.). *Controversy in Ophthalmology.* Philadelphia: Saunders, pp. 423–430.

PETRIG, B., JULESZ, B., KROPFL, W., BAUMGARTNER, G., AND ANLIKER, M. (1981). Development of stereopsis and cortical binocularity in human infants: electrophysiological evidence. *Science* 213, 1402–1405.

PETTIGREW, J. D. (1974). The effect of visual experience on the development of stimulus specificity by kitten cortical neurons. *J. Physiol.* 237, 49–76.

POGGIO, G. F., AND FISCHER, B. (1977). Binocular interaction and depth sensitivity of striate and prestriate cortical neurons of the behaving rhesus monkey. *J. Neurophysiol.* 40, 1392–1405.

PRATT-JOHNSON, J. A., AND TILLSON, G. (1983). Sensory results following treatment of infantile esotropia. *Can. J. Ophthalmol.* 18, 175–177.

RAKIC, P. (1976). Prenatal genesis of connections subserving ocular dominant columns in the rhesus monkey. *Nature* 261, 467–471.

RAKIC, P. (1981). *The Organization of the Cerebral Cortex.* Cambridge, MA: MIT Press, pp. 7–28.

REUSS, J. (1981). Human stereopsis: detection and development. *Dissert. Abstr. Int.* 42, 1961B.

ROBB, R. M., AND RODIER, D. W. (1987). The variable clinical characteristics and course of early infantile esotropia. *J. Pediatr. Ophthalmol. Strabismus* 24, 276–281.

SCARR, S., AND SALAPATEK, P. (1970). Patterns of fear development during infancy. *Merrill-Palmer Q.* 16, 53–90.

SHEA, S. L., FOX, R., ASLIN, R. N., AND DUMAIS, S. T. (1980). Assessment of stereopsis in human infants. *Invest. Ophthalmol. Vis. Sci.* 19, 1400–1404.

SHIMOJO, S., AND HELD, R. (1987). Vernier acuity is less than grating acuity in 2- and 3-month-olds. *Vision Res.* 77–86.

SHIMOJO, S., BAUER, J. A., JR., O'CONNELL, K. M., AND HELD, R. (1986). Pre-stereoptic binocular vision in infants. *Vision Res.* 26, 501–510.

SHIMOJO, S., BIRCH, E. E., GWIAZDA, J., AND HELD, R. (1984). Development of vernier acuity in infants. *Vision Res.* 24, 721–728.

SLATER, A. M., AND FINDLAY, J. M. (1975). Binocular fixation in the newborn baby. *J. Exp. Child. Psychol.* 20, 248–273.

STAGER, D. R., AND BIRCH, E. E. (1986). Preferential-looking acuity and stereopsis in infantile esotropia. *J. Pediatr. Ophthalmol. Strabismus* 23, 160–165.

SWINDALE, N. V., AND CYNADER, M. S. (1986). Vernier acuity of neurones in the cat visual cortex. *Nature* 319, 591–593.

TAKASHIMA, S., CHAN, F., BECKER, L. E., AND ARMSTRONG, D. L. (1980). Morphology of the developing visual cortex of the human infant. *J. Neurophysiol. Exp. Neurol.* 39, 487–501.

TAYLOR, D. M. (1974). Is congenital esotropia functionally curable? *J. Pediatr. Ophthalmol.* 11, 3–35.

THOMPSON, C., AND DRASDO, N. (1988). Clinical experience with preferential looking acuity tests in infants and young children. *Ophthalmic Physiol. Opt.* 8, 309–321.

TIMNEY, B. N. (1988). The development of depth perception. P. G. SHINKMAN (ed.). *Advances in Neural and Behavioral Development.* Norwood, NJ: Ablex, pp. 153–207.

TIMNEY, B. N. (1990). Effects of brief monocular occlusion on binocular depth perception in the cat: a sensitive period for the loss of stereopsis. *Vis. Neurosci.* 5, 273–280.

TYTLA, M. E., MAURER, D., LEWIS, T. L., AND BRENT, H. P. (1988). Contrast sensitivity in children treated for congenital cataract. *Clin. Vis. Sci.* 2, 251–264.

VAEGAN, AND TAYLOR, D. M. (1979). Critical period for deprivation amblyopia in children. *Trans. Ophthalmol. Soc. UK* 99, 432–493.

VON NOORDEN, G. K. (1973). Experimental amblyopia in monkeys: further behavioral observations and clinical correlations. *Invest. Ophthalmol. Vis. Sci.* 12, 721–726.

VON NOORDEN, G. K. (1976). Current concepts of amblyopia. In S. MOORE (ed.). *Orthoptics: Past, Present, and Future.* New York: Stratton, pp. 37–44.

VON NOORDEN, G. K. (1980). *Burian and von Noorden's Binocular Vision and Ocular Motility.* St. Louis: Mosby.

VON NOORDEN, G. K. (1981). New clinical aspects of clinical deprivation amblyopia. *Am. J. Ophthalmol.* 92, 416–421.

VON NOORDEN, G. K., AND CRAWFORD, M. L. J. (1979). The sensitive period. *Trans. Ophthalmol. Soc. UK* 99, 442–446.

VON NOORDEN, G. K., AND CRAWFORD, M. L. J. (1981). The effects of total unilateral occlusion vs. lid suture on the visual system of infant monkeys. *Invest. Ophthalmol. Vis. Sci.* 21, 142–146.

VON NOORDEN, G. K., AND MIDDLEDITCH, P. R. (1975). Histology of the monkey lateral geniculate nucleus after unilateral lid closure and experimental strabismus: further observations. *Invest. Ophthalmol. Vis. Sci.* 14, 674–683.

VON NOORDEN, G. K., CRAWFORD, M. L. J., AND MIDDLEDITCH, P. R. (1976). The effects of monocular deprivation: disuse or binocular interaction. *Brain Res.* 111, 277–285.

VON NOORDEN, G. K., DOWLING, J. E., AND FERGUSON, D. C. (1970). Experimental amblyopia in monkeys. I. Behavioral studies of stimulus deprivation amblyopia. *Arch. Ophthalmol.* 84, 206–214.

WALK, R. D., AND GIBSON, E. J. (1961). A comparative and analytical study of visual depth perception. *Psychol. Monogr.* 75, 1–44.

WALTERS, C. P., AND WALK, R. D. (1974). Visual placing by human infants. *J. Exp. Child Psychol.* 18, 34–40.

WESTHEIMER, G. (1975). Visual acuity and hyperacuity. *Invest. Ophthalmol. Vis. Sci.* 14, 570–572.

WIESEL, T. N. (1982). Postnatal development of the visual cortex and the influence of environment. *Nature* 299, 583–591.

WILSON, H. R. (1988). Development of spatiotemporal mechanisms in the human infant. *Vision Res.* 28, 611–628.

WORTH, C. (1903). *Squint. Its Causes, Pathology, and Treatment.* Philadelphia: Blakiston, pp. 59–62.

YESHURUN, Y., AND SCHWARTZ, E. L. (1987). An ocular dominance column map as a data structure for stereo segmentation. In *Proceedings, IEEE 1st Annual International Conference on Neural Networks,* pp. 369–377.

YOUDELIS, C., AND HENDRICKSON, A. E. (1986). A qualitative and quantitative analysis of the human fovea during development. *Vision Res.* 26, 847–855.

ZAK, R., AND BERKLEY, M. A. (1986). Evoked potentials elicited by brief vernier offsets: estimating vernier thresholds and properties of the neural substrate. *Vision Res.* 26, 439–451.

14 | Sensorimotor adaptation and development of the horopter

CLIFTON M. SCHOR

Perception of space is three-dimensional even though there is an optical transformation of a three-dimensional space onto a two-dimensional retinal image. The three-dimensional percept has a constancy or stability that gives us a spatial sense independent of our specific location or viewpoint at any given moment in time. For example, as we walk about and view objects from different vantage points, the objects appear to remain as rigid shapes despite the marked changes of the two-dimensional image formed on the retina. There is a loss of some information in the two-dimensional image that must be regained in order to perceive a three-dimensional space. Helmholtz (1866) proposed that unconscious inferences or assumptions were made about viewed objects that were not based on information contained in the retinal image. This inferential theory considers perception to be an intelligent process that reasons from experience. Some general examples, based on Euclidean geometry, are that (1) the size of the retinal image increases with object proximity, and (2) objects that are partially occluded or overlapped by another object must be farther away than the unoccluded object. In addition, there are many Euclidean static monocular "artist" cues to depth that are inferred from perspective distortions such as linear perspective, texture gradients, and shadow (Dember and Warm, 1979). Another approach to regaining information about three-dimensional space is to compute spatial relations of objects from two or more views from separate vantage points. These multiple views can be taken sequentially in time, such as in depth stimulated by motion parallax, or simultaneously by separate eyes located at slightly different viewing points. A comparison of these multiple views allows the computation of location and shape of objects in three-dimensional space using Euclidean geometry. This chapter is concerned with the influence of development of the eye on the derivation of differences between the two retinal images used in the spatial senses of stereoscopic depth, direction of motion in depth, and motor control of binocular eye alignment.

BINOCULAR DISPARITY

The slightly different perspective views that the two eyes have of the world yield two retinal images whose individual components have different relative positions. The position of each contour within the retinal image is described on the retina in reference to the fovea. For convenience, retinal locus has been represented in a polar plot as vectors having amplitude and direction. Amplitude or retinal eccentricity is quantified as a visual angle referenced to the nodal point of the eye so that the visual angle of a target in space is the same as the angular subtense of its image on the retina. The reference or origin of the visual angles is the visual axis, which includes the fovea and nodal point of the eye, and presumably the object of regard at which the fovea is directed. Although the direction of points in object space are described with reference to the visual axis at the nodal point of the eye, ultimately we are describing the retinal locus of their image points.

Retinal disparity, or difference in visual directions of a point viewed by the two eyes, is determined by a system of binocular correspondence. These disparities are of binocular, eye-centered, visual directions of objects seen by the two eyes (absolute disparity), and they are compared between multiple points to compute relative disparities (Westheimer, 1979). Absolute disparity can be thought of as the stimulus for change of convergence from one viewing distance to another, whereas relative disparity is the principal stimulus for relative depth perception (stereopsis).

The magnitude and direction of disparities are described in reference to zero retinal image disparity or the same disparity as the angle subtended by the intersection of the two visual axes. Zero disparity is described across the visual field as the *horopter*, or horizon of vision. The horopter describes the locus of points in space that subtend zero disparity or no binocular difference in perceived direction. This operational definition can be restated that the horopter describes the locus of points in space whose images are formed on corresponding retinal points. Hering (1868/1977) defined corresponding points in terms of their "local sign" or perceived direction. When stimulated simultaneously, corresponding points of the same local sign evoked a percept in identical visual directions. The topics of binocular correspondence, fusion, and stereopsis all hinge on the concept of perceived visual direction in reference to the visual axis of each eye. The horopter is used as an analytical tool to quantify disparity, but it also describes the isodisparity curve that the eyes attempt to align with objects in space using convergence and the region of space at which stereoscopic depth perception is most sensitive (Badcock and Schor, 1985).

THEORETICAL LONGITUDINAL HOROPTER

If retinal topography were such that corresponding points were equally spaced from their respective foveas, the horopter would be a circle, lying in the visual plane and passing through the fixation point and nodal points of the two eyes. The circular shape follows from a theory of geometry stating that any two points on a circle subtend equal angles with any other two points on the same circle. Consider two points to be the nodal points of the eyes and a third point to be the fixation point; any other point on the circle can then be imaged at an equal retinal eccentricity in the two eyes from their respective foveas. If retinal regions of approximately equal eccentricity were combined binocularly, as a reference for zero disparity, the horopter (Fig. 14-1) would have a circular shape (Veith-Muller circle, geometric horopter, or theoretical horopter).

Assuming that the nodal point and center of rotation of the eye are close together (0.5 cm), approximately the same circle can be used to describe an isovergence curve on which the visual axes converge during equal (conjugate) angular rotations of the eyes resulting from purely versional eye movements (Ono, 1983). Bifoveal fixation of targets along this circle requires equal versional eye movements, without a vergence component. If the empirical horopter equals this isovergence curve, binocular disparity stimuli and vergence responses are approximately the same. Usually, however, the empirical longitudinal horopter is less curved than the theoretical horopter. In this case an eccentric target on the isovergence circle stimulates a small convergence movement in addition to the horizontal versional movement. A precise motor response is independent of the shape of the horopter and should be a pure versional movement without a vergence component. This discrepancy between stimulus and response increases with stimulus eccentricity and proximity when the horopter deviates from the Vieth-Muller (V-M) circle. The discrepancy is

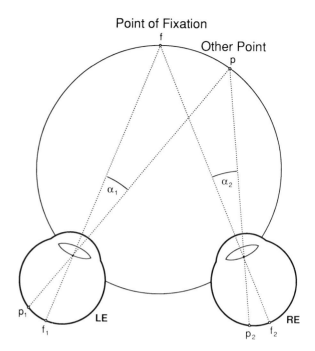

FIG. 14-1. Vieth-Muller circle, the locus of points determined when the included angles α_1 and α_2 are equal. (Adapted from Ogle, 1950, Fig. 3.)

compensated in part by a slight divergence of the eyes during normal saccadic eye movements (Collewijn et al., 1988). For example, during a 20 degree saccade, the eyes may initially diverge by 3 degrees (Maxwell, 1991) and then converge leaving a 0.3 degree divergence component at the end of the saccade (Collewijn et al., 1988). A 2.4 degree divergence error is predicted from Ogle's published measures of the horopter deviation from the V-M circle (Hering Hillebrand deviation = 0.12) (Ogle, 1950). During infancy this divergence compensation may be smaller than in the adult owing to the prismatic barrel distortion of the retinal image produced by angle α.

THEORETICAL VERTICAL HOROPTER

The vertical extent of the theoretical horopter is simply a straight vertical line passing through the V-M circle in the midline (Fig. 14-2). All other points in the visual plane that lie to the left or right of the midline are physically nearer to one eye. The unequal ocular magnification produced by this difference in proximity (Fig. 14-3) causes points above or below the visual plane to be imaged with a vertical disparity, and by definition they do not lie on the horopter or isozero disparity surface. These vertical disparities increase with convergence of the eyes to near targets, lateral displacement away from the midline, and elevation or depression of the test target from the visual plane. The magnitude of

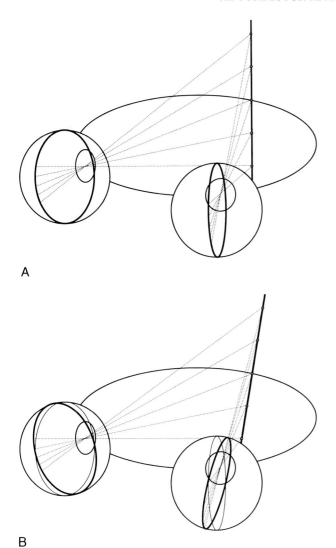

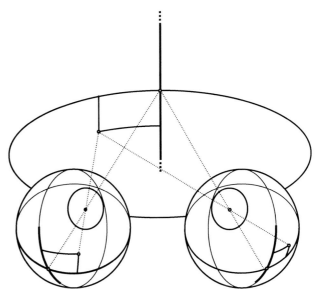

FIG. 14-3. For convergence at any distance other than infinity, all points that do not lie on the Vieth-Muller circle or the midline horopter project to the retina with either a vertical disparity or both a vertical and a horizontal disparity. Dashed lines show the geometric horopter for symmetrical fixation. Construction lines are dotted. Solid lines represent relevant light rays. The vertical disparity arises from the differential magnification that occurs when the point is closer to one eye than the other, as must occur with all points off the vertical axis. The three-dimensional point horopter is therefore not a surface but a line and a circle in space. (Adapted from Ogle, 1950, Fig. 7.4.)

FIG. 14-2. (A) Theoretical vertical horopter is a vertical line only if the corresponding retinal meridia are vertical. (B) Actual vertical horopter is a line slanting away from the observer, which implies that the corresponding retinal meridia (dashed lines) are extorted with respect to the vertical meridia (solid lines). (From Tyler and Scott, 1979. By permission.)

vertical aniseikonia equals the ratio of vertical angles, expressed as sines, subtended by the eccentric target at the entrance pupil of each eye. Normally, the potential diplopic appearance of targets above and below the visual plane is minimized by binocular sensory fusion as well as a slight declination of the empirical vertical horopter. The vertical disparities stimulate both versional and hypervergence motor responses to eccentric targets above or below the visual plane. Because these disparities result exclusively from geometry of horizontal eye placement in the cranium, they are predictable and the oculomotor system is capable of making preprogrammed vertical vergence adjustments to vertical versional movements (Schor et al., 1990). These vertical

vergence components of versional eye movements continue, even when one eye is occluded, which illustrates a form of neuromuscular adaptation. Similar preconditioned horizontal vergence adjustments are made during horizontal versional responses to compensate for deviations of the empirical longitudinal horopter from the V-M circle and isovergence curve (Henson and Dharamski, 1982). There may also be an orientation interaction between vertical disparity and horizontal versional eye movements. Vertical disparity is exclusively associated with eccentric targets that form larger images in the ipsilateral than the contralateral eye. In a Fick coordinate system, vertical vergence demand increases as the eyes move horizontally along a latitude above the visual plane. These horizontal versional movements require a concomitant vertical vergence adjustment to maintain binocular eye alignment. However, in a Helmholtz coordinate system, the vertical vergence stimulus is zero in all tertiary directions of gaze (Simonsz et al., 1990).

The presence of a vertical magnification of one eye's image may be associated with preconditioned larger horizontal and vertical movements of the eye with the larger ocular image. Although this prediction has not been tested, Morrison (1977) demonstrated a preconditioned vertical vergence component, described in a

Fick coordinate system, associated with versional movements to near targets displaced horizontally from the midline, whereby vertical versional movements of the abducted eye were larger than conjugate vertical movements of the adducted eye. Depending on the biological coordinate systems used by the ocular motor system, these observations could demonstrate a modification or continued recalibration of the yoking response described by Hering's law of versional movements. Any conditions that alter the predictable relation between target location and the versional motor response require recalibration of binocularly yoked eye movements. Recalibration is a neuromuscular adaptation in response to vertical and horizontal disparities produced by orbital geometry and the organization of binocular correspondence. Vertical disparities may also provide perceptual cues to disambiguate binocular stimuli for horizontal slant, which varies with target distance and eccentricity (Gillum and Lawergern, 1983). The influence of developmental factors on the interpretation of vertical disparity is discussed later in the chapter.

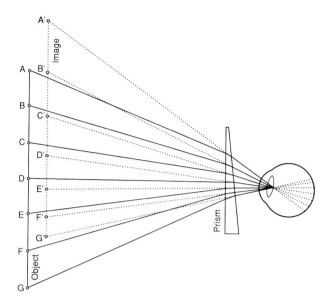

FIG. 14-4. Unsymmetrical angular magnification and distortion introduced by a flat ophthalmic prism. (Adapted from Ogle, 1950.)

EMPIRICAL LONGITUDINAL HOROPTER

The shape of the empirical longitudinal horopter (ELH) differs from the theoretical (geometrical) horopter in two ways. The curvature and slant symmetry of the ELH differ from the V-M circle at the point of fixation. There are many measures of the ELH based, for example, on disparity criteria such as singleness (haplopia), dichoptic vernier (nonius) alignment (identical visual directions), peak stereoacuity, and the null stimulus to vergence; or they may be based on perceived distance estimates such as the apparent frontoparallel plane, which are influenced by disparity as well as other distance cues (Ogle, 1950). All criteria result in measures of the ELH that are flatter, or less curved, than the V-M circle and that are tilted away from one eye. The degree of curvature change from the V-M circle is referred to as the Hering-Hillebrand deviation, which is quantified as a difference between nonuniform magnification of the two retinal images, such as that produced by an ophthalmic prism, which progressively minifies images seen through the prism base (Fig. 14-4) (Ogle, 1950).

If base-out prism is placed before both eyes, visual space is compressed in the temporal field of each eye. To stimulate identical visual directions (IVDs), targets must be placed at greater eccentricities in the temporal field than in their corresponding eccentricities in the nasal field of the other eye (Fig. 14-5). The locus of points in space that satisfy the IVD criterion, in the presence of base-out prism, is a curve that is flatter than the V-M circle. Normally, the curvature of the ELH is influenced by the alignment of the pupil and fovea with the optical axis of the eye. The symmetrical misalign-

ment of the pupil and fovea in the two eyes produces nonuniform vertical and horizontal disparities between the two ocular images.

The optic axis of the eye contains the center of curvature of both the lens and the corneal surface. Usually the eye pupil is displaced nasalward to the optic axis by 3 degrees in the adult eye (Bennett and Bavvetts, 1989). The pupillary axis contains the center of the

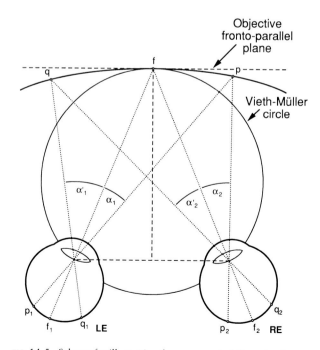

FIG. 14-5. Scheme for illustrating the asymmetrical distortion between the images in the two eyes for points lying on horopter curves that do not coincide with the Vieth-Muller circle. (Adapted from Davson, 1962, Fig. 9.)

entrance pupil, and it is perpendicular to the surface of the cornea. The locus of the fovea is described by the line of sight that contains the fovea and center of the exit pupil as well as the object of regard and center of the entrance pupil. The locus of the fovea is also described by the visual axis, which contains the fovea and posterior nodal point of the eye (Fig. 14-8).

Misalignment of the pupil from the line of sight is described clinically as angle λ (the angle between the pupillary axis and primary line of sight). Angle λ is sometimes referred to as angle kappa, which is the angle formed between the pupillary axis and the visual axis. The misalignment of the fovea from the optical axis is described by angle α, which is the angle formed between the visual axis and optic axis at the posterior nodal point of the eye. Angle λ is the only angle routinely measured clinically to quantify alignment of the pupil and line of sight (Alpern, 1969).

Shape distortion of the retinal image results from anterior sagittal and lateral displacement of the entrance pupil from the anterior nodal point of the eye. The anterior placement of the pupil from the nodal point is likely to produce a barrel distortion of the retinal image whereby small images are magnified more than large ones (Fincham, 1959). With barrel distortion, an object consisting of concentric rings of equal angular spacing is imaged as concentric rings whose separation diminishes with eccentricity or radius of curvature. With this type of distortion a square object is imaged as a bowed barrel shape. This barrel distortion can be skewed or made asymmetrical about the optic axis by lateral displacement of the pupil from the optic axis. Given the high dioptric power of the lens-cornea combination, these distortions may be considerable. Finally, the barrel distortion may be partially compensated for or corrected by the retinal (screen) curvature. The center of curvature of the retina is approximately 0.5 cm posterior to the nodal point of the eye, and this discrepancy tends to produce a pincushion distortion that partially cancels the barrel distortion caused by displacement of the entrance pupil from the anterior nodal point of the eye.

Barrel distortion would have no influence on binocular vision and the horopter if the fovea were aligned with the optic axis of the eye. Measures of angle λ, however, indicate that the fovea is displaced approximately 5 degrees temporalward on the retina from the optic axis of the adult eye. Assuming that the barrel distortion is symmetrical about the optic axis, angle λ displaces the foveas temporalward toward a compressed region of the retinal image that corresponds to the nasal visual field. The distortion that results is similar to that produced by base-in prism worn before the eyes. The nasal visual field before each eye can appear compressed (Ogle, 1950; Brown, 1953) and result in an increased curvature of the ELH with respect to the

V-M circle. Barrel distortion also produces vertical disparities between bowed or curved images of horizontal lines, viewed off-axis at the visual axis, and horizontal disparities between bowed images of vertical lines. For example, images of vertical lines passing through the foveas (temporal on the retina from the optic axis) are curved to produce variations of horizontal disparity along the vertical horopter, which has a concave distortion at the fixation point. Angle λ decreases during development from 10 degrees in the neonate to 5 degrees in the adult. This change should reduce shape distortion of the retinal image as well as the off-axis placement of the fovea from the optic axis and produce predictable changes in the curvature of the ELH during development of the optical parameters of the eye.

The slant, or tilt, of the ELH away from one eye is quantified as a uniform magnification of one ocular image (aniseikonia) produced, for example, by a difference in axial length or normally in asymmetrical convergence. When the horopter is tilted about a vertical axis, corresponding retinal points lie at greater eccentricities from the fovea of one eye than the other. The locus of points in space that satisfy the IVD criterion, in the presence of aniseikonia, is a curve that is tilted toward the eye with the optically magnified retinal image. For example, magnification of the left eye's image produces a counterclockwise rotation of the ELH (Fig. 14-6). In addition to optical factors, there are neurological sources of uniform and nonuniform binocular

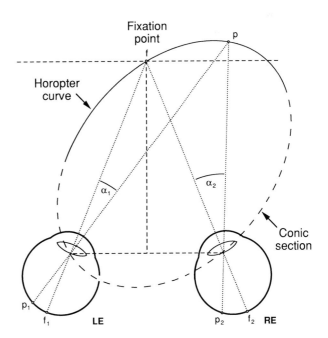

FIG. 14-6. Rotated position of a conic section corresponding to the ELH due to a difference in the magnifications of images in the two eyes. Here magnification of the dioptric image in the left eye (L.E.) is larger than that in the right (R.E.); therefore the sizes of the corresponding angles that null size differences are reversed. (Adapted from Ogle, 1950, Fig. 11.)

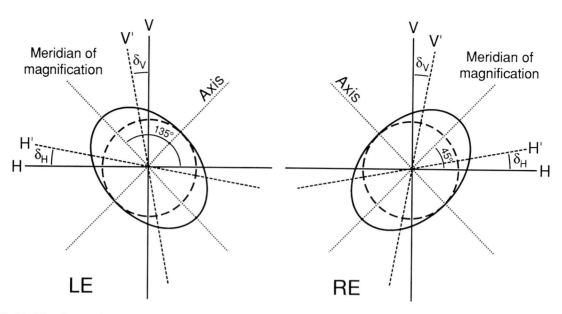

FIG. 14-7. Meridional magnification of images in the two eyes in oblique meridians cause "scissors" or rotary deviations of images of vertical (and horizontal) lines and affect stereoscopic spatial locali-zation in a characteristic manner. (From Ogle and Boeder, 1948. By permission.)

disparities (Brown, 1953) that are a product of the mapping the two ocular images onto binocular neurons in cortical hypercolumns.

EMPIRICAL VERTICAL HOROPTER

The empirical vertical horopter (EVH) as shown by Volkmann (1859) and Helmholtz (1866) is tilted backward or declinated from the theoretical vertical horopter as a result of an extorsion of corresponding vertical meridians by almost 2 degrees. No such tilt of corresponding meridians appears in the horizontal meridian, as would be expected if the tilt resulted from a binocular excyclotorsion eye movement. Consequently, the selective tilt of the vertical meridia is thought to result from a horizontal shear of retinal correspondence (Helmholtz, 1866; Nakayama, 1977; Tyler, 1983, 1991). The locus of points in space imaged on these extorted vertical meridia is a vertical line, tilted backward or declinated by an amount that would increase with viewing distance until at infinity the vertical horopter becomes horizontal (i.e., parallel to the ground plane). It also broadens from a thin line to a plane because at infinity points at all eccentricities are equidistant from the two eyes and there is no aniseikonia or image magnification asymmetry of peripheral targets above and below the visual plane. The relation between orientation of the vertical horopter with respect to the ground plane (β) and viewing distance (b) is tan β = IPD/(b * tan ɸ), where IPD = the interpupillary distance and ɸ = the excyclotorsion disparity of the two corresponding vertical meridia (Ogle, 1950; Howard, 1982).

The tilt of the vertical horopter is produced by an optical intorsion of the two retinal images or a neurological extorsion of the monocular components of a map of binocular correspondence. Oblique, mirror symmetrical astigmatism is one possible physiological optical source for the optical intorsion of the two retinal images. A mirror symmetrical intorsion of the axes of astigmatism (expressed as minus cylinder) causes a scissoring distortion or axis rotation of all meridians toward the axis of astigmatism (Fig. 14-7) (Ogle, 1950). An oculomotor source of tilt of the vertical horopter is ocular excyclotorsion, which normally increases by several degrees with convergence and depression of the eyes to a near viewing distance (Alpern, 1969; Nakayama, 1983). The advantage of the declinated vertical horopter is to allow single binocular views of the ground plane while locomoting and fixating on distant objects and to allow single binocular views of upright planes of near vertical objects. The magnitude of declination might be environmentally tuned; if so, it would be expected to decrease with the development of body height or distance of the eyes from the ground plane when gaze is directed downward toward the horizon or any other point on the ground plane.

DEVELOPMENT OF OCULAR PARAMETERS

This chapter considers the influence of the development of three ocular parameters—axial length, interpupillary distance (IPD), and retinal mosaic density—and their effect on the shape and orientation of the empirical horopter, as well as on binocular sensory functions (in-

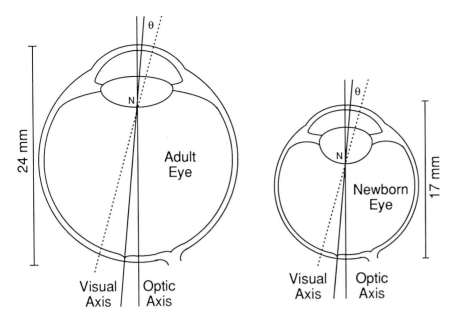

FIG. 14-8. Adult and newborn eyes showing the optic axis that passes through the center of the pupil and the visual axis that intersects the fovea on the retina (angle α). This angular discrepancy between the optic and visual axes is larger in the newborn than in the adult. The dashed line represents a constant angle (θ) with respect to the visual axis. Note that because of the difference in eye size the distance (in millimeters) on the retina between the visual axis and this dashed line is greater in the adult than in the newborn. N = posterior nodal point. (Adapted from Yonas, 1988, Fig. 5.1.)

cluding fusion, stereopsis, and direction of motion in depth) and binocular control of versional eye movements. All three developmental factors undergo marked changes during the first 1.5 years of life. The axial length of the neonate is 17 mm, and it increases to 24 mm during adulthood (Larsen, 1971). Most of the growth in axial length occurs during the first year of life (Hirano et al., 1979; Howland, 1982) and then increases gradually until the end of the second decade of life (Fig. 14-8). This change in axial length is correlated with a decrease in angle λ (Chavasse, 1939) from 10 degrees in the neonate to 5 degrees in the adult eye (Donders, 1864); 90% of this change takes place during the first 1.5 years (Slater and Findlay, 1972; London and Wick, 1982). The macula remains at a fixed distance temporal to the optic disc throughout life (Streeten, 1969), but the depth of both the anterior and posterior chambers increases. This combination produces changes in the position of the entrance pupil and angle λ (London and Wick, 1982) and brings the visual axis into closer alignment with the optical axis of the eye. Elongation of the eye reduces the physiological base-in prism distortion that magnifies corresponding features in the two retinal images nonuniformly in the region of the fovea. The interpupillary separation increases by 60% from 4.0 cm in the neonate to approximately 6.5 cm in the adult (Aslin and Jackson, 1979), with most of the change occurring during the first year of life (Larsen, 1971; Birnholtz, 1985). Finally, the density of foveal cones in the neonate increases as a result of centripetal cone

migration during the first 1.5 years of life (Yuodelis and Hendrickson, 1986). The result is an increase in retinal mosaic density at the fovea and presumably an improvement of spatial resolution. The migration of cones may not be uniform or coordinated in the two eyes such that both nonuniform and uniform magnification errors between the eyes may be changing abruptly during the first 1.5 years of life.

INFLUENCE OF GROWTH PARAMETERS ON THE EMPIRICAL HOROPTER

Angle λ

As mentioned earlier in the section describing the curvature of the ELH, nonuniform magnification errors, produced by developmental changes in prismatic distortion of angle λ, decrease the curvature of the horopter relative to the V-M circle. This change in curvature is quantified as the rate of change of magnification across the visual field (Hering-Hillebrand deviation, or H). The value of H increases from zero for the V-M circle to a normal value of approximately 0.12 in the adult eye (Ogle, 1950) where $H = \Delta \text{ mag}/\Delta \tan \phi$, where ϕ = the eccentricity from the fovea across the right eye's visual field and Δ mag equals ($\tan \alpha_R/\tan \alpha_L$). Because several optical factors of the infant eye are unknown, including the slant of the lens with respect to the retina, curvature of lenticular surfaces, index of refraction gradients, and center of retinal curvature, the exact distortions of the retinal image are unknown. However, qualitative predictions can be made about changes in distortion based on known changes in refractive state and axial length. The large angle λ suggests that the neonate horopter has a curvature similar to that of the V-M circle. As the axial length increases during development, the power of the lens and cornea decrease along with a reduction of angle λ. This optical growth reduces barrel shape distortions that produce vertical disparity and curvature of the vertical horopter and causes a flattening of the ELH from the V-M circle. Growth in interpupillary distance (IPD) also decreases the horopter curvature because as IPD increases the radius of curvature of the V-M circle increases. Because the Hering-Hillebrand deviation is described in reference to the curvature of the V-M circle, as IPD increases both the V-M circle and ELH are flattened during development. The influence of the IPD on the radius of curvature of the V-M circle is inversely related to the viewing distance. IPD has little or no effect on the radius of curvature of the V-M circle at optical infinity; but at near viewing distances, as the IPD approaches the diameter of the V-M circle it has its maximum influence during growth. For a viewing distance of 20 cm, the radius of curvature of the V-M circle increases from 10.10 cm in the infant to 10.26 cm in the adult. Together the development of axial length and IPD should reduce prismatic distortion and cause a decrease in horopter curvature (i.e., an increase in H).

IPD

Increased IPD also produces proportional increases in sensitivity to relative disparity and stereoscopic depth of static and moving targets. The increase in IPD may contribute to the postnatal appearance of stereoscopic vision at 3–4 months of age (Birch et al., 1982). In addition to depth perception, the rate and phase of horizontal retinal image motion provides information about the direction a moving target is traveling with respect to the head (Regan et al., 1989). As demonstrated in Figure 14-9, when the retinal image motion is equal in velocity and phase, the corresponding object is moving in the frontoparallel plane or more precisely along the V-M circle. So long as image motion is in phase, the corresponding target does not collide with the observer's head. If retinal image motion in the two eyes is in phase but they have unequal velocities, the corresponding target is moving at an oblique angle toward the eye with the lower image velocity. If the image motion is in antiphase, the object collides with the observer's head. The velocity of antiphase motion increases with IPD; however, the direction of motion, as interpreted from the phase relation of the two retinal

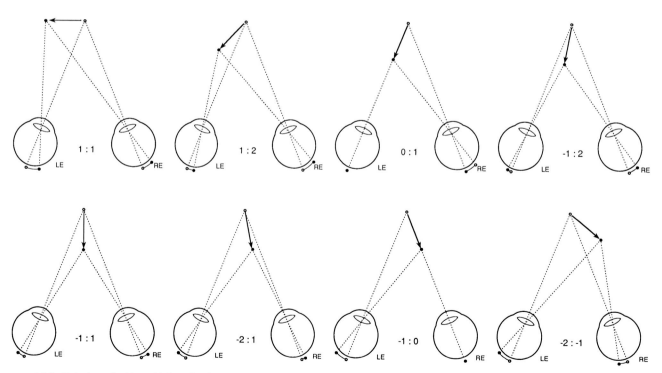

FIG. 14-9. Relative velocities of left and right retinal images for different target trajectories. When the target moves along a line passing between the eyes, its retinal images move in opposite directions in the two eyes; when the target moves along a line passing wide of the head, the retinal images move in the same direction, but with different speeds. The ratio of left-eye and right-eye image velocities (V_L/V_R) provides an unequivocal indication of the direction of motion in depth. (Adapted from Beverly and Regan, 1973.)

images, is unaffected by increasing IPD. The change in antiphase velocity produced by increasing the IPD requires some form of postnatal recalibration for veridical perception of the amplitude of motion in depth.

The increase in IPD also influences the empirical vertical horopter by increasing image size differences of eccentrically viewed targets and their vertical disparity, when they are positioned above or below the visual plane. The influence of IPD growth on vertical disparity increases with target proximity and eccentricity from the midline. The field of geometrical disparities of a flat (frontoparallel) plane viewed at 20 cm is shown in Figure 14-10 (Nakayama, 1977). The field size is 38 degrees from the center in each direction. Relatively large disparities (> 1 degree) occur at large eccentricities under conditions that emulate reading. These normal vertical disparities of eccentrically viewed targets may provide information about target slant or tilt about a vertical axis (Householder, 1943; Petrov, 1980, Morrison, 1977; Longuet-Higgens and Mayhew, 1982; Gillam and Lawergren, 1988); however, these benefits have not been verified (Cumming et al., 1991). Vertical disparity may also provide a retinal cue for viewing distance that is used to scale perceived depth from horizontal disparity (Rogers and Bradshaw, 1993). Slant about the vertical axis and overall image size differences between the two ocular images contribute to the horizontal disparity of eccentrically viewed targets. Overall size differences between the two ocular images introduce both horizontal and vertical disparities, whereas slant produces only horizontal disparity. The vertical disparity could pro-vide a baseline reference for uniform magnification differences between the two retinal images from which to gauge horizontal disparity caused by target slant. Development of IPD increases both sources of horizontal disparity; however, horizontal disparity from slant or tilt increases more than horizontal and vertical disparity from the overall size difference such that the increased vertical disparity would only partially compensate for exaggerations in stereotilt about the vertical axis caused by increasing the IPD. Consequently, as IPD increases with age, these potential perceptual functions may require recalibration.

Centripetal Cone Migration

Effects of changing retinal mosaic density on the shape and orientation of the empirical horopter are the most difficult to predict, as they may not be uniform and they may lack coordination between the eyes. However, centripetal cone migration along with increasing axial length predictably results in a doubling of foveal cone mosaic density at 15 months of age and a quadrupling of cone density by adulthood (Banks and Bennett, 1988). Accompanying these changes are an increase of spatial resolution and contrast sensitivity (Banks, 1988). Both stereopsis and binocular sensory fusion improve with spatial resolution, and stereoacuity improves with contrast sensitivity (Schor, 1985). Retinal disparities, which are quantified with respect to the horopter, are processed within spatial channels or filters whose dimensions limit the range of disparity that can be encoded by the visual system (Marr and Poggio, 1976). Both stereo thresholds and Panum's fusional limits increase proportionally with the size of detail or the spatial periods that are processed optimally by band-pass spatial channels. Stereo thresholds and Panum's fusional areas (PFAs) are lowest when measured with spatial frequencies higher than 2.5 cycles per degree (cpd) and they both increase to at least 6 degrees at the fovea when measured with spatial frequencies as low as 0.075 cpd (Fig. 14-11) (Schor et al., 1984). Clearly, the emergence of higher spatial frequency channels with development will influence both stereo acuity and the dimensions of the PFA. The peak of the contrast sensitivity function reaches 2.5 cpd at 5–6 months of age (Pirchio et al., 1978), which coincides approximately with the emergence and rapid development of stereopsis (Birch et al., 1982) and fusional vergence eye movements (Aslin, 1977). Prior to the development of spatial resolution and contrast sensitivity, enlarged Panum's areas associated with reduced visual acuity minimize the distortions of space perception that could result from distorted horizontal and vertical disparities caused by growth of IPD, axial length, and nonuniform variations in retinal mosaic density during the first year of development.

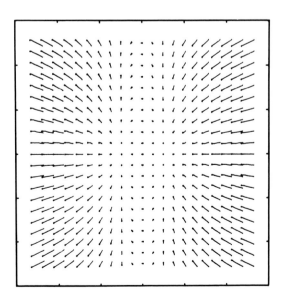

FIG. 14-10. Field of geometrical disparity of a flat plane viewed at 20 cm and slightly in front of the fixation point. Field size is ± 38 degrees in each direction. Relatively large disparity can occur in peripheral regions under conditions that might occur while reading or writing. (From Nakayama, 1977. By permission.)

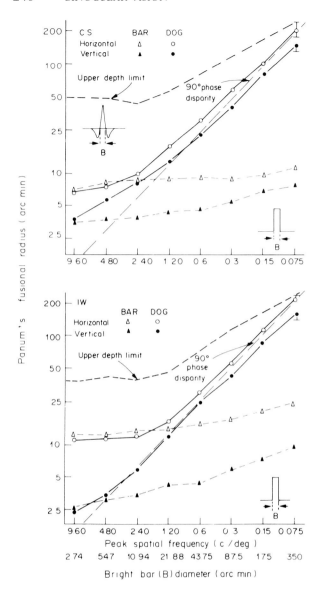

FIG. 14-11. Diplopia thresholds for two subjects are plotted as a function of the bright bar width (B) of the bar and the Difference Of two Gaussian functions (DOG). Luminance profiles of these two test stimuli are inset below and above the data, respectively. A constant phase disparity of 90 degrees is shown by the dashed diagonal line. Horizontal and vertical Panum's fusion ranges (solid lines) coincide with the 90-degree phase disparity for DOG widths greater than 21 arc minute. At the broadest DOG width, the upper fusion limit equals the upper disparity limit for stereoscopic depth perception (bold dashed line). The standard deviation of the mean is shown for the broadest DOG stimulus. At narrow DOG widths, both horizontal and vertical fusion limits approach a constant minimum threshold. Panum's fusion ranges remain fairly constant when measured with bar patterns (dotted lines) and resemble values obtained with high spatial frequency DOGs. (From Schor et al., 1984. By permission.)

Enlarged PFAs do not account for the lack of fusional vergence eye movements prior to 4 months of age. Panum's area does not set a lower limit to the size of disparity vergence responses, as clearly disparity vergence responses of adults are stimulated by disparities within the PFA (< 5 arc minute) (Riggs and Neihle, 1960;

Duwaer and van den Brink, 1981). The disparity vergence response, like optical reflex accommodation, is a fine adjustment mechanism that refines the coarse distance adjustments of gaze initiated by perceived distance (Schor et al., 1992). Large disparities (greater than several degrees) are ineffective stimuli for stereopsis (Schor and Wood, 1983) and disparity vergence (Rashbass and Westheimer, 1961; Schor et al., 1986; Erkelens, 1987). Vergence responses to large prismatic disparities (> 2 degrees) may be an acquired skill that infants do not learn until they gain experience adjusting vergence in response to smaller retinal image disparities. Prior to that age, vergence alignment of the eyes may be stimulated coarsely by accommodative vergence (Schor and Kotulak, 1986) and by proximal cues to distance (McLin et al., 1988) with extraretinal feedback used for maintaining binocular eye alignment (Schor et al., 1992). For a complete description of the development of accommodation and vergence see Chapter 3.

HERING'S LAW OF YOKED VERSIONAL EYE MOVEMENTS

In addition to convergence, which allows the eye to fuse objects binocularly at various viewing distances, binocular vision also relies on yoked conjugate eye movements to maintain a fixed vergence angle while shifting gaze with saccades and pursuits to peripheral regions of the visual field. Ling (1942) first observed conjugate binocular following eye movements of all types (fast and slow) and in all directions in 75 infants during the first 48 hours of life. She reported that the onset of convergence was delayed nearly 2 months in the same infants. There are sparse reports of an apparent lack of conjugacy or independent eye rotation in neonates (Guernsey, 1929), but these observations may have been of mixed versional and accommodative vergence movements, both of which are present in neonates (Aslin and Jackson, 1979). These observations demonstrate that the neural control mechanisms for conjugate eye movements are present at birth.

Hering's law describes this conjugacy as equal movements of the eyes guided by a common source of innervational control. As described above, deviations of the ELH from the V-M and isovergence circles produce a discrepancy between the versional stimulus and its motor response. For example, if the ELH were equal to the frontoparallel plane, a lateral target shift along the frontoparallel plane to an eccentric retinal locus would stimulate a pure versional tracking response along the isovergence circle and result in a noticeable convergence error (Fig. 14-5). This error is normally prevented by preprogramming a vergence component into the versional response (Schor et al., 1990; Schor, Gleason, Maxwell et al., 1993; Maxwell and Schor, 1993).

The vertical horopter also places demands on binocular vertical versional eye movements to near targets that are displaced in asymmetrical vergence, horizontally away from the midline. Because these targets are closer to one eye than the other, vertical movements of the closer eye must be greater than those of the more distant eye to maintain bifoveal fixation. This vertical disparity increases with target proximity, eccentricity, and height from the visual plane. The problem becomes exacerbated by the postnatal increase in IPD during the first 2 years of life, which produce a proportional increase in vertical disparity of off-midline targets. Accordingly, as IPD develops, Hering's yoking ratio for both vertical and horizontal eye movements must be recalibrated for near targets at large eccentricites.

Vertical disparity is described above in either Fick's Cartesian coordinate system, which has an earth referenced vertical axis, or Listing's polar coordinate system, whose single axis lies in Listing's plane and is perpendicular to both the primary and tertiary eye directions. When described in Helmholtz Cartesian coordinates, which have an earth referenced horizontal axis, targets in tertiary positions do not subtend vertical stimuli for vergence, or vertical disparity is not represented explicitly for vergence as it is in the other co-ordinate systems. Similarly, the innervational pattern to the extraocular muscles needed to bifoveally fixate these tertiary positions depends on the coordinate system used to control eye movements. Binocular fixation of a single point in tertiary gaze using either the Fick or Listing coordinate systems requires unequal vertical components of rotation by the two eyes, whereas the Helmholtz coordinate system requires equal vertical rotation of the two eyes (Lemij and Collewijn, 1992). Studies of ocular torsion in tertiary eye positions strongly suggest that it is appropriate to use Listing's coordinate system to describe movements of the eyes to tertiary positions (Nakayama, 1983). Accordingly, vertical components of binocular eye movements, using the same Listing coordinate system that describes ocular torsion, would require unequal binocular innervation for the vertical components of eye position to fixate targets in tertiary gaze. The vertical disparity subtended by tertiary targets would require nonconjugate vertical saccades and pursuits.

Preprogramming the vergence component of versional eye movements is more important for vertical than horizontal shifts of gaze because the vertical vergence system lacks the fast motor fusional response (<1 second) that characterizes horizontal disparity vergence

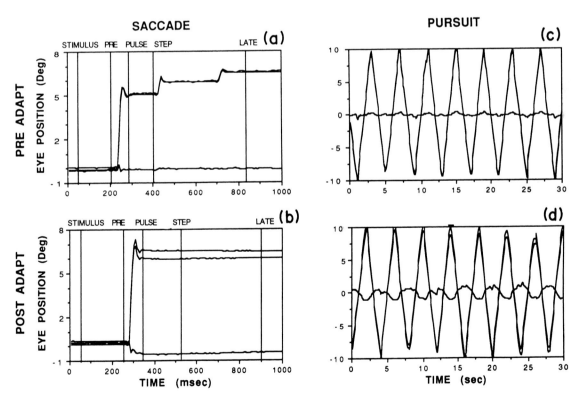

FIG. 14-12. Simultaneous vertical saccadic movements of the right and left eyes, stimulated monocularly, and their difference (right − left) (vergence − lower line) are shown before (A) and after (B) binocular adaptation to the 10% afocal magnifier worn over the left eye. (B) Post-adapted vergence component synchronized with the onset of the saccade. Simultaneous vertical pursuit movements of the right and left eyes, stimulated monocularly, and their difference (vergence-central line) are shown before (C) and after (D) binocular adaptation to the 10% afocal magnifier worn over the right eye. (D) Post-adapted vergence component that was evident after only 15 minutes of adaptation. (From Schor et al., 1990. By permission.)

(Rashbass and Westheimer, 1961). Vertical vergence responses to vertical disparity have limited amplitude (< 1 degree) and long durations (> 5 seconds) (Houtman et al., 1977; Kertesz, 1983). However, more rapid vertical vergence responses can occur when they are combined with vertical versional movements such as saccades (Enright, 1984) and pursuits (Schor et al., 1990; Schor, Gleason and Lunn, 1993; Gleason et al., 1993). Repeated exposure to vertically disparate versional stimuli for as little as 1 hour produces motor aftereffects that alter the yoking ratio (YR) of vertical eye movements. The YR is quantified with one eye occluded as the amplitude ratio of tracking movements of the seeing and occluded eye. This ratio of movements can be altered by placing an afocal overall magnifier over one eye and tracking the unequal image motion binocularly for approximately 1 hour. Vertical YRs are altered by as much as 10–15% as a result of aniseikonic image motion of the same magnitude. If during adaptation there is exclusive tracking of aniseikonic image motion by saccades or pursuits, aftereffects mainly influence the conjugacy of the adapted class of versional eye movements. For example, pursuit adaptation to aniseikonic image motion produces marked adaptation of the pursuit YR (Fig. 14-12C,D), whereas it has negligible effects on the saccade YR. Saccade adaptation to aniseikonic image displacements change the saccade YR (Fig. 14-12A,B) twice as much as the pursuit YR. These observations demonstrate independent adaptation of conjugate yoking of saccadic and pursuit versional eye movements.

In addition to these dynamic adjustments, vertical and horizontal eye alignment or phoria can adapt to static variations of prism across the visual field. This static adaptation of the phoria in one direction in the visual field spreads over a range of 12 degrees to other regions of the field (Schor, Gleason, Maxwell et al., 1993; Maxwell and Schor, 1993). Both the static and dynamic adaptable binocular motor mechanisms are needed to compensate for the motor responses to spatial distortions produced by rapid growth of axial length and IPD during the first year of life.

REFERENCES

ALPERN, M. (1969). Types of movements. In H. DAVSON (ed.). *The Eye*. Vol. 3. Orlando, FL: Academic Press, pp. 65–74.

ASLIN, R. N. (1977). Development of binocular fixation in human infants. *J. Exp. Child Psychol.* 23, 133–150.

ASLIN, R. N., AND JACKSON, R. W. (1979). Accommodative convergence in young infants: development of a synergistic sensory-motor system. *Can. J. Psychol.* 33, 222–231.

BADCOCK, D. R., AND SCHOR, C. M. (1985). Depth increment detection function for individual spatial channels. *J. Opt. Soc. Am.* 2, 1211–1216.

BANKS, M. S. (1988). Visual recalibration and the development of contrast and optical flow perception. In A. YONAS (ed.). *Perception Development in Infancy. The Minnesota Symposia on Child Psychology*. Vol. 20. Hillsdale, NJ: Erlbaum, pp. 145–196.

BANKS, M. S., AND BENNETT, P. (1988). Optical and photoreceptor immaturities limit the spatial and chromatic vision of human neonates. *J. Opt. Soc. Am.* [A] 5, 2059–2079.

BENNETT, A. G., AND BAVVETTS, R. B. (1989). *Clinical Visual Optics*. Boston: Butterworths.

BIRCH, E. E., GWIAZDA, J., AND HELD, R. (1982). Stereoacuity development for crossed and uncrossed disparities in human infants. *Vision Res.* 22, 507–514.

BIRNHOLZ (1985). Ultrasonic fetal ophthalmology. *Early Hum. Dev.* 12, 199–209.

BROWN, K. T. (1953). Factors affecting differences in apparent size between opposite halves of a visual meridian. *J. Opt. Soc. Am.* 43, 464–472.

CHAVASSE, F. B. (1939). *Worth's Squint: or the Binocular Reflexes and the Treatment of Strabismus*. Philadelphia: Blakiston, p. 449.

COLLEWIJN, H., ERKELENS, C. A., AND STEINMAN, R. M. (1988). Binocular co-ordination of human horizontal saccadic eye movements. *J. Physiol. (Lond.)* 404, 157–182.

CUMMING, B. G., JOHNSTON, E. B., AND PARKER, A. J. (1991). Vertical disparities and perception of three-dimensional shape. *Nature*. 349, 411–413.

DEMBER, W., AND WARM, J. (1979). *Psychology of Perception*. New York: Holt, Rinehart and Winston.

DONDERS, F. C. (1864). *On the Anomalies of Accommodation and Refraction of the Eye* (translated by W. D. MOORE). London: Sydenham Society.

DUWAER, A. L., AND VAN DEN BRINK, G. (1981). Diplopia thresholds and the initiation of vergence eye-movements. *Vision Res.* 21, 1727–1737.

ENRIGHT, J. T. (1984). Changes in vergence mediated by saccades. *J. Physiol. (Lond.)* 350, 9–31.

ERKELENS, C. J. (1987). Adaptation of ocular vergence to stimulation with large disparities. *Exp. Brain Res.* 66, 507–516.

FINCHAM, W. H. A. (1959). *Optics*. London: Hatton Press, p. 379.

GILLAM, B., AND LAWERGREN, B. (1983). The included effect, vertical disparity and stereoscopic theory. *Percept. Psychophys.* 34, 121–130.

GLEASON, G., SCHOR, C., LUNN, R., AND MAXWELL, J. (1993). Directionally selective short-term nonconjugate adaptation of vertical pursuits. *Vision Res.* 33, 65–71.

GUERNSEY, M. (1929). A quantitative study of the eye reflexes in infants. *Psychol. Bull.* 26, 160.

HELMHOLTZ, H. L., VON (1866). *Handbuck der Physiologische Optik*. Hamburg: Voss.

HENSON, D. B., AND DHARAMSKI, B. G. (1982). Oculomotor adaptation to induced heterophoria and anisometropia. *Invest. Ophthalmol. Vis. Sci.* 22, 234–240.

HERING, E. (1868/1977). *The Theory of Binocular Vision* (translated by B. BRIDGEMAN AND L. STARK). New York: Plenum Press.

HIRANO, S., YAMAMOTO, Y., TAKAYAMA, H., SUGATA, Y., AND MATSUO, K. (1979). Ultrasonic observation of eyes in premature babies. Part 6. *Acta Soc. Ophthalmol. Japon.* 83, 1679–1693.

HOUSEHOLDER, A. S. (1943). A theory of the induced size effect. *Bull. Math. Biophys.* 51, 155–160.

HOUTMAN, W. A., ROZE, J. H., AND SCHEPER, W. (1977). Vertical motor fusion. *Doc. Ophthalmol.* 44, 179–185.

HOWARD, I. P. (1982). Visual direction with respect to head and body. In *Human Visual Orientation*. New York: Wiley, pp. 275–341.

HOWLAND, H. C. (1982). *Infant Eyes: Optics and Accomodation*.

KERTESZ, A. (1983). Vertical and cyclofusional disparity vergence. In C. M. SCHOR AND K. CUIFFREDA (eds.). *Vergence Eye Movements: Basic and Clinical Aspects*. Boston: Butterworths, pp. 317–346.

LARSEN, S. J. (1971). Sagittal growth of the eye. II. Ultrasonic measures of the axial length of the eye from birth to puberty. *Acta Ophthalmol. (Copenh.)* 49, 873–886.

LEMIJ, H. G., AND COLLEWIJN, H. (1992). Nonconjugate adaptation of human saccades to anisometropic spectacles: meridian-specificity. *Vision Res.* 32, 453–464.

LING, B. C. (1942). A genetic study of sustained fixation and associated behavior in the human infant from birth to six months. *J. Genet. Psychol.* 61, 227–277.

LONDON, R., AND WICK, B. C. (1982). Changes in angle lambda during growth: theory and clinical application. *Am. J. Optom. Physiol. Opt.* 59, 560–572.

LONGUET-HIGGINS, H. C., AND MAYHEW, J. E. W. (1982). A computational model of binocular depth perception. *Nature* 297, 376–378.

MARR, D., AND POGGIO, T. (1976). A computational theory of human stereo version. *Proc. R. Soc.* 204, 310–328.

MAXWELL, J. (1991). The interaction of saccades and vergence eye movements and the effect of vergence angle on the discharge rate of abducens neurons in monkeys. PhD dissertation, University of Rochester, Center for Visual Sciences.

MAXWELL, J. S., AND SCHOR, C. M. (1993). Mechanisms of vertical phoria adaptations revealed by time course and two dimensional spatiotopic maps. *Vision Res.* In Press.

McLIN, L., SCHOR, C. M., AND KRUGER, P. (1988). Changing size (looming) as a stimulus to accommodation and vergence. *Vision Res.* 28, 883–898.

MORRISON, L. C. (1977). Stereoscopic localization with the eyes asymmetrically converged. *Am. J. Optom. Physiol. Opt.* 54, 556–566.

NAKAYAMA, K. (1977). Geometrical and physiological aspects of depth perception. *Proc. SPIE* 120, 1–8.

NAKAYAMA, K. (1983). Kinematics of normal and strabismic eyes. In C. M. SCHOR AND K. CUIFFREDA (eds.). *Vergence Eye Movements: Basic and Clinical Aspects.* Boston: Butterworths, pp. 543–564.

OGLE, K. N. (1950). *Researchers in Binocular Vision.* Philadelphia: Saunders.

OGLE, K. N., AND BOEDER, P. (1948). Distortion of stereoscopic spatial localization. *J. Opt. Soc. Am.* 38, 723–733.

ONO, H. (1983). The combination of version and vergence. In C. M. SCHOR AND K. CUIFFREDA (eds.). *Vergence Eye Movements: Basic and Clinical Aspects.* Boston: Butterworths, pp. 373–397.

PETROV, A. P. (1980). A geometrical explanation of the induced effect. *Vision Res.* 20, 407–413.

PIRCHIO, M., SPINELLI, D., AND FIORENTINI, A. (1978). Infant contrast sensitivity evaluated by evoked potentials. *Brain Res.* 141, 179–184.

RASHBASS, C., AND WESTHEIMER, G. (1961). Disjunctive eye movements. *J. Physiol. (Lond.)* 159, 339–360.

REGAN, D., FRISBY, J., POGGIO, G., SCHOR, C., AND TYLER, C. (1989). The perception of stereo-depth and stereo-motion: cortical mechanisms. In L. SPILLMAN AND J. WERNER (eds.). *Visual Perceptions. The Neurophysiological Foundations.* San Diego: Academic Press.

RIGGS, L. A., AND NIEHLE, W. (1960). Eye movements recorded during convergence and divergence. *J. Opt. Soc. Am. [A]* 50, 913–920.

ROGERS, B. J., AND BRADSHAW, M. F. (1993). Vertical disparities, differential perspective and binocular stereopsis. *Nature* 361, 253–255.

SCHOR, C. M. (1985). Development of stereopsis depends upon contrast sensitivity and spatial tuning. *J. Am. Optom. Assoc.* 56, 628–635.

SCHOR, C. M., ALEXANDER, L., CORMACK, L., AND STEVENSON S. (1992). Negative feedback control model of proximal convergence and accommodation. *Ophthal. Physiol. Optics.* 12, 307–318.

SCHOR, C. M., AND KOTULAK, J. (1986). Dynamic interactions between accommodation and convergence are velocity sensitive. *Vision Res.* 26, 927–942.

SCHOR, C. M., AND WOOD, I. C. (1983). Disparity range for local stereopsis as a function of luminance spatial frequency. *Vision Res.* 23, 1649–1654.

SCHOR, C. M., GLEASON, J., AND HORNER, D. (1990). Selective nonconjugate binocular adaptation of vertical saccades and pursuits. *Vision Res.* 30, 1827–1844.

SCHOR, C. M., ROBERTSON, K. M., AND WESSON, M. (1986). Disparity vergence dynamics and fixation disparity. *Am. J. Optom.* 63, 611–618.

SCHOR, C. M., WOOD, I. C., AND OGAWA, J. (1984). Binocular sensory fusion is limited by spatial resolution. *Vision Res.* 24, 661–665.

SCHOR, C. M., GLEASON, G., MAXWELL, J., AND LUNN, R. (1993). Spatial aspects of vertical phoria adaptation. *Vision Res.* 33, 73–84.

SCHOR, C. M., GLEASON, G., AND LUNN, R. (1993). Interactions between short-term vertical phoria adaptation and nonconjugate adaptation of vertical pursuit. *Vision Res.* 33, 55–63.

SIMONSZ, H. J., AND DEN TONKELAAR I. (1990). 19th century mechanical models of eye movements, Donder's Law, Listing's Law, and Helmholtz' direction circles. *Documenta Ophthalmologica* 74, 95–112.

SLATER, A. M., AND FINDLAY, J. M. (1972). The measurement of the fixation position in the newborn baby. *Exp. Child Psychol.* 14, 349–364.

STREETEN, B. W. (1969). Development of the human retinal pigment epithelium and the posterior segment. *Acta Ophthalmol. (Copenh.)* 81, 383–394.

TYLER, C. W. (1983). Sensory processing of binocular disparity. In C. M. SCHOR AND K. CUIFFREDA (eds.). *Vergence Eye Movements: Basic and Clinical Aspects.* Boston: Butterworths, pp. 119–287.

TYLER, C. W. (1991). The horopter and binocular fusion. In D. REGAN (ed.). *Binocular Vision. Vol. 9. Vision and Visual Dysfunction.* London: Macmillan, pp. 19–37.

TYLER, C. W., AND SCOTT, A. (1979). Binocular vision. In RECORDS, R. E. (ed.). *Physiology of the Human Eye and Visual System.* Hagerstown, MD: Harper & Row, pp. 643–671.

VOLKMANN, A. W. (1859). Die stereoskopischen Erscheinumgen in ihrer Beziehung zu der Lehre von den identischen Netzhautpunkten. *Arch. Ophthalmol.* 5 (pt. 2), 1–100.

WESTHEIMER, G. (1979). Cooperative neural processes involved in stereoscopic acuity. *Exp. Brain Res.* 36, 585–597.

YUODELIS, C., AND HENDRICKSON, A. (1986). A qualitative and quantitative analysis of the human fovea during development. *Vision Res.* 26, 847–855.

15 | Two stages in the development of binocular vision and eye alignment

RICHARD HELD

Increasing evidence supports the idea that there are two stages in the development of binocular vision during infancy (Held, 1985, 1991; Shimojo et al., 1986). During the earlier, primitive stage, little more than local summation of binocular signals from corresponding retinal loci may occur. During the later, mature stage, more complex processing in the form of disparity selectivity, interocular inhibition, and global processing can be inferred. Many investigators have claimed that maturing neuronal mechanisms at the level of the cerebral cortex account for the development of binocular vision (Atkinson, 1984; Held, 1985; Wilson, 1988). We have proposed a model, based on known cortical development, designed to account for a necessary step in the transition from primitive to mature binocularity (Held, 1985, 1988; Shimojo et al., 1986). Some of its implications have been examined. The following is a review and summary of results that bear on the two stages of development and the applicability of the proposed model of development. Birch (see Chapter 13) and Shimojo (see Chapter 12) have reviewed much of the work on testing binocular vision in infants, and Archer (see Chapter 22) has reviewed research on the development of eye alignment in infants that may be related to the development of binocularity. The following account amplifies the two-stage model and its implications for eye alignment.

ONSET OF STEREOPSIS

The early absence and abrupt onset of stereopsis at an average age of 10–15 weeks and the subsequent rapid development of stereoacuity (Held et al., 1980; Birch et al., 1982) have led to speculation as to the source of this striking change in binocular vision. Explanations have been proposed on the basis of change at any one of several levels of the visual system (Held, 1991; see also Chapter 13). I summarize here the arguments for the precortical levels. Aslin (1977) suggested that improvement in convergence accuracy (see below), which occurs during this age period, might account for the

onset of stereopsis. However, as outlined in Birch (see Chapter 13) and Held (1991), many arguments and experiments contradict this explanation.

On the basis of an ideal observer analysis, it has been argued that improvements in sensitivity and resolution at the retinal level could account for higher level changes in visual function and probably do (Banks and Bennet, 1988; Wilson, 1988). The fact that processing must occur at higher levels as in the case of stereopsis, as convergence of signals from the two eyes awaits this level, does not preclude this explanation. As Held (1992) has argued, such higher level processes may not be actuated until a threshold of signal strength is exceeded as a result of the increasing sensitivity at the lower level. In the case of stereopsis, this argument is countered by the fact that its onset may occur in the absence of any appreciable change in visual acuity, which can be regarded as a measure of retinal resolution (Held, 1991; see Chapter 13). More convincing is the change in preference for binocular fusion over rivalry (Birch et al., 1985; Shimojo et al., 1986), age-correlated with the onset of stereopsis (Gwiazda et al., 1989), which occurs with clearly suprathreshold stimuli and hence cannot be attributed to an increase in either sensitivity or resolution. In addition, no sex differences have been observed in the timing of the development of visual acuity (resolution), although they are found for stereopsis and binocular rivalry at their ages of onset (Bauer et al., 1986; Gwiazda et al., 1989) and during the development of vernier acuity over a similar range of ages (Held et al., 1984). This unexplained dimorphism serves as an indicator of different processing mechanisms.

Neuronal Model

Available evidence, then, suggests that the neuronal changes required for the development of mature binocularity do not occur prior to the cortical level. Our model was initially proposed to account for the early absence followed by the abrupt acquisition of stereopsis (Held, 1985). It was largely based on current accounts of the anatomy, single cell physiology, and developing

250

stereopsis of animals as reviewed by Birch (see Chapter 13). In brief, during the early stages of development the thalamocortical axons from each eye are topographically distributed in the entrance layer of striate cortex (Fig. 15-1). Distributed in layer 4 (4C in the monkey), they form maps of the retinas in correspondence with each other. In the early stage (Fig. 15-1A), axon terminals from the two eyes overlap extensively, and many are reported to synapse on the same cells. As a consequence, the address of the eye of origin is assumed lost for purposes of further processing. Unless processing for disparities is carried out at this entrance level, for which there is no good evidence, disparities cannot be extracted at any of the other cortical levels at which disparity sensitive neurons have been found. Only when the addresses of the eyes of origin are available can

NEONATE

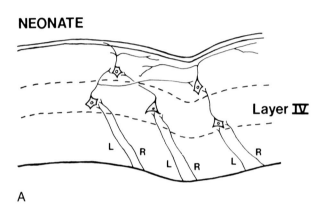

Layer **IV**

A

MATURE

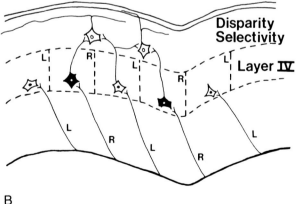

Disparity
Selectivity
Layer **IV**

B

FIG. 15-1. Model of transition from primitive (A) to mature (B) binocularity. (A) Geniculostriate afferents from both eyes (R and L) synapse on the same cells in layer IV, thereby losing information about the eye of origin. (B) Geniculostriate afferents are segregated on the basis of eye origin (R and L); consequently, recipient cells in layer IV may send their axons to cells outside that layer so as to synapse on cells that may be disparity selective. (From Held, 1985. By permission.)

further processing for interocular differences in stimulation be carried out. This latter state of affairs is presumed achieved when the segregation of the ocular dominance columns is completed as shown in Figure 15-1B. The stages of completion of such segregation and their timing are described in the literature for the cat (LeVay et al., 1978), monkey (LeVay et al., 1980), and human, for whom there is only fragmentary evidence (Hickey and Peduzzi, 1987). The late stages of segregation and the onset of stereopsis occur at roughly the same ages in the cat (Timney, 1981), monkey (O'Dell et al., 1991), and human (reviewed in Held, 1991). To the extent that the assumptions of the model are valid and the reasoning correct, one may conclude that segregation of the columns is a necessary but not sufficient condition for the onset of stereopsis. The model also accounts readily for the onset of sensitivity to rivalry by the same reasoning. Prior to the availability of eye-addressed signals beyond the thalamic entry level in visual cortex, no mutual inhibition can occur between signals exclusively from the left eye and exclusively from the right eye. Wilson (see Chapter 32) suggested that the general proliferation of synaptic connections during this period may account for both disparity detecting as well as mutually inhibitory circuitry. Be that as it may, eye-addressed information is essential to both these processes.

Prestereoptic Vision

The model has raised questions about the state of prestereoptic binocular vision. It implies that thalamocortical inputs from the two eyes are combined only by summation at the synapse of signals from corresponding retinal loci. In turn, that implication suggested the experiment in which interocularly orthogonal gratings (horizontal in one eye, vertical in the other) were paired with interocularly parallel gratings (either horizontal or vertical in both eyes) in a two-alternative preferential looking paradigm (Shimojo et al., 1986; see also Chapter 12). Young infants initially preferred the interocularly orthogonal to the parallel gratings but switched their preference to the parallel gratings at the average age at which stereopsis has its onset. The outcome implied nonselective combination of the interocularly orthogonal gratings into a central representation that would appear grid-like before but not after the onset of stereopsis. How is this result to be explained in relation to the known edge detection mechanisms at cortical levels?

Before segregation of the ocular dominance columns in both cat and monkey, cells are found that are selectively sensitive to oriented edges. Consequently, one can expect that even before segregation of the columns such sensitivity should be evident in the vision of those species as well as in the human infant. This presumption is confirmed by the demonstration in infants of orientational selectivity to edges by 6 weeks of age if not earlier (Held et al., 1989; Yoshida et al., 1990; see also Chapter 10). According to the model such cells should be largely binocular at this stage as we assume that most cortical cells are so. What happens at this stage when interocularly orthogonal gratings are presented paired with parallel gratings? The orthogonal gratings produce arrays of excited cells in layer 4 along both orientations and hence excite two classes of edge-responsive cells. The parallel gratings excite only one class. As mentioned above, young infants in fact preferred the orthogonal to the parallel gratings until the age of onset of stereopsis when they shifted preference to the parallel fused gratings. The authors (Shimojo et al., 1986) argued that this preference resulted from a preference for an interocularly combined grid over a grating, a claim consistent with their model.

With segregation of the ocular dominance columns preserving the address of the eye of origin, classes of connected cells outside of layer 4 can exist that are not merely summative of excitation from corresponding loci. They may now exhibit selective sensitivity to disparities and other noncorrespondences of spatial loci. It is only then that interocularly orthogonal gratings can induce rivalry and reverse the preference between orthogonal and fusible gratings. As with stereopsis, the age of onset of this reversal of preference occurs earlier in female than male infants (Gwiazda et al., 1989).

FURTHER TESTS OF THE TWO-STAGE MODEL

Visually Evoked Potentials

In the primitive stage, the system should be capable of selectively responding to certain binocular spatial differences by summation alone. Compare the outputs of in-phase (correlation 1.0) with out-of-phase (correlation -1.0) interocular patterns. In the former case inputs from both eyes to cells of layer 4 are all roughly equivalent and should show some summation, whereas in the latter case they differ and presumably show less summation. An analysis of the effects of interocular phase changes on single cells in the visual cortex of cat was presented by Ohzawa and Freeman (1986). They reported linearly reduced summation in the response of these cells as phase correspondence is reduced. Alternation of the phase of patterns can be expected to result in alternating voltage patterns in the visually evoked potentials (VEPs) generated by a mass of such neurons in visual cortex. In fact, potentials resulting from phase alternation have been reported from scalp electrodes on young infants at an earlier age than those produced by disparate stimuli by Eizenman et al. (1989). Previously,

Braddick et al. (1980) had raised this possibility but had not confirmed it.

Binocular Beats

By presenting dichoptic uniform fields modulated sinusoidally at different temporal frequencies, Baitch and Levi (1988) have demonstrated, with both psychophysical and evoked potential methods, a beat frequency generated by a nonlinearity at some level following summation between the two eyes. The nonlinearity is required, as mere superposition of the two frequencies would not produce the beat frequency. The beat frequency is either eliminated or markedly reduced in cases of loss of stereopsis, implying that signals from the two eyes remain independent. The beat was observed in each of a group of eight human infants ranging in age from 7 to 36 weeks of age (Baitch and Srebro, 1990). These authors argued that the presence of the binocular beat at such an early age indicates a primitive binocular interaction in cortex that can occur prior to the age of onset of stereopsis. This result is also consistent with our model of the neuronal summation process that occurs during the primitive stage of binocularity.

Binocular Summation

Binocular summation of brightness is a well known observation in normal adult observers. The same level of illumination observed by two eyes appears brighter than that observed with one eye. Increased pupillary contraction accompanies this change in apparent brightness and provides an objective measure of the effect. However, when measured in very young infants little or no summation is found. Birch and Held (1983) carried out a longitudinal study on binocular summation in infants aged 1–6 months. Although not detectable during the first few months, summation began to appear during the fourth month, and by 6 months most infants showed adult-like summation. When age of appearance of summation was correlated with the onset age for stereopsis, a Pearson r of 0.78 was found using 12 observers. The authors suggested that the appearance of binocular summation is related to the neuronal change that accounts for the onset of stereopsis [but see Shea et al. (1985) for an alternative account based on the low sensitivity of the infant's pupillary response].

Examination of the data of Figure 15-2 shows that summation (the increasing difference in pupillary contraction) appears to increase with age because monocular exposure produces less contraction (greater dilation). There is no increase in contraction with binocular exposure. Could it be the outcome of segregation of the dominance columns as detailed in the model? Yes, if

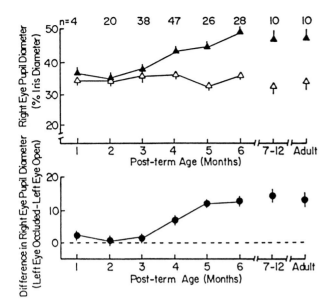

FIG. 15-2. Binocular summation of pupillary response. Mean right eye pupil diameter as a percentage of iris diameter with the left eye occluded (▲) and the left eye open (△). The number of infants tested in each age group is indicated along the top of the figure. Mean difference in pupil diameter under the two viewing conditions (●) is also shown. Vertical bars represent 1 standard error of the mean (SEM). (From Birch and Held, 1983. By permission.)

two conditions are satisfied. First, luminance changes extending over large areas must excite cells in layer 4. Second, the pupillary response must reflect the summation of cells excited in layer 4. Because according to the model most cells are innervated by each eye before segregation, monocular stimulation excites almost as many cells in layer 4 as does binocular stimulation. However, with the advent of segregation, monocular stimulation fails to stimulate half of these cells. The result should be a reduction in pupillary constriction, whereas the effect of binocular stimulation, continuing to excite all cells, should be unchanged. Parenthetically, I should mention that such a model was proposed by Doesschate and Alpern (1967) but was discarded on the grounds that it failed to account for the presumed effects of strabismus in increasing the percentage of monocular cells and reducing summation. Shea et al. (1985), however, using a much larger sample of strabismic patients, have not confirmed the results of Doesschate and Alpern.

Probability Summation at Threshold

Probability summation predicts that use of the two eyes will yield a lower threshold than the use of only one based on the assumption that each eye acts as an independent detector of equal sensitivity. Accordingly, Birch (1985) and Birch and Hale (1988) have found

such summation in measures of visual acuity in infants older than 4–6 months of age but not earlier. On the basis of these data, Birch and Swanson (1991) have argued that the assumption of two independent detectors, used in models of probability summation, must not hold for the very young infant. Instead they proposed that inputs from the two eyes are combined prior to detection with the consequence that the signal-to-noise ratio remains the same as that from the individual eyes. They reported that this result is consistent with the segregation model of the onset of binocularity. The primitive stage accounts for the initial lack of independent processing of inputs to the two eyes. In the mature stage segregation allows two independent detectors and probability summation.

CLINICAL RELEVANCE

Stereopsis and the Control of Vergence

Binocularly disparate stimuli drive vergence responses of the eyes of mature observers (Rashbass and Westheimer, 1961; Jones, 1983). Consequently, one may expect that the onset of stereopsis, indicating the initial presence of disparity processing, will influence the control of such eye movements (Held, 1988, 1991). Aslin (1977) has reported changes in the control of convergent eye movements that are in accord with this prediction. Infants 1 and 2 months old do not consistently follow a target moving in depth. Three-month-olds follow a slowly moving target. However, when convergence demand is increased abruptly and stepwise by applying a base-out wedge prism, vergent following of the target is ineffectual before 4.5 months. As has been pointed out (Held, 1988), efficient following of such a stepped displacement requires information about the angular misalignment and its direction. It is just this sort of information that is provided by disparities. Prior to the onset of disparity detection, rapid response to sizable stepped increments in target distance should be absent. Mitkin and Orestova (1988) reported an abrupt increase in the number of adequate vergence responses between 12 and 15 weeks of age. Most recently, Thorn et al. (1992) reported that the average age of full convergence to an approaching object occurred about 1 week after the onset of mature binocularity. The Pearson correlation between the two ages within individuals was 0.6 and highly significant. The authors inferred a causal relation between the onset of sensory binocularity and vergence control based on maturation of the neuronal mechanism for binocular vision.

The appearance of correct vergence before the onset of stereopsis may be produced by nonbinocular mechanisms such as accommodative control of vergence or by bifoveal fixation. Some degree of control of vergence by the primitive binocular system may be accomplished through the mediation of summation in layer 4, as has been suggested previously (Held, 1988). Binocular summation would normally be optimized when suprathreshold images in the two eyes are in binocular correspondence. During the primitive stage such optimization could drive vergence in response to small and slow changes in target distance. We expect, however, that the availability of disparity information should alter the dynamic properties of visually controlled vergent movements of the eyes in accord with the above reasoning.

Mature Binocularity, Esotropia, and Orthotropization

Assuming that the onset of stereopsis implies the availability of a set of detectors having a wide range of disparity selectivity, the necessary information for mature vergence control will have become available. We have speculated that the transition from the primitive mode of control to disparity control of vergence precipitates infantile esotropia: "[M]isconvergence does not occur chronically until this age. . . . Could it be that the transition period, when the vergence-maintaining mechanisms switch control is the time at which the eye movement system is most susceptible to that loss of alignment which characterizes infantile esotropia?" (Held, 1988). A preexisting defect in the interface (Fig. 15-3) between disparity signals and motor control of vergence may be expressed only when stereopsis becomes available. The curious fact that crossed stereopsis appears a few weeks earlier than uncrossed stereopsis (Held et al., 1980;

Birch et al., 1982) may also play a role in promoting esotropia, as during the intervening interval only convergence can be driven by disparity. The consequences for strabismus of such asymmetries in stereopsis are discussed by Richards (1970). In accord with these surmises, infantile esotropia is reported to first appear at the same average age as stereopsis (Nixon et al., 1985).

Archer (see Chapter 22) reports the average age of positive identification of orthotropia (straight eyes) at roughly 3 months of age. Prior to that age infants are reported to show high degrees of exotropia. Figure 22-1A displays the cumulated percentage of infants showing orthotropia, implying correct binocular convergence to target as a function of age. This agreement with the ages of onset of sensory binocularity suggests that the process of orthotropization is closely related to the achievement of mature binocularity. To follow up that suggestion we plotted the two sets of results together as follows.

Archer reported that 21.2% of infants have straight eyes shortly after birth "by chance," meaning that they are not functionally orthotropic but happened to have their eyes in a straight alignment at the time of examination. For present purposes it seems reasonable to eliminate this group and cumulate only those infants who have demonstrably achieved orthotropization. The result is shown in Figure 15-4 plotted together with the data of Figure 13-5 and the data of Gwiazda et al. (1989) on the onset of stereopsis. The agreement of the two curves of Figure 15-4, despite great differences in method and procedure, is striking. Their juxtaposition is consistent with our surmise that the onset of mature

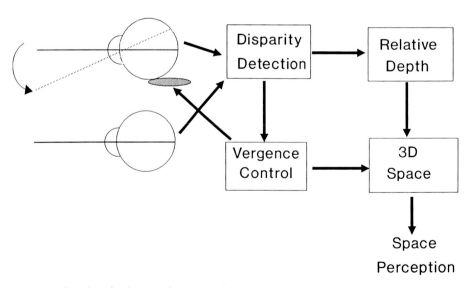

FIG. 15-3. Flow chart for disparity detection and consequences. When disparity signals become available, they contribute to vergence control at the same time as they allow stereopsis. Activation of vergence by disparity maintains orthotropy (solid lines of sight) in the normal infant but esotropy (dashed line of sight) in the at-risk infant. Stereopsis is presumed to include processing for relative depth and a metric for three-dimensional space when combined with an input from vergence control.

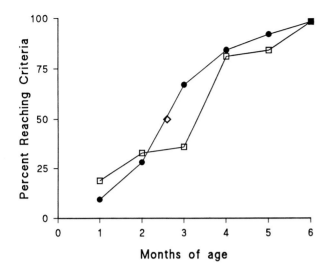

FIG. 15-4. Cumulative percent of infants achieving criterion for stereopsis (□: Birch, see Chapter 13; ◇: Gwiazda et al., 1989) and orthotropia (●, ■: Archer, see Chapter 22).

control of vergence, and now alignment, occurs when disparity processing becomes available (Held, 1988). However, when we attempted to replicate the findings of Archer and colleagues, using the conventional Hirschberg method, we failed to find either the large exotropic readings or the average age of 3 months for orthotropy.

Instead, most infants appeared orthotropic within the first few weeks after birth, and exotropic readings rarely exceeded 20 degrees (Thorn et al., 1992). The questions remain as to why our alignment results are so discrepant with theirs and yet Archer's curve approximates that for the onset of mature binocularity. The answer may derive in part from their assessment of eye alignment using reflections from the nearby examiner's face. Because very young infants do not converge to near targets (Thorn et al., 1992), an unsuspecting observer at a near distance sees the infant's eyes diverged—hence "exotropic." This divergence, however, lessens when mature binocularity emerges together with the ability to converge to near distances. As a result, the apparent exotropia lessens so as to make the eyes appear orthotropic. The cumulative reduction of "exotropia" (increase of orthotropy) with age should then parallel the cumulative curve of onset of mature binocularity, as is in fact shown in Figure 15-4.

If the above reasoning is correct, stereopsis should be present, at least briefly, at the age of onset of esotropia. Of course if stereopsis is to be measured during misalignment, special procedures must be used for maintaining interocular correspondence of images (Birch et al., 1983; Birch and Stager, 1985). Moreover, the degrading effects of chronic misconvergence, in time, cause the loss of mature binocularity. Notwithstanding

these difficulties, the results of attempts to study the development of stereopsis in infantile esotropes tend to bear out the prediction that stereopsis or other evidence of mature binocularity is present at the onset of infantile esotropia (Bechtoldt and Hutz, 1979; Birch and Stager, 1985; Mohindra et al., 1985; Wattam-Bell et al., 1987). Thus construed, infantile esotropia may be one consequence of achieving stereopsis. Chronic esotropia, in turn, destroys stereopsis by creating a chronic mismatch between the retinal images (Fig. 15-3).

Amblyopia and Loss of Stereopsis

Amblyopia and loss of stereopsis result from various types of chronic mismatch between retinal images such as are produced by monocular deprivation, occlusion, strabismus, and anisometropia during a susceptible period in development, which in children extends over the first few years (see Chapter 18). Amblyopia occurs as a result of interocular competition leading to the selective loss of cortical connections from the eye with weakened input. In cats (LeVay et al., 1978) and monkeys (LeVay et al., 1980), early monocular deprivation causes the thalamocortical afferents carrying signals from the occluded eye to lose their cortical connections beginning with cells in the entry layer 4 (layer 4c in the monkey). After completion of segregation of the ocular dominance columns, no further competition occurs in the entry layer, as few if any binocular cells remain. However, the competition continues in binocular units outside the entry layer. If esotropia does not occur prior to the mature stage of binocularity (segregation of the ocular dominance columns), amblyopia derived from esotropia must result from the competitive process that occurs outside the entry layer. This claim agrees with the reports that amblyopia, as measured by a significant difference in acuity between the eyes, has not been found prior to about 4 months of age in prospective studies (Jacobson et al., 1981; Birch and Stager, 1985). In agreement with these results are those coming from a retrospective analyses of cases of strabismus claiming that the critical period for loss of binocularity does not begin before several months after birth (Banks et al., 1975). Consequently, the stage of binocularity appears to play a role in susceptibility to amblyopia and loss of stereopsis as well as in eye alignment.

CONCLUSIONS

Current evidence appears to confirm a model incorporating two stages in binocular development. The importance of a model of the two stages lies in its ability to account for existing knowledge and to generate testable hypotheses. To some extent this situation has been the case. Confirmation has come from studies of the change in various interocular interactions during the transition from primitive to mature stages of binocular vision. In addition, the transition may have implications for the development of pathological eye alignment. On the basis of ages of onset, it is proposed that the transition to mature binocularity may trigger the manifestation of infantile esotropia in the at-risk infant. Esotropia in turn may cause a loss of stereopsis and amblyopia.

REFERENCES

ASLIN, R. N. (1977). Development of binocular fixation in human infants. *J. Exp. Child Psychol.* 23, 133–150.

ATKINSON, J. (1984). Human visual development over the first 6 months of life: a review and a hypothesis. *Hum. Neurol.* 3, 61–74.

BAITCH, L. W., AND LEVI, D. M. (1988). Binocular beat: psychophysical and electrophysiological correlates of binocular integration. *Invest. Ophthalmol. Vis. Sci.* 29 (suppl.), 10.

BAITCH, L. W., AND SREBRO, R. (1990). Binocular interactions in sleeping and awake human infants. *Invest. Ophthalmol. Vis. Sci.* 31 (suppl.), 251.

BANKS, M. S., AND BENNETT, P. J. (1988). Optical and photoreceptor immaturities limit the spatial and chromatic vision of human neonates. *J. Opt. Soc. Am.* 5, 2059–2079.

BANKS, M. S., ASLIN, R. N., AND LETSON, R. D. (1975). Sensitive period for the development of human binocular vision. *Science* 190, 675–677.

BAUER, J., SHIMOJO, S., GWIAZDA, J., AND HELD, R. (1986). Sex differences in the development of binocularity in human infants. *Invest. Ophthalmol. Vis. Sci.* 27 (suppl.), 265.

BECHTOLDT, H. P., AND HUTZ, C. S. (1979). Stereopsis in young infants and stereopsis in an infant with congenital esotropia. *J. Pediatr. Ophthalmol. Strabismus* 16, 49–54.

BIRCH, E. E. (1985). Infant interocular acuity differences and binocular vision. *Vision Res.* 25, 571–576.

BIRCH, E. E., AND HALE, L. A. (1988). Criteria for monocular acuity deficit in infancy and early childhood. *Invest. Ophthalmol. Vis. Sci.* 29, 636–643.

BIRCH, E. E., AND HELD, R. (1983). The development of binocular summation in human infants. *Invest. Ophthalmol. Vis. Sci.* 24, 1103.

BIRCH, E. E., AND STAGER, D. R. (1985). Monocular acuity and stereopsis in infantile esotropia. *Invest. Ophthalmol. Vis. Sci.* 26, 1624–1630.

BIRCH, E. E., AND SWANSON, W. H. (1991). Probability summation of grating acuity in the human infant. *Invest. Ophthalmol. Vis. Sci.* 32 (suppl.), 964.

BIRCH, E. E., GWIAZDA, J., AND HELD, R. (1982). Stereoacuity development for crossed and uncrossed disparities in human infants. *Vision Res.* 22, 507–513.

BIRCH, E. E., GWIAZDA, J., AND HELD, R. (1983). The development of vergence does not account for the onset of stereopsis. *Perception* 12, 331–336.

BIRCH, E. E., SHIMOJO, S., AND HELD, R. (1985). Preferential looking assessment of fusion and stereopsis in infants aged 1 to 6 months. *Invest. Ophthalmol. Vis. Sci.* 26, 366–370.

BRADDICK, O., ATKINSON, J., JULESZ, B., KROPFL, W., BODIS-WOLLNER, I., AND RABB, A. (1980). Cortical binocularity in infants. *Nature* 288, 363–365.

DOESSCHATE, J., AND ALPERN, M. (1967). Effect of photoexcitation of the two retinas on pupil size. *J. Neurophysiol.* 30, 562–576.

EIZENMAN, M., SKARF, B., AND McCULLOCH, D. (1989). Development of binocular vision in infants. *Invest. Ophthalmol. Vis. Sci.* 30 (suppl.), 313.

GWIAZDA, J., BAUER, J., AND HELD, R. (1989). Binocular function in human infants: correlation of stereoptic and fusion-rivalry discriminations. *J. Pediatr. Ophthalmol. Strabismus* 26, 128–132.

HELD, R. (1985). Binocular vision—behavioral and neural development. In J. MEHLER AND R. FOX (eds.). *Neonate Cognition: Beyond the Blooming, Buzzing Confusion.* Hillsdale, NJ: Erlbaum, pp. 37–44.

HELD, R. (1988). Normal visual development and its deviations. In G. LENNERSTRAND, G. VON NOORDEN, AND E. CAMPOS (eds.). *Strabismus and Amblyopia.* London: Macmillan, pp. 247–257.

HELD, R. (1991). Development of binocular vision and stereopsis. In D. REGAN AND J. R. CRONLY-DILLON (eds.). *Vision and Visual Dysfunction.* London: Macmillan, pp. 170–178.

HELD, R. (1992). What can rates of development tell us about underlying mechanisms? In C. GRANRUD (ed.). *Visual Perception and Cognition in Infancy.* Hillsdale, NJ: Erlbaum.

HELD, R., BIRCH, E. E., AND GWIAZDA, J. (1980). Stereoacuity of human infants. *Proc. Natl. Acad. Sci. USA* 77, 5572–5574.

HELD, R., SHIMOJO, S., AND GWIAZDA, J. (1984). Gender differences in the early development of human visual resolution. *Invest. Ophthalmol. Vis. Sci.* 25 (suppl.), 220.

HELD, R., YOSHIDA, H., GWIAZDA, J., AND BAUER, J. (1989). Development of orientation selectivity measured by a masking procedure. *Invest. Ophthalmol. Vis. Sci.* 30 (suppl.), 312.

HICKEY, J. L., AND PEDUZZI, J. D. (1987). Structure and development of the visual system. In P. SALAPATEK AND L. COHEN (eds.). *Handbook of Infant Perception.* Orlando, FL: Academic Press, pp. 1–42.

JACOBSON, S., MOHINDRA, I., AND HELD, R. (1981). Age of onset of amblyopia in infants with esotropia. *Doc. Ophthalmol.* 30, 210–216.

JONES, R. (1983). Horizontal disparity vergence. In C. M. SCHOR AND K. J. CIUFFREDA (eds.). *Vergence Eye Movements: Basic and Clinical Aspects.* Boston: Butterworths, pp. 297–316.

LEVAY, S., STRYKER, M. P., AND SHATZ, C. J. (1978). Ocular dominance columns and their development in layer IV of the cat's visual cortex: a quantitative study. *J. Comp. Neurol.* 179, 223–244.

LEVAY, S., WIESEL, T. N., AND HUBEL, D. H. (1980). The development of ocular dominance columns in normal and visually deprived monkeys. *J. Comp. Neurol.* 191, 1–51.

MITKIN, A., AND ORESTOVA, E. (1988). Development of binocular vision in early ontogenesis. *Psychol. Beitr.* 30, 65–74.

MOHINDRA, I., ZWAAN, J., HELD, R., BRILL, S., AND ZWAAN, F. (1985). Development of acuity and stereopsis in infants with esotropia. *Ophthalmology* 92, 691–697.

NIXON, R. B., HELVESTON, E. M., MILLER, K., ARCHER, S. M., AND ELLIS, F. D. (1985). Incidence of strabismus in neonates. *Am. J. Ophthalmol.* 100, 798–801.

O'DELL, C. D., QUICK, M. W., AND BOOTHE, R. G. (1991). The development of stereoacuity in infant rhesus monkeys. *Invest. Ophthalmol. Vis. Sci.* 32 (suppl.), 1044.

OHZAWA, I., AND FREEMAN, R. D. (1986). The binocular organization of simple cells in the cat's visual cortex. *J. Neurophysiol.* 56, 221–242.

RASHBASS, C., AND WESTHEIMER, G. (1961). Disjunctive eye movements. *J. Physiol. (Lond.)* 159, 339–360.

RICHARDS, W. (1970). Stereopsis and stereoblindness. *Exp. Brain Res.* 10, 380–388.

SHEA, S. L., DOUSSARD-ROOSEVELT, J. A., AND ASLIN, R. N. (1985). Pupillary measures of binocular luminance summation in infants and stereoblind adults. *Invest. Ophthalmol. Vis. Sci.* 26, 1064–1070.

SHIMOJO, S., BAUER, J. A., O'CONNELL, K. M., AND HELD, R. (1986). Prestereoptic binocular vision in infants. *Vision Res.* 26, 501–510.

THORN, F., GWIAZDA, J., CRUZ, A., BAUER, J., AND HELD, R. (1992). Eye alignment, sensory binocularity, and convergence in young infants. *Invest. Ophthalmol. Vis. Sci.* 33 (suppl.), 713.

TIMNEY, B. N. (1981). Development of binocular depth perception in kittens. *Invest. Ophthalmol. Vis. Sci.* 21, 493–496.

WATTAM-BELL, J., BRADDICK, O. J., ATKINSON, J., AND DAY, J. (1987). Measures of infant binocularity in a group at risk for strabismus. *Clin. Vis. Sci.* 1, 327–336.

WILSON, H. R. (1988). Development of spatiotemporal mechanisms in the human infant. *Vision Res.* 28, 611–628.

YOSHIDA, H., GWIAZDA, J., BAUER, J., AND HELD, R. (1990). Orientation selectivity is present in the first month and subsequently sharpens. *Invest. Ophthalmol. Vis. Sci.* 31 (suppl.), 8.

16 | On the development of the threshold nonlinearity, peripheral acuity, binocularity, and complex stereoscopic processing

CHRISTOPHER W. TYLER

Study of the developing infant brain and visual system has attained a high degree of sophistication. One of the features of the studies represented in this book is the diversity of assessment techniques that have been developed for use in infant studies. Most of these techniques, however, still rely on visually driven motor output to assess the properties of the neural processing that occurs when visual images are presented. The motor output may be in the form of eye movements (as in first-glance preferential looking, oculokinetic nystagmus, binocular vergence, and the visual-ocular reflex), or it may be motion of other muscle systems, such as head movements in preferential looking, eye blink, visually guided reaching, and avoidance responses. All such responses require the operation of the complete chain of neural processing, from retina to muscle. This chain is subject not only to development of each link in the process but also the attentional and motivational state of the infant at the time of testing. In many cases it has been possible to design paradigms to minimize contamination of the results by immaturities of the particular motor output in use. Nevertheless, this global susceptibility to immaturity at each link of the chain has often made it difficult to rely on any assignment of the effects to individual components of the neural pathway.

As a remedy for this shortcoming of behavioral studies of development, we have employed the visually evoked potential (VEP) as an essentially noninvasive method of measuring the visual response and its development at an early point in the visual processing stream (Tyler et al., 1979, 1987; Apkarian et al., 1981; Norcia and Tyler, 1985a,b, 1988, 1989, 1990; Tyler and Apkarian, 1985; Tyler and Norcia, 1986; Allen et al., 1986). These studies have focused on the idea of using VEP measures of sensory thresholds in a variety of stimulus dimensions and developed a rapid implementation that can be used effectively for infant studies. The key here is not to study the VEP waveform as such but to use it to define an

endpoint ("threshold") that can be compared with those from behavioral methods. As a balance to the predominantly behavioral emphasis of most of the chapters in this book, two empirical VEP studies are presented. The first is an analysis of the threshold behavior of the infant cortex by means of the VEP. The second study, which has relevance to several of the topics in other chapters, concerns the rate of development of peripheral vision.

The other main area addressed relates to the development of human binocular vision. One of the remarkable successes of infant psychophysics has been the measurement accuracy of the development of infant stereopsis. In Chapter 13 Birch reviews the evidence, much of which was generated in her own laboratory, for the sudden way that stereoscopic discrimination switches on during infancy, with a reliable gender difference in its timing. An earlier mean onset time of less than 1 week was reliably measurable for crossed versus uncrossed disparities. Shimojo (see Chapter 12) reviews studies on the development of binocular fusion and rivalry, which shows a different time course. The aim of my review is to emphasize that, although these two facets of binocular vision may be the most salient, there are many other stereoscopic and binocular functions that have been neglected in infant research. A great deal can be learned, not only about the developmental sequence of these functions during infancy but about the relation between them in adult vision, by comparing the developmental time courses of the identifiable binocular functions. The latter part of this review is designed to help stimulate and structure such developmental studies.

NATURE OF SENSORY THRESHOLD IN INFANTS

A basic tenet of much work in sensory development is that there is some limitation on the sensory response,

258

the "threshold," against which development of the response can be measured. There is a question of whether the threshold is, in fact, a stable criterion, or may have its own development. If the nature of threshold changed during development, it would confound the estimated development of the particular sensory function under study. It is therefore important to know whether response behavior in the threshold region shows any change with age, or exhibits the same properties regardless of developmental stage.

The simplest concept of a threshold in psychophysics is of a fixed limit below which there is no trace of stimulus-related event. However, even from the earliest days (e.g., Weber, 1834; Fechner, 1860) it was recognized that the threshold was a statistical concept, fluctuating over time around a mean value that had to be estimated from multiple measurements. Although the statistical description of such thresholds as being set by a noise-limited signal-detection process was not developed until about 100 years later (Tanner and Swets, 1954; Green and Swets, 1966), it is typically taken as an implicit assumption of the nature of psychophysical thresholds.

This statistical process is, however, a poor description of the behavior of cortical neurons, which do show a fixed threshold that operates differently from an optimal signal detection process. The nature of the functional threshold also affects the interpretation of psychophysical measures as revealing underlying physiological mechanisms. In particular, such interpretation in terms of the sensitivity profile of such mechanisms is distorted by probability summation within the detection process to the extent that the threshold is based on statistical properties.

True Threshold Model

An alternative model for detection behavior is that sensitivity has a genuine threshold below which there is no internal response to the stimulus, and that the d' measure of sensitivity of the internal response (Tanner and Swets, 1954) increases more or less linearly with stimulus intensity above this threshold. The true threshold model has been proposed in the past (e.g., Baumgardt, 1947; Bouman and van der Velden, 1947; Baumgardt and Smith, 1965), but these investigations operated at or close to zero false alarm rate and so were unable to assess the linearity of the internal response to the stimulus. When measured in a task with a well defined false alarm rate, such as the two-alternative forced-choice (2AFC) paradigm, the true threshold model can generate data whose d' function is fairly well fit with an exponent greater than 1.0, providing an adequate explanation for the observed exponents in the 2AFC ex-

periments. Nachmias and Kocher (1970), for example, found d' exponents averaging 2.5 for detecting a brief flash as a function of the luminance of a large adapting surround. Stromeyer and Klein (1974) found an exponent of about 2.0 for detection of contrast increments of a sinusoidal grating stimulus. The true threshold model, however, has a rather different interpretation from the high exponent model, and they can be distinguished empirically from one another.

Justification for true threshold behavior comes from consideration of the function of cortical neurons. Neurons in the cortex exhibit little spontaneous activity but may fire at high rates as soon as their optimal stimulus is present. Many neurons in the retina and optic tract, on the other hand, have a relatively high spontaneous activity level. This arrangement implies that cortical neurons must have a response threshold below which input from the noisy precortical cells evokes little output. Because it is to be expected that the cortical neurons would need to have as high a sensitivity as is compatible with the noise level in their inputs, the most efficient level to set the threshold is near the limit of the input noise, corresponding to some statistical criterion on the basis of the noise distribution (e.g., the 5% level for activation by the input noise).

Threshold Behavior in Infant Cortical Evoked Potentials

Tyler (1991a) has presented evidence supporting the idea that adult visual responses are limited by a true threshold, in both psychophysical detection tasks and the electrical response of the cortex represented by the VEP. Many VEP studies are analyzed under the assumption that there is a threshold in the response that can reasonably be compared with the psychophysical threshold estimate, especially with respect to the contrast of grating stimuli (e.g., Campbell and Maffei, 1970; Kulikowski, 1977; Cannon, 1983; Seiple et al., 1984; Tyler and Apkarian, 1985; Allen et al., 1986). In these and most other studies it was assumed that the VEP amplitude was proportional to the logarithm of the contrast above some threshold contrast level. Straight lines were therefore fit to the data on log contrast, linear VEP amplitude coordinates at the lower contrast levels and extrapolated to zero response voltage to provide the VEP threshold estimate.

The problem with this approach, which has proved effective in practice, is that it depends in principle on the twin assumptions that there is a true threshold and, less severely, that VEP amplitude increases with log contrast. This theoretical approach was examined in detail by Campbell and Kulikowski (1972), who also explored various other ways of analyzing VEP contrast functions and their thresholds but came to no convincing conclusion on the issue. Tyler (1991a) performed a detailed analysis of adult VEP responses to counterphasing grating stimuli in the region of psychophysical detection threshold. The contrast behavior was examined by means of a swept-contrast technique, in which the gratings were swept logarithmically in contrast over a 20-fold range during a 10-second epoch. This fine sampling ensured an accurate estimate of the point at which the VEP fell to the background noise level (Norcia et al., 1989). The evidence strongly supported the existence of a discrete threshold below which no hint of a signal could be recorded. The VEP amplitude also appeared to increase in proportion to log contrast, as was needed to support the cited VEP analyses.

The question of the development of visual threshold now may be addressed by determining whether the infant VEP shows the same kind of threshold behavior as the adult VEP. To do so, data were analyzed for 18 infants aged 6 months (26 ± 3 weeks) tested in the same swept contrast VEP paradigm. The analysis techniques [described fully by Norcia et al. (1989)] derived signal amplitude and phase for each infant every half-second during the 10-second contrast sweep. To obtain a homogeneous sample of contrast response functions, records were derived from the database of the responses at 1 cycle/degree (cpd) in a larger study (Norcia et al., 1990) on the criterion that the estimated contrast thresholds in these records were all in the range of 1.0% (± 0.4%). (Thresholds were estimated by extrapolation to 0 µV, as described in that study. That extrapolation was not used in the present analysis but was taken as a selection criterion for the homogeneous sample. To do so should not have prejudiced the outcome of the present analysis, as the extrapolations were performed on the portion of the data higher than 1.5 times the noise level and because the slope of the extrapolation was not considered in the present selection criterion.) The signal vectors for at each contrast were vector-averaged for all 18 infants to obtain a set of coherent mean estimates of the infant responses in the threshold region, to allow comparison with the predictions of the linear response model and a threshold model. In addition, contrast threshold was then estimated by extrapolation of the significant response at the highest spatial frequency down to 0 µV, as discussed below.

The means of the selected infant VEP responses to the contrast of the 1 cpd counterphasing grating are shown by the points plotted in terms of mean signal-to-noise ratio in Figure 16-1. The response amplitudes stayed close to the noise level (SNR = 1) up to a grating contrast of 1%. Beyond that value the response amplitude increased monotonically with contrast. The data are compared with three theoretical predictions in Figure 16-1: a linear + noise model, a threshold alone

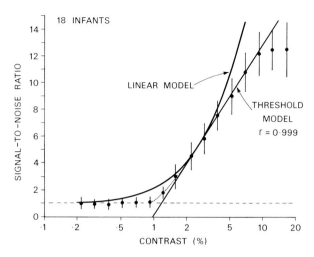

FIG. 16-1. Infant VEP responses close to contrast threshold. Dashed line = average estimate of noise level in the absence of stimulus. Filled circles = mean amplitudes of VEP second harmonic to counterphase reversal of a grating swept up in log contrast. Data are averaged for 18 infants after normalization of contrast axis relative to estimated threshold. Curved line = linear contrast response prediction; straight line = predicted signal for threshold model. Dotted line = predicted signal and noise for threshold model. Vertical bars = ±1 standard deviation of the error distributions.

model, and a threshold + noise model. On the linear + noise hypothesis, the VEP amplitude should be directly proportional to contrast except near the noise level, where the response should asymptote to the mean noise amplitude. The curved line in Figure 16-1 shows the expected value from a linear hypothesis, with the inclusion of additive noise at the level shown by the dashed line, drawn to fit the data in the midamplitude range. With Fourier analysis, noise combines with the signal on the basis of the Ricean distribution (Rice, 1945), but it is closely approximated by a square-root vector summation between the signal mean noise amplitudes (Norcia et al., 1989). Note that the linear hypothesis predicts a strongly curved function in the semilog coordinates of this plot.

The predicted signal function under the threshold hypothesis with a log-linear contrast response is shown as the thin straight line in Figure 16-1. Because the signal line cuts steeply through the mean noise level, the effect of additive noise (dotted line) is only a minor deviation from the straight line in the semilog plot. Thus the threshold prediction differs from the linear prediction mainly at low contrasts, where the threshold hypothesis predicts that the data should fall at the noise level, whereas they are progressively elevated on the linear hypothesis. Clearly the data favor the threshold hypothesis in this region, as they show no detectable deviation from the noise level. The data also fit the log-linear amplitude prediction with a correlation of 0.999

if the two datum points above the amplitude saturation level are excluded.

The VEP data of Figure 16-1 therefore support the idea that 6-month-old infants have a sensory threshold below which there is no detectable information about the stimulus (in contrast to a linear signal with additive noise, for example). *A fortiori*, this threshold nonlinearity must occur before the site of generation of the 12 Hz VEP response, which is probably early in the processing stream in the striate cortex. In this respect, the infant VEP at age 6 months is showing essentially the same response behavior as the adult VEP (Tyler, 1991a). Thus if the sensory threshold develops from an earlier state in which there is no threshold, for example, the threshold function must have developed prior to the age of 6 months. This information acts as a counterpoint to infant behavioral studies that might suggest infants have a higher noise level in the sensory pathway from which the signal must be extracted, as an explanation for their higher detection thresholds in behavioral paradigms. The presence of a discrete threshold, coupled with the surprisingly high contrast sensitivity values reported by Norcia et al. (1990), suggests that the initial cortical processing is nearly mature by 6 months of age.

VISUAL PROCESSING IN THE INFANT PERIPHERY

One recurring theme of this book is the role of peripheral vision in infant visual behavior. Evidence is accumulating that infants have poorly developed foveal anatomy at birth, whereas their peripheral retinal anatomy (beyond about 5 degrees eccentricity) is relatively mature (Mann, 1964; Yuodelis and Hendrickson, 1986). Such data suggest that peripheral vision function is likely to play a more important role in vision until the time that the foveal region develops to the same functional level as the periphery. This hypothesis implies that both the characterization of peripheral function and the measurement of the time at which it is overtaken by foveal function are relevant to understanding infant visual development.

Functional visual studies, however, do not fully validate the picture of development obtained from the anatomical studies. By varying the size of the test field in an evoked potential study of response amplitude, Spinelli et al. (1983) concluded that acuity already was highest in a small (2 degrees) retinal area by 3 months of age. This result implies that it is possible that the fovea is sufficiently mature to determine overall visual acuity, even though that acuity may be much lower than the adult value. In fact, even in newborns, the interreceptor spacing in the fovea is sufficient to support an acuity of about 15 cpd, which is substantially higher than the neonatal acuity from any measurement method

(Banks and Bennett, 1988; see Chapter 32). Thus the cortex and its magnification function, rather than retinal anatomy, may still be the factor limiting visual acuity.

This finding and other results suggest that it is still plausible that the infant has a functional fovea with higher resolution than the peripheral retina, perhaps because of the contribution of cortical development, rather than retinal limitations. Norcia, Allen, and I therefore designed a study to compare the developmental sequence of foveal and peripheral acuity in order to determine the role of peripheral sensitivity within the first year of life. The acuity for sinusoidal grating stimuli were determined by the sweep VEP method (Tyler et al., 1979; Norcia and Tyler, 1985a,b; Norcia et al., 1985a).

Experimental Methods

Vertical sinewave luminance gratings were presented on a triad of video monitors configured as in Figure 16-2. The dashed rectangles indicate the physical placement of the monitors together with their dimensions. The full line areas containing vertical bars indicate the regions of the monitors visible to the observers. These were configured as a central circular region with a radius of 2 degrees (at the viewing distance of 165 cm) and a peripheral region consisting of sectors of an annulus 8–16 degrees in extent. The annular sectors were set in the lower visual field to maximize the response from electrodes above the inion, and the sectors were as large as permitted by the screen configuration of the monitors (Fig. 16-2). The two monitors for the annular sectors were electrically yoked, so as always to present the same spatial pattern and temporal modulation signal. Mean luminance was 80 candelas (cd)/m^2 at a Michelson contrast of 80%. The display was carefully adjusted so as not to produce changes in mean luminance (flicker) correlated with pattern reversal, which was a temporal square wave avoiding potential even-order distortion products due to phosphor nonlinearities. The experiments were conducted in the low ambient illumination of an otherwise dark room.

The stimuli were presented in a version of the 10-second swept-parameter technique described previously (Norcia and Tyler, 1985a,b; Norcia et al., 1985a; Hamer et al., 1989). By recording continuously at a fixed analysis rate, the response profile may be obtained as a function of some stimulus parameter such as spatial frequency or contrast. For the present experiment the technique was enhanced by stimulating and recording simultaneously at two temporal frequencies. The two stimulus frequencies (6 and 8 Hz) were used to differentiate between the brain responses from macular and peripheral stimulus regions. Recording and Fourier

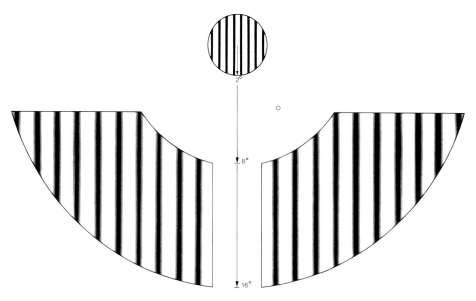

FIG. 16-2. Stimulus configuration for foveal/peripheral acuity comparison. Sinusoidal grating in peripheral 8- to 16-degree annular sectors was scaled to one-fourth the spatial frequency of that in the central disk of 2 degrees radius. Small circle shows an alternative fixation point.

waveform analysis were conducted at the second harmonics of the same two frequencies (12 and 16 Hz), allowing segregation of the response characteristics from the two stimulus regions. The advantage of this simultaneous recording method is that observer state changes, such as attention level, should affect the response at both frequencies similarly, allowing more accurate assessment of the relation between the two stimulus regions than would be possible with sequential analysis. The dual frequency method also speeds up the recording time by a factor of 2 (although the computer does take somewhat longer between trials for preanalysis and storage of the data).

Forty normal infants were recruited from parent education classes and newspaper announcements. Infants with eye turns and eye pathologies were excluded, as were infants whose birth date was not within 2 weeks of term. This latter restriction was important because visual experience variations caused by pre- and post-term birth dates have been shown to have a pronounced effect on infant VEP acuity (Tyler and Norcia, 1986). Five adults ranging from 25 to 43 years of age were tested in the same paradigm.

Except for the dual frequency analysis, the recording configuration and experimental procedure were similar to those used in our previous studies already reviewed. Electrodes were placed 3 cm above and 3 cm to the right of the reference electrode at 1 cm above the inion. The infants' attention was attracted to the fixation point shown in Figure 16-2 by a small bell or toy dangled in front of the screen throughout each 10-second recording. The experimenter judged whether the infant was fixating the toy. If eye position shifts or gross motor activity were noted, the trial was rejected. Presentation of a spatial frequency sweep was achieved by incrementing the spatial frequency linearly every 0.5 second for a period of 10 seconds. Sweep ranges for the foveal and periphery were set in a 4:1 frequency ratio. At 165 cm the full 20:1 frequency range, which was used for infants older than 6 months, gave a linear sweep from 1.6 to 37.0 cpd in the central field and from 0.4 to 9.2 cpd in the peripheral field. For younger infants the maximum value of the range was reduced to 24, 16, or 10 cpd in the central field (6.0, 4.0, or 2.5 cpd in the peripheral field) as appropriate to ensure that there was sufficient resolution for accurate estimation of lower acuities shown by these infants. [We have previously demonstrated that the sweep range has a negligible effect on the estimated detectability limits so long as the range is sufficient for the response to fall to the noise level within that range (Norcia et al., 1989).]

The experimental procedure was to test each infant under two conditions: one with the 6-Hz stimulus to the fovea and the 8-Hz stimulus to the peripheral location, and the other with the reverse assignment. The order of the tests was randomized across infants. After analysis of the sweep records by the methods described in our previous work, we could obtain two acuity estimates at each retinal location for each infant, one from each channel. (Only statistically reliable signal-to-noise ratios were used in the estimation procedure.) We selected all the infants ($n = 17$) who completed the conditions and gave significant acuity estimates at both temporal frequencies and both retinal locations. The best of the two acuity values on the two recording channels was taken as the final acuity estimate at each frequency for each retinal location. The 17 infants completing the procedure fell into four age groups, designated as 3, 4, 6, and 8 months of age (13, 17, 28, and 32 weeks ± 2 weeks).

Relative Development of Foveal and Peripheral Acuity

The mean acuity estimates for infants and adults are shown in Figure 16-3. For adults, acuities at the two temporal frequencies were not significantly different within the error of measurement (shown as the error bars indicating the standard error of the mean values for all subjects in each group). The mean estimate of adult acuity was 25 cpd in the fovea, comparable with previous values in the cited references under our recording conditions. It is also as should be expected at the relatively low luminance available from the display screens. The mean estimate of adult peripheral acuity was 6.6 cpd, which is close to one-fourth of the foveal value and well within the range expected from the literature for mean eccentricity of 12 degrees.

The mean estimates of infant acuity again showed no significant differences between the 6 and 8 Hz stimulation frequencies at any age. The mean estimates of infant foveal acuity increased from about 6.5 cpd at 3

months to 19.0 cpd by 8 months, showing a developmental time course similar to that in our previous VEP results (Norcia and Tyler, 1985a; Hamer et al., 1989).

The new result from this study is the development of infant peripheral acuity. The 8- to 16-degree field at 3 months gave a mean acuity estimate of 3.7 cpd, slightly more than half the foveal value. This value was significantly higher than one-fourth of the foveal estimate at the same age, implying that the functional acuity is more mature in the peripheral retina than the fovea at 3 months, as expected from the retinal anatomy results. The peripheral acuity was correspondingly closer (within a factor of 2) to the adult level at this point and consequently developed to the adult level in a shorter time. The data show mean peripheral acuity to have reached the adult level within measurement error by 6 months of age, where the foveal increase does not turn the corner until 8 months. Note, however, that this earlier asymptote point does not mean that peripheral development proceeded at a more rapid rate, merely that it was concluded sooner because it began from a level closer to the endpoint. The peripheral 8- to 16-degree location therefore showed, on the basis of the VEP measurements, greater maturity and earlier maturation than did the fovea.

DEVELOPMENT OF STEREOPSIS

Interocular Acuity Differences

During the course of Birch's discussion of the factors underlying the development of stereopsis, she appears to claim that reliable interocular competition may be operating to delay the onset of stereopsis. Using forced-choice preferential looking (FPL) techniques, Birch (1985) has reported unsigned differences in the measured acuity *averaging* almost 1.0 octave in infants up to 5 months of age, but there are no data establishing the reliability of these estimates. In fact, comparable intrasession differences are reported in Birch's (1985) original study and in the other FPL literature, consistent with the idea that the differences may be due entirely to measurement variability (given that the variability of a difference measure is 1.414 times larger than the variability of the underlying measure from which the difference was derived). Moreover, it seems inherently unlikely that binocular competition would occur coherently between the millions of afferent fibers from the two eyes to such an extent as noticeably to bias the measured acuity.

For interocular differences to affect the development of stereopsis, they must be present prior to the site of binocular combination in the primary visual cortex. A clear demonstration that interocular acuity differences

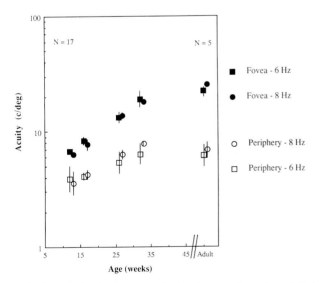

FIG. 16-3. Relative development of infant fovea and periphery. Filled symbols show means of the best estimate of foveal acuity (2 degrees radius) for each of 17 infants and 5 adults, at two temporal frequencies (■ 6 Hz; ● 8 Hz). Open symbols show comparable estimates for the 8- to 16-degree peripheral region (□ 6 Hz; ○ 8 Hz). Error bars show standard errors of the means. Note the similarity of results at the two frequencies and the relative maturity of the younger peripheries. Infants completing all four conditions showed no significant difference between 6 and 8 Hz.

at this level are much smaller than those measured behaviorally was provided by Hamer et al. (1989), who measured sweep VEP acuities for each eye in a group of infants 5–35 weeks of age. The unsigned acuity differences by this method averaged about 0.25 octaves up to 5 months of age, nearly four times smaller than those of Birch's study. These residual VEP acuity differences were well within the measurement noise of the technique, providing no evidence for any true interocular acuity difference.

There remains a question as to whether the VEP and FPL data were derived from the same region of the retina. Both studies used stimuli large enough to stimulate extrafoveal as well as foveal retina. It therefore would be difficult to argue that the immaturity of the fovea might have a differential effect in the two studies. In both cases, the most sensitive region of retina at each age is likely to have mediated performance. With this question answered, it seems safe to conclude that there are no significant differences in interocular acuity prior to the site of binocular combination in infants of any age, as the reported VEP differences fall within the measurement error of the techniques. In principle, it is possible that behavioral monocular acuities could still be different, mediated by differences in the monocular processing mechanisms beyond the site of the VEP generation. In practice, however, the behavioral differences also appear to be within the variability of the FPL technique, suggesting that the differences reported are an artifact of a noisy measurement method.

Dichoptic Fusion

It is interesting to ask whether, during the course of the development toward adult vision, infants pass through stages of perception of unique qualities that are no longer available to adults. If so, it would be analogous to the larval stage of insects or amphibia (e.g., caterpillars or tadpoles), which may possess physical capabilities unavailable to the adult stage. It has been suggested (Teller and Movshon, 1986) that this description applies to the responses of infants to dichoptic orthogonal gratings, which are perceived as rivalrous to adults. Shimojo et al. (1986) found that infants showed no preference for interocular orthogonal gratings over binocular grids up to the age of 3–4 months. This finding suggested that the infant cortex performed a nonselective combination of the inputs from the two eyes to produce a percept of a combined-orientation grid, even when the two orientations were presented to separate eyes. Beyond this age, the infants showed a pronounced preference for the binocular grids, suggesting that the dichoptic orthogonal gratings had become rivalrous and aversive. The full set of conditions is reviewed by Shimojo in Chapter 12.

The contention that the nonselective combination of orthogonal dichoptic gratings is a function unique to infants rests on the knowledge, dating back to Panum (1858) and other nineteenth century vision scientists, that adults perceive binocular rivalry under comparable stimulus conditions. Comparable stimulus conditions, however, do not necessary imply comparable neural responses, especially at a stage when the infant visual system is still relatively immature. Of particular interest is the fact that infant contrast sensitivity is immature at this age, so the neurons can be expected to respond as though the stimuli had a substantially lower effective contrast.

Until recently, the effect of contrast on binocular rivalry had not been explored. Our laboratory has looked at this question and found that binocular rivalry has a long latency at low contrast. Prior to the onset of rivalry, orthogonal dichoptic gratings show *complete perceptual summation* for periods of up to 0.5 minute after stimulus onset (Liu et al., 1990, 1991). The dichoptic summation lasted the longest for high spatial frequencies and near threshold contrasts, but at medium spatial frequencies (e.g., 3 cpd) and 10% contrast, dichoptic summation was still obtained for an average of 5 seconds, which might be a typical trial duration for a free-viewing task.

The discovery of dichoptic summation in adult vision removes from contention the idea that dichoptic summation is a process unique to the infant brain. It may instead suggest that if the retinal processing in infants had an immaturity corresponding to a lower effective contrast the signal going up to the infant cortex might be equivalent to that in adults, with the generation of dichoptic summation occurring at similar internal signal levels at both ages. It is also possible that the dichoptic summation process shows some immaturity in addition to that of the retinal signal, a quantitative question that can be approached by comparing the adult levels of rivalry induction with those predicted on the basis of the infant contrast sensitivity. Unfortunately, there is still a free parameter in this comparison: the equivalence of spatial frequency at the two ages. Because the infant's spatial frequency resolution is also immature relative to that of the adult, it is unclear how to equate spatial frequency to make a direct comparison of dichoptic summation at the two ages.

One can begin to approach the question of infant–adult equivalence by looking at the time course of development of contrast sensitivity. It is crucial to the hypothesis that the immaturity of the contrast signal occurs prior to the site of binocular combination. It is therefore arguable that the contrast response defined by early cortical VEP measures is a more appropriate index than the behavioral contrast response, which is subject to immaturities at all levels of the visual processing and response mechanisms. The development of infant VEP contrast thresholds described by Norcia et al. (1990) indicates that contrast sensitivity was about 1.0 log unit lower than adult levels at 1 month of age and reached its asymptotic level at the age of about 3 months for a stimulus of 1 cpd [roughly comparable with the width of the dark bars in the study of Shimojo et al. (1986)]. The infant immaturity is therefore in the right range of both depth and time course to allow an explanation in terms of the immaturity of the contrast response alone. A more specific test of the hypothesis, however, would require closer coordination between the experimental conditions between the three studies than is presently available.

Depth from Occlusion

One question raised by Shimojo in Chapter 12 is whether we develop types of depth perception different from those that can be characterized by conventional binocular disparity cues. One example may be provided by his interesting experiments with Nakayama on the type of depth perception they called "da Vinci stereopsis," deriving from monocular stimuli in relation to the occlusion geometry of the nearby objects. Such depth perception is a dramatic demonstration revealing a powerful effect of occlusion constraints in this type of depth perception. It is remarkable that this result has lain unsuspected for so long in the face of intensive exploration of depth perception for more than a century and a half.

However, before accepting the interpretation of the results presented by Nakayama and Shimojo (1990), several questions must be answered. An opposing viewpoint (the conventional disparity/suppression hypothesis) is that the depth perceived for the monocular object in the occlusion paradigm arises from the conventional disparity due to binocular correspondence of one of the edges of the monocular object with the adjacent edge of the occluder when those edges are of the same sign of contrast. (This and the following statements should be interpreted relative to Fig. 13 in Chapter 12.) Depth would then be perceived on the basis of the disparity of the veridical match between the occluder edges in the two eyes and the disparity of the false match between the monocular object and the occluder edge in the other eye. (There is no inherent contradiction in utilizing dual pairs of matches from three stimuli, as the cortex may well contain multiple parallel detectors ready to respond to any disparity presented to them. Only if there is inhibition between such detectors would they preempt such dual matches, but there seems to be no adaptive reason to expect such a restriction.)

The observed asymmetry of depth perception could then be obtained if the occlusion geometry acted as a gate to interdict depth perception when the monocular object was ecologically invalid (e.g., a monocular stimulus in the right eye to the left of an occluder). On this viewpoint, occlusion stereopsis would consist of depth perception derived from the conventional "Wheatstone" disparities in the configuration corresponding to Panum's (1858) limiting case. The role of occlusion constraints would be limited to the suppression of inappropriate depth signals, rather than to generation of depth perception per se.

The question raised by this alternative viewpoint is whether there is any information in the present data or further experiments that should be conducted before the hypothesis of da Vinci stereopsis is accepted. The conventional disparity/suppression hypothesis predicts that the matched depth should correspond to that derived from the disparity between the occluder edge and the same-sign monocular edge. It should provide veridical depth perception for each position of the monocular stimulus up to some critical disparity, with the depth declining beyond that point as the disparity exceeded the range analyzable by the stereoscopic system (Richards, 1971).

The da Vinci hypothesis, on the other hand, implies an occlusion constraint that predicts that the depth should fall in a range corresponding to the region of space behind the occlusion stimulus. The depth in this region extends from the veridical depth level down to a lower level determined by the other edge of the occluder. Because there is no further information as to where in this range the object would be, it seems that the occlusion hypothesis should predict that the perceived depth would be some form of average of the possible range of positions. Whatever the form of the average, the perceived depth on the occlusion hypothesis should therefore be less than the veridical depth predicted by the conventional disparity hypothesis, especially when the monocular point was close to the occluder. The data given by Shimojo (see Chapter 12) show that, up to about 20 minutes of disparity, the matched depths tend to fall close to the veridical disparity prediction. Over this range, therefore, they support the suppression hypothesis and do not show any systematic tendency to correspond to the lower depths predicted on the da Vinci hypothesis.

There are further experiments that could be performed to test the role of conventional disparity in the suppression hypothesis. No depth should be perceived if there is no possibility of a conventional disparity association between the monocular stimulus and the occluder in the other eye. In the configuration used by Nakayama and Shimojo (1990), the stimuli were the same sign of contrast, and both had elongated vertical edges. It therefore seems plausible that the depth could have arisen from conventional disparity relations in their stimuli. It is easy to design stimuli where depth from conventional disparity could not arise, based on what is known about interocular image matching. For example, no depth is reported if the two monocular stimuli are of opposite signs of contrast (Anstis, 1970) or if a monocular point in one eye must be matched to an elongated edge in the other eye (Tyler, 1971). The conventional disparity/suppression hypothesis would predict no difference in perceived depth with variations in the relative size or contrast sign of the monocular stimulus and the occluder. Such a test could act as a strong discrimination between the competing hypotheses.

Nakayama and Shimojo (1990) did report that when the occluder and the monocular test were of opposite luminance contrast relative to a gray background, as much depth was perceived as when they were of the same contrast. It should be noted, however, that a white square has an edge with the same sign of contrast as one of the edges of a dark line. This version of the test, which was designed for another purpose, is not therefore definitive in ruling out a conventional disparity explanation.

As a preliminary test, the demonstration of Figure 16-4 provides another test of the conventional disparity hypothesis. The figure is in the form of the triptych free-fusion type of stereogram developed by Nakayama and Shimojo (1990). Fusion across the image gives stereopairs with both signs of disparity, regardless of whether the observer is a crossed or an uncrossed fuser. The upper triptych reproduces the demonstration of Nakayama and Shimojo (1990), with a monocular test line on either side of the occluder. When free-fused, the stereopair in which the test lines on either side the occluder are in the right eye induces depth behind the occluder in the monocular line on the right but not for the line on the left. Conversely, when the lines are in the left eye, depth is seen for the line on the left but not for the line on the right. These observations are in accord with their data. The new result is shown in the lower triptych, which duplicates the configuration in the upper triptych except that the monocular stimuli are now dots instead of lines. This configuration is based on the assumption (Tyler, 1971) that depth perception is nonexistent or reduced when the disparity requires comparison of a dot in one eye with a line in the other.

When shown to a sample of observers naive to the hypothesis, depth perception appeared to be reduced in the new configuration (Fig. 16-5). Only 60% of the observers saw the same degree of depth in the dot case as in the line case, compared with 86% of the observers who saw depth according to the da Vinci hypothesis in the line targets, i.e., further back for the occlusion-valid configuration than the occlusion-invalid one. Because the occlusion hypothesis predicts no difference in the depth perceived in the line and dot variants of the monocular image configuration, the observations provide partial support for the conventional disparity hypothesis for the depth perceived in the line version. Full evaluation of the hypothesis would require determination of the degree to which depth perception from dot/line disparities is reduced relative to matched configurations, which is beyond the scope of this simple test.

Further light is shed on these supplementary depth perception processes by the depth observed in the occlusion-invalid case. According to the occlusion hy-

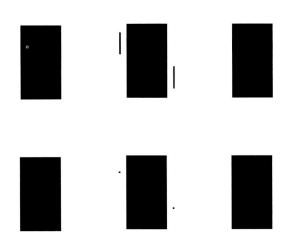

FIG. 16-4. Free-fusion stereogram in triptych form to demonstrate the relative weakness of the "occlusion cue" when dots (lower row) rather than lines (upper row) are used as the monocular stimuli. When the monocular line in the left eye is to the left of the occluder (or in the right eye is to the right of the occluder), it is generally seen behind. For reverse couplings, depth is usually weak or ambiguous. When monocular lines are replaced by dots (lower row), which allow less disparity pairing with the edge of the occluder, perceived depth is weaker for many observers.

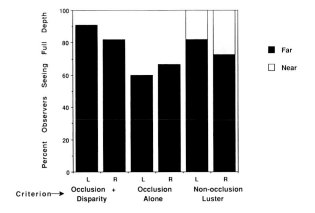

FIG. 16-5. Left pair of bars represent the percent of observers reporting farther perceived depth for the occlusion-valid line stimulus than the occlusion-invalid one in each eye. This condition contains disparity cues consistent with Panum's limiting case between the monocular lines and the occluder edge. Center pair of bars represent the corresponding condition with monocular dots instead of lines to minimize disparity cues and maximize occlusion cues. These bars show that only about 60% of observers saw depth to the same extent as for monocular lines. Right pair of bars represent the depth interpretation of binocular luster in occlusion-invalid dots. Most observers saw these stimuli behind the occluder (dark bars) or in front of the occluder (white bars), but not in the same plane as the occluder.

pothesis, this case should result in no perceived depth relative to the binocular occluder. In fact, none of the observers saw these stimuli in the same plane as the occluder. For 77% of the observers the occlusion-invalid stimuli appeared to be in front of the occluder, whereas the remainder saw them as behind the occluder (Fig. 16-5). I interpret this result as the perception of depth from the dichoptic luster cue that is seen around the monocular dots (cf. Julesz and Tyler, 1976). One possibility is that this depth is related to the "rival depth" mechanism proposed by O'Shea and Blake (1978) for depth in uncorrelated regions of random-dot stereograms. It is another depth process that is unrelated to the occlusion constraints but that needs to be taken into account in experiments on monocular stimuli.

MODES OF BINOCULAR PROCESSING

The current view of the visual cortex is that it consists of at least 28 visual representation areas organized along both a serial hierarchical principle and a parallel distributed principle, with interconnections within and between levels. This arrangement, which may be described as an interconnected serial-parallel heterarchy, appears to be a ubiquitous principle of neural organization. Unlike a hierarchy, which only has convergence from lower levels onto fewer elements at each higher level culminating in a single apical node, a heterarchy contains multiple parallel hierarchies, any one of which may dominate its local domain of the network at any given time by virtue of the lateral interactions between them. It is descriptive of the structure of the retina—of cortical hypercolumns in each representation area in each of the sensory systems (with the possible exception of olfaction, which may be just a homogeneous neural net). The local connectivity of arrays of individual neurons forms the same type of heterarchy within the visual system from the retina to the cerebellum. It would not be surprising, therefore, to find a similar arrangement within a particular sensory modality such as stereopsis. Although stereopsis is generally modeled as a single unified processing system, there is significant evidence that it has a number of independent subsystems, each specialized for extracting depth in a different manner.

It should be emphasized that stereopsis in this context is used to refer to any means of depth perception arising from differences between the images projecting to the two eyes, or binocular disparities. There are also many other monocular depth cues that can be used to generate dramatic depth impressions, such as differential motion cues, perspective, shape-from-shading, blur, and contrast. There are also nonvisual depth cues from such possible sources as convergence, accommodation, object familiarity, and auditory cues. These cues feed into the overall sense of depth in the real world situation. The present analysis, however, is limited to the role of binocular disparities of various types in the complex of depth phenomena constituting stereopsis.

Heterarchical Model

Reviewing the evidence for the mechanisms contributing to stereopsis, Tyler (1983) concluded that it was not possible to accommodate all the diverse results within single hierarchy models, which form the basis for all stereopsis models that have been proposed (e.g., Julesz, 1962; Sperling, 1970; Dev, 1975; Marr and Poggio, 1979; Pollard et al., 1985; Prazdny, 1985). However, depth perception has been demonstrated for a variety of stimulus dimensions that are incompatible with any single process for solving the binocular correspondence problem. The conceptual framework proposed here is concerned with a series of simple analyses by local cortical elements sensitive to the disparity field and similar processing at higher levels, in contrast to the inherently global models of such investigators as Julesz (1971). The region of space to be processed by this system is assumed to be optimized by means of both versional and vergent eye movements.

The point of departure is a parallel array of cortical disparity "detectors," each responding to the presence of a stimulus with a particular location in x, y, and z coordinates (represented by the first rectangle in Figure 16-6, with the y-axis omitted for clarity). The key feature of this approach is a reliance on arrays of specialized mechanisms to account for certain attributes of the stereoscopic process. Such mechanisms are represented by the sketched rectangles extending behind the first one in Figure 16-6. Examples of such attributes that are discussed here are the direction selectivity for motion in depth and selectivity of orientation of the stereoscopic figure in random-dot stereograms. Such selectivities are not predicted by inhibition or facilitation between simple disparity-selective neurons. Each specialized disparity array is assumed to operate in parallel with other such arrays at the same processing level, with the overall output being determined by either a combination of the processes or the most sensitive process under particular stimulus conditions.

The second feature of the analysis is to posit neural interactions in both the lateral (spatial) domain and the disparity domain. These inhibitory interactions introduce an element of "globality" into the model, in the sense that the processing of disparity at one point depends on the disparity relation in other regions of the image. Nevertheless, they are processes with great physiological plausibility, and because they operate with a few simple neural connections they are appropriate to

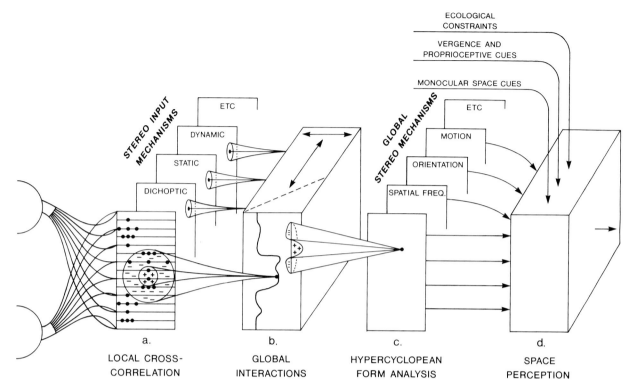

FIG. 16-6. Four stages (a–d) of the proposed model of stereoscopic space perception. Note that each slice at each stage is a two-dimensional representation of a three-dimensional array, and many possible interconnections are unknown. The parallel planes at stage a represent arrays of specialized mechanisms described in Fig. 16-7. Stage b represents the disparity-specific and interdisparity interactions (arrows) and disparity gradient limit (dashed line). Stage c shows arrays of hypercyclopean mechanisms for analysis of the form of the cyclopean image. Stage d shows input from nonstereoscopic depth cues to generate the final representation of the depth image. (Modified from Tyler, 1983.)

account for the rapidity of stereoscopic detection (Tyler, 1977).

This approach has the advantage of breaking down the global nature of stereopsis (Julesz, 1978) into a sequence of processes (Fig. 16-6) that are empirically separable. Within this serial structure is a further parallel organization for analyzing specialized global features of the stereoscopic image.

Specialized Disparity Mechanisms. There are numerous indications that specialized arrays of mechanisms might exist to process specific attributes of the field, in contrast to the unitary models that are often proposed for disparity processing. Examples are provided by neurons (or neural circuits) selectively sensitive to direction and velocity of retinal motion, color-opponent neurons, and neurons with orientation-specific excitation and inhibition. Each specialized mechanism for stereopsis is assumed to operate in parallel with the others, in a manner analogous to the "feature-specific" conception of neurons in striate cortex proposed by Hubel and Wiesel (1962). (Note that it is the processing arrays of neurons that are proposed to operate in parallel. Even unitary models postulate individual neurons that operate in parallel on the array of inputs from the retinas.)

Specialized disparity mechanisms may themselves exist in two classes according to whether specialization occurs at the local level (retinal-receptive-field characteristics) or global level (cortical interactions). Examples of local mechanisms that are discussed are those specialized for the detection of stimuli with specific sizes and orientations, orientational disparities, motion in depth, and spatial frequency differences between the eyes. Mechanisms in the second class (global mechanisms) may use either conventional positional disparity information from the two retinas or specialized disparity information, but they respond on the basis of some global aspect of the disparity field. Examples are global lateral inhibition, specificity for size and orientation of cyclopean depth figures, and processes specialized for sinusoidal stereograting detection. The evidence for each specialized mechanism is summarized in the individual sections following a general description of the model.

To show some of the range of specialized mechanisms that can be encompassed within the model of a binocular pair of oriented receptive fields, Figure 16-7 depicts the set discussed in the following sections. The top row depicts possible receptive field relations underlying binocular fusion into single vision, interocular rivalry between cells with monocular fields, the opposite contrast

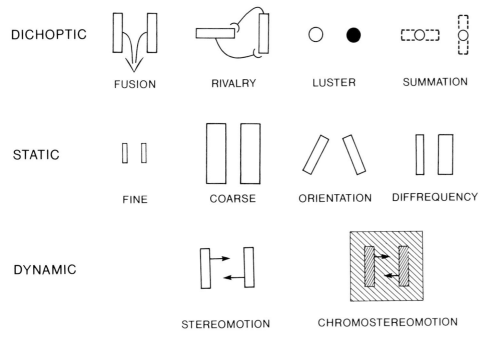

FIG. 16-7. Receptive field relations for specialized binocular mechanisms. (Top row) Binocular fusion for disparate images, interocular rivalry for noncongruent images, binocular luster for opposite contrast images, dichoptic summation in circularly symmetrical receptive fields for low contrast images with noncongruent features. (Second row) Specialized mechanisms for fine disparity, coarse disparity, orientational disparity, and interocular size differences. (Third row) Specialized mechanisms for luminance and chromatic stereomotion processing.

field relation for binocular luster, and the state of dichoptic summation of low contrast images, perhaps by circularly symmetrical receptive fields. The middle row shows binocular receptive fields for fine disparity processing, large fields for coarse disparity processing, interocular orientation differences for orientational disparities, and interocular size differences for disparities of spatial frequency. The final row contains only two types: the opposite directionally selective fields for stereomotion processing and the same arrangement for purely chromatic stereomotion conditions (the only chromatic case that has been shown to require a separate mechanism). Evidence for the existence of each of these mechanisms is reviewed in the following sections.

Structure of the Model. Stereoscopic space perception seems to involve at least four levels of processing beyond the retinal level (Fig. 16-6). At each level there may be parallel arrays of neurons processing specialized aspects of the previous level (although such arrays are needed at only the first and third levels to account for the evidence to be presented).

As depicted in Figure 16-6, the initial stage of binocular combination is a disparity detection process that might be achieved by the various types of neuron with facilitatory responses to particular disparities, as recorded in the visual cortex of the cat and monkey. This stage may be considered as a local cross-correlation process, performed by neurons tuned to different disparities, occurring at each location in the binocular visual field. As the eyes vary their vergence, cortical projections of the visual scene slide over one another to obtain the shift (or disparity) that produces the best match or correlation in each local region of the visual field. The images matched in this way are said to be in register. In practice there are, of course, two dimensions of field location, and there is no reason to suppose that the array is as regular as depicted here.

All disparities in the cortical image should give rise to a response somewhere in the neural disparity field, but they do not all necessarily produce veridical depth images because in complex stereograms there may be many disparities arising from spurious correlations between adjacent points (Julesz, 1960). Any degree of decorrelation in dynamic random-dot stereograms, such as that produced by images well out of register, tends to be visible as depth noise, a dynamic cloud of random depths (Julesz and Tyler, 1976). For static departures from register, such depth noise is not visible except with short-duration exposures; hence the depth image must involve processing beyond local disparity detection, as has been amply demonstrated by Julesz (1962, 1971). The further processing for depth is identified with the second, global processing level (Fig. 16-6), although it may not be physiologically distinct from the first level.

The result of the first two processing levels is a three-dimensional representation of the visual scene. Although some neural processing has been involved, this representation has advanced little beyond the form of a direct projection of the stimulus field into the brain. It is reasonable to suppose that there is a further stage of pattern processing that extracts specific features of this depth image for perceptual analysis, which has been called the hypercyclopean level (Tyler, 1975a), as shown in Figure 16-6. The studies described show that there are hypercyclopean processes operating on the stereoscopic depth images that are similar to some of the cortical processes operating on the two-dimensional retinal image. For example, there seems to be specific representation of the size and orientation of features of the stereoscopic image.

Even beyond the hypercyclopean level there may be a further level of abstract spatial representation in which stereoscopic information is integrated with other spatial representations, such as those from the motion vector field (Gibson, 1950; Nakayama and Loomis, 1974), the texture gradient field (Gibson, 1950), and accommodation, vergence, vestibular, and other nonstereoscopic cues. This level of integration is indicated by the fourth element of Figure 16-6 but is not considered in detail in the present analysis.

Dichoptic Mechanisms

Fusion. One of the basic facts of normal binocular vision is that disparate stimuli appear fused up to a particular disparity value, beyond which they give rise to diplopia (double vision), in which both monocular stimuli are seen simultaneously. This process must involve some kind of nonlinear combination rule because the fused image does not resemble the linear sum of the monocular images. In fact, the monocular components are suppressed and invisible in their former location. The elements of the fused image appear to be located spatially between the positions of the monocular elements, a phenomenon known as allelotropia.

For the present purpose, it is important to realize that fusion is a binocular mechanism distinct from stereoscopic depth perception. The fusion range is often treated as the limiting range for conventional disparity processing (e.g., Ogle, 1952; Julesz, 1971). In fact, the fusion range is neither limiting nor coextensive with the range of stereopsis (e.g., Richards, 1971). A straightforward demonstration that the fusion mechanism is entirely distinct from the stereoscopic mechanism is the demonstration of fusion for vertical disparities. No depth is perceived from vertical disparities [with the exception of certain indirect configurations related to the "induced effect" (Ogle, 1950)]. The existence of a fusion range for vertical disparities therefore indicates that fusion is a mechanism of binocular combination that can operate independently of the stereoscopic mechanism. Moreover, the range of fusion shows different temporal properties for vertical than for horizontal disparities. The vertical fusion range is approximately constant with temporal frequency, whereas the horizontal fusion range shows a pronounced reduction as temporal frequency is increased (Schor and Tyler, 1981).

Further evidence of the distinction between the fusion and stereoscopic mechanisms is based on the fact that fusion depends on the spatial extent of the stimulus. Schor et al. (1984a) compared the fusional range for bars with sharp edges and for blurred bars with a difference-of-Gaussian (DoG) luminance profile. The DoG bars showed progressively increasing fusion limits as bar width was increased, in contrast with the sharp-edged bars, which showed almost no dependence of the fusion range on bar width. Thus the fusion limit was not affected by size per se but by some aspect of the spatial frequency content of the image, which scaled concomitantly with the size of the stimuli to be fused.

The pronounced variation of fusion limits with the size of blurred images raises the question of the primitive feature controlling the behavior of the fusion limit. As the DoG profiles become wider, the luminance gradient on each side becomes shallower. The increased fusional range might therefore be attributable to either the shallower luminance gradient or the inherent width of the DoG profile. This issue can be decided by varying the luminance gradient without changing the width. Schor et al. (1989) showed that neither varying the contrast of the profile nor varying the phases of frequency components making up the luminance profiles had any detectable effect on the fusion limit. These results imply that the binocular fusion mechanism is completely insensitive to both the amplitude (or contrast) and phase relations between the frequency components of the image. The only primitive important for fusion therefore seems to be the actual frequency content of the features. With respect to the insensitivity to contrast, the stereoscopic system behaves differently, showing a variation in proportion to the square root of the image contrast (Halpern and Blake, 1988; Legge and Gu, 1989). For all the reasons enumerated, it is clear that the neural processes underlying fusion are distinct from those underlying stereopsis, even though the two perceptual properties may coexist for the same stimuli.

Luster. Binocular luster is a second class of percept that can occur with noncorresponding stimuli. It occurs with stimuli in which regions with corresponding borders have different luminances or colors in the two eyes. It was described by early investigators of visual science (e.g., Panum, 1858; Helmholtz, 1866) as a kind of lustrous or shimmering surface of indeterminate depth. In fact, the lustrous appearance of surfaces such as a waxed table top or a car body is essentially due to binocular luster. It results from the different position of partially reflected objects in the surface by virtue of the different position of the two eyes. This kind of lustrous appearance is distinct from both the shininess of a surface as seen by reflected highlights and from the clear depth image seen in a mirror.

The phenomenon of binocular luster has received little attention, despite the fact that it is qualitatively different from depth, diplopia, or rivalry. The lustrous region is not localizable in depth, but it seems unitary and does not fluctuate in the manner of binocular rivalry. More recent studies (Julesz, 1960; Julesz and Tyler, 1976; Tyler and Julesz, 1976) have demonstrated that binocular luster also may be observed in static and dynamic random-dot stereograms in which all the elements have opposite contrast in the two eyes. When the dots are identical in the two eyes they are perceived as fused; but when they are complemented in contrast in the two eyes the perception is of a lustrous surface. Changing between these states of identical and complemented contrast in the two eyes provides an opportunity to examine the speed of fusion and defusion in complex stimuli. Such changes in the interocular correlation are invisible to either eye alone when the noise is dynamically changing.

Julesz and Tyler (1976) used this paradigm to show that, for a large dynamic noise field, the average presentation time required for detection of a binocularly identical field interposed between two periods of lustrous stimuli (complemented fields) was 30 ms. Remarkably, the mean time required for detection of the complemented (lustrous) array between two periods of binocularly fused noise was only 4 ms. This anisotropy between correlation and decorrelation events held a constant ratio of about 1.0 log unit for all field sizes. The spatial integration area was about 2 degrees square for both tasks. Thus the anisotropy must involve differences in temporal processing, since the spatial integration properties are the same for the two phenomena.

The cyclopean correlation/decorrelation anisotropy is surprising in view of the fact that the change of information is mathematically identical for the two tasks. The only difference is which change came first. Because the neural processing of the binocular information was anisotropic, it did not conform to the mathematical properties of entropy and was instead given a new name, "neurontropy." This kind of temporal anisotropy was a particular property of the fusion/luster mechanism. No equivalent effect was found for a comparable stereoscopic task, which had a spatial integration area of only about 0.5 degree, or 1.2 log units less in area than for luster detection.

The detectability in a presentation time of only a few milliseconds, the neurontropic anisotropy and the much larger integration area combine to support the idea that the mechanism of luster perception is distinct from those of conventional disparity analysis. Because it occurs for unfused stimuli, luster is equally distinct from the fusion mechanism. Yet it must still be integrated into the global percept of the depth properties of the image, so it must be considered a low level mechanism of the same order of analysis as the other dichoptic mechanisms.

Interocular Rivalry and Suppression. If the binocular images are so different that the contours intersect through corresponding areas in the two eyes, conventional wisdom has been that there is always perceptual suppression the contours of one eye by those of the other (e.g., Panum, 1858; Blake and Fox, 1974a,b). If either the contours or the neural pathways are biased for one eye over the other, the suppression may be constant. If, on the other hand, the stimuli and pathways are well balanced, the suppression alternates between the two eyes to produce interocular (or "binocular") rivalry. This state of alternating suppression is distinct from the steady states of fusion of the two images into one, constant diplopia of two separate images, or the maintained lustrous depth impression of opposite dichoptic contrast. Although one can construct models in which the same cells are involved in some of these processes, the processes themselves are distinct properties of the arrays of cells. They may reasonably be regarded as providing qualitatively separate inputs into the overall structure of the three-dimensional image representation.

Dichoptic Summation. Part of the question of how signals in the two eyes combine to produce a unified impression concerns how they combine when stereopsis is not possible. Although dichoptic stimuli are generally thought to produce rivalry alternation, Liu et al. (1990) have found that it is not the case at low contrast or high-spatial frequency, where dichoptic stimuli of orthogonal orientations combine to form a fused plaid that is stable for many seconds or minutes. An example of the data obtained in this experiment is shown in Figure 16-8. The stimuli were sinusoidal gratings of orthogonal orientations in the two eyes, presented in a circular aperture containing six grating cycles at either frequency, with a dark surround. The mean duration of perception of a stable dichoptic plaid is plotted as a function of grating contrasts at two spatial frequencies (3 and 6 cpd). Dichoptic plaid durations fell on a roughly hyperbolic relation with stimulus contrast, from durations of the order of 1 second at high contrasts to about 30 seconds for the 6 cpd case at 10% contrast.

These data suggest that rivalry is a high-contrast, low-spatial-frequency phenomenon, not the universal result. The significance of these results lies in establishing a

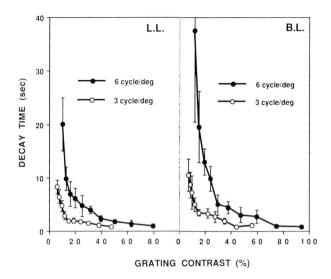

FIG. 16-8. Duration of stable dichoptic plaid percept as a function of contrast of orthogonal gratings for two spatial frequencies. Note dichoptic plaid durations as long as 10–40 seconds at low contrast.

perceptual role for the 60% of binocular cells in monkey cortex known to be approximately circularly symmetrical (Baizer et al., 1977). Such cells should permit dichoptic fusion of orthogonal orientations, as they have no means to respond selectively to different orientations. If there were no dichoptic fusion, this large group of circular, symmetrical binocular cells would appear to have no role in the ultimate perception.

Static Stereomechanisms

Fine Disparity. Stereoscopic processing of horizontal disparities has often been proposed to consist of two ranges with different properties, the fine and coarse disparity processes (Julesz, 1978). The distinction between processing of fine and coarse disparities is evidenced by the existence of different perceptual phenomena in the two disparity ranges. Schumer (1979) observed linear depth averaging of two interposed stereofigures in dynamic random-dot stereogram (RDS) stimuli up to disparities of about 20 arc minutes, but beyond this value the two interposed stereofigures were perceived separately and no averaging of the separate depth surfaces occurred. Mitchell and Baker (1973) found that the depth aftereffect produced by prolonged inspection of a disparate line target was optimal for a 5 arc minute adapting stimulus but could not be obtained for disparities greater than 15 to 20 arc minutes. A similar result was reported by Blakemore and Julesz (1971) for disparity adaptation in RDS. Both depth averaging and depth aftereffects thus seem to be restricted to the range of fine disparities, implying a different mechanism for the processing of coarse disparities. Similar distinctions have been observed in studies of vergence eye movements (Saye and

Frisby, 1975; Jones, 1977) and stereoscopic evoked potentials (Norcia et al., 1985b).

Schor et al. (1984b) characterized the disparity sensitivity of spatially tuned channels by means of stimuli with difference-of-Gaussian (DoG) luminance profiles. They found different spatial tuning properties for wide and narrow DoG stimuli. For coarse DoG centers, wider than about 20 arc minutes, their evidence suggested that static disparity was processed by a set of channels with a tuning approximating that of the DoG profile. (An alternative interpretation is that the measured narrow tuning reflects a sensitivity to differences in effective contrast between the eyes.) For fine DoG stimuli whose centers were narrower than about 20 arc minutes, however, a different picture was obtained. The disparity appeared to be processed by a single channel that was insensitive to the stimulus width (so long as it remained below 20 arc minutes). This behavior requires a complex mechanism to explain it. The channel must be able to accommodate DoG stimuli over an 8:1 ratio of sizes and disparities, yet exclude those beyond a center size of 20 arc minutes. The data seem to require a mechanism that can respond to small stimuli over a large range of disparities, as Schor and Wood (1983) showed that the upper disparity limit for depth detection in this range was about 50 minutes, even for DoGs as narrow as 3-minute center width (16:1 ratio). Such processing is reminiscent of a global mechanism of the type postulated by Julesz (1971).

A corresponding division has been described in neurophysiological studies of the neural response to disparity in monkey cortex (Poggio et al., 1985). Neurons that were predominantly binocular (in the classical sense of having identifiable receptive fields for monocular stimulation of each eye) tended to show a region of binocular facilitation (or, alternatively, of binocular occlusion) in a narrow range around zero disparity. The peak disparity range of such cells corresponds to the range of fine disparities reported in the psychophysical studies.

Coarse Disparity. In contrast to the cells tuned to fine disparities, Poggio's group found that cells with classically monocular receptive fields had a strikingly different disparity response profile from those with classically binocular receptive fields. Surprisingly, the "monocular" cells with a response to only one eye when tested separately nevertheless showed binocular facilitation under binocular testing, but it occurred for either crossed disparities only or uncrossed disparities only, with minimal response at zero disparity in either case. This lack of sensitivity near zero disparity implies that such cells are specialized for the processing of large disparities and comprise a distinct coarse disparity system.

Such neurophysiological data tend to support the psychophysical results of Schor's group, suggesting that coarse disparities are processed by mechanisms with properties different from those for fine disparities. Schor and Wood (1983) found a size-disparity correlation for static stimuli (as predicted by Tyler, 1973a), such that sensitivity for larger stimuli fell in direct proportion to their width. (Dynamic disparity changes gave a similar picture of a size-disparity correlation, but the sensitivity reduction was more gradual with size.) In this size-scaled regimen, the sensitivity could have been mediated by a set of local spatial channels with a fixed interocular phase relation, for example, the Gabor-shaped receptive fields on each retina with an interocular phase relationship of 90 degrees proposed by Ohzawa and Freeman (1986a,b).

If there is a relation of the psychophysical results to the coarse/fine disparity mechanisms, the data of Schor's group suggest that the coarse, local processing of these channels actually extends to the lower limits of the fine disparity range. Thus one could not expect to exclude local disparity processing by restricting stimuli to small disparities. One could only eliminate fine disparity processing by selecting stimuli with disparities that were large in relation to the horopteral zone.

Orientational Disparity. Blakemore et al. (1972) pointed out that the fact that cortical cells have oriented receptive fields implies that there may be orientational disparities between the receptive fields of the two eyes, in addition to a spatial binocular disparity. They found that such orientational disparities were present for cat neurons and hypothesized that they might be involved in the processing of inclination (depth slant). Detection of an inclination in this manner has the advantage that the orientational cues are independent of the distance (and hence the spatial disparity of the object).

Psychophysical support for this suggestion comes from an experiment by von der Heydt et al. (1977) using one-dimensional random visual noise with different orientations in the two eyes. The visual noise stimuli, which looked like bundles of straight sticks, were produced uncorrelated between the two eyes with the intention of precluding normal disparity relations. Although uncorrelated stimuli can give rise to random depth relations (Tyler 1974a, 1977; Julesz and Tyler, 1976), it does not seem to apply to static stimuli, when the uncorrelated images give rise to rivalry but not stereopsis (Julesz, 1971). If von der Heydt et al. (1977) thus succeeded in controlling the conventional disparity cues, the introduction of a difference in orientation between the two eyes should have no further effect. In fact, they observed a dramatic inclination in the median plane, providing a perceptual example of the use of orientational disparity cues when conventional disparity cues are inoperative.

Further experiments supporting the specific use of orientational disparity in human depth perception have been done by Cagenello and Rogers (1990), who showed that it played a strong role in peripheral vision when positional disparity cues were controlled. Mitchison and McKee (1990), however, did not find support for the idea that orientational disparity controlled slant perception in foveal presentations of line grids of various orientations, although they did obtain substantial slant perception when the only depth cue was the orientation difference between pairs of lines. They were not able definitively to partition the perceived depth between the orientation cue and the positional disparity gradient in these lines.

The possibility of a separate orientational disparity system is particularly interesting in light of the mathematical demonstration by Koenderink and van Doorn (1976) that orientational disparity can provide robust depth information. By analyzing the disparity vector field mathematically they found that the orientation disparity cue is less disturbed by various transformations, such as convergence, than are other aspects of the disparity vector field. Thus from the point of view of ecological optics, orientational disparity provides a relatively invariant perceptual depth cue.

Depth Tilt from Diffrequency. The presence of binocular spatial frequency differences between the images in the two eyes produces an impression of lateral depth tilt (Blakemore, 1970). The term "binocular spatial-frequency difference" is so unwieldy that we replace it with the term "diffrequency," by analogy with "disparity" for positional differences between the two eyes. That diffrequency as such might be a separate cue for stereopsis was first suggested by Blakemore (1970). He used vertical sinusoidal gratings in the frontal plane as stimuli and found that binocular diffrequencies gave rise to a horizontal depth tilt up to a ratio of 1.4 between the frequencies in the two eyes. The tilt persisted even when the grating in one eye was moving at velocities up to 1 degree/second, which seemed too fast to allow continuous rematching of the spatial disparity, leading Blakemore to suggest that the diffrequency was processed as a separate cue to depth tilt.

The suggestion was taken up by Tyler and Sutter (1979), who designed several stimulus paradigms to ensure that conventional disparity cues were not involved in the situation. The simplest consisted of sinusoidal gratings moving in opposite directions in the two eyes. When the velocity was slow, conventional disparity cues gave the perception of a flat plane moving toward the observer. Each time the gratings had moved the distance of a complete cycle, the plane flipped back and then continued to move toward the observer again. As the velocity was increased, a point was reached when the depth movement failed and was replaced by a perception of rivalry between the two monocularly moving images. At this rate (a velocity of 4 degrees/second) conventional disparity cues must have been eliminated, as the depth motion derived from those cues was no longer visible.

At this point the spatial frequency in one eye was varied by a small amount, and observers reported that the plane was simultaneously tilted into depth *and* rivalrous. Thus the rivalry within the conventional disparity system was maintained, superimposed on the depth attributable to the diffrequency between the two eyes, clearly demonstrating that diffrequency is a separate depth cue from disparity. Depth tilt was detectable up to surprisingly large diffrequency ratios of 2:1 between the two eyes.

A second experiment by Tyler and Sutter (1979) was fully cyclopean, in the sense that it utilized dynamic, one-dimensional visual noise (a random-bar stimulus) as the base stimuli. In the main experiment, the noise was uncorrelated between the two eyes in order to avoid conventional disparity cues. Nevertheless, horizontal depth tilt was readily visible, but only for diffrequency ratios in the high range between 1.2 and 2.0. For diffrequency ratios less than 1.2, depth tilt was not visible for uncorrelated one-dimensional noise, implying that the diffrequency system exhibits both a high threshold and a high range of frequency difference for producing sensations of depth tilt. In a control experiment, on the other hand, the same stimuli were presented with correlated noise in the two eyes, implying that bar-by-bar disparity correlations were now present. Depth tilt was easily seen throughout the diffrequency range, including values below a diffrequency ratio of 1.2. This low diffrequency range in correlated noise presumably needed conventional disparity cues for its operation, as depth was not visible in the uncorrelated case in this range.

Dynamic Stereomechanisms

Real Stereomotion Perception. Just as cortical receptive fields may exhibit a preferential response for one direction of lateral motion, so they may show directional specificity for motion in depth. Pettigrew (1973) has reported cells with opposite preferred directions in the two eyes. Such cells would be well suited to detect motion in depth toward or away from the observer. Cynader and Regan (1978) have shown that many cells, particularly those showing binocular occlusion, have a binocular interaction specific for motion in depth (i.e., motion in opposite directions on the two retinas).

Regan and Beverly (1973) and Beverley and Regan (1973, 1975, 1979) studied the psychophysical characteristics of the mechanisms for motion in depth. Using an adaptation paradigm, they showed that there are separately adaptable classes for different directions of motion in depth. The direction of motion in depth could be divided into four classes according to whether the motion passed outside the line of sight of the right eye, between the right line of sight and the midline, between the midline and the line of sight of the left eye, or outside the left line of sight.

Beverley and Regan (1973) found that prolonged stimulation with sinusoidal motion in a given direction in space produced adaptation throughout one or more of these direction ranges. For exposure to stimuli in the extreme leftward or rightward ranges, adaptation occurred only for the stimulated range. The adaptation was identical for a given test stimulus within the range, regardless of the adapting stimulus direction within the range. In summary, these results provide strong evidence for neural channels specific to the direction of motion in space.

Further evidence for the existence of separate processes for in-phase (lateral) and counterphase (depth) motion comes in the form of a substantial difference in psychophysical threshold for the two types of motion. It was originally found that the detection threshold for sinusoidal motion in depth was about three times higher than that for detection of each monocular component of the motion (Tyler, 1971, 1975b). Thus the depth motion system was not only less sensitive than the lateral motion system, indicating that the two systems have different motion-processing characteristics, but also less sensitive than each monocular motion system. This result suggests that activation of the stereomovement system causes suppression of some information that is otherwise available to the monocular and binocular lateral movement system.

This "stereomovement suppression" effect was not only operative to the same extent over a large range of temporal frequencies but also occurred for pulsed changes in depth (Tyler and Foley, 1974). Under certain stimulus conditions stereomovement suppression did not occur, and there can even be an enhancement of depth movement over lateral movement detection (Regan and Beverley, 1973b; Tyler and Foley, 1974) that operates for both horizontal and vertical changes in disparity (Tyler, 1975b). The latter fact implies that the suppression is occurring in the binocular fusion system, as vertical disparities do not generate stereoscopic depth per se. In this way, stereomovement suppression reveals much about the interactions between the three systems involved in binocular movement processing (binocular lateral movement, binocular depth movement, and binocular fusion).

Chromatic Stereomotion Perception. The concept of a sustained chromatic system and a transient stereoscopic system (Livingstone and Hubel, 1987) suggests that stereomotion should be much weakened with purely chromatic disparity stimuli, even in noncyclopean figural displays. However, because stereopsis is often enhanced by motion cues, Tyler and Cavanagh (1991) examined the detectability of purely chromatic stereomotion in red/green sinusoidal gratings. We found that it was not only a robust percept, but that under some conditions it was as well perceived as luminance stereomotion, although it exhibited different functional properties. This difference in functional properties gave a clear assurance that chromatic stereomotion processing was not just a degraded form of that for luminance stereomotion but an independent perceptual system.

Having first done experiments to ensure equiluminance of oscillating red/green gratings when viewed monocularly, oscillation thresholds were measured at the adjusted equiluminance point for monocular lateral motion and binocular stereomotion as a function of temporal frequency and compared with those for purely luminance gratings at the same contrast relative to threshold. For luminance gratings, both functions showed

a dramatic increase of oscillation phase threshold as temporal frequency was reduced below 3 Hz (Fig. 16-9A), implying that the thresholds were controlled by the velocity of the phase change rather than its absolute value. Figure 16-9A also shows that grating oscillation produced a stereomotion suppression effect similar to that reported by Tyler (1971).

The data for purely chromatic stereomotion had markedly different properties. At high temporal frequencies monocular chromatic motion thresholds were elevated by about a factor of 5 relative to monocular luminance motion thresholds in Figure 16-9B. On the other hand, within the chromatic condition there was no significant difference between monocular and stereomotion thresholds, so the stereomotion suppression seen in Figure 16-9A was absent. In addition, there was almost no low-frequency threshold elevation for chromatic stereomotion, so stereomotion thresholds became equal at 0.5 Hz for the two types of stimulation. We concluded that purely chromatic motion processing lacks the type of inhibitory mechanism necessary to produce

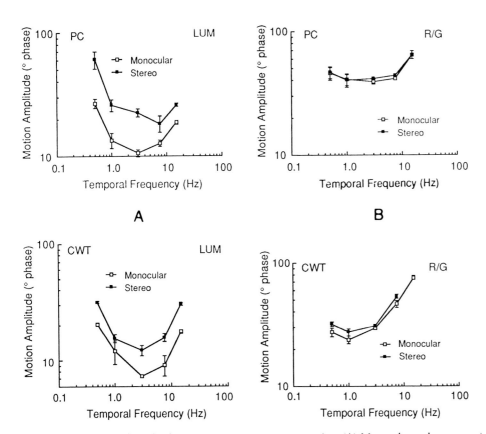

FIG. 16-9. Properties of purely chromatic stereomovement perception. (A) Monocular and stereoscopic thresholds for a 2 cpd luminance grating of 10% contrast as a function of temporal oscillation frequency for two observers. Both types of threshold are plotted in terms of the monocular amplitude of oscillation (i.e., no binocular summation is presumed). Amplitudes are given in terms of degrees of phase angle of the sinusoidal cycle. (B) Monocular and stereoscopic depth thresholds for purely chromatic red/green gratings with the same spatial configuration as the luminance gratings. Note similarity of monocular and stereoscopic thresholds and the lack of significant threshold elevation in the low frequency range from 3.0–0.5 Hz. (Modified from Tyler, 1990.)

an inhibitory falloff at low frequencies. Interestingly, for chromatic stimuli the visual system was as sensitive to depth motion as to lateral motion, which makes it relatively *more* sensitive to chromatic depth motion in comparison with the sensitivity ratio for luminance stimuli. The data of Figure 16-9 thus validate the concept of an independent mechanism for purely chromatic stereomovement, with both temporal and binocular combination properties different from those for luminance stereomotion.

Cyclopean Stereomotion Perception. In principle, it is possible to generate a stimulus that contains movement in depth without correlated monocular motion, if generated by means of a dynamic RDS. True cyclopean depth motion is obtained only when the monocular images change randomly between frames, so as to mask the temporal changes in disparity and require all aspects of the motion processing to occur at the cyclopean level or beyond. Norcia and Tyler (1984) showed for the first time that motion in depth is readily perceived in dynamic RDSs, and that it has similar temporal characteristics to those for nondynamic RDSs. Their stimulus was in fact the alternation of a dynamic RDS plane between two depth values, but stereomotion could be perceived up to frequencies of about 15 Hz, as is the case for monocular motion (Tyler and Torres, 1972; Tyler, 1973a,b).

It is feasible, though tricky, to make a distinction between cyclopean stereomotion detection and hypercyclopean stereomotion perception. Cyclopean stereomotion may be defined as motion that can be detected at the cyclopean level of binocular combination. To detect it, some disparity units must be alternately stimulated and not stimulated (while the change remains monocularly invisible). In this sense, cyclopean motion detection does not involve cognizance of the abstracted form of the motion. It would not, for example, involve discrimination of the direction of motion. The processes of encoding motion direction and the smooth sense of change of position through the cyclopean retina, however, are regarded as hypercyclopean processes of temporal form analysis. They are discussed in a subsequent section.

Global Interactions

The second cortical stage of the model is the site of the global interactions between the local disparity detectors that serve to refine the representation of the disparity image from its initial crude array of stimulated points to a coherent representation of the three-dimensional surfaces present in the field of view. A variety of such processes have been proposed over the years, many summarized by Tyler (1983, 1991b). They include dis-

parity-specific facilitation, pooling, and inhibition, occlusion between different disparities, disparity gradient limitation, coarse-to-fine matching, search for dense surfaces, and so on.

This chapter is not, however, the forum to review such material, as most of it requires extensive experimentation to establish in adults; and the findings are too premature to consider for infant research. The emphasis for the infant studies proposed later in the chapter is on study of some of the input variables for stereopsis reviewed in the preceding pages. However, it is also feasible to study higher level form analysis of the stereoscopic image by standard techniques for infant behavior. For this reason, the basic properties of this level of stereopsis are reviewed in the next section.

Hypercyclopean Perception

The concept of hypercyclopean analysis refers to the third level of processing of stereoscopic images described in Figure 16-6. By analogy with the cortical neurons with receptive fields selective for particular properties of the retinal image, there could be neurons at a higher level in cortex having "receptive fields" at the level of the "cleaned" cyclopean depth image. These receptive fields would have a cyclopean basis, in the sense of having properties specific to the disparity selective neurons in the cyclopean retina, but they would perform a hypercyclopean analysis of the spatial and temporal *form* of the depth image. Hypercyclopean receptive fields would have characteristics defined in terms of the figural properties of the cyclopean image but independent of its specific disparity characteristics (i.e., which particular disparity is stimulated at any given retinal location).

The existence of such a hypercyclopean level of processing can be demonstrated by means of an adaptation paradigm (Tyler, 1975a). The analogy is with the demonstration of cortical involvement in the processing of luminance gratings by adaptation to drifting gratings on the retina (Blakemore and Campbell, 1969; Kelly and Burbeck, 1980). Because the grating is drifting, there can be no retinal afterimage; hence the threshold elevation, which is specific to both spatial frequency and orientation of the adapting grating, must be occurring at a higher, presumably cortical, level of processing. In the same way, if adaptation is found for a cyclopean stereograting that is moving across the retina, it represents the activity of a level of form processing beyond that of the cyclopean processing for depth per se. Although there is no particular reason to expect a neural specificity for this type of stimulus, there are nevertheless several lines of evidence that suggest the existence of channels selective for cyclopean form.

Hypercyclopean Spatial Frequency Specificity. The first demonstration of a hypercyclopean aftereffect (Tyler, 1975a) was based on the Blakemore and Sutton (1969) experiment showing a perceived spatial frequency shift in a luminance grating after adaptation to one of a slightly different spatial frequency. In the hypercyclopean experiment, adaptation to a random-dot *stereograting* of one spatial frequency produced the perception of an increased spatial frequency of disparity modulation in a *stereograting* of slightly higher spatial frequency and a corresponding decrease after adaptation to a slightly lower spatial frequency. The use of scanning eye movements during adaptation ensured that this result was not due to local disparity adaptation but was a hypercyclopean effect. The result is suggestive of the existence of channels selective to the spatial frequency of disparity modulation.

Schumer and Ganz (1979) used an adaptation paradigm to investigate stereograting specificity. They adapted for 8 minutes to one spatial frequency of disparity modulation and measured the threshold elevation for stereograting across a range of spatial frequencies. Adaptation was maximal at the spatial frequency of the adapting stereograting and showed a rather broad function with a bandwidth of about ± 1.0 octave around each adapting frequency. It is important to note, however, that only those channels that are adaptable may be revealed by this technique. Other channels may exist that are not adaptable by the stimulus exposure used. Furthermore, the adaptation might not have a linear characteristic and thus might distort the apparent shape of the channels when measured by this method.

An alternative approach to measurement of stereograting channel bandwidth is based on the narrow-band masking paradigm introduced by Stromeyer and Julesz (1972) for contrast gratings. By masking the test grating with a 1.0-octave band of noise at various center frequencies, they showed that frequency-selective channels in the contrast domain extended throughout the suprathreshold range, with bandwidths similar to those found by the threshold adaptation paradigm. Using a comparable technique, Tyler and Julesz (1980b) (see Tyler, 1983) found that a frequency selectivity for stereogratings that was much narrower than that obtained with the adaptation paradigm. At each test stereograting spatial frequency, the threshold elevation function had a bandwidth of about 0.25 octave on the low side and 0.5 octave on the high side. These narrow bandwidths seem to imply the existence of specialized mechanisms for the processing of repetitive patterns of disparity modulation on the cyclopean retina.

Hypercyclopean Orientation Specificity. An argument similar to that adduced for spatial frequency can be developed for the existence of orientation specificity in the hypercyclopean domain. An experiment in support of this idea (Tyler, 1975a) was based on the well known tilt aftereffect paradigm (Gibson and Radner, 1937; Campbell and Maffei, 1971). Adaptation to a stereograting with an orientation at some angle away from horizontal produced a perceived tilt in a horizontal test stereograting. The magnitude of tilt aftereffect had the conventional S-shaped form but peaked at about 25 degrees orientation of the adapting plane from the test plane, in comparison to the 12 degrees peak obtained for contrast gratings (Campbell and Maffei, 1971).

One can ask whether the hypercyclopean and contrast tilt aftereffects are independent or there is cross-adaptation between them. The relative degree of cross-adaptation indicates the extent to which the two systems share a common pathway. Cross-adaptation was tested by adapting to a contrast grating of the same spatial frequency and measuring the tilt aftereffect obtained in a stereograting (which, it should be emphasized, had no orientation specificity in the contrast domain, i.e., the random-dot matrix). A cross-adaptation tilt aftereffect was obtained but with about half the magnitude of the pure hypercyclopean effect (or indeed the pure contrast effect). It was therefore concluded that there are some oriented elements common to the two systems. Because the stimulus specification essentially precludes a common basis at the early stages of visual processing, it seems likely that this common orientation specificity occurs even beyond the hypercyclopean level. A high level oriented "map" of the visual world can be hypothesized to draw together the orientation information from previous levels and to be slightly rotated by adaptation to either contrast or cyclopean form information (stage D in Fig. 16-6).

Hypercyclopean Stereomotion Perception. The study by Norcia and Tyler (1984) used a dynamic RDS stimulus that contained the alternation of a dynamic RDS plane between two discrete depth values, but it was perceived at low frequencies as a smooth, sinusoidal motion in depth. Thus there must be some hypercyclopean process of interpolation that allows smooth phi (ϕ) movement to be seen between disparity planes generated at the cyclopean level of processing similar to that operating between pairs of flashing lights separated laterally in space. The fact that smooth cyclopean motion is limited to the same temporal frequency range as monocular apparent motion processing (about 5 Hz with a large separation) (Tyler, 1973b) suggests that the limit for both may be identical and may lie at the hypercyclopean level. It may require a perceptual interpolation process rather than a direct linkage between motion selective units at the cyclopean representation level.

Further support for the idea that the interpolation is a higher-level process comes from the fact that Norcia and Tyler (1984) found that detection of changes in depth was not limited to the same 5 Hz range in dynamic RDS. Instead, they found that alternation between the two depth planes was detectable both psychophysically and electrophysiologically up to frequencies almost three times higher. Thus the limit on processing for disparity change was not set by the hypercyclopean process for smooth interpolation of disparity motion between the discrete disparity planes. Presumably, the initial cyclopean disparity detection process was giving rise to these rapid signals early in the neural chain, which then served as input to both a disparity level detector and the hypercyclopean depth motion interpolator. To my knowledge, however, there have been no studies of smooth dynamic RDS motion that would allow a clearer distinction to be drawn as to the functional properties of these two processing levels.

Hypercyclopean Object Constancy.   To extend the analysis to more complex space perception, one can approach the question of object constancy from the point of view of stereoscopic processing. Object constancy is the ability to perceive an object as having a rigid three-dimensional structure even while the retinal image is distorted as the object rotates or moves about in space. Although the contours of the object are undergoing continuous transformation, the brain often has the capability to reduce the motions to a single projective transformation, within which the object retains its rigid form.

This concept can be applied to transformations of stereoscopic images. When an RDS is rotated or the observer moves around with respect to the stereogram, the cyclopean form is perceived as undergoing shape distortions in the form of relative motion between the various disparity planes (Julesz, 1971). This percept occurs even though the monocular half-images consist of flat planes in which there is no objective relative motion. This induced stereomovement has been attributed to the operation of object constancy (Tyler, 1974b), as it occurs at depth edges where the planes at different depths should move past each other if the stereoscopic form were a rigid object undergoing rotation. When the object does not behave as expected, the stereoscopic object seems to become distorted in a nonrigid fashion, inducing relative movements of the stereoscopic planes.

The dynamic characteristics of the object constancy system were measured by determining the sensitivity limits for induced stereomovement as a function of temporal frequency of rotation (Tyler, 1974b). At low frequencies the object constancy mechanism, as evinced from the induced stereomovement effect, operated down to about twice the amplitude of stereomovement threshold itself. As frequency was increased, the object constancy mechanism progressively failed, and no induced stereomovement was seen above about 5 Hz, which was still close to the peak sensitivity for binocular movement

perception. A remarkable observation was that, in the region where induced stereomovement was absent, substantial stereoscopic rotation could be perceived, whereas the stereoscopic form appeared to be a rotating rigid object. Thus there seems to be a clear perceptual dissociation of the stereomovement system, which was reporting depth motion, and the more sluggish object constancy system, which was signaling no change in the shape of the object.

PROPOSED EXPERIMENTS FOR INFANT BINOCULAR VISION

The demonstrable diversity and richness of stereoscopic disparity processing suggests that it may be a fertile source of interaction between infant and adult visual studies. From the developmental perspective, it would be of great interest to extend the study of infant stereopsis to the additional stereoscopic depth cues elaborated in the previous sections and determine whether they all have similar time courses or some mature at different times than others. It has been suggested, for example, that the perception of depth tilt from diffrequency might be a more elementary form of stereopsis than the point-to-point disparity mechanism (Tyler and Sutter, 1979). If so, this result might be taken to predict that diffrequency depth tilt would exist at an earlier developmental stage than the onset of disparity detection. Such a result would, in turn, provide supportive evidence that the two mechanisms are different in adults. Of course, the experiments would always have to be performed with sufficient controls to ensure that the differences were not due to ancillary processes such as the development of contrast sensitivity (discussed earlier in this review) or patterns of eye movement behavior that could discriminate between the stimulus conditions under comparison.

In general, reliable differences in developmental time courses would not only provide evidence for separation of such mechanisms but would suggest grouping of such mechanisms into categories that developed at about the same time. Such groupings should generate hypotheses as to how the mechanisms are connected (e.g., by being in the same level of cortical representation), as different parts of the visual system reach maturity at different times. In this way the developmental results could contribute to a deeper understanding of adult stereopsis, as well as the converse.

Development of Coarse Disparity Processing

An obvious experiment in infants would be to study the development of depth perception for the coarse disparity system (as oppposed to detection threshold for the smallest visible disparities, which has been well studied). Adult data have been fully specified, for example, by Schor and Wood (1983) for single targets (both hard-edged bars and bars with difference-of-Gaussian profiles) and by Tyler and Julesz (1980a) for cyclopean stimuli. The maximum disparity for depth detection ranged as high as 4 degrees in the single targets and 2 degrees in the cyclopean ones.

An interesting paradigm would be to perform FPL experiments in infants as a function of disparity, with the null target being a disparity beyond the range of adult depth perception. The positional information could be masked in cyclopean fashion by using targets consisting of a small set of randomly spaced vertical lines, each on a different vertical level. All the lines except one would have large disparities, causing them to be seen as diplopic and at the depth of the horopter. One line would have the smaller test disparity, allowing it to be seen as standing out in depth if the disparity could be processed, but still diplopic if the disparity was beyond the Panum range of about 10 minutes. The largest disparity eliciting reliable FPL would be regarded as the upper depth limit for an infant of a particular age. It would then be possible to map the development of that limit and determine if it had the same time course as that for stereoacuity (reviewed in Chapter 13).

It might further be possible to obtain an estimate of the range of maximum perceived depth by FPL. Presumably the preference would be proportion to perceived depth in the display. If so, the proportion of correct responses and perhaps other measures (e.g., the delay to first look or time to disengage fixation) might provide estimates of the strength of the depth perceived by the infants. It would then be straightforward to estimate the perceived depth as a function of disparity to obtain comparisons of the full depth range with that of adults.

Interocular Rivalry and Suppression

Interocular suppression occurs when there are different images projecting in the same direction in visual space. If the image in one eye is of a higher contrast or otherwise more salient than the image in the other eye, the less salient image is suppressed from consciousness. If the two images are of equal salience (but still different in spatial properties, such as local orientation or direction of motion), the interocular suppression alternates between the two eyes to generate interocular rivalry (often known as "binocular rivalry"). Such interocular rivalry is aperiodic, with alternation intervals of a range of durations forming a Poisson distribution (Blake et al., 1971). This situation is curious, as most unstable physical systems tend to go into oscillation at some

resonant frequency. It suggests that interocular rivalry is governed not by some fatigue process with a stable decay function but by the random arrival of neural events tending to induce a switch between the two eyes. Nevertheless, it is relevant to note that the Poisson distribution has a mean value that characterizes the average length of dominance in each eye.

The interocular suppression process, and the ensuing alternation when the images are balanced, are clearly distinct from the processes of binocular fusion and stereopsis. If rivalry suppression were occurring for a similar image with a small binocular disparity, stereopsis would be impossible, as only one eye's image would be available at any time. That the fusion process is not a miniature version of rivalry suppression can be demonstrated by viewing a stimulus with a disparity near the limit of the fusional range (e.g., 5 minutes). If rivalry alternation were occurring, the stimulus should be visibly alternating between two spatial positions separated by 5 minutes. Interocular apparent motion is readily visible at this separation, but none is seen during binocular fusion (Tyler, 1983). Instead, the stimulus appears at a stable position intermediate between the two monocular positions (Sheedy and Fry, 1979). Evidently, therefore, the processes of interocular suppression and rivalry are distinct from those of binocular fusion. Nevertheless, rivalry suppression is part of the process generating the final full-dimensional percept from the retinal light arrays.

The interpretation of the dichoptic plaid result discussed in Chapter 12 is that there is a period of early vision prior to stereopsis during which infants experience not binocular rivalry but direct summation of the images in the two eyes. It is possible to test this interpretation directly in a 2AFC paradigm by generating a comparison stimulus that contains alternations between orthogonal gratings on the same kind of aperiodic schedule that has been established to occur in adult binocular rivalry (Blake et al., 1971). If the targets are small, it should be sufficient for the comparison stimulus to consist of the entire monocular patch alternating between one orientation and the other because rivalry is homogeneous for small targets. The other eye should contain a blank stimulus, as this coupling has been shown to induce the same type of binocular luster as occurs in the dichoptic orthogonal gratings to be used for the test stimulus. The basic test would be to find the mean alternation rate at which the infants no longer discriminated between the two stimuli, presumably the alternation rate at which it matched the alternation distribution in the dichoptic stimulus. Thus one would predict that the forced-choice discrimination function for infants would show clear discriminability for lower and higher mean alternation rates but show a minimum of nondiscrimination when the stimulus alternation rate and rivalry alternation rate were equal.

Infant Stereopsis from Nonconventional Disparity Cues

There are interocular cues that have been shown to yield depth perception in adults despite the absence of conventional horizontal disparities. Two examples are orientational disparity and interocular diffrequency. In each case, there is information that depth perception occurs independently of the horizontal disparity information, as already reviewed. The existence of an early period of a few months when infant acuity and contrast sensitivity may be too poor to support conventional stereopsis makes it interesting to test whether these less-refined cues may allow a more basic level of depth perception.

In particular, both orientation disparity and diffrequency are cues involving disparity gradients, which are absent in conventional depth stimuli of a square or a bar standing out from its background. It is therefore necessary to test for these cues with stimuli containing depth gradients rather than abrupt edges. In doing so, however, the stimuli should be designed to avoid the problem that gradients of broad extent provide only weak cues to their depth orientation (as is the case for simple tilts of the entire depth plane, for example). A straightforward solution to this problem is to use sinusoidal modulations of disparity, or stereogratings (Tyler, 1974c). The repeated bars of a stereograting form a more interesting (and more discriminable) stimulus than a flat tilted plane or a single bulge.

Development of Hypercyclopean Processing

A final suggestion is to take a look at the onset and development of hypercyclopean processing in infants. Infants can discriminate depth well enough by 6 months, but do they have the apparatus to process the form of cyclopean depth images? The answer may already be "yes" to one type of cyclopean form: lateral motion of a cyclopean target. Fox et al. (1980) showed that infants could track the direction of a set of depth bars visible only in dynamic RDS, suggesting that the infants could discriminate the direction of motion of the cyclopean bars—a hypercyclopean ability. An alternative explanation, however, is that the infants were tracking by detecting the position error between their fixation point and the nearest cyclopean edge, then randomly hunting until that position error was minimized at each moment in time. This explanation appears far-fetched, particularly in light of the relatively smooth tracking movements shown by some infants. It seems much more likely that the infant visual systems were able to code the velocity error (a motion signal) and use this code as an input to control the direction and speed of the required eye movements.

The simplest type of hypercyclopean infant experiment is perhaps the satiation type. Here the infant repeatedly views a target that has one cyclopean feature (e.g., left oblique bars) until the fixation time is reduced close to zero, then is shown a target with a different cyclopean feature (e.g., right oblique bars) to determine if renewed interest is implied by increased fixation to the novel cyclopean form. This change would imply a hypercyclopean discrimination of the bar orientation (in contrast to simple awareness that the image was not flat, for example). The same paradigm could be used to determine the onset and development of hypercyclopean processing of such depth features as the orientation, spatial frequency, and direction of motion for cyclopean depth images.

Acknowledgments. The visual evoked potential studies described in this chapter were performed in collaboration with Anthony Norcia, Russell Hamer, and Dale Allen. Supported by NIH grants 1P30 EY 6883, RR 5981, and RO1 EY 7890.

REFERENCES

ALLEN, D., NORCIA, A. M., AND TYLER, C. W. (1986). A comparative study of electrophysiological and psychophysical measurement of the contrast sensitivity function in humans. *Am. J. Optom. Physiol. Opt.* 63, 442–449.

ANSTIS, S. M. (1970). Phi movement as a subtraction process. *Vision Res.* 20, 1411–1430.

APKARIAN, P. A., NAKAYAMA, K., AND TYLER, C. W. (1981). Binocularity in the human visual evoked potential: facilitation, summation and suppression. *Electroencephalogr. Clin. Neurophysiol.* 51, 32–48.

BAIZER, J. S., ROBINSON, D. L., AND DOW, B. M. (1977). Visual responses of area 18 neurons in awake, behaving monkey. *J. Neurophysiol.* 40, 1024–1037.

BANKS, M. S., AND BENNETT, P. J. (1988). Optical and photoreceptor immaturities limit the chromatic and spatial vision of human neonates. *J. Opt. Soc. Am. [A]* 5, 2059–2079.

BAUMGARDT, E. (1947). Sur les mécanismes de l'excitation visuelle. *Arch. Sci. Physiol.* 1, 257–274.

BAUMGARDT, E., AND SMITH, S. W. (1965). Facilitation effect of a background light on target detection: a test of theories of absolute threshold. *Vision Res.* 5, 299–312.

BEVERLEY, K. I., AND REGAN, D. (1973). Evidence for the existence of neural mechanisms selectively sensitive to the direction of movement in space. *J. Physiol. (Lond.)* 235, 17–29.

BEVERLEY, K. I., AND REGAN, D. (1975). The relation between sensitivity and discrimination in the perception of motion-in-depth. *J. Physiol. (Lond.)* 249, 387–398.

BEVERLEY, K. I., AND REGAN, D. (1979). Separable aftereffects of changing-size and motion-in-depth: different neural mechanisms? *Vision Res.* 19, 727–732.

BIRCH, E. E. (1985). Infant interocular acuity differences and binocular vision. *Vision Res.* 25, 571–576.

BLAKE, R., AND FOX, R. (1974a). Binocular rivalry suppression: insensitive to spatial frequency and orientation change. *Vision Res.* 14, 687–692.

BLAKE, R., AND FOX, R. (1974b). Adaptation to invisible gratings and the site of binocular rivalry suppression. *Nature* 249, 488–490.

BLAKE, R., FOX, R., AND McINTYRE, C. (1971). Stochastic properties of stabilized-image binocular rivalry alternations. *J. Exp. Psychol.* 88, 327–332.

BLAKEMORE, C. (1970). A new kind of stereoscopic vision. *Vision Res.* 10, 1181–1200.

BLAKEMORE, C., AND CAMPBELL, F. W. (1969). On the existence of neurones in the human visual system selectively sensitive to the orientation and size of retinal images. *J. Physiol. (Lond.)* 203, 237–260.

BLAKEMORE, C., AND JULESZ, B. (1971). Stereoscopic depth aftereffect produced without monocular cues. *Science* 171, 286–288.

BLAKEMORE, C., AND SUTTON, P. (1969). Size adaptation: a new aftereffect. *Science* 166, 245–247.

BLAKEMORE, C., FIORENTINI, A., AND MAFFEI, L. (1972). A second neural mechanism of binocular depth discrimination. *J. Physiol. (Lond.)* 226, 725–749.

BOUMAN, M. A., AND VAN DER VELDEN, H. A. (1947). The two-quantum explanation of the dependence of threshold values and visual acuity on the visual angle and the time of observation. *J. Opt. Soc. Am.* 37, 908.

CAGENELLO, R. B., AND ROGERS, B. J. (1990). Orientation disparity, cyclotorsion and the perception of surface slant. *Invest. Ophthalmol. Vis. Sci.* 31 (suppl.), 97.

CAMPBELL, F. W., AND KULIKOWSKI, J. J. (1972). The visual evoked potential as a function of the contrast of a grating pattern. *J. Physiol. (Lond.)* 222, 345–356.

CAMPBELL, F. W., AND MAFFEI, L. (1970). Electrophysiological evidence for the existence of orientation and size detectors in the human visual system. *J. Physiol. (Lond.)* 207, 635–652.

CAMPBELL, F. W., AND MAFFEI, L. (1971). The tilt aftereffect: a fresh look. *Vision Res.* 11, 833–840.

CANNON, M. W. (1983). Contrast sensitivity: psychophysical and evoked potential methods compared. *Vision Res.* 23, 87–95.

CYNADER, M., AND REGAN, D. (1978). Neurons in cat parastriate cortex sensitive to the direction of motion in three-dimensional space. *J. Physiol. (Lond.)* 274, 549–569.

DEV, P. (1975). Perception of depth surfaces in random-dot stereograms. *Int. J. Man Machine Stud.* 7, 511–528.

FECHNER, G. T. (1860). *Elemente der Psychophysik.* Leipzig: Breitkopf & Hertel.

FOX, R. L., ASLIN, R. N., SHEA, S. L., AND DUMAIS, S. T. (1980). Stereopsis in human infants. *Science* 207, 323–324.

GIBSON, J. J. (1950). *The Perception of the Visual World.* Boston: Houghton, Mifflin.

GIBSON, J. J., AND RADNER, M. (1937). Adaptation, aftereffect and contrast in the perception of tilted lines. I. Quantitative studies. *J. Exp. Psychol.* 20, 453.

GREEN, D. M., AND SWETS, J. A. (1966). *Signal Detection Theory and Psychophysics.* Huntington, NY: Krieger.

HALPERN, D. L., AND BLAKE, R. (1988). How contrast affects stereoacuity. *Perception* 17, 483–495.

HAMER, R. D., NORCIA, A. M., TYLER, C. W., AND HSU-WINGES, C. (1989). The development of monocular and binocular VEP acuity. *Vision Res.* 29, 397–408.

HELMHOLTZ, H. L. VON (1866). *Handbuch der Physiologische Optik.* Hamburg: Voss.

HUBEL, D. H., AND WIESEL, T. N. (1962). Receptive fields, binocular interaction and functional architecture in the cat's visual cortex. *J. Physiol. (Lond.)* 160, 106–154.

JONES, R. (1977). Anomalies of disparity detection in the human visual system. *J. Physiol. (Lond.)* 264, 621–640.

JULESZ, B. (1960). Binocular depth perception of computer-generated patterns. *Bell Syst. Tech. J.* 39, 1125–1162.

JULESZ, B. (1962). Towards the automation of binocular depth perception (AUTOMAP-I). In C. M. POPPLEWELL (ed.). *Proceedings of the IFIPS.* Amsterdam: North Holland.

JULESZ, B. (1971). *Foundations of Cyclopean Perception.* Chicago: University of Chicago Press.

JULESZ, B. (1978). Global stereopsis: cooperative phenomena in stereoscopic depth perception. In R. HELD, H. W. LEIBOWITZ, AND H-L. TEUBER (eds.). *Handbook of Sensory Physiology. Vol. VII. Perception.* Berlin: Springer-Verlag.

JULESZ, B., AND TYLER, C. W. (1976). Neurontropy, an entropy-like measure of neural correlation in binocular fusion and rivalry. *Biol. Cybern.* 22, 107–119.

KELLY, D. H., AND BURBECK, C. A. (1980). Motion and vision. III. Stabilized pattern adaptation. *J. Opt. Soc. Am.* 70, 1283–1289.

KOENDERINK, J. J., AND VAN DOORN, A. J. (1976). Geometry of binocular vision and a model for stereopsis. *Biol. Cybern.* 21, 29–35.

KULIKOWSKI, J. J. (1977). Visual evoked potentials as a measure of visibility. In J. E. DESMEDT (ed.). *Visual Evoked Potentials in Man.* Oxford: Clarendon, pp. 184–196.

LEGGE, G. E., AND GU, Y. (1989). Stereopsis and contrast. *Vision Res.* 29, 989–1004.

LIU, L., TYLER, C. W., SCHOR, C. M., AND LUNN, R. (1990). Dichoptic plaids: no rivalry for lower contrast orthogonal gratings. *Invest. Ophthalmol. Vis. Sci.* 31, 526.

LIU, L., TYLER, C. W., AND SCHOR, C. M. (1991). Linear summation of binocular contrast with dichoptic stimuli—failure of Fechner's paradox. *Invest. Ophthalmol. Vis. Sci.* 32, 708.

LIVINGSTONE, M. S., AND HUBEL, D. H. (1987). Psychophysical evidence for separate channels for the perception of form, color, movement and depth. *J. Neurosci.* 7, 3416–3468.

MANN. I. (1964). *The Development of the Human Eye.* 3rd Ed. London: British Medical Association.

MARR, D., AND POGGIO, T. (1979). A theory of human stereopsis. *Proc. R. Soc. Biol.* 204, 301–328.

MITCHELL, D. E., AND BAKER, A. G. (1973). Stereoscopic aftereffects: evidence for disparity specific neurones in the human visual system. *Vision Res.* 13, 2273–2288.

MITCHISON, G. J., AND McKEE, S. P. (1990). Mechanisms underlying the anisotropy of stereoscopic tilt perception. *Vision Res.* 30, 1781–1792.

NACHMIAS, J., AND KOCHER, E. C. (1970). Visual detection and discrimination of luminance increments. *J. Opt. Soc. Am.* 60, 382–389.

NAKAYAMA, K., AND LOOMIS, J. M. (1974). Optical velocity patterns, velocity sensitive neurons and space perception: a hypothesis. *Perception* 3, 63–80.

NAKAYAMA, K., AND SHIMOJO, S. (1990). Da Vinci stereopsis: depth and subjective occluding contours from unpaired image points. *Vision Res.* 30, 1811–1825.

NORCIA, A. M., AND TYLER, C. W. (1984). Temporal frequency limits for stereoscopic apparent motion processes. *Vision Res.* 24, 395–401.

NORCIA, A. M., AND TYLER, C. W. (1985a). Spatial frequency sweep VEP: visual acuity during the first year of life. *Vision Res.* 25, 1399–1408.

NORCIA, A. M., AND TYLER, C. W. (1985b). Infant VEP acuity measurements: analysis of individual differences and measurement error. *Electroenceph. Clin. Neurophysiol.* 61, 359–369.

NORCIA, A. M., CLARKE, M., AND TYLER, C. W. (1985a). Digital filtering and robust regression techniques for estimating sensory thresholds from the evoked potential. *IEEE Eng. Med. Biol.* 4, 26–32.

NORCIA, A. M., SUTTER, E. E., AND TYLER, C. W. (1985b). Electrophysiological evidence for the existence of coarse and fine disparity mechanisms in human vision. *Vision Res.* 25, 1603–1611.

NORCIA, A. M., TYLER, C. W., AND HAMER, R. D. (1988). High contrast sensitivity in the young human infant. *Invest. Ophthalmol. Vis. Sci.* 29, 44–49.

NORCIA, A. M., TYLER, C. W., AND HAMER, R. D. (1990). Development of contrast sensitivity in the human infant. *Vision Res.* 30, 1475–1486.

NORCIA. A. M., TYLER, C. W., HAMER, R. D., AND WESEMANN, W. (1989). Measurement of spatial contrast sensitivity with the swept contrast VEP. *Vision Res.* 29, 627–637.

OGLE, K. N. (1950). *Researches in Binocular Vision.* Philadelphia: Saunders.

OGLE, K. N. (1952). On the limits of stereoscopic vision. *J. Exp. Psychol.* 44, 253–259.

OHZAWA, I., AND FREEMAN, R. D. (1986a). The binocular organization of simple cells in the cat's visual cortex. *J. Neurophysiol.* 56, 221–242.

OHZAWA, I., AND FREEMAN, R. D. (1986b). The binocular organization of complex cells in the cat's visual cortex. *J. Neurophysiol.* 56, 243–249.

O'SHEA, R. P., AND BLAKE, R. (1987). Depth without disparity in random-dot stereograms. *Percept. Psychophys.* 42, 205–214.

PANUM, P. L. (1858). *Physiologische Untersuchungen über das Sehen mit zwei Augen.* Kiel: Schwerssche Buchhandlung.

PETTIGREW, J. D. (1973). Binocular neurones which signal change of disparity in area 18 of cat visual cortex. *Nature [New Biol.]* 241, 123–124.

POGGIO, G. F., MOTTER, B. C., SQUATRITO, S., AND TROTTER, Y. (1985). Responses of neurons in visual cortex (V1 and V2) of the alert macaque to dynamic random-dot stereograms. *Vision Res.* 25, 397–406.

POLLARD, S. B., MAYHEW, J. E. W., AND FRISBY, J. P. (1985). PMF: a stereo correspondence algorithm using disparity gradient. In *Proceedings of the 3rd International Symposium on Robotics Research.* Cambridge, MA: MIT Press, pp. 19–26.

PRAZDNY, K. (1985). Detection of binocular disparities. *Biol. Cybern.* 52, 93–99.

REGAN, D., AND BEVERLEY, K. (1973a). Disparity detectors in human depth perception: evidence for directional selectivity. *Science* 181, 877–879.

REGAN, D., AND BEVERLEY, K. I. (1973b). The dissociation of sideways movements from movements in depth: psychophysics. *Vision Res.* 13, 2403–2415.

RICE, S. O. (1945). Mathematical analysis of random noise. *Bell Syst. Tech. J.* 24, 46–156.

RICHARDS, W. (1971). Anomalous stereoscopic depth perception. *J. Opt. Soc. Am.* 61, 410–414.

SAYE, A., AND FRISBY, J. P. (1975). The role of monocularly conspicuous features in facilitating stereopsis from random-dot stereograms. *Perception* 4, 159–171.

SCHOR, C. M., AND TYLER, C. W. (1981). Spatio-temporal properties of Panum's fusional area. *Vision Res.* 21, 683–692.

SCHOR, C. M., AND WOOD, I. (1983). Disparity range for local stereopsis as a function of luminance spatial frequency. *Vision Res.* 23, 1649–1654.

SCHOR, C. M., HECKMANN, T., AND TYLER, C. W. (1989). Binocular fusion limits are independent of contrast, luminance gradient and component phases. *Vision Res.* 29, 821–836.

SCHOR, C. M., WOOD, I., AND OGAWA, J. (1984a). Binocular sensory fusion is limited by spatial resolution. *Vision Res.* 24, 661–665.

SCHOR, C. M., WOOD, I., AND OGAWA, J. (1984b). Spatial tuning of static and dynamic local stereopsis. *Vision Res.* 24, 573–578.

SCHUMER, R. A. (1979). Mechanisms in human stereopsis. Ph.D. thesis, Stanford University.

SCHUMER, R. A., AND GANZ, L. (1979). Independent stereoscopic channels for different extents of spatial pooling. *Vision Res.* 19, 1303–1314.

SEIPLE, W. H., KUPERSMITH, M. J., NELSON, J. I., AND CARR, R. E. (1984). The assessment of evoked potential contrast thresholds using real-time retrieval. *Invest. Ophthamol. Vis. Sci.* 25, 627–635.

SHEEDY, J. E., AND FRY, G. A. (1979). The perceived direction of the binocular image. *Vision Res.* 19, 201–211.

SHIMOJO, S., BAUER, J., O'CONNELL, K. M., AND HELD, R. (1986). Prestereoptic binocular vision in infants. *Vision Res.* 26, 501–510.

SPERLING, G. (1970). Binocular vision: a physical and neural theory. *J. Am. Psychol.* 83, 461–534.

SPINELLI, D., PIRCHIO, M., AND SANDINI, G. (1983). Visual acuity in the young infant is highest in a small retinal area. *Vision Res.* 23, 1133–1136.

STROMEYER III, C. F., AND JULESZ, B. (1972). Spatial frequency in vision: critical bands and spread of masking. *J. Opt. Soc. Am.* 62, 1221–1232.

STROMEYER III, C. F., AND KLEIN, S. A. (1974). Spatial frequency channels in human vision as asymmetric (edge) mechanisms. *Vision Res.* 14, 1409–1420.

TANNER JR., W. P., AND SWETS, J. A. (1954). A decision-making theory of visual detection. *Psychol. Rev.* 61, 401–409.

TELLER, D. Y., AND MOVSHON, J. A. (1986). Visual development. *Vision Res.* 26, 1483–1506.

TYLER, C. W. (1971). Stereoscopic depth movement: two eyes less sensitive than one. *Science* 174, 958–961.

TYLER, C. W. (1973a). Stereoscopic vision: cortical limitations a disparity scaling effect. *Science* 181, 276–278.

TYLER, C. W. (1973b). Temporal characteristics in apparent movement: omega movement versus phi movement. *Q. J. Exp. Psychol.* 25, 182–192.

TYLER, C. W. (1974a). Stereopsis in dynamic visual noise. *Nature* 250, 781–782.

TYLER, C. W. (1974b). Induced stereomovement. *Vision Res.* 14, 609–613.

TYLER, C. W. (1974c). Depth perception in disparity gratings. *Nature* 251, 140–142.

TYLER, C. W. (1975a). Stereoscopic tilt and size aftereffects. *Perception* 4, 187–192.

TYLER, C. W. (1975b). Characteristics of stereomovement suppression. *Percept. Psychophys.* 17, 225–230.

TYLER, C. W. (1977). Spatial limitations in stereopsis. *Proc. S.P.I.E.* 120, 36–42.

TYLER, C. W. (1983). Sensory processing of binocular disparity. In C. M. SCHOR AND K. J. CIUFFREDA (eds.). *Vergence Eye Movements: Basic and Clinical Aspects.* London: Butterworths.

TYLER, C. W. (1991a). Some tacit assumptions in visual psychophysics. In A. GOREA (ed.). *Representations of Vision.* Cambridge: Cambridge University Press, pp. 251–278.

TYLER, C. W. (1991b). Cyclopean vision. In D. REGAN (ed.). *Vision and Visual Dysfunction. Vol. 9. Binocular Vision.* London: Macmillan, pp. 38–74.

TYLER, C. W., AND APKARIAN, P. A. (1985). Effects of contrast, orientation and binocularity on the pattern evoked potential. *Vision Res.* 25, 755–766.

TYLER, C. W., AND CAVANAGH, P. (1991). Purely chromatic perception of motion in depth: two eyes as sensitive as one. *Percept. Psychophys.* 49, 53–61.

TYLER, C. W., AND FOLEY, J. (1974). Stereomovement suppression for transient disparity changes. *Perception* 3, 287–296.

TYLER, C. W., AND JULESZ, B. (1976). The neural transfer characteristic (neurontropy) for binocular stochastic stimulation. *Biol. Cybern.* 23, 33–37.

TYLER, C. W., AND JULESZ, B. (1980a). On the depth of the cyclopean retina. *Exp. Brain Res.* 40, 196–202.

TYLER, C. W., AND JULESZ, B. (1980b). Narrowband spatial frequency tuning for disparity gratings in the cyclopean retina. *J. Opt. Soc. Am.* 70, 1584.

TYLER, C. W., AND NORCIA, A. M. (1986). Plasticity of human acuity development with variations in visual experience. In E. L.

KELLER AND D. S. ZEE (eds.). *Adaptive Processes in Visual and Oculomotor Systems*. Oxford: Pergamon, pp. 95–100.

TYLER, C. W., AND SUTTER, E. E. (1979). Depth from spatial frequency difference: an old kind of stereopsis? *Vision Res.* 19, 859–865.

TYLER, C. W., AND TORRES, J. (1972). Frequency response characteristics for sinusoidal movement in the fovea and periphery. *Percept. Psychophys.* 12(B), 232–236.

TYLER, C. W., APKARIAN, P., LEVI, D. M., AND NAKAYAMA, K. (1979). Rapid assessment of visual function: an electronic sweep technique for the pattern VEP. *Invest. Ophthalmol. Vis. Sci.* 18, 703–713.

TYLER, C. W., NORCIA, A. M., AND HAMER, R. D. (1987). Two mechanisms revealed by sweep VEP contrast functions in infants. *OSA Tech. Dig.* 87-4, 24–27.

VON DER HEYDT, R., ADORJANI, C., AND HANNY, P. (1977). Neural mechanisms of stereopsis: sensitivity to orientational disparity. *Experientia* 33, 786.

WEBER, E. H. (1834). *De Pulsu, Resorptione, Auditu et Tactu. Annotationes anatomicae et physiologicae.* Leipzig: Koehler.

YUODELIS, C., AND HENDRICKSON, A. (1986). A qualitative and quantitative analysis of the human fovea during development. *Vision Res.* 26, 847–855.

V. Retinal and Cortical Development
Introduction

MICHAEL P. STRYKER

Human visual development rests on the changing biology of both peripheral and central visual structures. On the one hand, developmental changes in the spacing of retinal cones provide an absolute limit to the spatial resolving power of the visual system. On the other hand, high resolution in the retina is of little use unless the precision of connections within central visual structures, particularly the lateral geniculate nucleus and primary visual cortex, is adequate to process visual inputs with high resolution. One major question addressed experimentally in the papers of this section is—which stage sets the limits to visual performance at various periods in development?

Abnormal development can result from a variety of causes. Many of these causes are postnatal abnormalities in early visual experience. Abnormal experience produces abnormal patterns of neural activity, which can cause the mechanisms of plasticity that normally refine central neural connections to disrupt them instead. Other abnormalities in visual development can appear prenatally. Similar mechanisms of neural plasticity may operate in both pre- and postnatal development, and the disruption of neural activity at either stage of development can have serious consequences.

The early development of the retina and its specializations is reviewed by Hendrickson. It is worth considering as well as the events and mechanisms that give rise to the central portions of the visual brain, along with much of the rest of the nervous system, for an appreciation of the processes with which central visual development interacts.

The early events in central nervous system neurogenesis appear in general to be regulated by biochemical mechanisms that operate independent of neural activity. To produce the central visual system, it is first necessary to generate appropriate numbers of cells at appropriate times and places: retinal ganglion cells and their targets in the lateral geniculate nucleus, as well as visual cortical target cells for the geniculate afferents. Cell generation need be only approximately correct, since it is later refined during a period of natural cell death, but it must

certainly be sufficient (Rakic, 1988; McConnell, 1991). The molecular mechanisms that govern the production of appropriate numbers and types of cells are not yet understood.

In many cases, cells are generated far from the sites they will ultimately occupy and must migrate over long distances to assume their appropriate positions. While some important cellular interactions have been uncovered, the mechanisms that regulate cell migration are also not yet understood at the molecular level (McConnell, 1992).

Retinal ganglion cells and lateral geniculate nucleus principal cells then produce axons that find their way along defined pathways to their respective target structures, the lateral geniculate nucleus and visual cortex. The recognition of both pathway and target appear to result from both positive and negative interactions between the growing axons and the substrates through which they grow. Again, the specific molecular mechanisms responsible have eluded full characterization to date.

Upon arrival at the targets, retinal and geniculate axons form at least a coarse topographic map. All of the events in the development of the central visual system up to this point appear to proceed normally in animals in which the discharge activity of neurons is blocked (Shatz and Stryker, 1988; Shatz, 1990).

After the basic regional connectivity of the central visual system is established, a period of refinement of connections ensues, during which patterns of neural activity appear to play a crucial organizing role. The first event that takes place in the lateral geniculate nucleus is the stratification and segregation of the input fibers from the two eyes, a process that ends in the formation of eye-specific layers in this nucleus. This process takes place *in utero* at a time at which there is substantial maintained discharge of the retinal ganglion cells, and it does not take place if retinogeniculate discharge activity is experimentally blocked (Shatz and Stryker, 1988).

In the visual cortex, afferent fibers from the lateral-geniculate nucleus then rearrange their terminal arbors

285

into precise maps and columns of various sorts, most commonly orientation and then (in many species) ocular dominance columns (reviewed in Stryker, 1991). These rearrangements all require neural activity for their success. Corticocortical as well as geniculocortical connections to these columns are also rearranged by processes that depend on neural activity. There are tremendous similarities in the basic outlines of these processes among all mammalian species studied, from mouse to human, as well as among vertebrates in general, including fish, reptiles, and amphibians. Surprisingly, the time of birth appears not to be very significant. Insofar as we understand them, the same events take place in species such as the ferret, in which much of the geniculate and practically all the cortical events take place postnatally; the cat, in which the geniculate events are prenatal but the cortical ones are perinatal and postnatal; and the macaque monkey, in which, as apparently in the human, both geniculate and primary visual cortical organization is largely achieved prenatally. Perhaps this similarity should not be surprising, since similar locally correlated or wave-like discharges of neighboring ganglion cells are present pre- and postnatally in different species (Meister et al., 1991).

The basic organization of the retinogeniculocortical visual system is thus produced independent of visual experience by early activity-independent and later activity-dependent mechanisms. Visual experience then plays a further role in shaping the development of binocular vision and stereopsis (see section IV) and, as reviewed by Movshon and Kiorpes in this section, spatial vision and acuity.

Visual deprivation can powerfully affect this later development, and the mechanisms responsible for these effects, as well as their detailed consequences for the anatomy, physiology, and behavior of experimental animals have been studied and are reviewed by Movshon and Kiorpes. It is now possible to apply some of the same techniques used in experimental animals to investigate the anatomical abnormalities that underlie the common forms of amblyopia in human patients (Horton and Stryker, 1993).

In considering the consequences of visual deprivation, it is necessary to distinguish between the effects of disuse *per se* and those of unequal competition between the two eyes. The same cellular mechanisms that mediate profound, rapid, and irreversible deprivation effects when the two eyes are put in unequal competition, are remarkably insensitive to binocular disuse and allow normal development with only minimal visual stimulation. One may wish to regard the extreme sensitivity of the developing visual system to unequal binocular competition as the price that must be paid for mechanisms that refine neural connections to high precision by the use of patterns of activity.

Little experimental attention has been given to date to the development of the primate visual system beyond the striate cortex. Much of the cortical machinery for object location and recognition must develop postnatally in relation to visual and visual-motor experience. With the basic outlines of early development in hand, at least as far as the input layer of striate cortex, the next decade of research on infant vision may bring an understanding of these stages beyond.

REFERENCES

HORTON, J., AND STRYKER, M. P. (1993). Amblyopia induced by anisometropia without shrinkage of ocular dominance columns in human striate cortex. *Proc. Nat. Acad. Sci. USA* 90, 5494–5498.

McCONNELL, S. K. (1992). The control of neuronal identity in the developing cerebral cortex. *Curr. Opin. Neurobiol.* 2, 23–27.

McCONNELL, S. K. (1991). The generation of neuronal diversity in the central nervous system. *Ann. Rev. Neurosci.* 14, 269–300.

MEISTER, M., WONG, R. O., BAYLOR, D. A., AND SHATZ, C. J. (1991). Synchronous bursts of action potentials in ganglion cells of the developing mammalian retina. *Science* 252, 939–943.

RAKIC, P. (1988). Specification of cerebral cortical areas. *Science* 241, 170–176.

SHATZ, C. J. (1990). Impulse activity and the patterning of connections during CNS development. *Neuron* 5, 745–756.

SHATZ, C. J., AND STRYKER, M. P. (1988). Prenatal tetrodotoxin infusion blocks segregation of retinogeniculate afferents. *Science* 242, 87–89.

STRYKER, M. P. (1991). Activity-dependent reorganization of afferents in the developing mammalian visual system. In D. M. K. LAM AND C. J. SHATZ (eds.) *Development of the Visual System.* Cambridge, MA: MIT Press, pp. 267–287.

17 | Morphological development of the primate retina

ANITA E. HENDRICKSON

This chapter emphasizes human retinal development, but *Macaca* retinal development is included because monkey retina can be used for experimental procedures, and generally the tissue obtained is in better condition than that from the human. The different gestational periods of the two species [human, 40 fetal weeks (Fwk); monkey, 168 fetal days (Fd)] can be corrected by giving percent gestation in addition to fetal age. Postnatal ages are given directly, e.g., 5 days, 20 weeks. When postnatal development of acuity is compared for monkeys and humans, there is a consistent relation of 1 monkey postnatal week = 1 human postnatal month (Boothe et al., 1985), which can be used as a postnatal correction factor. Earlier reviews on primate retinal development have covered some of this material (Hendrickson, 1988, 1992a; Curcio and Hendrickson, 1991).

DEVELOPMENT OF CELL POPULATIONS IN PRIMATE RETINA

The first neurons to undergo terminal mitosis and to differentiate morphologically are found in or near the future fovea (Barber, 1955; Mann, 1964; Hendrickson and Kupfer, 1976; Provis et al., 1985, Lindberg and Fisher, 1990; LaVail et al., 1991). Each type of neuron and the Müller glia appear first in central retina and last at the far periphery, indicating a generalized central to peripheral gradient characteristic of mammalian retinas.

When dividing cells are marked by tritiated thymidine in monkey retina (LaVail et al., 1991), ganglion cells (GCs) and horizontal cells are the first neurons to become postmitotic at 30 Fd (18%), closely followed by cones at 33–36 Fd. Central rods and Müller glial cells first appear at 45 Fd (27%), and amacrines and bipolars first appear at 43 Fd. Thus there is a distinct time gap between GCs, horizontal cells, and cone generation and that of the other retinal cells. A fovea, including cones, can be morphologically distinguished at 51 Fd (30%) (Hendrickson, 1992b).

In humans, cell generation has been studied by analyzing whole-mounted retinas for the distribution of mitotic figures in the germinal layer (Provis et al., 1985). Mitosis stops by 14 Fwk (35%) in the region of the future fovea so that all foveal cells must be generated by this age.

Given the above sequence for the monkey, it is likely that human GCs, horizontal cells, and cones are generated much earlier, certainly before they can be morphologically identified at 11–12 Fwk (28–30%) (Hollenberg and Spira 1972, 1973; Provis et al., 1985; Lindberg and Fisher, 1990). In the monkey the most peripheral GCs are generated on 70 Fd (41%) and the most peripheral cones on 110 Fd (65%). Mitoses are still present in human far peripheral retina at 29 Fwk (73%) (Provis et al., 1985). In the monkey (LaVail et al., 1991) a few bipolar cells, rods, and Müller cells in the far retinal periphery label with tritiated thymidine on the day of birth and even a few rods label at 32 days, suggesting that some peripheral cells are generated for several weeks after birth in monkeys and for several months after birth in humans.

Information about the second important developmental factor, cell death, is much less available. In both humans (Provis, 1987; Provis and Penfold, 1988) and monkeys (Rakic and Riley, 1983) more than half of the GCs generated eventually die as judged by adult optic nerve axon counts. Determining cell death in other retinal populations is more difficult. One of our studies (Packer et al., 1990) found that up to 25% of the cones may die during postnatal development, but no consistent trend was found for rods. Penfold and Provis (1986) found cell death in the germinal zone of fetal human retina but no evidence for massive cell death in differentiated photoreceptors, although in cat retina (Robinson, 1988) cell death is coincident with differentiation. Thus the role for cell death in retinal development remains unclear except for the GC layer.

DEVELOPMENT OF THE FOVEA

The developing fovea in primate retina was first identified as the region where the GC layer was thickest

(Bach and Seefelder, 1914; Mann, 1964); but Barber (1955) pointed out that this region also was characterized by the presence of a single layer of immature cones with few rods present. This "rod-free zone" has been found in humans by 11–12 Fwk (28–30%) (Hollenberg and Spira, 1972, 1973; Rhodes, 1979, Lindberg and Fisher, 1990) and in monkeys at 51 Fd (30%) (Hendrickson, 1992b). The foveal pit appears in humans at 24–26 Fwk (63%) (Mann, 1964; Hendrickson and Yuodelis, 1984) and 100 Fd in monkeys (Hendrickson, 1992b), although counts show that the human GC layer begins to thin as early as 14 Fwk (Provis et al., 1985). During the last third of gestation foveal development proceeds more rapidly in monkeys than humans. By birth the monkey foveal pit contains only a single layer of inner retinal neurons, and foveal cones are thin and packed two or three cells deep in the foveal center (Hendrickson, 1992b), whereas the human fovea at birth still has one or two layers of GC, most of the inner nuclear layer neurons, and only a single layer of large cones (Hendrickson and Kupfer, 1976; Hendrickson and Yuodelis, 1984; Hendrickson, 1992b). Superficially, the appearance of the fovea is mature by 12 weeks in monkeys and 11–15 months in humans, but in both species cone density continues to increase for some time (see below). Table 17-1 summarizes the overall development of monkey and human foveal morphology.

The distance across the photoreceptor-layer rod-free zone from first nasal rod inner segments to first temporal rod inner segments was measured in *Macaca* monkeys during fetal and postnatal development (Hendrickson and Kupfer, 1976). This distance decreased from more than 1600 μm at 70 Fd (41%) to 200 μm in adults, with a rapid decrease in diameter just after birth. A similar but more prolonged decrease in the diameter of the human rod-free zone also has been found (Yuodelis and Hendrickson, 1986). (Table 17-2). The area of the rod-free zone decreases from 2.00 mm^2 at 22 Fwk to 0.95 mm^2 at birth to less than 0.40 mm^2 at 45 months. If only the retina inside the disc is considered, the newborn human fovea covers 5.6 visual degrees and is 2.4% of the retinal area inside the disc. By 45 months it has decreased to 2.6 visual degrees and is 0.8% of the central retinal area (Mohn and van Hof-van Duin, 1990; Hendrickson, 1992a) (Table 17-2). This finding means that the neonatal fovea offers a much larger visual target relative to the size of the eye.

At the same time the size of the rod-free zone is decreasing, there is a marked change in the spatial density of foveal cones. Bach and Seefelder (1914) illustrated the progressively smaller size of the human foveal cones, but the first quantitative study of this process was done in the monkey (Hendrickson and Kupfer, 1976) where a fourfold increase in cone density between birth and 2 years was found. More recently, retinal whole mounts have been analyzed from 152 Fd to adulthood (Packer et al., 1990). At 152 Fd (90%) peak cone density was 43,000 cones/mm^2, which increased to 65,000 cones/mm^2 by 3 weeks and doubled to 133,000 cones/mm^2 by 13 months, a value that is still only 63% of the adult level (210,000 cones/mm^2) (Packer et al., 1989). The increase of cone density in human retina has been studied in vertical plastic sections (Yuodelis and Hendrickson, 1986). At 22 Fwk (55%) cone density is 18,000 cones/mm^2, rising to 36,000 cones/mm^2 at 5 days and 108,000 cones/mm^2 at 45 months, a value about half that of the average adult human (208,000 cones/mm^2) (Curcio et al., 1990). Foveal cone density increase occurs within an existing population of photoreceptors because photoreceptor generation has long since ceased

TABLE 17-1. *Comparative development of foveal morphology in monkey and human.*

Foveal morphology	Monkey	Human
PRENATAL	Birth to 168 days (%)	Birth to 40 weeks (%)
Cones form a continuous row; OPL present	30	26
Cones begin IS	46	53
Cones tilt toward fovea center; fibers of Henle appear	53	63
Shallow foveal pit in GCL; OS appear	65	63
GCL 1–2 cells thick; INL thinned; single layer cones elongated with thick, tapered IS and clear OS	78–88	1–5 days
GCL/INL fused in foveola; cones 3 deep; IS thinner, elongated and tapered; OS 30–50% of IS length	92–98	2 Months
POSTNATAL	Weeks	Months
Scattered GCL/INL layer; very elongated IS; OS 100% + of IS length	2–6	11–15
Cones 4–5 deep; OS 150% IS length; IS much thinner; foveola mainly cone axons and glial cells	12	45
Nearly adult cone density; scattered GCL/INL layer; OS 200% of IS length	39	156

OPL = outer plexiform layer; IS = inner segment; GCL = ganglion cell layer; OS = outer segment; INL = inner nuclear layer.

TABLE 17-2. *Development of human fovea.*

Age[a]	Foveal cones/mm²	Central foveal cones/100 μm	Rod-free area (diameter, μm)	% Retina inside disc covered by rod-free area
F22wk	18,472	11	1605	
F26wk	21,268	12	1400	
P5d	36,294	13	1100 (5.6 degrees[b])	2.4
P15mo	52,787	19	725 (<3.0 degrees[b])	1.0
P45mo	108,439	31	620 (<2.6 degrees[b])	0.8
37 Years	208,203	43	683 (<2.0 degrees[b])	0.9
20–40 Years[c]			350	0.2[b]

Most data are from Yuodeles and Hendrickson (1986) except: [b]from Mohn and van Hof-van Duin (1990); [c]from Curcio et al. (1990).
[a]F22wk = fetal age 22 weeks; P5d = postpartum day 5; P15mo = postpartum month 15.

in central retina (LaVail et al., 1991); and cone death, if it exists, would lower density. The area of central retina inside the disc is unchanged after the first third of gestation (Lia and Chalupa, 1988; Steineke and Kirby, 1989), so areal or growth effects are not a major factor. Therefore we have argued that postnatal foveal cone density increases can be due only to a centralward migration or redistribution of cones (Hendrickson and Kupfer, 1976; Yuodelis and Hendrickson, 1986; Packer et al., 1990).

It has proved difficult to determine reliably when human foveal cone density is fully adult because cone density shows a three-fold variation in normal young adults (Curcio et al., 1990). Often only one eye is available at a given age for fetal or infant studies, making individual developmental variability unclear but very likely. For instance, a longitudinal study of contrast sensitivity and acuity development in colony-born *Macaca nemestrina* monkeys (Boothe et al., 1988) found that the seven animals varied in age from 20 to 38 weeks for when they achieved adult acuity levels, and the shape of each animal's longitudinal developmental curve also varied widely. A visual evoked potential study of human infant grating acuity development (Norcia et al., 1990) showed a marked variation in the shape of longitudinal developmental curves for 15 infants, as well as a final acuity at 35 weeks that varied from 8 cycles/degree (cpd) to more than 20 cpd. Given the current limited data, it appears that monkeys at 13 months are about 70% and humans at 45 months are about 50% of adult peak foveal cone density. Table 17-3 shows a comparison of cone density development, plotted as percent of the adult value in humans and monkeys. Around birth the monkey has 31–41% of adult cone density, but the human has only 17%. Even at roughly comparable ages of 13 weeks and 15 months, the monkey still has 39% and the human 25%. Thus our data show that monkey fovea is much more mature than human fovea at birth for both overall morphology (Table 17-1) and cone density (Tables 17-2, 17-3). Human fovea develops rapidly after birth so that by 15 months it is roughly equal

to monkey fovea, although both species continue to show increases in cone density well into early childhood.

Foveal maturation is accompanied by a profound change in cone morphology, summarized in Figure 17-1 for the human. At 22 Fwk (55%) in humans [74–90 Fd (44–54%) in monkeys] the future foveal cones are thick, columnar epithelial cells, with a short, thick, rounded apical end that is the developing inner segment. There are no outer segments at this age, although a cilium is present on cones at 12–15 Fwk (Hollenberg and Spira, 1973; Johnson et al., 1985). Monkey cones have a tiny outer segment at 110 Fd (65%) that lengthens slowly until a month before birth (Samorajski et al., 1965; Hendrickson and Kupfer, 1976). The outer segment appears on human foveal cones at 24–26 Fwk (63%) but remains short up to birth (Hendrickson and Yuodelis, 1984). During the last third of gestation the entire cone lengthens and thins. The inner segment fills with mitochondria and endoplasmic reticulum, grows beyond the external limiting membrane, and becomes more tapered. This process is more advanced at birth in monkeys than in humans (Hendrickson, 1992b). In humans at 5 days (Table 17-4), foveal cone inner segments are about 6 μm in diameter and less than 10 μm

TABLE 17-3. *Comparative development of foveal cone density in monkey and human.*

Monkey[a]		Human[b]	
Age	% Adult density	Age	% Adult density
Fetal		Fetal	
90%	20	53%	9
98%	41	63%	11
After birth		After birth	
3 weeks	31	5 days	17
6 weeks	31		
13 weeks	39	15 Months	25
26 Weeks	75		
		45 Months	52
52 weeks	63		

[a]Data modified from Hendrickson (1992b).
[b]Data modified from Yuodelis and Hendrickson (1986).

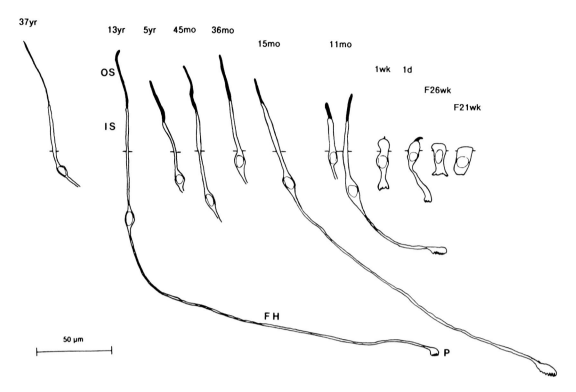

FIG. 17-1. Development of the foveola, as shown by cone photoreceptors from the center of the human fovea (foveola). All cells are drawn from histological sections and represent "typical" foveolar cones for a given age. The dotted line is the external limiting membrane. OS = outer segments; IS = inner segments; FH = fiber of Henle; P = cone pedicle.

long, whereas the adult inner segment is about 2 μm in diameter and 30–35 μm long. Outer segments increase seven-fold in length from birth to 15 months and are doubled again by adulthood. This decrease in cone inner segment diameter allows many more cells to pack into the foveal center, providing the substrate for the adult primate high visual acuity.

The synaptic region of foveal cones also changes markedly during development. Foveal cones make synapses at 11–12 Fwk (30%) in humans (Hollenberg and Spira, 1973; Lindberg and Fisher, 1990) and 74 Fd (44%) in monkeys (Smelser et al., 1974) with postsynaptic processes that resemble both horizontal and bipolar dendrites. In human inner retina at 15 Fwk (van Driel et al., 1990) immature amacrine conventional and bipolar ribbon synapses are present, suggesting that even at this young stage the retinal circuitry is present to

carry information from cones to the GCs. By midgestation (Fig. 17-1) the basal end of the cone begins to elongate, forming the fiber of Henle, and the entire cell "tips" toward the foveal center, indicating the beginning of the two major neuronal migrations in the fovea. The earlier migration is in the inner retina. The synaptic pedicle remains in contact with horizontal and bipolar cells, which are migrating toward the periphery to form the foveal pit, so the fiber of Henle must elongate to accommodate this process. The foveal pit is complete by 12 weeks in monkeys and 11–15 months in humans (Table 17-1). The later migration is in the outer retina. The cone cell body and inner segment are moving centrally toward the foveal center, also requiring elongation of the fiber of Henle. Cones originally in the center of the rod-free zone change their cell body position relatively little, but their bipolars move the farthest pe-

TABLE 17-4. *Development of human foveal cones.*

	Foveal cones (avg. μm)					Nyquist limit (cpd)		
	Inner segment		Outer segment					
Human age	Width	Length	Width	Length	Avg. no. cones/100 μm	a	b	Spatial acuity[c] (cpd)
5 Days	6.3	8.8	1.5	3.0	13	14	15	6.7
15 Months	2.6	22.5	1.2	22.5	19	25	27	13.6
45 Months	2.0	26.3	1.0	29.5	31	44	—	23.4
37+ Years	1.9	32.3	1.0	45.5	43	72	60	35.2

All data from Yuodelis and Hendrickson (1986) except: [a]calculated by Mohn and van Hof-van Duin (1990); [b]calculated by Banks and Bennett (1988); [c]calculated by Wilson (1988).

ripherally. The maximum distance monkey cone inner segments migrate has been calculated to be 230 μm for cones originally located at 1 mm eccentricity at 152 Fd, near the edge of the rod-free zone (Packer et al., 1990). More peripheral to this point the inner retinal neurons show little displacement; thus the more peripheral fibers of Henle, which are seen on both rods and cones out to the disc, are mainly responses to photoreceptor centralward migration.

In addition to inner retinal neurons and photoreceptors, the pigment epithelium also shows an altered distribution with age. Over the same period that the fovea forms, the number of central pigment epithelial cells increases while peripheral density decreases (Robb, 1985). Because mitotic activity has stopped well before this time (Rapaport et al., 1987), it is likely that migration also is responsible for this redistribution.

DEVELOPMENT OF PERIPHERAL RETINA

The adult midcentral retina (2−12 degrees or from the foveal slope to the disc) contains a mixture of rods and cones. There is a sharply decreasing number of cones, moving from the foveal slope to the optic disc. Density decreases from 100,000 cones/mm^2 at 750 μm from the fovea center to 6000−8000 cones/mm^2 at the disc. Over the same distance rod density rises sharply, so the peak density of rods is found at the level of the optic disc in monkeys (Packer et al., 1990; Wickler et al., 1990) and humans (Osterberg, 1935; Curcio et al., 1990). In the human there is a complete "rod ring" centered on the fovea with a mean density of 95,000 rods/mm^2. The peak rod density, the "hot spot" at 176,000 rods/mm^2, is usually found on or near the superior vertical meridian. The lowest rod ring density occurs where it crosses the nasal horizontal meridian. In the monkey retina, the ring is incomplete, with a much higher rod density and a rod hot spot (176,000 rods/mm^2) in superior retina. This difference gives rise to an overall cone/rod density of 1:20 in humans and 1:15 in *Macaca* monkeys (Curcio and Hendrickson, 1991). There also is a difference in cone density on the nasal horizontal meridian compared to temporally (cone streak), so that by the level of the disc the nasal/temporal cone ratio is 1.4:1.0. In the retinal periphery, cone density continues to be higher along the nasal horizontal meridian (3:1 nasal/temporal cone ratio at 9 mm) (Curcio and Hendrickson, 1991), but it declines regularly along other meridia into the far periphery to reach 2000−4000 cones/mm^2. Rod density declines symmetrically into the far periphery along all meridia to 50,000−75,000 rods/mm^2.

Outside the disc the area of the retina increases dramatically over development, so areal growth must be considered as a major mechanism in photoreceptor development. Human retinal area increases 6.6 times from 14 Fwk to 40 Fwk (Provis et al., 1985) and 1.8 times from birth to 6 years (Robb, 1982). Monkey retina enlarges 1.7 times from 152 Fd to 13 months and 1.4 times again to adulthood (Packer et al., 1990). These numbers do not take into account the areal stability of the central retina (Lia and Chalupa, 1988; Steineke and Kirby, 1989), so the actual peripheral growth is even larger.

Current evidence suggests that photoreceptor topographical differences are apparent early. At all points cones are generated before rods (LaVail et al., 1991). Even at the youngest stages of development, only cones are found in the future fovea (Barber, 1955; Hollenberg and Spira, 1972, 1973; Hendrickson and Kupfer, 1976; Provis et al., 1985; Lindberg and Fisher, 1990; Hendrickson, 1992b), but rods appear intermixed with cones just outside this zone. There are more mitotic figures in fetal human nasal retina compared to those in temporal retina (Provis et al., 1985) especially after 18 Fwk when the peripheral cone streak is being generated. In monkeys (Packer et al., 1990) a primitive but characteristic cone streak and rod ring are present at 152 Fd. The cone density ratio at equal nasal and temporal eccentricities remains the same from this age to adulthood, despite a four-fold drop in absolute cone density. These data suggest that characteristic rod and cone topographic patterns are initiated by differential cell generation early in development.

Retinal areal growth also plays a major role in peripheral retinal topographic development. Retinal growth in nonprimates has been explained by a balloon model in which, as the retinal area increases, a stable population of cells is expanded in such a way that its density is uniformly decreased (discussed by Stone et al., 1984; Robinson et al., 1989). Nonuniformities in the topography of cat GC development prompted the formulation of a more complex, radially symmetrical but nonuniform balloon model in which the central retina remains relatively fixed and the far periphery grows the most (Mastronarde et al., 1984). This model also helps explain the quantitative development of peripheral rod and cone topography in monkeys (Packer et al., 1990); quantitative data of peripheral retinal development are not available for humans. The retina inside the disc does not change in area after early gestation and so the five-fold postnatal increase in foveal cone density must be due to such mechanisms as cell migration. The large postnatal decrease in peripheral rod and cone density is mainly due to a large increase in peripheral retinal area. For instance, mean cone density in the far periphery of monkey retina decreases from 10,000 cones/mm^2 at 152 Fd to 2700 cones/mm^2 in the adult. Rod density decreases from 150,000 rods/mm^2 at 3 weeks to 50,000 rods/mm^2 in the adult. Over the same period near the disc the decrease is less, with cones decreasing from 12,500 to 7,500 cones/mm^2 and rods from 170,000 to 110,000 rods/mm². These decreases can be explained if it is assumed that cell number is stable and there is a 3.1-fold increase in retinal area with a proportionately greater increase in the far periphery (nonuniform expansion). The end result of peripheral retinal growth is a change in the central/peripheral cone ratio from 4:1 at 152 Fd to 78:1 in the adult (Curcio and Hendrickson, 1991). The monkey rod ring is present at 3 weeks but almost covers the entire peripheral retina where densities barely go below 100,000 rods/mm². Retinal growth cuts peripheral rod density in half by 13 weeks and in half again by 13 months, although these levels are still twice as high as those in the adult. The rod hot spot density averages 215,000 rods/mm² around birth and then decreases to 170,000 rods/mm² by 13 months. Both rod and cone topography are immature at 13 months and do not become adult until near 2 years (104 weeks) in monkeys. Applying the 1 week = 1 month rule, this finding suggests that peripheral retinal photoreceptor topographic development could continue until 8.7 years in humans.

There are surprisingly few morphological studies of developing peripheral primate retina. Johnson et al. (1985) have compared the same three points in central, midperipheral, and far peripheral human nasal retina (10%, 40%, and 70%, respectively, of the distance between disc and ora) at 22, 24, and 28 Fwk. At 22 Fwk

central and midperipheral rods and cones are beginning to differentiate, whereas far peripheral photoreceptors are still in a neoblastic mitotic zone. By 24 Fwk the outer plexiform layer has reached the midperiphery, both rods and cones have appeared in the far periphery, and central photoreceptors have tiny outer segments. Outer segments and a thin outer plexiform layer are present throughout the 28 Fwk retina, although both are less mature in the far periphery. There was a good correlation between the immunocytochemical detection of interstitial retinal binding protein and the appearance of outer segments. Using plastic-embedded vertical sections, we have examined the morphological development of foveal center and slope (Hendrickson and Yuodelis, 1984), parafoveal (1.5 mm to fovea), and midperipheral rod ring (4 mm temporal to the fovea) human retina (Hendrickson and Drucker, 1992) (Figs. 17-2, 17-3) in an attempt to determine the differential maturation of central and peripheral points. The development of the fovea is described in the previous section. All layers and neuronal types are present across the peripheral retina at 24–26 Fwk (63%). In parafoveal retina photoreceptors have only a rudimentary inner segment and no outer segments, but outer segments are present on rods in midperipheral retina. Outer segments are present on both rods and cones in parafovea and cones in midperiphery at 36 Fwk. By 5–8

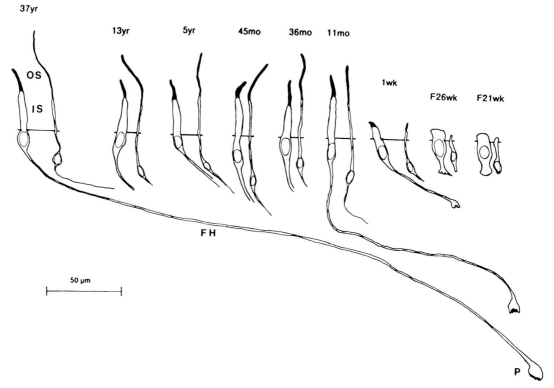

FIG. 17-2. Development of the parafovea, as shown by cone and rod photoreceptors taken from the human parafovea approximately 1 mm from the foveal center. All cells are drawn from histological sections and represent "typical" photoreceptors for a given age. The dotted line is the external limiting membrane. OS = outer segments; IS = inner segments; FH = fiber of Henle; P = cone pedicle.

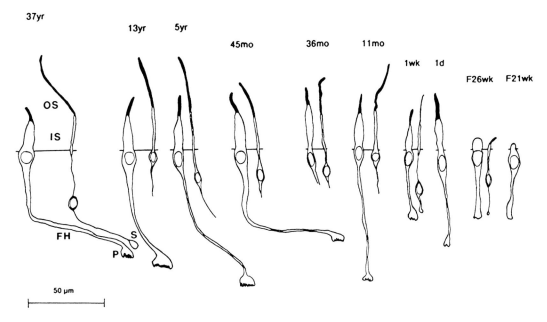

FIG. 17-3. Development of rod ring, as shown by cone and rod photoreceptors taken from the human midperipheral retina 4 mm from the foveal center, which would be within the "rod ring." All cells are drawn from histological sections and represent "typical" photoreceptors for a given age. The dotted line is the external limiting membrane. OS = outer segments; IS = inner segments; FH = fiber of Henle; P = cone pedicle; S = rod spherule.

days the inner retina is mature at both points, but a larger percentage of total retinal thickness is occupied by the photoreceptors owing to elongation of the inner segments and fiber of Henle. In parafovea at birth cone inner segments are untapered, but rod inner segments have already reached their adult width of 2 μm. Both rod and cone inner and outer segments are 30–50% adult length. In midperiphery at birth both rod and cone inner segments are slightly longer and appear more mature than in the parafovea, and outer segments are 50% longer. By 13 months the parafoveal retina appears mature, with the photoreceptors accounting for 50% of the retinal thickness, although cone outer segments continue to elongate up to 5 years and rod outer segments up to 13 years. Midperipheral photoreceptor outer segments continue to be slightly longer than in more central retina and appear mature by 5 years. These studies have found that rod ring photoreceptors are morphologically more mature at birth than those in parafoveal or foveal retina, and in turn parafoveal photoreceptors develop well in advance of foveal cones, suggesting that human neonates may utilize more peripheral retinal regions for some aspects of visual function before foveal cone vision becomes dominant.

RELATION OF FOVEAL MATURATION AND SPATIAL VISUAL ACUITY DEVELOPMENT

Contributors to this book have discussed various aspects of human infant visual psychophysical testing. It is clear that contrast sensitivity, grating acuity, orientation detection, and color vision are relatively poor in the newborn, and that they improve rapidly over the first year. Four groups of authors (Brown et al., 1987; Banks and Bennett, 1988; Wilson, 1988; Mohn and van Hof-van Duin, 1990) have addressed the issue of whether the postnatal improvement in spatial acuity can be explained entirely or in part by the striking postnatal maturational changes in size, packing density, and shape of human foveal cones. These groups have based their models on the quantitative anatomical data of Yuodelis and Hendrickson (1986), which is the only existing study in neonatal humans. It should be pointed out that this study contains no eyes between 5 days and 13 months, and only one eye was counted at each age. All groups agree that the physiology of the anterior neonatal eye and its optics can be eliminated as a major contributor to the difference between neonatal and adult acuity.

Banks and Bennett (1988) created an ideal observer (Geisler and Davila, 1985) based on the optics and the characteristics of the foveal cone mosaic of the neonatal human eye. Because the neonatal eye is smaller and has more widely spaced cones, its Nyquist frequency is calculated to be 15 cpd, compared to 60 cpd achieved by an adult ideal observer. Adult cone inner segments are thin and tapered and function as wave guides to funnel photons into the outer segment; this structure is called the cone aperture (Miller and Bernard, 1983). Neonatal cones have much larger untapered inner segments that may not act as efficient wave guides, so Banks and Bennett postulated that the much smaller diameter (2–

3 μm) outer segment actually functions as the effective cone aperture in neonates. This postulate means that only 2% of the neonatal foveal surface is covered by cone apertures, compared to more than 65% in the adult, which causes the neonatal fovea to absorb 350 times fewer photons than adults, markedly reducing sensitivity. These factors have been incorporated into neonatal and adult ideal observers. If these retinal factors were the major limitation for the ideal observer, the shapes of adult and infant acuity or contrast sensitivity functions should be the same, except the infant would have reduced sensitivity. Behavioral measurements of these visual functions in neonates and adults, however, reveal different shapes, with large divergence at high spatial frequencies. Banks and Bennett suggested that photoreceptor immaturities in the newborn human fovea contribute 40–55% of the neonatal acuity difference, with the remainder caused by poorly specified "postreceptoral mechanisms."

Mohn and van Hof-van Duin (1990) also assumed wider cone spacing and lower sensitivity owing to short outer segments. They calculated a Nyquist limit of 14 cpd for the neonatal human fovea and concluded that the photoreceptor mosaic cannot be the limiting factor for neonatal acuity. They pointed out, however, that the larger size of the neonatal rod-free zone may compensate somewhat for its immature cells.

Brown et al. (1987) proposed that reduced neonatal acuity derives from reduced sensitivity caused by the shorter outer segments and larger diameter inner segments found in neonatal cones. They used behavioral psychophysics to measure how different levels of retinal illuminance affected grating acuity in 2-month-old human infants and in adults. Infants had poorer acuity over a wide range of luminance, suggesting that decreased sensitivity was not the only factor. To test the possibility that neonates had poor optics or were using their more peripheral retina, adult observers were tested with blurring lenses and at parafoveal locations. Only one combination reduced adult performance to that of the neonate, suggesting that refractive error, foveal immaturity, use of rods instead of cones, eccentric fixation, or overall reduced sensitivity cannot account for poor neonatal acuity. The authors concluded that retinal factors contribute to the low level of infant vision, but that most of the cause(s) are central to the photoreceptors.

Wilson (1988) created a composite whole visual system model involving anatomical, electrophysiological, and behavioral measures. Three processes were proposed to underlie development of the adult contrast sensitivity function. First, a combination of postnatal eye growth and migration of cones toward the center of the fovea reduces the angular subtense of each foveal cone, which in turn decreases receptive-field size at GC,

thalamic, and cortical levels, shifting peak sensitivity to higher spatial frequencies with age. Second, the elongation of outer segments adds photopigment and increases sensitivity with time. Third, receptive field mechanisms to sharpen orientation and spatial frequency are refined as cortical synaptic density reduces after 10 months (Huttenlocher et al., 1982). A quantitative model of adult visual system parallel processing mechanisms for orientation and spatial acuity (Wilson and Gelb, 1984) was then applied to the neonate. A neonatal acuity of 6.7 cpd was predicted by this model, close to the 4.5 cpd acuity found for 1-week-old infants with visual evoked potential measurements (Norcia and Tyler, 1985), which led Wilson to conclude that foveal cone immaturities are the major limiting factor for visual evoked potential measurements of grating acuity. Neonatal forced-choice preferential looking measures of grating acuity (Dobson and Teller, 1978), however, are far worse than the predicted acuity in the model, so Wilson suggested that this method is limited more by postreceptoral factors, similar to the conclusions of the other three groups.

Although the calculated values differ somewhat in these four groups, they all come to a similar conclusion: Neonatal grating acuity *is* affected by immaturities in the foveal cone mosaic, but immature circuitry in the inner retina, thalamus, or visual cortex poses equal or greater limitations to neonatal human visual acuity performance. Our anatomical results, which found that the parafoveal and midperipheral retina are significantly more mature than foveal cones, need to be examined experimentally and by similar models to test whether some aspects of early infant visual function might not be subserved by these retinal areas.

REFERENCES

BACH, L., AND SEEFELDER, R. (1914). *Atlas zur Entwicklungsgeschichte des Menschlichen Auges*. Leipzig: Verlag von Wilhelm Engelmann.

BANKS, M., AND BENNETT, P. (1988). Optical and photoreceptor immaturities limit the spatial and chromatic vision of human neonates. *J. Opt. Soc. Am. [A]* 5, 2059.

BARBER, A. (1955). *Embryology of the Human Eye*. St. Louis: Mosby.

BOOTHE, R. G., DOBSON, V., TELLER, D. Y. (1985). Postnatal development of vision in human and nonhuman primates. *Annu. Rev. Neurosci.* 8, 495–545.

BOOTHE, R. G., KIORPES, L., WILLIAMS, R. A., AND TELLER, D. Y. (1988). Operant measurements of contrast sensitivity in infant macaque monkeys during normal development. *Vision Res.* 28, 387–396.

BROWN, A., DOBSON, V., AND MAIER, J. (1987). Visual acuity of human infants at scotopic, mesopic and photopic luminances. *Vision Res.* 27, 1845.

CURCIO, C. A., AND HENDRICKSON, A. E. (1991). Organization and development of the primate photoreceptor mosaic. In N. Os-

BORNE AND J. CHADER (eds.). *Progress in Retinal Research*. Vol. 10. Oxford: Pergamon, pp. 89–120.

CURCIO, C., SLOAN, K., KALINA, R., AND HENDRICKSON, A. (1990). Human photoreceptor topography. *J. Comp. Neurol.* 292, 497.

DOBSON, M. V., AND TELLER, D. Y. (1978). Visual acuity in human infants: a review and comparison of behavioral and electrophysiological studies. *Vision Res.* 18, 1469–1483.

GEISLER, W. S., AND DAVILA, K. D. (1985). Ideal discriminators in spatial vision: two point stimuli. *J. Opt. Soc. Am. [A]* 2, 1483–1492.

HENDRICKSON, A. E. (1988). Development of the primate retina. In E. MEISAMI AND P. S. TIMIRAS (eds.). *Handbook of Human Growth and Developmental Biology*. Vol. 1, Part B. Boca Raton, FL: CRC Press, pp. 165–178.

HENDRICKSON, A. (1992a). The morphological development of human and monkey retina. In D. ALBERT AND F. JAKOBIEK (eds.). *Principles and Practice of Ophthalmology. Vol. 1*. Development (A. FULTON AND J. WRIGHT, eds.). Philadelphia: W. B. Saunders.

HENDRICKSON, A. (1992b). A morphological comparison of foveal development in man and monkey. *Eye* 6, 136–144.

HENDRICKSON, A., AND DRUCKER, D. (1992). The development of parafoveal and mid-peripheral human retina. *Behav. Brain Res.*. 49, 21–32.

HENDRICKSON, A. E., AND KUPFER, C. (1976). The histogenesis of the fovea in the macaque monkey. *Invest. Ophthalmol.* 15, 746–756.

HENDRICKSON, A., AND YOUDELIS, C. (1984). The morphological development of the human fovea. *Ophthalmology* 91, 603.

HOLLENBERG, M., AND SPIRA, A. W. (1972). Early development of the human retina. *Can. J. Ophthalmol.* 7, 472–491.

HOLLENBERG, M., AND SPIRA, A. W. (1973). Human retinal development: ultrastructure of the outer retina. *Am. J. Anat.* 137, 357–386.

HUTTENLOCHER, P. R., DECOURTEN, C., GAREY, L. J., AND VAN DER LOOS, H. (1982). Synaptogenesis in human visual cortex—evidence for synapse elimination during normal development. *Neurosci. Lett.* 33, 247–252.

JOHNSON, A. T., KRETZER, F. L., HITTNER, H. M., GLAZEBROOK, P. A., BRIDGES, C. D., AND LAM, D. M. K. (1985). Development of the subretinal space in the preterm human eye: ultrastructural and immunocytochemical studies. *J. Comp. Neurol.* 233, 497–505.

LAVAIL, M. M., RAPAPORT, D. H., AND RAKIC, P. (1991). Cytogenesis in the monkey retina. *J. Comp. Neurol.* 309, 86–114.

LIA, B., AND CHALUPA, L. (1988). Prenatal development of regional specialization in the infant primate retina. *Invest. Ophthalmol. Vis. Sci.* 29 (suppl.), 378.

LINDBERG, K. A., AND FISHER, S. K. (1990). A burst of differentiation in the outer posterior retina of the eleven-week human fetus: an ultrastructural study. *Vis. Neurosci.* 5, 43–52.

MANN, I. (1964). *The Development of the Human Eye*. 3rd Ed. New York: Grune & Stratton.

MASTRONARDE, D., THIBEAULT, M., AND DUBIN, M. (1984). Nonuniform postnatal growth of the cat retina. *J. Comp. Neurol.* 228, 598.

MILLER, W. H., AND BERNARD, G. (1983). Averaging over the fovea receptor aperture curtails aliasing. *Vision Res.* 23, 1365–1369.

MOHN, G., AND VAN HOF-VAN DUIN, J. (1990). Development of spatial vision. In C. DILLON (ed.). *Vision and Visual Dysfunction. Vol. 10. Spatial Vision* (D. M. REGAN, ed.). London: Macmillan.

NORCIA, A. M., AND TYLER, C. W. (1985). Spatial frequency sweep VEP: visual acuity during the first year of life. *Vision Res.* 25, 1399–1408.

NORCIA, A. M., TYLER, C. W., AND HAMER, R. D. (1990). Development of contrast sensitivity in the human infant. *Vision Res.* 30, 1475–1486.

OSTERBERG, G. A. (1935). Topography of the layer of rods and cones in the human retina. *Acta Ophthalmol. (Copenh.)* 13, 1–97.

PACKER, O., HENDRICKSON, A., AND CURCIO, C. (1989). Photoreceptor topography of the retina in the adult pigtail macaque (*Macaca nemestrina*). *J. Comp. Neurol.* 288, 165–183.

PACKER, Q., HENDRICKSON, A., AND CURCIO, C. (1990). Developmental redistribution of photoreceptors across the *Macaca nemestrina* (pigtail macaque) retina. *J. Comp. Neurol.* 298, 472–493.

PENFOLD, P. L., AND PROVIS, J. M. (1986). Cell death in the development of the human retina: phagocytosis of pyknotic and apoptotic bodies by retinal cells. *Graefes Arch. Clin. Exp. Ophthalmol.* 224, 549–553.

PROVIS, J. M. (1987). Patterns of cell death in the ganglion cell layer of the human fetal retina. *J. Comp. Neurol.* 259, 237–246.

PROVIS, J. M., AND PENFOLD, P. L. (1988). Cell death and elimination of retinal axons during development. *Prog. Neurobiol.* 31, 331.

PROVIS, J. M., VAN DRIEL, D., BILLSON, F. A., AND RUSSELL, P. (1985). Development of the human retina: patterns of cell distribution and redistribution in the ganglion cell layer. *J. Comp. Neurol.* 233, 429–451.

RAKIC, P., AND RILEY, K. P. (1983). Overproduction and elimination of retinal axons in the fetal rhesus monkey. *Science* 219, 1441–1444.

RAPAPORT, D. H., YASUMURA, D., LAVAIL, M. M., AND RAKIC, P. (1987). Cytogenesis of monkey retina: comparison of the generation of retinal pigment epithelium and neural retina. *Soc. Neurosci. Abstr.* 13, 238.

RHODES, R. H. (1979). A light microscopic study of the developing human neural retina. *Am. J. Anat.* 154, 195–210.

ROBB, R. (1982). Increase in retinal surface area during infancy and childhood. *J. Pediatr. Ophthalmol. Strabismus* 19, 16.

ROBB, R. M. (1985). Regional changes in retinal pigment epithelium cell density during ocular development. *Invest. Ophthalmol. Vis. Sci.* 26, 614–620.

ROBINSON, S. R. (1988). Cell death in the inner and outer nuclear layers of the developing cat retina. *J. Comp. Neurol.* 267, 507–515.

ROBINSON, S., DREHER, B., AND McCALL, M. (1989). Nonuniform retinal expansion during the formation of the rabbit's visual streak: implications for the ontogeny of mammalian retinal topography. *Vis. Neurosci.* 2, 201.

SAMORAJSKI, T., KEEFE, J. R., AND ORDY, J. M. (1965). Morphogenesis of photoreceptor and retinal ultrastructure in a sub-human primate. *Vision Res.* 5, 639–648.

SMELSER, G. K., OZANICS, V., RAYBORN, M., AND SAGUN, D. (1974). Retinal synaptogenesis in the primate. *Invest. Ophthalmol.* 13, 340–361.

STEINEKE, T., AND KIRBY, M. (1989). Early axon outgrowth of retinal ganglion cells in the retina of the rhesus macaque. *Invest. Ophthalmol. Vis. Sci.* 30 (suppl.), 26.

STONE, J., MASLIM, J., AND RAPAPORT, D. (1984). The development of the topographical organization of the cat's retina. In J. STONE, B. DREHER, AND D. RAPAPORT (eds.). *Development of Visual Pathways in Mammals*. New York: Alan R. Liss, pp. 3–21.

VAN DRIEL, D., PROVIS, J. M., AND BILLSON, F. A. (1990). Early differentiation of ganglion, amacrine, bipolar and Müller cells in the developing fovea of human retina. *J. Comp. Neurol.* 291, 203.

WICKLER, K. C., WILLIAMS, R. W., AND RAKIC, P. (1990). Photoreceptor mosaic: number and distribution of rods and cones in the rhesus monkey retina. *J. Comp. Neurol.* 297, 499–508.

WILSON, H. (1988). Development of spatiotemporal mechanisms in infant vision. *Vision Res.* 28, 611.

WILSON, H. R., AND GELB, D. J. (1984). Modified line element theory for spatial frequency and width discrimination. *J. Opt. Soc. Am. [A]* 1, 124–134.

YOUDELIS, C., AND HENDRICKSON, A. (1986). A qualitative and quantitative analysis of the human fovea during development. *Vision Res.* 26, 847.

18 | Biological limits on visual development in primates

J. ANTHONY MOVSHON AND LYNNE KIORPES

The goal of this chapter is to explore the factors that limit the development of spatial visual performance in nonhuman primates. We first consider the factors that govern the development of normal visual performance, with a particular view to exploring those factors that are relatively inaccessible in the human subjects whose vision is the subject of the greater part of this volume. Second, we examine the limits on performance when abnormal visual development is used to induce experimental amblyopia in nonhuman primates. In each part, we first summarize the behavioral data that document the similarities between the development of vision in monkeys and humans, because it is these similarities that justify the use of the monkey model for human visual development. We then present neuroanatomical and neurophysiological evidence that allows us to deduce (or surmise) the particular sites in the visual system whose function changes during development, and the nature of those changes. We conclude that in normal development a great part of the change in visual performance from infancy to adulthood is attributable to improvements in the capacity of peripheral visual mechanisms, though perhaps not the photoreceptors themselves. Abnormal development produced by visual deprivation, anisometropia, or strabismus, however, appears to result in changes in the primary visual cortex, which ceases to be a faithful relay of visual signals from the periphery.

Many of the questions that arise when considering visual development in monkeys are, of course, the same as those that apply in humans. This volume contains thorough reviews of many of these topics, particularly the chapters by Banks and Crowell, Birch, Braddick, Hainline, Held, and Wilson. As we shall see, much interest centers on the role of retinal maturation, reviewed here by Hendrickson, and of central nervous system development.

DEVELOPMENT OF SPATIAL VISION

There are two distinct kinds of developmental change that contribute to changes in visual performance during development, which we can term changes of *scale* and changes of *sensitivity*. By changes of scale we mean changes in the spatial filtering or integration properties of elements of the visual system. The visual system of infants operates on a much coarser spatial scale than that of adults; and it may be that if allowance is made for this point, the infant's visual capacity is otherwise more or less adult-like. We use the term sensitivity to describe the efficiency or accuracy with which the visual system can process targets adjusted for changes in spatial scale. Thus, the sensitivity of an immature observer cannot be properly estimated if performance is measured with targets selected for adults—it is often necessary to adapt the characteristics of the display to the scale of the system under study.

Changes in both scale and sensitivity can be simply documented by measuring the development of the *spatial contrast sensitivity function*, which describes the performance of the visual system in terms of the minimal detectable contrast for sinusoidal grating patterns of varying spatial frequency (Campbell and Green, 1965). Figure 18-1 shows the development of contrast sensitivity for two individual monkey infants (Boothe et al., 1988). At each age, these functions show the usual bandpass shape, with a range of intermediate spatial frequencies being detectable at lower contrasts than at either lower or higher frequencies. Contrast sensitivity functions from monkeys at the earliest test ages were considerably reduced in overall amplitude as well as in the range of resolvable spatial frequencies. Examination of the longitudinal development of contrast sensitivity in infant monkeys reveals that the observed changes in contrast sensitivity are the result of the function shifting upward in sensitivity and rightward toward higher spatial frequencies concurrently. A subsequent analysis of these data shows that the full developmental change in spatial contrast sensitivity can be accounted for by the hypothesis that the function does not change shape, but undergoes changes in *only* scale and sensitivity during development (Movshon and Kiorpes, 1988). Although behavioral contrast sensitivity data from human infants are sparse, human contrast sensitivity seems also to develop according to the same rules as in monkeys, albeit more slowly (Banks and Salapatek, 1981; Movshon and Kiorpes, 1988). An analysis of human development using evoked potential measurements confirmed this impression (Norcia et al., 1990).

More traditional measures of visual acuity, such as spatial resolution, are also captured by the contrast sensitivity function: The spatial frequency at which contrast sensitivity falls to 1 corresponds to the resolution limit for grating targets. It can readily be appreciated from Figure 18-1 that the development of spatial resolution depends jointly on changes in scale and sensitivity. Nonetheless, the value of spatial resolution succinctly captures an important limit on visual performance; because it is more easily measured than the entire contrast sensitivity function, it has been widely studied. The development of resolution shows a similar developmental profile in all species examined. Spatial resolution in newborns is at least 10-fold poorer than in adults; it improves rapidly over the early weeks or months of life, then continues to develop at a slower rate to adult levels. Adult levels are reached by the end of the first year in monkeys (Boothe et al., 1988) and between 3 and 5 years in humans (Mayer and Dobson, 1982; Birch et al., 1983). Comparison of the time courses for the development of human and monkey spatial resolution reveals several similarities. Spatial resolution is comparable in newborn human and monkey infants, both measuring between 1 and 2 cycles/degree (cpd). Adult levels of resolution are in the range of 30–50 cpd. The time courses for the development of resolution in monkeys and humans superimpose fairly well if human age is plotted in postnatal months and monkey age in postnatal weeks (Teller and Boothe, 1979).

The open circles in Figure 18-2 show the development of grating resolution in seven longitudinally tested infant monkeys, as measured behaviorally using a combination of preferential-looking and operant techniques (Kiorpes and Movshon, 1989a). Development proceeds smoothly and regularly until adult levels are approached after the age of 1 year.

The development of various other visual functions has been studied in human and monkey infants. Direct comparisons are possible only for the development of vernier acuity, which occurs during roughly the same period as the development of spatial resolution but which takes place at a substantially higher rate (Shimojo et al., 1984; Kiorpes and Movshon, 1989a).

LIMITS ON NORMAL VISUAL DEVELOPMENT

Analysis of the factors that limit the development of visual performance has attracted considerable attention. In humans, it is of course not possible to make physiological measurements of the properties of individual visual mechanisms during development, whereas such measurements can be, and have been, made in monkeys.

Physiological Optics

The first issue is whether development is limited by the mechanisms that lead to the formation of the clear, focused, stable retinal image needed for good vision. Much of the best evidence here comes from humans and is reviewed elsewhere in this volume (see Chapters 4, 6, 30, 32).

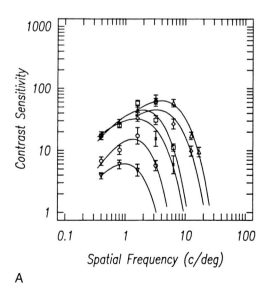

A

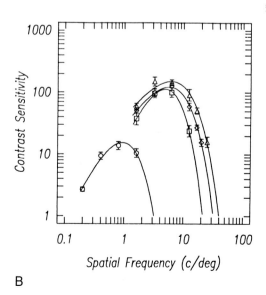

B

FIG. 18-1. Development of spatial contrast sensitivity in two macaque monkeys. Note the regular translation of the contrast sensitivity function upward and to the right during the course of development. (From Boothe et al., 1988. By permission.)

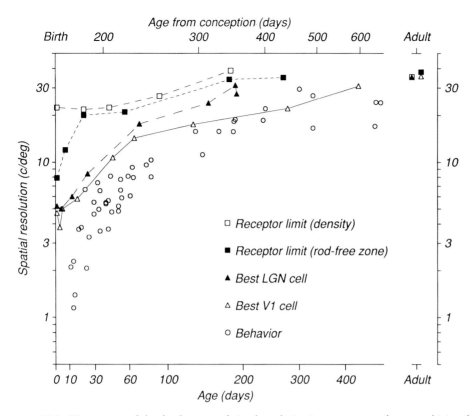

FIG. 18-2. Time course of the development of visual resolution in macaque monkeys, combining data on different functions from several sources. □ = Nyquist frequency for the retinal cone mosaic, calculated from the retinal density data of Packer et al. (1990). ■ = Nyquist frequency for the cone mosaic, calculated by Jacobs and Blakemore (1988) from measurements of Hendrickson and Kupfer (1976) of the size of the rod-free zone. Both Nyquist calculations assume that the central cone mosaic is a perfect hexagonal lattice; the Nyquist frequency is calculated from the cone spacings in such a lattice. Growth of the eye and associated retinal magnification is assumed to follow the function suggested by Jacobs and Blakemore (1988). ▲ = visual resolution of the best LGN neuron recorded from suitable populations in normally reared monkeys (Blakemore and Vital-Durand, 1986a). △ = visual resolution of the best neuron recorded from the striate cortex in normally reared monkeys of different ages (Blakemore and Vital-Durand, 1983a, b; Blakemore, 1990). ○ = behavioral measurements of visual resolution for seven macaque monkeys studied longitudinally (Kiorpes and Movshon, 1989a). The abscissa indicates the approximate postconceptional age at the top and conventionally at the bottom.

The quality of the retinal image in the infant monkey eye is remarkably good and quickly approaches adult levels (Williams and Boothe, 1981). Quantitatively, the developmental improvement in contrast modulation transfer is negligible over the range of frequencies visible to the infant monkey.

An aspect of optical development that is quantitatively important when considering the development of spatial properties in the visual system is the change in retinal image magnification that accompanies the growth of the eye. For example, the axial length of the monkey eye increases by about two-thirds between birth and adulthood (Blakemore and Vital-Durand, 1986a). This has no direct effect on the quality of the retinal image, but it alters the effect of that image on the subsequent neural elements of the visual system. All other things being equal, visual resolution should grow by about

two-thirds as the eye grows, simply because the size of the retinal image increases while the size of the neural elements used to analyze the image does not.

Although young infants often demonstrate the ability to accommodate correctly to a range of target distances, they do so less consistently than older infants. A similar trend is apparent in infant monkeys (Howland et al., 1982). Accommodative accuracy is poor in infant monkeys prior to about 5 postnatal weeks. Infants older than 5 weeks show consistently high accommodative accuracy over a range of target distances from 20 to 100 cm, corresponding to a 1–5 diopter (D) range of accommodative power. It appears that accommodative control in monkey infants is no worse than is needed to maintain an image of good apparent quality (cf. Green et al., 1980).

Data on the quality of oculomotor control in infant

monkeys are sparse but consistent with the available data on humans (Shupert and Fuchs, 1986). As in the case of accommodation, oculomotor performance is likely to be sufficiently good at all ages to impose no limit to visual performance.

In summary, it appears that neither the quality of the optics of the infant eye, the ability of infants to accommodate, nor their ability to fixate and track visual targets accurately imposes significant limits on performance. Indeed in appears that these physiological mechanisms develop at a pace that just comfortably *prevents* them from becoming an impediment to clear vision (Kiorpes and Movshon, 1990).

Photoreceptors

The next question is whether the retinal image, once formed, can be adequately captured and encoded by the photoreceptors (see Chapter 17 for a detailed review of retinal development). Yuodelis and Hendrickson (1986) provided evidence of two significant immaturities in the retinas of human infants. First, cones in the central retina of infants are abnormally shaped in a way that probably significantly impedes their light-gathering power; second, the density of cones in the infant's central retina is low, resulting in a limit to the resolution with which the retinal image can be adequately sampled. Based on an analysis of these data using an "ideal detector" model (Geisler, 1984), Banks and Bennett (1988) suggested that spatial visual development during the early postnatal months in human infants may largely be due to the maturation of foveal cone position and morphology (see Chapter 6 for a more recent recapitulation of this analysis). Their analysis readily accounts for a good part of the improvement in sensitivity seen during development, and modeling of the effects of cone migration by Wilson (see Chapter 32) suggests that a portion of the change in spatial scale can be attributed to retinal changes as well.

Development of the monkey retina has been studied by Hendrickson and Kupfer (1976) and Packer et al. (1990). Qualitatively, the changes in retinal organization are similar to those seen in humans, but quantitatively they seem to be somewhat less pronounced. The upper two curves in Figure 18-2 plot the development of the theoretical resolution limit for the cones of the central retina in monkeys, assuming that the limit of vision corresponds to the limit of retinal sampling (in theory, undersampled "aliased" images of frequencies higher than the resolution limit could be seen because the capacity of the optics exceeds the capacity of the receptors). The uppermost curve (open squares) is calculated from the cone densities measured by Packer et al. (1990); the subadjacent curve (filled squares) is based on densities calculated by Jacobs and Blakemore (1988)

from the size of the central rod-free zone reported by Hendrickson and Kupfer (1976). The change in the size of the rod-free zone should predict density under the assumption that all the cones within that zone remain within it as they migrate across the retina; this assumption seems to be consistent with the values reported by Packer et al. (1990). The wide variation between the two curves at ages less than 20 days seems to reflect real differences in the maturity of different monkeys at birth and makes it difficult to draw straightforward conclusions about the limits imposed by the receptors. It appears, however, that beyond the age of 20 days the resolution of the retinal mosaic significantly exceeds the behavioral resolution (open circles); for example, behavioral resolution between 20 and 30 days does not exceed 4–6 cpd, yet retinal resolution is four times greater.

The other important component of photoreceptor development is the change in sensitivity attributable to increased light capture. As noted above, increasing sensitivity ought to increase spatial resolution simply by raising the contrast sensitivity function and exposing more of its "shoulder" above the limiting value of 1. We are aware of no calculations comparable to those of Banks and Bennett that are based on Packer et al.'s monkey data, but the relatively modest postnatal maturation of the outer segment morphology of monkey cones suggests that the contribution of this change to monkey visual development is small.

Neural Mechanisms

In monkeys it is possible to study the spatial resolution of the neural elements that intervene between phototransduction and behavior. It is technically difficult to record retinal activity in infant monkeys, and we are not aware of physiological data on monkey retinal development. Ample data exist, however, for more central neural processing. The two last curves (filled and open triangles) in Figure 18-2 show data of this kind collected by Blakemore and Vital-Durand (1983a,b, 1986a; Blakemore, 1990), reporting the highest spatial resolution encountered in single-unit recordings from the lateral geniculate nucleus (LGN) and primary visual cortex of normally reared monkeys of various ages. It is evident from these data that the visual resolution of neurons in these structures barely, but reliably, exceeds behavioral resolution throughout most of development. Like behavioral resolution, it appears that the resolution of central neurons does not begin to approach the photoreceptor sampling limit until about 6 months of age. Although not pictured in Figure 18-2, Blakemore and Vital-Durand (1983a, 1986a; Blakemore and Hawken, 1985) also reported that the responsiveness and sensitivity of LGN and V1 neurons in young monkeys is reduced in comparison with those in adults; the improvement in neuronal responsiveness takes place over the period during which behavioral sensitivity also improves.

It may be that the performance of LGN neurons, at least, is better in young monkeys than reported by Blakemore and Vital-Durand (1986a). Blakemore and Hawken (1985, unpublished observations) studied the resolution and contrast sensitivity of neurons in infant monkey LGN, and showed that even near the time of birth resolution may approach 10 cpd, and contrast sensitivity (defined by a statistical criterion) may exceed 10. It is possible that a more quantitative examination of cortical unit properties would reveal similar subtle improvements over the data reproduced in Figure 18-2. It appears unlikely, however, that new measurements of the resolution of central neurons would alter the conclusion that they do not approach the sampling limit set by the retinal mosaic.

In summary, it appears that peripheral optical and receptoral mechanisms account for only a modest part of the improvement in visual resolution seen during development in monkeys. It seems that the greatest part of the developmental change is captured by considering the fidelity with which LGN neurons approach the retinal limits. Two important unexplored processing stages could account for this improvement. First, it might be that signal transmission within the retina is impeded early in development, and that the retina's functional properties develop importantly over the first 2 months of life. Alternatively, it might be that retinal processing is normal in young monkeys, but that the relay of signals from retinal ganglion cells to the LGN is of low fidelity. This question could be resolved with data on the function of retinal ganglion cells, but no data are presently available for monkeys (but see Tootle and Friedlander (1989) for data on kittens). It *is* possible to conclude that the development of resolution in visual cortex and the development of behavioral resolution are only slightly worse than the signals presented by the LGN permit.

ENVIRONMENTAL INFLUENCES ON VISUAL DEVELOPMENT

The development of the visual system is not a simple maturation; rather, it is susceptible to modification by the visual environment within which the system grows. Such modification can be produced within an early *sensitive period* whose duration varies from species to species and possibly from function to function within a species (Movshon and Van Sluyters, 1981; Harwerth et al., 1986). In humans, the sensitive period lasts between 2 and 5 years from birth; in monkeys, it is complete within a year, perhaps less.

During the sensitive period, deprivation of form or light experience has a globally disruptive effect on visual performance; various aspects of vision can be disrupted in a more specific fashion by arranging partial deprivation of specific kinds (for reviews see Movshon and Van Sluyters, 1981; Movshon and Kiorpes, 1990). Vivid evidence of the visual consequences of this deprivation is shown in Figure 18-3, which shows the effect of monocular eye closure for varying periods on the spatial contrast sensitivity of four monkeys (Harwerth et al., 1983). It is evident that the deprivation (which in case D was only of 2 weeks' duration) almost totally abolished the visual resolution and sensitivity in the deprived eye; in fact, the "contrast sensitivity functions" measured in the deprived eye may reflect nothing more than the monkey's ability to discriminate the brightness of diffuse lights when viewed through that eye.

The consequences of less radical forms of visual deprivation on visual development can also be substantial. We have explored the consequences of unilateral blur and strabismus—two forms of abnormal early visual experience designed to mimic the anisometropia and strabismus that often lead to amblyopia in human subjects. We created early unilateral blur using one of two methods: (1) continuous instillation of atropine in one eye for the first 6 months of life—the resulting dilation of the pupil and paralysis of accommodation substantially degrade the retinal image (Kiorpes et al., 1987); and (2) extended-wear soft contact lenses of − 10 D

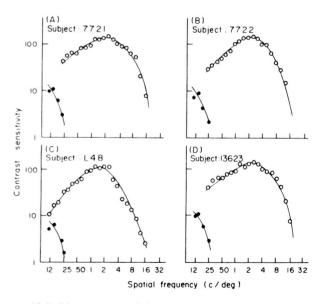

FIG. 18-3. Measurements of the spatial contrast sensitivity of four monkeys deprived of vision in one eye from birth to the ages of 22 months (A), 18 months (B), 8 weeks (C), and 2 weeks (D). At the end of the deprivation the lids were opened and visual experience permitted until the animals were fully mature. ● = data obtained using the deprived eye; ○ = data obtained using the nondeprived eye. (From Harwerth et al., 1989. By permission.)

(Kiorpes and Movshon, 1989b). We have also explored the effect of early strabismus, produced by either surgical alteration of the extraocular muscles (Kiorpes and Boothe, 1980; Kiorpes et al., 1989) or injection of a neurotoxin into a muscle (Kiorpes and Movshon, 1989b). Behaviorally, strabismus and anisometropia produce similar effects: loss of visual resolution and contrast sensitivity in the treated eye compared to its normal fellow. The loss, however, is always much more modest than that produced by total deprivation. Figure 18-4 shows behavioral contrast sensitivity data for two monkeys that developed amblyopia as the result of abnormal experience. Figure 18-4A shows data from an animal raised with blurred vision induced by contact lenses; Figure 18-4B shows data from an animal made strabismic by injection of botulinum A neurotoxin into the lateral rectus muscle. In both cases, the treated eye shows reliable losses of resolution and sensitivity compared to the fellow eye, but it retains a sizable fraction of its sensitivity and resolving power.

These results and others from other laboratories show that the visual performance measures obtained in animal models of deprivation are in substantial agreement with those from amblyopic humans (see Chapter 24 for a review). As in the course of normal development, it is therefore reasonable to seek explanations for the neural foundations of human visual function in neurobiological data from an animal model.

LIMITS ON VISUAL PERFORMANCE AFTER VISUAL DEPRIVATION

It is possible to draw an unambiguous conclusion from the available data on the effects of visual deprivation on central visual processing in primates. This conclusion—that the only substantial effects of visual deprivation are expressed in the visual cortex—is wholly different from our conclusion that the cortex does *not* limit normal visual development.

Physiological Optics

It is relatively easy to rule out the peripheral factors that influence normal development because it seems that the optical quality of the eye and the maturation of the morphology and distribution of photoreceptors (Hendrickson and Boothe, 1976) are unaffected by any of the forms of visual deprivation discussed here. Visual deprivation, either complete or partial, can alter the normal development of the refractive state of the eye (Wiesel and Raviola, 1977; Kiorpes et al., 1987). This change, however, has no practical consequence for vision once corrected with suitable lenses.

Neural Mechanisms

Figure 18-5 presents four sets of data obtained by Blakemore and Vital-Durand (1983a, 1986a,b; Blakemore,

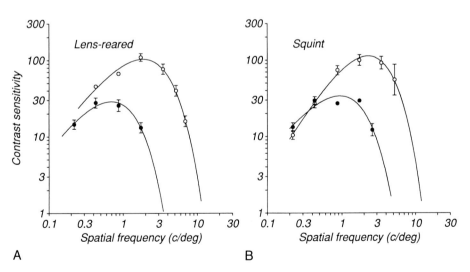

FIG. 18-4. Spatial contrast sensitivity of two macaque monkeys subjected to mild forms of visual deprivation. (A) Data from a monkey raised from birth to the age of 6 months with unilaterally blurred vision resulting from wearing extended-wear contact lenses of − 10 D in one eye and zero power in the other. (B) Data from a monkey made strabismic by injection of botulinum A neurotoxin into the lateral rectus muscle of one eye at the age of 26 days. ● = data obtained from the treated eye; ○ = data obtained from the untreated eye.

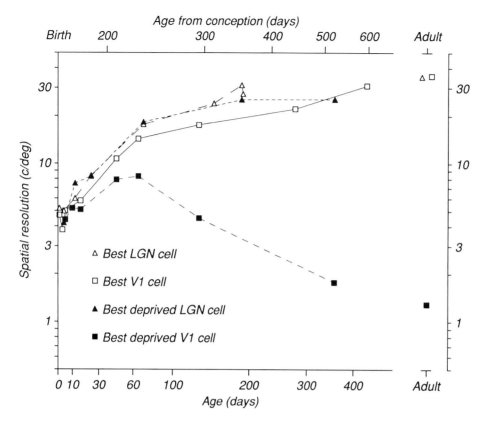

FIG. 18-5. Development of neural visual resolution in normally reared and deprived monkeys. △ = visual resolution of the best LGN neuron recorded from suitable populations in normally reared monkeys (Blakemore and Vital-Durand, 1986a). □ = visual resolution of the best neuron recorded from the striate cortex in normally reared monkeys of different ages (Blakemore and Vital-Durand, 1983a; Blakemore, 1990). ▲ = visual resolution of the best LGN neuron recorded from layers innervated by the deprived eye in monkeys subjected to unilateral eye closure from birth to the time of recording (Blakemore and Vital-Durand, 1986b). ■ = visual resolution of the best neurons recorded from the striate cortex of monkeys binocularly deprived from birth to the age of recording by bilateral eyelid suture (Blakemore and Vital-Durand, 1983b, unpublished observations; Blakemore, 1990).

1990, unpublished observations). The upper two curves (open symbols) are transferred from Figure 18-2 and show the development of visual resolution in the LGN and primary visual cortex, as measured by the resolution of the best cell encountered in animals of particular ages. The data represented by filled triangles show the development of visual resolution of cells in the deprived layers of the LGN of animals subjected to monocular eyelid suture from birth to the age of recording. Comparison of these data with data from normals (filled triangles) or from the nondeprived layers of the LGN in the same animals (not shown) (Blakemore and Vital-Durand, 1986b) shows that deprivation appears to be without effect on the resolution of these cells. In a more exhaustive analysis, Levitt et al. (1989) showed that the quantitatively measured spatial and temporal properties of LGN neurons in long-term deprived monkeys are almost indistinguishable from those of normal or nondeprived cells. This lack of effect of monocular deprivation on properties in the LGN is in stark contrast to

the devastating behavioral consequences of this deprivation (Fig. 18-3).

The bottom curve in Figure 18-5 shows the data of Blakemore and Vital-Durand on the development of visual resolution in deprived cortical neurons. In this case, the monkeys were binocularly deprived of vision because monocular deprivation removes almost all detectable influence of the deprived eye from the visual cortex (LeVay et al., 1980). It is evident that, although neuronal properties develop roughly normally for the first month or so, neuronal performance falls dramatically thereafter. The best neuronal resolution is deprived animals older than a year or so is actually worse than it is at birth.

The results in Figure 18-5 speak largely for themselves. In animals deprived of patterned visual experience, the relay of neuronal signals up to the LGN appears unimpeded. These signals do not transfer effectively to the cortex. It is thus safe to conclude that the failure in these cases arises at the geniculocortical synapse or perhaps among the earliest synaptic relays within the cortex itself.

Although the previous results strongly implicate cortical mechanisms in the visual effects of deprivation, it may be that these "blockbuster" environmental manipulations are too overwhelming to reveal more subtle changes that might be produced under less extreme conditions. We therefore also explored the effects of early blur-rearing and strabismus on the properties of neurons in the LGN and V1. Figure 18-6 shows summary scatter diagrams of the joint distribution of optimal spatial frequency and peak contrast sensitivity for populations of neurons from four monkeys raised with unilateral blur by means of atropinization (Fig. 18-6A) (Movshon et al., 1987) and from three monkeys raised with esotropic strabismus induced surgically (Fig. 18-6B) (Eggers et al., 1984). In each part of the figure, data represented as points are for neurons dominated by and tested through the untreated eye, and data represented as squares are for neurons tested through the blurred or deviated eye. Inspection reveals that in both cases neurons driven through the treated eye have poorer contrast sensitivity and spatial resolution than neurons driven through the fellow eye; the shifts in sensitivity and scale are comparable to those seen behaviorally in similarly reared animals (e.g., Fig. 18-4). In the case of the blur-reared monkeys, control experiments show that, as in the case of monocular visual deprivation, the res-

olution and sensitivity of neurons in the LGN is unaffected by the early rearing conditions. We conclude that the effects of these two modest forms of visual penalization, like those of complete deprivation, are expressed in the cortex, and that the peripheral optical and neural mechanisms of the visual system are unaffected.

CONCLUSIONS

We explored the limits on visual performance in two domains: during early development and following abnormal early experience. Our conclusions from these two sets of studies are wholly different from each other. In agreement with others considering the human literature, we believe that the main limits to visual performance in young developing animals are peripheral. Perhaps because they are accessible to anatomical investigation, much attention has been focused in the human literature on the development of retinal photoreceptors. Our consideration of the data from nonhuman primates suggests that although their photoreceptor development in some respects mirrors that of humans, it does not account in quantitative terms for the improvement in visual performance seen during early development. Instead, it appears that peripheral neural processing of photoreceptor signals—either in the retina or between the retina

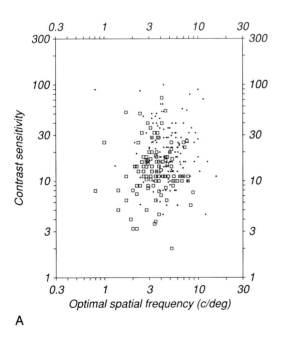

A

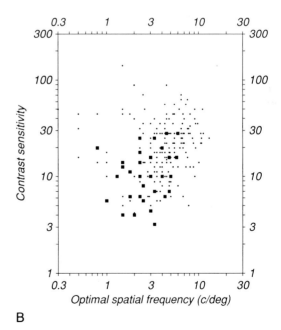

B

FIG. 18-6. Spatial properties of neurons recorded from the primary visual cortex of monkeys with experimentally induced amblyopia. (A) Data from 256 neurons from four monkeys raised with blurred vision produced by unilateral instillation of atropine from birth to the age of 6 months (Movshon et al., 1987). (B) Data from 234 neurons from three monkeys made strabismic by surgical alteration of the medial and lateral rectus muscles before the age of 3 weeks (Eggers et al., 1984). (A,B) Each datum represents the optimal spatial frequency and contrast sensitivity of a single neuron. Points = data for neurons dominated by (and measured through) the untreated eye; squares = data for neurons dominated by the treated eye.

and the LGN—is the stage of the visual process that limits performance in young monkeys. It seems clear that once signals reach the LGN they are faithfully relayed and processed by the primary visual cortex and subsequent centers.

When development is disrupted by abnormal early experience, however, a different picture emerges. There is little evidence in the literature for significant functional changes in the image-forming machinery of the eye or for changes in the peripheral components of the visual nervous system. Indeed, it is striking that the visual periphery is so utterly indifferent to its early visual input. On the other hand, with deprivation, the cortex, which responds properly to its input in the young animal, now fails to process the rich array of visual information forwarded to it from the LGN. Evidence from several kinds of abnormal visual experience discussed here, and many others not mentioned, points with regularity to the cortex as the site of the deficit. Indeed, because *all* signals afferent to the cortex seem normal and *no* signals within the cortex survive deprivation with a semblance of normality, it may be that the developmental anomaly can be pinned down in many cases to be a single set of synapses—those that link geniculate afferents to their cortical target neurons.

It should be noted that significant differences may exist between species; considerable evidence (not all of it uncontested) suggests that abnormalities may develop in the peripheral visual system of cats following deprivation (Movshon and Van Sluyters, 1981; Friedlander and Tootle, 1990). One must assume, however, that the factors acting in humans are more similar to those in monkeys than in cats. On this basis we conclude that the factors limiting human visual development are in the peripheral visual pathway, whereas those affected by abnormal experience are within the central nervous system.

REFERENCES

BANKS, M. S., AND BENNETT, P. J. (1988). Optical and photoreceptor immaturities limit the spatial and chromatic vision of human neonates. *J. Opt. Soc. Am.* [A] 5, 2059–2079.

BANKS, M. S., AND SALAPATEK, P. (1981). Infant pattern vision: a new approach based on the contrast sensitivity function. *J. Exp. Child Psychol.* 31, 1–45.

BIRCH, E. E., GWIAZDA, J., BAUER JR., J. A., NAEGELE, J., AND HELD, R. (1983). Visual acuity and its meridional variations in children aged 7–60 months. *Vision Res.* 23, 1019–1024.

BLAKEMORE, C. (1990). Maturation of mechanisms for efficient spatial vision. In C. BLAKEMORE (ed.). *Vision: Coding and Efficiency.* Cambridge: Cambridge University Press.

BLAKEMORE, C., AND HAWKEN, M. (1985). Contrast sensitivity of neurones in the lateral geniculate nucleus of the neonatal monkey. *J. Physiol.* (Lond.) 369, 37P.

BLAKEMORE, C., AND VITAL-DURAND, F. (1983a). Development of contrast sensitivity by neurones in monkey striate cortex. *J. Physiol.* (Lond.) 334, 18–19P.

BLAKEMORE, C., AND VITAL-DURAND, F. (1983b). Visual deprivation prevents the postnatal maturation of spatial resolution and contrast sensitivity for neurones of the monkey's striate cortex. *J. Physiol.* (Lond.) 345, 40P.

BLAKEMORE, C., AND VITAL-DURAND, F. (1986a). Organization and postnatal development of the monkey's lateral geniculate nucleus. *J. Physiol.* (Lond.) 380, 453–491.

BLAKEMORE, C., AND VITAL-DURAND, F. (1986b). Effects of visual deprivation on the development of the monkey's lateral geniculate nucleus. *J. Physiol.* (Lond.) 380, 493–511.

BOOTHE, R. G., KIORPES, L., WILLIAMS, R. A., AND TELLER, D. Y. (1988). Operant measurements of spatial contrast sensitivity in infant macaque monkeys during normal development. *Vision Res.* 28, 387–396.

CAMPBELL, F. W., AND GREEN, D. G. (1965). Optical and retinal factors affecting visual resolution. *J. Physiol.* (Lond.) 181, 576–593.

EGGERS, H. M., GIZZI, M. S., AND MOVSHON, J. A. (1984). Spatial properties of striate cortical neurons in esotropic macaques. *Invest. Ophthalmol. Vis. Sci.* 25 (suppl.), 278.

FRIEDLANDER, M. J., AND TOOTLE, J. S. (1990). Postnatal anatomical and physiological development of the visual system. In J. R. COLEMAN (ed.). *Development of Sensory Systems in Mammals.* New York: Wiley.

GEISLER, W. S. (1984). Physical limits of acuity and hyperacuity. *J. Opt. Soc. Am.* [A] 1, 775–782.

GREEN, D. G., POWERS, M. K., AND BANKS, M. S. (1980). Depth of focus, eye size, and visual acuity. *Vision Res.* 20, 827–835.

HARWERTH, R. S., SMITH III, E. L., BOLTZ, R. L., CRAWFORD, M. L. J., AND VON NOORDEN, G. K. (1983). Behavioral studies on the effect of abnormal early visual experience in monkeys: spatial modulation sensitivity. *Vision Res.* 23, 1501–1510.

HARWERTH, R. S., SMITH III, E. L., DUNCAN, G. C., CRAWFORD, M. L. J., AND VON NOORDEN, G. K. (1986). Multiple sensitive periods in the development of the primate visual system. *Science* 232, 235–238.

HENDRICKSON, A., AND BOOTHE, R. (1976). Morphology of the retina and dorsal lateral geniculate nucleus in dark-reared monkeys *(Macaca nemestrina). Vision Res.* 16, 517–521.

HENDRICKSON, A. E., AND KUPFER, C. (1976). The histogenesis of the fovea in the macaque monkey. *Invest. Ophthalmol.* 15, 746–756.

HOWLAND, H. C., BOOTHE, R. G., AND KIORPES, L. (1982). Accommodative defocus does not limit development of acuity in infant *Macaca nemestrina* monkeys. *Science* 215, 1409–1411.

JACOBS, D. S., AND BLAKEMORE, C. (1988). Factors limiting the postnatal development of visual acuity in the monkey. *Vision Res.* 28, 947–958.

KIORPES, L., AND BOOTHE, R. G. (1980). The time course for the development of strabismic amblyopia in infant monkeys *(Macaca nemestrina). Invest. Ophthalmol. Vis. Sci.* 19, 841–845.

KIORPES, L., AND MOVSHON, J. A. (1989a). Differential development of two visual functions in primates. *Proc. Nat. Acad. Sci. USA* 86, 8998–9001.

KIORPES, L., AND MOVSHON, J. A. (1989b). Vernier acuity and spatial contrast sensitivity in monkeys with experimentally induced strabismus or anisometropia. *Invest. Ophthalmol. Vis. Sci.* 30 (suppl.), 327.

KIORPES, L., AND MOVSHON, J. A. (1990). Behavioral analysis of visual development. In J. R. COLEMAN (ed.). *Development of Sensory Systems in Mammals.* New York: Wiley.

KIORPES, L., BOOTHE, R. G., HENDRICKSON, A. E., MOVSHON, J. A., EGGERS, H. M., AND GIZZI, M. S. (1987). Effects of early unilateral blur on the macaque's visual system. I. Behavioral observations. *J. Neurosci.* 7, 1318–1326.

KIORPES, L., CARLSON, M. R., AND ALFI, D. (1989). Development of visual acuity in experimentally strabismic monkeys. *Clin. Vis. Sci.* 4, 95–106.

LeVay, S., Wiesel, T. N., and Hubel, D. H. (1980). The development of ocular dominance columns in normal and visually deprived monkeys. *J. Comp. Neurol.* 191, 1–51.

Levitt, J. B., Movshon, J. A., Sherman, S. M., and Spear, P. D. (1989). Effects of monocular deprivation on macaque LGN. *Invest. Ophthalmol. Vis. Sci.* 30 (suppl.), 296.

Mayer, D. L., and Dobson, M. V. (1982). Visual acuity development in infants and young children, as assessed by operant preferential looking. *Vision Res.* 22, 1141–1151.

Movshon, J. A., and Kiorpes, L. (1988). Analysis of the development of spatial contrast sensitivity in monkey and human infants. *J. Opt. Soc. Am.* [A] 5, 2166–2172.

Movshon, J. A., and Kiorpes, L. (1990). The role of experience in visual development. In J. R. Coleman (ed.). *Development of Sensory Systems in Mammals.* New York: Wiley.

Movshon, J. A., and Van Sluyters, R. C. (1981). Visual neural development. *Annu. Rev. Psychol.* 32, 477–522.

Movshon, J. A., Eggers, H. M., Gizzi, M. S., Hendrickson, A. E., Kiorpes, L., and Boothe, R. G. (1987). Effects of early unilateral blur on the macaque's visual system. III. Physiological observations. *J. Neurosci.* 7, 1340–1351.

Norcia, A. M., Tyler, C. W., and Hamer, R. D. (1990). Development of contrast sensitivity in the human infant. *Vision Res.* 30, 1475–1486.

Packer, O., Hendrickson, A. E., and Curcio, C. A. (1990). Developmental redistribution of photoreceptors across the *Macaca nemestrina* (pigtail macaque) retina. *J. Comp. Neurol.* 298, 472–493.

Shimojo, S., Birch, E. E., Gwiazda, J., and Held, R. (1984). Development of vernier acuity in human infants. *Vision Res.* 24, 721–728.

Shupert, C. L., and Fuchs, A. F. (1986). Preliminary studies on the development of reflexive eye movements in infant monkeys. *Invest. Ophthalmol. Vis. Sci.* 27 (suppl.), 154.

Teller, D. Y., and Boothe, R. G. (1979). The development of vision in infant primates. *Trans. Ophthalmol. Soc. UK* 99, 333–337.

Tootle, J. S., and Friedlander, M. J. (1989). Postnatal development of the spatial contrast sensitivity of X- and Y-cells in the kitten retinogeniculate pathway. *J. Neurosci.* 9, 1325–1340.

Wiesel, T. N., and Raviola, E. (1977). Myopia and eye enlargement after neonatal lid fusion in monkeys. *Nature* 266, 66–68.

Williams, R. A., and Boothe, R. G. (1981). Development of optical quality in the infant monkey (*Macaca nemestrina*) eye. *Invest. Ophthalmol. Vis. Sci.* 21, 728–736.

Yuodelis, C., and Hendrickson, A. E. (1986). A qualitative and quantitative analysis of the human fovea during development. *Vision Res.* 26, 847–855.

VI. Abnormal Visual Development
Introduction

MARK J. GREENWALD

Throughout neurobiology and sensory psychology, the study of people with disordered function has proved rewarding for both basic researchers and clinicians. Because of the evolutionary uniqueness of the human nervous system, understanding of fundamental mechanisms derived through familiarity with and investigation of its naturally occurring defects provides an essential complement to knowledge gained from experimental work in animals. On the other hand, evidence of homology between human disorders and well-studied laboratory models can and frequently does lead to valuable new treatments and diagnostic techniques. No area shows this better than visual development.

The modern history of clinical/laboratory symbiosis in visual development research began in the 1960s, when David Hubel and Torsten Wiesel first encountered striking and apparently irreversible physiological changes in the brains of kittens subjected to monocular visual deprivation. Confirmation that they were on the track of a real and important phenomenon came quickly from clinicians familiar with the very poor visual prognosis of infants who suffered from unilateral cataract. The therapeutic challenge posed by these patients provided stimulation for subsequent work of Hubel and Wiesel and others, which led in turn to recognition of a major truth clinical experience had failed to reveal: that intervention during the first few weeks of life ("the critical period") could reverse many of the profound effects of deficient early visual experience. Armed with this knowledge, pediatric ophthalmologists in the 1980s were able to make successful visual rehabilitation the rule rather than the exception for infantile cataracts. Further analysis of such clinical experience is now again providing important insight into basic issues of visual development, as the work of Lewis and Maurer described in this section beautifully illustrates.

Cataracts that may induce severe developmental visual loss occur relatively rarely, but amblyopia (defective monocular vision due to abnormal early visual experience) from other causes is one of the most common chronic pediatric disorders, affecting 2 to 4 percent of the population and responsible for a majority of all visual impairment in children and young adults. The existence of this vast and youthful population of developmentally abnormal humans has very significant implications for vision research.

For one, the potential social and economic impact of advances in knowledge that benefit these people is enormous because of their age as well as their number. When a child's level of function is elevated, the quality of an entire productive life span is enhanced. Children may not express much gratitude for small increments in performance capability, but they *use* them. The 1990s have been proclaimed the "Decade of the Child," in belated recognition of the fact that investing health care and medical research dollars in the problems of children (who, unfortunately for themselves, don't vote or pay taxes) makes great sense even in times of tight money. Isolated disturbances of vision rank high in importance among the causes of disability in childhood. Visual issues also increasingly demand attention in the context of more global developmental disorders, the subject of chapters by Fielder and Hoyt and their colleagues in this section.

The need to provide care for large numbers of amblyopic children has been a principal stimulus to the growth of pediatric ophthalmology as a medical subspecialty, and to growing emphasis on abnormal visual development in optometric institutions. In nearly every North American region, these patients can now be found concentrated in a relatively small number of subspecialty practices, affording their care providers invaluable opportunity to acquire clinical insight into the nature of their disorders. These clinicians, mostly now well schooled in the work of the pioneering investigators of visual development, increasingly are making their expertise and patients available to laboratory based researchers. The fruit of such collaborations is represented by many of the chapters in this volume. A few individuals, among them chapter authors Fulton, Levi, and Tychsen, have brought strong personal backgrounds in both clinical and laboratory disciplines to the investigation of disordered visual development in recent years.

With greater involvement of clinicians in vision research has come long overdue recognition of the need to elucidate the physiological bases of essential strabismus (misalignment of the eyes, with associated disturbance of binocular visual function, that cannot be attributed to muscle weakness, nerve palsy, or the effects of accommodation). Esotropia (excessive convergence or inturning of the deviating eye), exotropia (divergence or outward deviation), and/or hypertropia (vertical misalignment) may be seen in patients with this condition, which commands an even greater share of clinical resources than amblyopia, yet has been almost totally neglected by laboratory investigators in the past. The work reviewed by Archer and by Tychsen in this section represents significant progress toward a most worthy goal, and the thought-provoking chapter by Simons shows how rich are the opportunities for future research.

The high incidence of developmental vision disorders, and the frequency with which they occur in asymptomatic children, makes it both feasible and necessary to consider screening of the entire population at risk as a primary means of reducing morbidity. Photorefraction, a tool developed in the laboratories of chapter author Howland and others, has reached the threshold of use on a scale that could significantly influence public health in a remarkably short time. With future widespread application, this modality is likely to provide information much needed by both clinicians and researchers concerning the natural history of amblyopiogenic refractive abnormalities, in addition to helping insure that children in need of care receive it on a timely basis. Education of primary health care workers and others who interact with large numbers of children should also be recognized as a priority by the vision research community: the improved prognosis of pediatric cataract patients in the past decade has been due in large part to growing awareness by pediatricians of the importance of early recognition and referral of affected infants.

Preferential looking acuity measurement is another technological innovation that has quickly found application outside the vision laboratory. With exemplary dedication and effort, chronicled in Dobson's chapter in this section, the developers of this research tool personally guided it into the offices of a host of clinicians, where it has in just a few years come to be viewed as an indispensable aid to the care of infants with sight threatening problems. Here too, reciprocal contributions to scientific progress are likely to be forthcoming, as data on the infantile history of numerous uncommon but interesting disorders from pediatric ophthalmological and optometric clinics round the world is accumulated and analyzed.

With early diagnosis, present day treatment of amblyopia and strabismus is generally quite effective, but for the most part involves modalities that are decades or even centuries old. Given the numbers of affected individuals, even a relatively small increase in success rate can be expected to benefit many thousands of people. Unfortunately, progress on the therapeutic front remains a much hoped for but largely unrealized end of research in visual development. One recent effort to apply knowledge gained from the laboratory study of vision directly to amblyopia treatment (the CAM stimulator) was heralded by its developers as a possible breakthrough before critical testing by others showed that it provided no significant benefit. This experience highlighted an important truth: that while the vision laboratory can and should point the way toward new therapies, they must be approached cautiously in collaboration with the clinical researcher, using controlled prospective studies.

The reader of this section will be impressed by the diversity of background, interest, and style its contributors bring to bear on its vast and still largely uncharted topic. Their differing approaches may seem confusing at first, but as the concepts presented settle in the reader's mind, a coherent picture will begin to form, made all the more intriguing by its many obscure and hazy patches. Taken together, these chapters provide a rich introduction to one of the major frontiers for vision research in the years to come.

19 | Clinical examination of infant visual status

ANNE B. FULTON, RONALD M. HANSEN,
D. LUISA MAYER, AND DOROTHY W. RODIER

In recent years the clinical examination of infant visual status has been supplemented by vision test procedures that originated as laboratory methods to study human visual development. Commonly, laboratory studies report data from groups of infants, and from the group data a description of the developmental course of an entire visual function is sketched. Sometimes a single visual function, such as scotopic spectral sensitivity (Powers et al., 1981) or spatial summation of dark-adapted infants (Hamer and Schneck, 1984; Schneck et al., 1984) has been derived from cross-sectional data.

When these test procedures that were born in the laboratory are used to address clinical issues that arise during management of a patient, the test results must deliver information about the individual patient. Abnormal and normal vision for age are to be distinguished, of course. Furthermore, longitudinal measures of an individual's vision, done for the purpose of identifying significant change over time, are destined to have a bumpy course atop the countercurrents of development, generally improving vision, and disease that may be impairing vision progressively. Add to development and disease the perturbation of treatment effect, and the Bermuda triangle of infant vision testing in the clinic is complete. In light of these considerations, the aim of the selective review presented herein is to comment on the present state of clinical examination of infant visual status.

This chapter (1) defines a preverbal patient population that presents for evaluation of visual status and (2) describes the pediatric ophthalmologist's examination, emphasizing those maneuvers aimed at defining the infant's visual capacities. The general features of infant visual function tests that have withstood clinical trial include practicability and efficiency; these factors are discussed using psychophysical measures of grating acuity and dark-adapted threshold tests as examples. A discussion of specificity and sensitivity examines the efficacy of particular tests for the diagnosis of pediatric vision disorders. The diagnoses of amblyopia and pediatric retinal degenerations are selected to illustrate these points. Variability of clinical measures of infant patients' visual function are considered from the perspective of the clinician's compelling need to disentangle significant from nonsignificant variations in vision over time.

PATIENTS

Who are the patients who come in for clinical examination of infant visual status? A survey of the last 350 children, ages 0–36 months at their first visit to the pediatric ophthalmologist (A.F.), provides one answer to this question. A.F. works in a department situated at a major medical center, but she also accepts referrals from any source, not only ophthalmologists. Of the 350 patients, the largest proportion are seen before age 12 months (Fig. 19-1). Throughout the 0–36 months age range many young children must be enticed to reveal their visual capabilities using infant test procedures.

Pediatricians refer most (60%) of the patients (Fig. 19-2A), the largest proportion of whom are suspected of having strabismus. Specialists, including neurologists, geneticists, and otolaryngologists, request ophthalmic examination and special tests to look for ocular signs of a generalized, systemic disorder (Fig. 19-2A). All patients referred by other ophthalmologists have eye problems and are referred for additional information about visual or retinal function and diagnosis (Fig. 19-2A).

Overall (Fig. 19-2B), about one-third of the patients from the combined referral sources are suspected of being strabismic. The second group is sent because the eyes or adnexae appear abnormal, and the children in the last group have systemic disorders with possible ocular involvement. The pediatric ophthalmologist, using a combination of clinical examination techniques, and, as indicated by the clinical issues, a variety of psychophysical and electrophysiological tests determined that 61% of the 350 patients have abnormalities of the globes or visual function, or both. The other 39%,

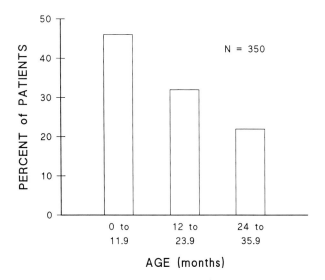

FIG. 19-1. Distribution of patient's ages at first visit to the pediatric ophthalmologist (A.F.). These patients are the last 350 children who came for their initial visit at age 36 months or younger. The largest proportion is less than 12 months old.

sent because of suspected eye problems, have perfectly normal eyes and visual function.

An abnormal appearance of the eyes, other than strabismus, prompts the largest percentage (41%) of referrals (Fig. 19-2B). Most of these patients do indeed have abnormalities, many of which are recognized amblyopiagenic entities such as cataracts. The overreferral rate for these patients is low. Nevertheless, the possibility that special tests of vision could enable earlier detection of eye abnormalities cannot be ruled out. For other infants with abnormal appearing eyes, assessment of retinal or visual function is critical for securing the final diagnosis (e.g., the electroretinogram for diagnosis of Leber's congenital amaurosis).

Suspected strabismus, a known risk factor for amblyopia, accounted for 109 (31%) of the referrals. However, 51 (47%) of these patients had perfectly normal eyes (false positives). Only about half ($n = 58$; 53%) were actually diagnosed as having strabismus, and only half of those patients were judged, mainly by fixation preference, to be amblyopic. Does it mean that appropriate referral for strabismus is a matter of chance? Perhaps. But we have no information as to how many children who truly had strabismus were not referred (false negatives). Of course, pediatricians would much rather overrefer than have the child suffer the consequences of delayed diagnosis of strabismus and amblyopia or, worse yet, a serious disease of the posterior pole. This conservative stance is balanced by reports of limited benefits afforded by early identification and treatment of amblyopia (Abrahamson et al., 1989; Ingram, 1989; Ingram et al., 1990a,b). At any rate, for this sample (Fig. 19-2) and perhaps others, the biggest unmet need at the referral end is for an improved strategy for detecting strabismus and associated vision problems. Clearly, more information about amblyopiagenic

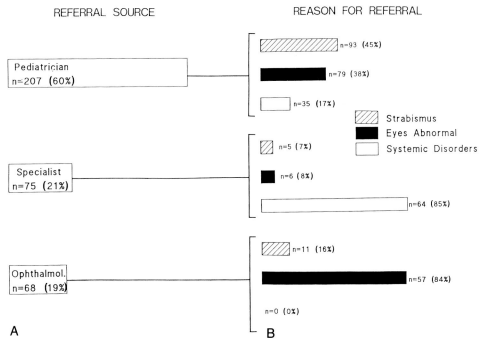

FIG. 19-2. Referral sources and reasons for referral. Note the proportions of patients referred by general pediatricians, pediatric subspecialists, and other ophthalmologists because of suspected strabismus, abnormalities of the eyes, or systemic disorders.

factors and their relation to the onset of strabismus and amblyopia as well as age-dependent variations of the response to therapies of strabismus and amblyopia are needed. From such information, one can envision emergence of improved guidelines for dealing with the issue of preverbal amblyopia at all points along the referral chain.

The presence of a systemic disorder, including neurological disease, motivates referral of the smallest percentage (28%) of patients. For these patients definition of visual capabilities is of interest (e.g., visually inattentive infants), or a test of visual or retinal function is needed to narrow the differential diagnosis.

OFFICE EXAMINATION BY PEDIATRIC OPHTHALMOLOGIST

The clinician customarily appraises an infant's vision using a cluster of nonquantitative or semiquantitative assessments. Information is gleaned from the clinical history, observations of the infant's visual behavior and fixation, the pupils and pupillary responses, motility, cycloplegic retinoscopy, and inspection of the structures in the anterior and posterior segments of the eyes.

The family's description of the infant's visual behavior is sought. By age 6 weeks, one expects a young infant to respond to visual stimuli, a smile for a smile and so forth. Both eyes are usually aimed in the same direction at this age. For those whose visual behavior departs from the norm, inquiry as to the stimuli that provoke vision-mediated responses is made. For example, apparent photophobia suggests achromatopsia, a stationary congenital condition in which the retina contains few if any functioning cones, or a hypopigmentation (albinism) syndrome. What are the eye movements like? Wandering, apparently purposeless eye movements are seen in infants with profound visual deficits. Nystagmus, rhythmic to-and-fro movements of the eyes, is associated with disorders that decrease acuity. Moreover, nystagmus has a disconcerting effect on parents; infants with nystagmus do not make the eye contact parents expect.

A family history of heritable visual disorders may orient the interview of the infant's parents. Hints of heritable eye disorders, even within a diagnostic category, may be elusive. For example, an infant with visual inattention and nystagmus due to a hypopigmentation syndrome may not have an obvious, long lineage of albinism but may have a several-generation background of relatives with inconspicuous nystagmus who are found on specific questioning to be the most lightly pigmented of their siblings.

Some observations made during the office examination are graded, and more could be. Perhaps most commonly used is gradation of the quality of fixation (e.g., Frank, 1983) on a scale 1 to 4:

1. Alternates spontaneously
2. Holds fixation well with each eye through a blink
3. Holds fixation briefly but not through a blink
4. Does not hold fixation

When used in conjunction with prism displacement, fixation preference can be evaluated in nonstrabismic children (Zipf, 1976; Wright et al., 1986).

Pupillary responses can be graded from brisk to absent. Metrics based on such observations yield information correlated with that gained from some of the infant vision tests. For example, the pupillary response (Fig. 19-3) of youngsters with generalized retinal degenerations is correlated with grating acuity measured using 9-degree fields of square-wave gratings [Spearman's rho $(\rho) = -0.654; p < 0.01$]. The more sluggish the pupil, the coarser the grating acuity. Thus standardization and validation of some graded measures obtained using routine clinical procedures may be warranted.

Refraction, commonly measured using retinoscopic techniques, is a controller of visual development because it is one of the determinants of inputs to the developing visual system. Normal, age-dependent variations in refractions are recognized (e.g., Howland et al., 1978; Mohindra et al., 1978; Banks, 1980; Fulton et al., 1980; Mohindra and Held, 1980). Astigmatism is frequently found in infants but becomes less frequent with age (Dobson et al., 1984; Gwiazda et al., 1984; Howland and Sayles, 1984). Anisometropia deserves

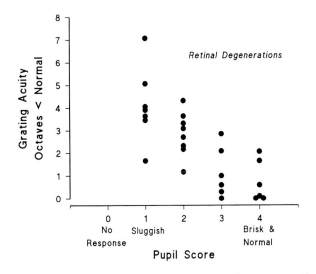

FIG. 19-3. Pupillary responses and grating acuities of 36 patients with retinal degenerative disorders of early onset: Leber's congenital amaurosis ($n = 11$); Bardet-Biedl syndrome ($n = 10$); retinitis pigmentosa ($n = 15$). Normal control subjects have pupil scores of 4. The patients' scores are distributed from 1 to 4 (poor = 1; fair = 2; good = 3; brisk = 4). Normal mean acuity is indicated by zero on the vertical axis.

attention when evaluating an infant for amblyopia. However, anisometropia varies or disappears with increasing age (Abrahamsson et al., 1989; Almeder et al., 1990).

Alternatively, refractive errors may be the consequence of abnormal ocular development and thus yield diagnostic clues. For example, hyperopia and congenital retinal disorders are associated (Foxman et al., 1983; Evans et al., 1989; Dagi et al., 1990), and prematurely born infants with otherwise normal eyes have a significantly higher proportion of refractive errors (e.g., Dobson et al., 1981).

CLINICAL MEASURES OF VISUAL FUNCTION

Short-Cut Procedures

The tests in current, routine clinical use are extant because they are quick, relatively inexpensive, and, at least for certain patient groups, sensitive and specific. Tests of grating acuity using psychophysical or evoked potential techniques and scotopic retinal function using psychophysical and electroretinographic techniques have been tried sufficiently in the clinical crucible that comment on some of their general and particular properties is possible.

Test efficiency, which is seldom a prime issue with adults, is always an issue with infants. If infant results cannot be obtained at one session, the duration of which is bounded by the infant's behavior, the impact vision data can have on the management of the individual infant patient diminishes—sometimes vanishes. Preston and coworkers' (1987) comparison of preferential looking performance of the quick Acuity Cards (AC) procedure and a two-alternative forced-choice method of constant stimuli (MCS) procedure (5 points; 20 trials per point) for estimating the grating acuities of twenty 2- to 8-month-old patients demonstrates that the quick procedure has the features necessary for clinical testing. The MCS procedure took, on average, 3.6 sessions, each 45–60 minutes long, to obtain an acuity from each eye and binocularly. The AC procedure accomplished the same in 36 minutes. Happily, the AC and MCS acuities were similar. In fact, mean acuities were not significantly different if the MCS threshold of the probit fit was taken to be 70% correct. These results indicate little is lost and all is gained by using an abbreviated procedure for acuity measures. Of course, it is only fair to mention that speedy MCS testing (total of 60 trials) has been accomplished by Birch and colleagues in an important study of infant esotropes (Birch and Stager, 1985). Another important observation of Preston et al. (1987) deserves reiteration here; it takes longer to evaluate patients with abnormalities than normal infants in the laboratory.

Measures of dark-adapted thresholds are almost always done on patients suspected of having symmetrical peripheral retinal disease (Fulton and Hansen, 1983a,b). Therefore one measure of threshold with binocular viewing obtained used a two-alternative forced-choice procedure yields the relevant clinical information. Conceivably, one threshold, determined using a method of constant stimuli (MCS) procedure with 100–120 trials, could be completed in a 60-minute session. Does the MCS approach upgrade the information over that obtained using a short-cut staircase procedure (Wetherill and Levitt, 1965), which can ordinarily be completed in less than 15 minutes?

A comparison of the MCS and staircase thresholds of normal 10-week-old infants for detecting 50 ms, 10 degrees diameter blue flashes shows that the MCS thresholds (75%) are on average 0.2 log units higher than the staircase estimate of threshold. Choosing a 71% criterion for threshold to match the 71% used for the staircase threshold estimate reduces the disparity between MCS and staircase results to 0.04 log units. As for variability, the standard deviations for staircase (0.11; $n = 15$) and MCS (0.13 at 75% correct; 0.18 at 71% correct; $n = 9$) thresholds are similar (F = 2.68; df 8,14; not significant). Therefore little is lost by using the staircase rather than the MCS procedure. Short-cut procedures such as the AC and staircase procedures are, in summary, reliable and necessary for these and presumably other clinical applications.

Evaluation of the Infant Tests in Clinical Use: Trade-Off of Sensitivity and Specificity

An ideal test would never miss disease (Fig. 19-4A), and it would correctly label any patient with a score above the cutoff point as having disease. This hypothetical test (Fig. 19-4A) is perfectly sensitive to disease. An ideal test would never mistake an individual with normal function for one with disease. This test correctly identifies anyone below the cutoff, a score of 5 or lower, as having normal function. Specificity is high. The ideal test cleanly distinguishes normals from individuals with disease.

Ideal is not real, however, and test sensitivity and specificity seldom attain perfect, 100% scores. Rather than a clean separation of normal from abnormal function, one is likely to find an overlap, as the simulated distributions of Figure 19-4B illustrate. Above the zero line is a hypothetical distribution of the interocular differences in the preferential looking grating acuities of infant amblyopes. Below the zero line is a simulated distribution of interocular differences in acuity of infants with normal function. Given the overlap, the choice of any cutoff involves some compromises. Given that neither test sensitivity nor specificity can be perfect, a

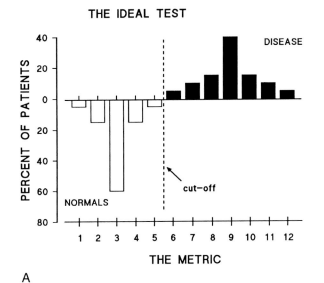

THE IDEAL TEST

THE METRIC

A

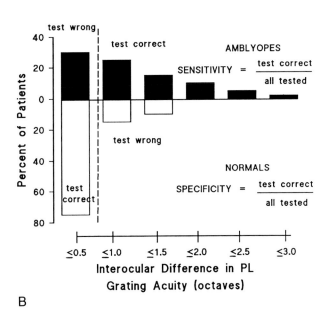

AMBLYOPES

SENSITIVITY = $\dfrac{\text{test correct}}{\text{all tested}}$

NORMALS

SPECIFICITY = $\dfrac{\text{test correct}}{\text{all tested}}$

B

FIG. 19-4. Sensitivity and specificity. (A) Ideal test has 100% sensitivity and 100% specificity. Such a test cleanly distinguishes individuals with disease from normal, disease-free individuals. (B) These simulated distributions demonstrate the overlap of test results typically encountered.

cutoff score that balances sensitivity and specificity is selected (Fletcher et al., 1982; Ingelfinger et al., 1987). Selection is tempered by factors inherent to the test, such as the variance and reliability of the measure, as well as disease prevalence and the burden of missing disease. Among infants and preverbal children, a question to answer is how costly of visual potential is it to miss an infant amblyope? If a cutoff of 0.5 octave in interocular difference is selected (Fig. 19-4B), for the known amblyopes the test comes up with the wrong

answer (misses amblyopia) for 30% and the correct answer for 70%. Sensitivity, the true positive rate, is 70%. For those with certified normal function, the test, using the 0.5-octave cutoff, is correct for 75%, and the false-positive rate is 25%. Specificity is 75%.

The analyses of clinical data shown in the next graphs use these concepts to, in effect, test the infant vision tests. Tests for amblyopia that are suitable for preverbal children (preferential looking grating acuities, fixation preference, and sweep VEP grating acuities) are analyzed (Figs. 19-5, 19-6, 19-7). The visual impairment of amblyopia is chosen as one example because it pervades many diagnostic categories whether it be strabismus, cataracts, or other entities; and it affects a larger number of children than any other visual deficit. Also assessed are the dark-adapted threshold and scotopic electroretinographic (ERG) tests for retinal degenerations (Figs. 19-8, 19-9). Retinal degenerations are relatively rare: but, in contrast to the amblyopia complex, their primary pathophysiology of the visual system is limited to the retina.

The relation of sensitivity and specificity of preferential looking (PL) grating acuities for amblyopia is shown in Figure 19-5. Data from the esotropic amblyopes found in the patient survey (Figs. 19-1, 19-2) and in Birch et al. (1990) are analyzed. The metric used

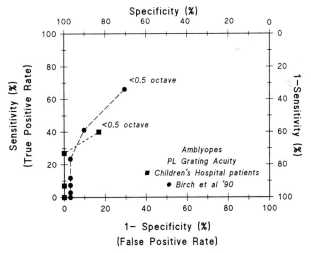

FIG. 19-5. Sensitivity and specificity of interocular differences in preferential looking (PL) grating acuities for amblyopia. The circles plot data taken from the study reported by Birch et al. (1990). The patients ($n = 68$) are infantile esotropes; each had a fixation preference. Acuities obtained on their initial visit are used in this analysis. The controls are 61 normal, age-matched infants. The squares plot the results from esotropic amblyopes in the survey (summarized in Figures 19-1 and 19-2) who had a PL acuity measure for each eye ($n = 15$). The control group ($n = 31$) was composed of infants who were referred because of suspected strabismus but were found to have perfectly normal eyes. The sensitivity-specificity relation for a series of cutoff scores from less than 0.5 octave (topmost circle and square) to less than 2.0 octaves interocular difference are shown.

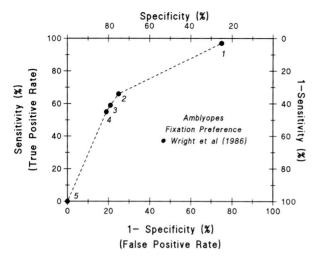

FIG. 19-6. Sensitivity and specificity of fixation preference for amblyopia. The sensitivity-specificity relations for fixation grades 1 (alternates) through 5 (will not hold) are shown.

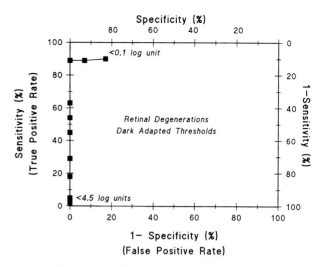

FIG. 19-8. Sensitivity and specificity of the dark-adapted threshold test for pediatric retinal degenerations. In this example sensitivity and specificity are calculated for cutoff scores from 0.1 to 4.5 log units.

is the interocular difference in acuity. Both data sets, as do other sets of PL grating acuities (Birch and Stager, 1985; Harris et al., 1986; Birch and Hale, 1988; Rodier et al., 1989) show a high specificity. That is, the PL grating acuity test is unlikely to label a normal infant amblyopic; there is a low false-positive rate. However, sensitivity, the true positive rate, is only moderately good. Even if the most favorable cutoff (<0.5 octave) is chosen, PL has sensitivities of only 40% and 65%, respectively, in these examples (Fig. 19-5). Similar PL grating acuity sensitivity-specificity relations are found among older patients whose diagnosis of amblyopia is

based on recognition acuities rather than fixation preference (Harris et al., 1986). Grating acuities, measured psychophysically, are known to be less affected by amblyopia than are recognition acuities (e.g., Levi and Klein, 1982, 1985). High pass stimuli used in conjunction with PL procedures have not been a breakthrough (Harris et al., 1984, 1986; Rodier et al., 1989).

The analysis of Figure 19-6 evaluates the efficacy of fixation preference, the clinician's common standard for deciding if amblyopia is present. The data published by

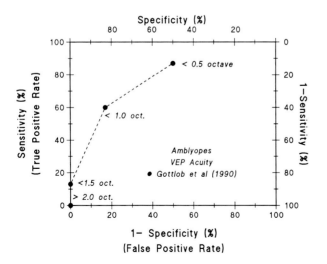

FIG. 19-7. Sensitivity and specificity of sweep VEP acuities for amblyopia. The difference in acuity between eyes is the metric used. The data are from Gottlob et al. (1990). Acuity of each eye was measured in 15 amblyopes and 6 normal subjects. Sensitivity is higher than that found for PL grating acuities, but specificity is somewhat low; half of the normals had 1.0 octave or more interocular acuity difference.

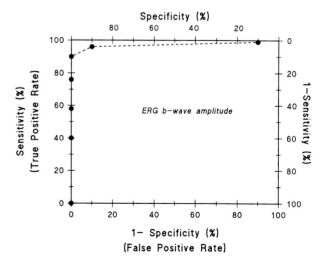

FIG. 19-9. Sensitivity and specificity of scotopic b-wave amplitudes for pediatric retinal degenerations. The amplitude of the ERG b-wave response to a blue flash (Wratten 47B; 10 μs, producing about zero log scotopic troland seconds) is the metric used. This flash elicits a 266 μV (SD 25) b-wave response from a normal eye. Cutoff scores in 50-μV steps between 350 and 100 μV are used to calculate the dashed curve.

Wright and coworkers (1986) are used to construct this display. Amblyopes ($n = 116$) were defined by an interocular difference of at least one line in recognition acuities. Amblyopia-free patients, 95 children with no interocular difference in recognition acuity, constituted the control group. The results of the test, fixation preference, were graded 1 to 5; 1 is for alternators, 5 for those who would not fix and hold with one eye; 2, 3, and 4 are for those in between. Sensitivity appears better than PL sensitivity (Fig. 19-5), although specificity is somewhat lower. Only patients with a fixation preference (the 5s, 4s and possibly 3s), however, are included in the PL analysis (Fig. 19-5). Perhaps fixation preference does not gain much in sensitivity and loses specificity compared to PL. The results of a cluster of tests on the same individual might clarify this point.

Grating acuities measured using sweep VEP procedures are another test for amblyopia in preverbal patients. The VEP data shown in Figure 19-7 are drawn from the study reported by Gottlob et al., (1990). Fifteen amblyopes and six normal subjects had acuities of each eye measured. The metric used for this analysis is the interocular difference in acuity. For a cutoff of 0.5 octave, sensitivity is higher than for PL. However, specificity is low. Half of the normals had an octave or more interocular difference in acuity. Orel-Bixler and Norcia's (personal communication) report of higher specificity does hold promise that the sweep VEP is a good clinical test for amblyopia.

Taken as a whole, these analyses of the tests—PL, fixation preference, and VEP—indicate that better tests for preverbal amblyopia are needed. Maybe amblyopia needs definition.

In contrast to the tests for amblyopia, tests for pediatric retinal degenerations have high specificity and sensitivity. When dark-adapted threshold and scotopic ERG parameters are examined, the following sensitivity-specificity relations are found. For the dark-adapted threshold test (Fulton et al., 1991) cutoff scores from 0.1 to 4.5 log units were calculated (Fig. 19-8). Patients ($n = 57$) with a variety of retinal degenerations and 31 normal subjects contributed data; diagnoses were made on the basis of a cluster of clinical observations and standard ERG criteria. Dark-adapted thresholds for detecting 50 ms, 10 degrees diameter, blue ($\lambda < 510$ nm) flashes of light presented 20 degrees from central fixation were measured. The patients had threshold elevations of 0–4.5 log units above normal. The thresholds of normal control subjects were distributed from 0.11 log units below to 0.29 log units above the mean. For threshold elevations of 0.5 log units or more, the dark-adapted threshold test has a sensitivity of 91% and a false alarm rate (1 minus specificity) of zero. Thus for a more than 0.5 log unit threshold elevation, the test is sensitive to the effects of generalized retinal de-

generations and highly specific. In other words, for this threshold test there is little chance that a normal subject will be mistakenly diagnosed as having a retinal degeneration. Scotopic b-wave amplitudes, an indicator of distal retinal function, offer another test that is highly specific and sensitive to pediatric retinal degenerations that affect primarily the photoreceptors (Fig. 19-9). When the nature of the disease to be detected is well defined, as in retinal degenerations, good tests can be designed.

Longitudinal Measures

The clinician makes serial measures to monitor the patient's vision for significant change over time. For example, the aim might be to find out if treatment, such as patching of an amblyope, had caused a significant improvement in acuity. In the case of a retinal degeneration, the purpose might be to find out if a child's night vision, the dark-adapted threshold, had shown a significant change for the worse. The short-term, intervisit variation is used to define significant change over the long haul.

Consider the dark-adapted threshold, which has high specificity and sensitivity for retinal degenerations, and for normals low intersubject variability. For test-retest of normal infants the differences in dark-adapted threshold between first and second tests are distributed as shown in Figure 19-10A. For patients with retinal degenerations the distribution is somewhat broader (Fig. 19-10B) than that of the normal subjects. From these distributions confidence intervals can be calculated (Berson et al., 1985). The 99% confidence interval for the normals is smaller ($\pm$ 0.66 log unit) and of course not appropriate for the patients whose 99% confidence interval is $\pm$ 1.06 log units (Fig. 19-10C). A significant change in a patient's threshold is large—about 1.0 log unit.

SUMMARY

Clinical infant vision tests are, unequivocally, feasible and show promise as diagnostic tools. Better tests for infantile amblyopia, a cause of visual impairment that pervades all diagnostic categories, would be welcome. Preverbal amblyopes do not yet enjoy the benefits of a metric as refined as optotype acuity, whatever the shortcomings of the optotype tests. On the other hand, as the recent clinical literature attests, numerous infant patients with a variety of other ocular disorders have benefited from preferential looking and evoked potential measures of acuity that a decade ago would not have been offered in routine clinical testing. In contrast to the amblyopia complex, it appears to be a more straightforward matter to test efficaciously for the path-

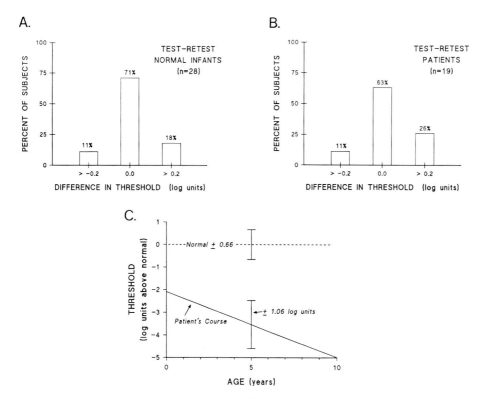

FIG. 19-10. Dark-adapted threshold test-retest reliability and assessment of significant change in threshold over time. (A) Distribution of the differences between thresholds obtained at test 1 and after a short (1 week) intervisit interval at test 2 is shown for normal subjects (*n* = 28). (B) Distribution of differences in test 1 and test 2 thresholds for pediatric patients (*n* = 19) with retinal degenerations is shown. (C) The 99% confidence intervals for normal subjects and patients, calculated based on the distribution shown in (A) and (B) are shown. The sloping line is the average course of threshold change for 13 patients with Bardet-Biedl syndrome, a rare, heritable disorder in which retinal degeneration is a component.

ophysiology of retinal degenerations. The exercise of evaluating these acuity and retinal tests heighten one's awareness that, as clinical infant vision testing moves forward with the development of new and promising measures of infants' visual capacities, the choice of appropriate control groups—appropriate definers of specificity—will be important.

Longitudinal measures to identify significant change over time as well as the problem of predictive validity of tests of the developing visual system's function warrant considerable additional work. Some vision tests, such as preferential looking grating acuity, are predictive of later visual performance in low vision infant patients with nystagmus (Mayer et al., 1988) and severe, bilateral ocular disorders (Fielder et al., 1991). These tests begin to meet the frequent and justifiable demands for prognostic information about infant and young child patients.

Efforts to develop new tests of infants' vision, even if the particular test is not destined to become a routine clinical procedure, deserve encouragement mainly because the tests can potentially probe anomalous visual processing in pediatric diseases. It is a route to under-

standing disease mechanisms and so provides a foundation on which logical approaches to diagnosis and therapy can be built. As clinicians contend with the development—disease—treatment triangle, the advice and input of basic scientists will be critical. All the same, clinical judgments will certainly continue to depend also on the nonquantitative information collected during the course of clinical examination, and ongoing surveillance of a child's vision and visual system health will be important to ensure the best possible visual outcome for that child.

Acknowledgments. Dr. Eileen Birch made raw data available to us for the analysis presented in Figure 19-5. Dr. Robert D. Reinecke made the raw data used for the analysis presented in Figure 19-7 available. We are grateful for these generous contributions.

REFERENCES

ABRAHAMSSON, M., SJOSTROM, A., AND SJOSTRAND, J. (1989). A longitudinal study of changes in infantile anisometropia. *Invest. Ophthalmol. Vis. Sci.* 30 (suppl.), 141.

ALMEDER, L. M., PECK, L. B., AND HOWLAND, H. C. (1990). Prevalence of anisometropia in volunteer laboratory and school screening populations. *Invest. Ophthalmol. Vis. Sci.* 31, 2448–2455.

BANKS, M. S. (1980). Infant refraction and accommodation. *Int. Ophthalmol. Clin.* 20, 205–232.

BERSON, E. L., SANDBERG, M. A., ROSNER, B., BIRCH, D. G., AND HANSON, A. H. (1985). Natural course of retinitis pigmentosa over a three-year interval. *Am. J. Ophthalmol.* 99, 240–251.

BIRCH, E. E., AND HALE, L. A. (1988). Criteria for monocular acuity deficit in infancy and early childhood. *Invest. Ophthalmol. Vis. Sci.* 29, 636–643.

BIRCH, E. E., AND STAGER, D. (1985). Monocular acuity and stereopsis in infantile esotropia. *Invest. Ophthalmol. Vis. Sci.* 26, 1624–1630.

BIRCH, E. E., STAGER, D. R., BERRY, P., AND EVERETT, M. E. (1990). Prospective assessment of acuity and stereopsis in amblyopic infantile esotropes following early surgery. *Invest. Ophthalmol. Vis. Sci.* 31, 758–765.

BROWN, A. M., AND TELLER, D. Y. (1989). Chromatic opponency in 3-month-old human infants. *Vision Res.* 29, 37–45.

DAGI, L. R., LEYS, M. J., HANSEN, R. M., AND FULTON, A. B. (1990). Hyperopia in complicated Leber's congenital amaurosis. *Arch. Ophthalmol.* 108, 709–712.

DOBSON, V. L., FULTON, A. B., MANNING, D., SALEM, D., AND PETERSEN, R. (1981). Cycloplegic refractions of premature infants. *Am. J. Ophthalmol.* 91, 490–495.

DOBSON, V., FULTON, A. B., AND SEBRIS, S. L. (1984). Cycloplegic refractions of infants and young children: the axis of astigmatism. *Invest. Ophthalmol. Vis. Sci.* 25, 83–97.

EVANS, N. M., FIELDER, A. R., AND MAYER, D. L. (1989). Ametropia in congenital cone deficiency—achromatopsia: a defect of emmetropisation. *Clin. Vis. Sci.* 4, 129–136.

FIELDER, A. R., FULTON, A. B., AND MAYER, D. L. (1991). The visual behavior of infants with severe ocular disorders. *Ophthalmology* 98, 1306–1309.

FLETCHER, R. H., FLETCHER, S. W., AND WAGNER, E. H. (1982). *Clinical Epidemiology.* 2nd Ed. Baltimore: Williams & Wilkins, pp. 46–51.

FOXMAN, S. G., WIRTSCHAFTER, J. D., AND LETSON, R. D. (1983). Leber's congenital amaurosis and high hyperopia: a discrete entity. In P. HENKIND (ed.). *Acta 25th International Congress of Ophthalmology.* Philadelphia: Lippincott, pp. 55–58.

FRANK, J. W. (1983). The clinical usefulness of the induced tropia test for amblyopia. *Am. Orthoptic J.* 33, 60–69.

FULTON, A. B., AND HANSEN, R. M. (1983a). Retinal adaptation in infants and children with retinal degenerations. *Ophthalmic Pediatr. Genet.* 2, 69–81.

FULTON, A. B., AND HANSEN, R. M. (1983b). Retinal sensitivity and adaptation in pediatric patients. *Behav. Brain Res.* 10, 59–70.

FULTON, A. B., DOBSON, V., SALEM, D., MAR, C., PETERSEN, R. A., AND HANSEN, R. M. (1980). Cycloplegic refractions in infants and young children. *Am. J. Ophthalmol.* 90, 239–247.

FULTON, A. B., HANSEN, R. M., YEH, Y-L., AND TYLER, C. W. (1991). Temporal summation in 10-week-old infants. *Vision Res.* 31, 1259–1269.

GOTTLOB, I., FENDICK, M. G., GUO, S., ZUBCOV, A. A., ODOM, J. V., AND REINECKE, R. D. (1990). Visual acuity measurements by swept spatial frequency visual-evoked-cortical potentials (VECPs): clinical application in children with various visual disorders. *J. Pediatr. Ophthalmol. Strabismus* 27, 40–47.

GWIAZDA, J., SCHEIMAN, M., MOHINDRA, I., AND HELD, R. (1984). Astigmatism in children: changes in axis and amount from birth to six years. *Invest. Ophthalmol. Vis. Sci.* 25, 88–92.

HAMER, R. D., AND SCHNECK, M. E. (1984). Spatial summation of dark adapted human infants. *Vision Res.* 24, 77–85.

HARRIS, S. J., HANSEN, R. M., AND FULTON, A. B. (1984). Assessment of acuity in human infants using face and grating stimuli. *Invest. Ophthalmol. Vis. Sci.* 25, 782–786.

HARRIS, S. J., HANSEN, R. M., AND FULTON, A. B. (1986). Assessment of acuity in amblyopic subjects using face, grading and recognition stimuli. *Invest. Ophthalmol. Vis. Sci.* 27, 1184–1187.

HOWLAND, H. C., AND SAYLES, N. (1984). Photorefractive measurements of astigmatism in infants and young children. *Invest. Ophthalmol. Vis. Sci.* 25, 93–102.

HOWLAND, H. C., ATKINSON, J., BRADDICK, O., AND FRENCH, J. (1978). Infant astigmatism measured by photorefraction. *Science* 202, 331–333.

INGELFINGER, J. A., MOSTELLER, F., THIBODEAU, L. A., AND WARE, J. H. (1987). *Biostatistics in Clinical Medicine.* New York: Macmillan, pp. 7–9.

INGRAM, R. M. (1989). Amblyopia editorial: neither screening nor treatment is satisfactory. *BMJ* 298, 204.

INGRAM, R. M., ARNOLD, P. E., DALLY, S., AND LUCAS, J. (1990a). Results of a randomized trial of treating abnormal hypermetropia from the age of 6 months. *Br. J. Ophthalmol.* 74, 158–159.

INGRAM, R. M., WALKER, C., BILLINGHAM, B., LUCAS, J., AND DALLY, S. (1990b). Factors relating to visual acuity in children who have been treated for convergent squint. *Br. J. Ophthalmol.* 74, 82–83.

LEVI, D. M., AND KLEIN, S. (1982). Differences in vernier discrimination for gratings between strabismic and anisometropic amblyopes. *Invest. Ophthalmol. Vis. Sci.* 23, 398–407.

LEVI, D. M., AND KLEIN, S. (1985). Vernier acuity, crowding and amblyopia. *Vision Res.* 25, 979–991.

MAYER, D. L., RODIER, D. R., AND FULTON, A. B. (1988). Grating acuity differentiates good from poor prognosis for vision in infants with nystagmus. *Invest. Ophthalmol. Vis. Sci.* 29 (suppl.), 435.

MOHINDRA, I., AND HELD, R. (1980). Refractions in humans from birth to five years. *Doc. Ophthalmol. Proc. Ser.* 28, 19–27.

MOHINDRA, I., HELD, R., GWIAZDA, J., AND BRILL, J. S. (1978). Astigmatism in infants. *Science* 202, 329–331.

POWERS, M. K., SCHNECK, M., AND TELLER, D. Y. (1981). Spectral sensitivity of human infants at absolute visual threshold. *Vision Res.* 21, 1005–1016.

PRESTON, K. L., MCDONALD, M. A., SEBRIS, S. L., DOBSON, V., AND TELLER, D. Y. (1987). Validation of the acuity card procedure for assessment of infants with ocular disorders. *Ophthalmology* 94, 644–653.

RODIER, D. W., SCHREINER, L. A., PELLI, D. G., HANSEN, R. M., MAYER, D. L., AND FULTON, A. B. (1989). New "face" and grating stimuli to test acuity of pediatric eye patients. *Invest. Ophthalmol. Vis. Sci.* 30 (suppl.), 142.

SCHNECK, M. E., HAMER, R. D., PACKER, O. S., AND TELLER, D. Y. (1984). Area threshold relations at controlled retinal locations in 1-month-old human infants. *Vision Res.* 24, 1753–1763.

WETHERILL, G. B., AND LEVITT, H. (1965). Sequential estimation of points on a psychometric function. *Br. J. Math. Statist. Psychol.* 18, 1–10.

WRIGHT, K. W., EDELMAN, P. M., WALONKER, F., AND YIU, S. (1986). Reliability of fixation preference testing in diagnosing amblyopia. *Arch. Ophthalmol.* 104, 549–553.

ZIPF, R. F. (1976). Binocular fixation pattern. *Arch. Ophthalmol.* 94, 401–405.

20 | Visual acuity testing in infants: from laboratory to clinic

VELMA DOBSON

A frequent part of many basic science grant proposals is a section describing the clinical relevance of the proposed research. It may describe how the proposed research will aid in diagnosing a disorder, in understanding the underlying causes of a disorder, or in the development of new means of treating a disorder. In some cases, the potential clinical benefits of the research are largely hypothetical and are constrained by practical and scientific limitations that prevent the benefits from reaching the clinic for years or decades. In other cases, however, the research produces developments that have the potential to be incorporated into clinical settings almost immediately.

One area in which attempts have been made to apply the results of laboratory research to clinical problems is the area of behavioral assessment of visual acuity of human infants.[1] Initially, basic science researchers tested individual infants with ocular pathology in their laboratories (e.g., Teller et al., 1978; Thomas et al., 1979; Atkinson et al., 1982; Jacobson et al., 1982; Birch and Stager, 1985) or took their laboratory-based techniques into clinical settings to test infants (e.g., Mayer et al., 1982; Catalano et al., 1987). In general, the basic science researchers were successful in assessing acuity in clinical populations. A number of features of laboratory-based behavioral assessment techniques, however, made the techniques ill-suited for widespread clinical use. First, statistical limitations of the forced-choice laboratory-based procedures required repeated stimulus presentations to obtain an accurate acuity estimate (McKee et al., 1985). As a result, acuity testing was too time-consuming to be incorporated easily into busy clinic settings. Second, each group of researchers used their own individualized apparatus, so no standardized equipment was available. Finally, because research groups differed regarding the testing procedures used and the methods

by which acuity results were scored, neither standardized instructions for conducting the procedures nor clear guidelines for interpreting acuity results from laboratory-based procedures were available.

A technique has been developed that appears to be successfully bringing laboratory-base technology for behavioral assessment of grating acuity of infants into widespread clinical use. This technique is the acuity card procedure (McDonald et al., 1985), which was developed through the efforts of a group of researchers based at the University of Washington, Seattle. The procedure is currently being used in more than 100 clinical locations. The goal of the present chapter is to: (1) review the research that led to the development of the acuity card procedure; (2) describe acuity card studies that have been conducted to validate the procedure, study its clinical utility, explore effects of variations in stimuli and procedure, and define the limitations of the procedure; and (3) speculate on the possible reasons the procedure appears to be successfully making the transition from the laboratory to the clinic.

ACUITY CARD PROCEDURE

The acuity card procedure (Fig. 20-1) is a rapid, subjective method for measuring grating acuity in infants and young children. In the procedure, the infant is shown a series of gray cards, each 25.5×51.0 cm. Each card contains a 12.5×12.5 cm square patch of black-and-white grating located to the left or right of a small, 4 mm diameter, central aperture. The spatial frequency of the grating varies from card to card, from 0.23 to 38 cycles/cm, in approximately 0.5-octave[2] steps. During testing the cards are placed face-down on a table beside the tester, arranged in order of increasing spatial frequency. The tester, who does not know whether the grating is located on the left or right side of each card,

---

1. Electrophysiological methods for measuring visual acuity in infants are also making the transition from the laboratory to clinical use (e.g., Sokol, 1980; Odom et al., 1981; Norcia et al., 1987). A review of electrophysiological methods for acuity assessment of infants, however, is beyond the scope of this chapter.

2. One octave is a halving or doubling of spatial frequency, e.g., from 4 to 8 cycles/cm or from 4 to 2 minutes of arc per stripe.

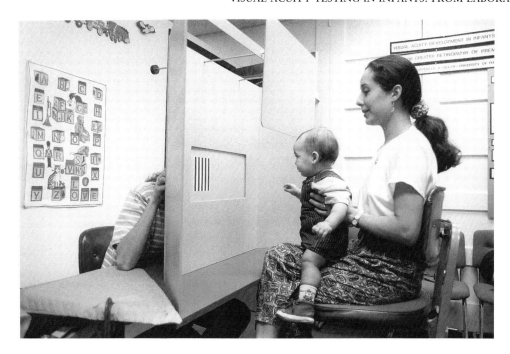

FIG. 20-1. Measurement of grating acuity with the Teller Acuity Card apparatus and procedure. Infant is seated on parent's lap with eyes 38 cm from the viewing aperture in the center of the acuity card. The tester (behind the screen) presents a series of Acuity Cards (the 0.43 cycle/cm card is shown here) and watches the infant's eye and head movements through the viewing aperture. Based on the infant's preferential fixation of the gratings on the acuity cards, the tester estimates acuity as the finest grating that the infant gives evidence of being able to resolve.

watches the infant's eye and head movements during repeated presentations of each card. Based on the infant's looking behavior, the tester decides which cards contain gratings that can be resolved by the infant. Cards for which the infant shows consistent looking behavior toward one side and a switch in direction of looking when the left-right position of the grating is switched are judged to contain gratings the infant can resolve. Cards that do not elicit consistent looking behavior are judged to contain gratings that cannot be resolved by the infant. Acuity is estimated as the spatial frequency of the finest grating the tester judges the infant can resolve.

Two aspects of the acuity card procedure enhance its suitability for use in clinical settings. First, test duration is short. Average test duration for a monocular or a binocular acuity card test is 3–5 minutes for normal infants and young children 4 weeks to 36 months of age (McDonald et al. 1985, 1986a,b) and approximately 8 minutes for infants with eye disorders (Preston et al., 1987). Second, the equipment and procedure are easy to use. The equipment is portable and has no moving or electrical parts to break down. The procedure requires training and practice, but no technical expertise or scientific knowledge is needed for an individual to become an accomplished tester.

RESEARCH BASE

The acuity card procedure is based on 30 years of laboratory investigations. The goals of the laboratory investigations were, first, to create methodologies for assessing vision in infants and, second, to define parameters that affect the results obtained with those methodologies.

Methodological Research Base

The acuity card procedure grew out of laboratory-based preferential looking (PL) techniques for the assessment of visual function in infants. The PL techniques were based on independent observations by Berlyne (1958) and Fantz (1958) that an infant's looking behavior in the presence of two stimuli can be used to indicate whether the infant can discriminate between the two stimuli. Berlyne and Fantz proposed that if an infant looks more toward one stimulus than toward the other, regardless of where the stimuli are located with respect to one another, the infant must be able to tell that the stimuli are different.

The PL testing of visual acuity began in 1962, when Fantz and his colleagues showed infants black and white gratings of various spatial frequencies paired with a homogeneous gray field of equal space-average luminance. Fantz et al. (1962) noted which spatial frequencies produced more looking behavior toward the grating than toward the homogeneous field in infants at several ages between birth and 6 months, and they used this information to describe acuity development in young infants.

One of the difficulties Fantz had to overcome when developing the PL procedure was infants' inability to cooperate for long periods. Fantz overcame this difficulty by showing each infant only 10 grating-versus-homogeneous-field pairings and then combining the data from infants of the same age to produce a mean acuity for each test age. This method was acceptable to Fantz, because, as a developmental psychologist, he was interested in the visual perceptual capabilities of various groups of infants, including normal infants at different ages, preterm infants, and infants with Down syndrome (reviewed in Fantz et al., 1975).

When Davida Teller entered the field of infant vision testing during the early 1970s, her background was in visual psychophysics, where the emphasis is on collecting large amounts of data on a small number of subjects, rather than a small amount of data from a large number of subjects. As a result, Teller modified Fantz's PL procedure to make it more like psychophysical procedures used with adults (Teller et al., 1974; Teller, 1979). Each infant was presented with many pairings of gratings and homogeneous fields, with the spatial frequency and the left-right position of the grating varying from pairing to pairing. Instead of timing the duration of the infant's looking toward the stimuli or the direction of the infant's first fixation, as did Fantz's testers, testers in Teller's procedure were required to make a forced-choice judgment as to whether each grating was located to the left or to the right of center, based on all aspects of the infant's looking behavior. This change in the tester's task resulted in data that were scorable in a manner similar to that used to score forced-choice psychophysical data from adults. The percentage of trials on which the tester correctly judged the location of the grating was plotted as a function of grating spatial frequency. This method yielded a psychometric function that ranged from nearly 100% correct (for low spatial frequency gratings that elicited clear looking behavior from the infant) to chance, or 50% correct (for higher spatial frequency gratings to which the infant showed no preferential fixation). As in adult psychophysics, acuity threshold was estimated as the spatial frequency that produced 75% correct, the score that is halfway between chance and 100%.

Teller's modification of the PL procedure into the *forced-choice* preferential looking (FPL) procedure was a major step toward the development of a clinical tool for infant acuity testing because: (1) it shifted the emphasis from group acuity data to acuity testing of individual infants; and (2) it launched an era of research into the parameters that influence acuity results in infants.

Parametric Research Base

An important precursor to incorporation of the acuity card procedure into clinical settings was the body of parametric research that was produced using the FPL technique during the 1970s and 1980s. These parametric studies produced data on the effect of stimulus luminance, target distance, grating orientation, and monocular versus binocular test conditions on acuity; moreover, the studies alerted investigators to the importance of correcting for gestational age when comparing a preterm infant's acuity with norms based on the data of term infants.

Stimulus Luminance. During the 1980s, the effect of stimulus luminance on grating acuity in 2-month-olds was assessed in two FPL studies (Dobson et al., 1983; Brown et al., 1987). These studies were conducted primarily to test hypotheses about the nature of the mechanisms underlying infant vision. They also gave rise, however, to information important to the development of clinical acuity test procedures for infants. The most important piece of information was that the visual acuity of the 2-month-old varies little, if any, with variations in luminance above about 10 candelas (cd)/m^2. This result is similar to that found for adults and suggests that for infants, as for adults, cross-clinic variations in luminance have little effect on acuity results so long as luminance is above 10 cd/m^2. The finding that infants' acuity becomes poorer as luminance is reduced below 10 cd/m^2, however, indicates that care must be taken to maintain target luminance above that value.

Target Distance. In adults, acuity is typically measured at 20 feet (6 meters). Most studies of acuity in infants, however, have used test distances closer than 1 meter, because it is easier to get infants to pay attention to near than to distant targets. Several pieces of evidence suggest that the precise target distance used has little if any effect on infants' acuity. First, there is good agreement among acuity results obtained across studies from infants of the same age, even though test distance has varied across studies (for review see Dobson and Teller, 1978). Second, Salapatek et al. (1976) found that acuity did not vary across test distances from 30 to 150 cm in 2-month-olds. Finally, Cornell and McDonell (1986) reported that acuity results obtained from 6- to 36-week-old infants tested at 6 meters were similar to those obtained in FPL studies using near test distances.

These studies, then, suggested that the precise distance at which infants' acuity is tested clinically is not crucial to the test results so long as test results are reported in a unit of measure (e.g., cycles/degree) that takes into account test distance. It is important to remember, however, that because tests of infants' acuity are typically conducted at a near distance, test results are not as sensitive to myopic (near-sighted) refractive errors as are the distance acuity tests used with adults.

Grating Orientation. In adults, acuity for vertical and horizontal gratings is typically slightly better than acuity for oblique gratings (Appelle, 1972). This finding is known as the oblique effect. Evidence for the oblique effect has also been found in infants and young children (Gwiazda et al., 1978, 1984; Birch et al., 1983), which indicates that it would be advisable to standardize grating orientation across clinical settings or at least limit grating orientation to vertical and horizontal.

Another factor that can affect an infant's acuity for gratings of different orientations is the refractive error of the infant. In adults and children, a history of uncorrected astigmatism is correlated with the presence of meridional amblyopia, in which acuity for orthogonal orientations (vertical versus horizontal or right-oblique versus left-oblique) is unequal, even when the astigmatism is optically corrected (Freeman et al., 1972; Mitchell et al., 1973). Infants do not appear to develop meridional amblyopia until they reach early childhood (Teller et al., 1978; Gwiazda et al., 1985a,b, 1986); however, uncorrected astigmatism can differentially affect acuity for gratings of different orientations (Teller et al., 1978; Gwiazda et al., 1985a,b). Thus an uncorrected, astigmatic infant can show either normal acuity or below-normal acuity, depending on the orientation of the grating used to assess acuity. This finding emphasizes the importance of correcting an infant's refractive error prior to acuity testing, as well as the importance of interpreting an infant's acuity results in the context of that infant's refractive error.

Monocular Versus Binocular Acuity. In adults, acuity tested binocularly is better than acuity tested monocularly by a factor of 0.1–0.2 octave. This difference is due to a combination of probability summation and neural summation that occurs under binocular test conditions (for review see Blake et al., 1981). Infants have been shown to have an acuity difference of approximately 0.5 octave between monocular and binocular acuity results (Atkinson et al., 1982; Birch, 1985; McDonald et al., 1986b; Birch and Hale, 1988). It is not known whether this larger monocular versus binocular difference shown by infants is due to sensory factors or to the distracting effect the patch used for monocular testing may have on the infant. The fact that a measurable difference in monocular versus binocular acuity results exists in infants indicates that both monocular and binocular norms

are needed for the correct interpretation of acuity results from infants with unilateral and bilateral visual system abnormalities.

Gestational Age. A preterm infant and a term infant of the same *postnatal* age have had similar amounts of visual experience, but because of their differing gestational ages the maturational status of the preterm infant is less than that of the term infant. Developmental psychologists have long been interested in comparing acuity development in preterm and term infants to define the relative influence of maturational versus environmental factors on visual development.

The results of FPL studies indicate that visual acuity development in preterm infants is more similar to that of term infants of the same age from conception than to that of term infants of the same postnatal age (Fantz et al., 1975; Dobson et al., 1980; van Hof-van Duin et al., 1983; Shepherd et al., 1985; van Hof-van Duin and Mohn, 1986; Birch and Spencer, 1991). This finding suggests that the time course of visual acuity development in infants with a normal visual environment is controlled more by maturational factors than by environmental factors. It also suggests that if one wishes to know whether a preterm infant's acuity is developing normally the comparison of acuity results with norms from term infants should be made on the basis of the preterm infant's corrected age (age from due date). Clinically, this point is of considerable importance because preterm infants are more likely than term infants to have eye disorders (Fledelius, 1976), and therefore preterm infants are often seen for clinical evaluation.

ACUITY CARD STUDIES

Validation Studies

Although the acuity card procedure grew out of a body of basic science research, the procedure is less rigorous and therefore more subject to observer bias than the procedures used in basic science studies of infant vision. For this reason, the developers of the acuity card procedure have conducted a number of studies to examine the procedure's validity. The validation studies have helped to define the strengths and limitations of the acuity card procedure and have helped to indicate the extent to which the large body of basic science FPL research is applicable to the modified version of FPL that is used with the acuity cards.

As indicated in the American Psychological Association's *Standards for Educational and Psychological Testing* (APA, 1974), there are several types of validity, the most important of which are construct validity, content validity, and the criterion-related validities (concurrent and predictive).

Construct Validity. Construct validity implies that a test is an accurate estimator of an underlying construct or set of theoretical constructs. In the case of the acuity cards, the underlying construct is assumed to be grating acuity, as measured with FPL techniques. Two types of evidence support the construct validity of the acuity card procedure.

First, the acuity card procedure yields results that are consistent with what are believed to be the underlying characteristics of grating acuity in infants. Acuity card studies, like FPL, show an increase in mean acuity with age in infants and young children (McDonald et al., 1985, 1986a,b; Kohl et al., 1986; Mohn and van Hof-van Duin, 1986; Chandna et al., 1988; Kohl and Samek 1988; Mohn et al., 1988; Vital-Durand and Hullo, 1989; Chandna and Doran, 1990; Heersema and van Hof-van Duin, 1990; Katz and Sireteanu, 1990). Also, acuity card results, like FPL results, show better acuities for infants and young children tested binocularly than for those tested monocularly (McDonald et al., 1986a,b; Vital-Durand and Hullo, 1989; Heersema and van Hof-van Duin, 1990). Finally, acuity card results show poorer-than-normal acuity in infants with visual disorders that are known to produce poor FPL acuity, e.g., aphakia or prolonged eyelid closure (Mayer et al., 1986; Preston et al., 1987; Sebris et al., 1987; Katz and Sireteanu, 1990).

A second piece of evidence in support of the construct validity of the acuity card procedure is that there is good agreement between results when the acuity card procedure and the FPL procedure are used to test the same group or similar groups of infants. A number of researchers (McDonald et al., 1985, 1986a,b; Brown and Yamamoto, 1986; Kohl et al., 1986; Mohn and van Hof-van Duin, 1986; Teller et al., 1986; Dobson et al., 1987; Kohl and Samek, 1988; Mohn et al., 1988) have shown that when *normal* infants and young children are tested group mean acuity scores obtained with the acuity cards agree closely with previously reported FPL group mean acuities for *normal* infants and young children of the same ages. The good agreement between acuity card and FPL results in normal infants and children is illustrated in Figure 20-2.

Not only is there good agreement between mean acuities for FPL and acuity card results, there is also good agreement between the standard deviations of the acuity estimates obtained. The standard deviation of acuity estimates for *normal* infants and young children range from 0.5 to 1.0 octave for both acuity card (McDonald et al., 1985, 1986a,b; Brown and Yamamoto, 1986; Kohl et al., 1986; Mohn and van Hof-van Duin, 1986; Teller et al., 1986; Dobson et al., 1987; Kohl and Samek, 1988) and FPL studies (Gwiazda et al., 1978; Allen, 1979; Atkinson et al., 1982; Mayer and Dobson, 1982).

Finally, when individual infants with *ocular or neurological abnormalities* are tested with *both* the acuity

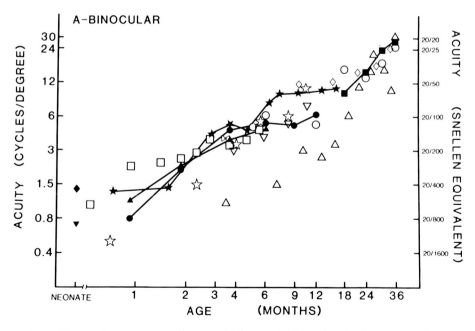

FIG. 20-2. Mean grating acuity scores for normal infants and children from birth to 3 years of age tested binocularly with preferential looking (open symbols) and acuity card (filled symbols) procedures. ▲ McDonald et al. (1985); ▼ Yamamoto and Brown (1985); ■ McDonald et al. (1986a); ● McDonald et al. (1986b); ★ Mohn and van Hof-van Duin (1986); ◆ Dobson et al. (1987); ▽ Gwiadza et al. (1978); □ Allen (1979); ☆ Gwiazda et al. (1980); ⋈ Atkinson et al. (1982); ○ Mayer and Dobson (1982); ◇ Birch et al. (1983); △ Yamamoto et al. (1984). (From Teller et al., 1986. By permission.)

card and FPL procedures, there is usually agreement to within 1.0 octave between the results of the two techniques. Mohn and van Hof-van Duin (1986) found agreement of 1.0 octave or better in 22 of 23 comparisons of binocular FPL versus acuity card acuities in visually impaired, neurologically impaired, and normal children 6–36 months of age. Preston et al. (1987), in a study of twenty 2- to 8-month-old infants with ocular disorders, found agreement of 1.0 octave or better in 98% of binocular tests and 91% of monocular tests.

Content Validity. Content validity implies that the results of the test being evaluated are representative of the type of behaviors in the performance domain being evaluated. In the context of the acuity card procedure, content validity implies that the type of visual responses the observer uses to obtain an acuity estimate are similar to the response the infant shows in the FPL procedure. The good agreement between FPL and acuity card results, shown for normal infants (summarized in Dobson et al., 1985; Teller et al., 1986) and infants with ocular or neurological abnormalities (Mohn and van Hof-van Duin, 1986; Preston et al., 1987; Mohn et al., 1988), suggests that either the same type of behavioral response(s) that correlate highly with one another are present in the acuity card and FPL procedures.

Criterion-Related Validity. Criterion-related validity implies that an individual's score on the test in question is systematically related to the individual's standing on some other variable called a criterion. Criterion-related validity can be broken down into concurrent validity and predictive validity.

Concurrent Validity. Concurrent validity refers to the extent to which the measure in question estimates an individual's present standing on the criterion. In the case of the acuity cards, concurrent validity implies that the cards provide a true estimate of the infant's grating acuity. It would be reflected by: (1) high *intra*observer test-retest reliability; (2) high *inter*observer test-retest reliability; and (3) good agreement with the results of other measures of the same underlying characteristic (grating acuity) of the individual.

1. *Intraobserver reliability.* In the study in which development of the acuity card procedure was first reported, McDonald et al. (1985) examined the intraobserver test-retest reliability of the procedure for binocular assessment of normal infants 1–6 months of age. The results showed agreement of 1.0 octave or better in 56 of 64 (88%) test-retest comparisons. Mean intraobserver test-retest difference was 0.7 octave. Mean FPL test-retest differences reported by Birch (1985) for infants less than 1 year of age ranged from 0.4 to 0.6 octave, and mean FPL test-retest differences for infants and children 1 month to 5 years of age ranged from 0.2 to 0.4 octave (Birch and Hale, 1988).

The only other studies of intraobserver reliability with the acuity cards are a study by Marx et al. (1990), who reported intraobserver agreement of 0.5 octave or better in 100% of 11 noncommunicating elderly patients, and a series of studies by Hertz and colleagues on mentally and physically handicapped older children and adults. In her initial study, Hertz (1987) examined intraobserver test-retest agreement across days in a sample of mentally retarded patients and found agreement of 1.0 octave or better in 20 of 25 binocular (80%) and 14 of 22 monocular (64%) test-retest comparisons. In a subsequent study of retarded individuals in special schools, Hertz (1988) found day-to-day intraobserver agreement of 1.0 octave or better in 35 of 42 (83%) of binocular tests. For mildly handicapped children with cerebral palsy, intraobserver agreement of 1.0 octave or better was found in 83% of test-retest comparisons but in only 65% of test-retest comparisons of severely retarded individuals (Hertz and Rosenberg, 1988). The day-to-day intraobserver agreement reported in the various studies by Hertz and colleagues was poorer than the within-day *inter*observer agreement found for the same populations. Hertz suggested that the day-to-day variability in intraobserver agreement may reflect variations in attention and cooperation, as well as possible variations in sensory processing capabilities, in severely mentally handicapped individuals.

2. *Interobserver reliability.* Another test characteristic implied by concurrent validity is high interobserver test-retest reliability. As shown in Table 20-1, many studies have examined the interobserver reliability of the acuity card procedure, and all have reported it to be similar to the interobserver reliability reported for the FPL procedure. In the earliest acuity card study, McDonald et al. (1985) reported that 59 of 64 interobserver comparisons of binocular acuity (92%) in 1- to 6-month-olds differed by 1.0 octave or less. In their next study, McDonald et al. (1986b) found that 97% of interobserver comparisons of binocular acuity and 86% of interobserver comparisons of monocular acuity in 1- to 12-month-olds differed by 1.0 octave or less. As shown in Table 20-1, these results are similar to the interobserver agreement reported by Atkinson et al. (1982) for 12 normal 4-month-olds and by Maurer et al. (1989a) for 57 normal 6- to 12-month-olds tested with FPL procedures.

In tests of young children 18–36 months of age, McDonald et al. (1986a) found that 92% of interobserver comparisons of binocular acuity and 88% of comparisons of monocular acuity differed by 0.5 octave or less. Heersema and van Hof-van Duin (1990) reported that 82% of binocular test-retest comparisons in normal 1- to 4-year-olds differed by 0.33 octave or less and 92% differed by 1.00 octave or less. These results are similar to the FPL results of Maurer et al.

TABLE 20-1. *Interobserver agreement in acuity card and FPL studies.*

Study	Condition	Age	No.[a]	≤ 1.0 Octave (%)
Acuity card studies				
McDonald et al. (1985), normals	Binocular	1 month	15	87
Dobson et al. (1990a), NICU-treated	Binocular	7–31 days	54	85
McDonald et al. (1986b), normals	Binocular	1–12 months	36	97
Preston et al. (1987), visual abn.	Binocular	2–8 months	20	100
McDonald et al. (1986a), normals	Binocular	18–36 months	36	92[b]
Heersema & van Hof-van Duin (1990), normals	Binocular	1–4 years	50	82[c]
Hertz & Rosenberg (1988), cerebral palsy	Binocular	2–7 years	59	83
Hertz (1988), mentally retarded	Binocular	8–17 years	44	89
Hertz et al. (1988), mentally retarded, cortically visually impaired	Binocular	2–12 years	8	75
Marx et al. (1990), noncommunicative, elderly	Binocular	74–96 years	15	100[b]
McDonald et al. (1986b), normals	Monocular	1–12 months	66	86
Dobson et al. (1990a), NICU-treated	Monocular	4–12 months	382	80
Preston et al. (1987), visual abn.	Monocular	2–8 months	40	95
Dobson & Carpenter (1991), NICU-treated	Monocular	4–24 months	1013	85
McDonald et al. (1986a), normals	Monocular	18–36 months	36	88[b]
FPL studies				
Atkinson et al. (1982), normals	Monocular	4 months	12	100
Maurer et al. (1989a), normals	Monocular	6–12 months	57	93
Maurer et al. (1989a), normals	Monocular	18–36 months	135	86[b]
Maurer et al. (1989a), aphakes	Monocular	6–36 months	101	79

Adapted from Dobson et al. (1990a).
[a]Number of interobserver test-retest pairs.
[b]Percent ≤ 0.5 octave.
[c]Percent ≤ 0.3 octave.

(1989a), who reported differences of 0.5 octave or less in 86% of test-retest comparisons conducted with 18- to 36-month-olds.

Interobserver agreement has also been examined for acuity card testing of clinical populations. Preston et al. (1987) found interobserver agreement of 1.0 octave or better in 100% of binocular and 95% of monocular test-retest comparisons of a group of young infants with ocular abnormalities. Dobson and colleagues (Dobson et al., 1990a; Dobson and Carpenter, 1991) tested infants and young children who had been treated in a neonatal intensive care unit for preterm birth or perinatal complications. The results showed agreement of 1.0 octave or better in 80% of 382 monocular test-retest comparisons of 4- to 12-month-olds tested with an early version of the acuity cards (Dobson et al., 1990a) and in 85% of 1013 monocular test-retest comparisons of 4- to 24-month-olds tested with Teller Acu-

ity Cards (Dobson and Carpenter, 1991). Marx et al. (1990) found interobserver agreement of 0.5 octave or better in 100% of noncommunicative elderly patients. The final clinical sample in which interobserver agreement was examined was a group of older children suffering from mental retardation or cerebral palsy, who were tested in a series of studies by Hertz and colleagues (Hertz, 1988; Hertz and Rosenberg, 1988; Hertz et al., 1988). Interobserver reliability data indicated interobserver agreement of 1.0 octave or better in only 75–89% of test-retest comparisons, suggesting that it would be advisable to conduct repeated testing to verify acuity results in older, institutionalized patients with mental retardation or cerebral palsy.

The only FPL study of test-retest reliability of clinical patients against which these clinical studies of acuity card reliability can be compared is one by Maurer et al. (1989a). These researchers reported interobserver test-retest agreement of 1.0 octave or better in 79% of monocular tests of 6- to 36-month-old children with aphakia.

The good agreement between interobserver test-retest results obtained with the acuity card and FPL procedures indicates that the criterion validity of the acuity card procedure is equivalent to the criterion validity of the FPL procedure as a measure of grating acuity in infants and young children. However, the finding that test-retest reliability is less than 100% for either the FPL or the acuity card procedure indicates that there are times when an acuity estimate obtained with either procedure is not an accurate estimate of grating acuity. Dobson et al. (1990a) found that, in some instances, tests yielding inaccurate estimates of acuity have long test times or low tester confidence in the acuity estimate. However, Dobson et al. (1990a) also reported that there were many instances in which an inaccurate estimate of acuity (evidenced by a large interobserver test-retest difference) was obtained with short test times and high tester confidence ratings. These results indicate that behavioral measures of grating acuity in infants: (1) should be interpreted in the context of the entire clinical picture of the infant; and (2) should be repeated for confirmation of the accuracy of the acuity results.

3. *Good agreement among acuity measures.* In addition to implying good intra- and interobserver reliability, concurrent validity also implies good agreement among various measures of the underlying function. As described in the section on content validity (above), acuity results obtained using the acuity card procedure show good agreement with the acuity results obtained using the FPL procedure for both normal infants and infants with ocular or neurological abnormalities.

Predictive Validity. The second type of criterion-related validity is predictive validity. Predictive validity implies that a measurement taken in the present is predictive of an individual's status on the same measure in the future. Only one study has examined the predictive validity of the acuity card procedure (Dobson et al., 1989). This study looked at acuity development between birth and 1 year in 174 infants who were treated in a neonatal intensive care unit for preterm birth or perinatal complications. The results indicated that more than 90% of infants who had monocular acuity in the normal range during early infancy continued to show normal monocular acuity at age 1 year. However, only about 35% of infants who showed below-normal acuity during early infancy continued to show below-normal acuity at age 1 year, and only 21% of infants who showed below-normal acuity at age 1 year had shown below-normal acuity during early infancy. Unfortunately, this study of the predictive validity of the acuity cards had several significant limitations: (1) the period between the initial and the final acuity measures was brief (<1

year); (2) the number of infants with below-normal acuity results was much smaller than the number with acuity results in the normal range; and (3) only limited information was available to indicate whether infants experienced ocular changes between the initial and final tests that would have been expected to affect acuity results. A better study of predictive validity would follow infants for a longer period, would include a substantial proportion of infants with below-normal acuities, and would screen out infants who, during the time between the initial and final acuity tests, developed ocular or neurological conditions known to produce abnormal visual acuity.

An FPL study that meets these three criteria was reported by Maurer et al. (1989b). These researchers compared grating acuity at 12, 18, 24, 30, and 36 months with Snellen acuity after age 5 years in children treated for unilateral or bilateral cataracts, who would be expected to show a wide range of acuities depending on the success of treatment. Children underwent frequent eye examinations, so the data of those who developed glaucoma or a detached retina between test sessions could be eliminated from the study. The results indicated that FPL acuity at 12, 30, and 36 months was predictive of later Snellen acuity, but that FPL acuity at 18 and 24 months, when children are especially difficult to test, was not predictive of later Snellen acuity.

The similarity between acuity card and FPL acuity results obtained in cross-sectional studies of different populations of infants suggests that the predictive validity of the acuity card procedure is similar to that of the FPL procedure. Further studies of the predictive validity of both the acuity card and the FPL procedures are needed.

Reports of Testability Rates

To be useful clinically, a procedure must allow successful assessment of a high percentage of the population on whom it will be used. Initial acuity card studies showed success rates of 90–100% for both monocular and binocular testing of all but one age group of *normal* infants and children between 4 weeks and 36 months of age tested in the laboratory. The exception occurred with 24-month-old children, who showed a success rate of only 75% for monocular testing (McDonald et al., 1986a,b). The success rate for a group of twenty 2- to 8-month-old infants *with eye problems* tested in the laboratory was 100% for both monocular and binocular testing (Preston et al., 1987).

Success rates in the first study in which acuity cards were used in clinical settings showed an overall success rate of 94% for 842 binocular tests and 83% for 1068 monocular tests (Sebris et al., 1987). Success rates varied with age, with binocular success rates ranging from

86% for 22 preterm infants tested prior to their due date to 93–97% at all other test ages. Monocular success rates ranged from 64% for 1- to 3-month-olds and 66% for 18- to 24-month-olds to 90% for 3- to 6-month-olds and 96% for 4- to 5-year-olds. Little variation in success rate was found when patients were categorized by the presence versus the absence of ocular disorder, presence versus absence of preterm birth, and presence versus absence of developmental delay.

More recently, Mohn et al. (1988) reported success rates ranging from 81% in severely retarded children 14 months to 24 years of age to more than 95% in normal and neurologically at-risk infants. Hertz (1987) reported success rates of 97% (32/33) and 85% (28/33) for binocular and monocular testing, respectively, of children with Down syndrome and 95% (18/19) for binocular testing of severely retarded patients. Hertz et al. (1988) were able to obtain an acuity estimate in 9 of 11 multiply handicapped patients with cortical visual impairment. One of the untestable patients refused to cooperate during testing, and the other had such poor acuity that he did not fixate even the lowest spatial frequency grating. Marx et al. (1990) reported that an acuity estimate was obtained in 13 of 15 (87%) non-communicative elderly adults. Finally, results from 814 twelve-month-old preterm infants tested in the Multicenter Study of Cryotherapy for Retinopathy of Prematurity indicated that monocular acuity estimates were obtained from each eye of 95% of the infants, and at least one monocular or one binocular acuity test was completed by all infants, even though many of the infants had significant visual or neurological abnormalities (Dobson et al., 1990b).

These results indicate that success rates with the acuity card procedure are high enough to be useful clinically, even when patients are difficult to test, multiply handicapped individuals.

Studies of the Effects of Stimulus and Procedural Variations

Stimulus Configuration. In the initial acuity card studies (e.g., McDonald et al., 1985, 1986a,b; Brown and Yamamoto, 1986; Dobson et al., 1986, 1987; Kohl et al., 1986; Mohn and van Hof-van Duin, 1986; Hertz, 1987; Sebris et al., 1987), the stimulus configuration of the acuity cards was similar to that used in most FPL acuity studies: A test grating stimulus was located to one side of a small central aperture, and a "blank" stimulus consisting of a high spatial frequency grating was located on the other side. Both the test grating and the "blank" stimulus were located behind circular 9 cm diameter openings in the acuity cards. Care was taken to match the space-average luminance and the perceived hue of the two stimuli to ensure that any preferential

looking shown by the infant toward the test grating was due to discrimination of the grating and not to a brightness or hue mismatch between the two stimulus positions.

Commercial production of the acuity cards resulted in a change in the stimulus configuration. The test grating was printed on the card, flush with the background, and there was no "blank" stimulus on the side of the card opposite the test grating. Instead, the test grating was matched as closely as possible in hue and space-average luminance to the gray background of the entire card. This configuration had the advantage that the edges of the stimulus apertures, which some people thought were distracting to infants, were eliminated. However, the configuration had the disadvantage that any imperfections in the match between the test grating and the background were not controlled for by having a "blank" stimulus on the opposite side of the card.

Adults who viewed the commercially produced acuity cards (Teller Acuity Cards, Vistech, Inc., Dayton, Ohio) could perceive slight mismatches in brightness between the grating and background, as well as "edge artifacts" between the edge of the grating and the background. These brightness and edge artifacts made it possible for adults to identify the location of gratings that were too fine to be resolved. Two groups of researchers (Robinson et al., 1988; Hainline et al., 1989) found that the brightness and edge artifacts in the Teller cards could lead to overestimation of acuity in adults. These researchers suggested that such artifacts might also lead to overestimation of acuity in infants. Robinson et al. (1988) and Hainline et al. (1989) found that when a border was placed around the test grating and around a corresponding area on the side of the card opposite the grating, overestimation of acuity in *adults* was reduced. As a result, these researchers proposed the development of modified acuity cards containing two stimulus positions delineated by borders.

In a reply to Robinson et al. (1988), Teller (1990) pointed out that the finding that Teller Acuity Cards overestimate grating acuity in *adults* does not necessarily imply that they overestimate acuity in *infants*. Infants are less sensitive to contrast than are adults (Atkinson et al., 1977; Teller, 1979), and their acuity is poorer than that of adults (for review see Dobson and Teller, 1978). Therefore the brightness and edge artifacts in the Teller Acuity Cards would be expected to have little if any effect on an infant's response to the acuity cards.

Empirical evidence in support of Teller's observation was reported by Dobson and Luna (1990, 1991). Dobson and Luna compared monocular acuity results obtained from 4-, 12-, and 36-month-old children tested with the two-aperture prototype acuity cards to monocular acuity results obtained from the same subjects tested with Teller Acuity Cards. The results showed no differences between acuity scores obtained with the two stimulus configurations at any of the three test ages, indicating that the brightness and edge artifacts that adults can detect in the acuity cards have no measurable effect on acuity results in infants and children up to 3 years of age.

Stimulus Orientation. The gratings on the acuity cards are oriented vertically, as has been the case in almost all studies of infants' acuity conducted over the past 30 years. Use of vertical gratings with the acuity cards is supported by results of FPL studies of stimulus orientation, which have shown that, for most infants, vertical gratings produce an acuity estimate that is equal to or better than acuity estimates for all other grating orientations (Teller et al., 1974; Gwiazda et al., 1978, 1980; Birch et al., 1983).

Although vertical gratings are adequate for most clinical testing, there are at least two clinical conditions where vertical gratings may underestimate acuity. The first is astigmatism, in which the grating orientation that produces the best acuity is dependent on the optical properties of the cornea and lens. Astigmatism occurs frequently in infants (Howland et al., 1978; Mohindra et al., 1978; Ingram and Barr, 1979; Fulton et al., 1980). Therefore to obtain an estimate of the infant's best acuity, acuity card testing should be conducted *after* the infant's refractive error has been measured and corrected.

The second clinical condition in which vertical gratings may underestimate acuity is in the case of patients who have horizontal nystagmus. Raye et al. (1991) compared acuity card results for vertical versus horizontal gratings in eight infants and young children with horizontal nystagmus. In all cases, better acuity was obtained with horizontal than with vertical gratings. For the three patients with fine nystagmus, the orientation of the acuity card itself (vertical versus horizontal) did not affect acuity results for horizontal gratings. The five patients with coarse nystagmus, however, showed better acuity for horizontal gratings when the cards were held vertically than when they were held in the standard horizontal position, probably because it was easier for the tester to judge the infant's fixation preference when stimulus position varied along the vertical dimension than when it varied along the horizontal dimension. Thus patients with nystagmus should be tested with horizontally oriented gratings, and the easiest and most appropriate way to do it is to hold the standard acuity cards vertically during testing.

Testing Procedure. The task of the tester using the acuity cards is to determine the finest grating the infant or child can resolve. The procedure by which the tester accomplishes this task, however, has varied from study to study. In the initial acuity card studies of normal infants, testers were kept masked to the absolute spatial frequencies of the gratings used during testing but were aware of the relative order of spatial frequencies (from lower to higher) and the left-right location of the grating on each card (McDonald et al., 1985, 1986a,b). In the initial *clinical* studies, cards continued to be presented in order from lower to higher spatial frequencies, but the tester was aware of both the absolute spatial frequency and the location of the grating on each card (Preston et al., 1987; Sebris et al., 1987). More recently, acuity card procedures used with clinical populations have included (1) presentation of the cards in random order with respect to spatial frequency (Reed et al., 1989); (2) presentation of the cards in order from lower to higher spatial frequencies with the tester masked to both absolute spatial frequency and location of the grating (Scher et al., 1989; Luna et al., 1990; Dobson et al., 1990a); (3) a staircase procedure similar to that used for FPL testing in which the tester, who is unaware of grating spatial frequency and location, makes a left-right judgment concerning grating location after a single presentation of the card (Hertz, 1987; Chandna et al., 1988); and (4) the clinical procedure recommended in the *Teller Acuity Card Manual* (1990) in which the tester is aware of the absolute spatial frequency but masked to the location of the grating on each card.

Despite the many variants of the acuity card procedure, there have been only two studies that have compared acuity outcomes with more than one procedure. In one study, Hartmann et al. (1989) compared acuity results from testers masked to grating location with those from testers unmasked to grating location for a group of sixteen 8- to 12-month-old infants. Testers presented the cards in order from lower to higher spatial frequencies, and all were aware of the absolute spatial frequencies of the gratings. The results showed no difference between acuity results of testers who were masked versus results of testers who were unmasked to grating location.

In the second study of the effects of procedural variations, Reed et al. (1989) tested 15- to 33-month-old children suspected of being amblyopic. Children were tested with the FPL procedure and with three variants of the acuity card procedure: (1) random ordering of acuity cards with the tester informed as to grating location; (2) ordered presentation of acuity cards with the tester informed of both grating spatial frequency and location; and (3) ordered presentation of acuity cards with the tester informed of neither grating spatial frequency nor location. The results showed poor agreement between FPL results and the results of the random ordering procedure, but there was a significant correlation between the results of each of the other two procedures and the results of FPL testing. The procedure that produced results most similar to the FPL results was the third procedure (ordered presentation of cards with the tester uninformed about grating frequency and location). Acuity results obtained with the third procedure were within 1.0 octave of FPL results in more than 75% of comparisons and within 0.5 octave of FPL results in 54% of comparisons. These percentages are similar to those found by the same researchers for FPL test-retest comparisons of aphakic children (Maurer et al., 1989a), indicating that the between-procedure variability was no greater than the within-procedure variability of FPL acuity results.

The finding of Reed et al. (1989) that procedural variations in the use of the acuity cards can affect acuity results suggests that further empirical work is needed in this area. Especially interesting would be a comparison of the acuity results of the clinical testing procedure recommended in the *Teller Acuity Card Manual* (1990) with the acuity results of either the FPL procedure or the third procedure (ordered cards, tester uninformed of spatial frequency and grating location) of Reed et al. (1989).

Special Populations

A number of studies have investigated the applicability of the acuity card procedure in special populations of patients. The populations studied most frequently are amblyopes, infants born prior to term, and nonverbal adults.

Amblyopes. Infants who have strabismus, anisometropia, unilateral cataracts, or any of a variety of other problems that affect the two eyes unequally are at risk for the development of amblyopia, a neurally based difference in acuity between the two eyes. Clinicians are therefore interested in techniques, such as the acuity card procedure, that allow them to test for acuity differences between infants' eyes and to monitor changes in acuity that occur during treatment.

Several studies have reported results from strabismic infants and young children tested with the acuity card procedure (Hertz, 1987; Moskowitz et al., 1987; Ellis, et al., 1988; Moseley et al., 1988; Tomlinson and Martinez, 1988; Chandna and Doran, 1990, 1991; Hartmann et al., 1990; Katz and Sireteanu, 1990). The results of these studies indicate that monocular acuity can be measured in strabismic amblyopes with the acuity card procedure and that an estimate of the patient's interocular acuity difference can be obtained. However, several of the studies indicated that the acuity card procedure, like all measures of *grating* acuity (Levi and Klein, 1982a,b), underestimates the magnitude of the difference in *letter* acuity between eyes in strabismic amblyopes (Hertz, 1987; Moskowitz et al., 1987; Katz and Sireteanu, 1990). Thus clinicians must be aware that acuity card results from strabismic infants may fail to reveal amblyopia that would be present if these in-

fants could be tested with a letter or other form of recognition acuity task.

Adult patients with anisometropia and other forms of nonstrabismic amblyopia tested with gratings typically show interocular acuity differences similar to those found with measures of recognition acuity (Levi and Klein, 1982a,b). Results for nonstrabismic amblyopes tested with Teller Acuity Cards are mixed. Katz and Sireteanu (1990) found good agreement between acuity estimates obtained with Teller Acuity Cards and those obtained with the Landolt C recognition acuity test in children with anisometropic amblyopia or other structural eye disorders. On the other hand, Friendly et al. (1990) reported that Teller Acuity Cards underestimated interocular acuity differences in comparison with the results of letter acuity charts in children with anisometropic amblyopia without strabismus. Thus more research is needed to determine the usefulness of the acuity cards in the evaluation of the nonstrabismic amblyope.

Preterm Infants. Infants born prior to term are at higher risk than term infants for abnormal visual development (Fledelius, 1976). As a result, clinicians have become interested in acuity card screening of preterm infants.

Before acuity card screening could be conducted, it was necessary to establish norms against which acuity results from individual preterm infants could be compared. The question was: Could norms based on data from term infants (Sebris et al., 1987; *Teller Acuity Card Manual*, 1990) be used for preterm infants, or do healthy preterm infants have a course of acuity development different from that of term infants? Mohn and van Hof-van Duin (1986) compared the acuity card results from a group of healthy preterm infants with those of term infants between birth and 12 months of age. The results indicated that, when acuity results were compared for infants of the same *corrected age* (age from due date), the acuity development of preterm and term infants was similar. These results are in agreement with previously reported FPL comparisons of acuity development in healthy preterm and term infants (Fantz et al., 1975; Dobson et al., 1980; van Hof-van Duin et al., 1983; van Hof-van Duin and Mohn, 1986) and indicate that acuity card norms obtained from term infants are an appropriate standard against which to compare the data of a preterm infant so long as the preterm infant's corrected age is used for the comparison. Getz et al. (1992) extended the age range over which healthy preterm infants were tested to 36 months and showed that normative data from term infants are an appropriate standard against which to compare the results of preterm infants across the entire age range from birth to 30 months of age. At 36 months, however, the healthy preterm children showed acuity values at the low end of the normal range found for term children of the same age. These results are in agreement with

FPL acuity results reported previously by Sebris et al. (1984) in 3- to 4-year-old preterm children and suggest caution when comparing acuity results from 3-year-old preterm children with those of term children of the same age.

The acuity card procedure has also been used to measure acuity in preterm infants who suffered perinatal complications including birth weight less than 1500 g (van Hof-van Duin et al., 1989; Hermans and van Hof-van Duin, 1991), hypoxia (Mohn and van Hof-van Duin, 1986; Mohn et al., 1988; Groenendaal et al., 1989), retinopathy of prematurity (Cryotherapy for Retinopathy of Prematurity Cooperative Group, 1990; Dobson et al., 1990b; Luna et al., 1990), and periventricular leukomalacia (Scher et al., 1989). The results indicated that the preterm infants at highest risk for below-normal acuity were those who had significant neurological abnormalities or structural neural changes.

Nonverbal Adults. Hertz and colleagues have conducted several studies of older children and adults with cerebral palsy or mental retardation (Hertz, 1987, 1988; Hertz and Rosenberg, 1988; Hertz et al., 1988). The results indicate that the acuity cards can be used with these patients satisfactorily, especially if the cards are presented in the absence of the screen, which seems to distract this population. Hertz was able to test some members of her sample with a recognition (picture) acuity task and reported good agreement between acuity card and picture acuity results, except in strabismic patients, for whom the acuity cards underestimated the acuity loss found with the picture acuity task.

Marx et al. (1990) reported the use of the acuity card procedure with a sample of elderly nonverbal patients. Success rates were high (13 of 15 patients could be tested) and interobserver test-retest agreement was 0.5 octave or better in all cases. These results indicate that the acuity card procedure can provide a reliable measure of acuity in the elderly, nonverbal population.

LIMITATIONS OF THE ACUITY CARD PROCEDURE

This chapter has concentrated on the strengths of the acuity card procedure as a tool for clinical assessment of grating acuity. It is also important, however, to define the limitations of the technique. These limitations can be categorized under four headings: accuracy of acuity measurements, potential for observer bias, insensitivity to myopic refractive errors, and lack of durability of the cards.

Accuracy of Measurement

When Snellen (letter) acuity is tested in adults, measurement is considered accurate to within a line of letters on the chart. Because each line on a logMAR acuity chart represents 0.3 octave, clinicians are accustomed to behavioral acuity estimates being accurate to within 0.3 octave. With infants, acuity estimates are much less precise, regardless of whether the measurements are made in the laboratory or in the clinic and regardless of whether the FPL or the acuity card procedure is used.

In the first acuity card study, McDonald et al. (1985) examined *intraobserver* test-retest agreement for tests of binocular acuity of 1- to 6-month-old infants. The cards used contained gratings spaced in 1.0-octave steps. The results indicated that only 28 (44%) of 64 *intraobserver* test-retest comparisons agreed to within 0.3 octave. Furthermore, only 56 (88%) of 64 comparisons agreed to 1.0 octave or better. The average test-retest difference was 0.7 octave.

The variability of acuity card results is also apparent in the studies of *interobserver* test-retest reliability shown in Table 20-1, most of which reported interobserver agreement of 1.0 octave or better in only 80–90% of test-retest pairs. The two exceptions are a study by Preston et al. (1987), in which the tester's knowledge of the location and spatial frequencies of the gratings may have improved reliability, and a study by Heersema and van Hof-van Duin (1990), in which gratings on the acuity cards were spaced in 0.3-octave steps, instead of the 0.5- to 1.0-octave steps used in all other studies.

The improved test-retest agreement found by Heersema and van Hof-van Duin (1990) with gratings spaced in 0.3-octave steps suggests that the accuracy of acuity estimation of infants in clinical settings might be improved by reducing the step size between adjacent cards in the set of commercially available Teller Acuity Cards. Before increasing the number (and expense) of the Teller Acuity Cards, however, it would be wise to determine whether the increased accuracy afforded by a smaller step size between cards would be offset by the disadvantage of the added test time required to show the infant the additional cards.

In summary, the accuracy of the acuity card procedure is less than that for older children and adults tested with a Snellen letter chart. Because of the variability of acuity card results, repeat acuity card testing must be conducted to verify interocular acuity differences of less than about 1.5 octaves and to validate acuity scores that fall less than 1.5 octaves below the normal range. Also, repeat acuity card testing must be conducted to determine whether acuity card results that do not fit with other clinical information on the patient's ocular status are an accurate or an inaccurate estimate of the patient's grating acuity.

Potential for Bias

Many procedures used in clinical settings can be influenced, or biased, by the person performing the examination. For example, retinoscopic measurement of refractive error can be influenced by the retinoscopist's knowledge of the patient's previous refractive error, and measurement of visual fields by confrontation can be influenced by the examiner's knowledge of the patient's neurological status. The recent development of automated refractometers for measuring refractive errors and automated perimeters for measuring visual fields has helped to eliminate problems of examiner bias from the clinical evaluation of vision in adults.

It is difficult to assess infants with automated equipment, and so the clinician working with infants must be alert to the possibility of examiner bias in all procedures, including the acuity card procedure. To minimize tester bias in the acuity card procedure, the tester must be kept as unaware as possible of the patient's medical history. In addition, bias can be reduced by masking the tester to the spatial frequencies of the gratings on the acuity cards and by having the patient tested by two independent testers.

An excellent method of avoiding tester bias is to use the "scrambled cards" procedure (Reed et al., 1989), in which the acuity cards are presented with spatial frequencies ordered randomly. The tester, who is masked to the spatial frequency of the grating on each card, must show all cards to the infant and must sort the cards into two stacks ("seen" and "not seen") based on the infant's response to each card. This method prevents bias by keeping the tester masked to both absolute and relative spatial frequency of the grating on each card. This method is time-consuming, however, because all cards must be presented to the infant, in contrast to the standard acuity card technique in which cards containing gratings well above threshold are not presented. Therefore the "scrambled cards" procedure is probably more useful as a training technique than for everyday assessment of grating acuity.

Insensitivity to Myopic Refractive Errors

The recommended test distances for Teller Acuity Card testing are 38 cm for infants between birth and 6 months of age, 55 cm for children between 7 months and 3 years, and 84 cm for children older than 3 years (*Teller Acuity Card Manual*, 1990). Because the acuity card procedure is conducted at these relatively near distances, it is less sensitive to myopic refractive errors than are the 10- and 20-feet picture and letter acuity tests used with older children. The insensitivity of the acuity card procedure to myopic refractive errors suggests that if the procedure is used as a screening instrument in infants and young children (e.g., Wyngaarden et al., 1990), it should be accompanied by screening of refractive errors in these patients.

Lack of Durability of the Acuity Cards

A critical aspect of the design of the acuity cards is that the face of the card should appear uniformly gray when the grating cannot be resolved. Blemishes on a card can produce consistent looking behavior by the patient, which could be interpreted by the observer to indicate that the child could resolve the grating. Unfortunately, the surface of the cards is such that the cards can be marred by dirt, fingerprints, or rough surfaces, which means that each acuity card must be examined frequently and marred cards replaced.

NONSCIENTIFIC CONSIDERATIONS RELATED TO TRANSITION FROM LABORATORY TO CLINIC

The preceding pages have described the history and current status of the acuity card procedure as a clinical assessment tool. In addition to the body of research described, a variety of nonscientific activities were required to bring the acuity card procedure from its development in the laboratory to its incorporation into clinical settings. The purpose of this section is to describe some of these nonscientific activities, many of which involve skills not usually required of basic scientists.

Construction and Marketing of the Equipment

An important nonscientific aspect of bringing a technique into the clinic is to find a company to manufacture the equipment. During the development of the acuity card procedure, the cards were constructed by cutting gray cardboard to the appropriate size and mounting photographically produced gratings behind hand-cut apertures in the cards. This method of constructing cards was time-consuming and resulted in cards with a homemade appearance that was inappropriate for general clinical use. Therefore through the Washington Research Foundation, an agency that serves as an interface between the University of Washington and commercial businesses, production of the acuity cards was licensed to Vistech, Inc. (Dayton, Ohio), a company skilled in the production of high-quality printed gratings and in the marketing of equipment for the assessment of vision in clinical settings. This disposition solved the problem of producing acuity card equipment for clinical use. It did not, however, relieve the developers of the technique of the need to continue nonscientific activities.

Other Nonscientific Activities

Other nonscientific activities involved ensuring that the information disseminated about the acuity card procedure was accurate and then monitoring the quality of the cards that were produced. Ensuring accuracy of information about the acuity card procedure meant that the developers had to write, and then periodically update, a detailed manual of procedures (*Teller Acuity Card Manual*, 1990). It also meant that there must be monitoring of the advertisements produced by the manufacturer. Ensuring the quality of the acuity cards themselves meant talking with new purchasers of the cards to check that quality control was maintained and to determine that the manufacturer had not made "minor" changes to the cards that might compromise their effectiveness as a clinical tool. Other nonscientific activities included answering phone calls and letters about the procedure and conducting hands-on training sessions to instruct new users in the use of the procedure.

SUMMARY AND SPECULATION ABOUT TRANSITION OF ACUITY CARDS FROM LABORATORY TO CLINIC

Most researchers would like to believe that their efforts benefit society in some way. Often the benefit is largely hypothetical or occurs at some time in the future, which means that the researcher concentrates primarily on the laboratory-based, scientific aspects of the research. Sometimes, however, the researcher develops a procedure or tool that has immediate applicability to some portion of society. When this happens, the researcher must concentrate on how to move the procedure or tool from the laboratory to a position where it can benefit the segment of the population for which it is intended.

In the case of visual acuity testing of infants, laboratory methods for quantifying infants' visual acuity have been available for 25 years. Until recently, however, procedures for testing acuity in infants were too complicated and too time-consuming to be used for widespread testing of infants. The acuity card procedure, conceptualized by Teller in 1984, provided a method sufficiently simple and rapid that it had the potential to fit into routine clinical practice. The goal of this chapter has been to review the many studies and the considerable effort required to allow the acuity card procedure to make the transition from its laboratory conceptualization to its routine use in clinical settings.

Initially, the acuity card procedure was tested under controlled conditions in the laboratory. Validation studies were conducted to ensure that the procedure yielded acuity results comparable to those obtained with standard laboratory procedures, and success rates and test times were evaluated for various ages and ocular conditions. The introduction of the acuity card procedure to clinical settings was done in a limited fashion, with 10 centers selected to represent a cross section of the types of setting in which knowledge of acuity results in

infants and young children would be expected to be useful. After the initial, controlled studies, the acuity cards were made available to researchers and clinicians through commercial production. Widespread acceptance of the acuity card procedure as a useful clinical tool has been aided by the continued interest of the developers of the procedure in communicating with the clinical users, studies conducted by numerous other researchers in the field of infant vision testing, and incorporation of the procedure into a multicenter study involving more than 100 ophthalmologists (Cryotherapy for Retinopathy of Prematurity Cooperative Group, 1990).

Limitations in the acuity card procedure exist, including underestimation of the depth of amblyopia of strabismic patients, imprecision in acuity estimates, the possibility of bias in the acuity results, and lack of durability of the acuity cards. Furthermore, the acuity card procedure is less sensitive to myopia than are distance-acuity letter charts, and so it cannot be used to screen for refractive errors in the way that letter charts are used as a screening tool with school-age children.

Despite its limitations, the acuity card procedure appears to be making the transition into ophthalmologists' offices, optometrists' offices, follow-up clinics for infants treated in neonatal intensive care units, and institutions for mentally and physically handicapped individuals. As the acuity cards are used in more varied clinical populations, knowledge will be gained about which populations benefit most from testing, and modifications will be developed that increase the utility of the procedure.

Eventually, the acuity card procedure will probably be replaced by an automated infant vision tester or a technique for measuring recognition acuity in infants. Until that time, however, it appears that the acuity card procedure will be the most widespread behavioral method for testing acuity in infants and nonverbal individuals, and that the considerable effort expended to bring the procedure from the laboratory to the clinic was worthwhile.

Acknowledgments. The writing of this chapter and much of the research reported therein was supported by grant R01 EY05804 from the National Eye Institute. The author thanks Dr. Davida Teller for helpful comments on earlier drafts of the manuscript.

REFERENCES

ALLEN, J. L. (1979). The development of visual acuity in human infants during the early postnatal weeks. Unpublished doctoral dissertation, University of Washington, Seattle.
AMERICAN PSYCHOLOGICAL ASSOCIATION (1974). *Standards for Educational and Psychological Tests*. Washington, DC: American Psychological Association.

APPELLE, S. (1972). Perception and discrimination as a function of stimulus orientation: the "oblique effect" in man and animals. *Psychol. Bull.* 78, 266–278.

ATKINSON, J., BRADDICK, O., AND MOAR, K. (1977). Development of contrast sensitivity over the first 3 months of life in the human infant. *Vision Res.* 17, 1037–1044.

ATKINSON, J., BRADDICK, O., AND PIMM-SMITH, E. (1982). 'Preferential looking' for monocular and binocular acuity testing of infants. *Br. J. Ophthalmol.* 66, 264–268.

BERLYNE, D. E. (1958). The influence of the albedo and complexity of stimuli on visual fixation in the human infant. *Br. J. Psychol.* 49, 315–318.

BIRCH, E. E. (1985). Infant interocular acuity differences and binocular vision. *Vision Res.* 25, 571–576.

BIRCH, E. E., AND HALE, L. A. (1988). Criteria for monocular acuity deficit in infancy and early childhood. *Invest. Ophthalmol. Vis. Sci.* 29, 636–643.

BIRCH, E. E., AND SPENCER, R. (1991). Monocular grating acuity of healthy preterm infants. *Clin. Vis. Sci.*

BIRCH, E. E., AND STAGER, D. R. (1985). Monocular acuity and stereopsis in infantile esotropia. *Invest. Ophthalmol. Vis. Sci.* 26, 1624–1630.

BIRCH, E. E., GWIAZDA, J. A., NAEGELE, J., AND HELD, R. (1983). Visual acuity and its meridional variations in children aged 7 to 60 months. *Vision Res.* 23, 1019–1024.

BLAKE, R., SLOANE, M., AND FOX, R. (1981). Further developments in binocular summation. *Percept. Psychophys.* 30, 266–276.

BROWN, A. M., AND YAMAMOTO, M. (1986). Visual acuity in newborn and preterm infants measured with grating acuity cards. *Am. J. Ophthalmol.* 102, 245–253.

BROWN, A. M., DOBSON, V., AND MAIER, J. (1987). Visual acuity of human infants at scotopic, mesopic, and photopic luminances. *Vision Res.* 27, 1845–1858.

CATALANO, R. A., SIMON, J. W., JENKINS, P. L., AND KANDEL, G. L. (1987). Preferential looking as a guide for amblyopia therapy in monocular infantile cataracts. *J. Pediatr. Ophthalmol. Strabismus* 24, 56–63.

CHANDNA, A., AND DORAN, R. M. L. (1990). Observations on grating acuity measures of children in clinical practice using Teller acuity cards. In E. C. CAMPOS (ed.). *Strabismus and Ocular Motility Disorders.* London: Macmillan, pp. 85–94.

CHANDNA, A., AND DORAN, R. M. L. (1991). Criteria for amblyopia in infants: sensitivity of grating acuity and interocular acuity difference. *Invest. Ophthalmol. Vis. Sci.* 32 (suppl.), 1239.

CHANDNA, A., PEARSON, C. M., AND DORAN, R. M. L. (1988). Preferential looking in clinical practice: a year's experience. *Eye* 2, 488–495.

CORNELL, E. H., AND MCDONNELL, P. M. (1986). Infants' acuity at twenty feet. *Invest. Ophthalmol. Vis. Sci.* 27, 1417–1420.

CRYOTHERAPY FOR RETINOPATHY OF PREMATURITY COOPERATIVE GROUP (1990). Multicenter trial of cryotherapy for retinopathy of prematurity—one year outcome: structure and function. *Arch. Ophthalmol.* 108, 1408–1416.

DOBSON, V., AND CARPENTER, N. (1991). Interobserver agreement and observer bias in the acuity card procedure. In *Digest of Topical Meeting on Noninvasive Assessment of the Visual System.* Vol. 1. Washington, DC: Optical Society of America, pp. 20–23.

DOBSON, V., AND LUNA, B. (1990). Grating acuity in infants: Prototype vs Teller acuity cards. In *Digest of Topical Meeting on Noninvasive Assessment of the Visual System.* Vol. 3. Washington, DC: Optical Society of America, pp. 10–13.

DOBSON, V., AND LUNA, B. (1991). Prototype and Teller acuity cards yield similar acuities despite stimulus differences. *Invest. Ophthalmol. Vis. Sci.* 32 (suppl.), 961.

DOBSON, V., AND TELLER, D. Y. (1978). Visual acuity in human infants: a review and comparison of behavioral and electrophysiological studies. *Vision Res.* 18, 1469–1483.

DOBSON, V., CARPENTER, N. A., BONVALOT, K., AND BOSSLER, J. (1990a). The acuity card procedure: interobserver agreement in infants with perinatal complications. *Clin. Vis. Sci.* 6, 39–48.

DOBSON, V., D'ANTONIO, J. A., AND BONVALOT, K. (1989). Grating acuity in early infancy predicts grating acuity at age 1 year in infants with perinatal complications. *Invest. Ophthalmol. Vis. Sci.* (suppl.), 142.

DOBSON, V., MAYER, D. L., AND LEE, C. P. (1980). Visual acuity screening of preterm infants. *Invest. Ophthalmol. Vis. Sci.* 19, 1498–1505.

DOBSON, V., MCDONALD, M. A., AND TELLER, D. Y. (1985). Visual acuity of infants and young children: forced-choice preferential looking procedures. *Am. Orthoptic J.* 35, 118–125.

DOBSON, V., MCDONALD, M. A., KOHL, P., STERN, N., SAMEK, M., AND PRESTON, K. (1986). Visual acuity screening of infants and young children with the acuity card procedure. *J. Am. Optom. Assoc.* 27, 284–289.

DOBSON, V., QUINN, G. E., BIGLAN, A. W., TUNG, B., FLYNN, J. T., AND PALMER, E. A. (1990b). Acuity card assessment of visual function in the cryotherapy for retinopathy of prematurity trial. *Invest. Ophthalmol. Vis. Sci.* 31, 1702–1708.

DOBSON, V., SALEM, D., AND CARSON, J. B. (1983). Visual acuity in infants—the effect of variations in stimulus luminance within the photopic range. *Invest. Ophthalmol. Vis. Sci.* 24, 519–522.

DOBSON, V., SCHWARTZ, T. L., SANDSTROM, D. J., AND MICHEL, L. (1987). Binocular visual acuity in neonates: the acuity card procedure. *Dev. Med. Child Neurol.* 29, 199–206.

ELLIS, G. S., JR., HARTMANN, E. E., LOVE, A., MAY, J. G., AND MORGAN, K. S. (1988). Teller acuity cards versus clinical judgment in the diagnosis of amblyopia with strabismus. *Ophthalmology* 95, 788–791.

FANTZ, R. L. (1958). Pattern vision in young infants. *Psychol. Rec.* 8, 43–47.

FANTZ, R. L., FAGAN III, J. F., AND MIRANDA, S. B. (1975). Early visual selectivity. In L. B. COHEN AND P. SALAPATEK (eds.). *Infant Perception: From Sensation to Cognition. Vol. 1. Basic Visual Processes.* Orlando, FL: Academic Press, pp. 249–345.

FANTZ, R. L., ORDY, J. M., AND UDELF, M. S. (1962). Maturation of pattern vision in infants during the first six months. *J. Comp. Physiol. Psychol.* 55, 907–917.

FLEDELIUS, H. (1976). Prematurity and the eye. *Acta Ophthalmol. Suppl. (Copenh.)* 128, 3–245.

FREEMAN, R. D., MITCHELL, D. E., AND MILLODOT, M. (1972). A neural effect of partial visual deprivation in humans. *Science* 175, 1384–1386.

FRIENDLY, D. S., JAAFAR, M. S., AND MORILLO, D. L. (1990). A comparative study of grating and recognition visual acuity testing in children with anisometropic amblyopia without strabismus. *Am. J. Ophthalmol.* 110, 293–299.

FULTON, A., DOBSON, V., SALEM, D., MAR, C., PETERSEN, R. A., AND HANSEN, R. M. (1980). Cycloplegic refractions in infants and young children. *Am. J. Ophthalmol.* 90, 239–247.

GETZ, L., DOBSON, V., AND LUNA, B. (1992). Grating acuity development in 2-week-old to 2-year-old children born prior to term. *Clin. Vis. Sci.* 7, 251–256.

GROENENDAAL, F., VAN HOF-VAN DUIN, J., BAERTS, W., AND FETTER, W. P. F. (1989). Effects of perinatal hypoxia on visual development during the first year of (corrected) age. *Early Hum. Dev.* 20, 267–279.

GWIAZDA, J., BAUER, J., THORN, F., AND HELD, R. (1986). Meridional amblyopia *does* result from astigmatism in early childhood. *Clin. Vis. Sci.* 1, 145–152.

GWIAZDA, J., BRILL, S., MOHINDRA, I., AND HELD, R. (1978). Infant visual acuity and its meridional variation. *Vision Res.* 18, 1557–1564.

GWIAZDA, J., BRILL, S., MOHINDRA, I., AND HELD, R. (1980).

Preferential looking acuity in infants from two to fifty-eight weeks of age. *Am. J. Optom. Physiol. Opt.* 57, 428–432.

GWIAZDA, J., MOHINDRA, I., BRILL, S., AND HELD, R. (1985a). The development of visual acuity in infant astigmats. *Invest. Ophthalmol. Vis. Sci.* 26, 1717–1723.

GWIAZDA, J., MOHINDRA, I., BRILL, S., AND HELD, R. (1985b). Infant astigmatism and meridional amblyopia. *Vision Res.* 25, 1269–1276.

GWIAZDA, J., SCHEIMAN, M., AND HELD, R. (1984). Anisotropic resolution in children's vision. *Vision Res.* 24, 527–531.

HAINLINE, L., EVELYN, L., AND ABRAMOV, I. (1989). Acuity cards—what do they measure? *Invest. Ophthalmol. Vis. Sci.* 30 (suppl.), 310.

HARTMANN, E. E., CALL, W., AND ELLIS JR., G. S. (1989). Acuity card procedure: masked versus unmasked observer: does it make a difference? *Invest. Ophthalmol. Vis. Sci.* 30 (suppl.), 142.

HARTMANN, E. E., ELLIS JR., G. S., MORGAN, K. S., LOVE, A., AND MAY, J. G. (1990). The acuity card procedure: longitudinal assessments. *J. Pediatr. Ophthalmol. Strabismus* 27, 178–184.

HEERSEMA, D. J., AND VAN HOF-VAN DUIN, J. (1990). Age norms for visual acuity in toddlers using the acuity card procedure. *Clin. Vis. Sci.* 5, 167–174.

HERMANS, J., AND VAN HOF-VAN DUIN, J. (1991). Visual acuity of preterm and fullterm infants during the neonatal period. *Invest. Ophthalmol. Vis. Sci.* 32 (suppl.), 961.

HERTZ, B. G. (1987). Acuity card testing of retarded children. *Behav. Brain Res.* 24, 85–92.

HERTZ, B. G. (1988). Use of the acuity card method to test retarded children in special schools. *Child Care Health Dev.* 14, 189–198.

HERTZ, B. G., AND ROSENBERG, J. (1988). Acuity card testing of spastic children: preliminary results. *J. Pediatr. Ophthalmol. Strabismus* 25, 139–144.

HERTZ, B. G., ROSENBERG, J., SJO, O., AND WARBURG, M. (1988). Acuity card testing of patients with cerebral visual impairment. *Dev. Med. Child Neurol.* 30, 632–637.

HOWLAND, H. C., ATKINSON, J., BRADDICK, O., AND FRENCH, J. (1978). Infant astigmatism measured by photorefraction. *Science* 202, 331–332.

INGRAM, R. M., AND BARR, A. (1979). Changes in refraction between the ages of 1 and 3½ years. *Br. J. Ophthalmol.* 63, 339–342.

JACOBSON, S. G., MOHINDRA, I., AND HELD, R. (1982). Visual acuity of infants with ocular diseases. *Am. J. Ophthalmol.* 93, 198–209.

KATZ, B., AND SIRETEANU, R. (1990). The Teller acuity card test: a useful method for the clinical routine? *Clin. Vis. Sci.* 5, 307–323.

KOHL, P., AND SAMEK, B. M. (1988). Refractive error and preferential looking visual acuity in infants 12–24 months of age: year 2 of a longitudinal study. *J. Am. Optom. Assoc.* 59, 686–690.

KOHL, P., ROLEN, R. D., BEDFORD, A. K., SAMEK, M., AND STERN, N. (1986). Refractive error and preferential looking acuity in human infants: a pilot study. *J. Am. Optom. Assoc.* 57, 290–296.

LEVI, D. M., AND KLEIN, S. (1982a). Differences in Vernier discrimination for gratings between strabismic and anisometropic amblyopes. *Invest. Ophthalmol. Vis. Sci.* 23, 398–407.

LEVI, D. M., AND KLEIN, S. (1982b). Hyperacuity and amblyopia. *Nature* 298, 268–270.

LUNA, B., DOBSON, V., AND BIGLAN, A. W. (1990). Development of grating acuity in infants with regressed stage 3 retinopathy of prematurity. *Invest. Ophthalmol. Vis. Sci.* 31, 2082–2087.

MARX, M. S., WERNER, P., COHEN-MANSFIELD, J., AND HARTMANN, E. E. (1990). Visual acuity estimates in noncommunicative elderly persons. *Invest. Ophthalmol. Vis. Sci.* 31, 593–596.

MAURER, D., LEWIS, T. L., AND BRENT, H. P. (1989a). The effects of deprivation on human visual development: studies of children treated for cataracts. In F. J. MORRISON, C. E. LORD, AND D. P. KEATING (eds.). *Applied Developmental Psychology, Vol. 3. Psychological Development in Infancy.* Orlando, FL: Academic Press, pp. 139–227.

MAURER, D., LEWIS, T. L., AND BRENT, H. P. (1989b). Preferential looking and optokinetic nystagmus: concurrent and predictive validity. *Invest. Ophthalmol. Vis. Sci.* 30 (suppl.), 408.

MAYER, D. L., AND DOBSON, V. (1982). Visual acuity development in infants and young children, as assessed by operant preferential looking. *Vision Res.* 22, 1141–1151.

MAYER, D. L., FULTON, A. B., AND HANSEN, R. M. (1982). Preferential looking acuity obtained with a staircase precedure in pediatric patients. *Invest. Ophthalmol. Vis. Sci.* 23, 538–543.

MAYER, D. L., MORRELL, A. S., AND RODIER, D. W. (1986). Breakthrough acuity test for the pediatric eye clinic: the acuity card procedure. *Invest. Ophthalmol. Vis. Sci.* 27 (suppl.), 147.

McDONALD, M. A., ANKRUM, C., PRESTON, K., SEBRIS, S. L., AND DOBSON, V. (1986a). Monocular and binocular acuity in 18- to 36-month-olds: acuity card results. *Am. J. Optom. Physiol. Opt.* 63, 181–186.

McDONALD, M. A., DOBSON, V., SEBRIS, S. L., BAITCH, L., VARNER, D., AND TELLER, D. Y. (1985). The acuity card procedure: a rapid test of infant acuity. *Invest. Ophthalmol. Vis. Sci.* 26, 1158–1162.

McDONALD, M. A., SEBRIS, S. L., MOHN, G., TELLER, D. Y., AND DOBSON, V. (1986b). Monocular acuity in normal infants: the acuity card procedure. *Am. J. Optom. Physiol. Opt.* 63, 127–134.

McKEE, S. P., KLEIN, S. A., AND TELLER, D. Y. (1985). Statistical properties of forced-choice psychometric functions: implications of probit analysis. *Percept. Psychophys.* 37, 286–298.

MITCHELL, D. E., FREEMAN, R. D., MILLIDOT, M., AND HAEGERSTROM, G. (1973). Meridional amblyopia: evidence for modification of the human visual system by early visual experience. *Vision Res.* 13, 535–558.

MOHINDRA, I., HELD, R., GWIAZDA, J., AND BRILL, S. (1978). Astigmatism in infants. *Science* 202, 329–331.

MOHN, G., AND VAN HOF-VAN DUIN, J. (1986). Rapid assessment of visual acuity in infants and children in a clinical setting, using acuity cards. *Doc. Ophthalmol. Proc. Ser.* 45, 363–372.

MOHN, G., VAN HOF-VAN DUIN, J., FETTER, W. P. F., DE GROOT, L., AND HAGE, M. (1988). Acuity assessment of non-verbal infants and children: clinical experience with the acuity card procedure. *Dev. Med. Child Neurol.* 30, 232–244.

MOSELEY, M. J., FIELDER, A. R., THOMPSON, J. R., MINSHULL, C., AND PRICE, D. (1988). Grating and recognition acuities of young amblyopes. *Br. J. Ophthalmol.* 72, 50–54.

MOSKOWITZ, A., SOKOL, S., AND HANSEN, V. (1987). Rapid assessment of visual function in pediatric patients using pattern VEPs and acuity cards. *Clin. Vis. Sci.* 2, 11–20.

NORCIA, A. M., TYLER, C. W., PIECUCH, R., CLYMAN, R., AND GROBSTEIN, J. (1987). Visual acuity development in normal and abnormal preterm human infants. *J. Pediat. Ophthalmol. Strabismus* 24, 70–74.

ODOM, J. V., HOYT, C. S., AND MARG, E. (1981). Effect of natural deprivation and unilateral eye patching on visual acuity of infants and children. *Arch. Ophthalmol.* 99, 1412–1416.

PRESTON, K. L., McDONALD, M. A., SEBRIS, S. L., DOBSON, V., AND TELLER, D. Y. (1987). Validation of the acuity card procedure for assessment of infants with ocular disorders. *Ophthalmology* 94, 644–653.

RAYE, K., PRATT, E., RODIER, D., PALAFOX, G., AND MAYER, D. L. (1991). Acuity card and grating orientation: acuity of normals and patients with nystagmus. *Invest. Ophthalmol. Vis. Sci.* 32 (suppl.), 960.

REED, M. J., LEWIS, R. L., MAURER, D., WYNGAARDEN, P., AND BRENT, H. P. (1989). A comparison of three acuity card procedures. *Invest. Ophthalmol. Vis. Sci.* 30 (suppl.), 143.

ROBINSON, J., MOSELEY, M. J., AND FIELDER, A. R. (1988). Grating acuity cards: spurious resolution and the 'edge artifact.' *Clin. Vis. Sci.* 3, 285–288.

SALAPATEK, P., BECHTOLD, A. G., AND BUSHNELL, E. W. (1976). Infant visual acuity as a function of viewing distance. *Child Dev.* 47, 860–863.

SCHER, M. S., DOBSON, V., CARPENTER, N. A., AND GUTHRIE, R. D. (1989). Visual and neurological outcome of infants with periventricular leukomalacia. *Dev. Med. Child Neurol.* 31, 353–365.

SEBRIS, S. L., DOBSON, V., AND HARTMANN, E. E. (1984). Assessment and prediction of visual acuity in 3- to 4-year-old children born prior to term. *Hum. Neurobiol.* 3, 87–92.

SEBRIS, S. L., DOBSON, V., McDONALD, M. A., AND TELLER, D. Y. (1987). Acuity cards for visual acuity assessment of infants and children in clinical settings. *Clin. Vis. Sci.* 2, 45–58.

SHEPHERD, P. A., FAGAN III, J. F., AND KLEINER, K. A. (1985). Visual pattern detection in preterm neonates. *Infant Behav. Dev.* 8, 47–63.

SOKOL, S. (1980). Pattern visual evoked potentials: their use in pediatric ophthalmology. *Int. Ophthalmol. Clin.* 20, 251–268.

Teller Acuity Card Manual (1990). Dayton, Ohio: Vistech.

TELLER, D. Y. (1979). The forced-choice preferential looking procedure: a psychophysical technique for use with human infants. *Infant Behav. Dev.* 2, 135–153.

TELLER, D. Y. (1990). The design of acuity cards: a reply to Robinson, Moseley and Fielder (1988). *Clin. Vis. Sci.* 6, 81–83.

TELLER, D. Y., ALLEN, J. L., REGAL, D. M., AND MAYER, D. L. (1978). Astigmatism and acuity in two primate infants. *Invest. Ophthalmol. Vis. Sci.* 17, 344–349.

TELLER, D. Y., McDONALD, M. A., PRESTON, K., SEBRIS, S. L., AND DOBSON, V. (1986). Assessment of visual acuity in infants and children: the acuity card procedure. *Dev. Med. Child Neurol.* 28, 779–789.

TELLER, D. Y., MORSE, R., BORTON, R., AND REGAL, D. (1974). Visual acuity for vertical and diagonal gratings in human infants. *Vision Res.* 14, 1433–1439.

THOMAS, J., MOHINDRA, I., AND HELD, R. (1979). Strabismic amblyopia in infants. *Am. J. Optom. Physiol. Opt.* 56, 197–201.

TOMLINSON, E., AND MARTINEZ, D. (1988). The measurement of visual acuity: comparison of Teller acuity cards with Snellen and MBL results. *Am. Orthoptic J.* 38, 130–134.

VAN HOF-VAN DUIN, J., AND MOHN, G. (1986). The development of visual acuity in normal fullterm and preterm infants. *Vision Res.* 26, 909–916.

VAN HOF-VAN DUIN, J., EVENHUIS-VAN LEUNEN, A., MOHN, G., BAERTS, W., AND FETTER, W. P. F. (1989). Effects of very low birth weight (VLBW) on visual development during the first year after term. *Early Hum. Dev.* 20, 255–266.

VAN HOF-VAN DUIN, J., MOHN, G., FETTER, W. P. F., METTAU, J. W., AND BAERTS, W. (1983). Preferential looking acuity in preterm infants. *Behav. Brain Res.* 10, 47–50.

VITAL-DURAND, F., AND HULLO, A. (1989). La mesure de l'acuite visuelle du nourrisson en six minutes: les Cartes d'Acuite de Teller. *J. Fr. Ophtalmol.* 3, 221–225.

WYNGAARDEN, P. A., MAURER, D., LEWIS, T. L., HARVEY, P., AND ROSENBAUM, P. (1990). Preferential looking and Teller acuity cards as screening instruments. *Invest. Ophthalmol. Vis. Sci.* 31 (suppl.), 607.

YAMAMOTO, M., AND BROWN, A. M. (1985). Vision testing of premature infants using grating acuity cards. *Folia Ophthalmol. Jpn.* 36, 796–799.

YAMAMOTO, M., KANAGAWA, J., AND OKUDA, T. (1984). Preferential looking of infants and younger children with ocular diseases. *Acta Soc. Ophthalmol. Jpn.* 88, 885–890.

21 | Infant vision screening: Prediction and prevention of strabismus and amblyopia from refractive screening in the Cambridge Photorefraction Program

JANETTE ATKINSON

The visual disorders with which we have been primarily concerned are strabismus and amblyopia. These conditions have also received a great deal of scientific attention because of their significance for general understanding of visual plasticity in man and animals (von Noorden, 1974; Mitchell, 1981; Jacobson et al., 1982; Booth et al., 1985).

Amblyopia is a functional loss of visual performance that is not improved by optical correction of image blur and is not due to pathology of the eye. Rather it is believed to be a disruption of the normal development of the visual pathway due to abnormal input. The best understood form is *deprivation amblyopia*, where one eye's vision is temporarily obstructed (e.g., by a cataract) and in consequence its input to the visual cortex becomes largely disconnected (Blakemore, 1978). Anisometropia, a difference in refractive power between the eyes, causes one eye to have a more blurred image than the other, and so *anisometropic amblyopia* is generally accepted to be a less extreme form of deprivation amblyopia. *Strabismic amblyopia* occurs when the axes of the two eyes are not maintained parallel and the child comes to use one eye consistently for fixation; the nonfixing eye becomes amblyopic. Because both eyes are still receiving visual input, the neural basis of this amblyopia is currently less well understood in terms of animal models.

Strabismus is a deviation of the optic axes so they are not directed at the same point of fixation. The deviation may be either divergent or convergent, though in the population discussed here most of the manifest strabismus was convergent (or esotropic). Manifest strabismus means that the deviation is apparent even with normal binocular viewing; clinically, it is also possible to detect latent strabismus (often a stage in the development of manifest strabismus), in which the eyes can be held straight with normal viewing but deviate when their views are dissociated.

Normally, accurate convergence and binocular fixation are maintained by the detection of binocular disparity. Evidently with manifest strabismus the mechanism is failing. In principle, it could be for either (or both) of two broad reasons. (1) The strabismic child might lack the neural mechanisms necessary to detect binocular disparity (believed to be disparity-selective binocular neurons in striate and extrastriate visual cortex). (2) Disparity processing might be intact but its control over vergence overwhelmed by some other factor; a muscular paralysis would be the most obvious and extreme example.

If lack of binocular disparity detection is not the cause of strabismus but only secondary to it, what are the forces that can override the control of vergence by disparity? Clinically, a large proportion of children with convergent strabismus are considered to be accommodative esotropes associated with hyperopia. This idea is based on the fact that the control systems for vergence and accommodation are closely coupled. Even in the absence of any stimulus from binocular disparity, accommodation on a near target is accompanied by a degree of convergence of the eyes (accommodative vergence). A hyperopic child has to accommodate more strongly than normal. According to the theory of accommodative esotropia, *accommodative* vergence would therefore be a stronger force than normal in such a child; in some cases it is so strong it breaks down the maintenance of convergence on the target by disparity control and the child overconverges.

This theory leaves several questions unanswered. First, why do some hyperopic children become strabismic whereas others do not? In adults, it is possible to measure the strength of accommodative convergence, expressed as the AC/A ratio, which shows large variations from one individual to another. Presumably a large AC/A ratio in a hyperope disposes the child toward accommodative esotropia; but the developmental foundations of this ratio are unknown, and unfortunately we do not have at present any means of measuring it in infants at the stage when the strabismus may be originating. This problem leads to a second question, which is why should the hyperopic child's accommodative vergence not adjust to the particular amount required given the refractive error present? Visuomotor systems are generally highly flexible when adjusting to the relation between sensory input and required output. Why should this system not be sensitive to the individual's particular correspondence between the amount of vergence required to null a target's disparity and the amount of accommodation required to minimize its blur? It is made more surprising by the expectation that plasticity of the system would be required to cope with the changes in vergence requirements caused by the changing interocular separation during growth of the head. Furthermore, the accommodation–vergence relation has been shown experimentally to be plastic during adulthood (Miles and Judge, 1982). An interesting feature of this last evidence is that plasticity has been demonstrated in the direction of increasing the required vergence (the kind of change that would be demanded to cope with a growing head) but not yet in the opposite direction (the change that would be demanded to cope with hyperopia).

The idea of accommodative esotropia derives from the fact that the child who presents to an ophthalmologist with convergent strabismus is often hyperopic, and that spectacle correction of this error can sometimes reduce the angle of strabismus. In clinical practice, however, the child's refraction before the onset of the strabismus is usually unknown. It is possible that some strabismics, who are initially hyperopic, have lost this refractive error by the time they present clinically. This possibility is supported by both Ingram's study (1979) and that described below.

The large-scale Cambridge study described here was designed to test this possibility further using a relatively new refractive screening method to detect hyperopia and other refractive errors during infancy. If the theory of accommodative esotropia is correct, it should be possible not only to detect the hypermetropia but also, by prescribing spectacles that relieve the accommodative effort the child has to make, help to prevent the later onset of strabismus. Our study therefore includes a trial of this intervention strategy.

REVIEW OF SCREENING PROCEDURES

Strabismus and amblyopia are not necessarily the most individually serious visual problems during childhood, but they are important because they are the most prevalent in developed countries. Estimates of incidence from different studies and different populations have been variable, but in the United Kingdom an estimate of 3% of preschool children is conservative.

Screening procedures vary from country to country (for examples see reviews by Ehrlich et al., 1983; Hyvarinen, 1988; van der Lem et al., 1990). Most procedures on children below 3 years of age have attempted to identify strabismus alone; the most common procedures for 3–5 year olds involve a measure of orthoptic status and monocular visual acuity (usually with attempts to identify cases of amblyopia). As many procedures do not involve measures of refraction, however, the distinction of an acuity deficit due to optical defocus and one due to amblyopia is often incomplete, which tends to increase the apparent incidence of amblyopia. Many of the studies with "screening" in their title state an incidence and prevalence of strabismus and amblyopia for the screened population with no description of the method of population selection, compliance for attendance at screening and with the tests, socioeconomic and ethnic status of the population, or clear definitions of amblyopia. Without these data it is often difficult to decide which factor or interaction of factors is responsible for the variation in the cited values of incidence of visual disorders between one study and another. Even more remarkably, few screening studies mention the effectiveness of screening in relation either to the detection of true cases of strabismus and amblyopia (i.e., data on true positives and negatives on follow-up of those identified) or to the effectiveness of intervention in preventing visual disability; most studies regard identification of strabismus and amblyopia as an outcome in itself and do not concern themselves with effectiveness of treatment.

Holland, an authority on screening, has stated (Holland and Stewart, 1990):

> "Screening stands apart from traditional medicine in that it seeks to detect disease before symptoms present and before an individual decides to seek medical advice. Screening therefore carries considerable ethical responsibilities since it contains the potential to move an individual from a state of supposing himself or herself to be healthy to the state of having some disorder or potential disorder. But we must be sure that screening is not being used to identify conditions that are either *untreatable* or *insignificant* since at either end of this spectrum lie anguish and anxiety. Screening is costly in terms of man hours required to run the programmes, carry out the tests, and act on the results. It is vital, therefore, that there is proper assessment of the resource implications of any screening or prevention proposal both in terms of primary and of secondary workload, and that screening is included in medical audit."

Considering this definition of screening applied to strabismus and amblyopia, we can see that the following four questions need to be addressed:

1. Which vision screening tests are reliable, sensitive, and specific for identifying the presymptomatic indicators of these visual defects?

2. How significant are these defects, if not successfully treated, in causing visual disability and wider developmental problems (e.g., visuomotor, visuocognitive, behavioral)?

3. How effective are treatment regimens for these defects?

4. How cost-effective are existing vision screening programs?

These questions are briefly addressed below, although the financial aspects are not covered, as they are likely to vary greatly from one situation to the next, depending on the resources and manpower available for screening.

Which Vision Screening Tests are Reliable, Sensitive, and Specific for Identifying the Presymptomatic Indicators of these Visual Defects?

Two alternative screening strategies have been pursued: (1) screening subgroups at high overall risk of visual defects on the basis of current scientific and epidemiological knowledge; and (2) screening whole populations at a particular age. The former may turn out to be the most cost-effective but contravenes geographic and ethnic equity. These grounds can be used to justify screening whole populations.

Screening Programs for High Risk Groups.

1. *Very low birth weight/extremely premature infants.* A study commissioned by the Scottish Home and Health Department (1991) found moderate to severe disability, often including vision, in 15% of very low birth weight (VLBW) survivors at 2 years, with an additional 15% having more minor defects including strabismus. Neonatal screening programs exist to identify ophthalmological problems such as retinopathy of prematurity (ROP) in the VLBW population, and here the long-term prognosis for permanent visual disability would benefit from more detailed investigation in longitudinal studies. For example, in many studies to date, ROP has been identified and graded without any long-term follow-up to evaluate the consequences to health and education of these neonatal problems. More sophisticated screening programs, to identify visual defects with or without other neurological defects during the first year of life, must be devised and carefully evaluated to allow early reliable diagnosis and intervention. Some attempts are already under way in a number of centers (e.g., Dobson, 1991; Atkinson and van Hof-van Duin, in press).

2. *Infants and children identified with major neurological disability* (e.g., cerebral palsy). At present there is no consistent vision screening program for children with multiple disabilities, although most of these children are likely to have one or more visual defects (e.g., Atkinson, 1985). The interplay between screening programs, detailed assessments (usually carried out in specialized centers), and rehabilitation and special teaching programs needs to be clarified. Considerable basic research is needed specifically on these groups, as it is more generally, to clarify the relation between a technically defined loss of vision and its impact on everyday living skills, taking into account the other disabilities present. Consideration of the value of specialized regional centers, with multidisciplinary teams covering health and education to visually screen and assess this special population at an early age, is vitally needed. Major reports (Hall, 1989; RNIB, 1990; van der Lem et al., 1990) have highlighted the research need for reliable screening tests to be devised for both infants (under age 2 years) with normal development and older children whose physical and mental delays make their response repertoire and skills comparable to those of normal children under 2 years old. Here photo- and videorefractive screening can be seen as useful possibilities.

There is some debate as to whether simple single screening tests, or batteries of tests, would be most effective for identifying visual defects in multiply disabled children. Some have argued that because of variable performance and uneven profiles, it is only from extensive testing of these children in a number of visual domains that the more subtle visual defects can be identified (Atkinson et al., 1989). For example, research using specialized tests has pinpointed a dissociation between attentional visual defects and sensory loss of resolution acuity in some neurologically impaired children (Hood and Atkinson, 1990). A second example is the relative sparing of basic visual capacities in Williams syndrome children accompanied by extensive visuospatial deficits (Bellugi et al., in press). Single simple screening procedures of one visual function (e.g., acuity measures) may yield valuable information but may fail to identify important visuocognitive deficits. Comparisons of the effectiveness of multiple test batteries against single screening tests for different multiply impaired groups is necessary before conclusions can be reached.

3. *High risk groups with a family history of a visual defect* (e.g., family history of strabismus, genetic disorders such as retinitis pigmentosa, albinism). Although children with a history of strabismus in a first-degree relative show a higher than normal incidence of strabismus and refractive errors (Anker et al., 1991), it is unlikely that screening this population alone would identify most of these problems in the whole population. Selective screening once genetic links have been identified, however, may lead to early diagnosis of many forms of albinism and retinitis pigmentosa.

Population Screening Program. There is still some debate about what constitutes surveillance, in contrast to screening of child vision. Holland (1990) defined screening as a more specific tool within more general programs of health surveillance, to be used for particular conditions or in particular high risk groups. In the United Kingdom the Hall Report (1989) recommended a core program of surveillance (including vision at 21 and 39 months and at 5, 8, and 11 years) to be undertaken by primary health care teams (often the family practice nurse), with no specific vision screening tests included. Visual defects were to be detected largely by questioning parents about worries and family history. Doubts have been expressed as to how effective this emphasis on parental reporting can be for detecting visual defects (Bax and Whitmore, 1990); and of course many cases of amblyopia without accompanying strabismus, most refractive errors, and less apparent ophthalmological defects would go undetected during the preschool years and in children with developmental delay.

At present in the United Kingdom and most other European countries, widely varied preschool screening programs are in use (van de Lem et al., 1990), but there have been few detailed measures of the effectiveness of these programs. In many where evaluation has been attempted, the population screened has been preselected (e.g., McClellan, 1977), or analysis has been carried out on relatively small samples (e.g., Beardsell, 1989). The Hall Report (1989) doubted the value of any of the present preschool screening schemes in the United Kingdom and recommended that they be discontinued until proved effective. Many clinical professionals state anecdotally, however, that they believe screening makes a valuable contribution to detecting vision problems at an early age.

At present there are two points during the preschool period in the United Kingdom (and in many other European countries, e.g., Germany, Finland, France) when vision is screened in most of the population.

1. *Neurological neonatal discharge examination.* Here there is examination of the red reflex to detect severe ophthalmological visual defects, the most common of which is cataract (Taylor and Rice, 1982). Although severe visual defects at birth are rare, it is essential that this test is adequately carried out to produce a high specificity and sensitivity. Many personnel carrying out this examination, however, need additional training in the techniques and in counseling parents about possible future visual development and impairment. All too often a comment such as "the eyes are fine" gives parents a false sense of security, leading them to ignore even an obvious visual defect such as strabismus, at a later age.

2. *Orthoptic examination for binocularity, and acuity testing of each eye with a single optotype matching test at 3.5–4.0 years of age.* In European countries there are several single optotype tests in use (e.g., LH-test in Finland; Sheridan-Gardiner in the United Kingdom; illiterate E test and R4 test in Germany. It is well recognized that there are several inadequacies in single optotype tests for preschool acuity measures (e.g., the practical difficulties of testing young children at 6 meters testing distance specified for many tests such as the Sheridan-Gardiner Test and inadequate sensitivity to amblyopia). Tests that overcome these problems have now been devised (e.g., Cambridge Crowding Cards), although their effectiveness in comparison to current standard clinical screening procedures must still be measured. Although several small-scale projects to evaluate orthoptic preschool screening have been undertaken (e.g., Beardsell, 1989) a multicenter approach with standardized protocols and registration of results is necessary before the true value of these widespread programs can be determined.

A report comparing pediatric screening in a number of European countries shows that not only are there marked differences in approaches to screening between one country and another but that different domains of development (vision, hearing, and language) receive different degrees of evaluation, for example, relatively sophisticated analysis of screening tests for hearing compared to visual deficits (van der Lem et al., 1990). For vision, it appears that pediatric screening is undertaken by a wide variety of professionals in different European countries and those outside Europe, with marked differences in training. In many countries "quality control" and central collation of screening data are not routinely undertaken at present.

NEW SCREENING TECHNIQUES

In recent years several methods, such as photorefraction techniques, Teller/Keeler acuity cards, and Cambridge Crowding Cards, have been developed that may be applicable to preschool vision screening. Here, only refractive screening is considered, as it is directly relevant to the program described in this chapter.

To date, two groups in the United Kingdom have carried out population screening programs for infant refractive errors. Both have aimed not only to detect refractive errors but to assess their predictive value for later preschool vision defects (strabismus and amblyopia). Ingram et al. (1985) used *retinoscopy* as the screening technique, a technique that requires skilled personnel and a certain degree of cooperation on the part of the child. It is consequently costly and not optimal for widespread screening. Atkinson et al. (1984, 1987b) have used another technique, *isotropic photorefraction*, which is carried out by trained orthoptists and has been previously validated against retinoscopy. Further independent validations of isotropic videorefraction against retinoscopy have been carried out by Spanish and Russian clinical teams (Castenera de Molina et al., 1989; Somov, 1989). Compared to retinoscopy, isotropic photorefraction requires less highly trained personnel and less cooperation on the child's part; it is therefore a relatively robust and inexpensive method.

Both refractive trials have shown a high predictive value for identifying children at risk of strabismus and amblyopia from their cycloplegic refraction, with acceptably high specificities and sensitivities for identification of both strabismus and abnormal refractive errors. Several other studies have attempted to specify ambylogenic precursors and to identify them (Castenera de Molina et al., 1989; Angi, 1991). The importance of these programs can be realized only if treatment of refractive precursors reduces the incidence of long-term visual defects. A number of photo- and videorefractive instruments, based on related optical principles, are available either commercially or in prototype form and are now being compared (Braddick and Atkinson, 1983; Howland, 1991).

How Significant Are these Defects, If Not Successfully Treated, in Causing Disability and Developmental Problems in Areas Other than Vision (e.g., Visuomotor, Visuocognitive, Social)?

Apart from a limited number of well documented syndromes (e.g., congenital cataracts), we have no precise measures of the degree of disability likely to evolve from a visual defect, nor do we have detailed scales of changes regarding the extent of disability with increasing age. For example, it is unlikely that the reduced acuity associated with infantile idiopathic congenital nystagmus leads to extensive disability at the time the condition is identified during infancy. This defect, however, is likely to be related to disability during later childhood (inability to read the blackboard) and adulthood (exclusion from certain professions and car driving).

Some would argue that no disability is associated with mild defects (strabismus, amblyopia, color blindness). Amblyopia as a unilateral condition leads to significant disability only if the use of the good eye is lost, and it has been argued that this risk is low. The increase in life expectancy in recent decades, however, has increased the significance of cataract as a visual problem of the elderly. It would be illuminating to know what proportion of first eye cataracts are in the good eye of

unilateral amblyopes, leaving the patient with a relatively severe visual disability of rapid onset.

There is a need for much more detailed longitudinal analysis of the defect/disability relation to serve as the basis for clearer guidelines for both parents and health counseling professionals. Although these issues are not directly related to screening procedures, they are pertinent to considering the effectiveness of screening programs on a wider scale and as such deserve much more research effort than at present.

A second issue is the extent of subsequent nonvisual problems as a result of a primary visual deficit. The problem is to differentiate between correlation and causality. Two areas where these issues are of current interest are (1) in multiply handicapped visually impaired (MHVI) children, and (2) concerning visual precursors of certain learning disabilities (e.g., dyslexia) in otherwise normal preschool children.

Many believe that a visual defect (either severe or mild) during early life limits visuomotor, visuosocial, and visuocognitive development, although there is scant evidence for these causal relations and much evidence for clusters of correlated defects within a single individual. Only randomized control trial studies of early intervention, with diverse outcome measures of motor, social, and cognitive competence, would be able to give clear answers to these questions.

How Effective are Treatment Regimens for These Defects?

There are few published data on the effectiveness of any preschool vision screening programs for identifying precursors of visual defects that may lead to disability. In addition, there is long-standing controversy on the effectiveness of treatment for both strabismus and amblyopia.

Probably the most debated issue is occlusion therapy for treatment of amblyopia (a procedure that has been advocated for 200 years without extensive control trials). Some have claimed a high failure rate for occlusion therapy, which is likely to be due to a combination of factors such as the delay between onset of amblyopia, referral time, and treatment onset, poor compliance with treatment, and confounding additional factors of other disabilities. A second major issue is the degree of success of strabismus treatment in restoring binocularity and preventing amblyopia. It is generally believed that surgery during the first year of life for early-onset strabismus provides the best outcome in terms of binocular vision. Some studies, however, have suggested that even in this case the outcome in terms of stereoscopic vision is frequently poor (e.g., Atkinson et al., 1991) and that the primary justification for early treatment (surgery, occlusion, and sometimes spectacle correction) must be the reduction of amblyopia and cosmetic improvement. There is a need for controlled trials of late and early surgery with careful longitudinal outcome measures, although such studies would present considerable problems of ethical acceptability.

The trials of infant refractive screening discussed above have been linked to evaluations of refractive correction by spectacles. The results, however, show some disagreement on whether such correction can successfully prevent later amblyopia and strabismus. The two studies (Ingram, 1979; Ingram et al., 1985; Atkinson et al., 1984, 1987b) discussed in more detail below, differed in the exact criteria and protocol for spectacle prescription and the compliance level achieved, and these factors may be critical when deciding on effectiveness.

CAMBRIDGE INFANT SCREENING PROGRAM

In our refractive screening program, every infant living in the City of Cambridge over a 2-year period was sent an appointment to attend a local well-baby clinic when the infant was between 6 and 8 months of age. A trained orthoptist conducted the screening tests, which consisted of a basic orthoptic examination (Hirschberg test, cover test, ability to overcome 20 diopter prisms) and isotropic photorefraction following cycloplegia with 1% cyclopentolate (Atkinson et al., 1981; Atkinson and Braddick, 1983a,b; Howland et al., 1983). Three photographs with different camera focus settings were taken. Photorefraction was on 35 mm film. Infants were referred for follow-up if the photorefraction revealed marked hyperopia, myopia, or anisometropia or if strabismus or any ocular pathology was evident. Further details of the procedures for screening and follow-up and of the validation of the photorefraction measure have been reported by Atkinson et al. (1984).

The first follow-up occurred by age 9 months and included a fuller orthoptic examination, photorefraction or videorefraction (using the Cambridge Videorefractor VPR-L) prior to cycloplegia to examine accommodative performance, acuity testing by forced-choice preferential looking (FPL), cycloplegic refraction by both photorefraction and retinoscopy, and an ophthalmological examination of the fundi. For children in whom a refractive error was confirmed, there were repeated follow-ups at regular intervals up to age 4 years, primarily concerned with monitoring the development of the child's refraction, acuity, and any changes in orthoptic status. Figure 21-1 outlines our follow-up protocol. At 4 years there were careful tests of the child's acuity and binocular vision. These tests represent measures of the main outcome of the study. Children who at any stage in the screening or follow-up showed man-

ifest strabismus, demonstrable amblyopia, or ocular pathology were referred directly to the regular hospital eye clinic; and follow-up information was derived from their examinations there.

Our most extensive study is of the group who were found during the screening to have a hyperopic refractive error of 4 diopters (D) or more at 6–8 months. This part of the study had two aspects.

1. *Emmetropization.* We were concerned with the "natural history" of the group: How does their refractive error change, and is it a precursor of later strabismus, poor vision, or both? To examine this question, they had to be compared with a control group; for each hyperopic child we followed a child with none of our categories of refractive error who was screened at the same clinic at the same time.

2. *Randomized control trial of spectacle correction.* We tested whether any effects of early hyperopia on visual development could be countered by a spectacle correction, which would reduce the accommodation the child was habitually exerting, the image blur, or both. For this purpose infants in the hyperopic group were randomly assigned to "spectacles" and "nonspectacles" groups. The prescription protocol was as follows
a. Sphere: 1.0 D less than least hyperopic meridian (corrections under 1.5 D were not prescribed)
b. Cylinder: up to 2 years of age—half of astigmatic error if over 2.5 D; at 2.0–3.5 years—half of any astigmatic refractive error; over 3.5 years—full correction

Prescriptions were checked frequently, at which times the child's wearing of the spectacles was monitored by close, sympathetic questioning of the parents. This technique enabled us to measure compliance. We took as our working definition of "compliant" any infant who wore the spectacle correction for 50% or more of their waking hours throughout the period of infancy when they were prescribed spectacles. Our compliance level was around 70% of those prescribed.

Results of the Study

Early Detection of Refractive Errors and Strabismus. A group of 3166 infants were screened (an average of 74% of the total population) during the period of the study, and 9.3% of them were referred for follow-up because of the screening findings. Figure 21-2 illustrates the distribution of these patients among the various categories and shows that most of the screening findings were confirmed on the fuller examination at follow-up. There was good agreement between photorefraction and retinoscopy, with retinoscopy being taken as the "gold standard." The largest single category of refractive errors was the hyperopes (4.6%). It should be noted that we have not included a separate category for astigma-

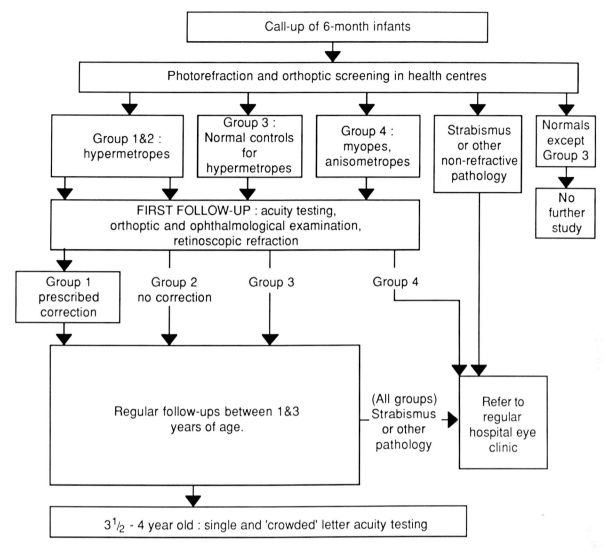

FIG. 21-1. Follow-up protocol.

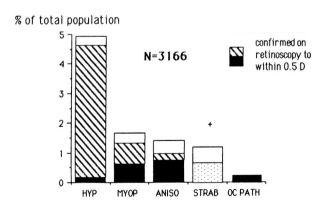

FIG. 21-2. Results from screening 3166 infants and at retinoscopy follow-up. HYP = hyperopes; MYOP = myopes; ANISO = anisotropes; STRAB = strabismus; OC PATH = ocular pathology.

tism. Substantial degrees of astigmatism are common at the age we screened, with more than 50% of infants having more than 1 D of astigmatism (Howland et al., 1978; Mohindra et al., 1978; Atkinson and Braddick, 1983a,b), which in most cases largely disappears over the first 2 years of life (Atkinson et al., 1980). Because the criterion for our hyperopic group was a refraction over 3.5 D in any meridian, and because even our normal group is on average more than 1 D hyperopic, infants with large astigmatisms are likely to appear in the hyperopic group.

We should also note the small size of the group found to be already strabismic at this age: 1.2%, of whom only 0.7% were showing a clear manifest strabismus. We were concerned that our screening might be omitting a strabismic group who had already seen an ophthalmologist before 6 months and who therefore did not attend screening. We then investigated a group of 100 infants chosen from the approximately 25% who had not attended their appointments; only 2 were found to have been referred to a hospital eye clinic with possible strabismus, and in neither case was this abnormality confirmed. Any bias arising from differential attendance must therefore be small, and the true figure for manifest strabismus before 6 months in this population is almost certainly below 1%. It is of course possible that this group of early-onset strabismics differ fundamentally from those of later onset in terms of their etiology and precipitating mechanisms. Some workers have argued that a fundamental lack of the ability to develop disparity detectors may characterize the early-onset group (possibly a lack of uncrossed pathway as in ocular albinism). However, we were unable to find any substantial evidence for this idea in another longitudinal study of infants with a familial strabismus history (Wattam-Bell et al., 1987).

Changes in Refraction with Age. How far do refractive errors identified at 6–8 months persist? From data analyzed so far (Fig. 21-3) it appears that the control children are showing, overall, little change in their refraction between 9 months and 3.5 years, although there is some reduction in the level of astigmatism (note here that we have plotted the least hyperopic axis). These results are in line with data showing little average change

in refraction over the first 3 years (reviewed by Banks, 1980a,b), as the group represented by our controls dominates any population data. Insofar as changes in this age range are generally in the direction of emmetropia, they have of course relatively little scope for change, as the control group's average refraction at 9 months is close to emmetropic.

The hyperopic groups, however, present a different picture. Overall there is a strong trend for their hyperopia to decline. There is no marked difference in the rate of decline between the hyperopes who wore a partial correction and those who were uncorrected. However, this decline is most marked among the children whose hyperopia is not accompanied by marked astigmatism; a substantial fraction of the astigmatic infants show no reduction or even a small increase in the amount of astigmatism over the preschool years—due to reduction in hyperopia in one axis with the opposing axis remaining unchanged. Figure 21-4 summarizes how the infants' astigmatisms changed in the uncorrected hyperopic group. It is apparent that the rate of reduction in astigmatism depends on the axis of astigmatism; if the most hyperopic axis is vertical, there is likely to be a smaller reduction in the level of astigmatism than if the greatest hyperopia is in the horizontal axis. Oblique astigmatisms show an intermediate pattern.

There has been some speculation as to whether there may be an active visual feedback control of the development of the eye that acts to optimize image quality (see discussion by Banks, 1980a,b). If there were such a thing as an active process of emmetropization, the correction of image defocus by spectacles would reduce the error signal in this feedback loop and therefore reduce the developmental trend toward emmetropia. At present our data show no consistent difference between the average rate of emmetropization in the spectacle wearers and the nonspectacle wearers, which provides no support for the idea of an active feedback loop. It should be remembered, however, that we gave a partial spectacle correction with cylinder corrections only for only the largest astigmatisms, which means that there was probably scope even in the corrected hyperopes for some *accommodative* adjustments to be made and for activation of a feedback loop.

If there was an active corrective process, however, it is difficult to see why it should act better in the vertical than the horizontal meridian, or vice versa, in the case of astigmatism. The marked difference between the rates at which hyperopia astigmatism declines in these two meridia seems more plausibly explained on the basis of maturational processes, which are anisotropic (perhaps constrained by mechanical forces of the eyelid on the cornea, for instance) and which proceed without influence from the visual input. On this view, the eye is programmed to have equal refractive power in different

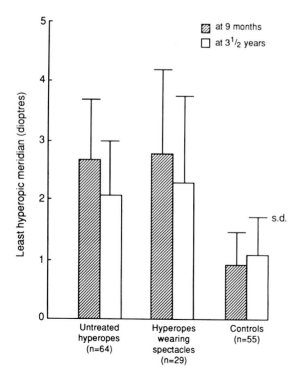

FIG. 21-3. Changes in refraction in infants at 9 months to 3.5 years of age.

Most hyperopic axis :   horizontal   vertical   oblique

Shaded area :
proportion still
astigmatic at
18 months

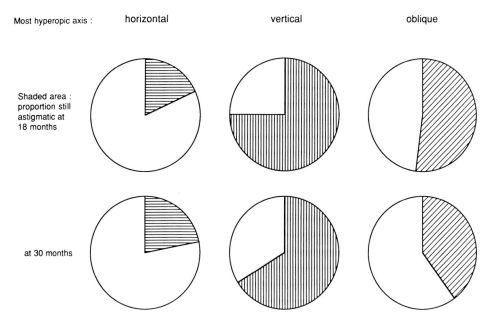

at 30 months

FIG. 21-4. Changes in astigmatism in infants in the hyperopic group (untreated) who showed at least 1 D astigmatism at 6–9 months. The difference in proportions between axes is significant at the 1% level.

meridia, but one meridian may lag behind another in achieving this goal at different stages of development.

Predictive Value of Refractive Screening for Later Onset of Strabismus and Amblyopia. We should not assume that an early refractive error of itself necessarily represents a visual deficit. Rather, we must ask how far can identification of early refractive errors predict lasting, functionally significant, vision problems? We have two main outcome measures at 4 years: one of binocularity and one of preschool acuity. The main measure of binocularity is the presence or absence of strabismus, although all children were also given the TNO random-dot stereo test. The two acuity tests were both conducted with the child wearing any appropriate refractive correction (in particular correcting any remaining astigmatism) even if the child was not wearing spectacles regularly as part of the trial, so failures would not be expected simply as consequences of optical blur at the time of testing. Each eye was tested separately. The "single-letter acuity" was obtained using the Sheridan-Gardiner letter matching test (Sheridan, 1976), modified by us for a testing distance of 3 meters rather than the standard 6 meters. "Failure" was defined as 6/9 or poorer with either eye. However, it is well known that testing with single optotypes does not satisfactorily reveal problems of amblyopia, where "crowding" effects can be marked (Hilton and Stanley, 1972). Because a conventional Snellen chart is not practical at this age, we have devised a letter-matching task analogous to the Sheridan-Gardiner test but that presents the letters in a "crowded" context (the Cambridge Crowding Cards)

(Atkinson et al., 1987a, 1989; Anker et al., 1991). Acuity estimates using the Cambridge Crowding Cards agree well with Snellen measures of acuity for adults. On the basis of testing visually normal children, we set 6/12 or poorer as the criterion of failure on this multiple-letter test.

The data were analyzed in two ways: (1) in terms of a "treated" (T) group, i.e., those who were offered treatment and complied by wearing their correction, compared to those who had not been treated (NT), i.e., those who did not comply plus those not given spectacles; (2) in terms of those who were "offered treatment" (OT), compliers and noncompliers being deemed to be in the same outcome group, compared to those not offered treatment (NOT).

Comparison of Control, Treated, and Nontreated Groups. Figure 21-5 shows the proportion of children in the control, NT, and T hyperopic groups who developed strabismus after the initial screening but before 4 years of age. Twenty-one percent (16 of 76) of the children who had been hyperopic initially and had not worn a correction throughout infancy (NT) became strabismic, compared to 1.6% (2 of 123) of the control group (emmetropic in infancy) and 6.3% (3 of 48) of the T group. The difference between incidence in the T and NT groups is significant on the chi squared (χ^2) test ($p < 0.05$), but there is no significant difference between the control and T hyperopic groups (although the incidence is higher in the latter group).

The pass/failure rates for these two tests are shown

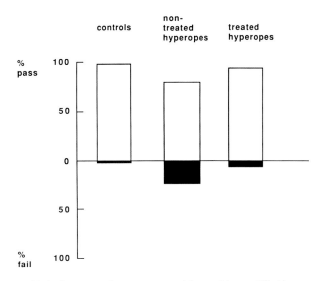

FIG. 21-5. Outcome of groups screened for strabismus. Filled bars = those who became strabismic.

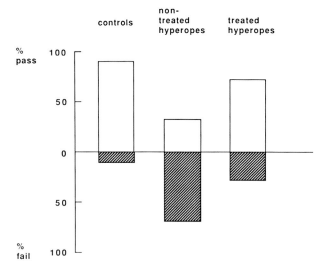

FIG. 21-7. Outcome of screened groups: pass/failure rates for acuity using the crowded letters matching test.

for the three groups in Figures 21-6 and 21-7. On the single letter matching test 37.5% (27 of 72) of the NT group failed in one or both eyes, compared to 9.5% (4 of 42) of the T hyperopes and 5.6% (7 of 123) of the control group. On the χ^2 test the NT group were significantly worse than the other two groups ($p < 0.001$ in both cases). On the crowded letters test 68% (47 of 69) of the NT group, 28.6% (12 of 42) of the T group, and 11.1% (11 of 99) of the controls failed to obtain 6/9 equivalent in one or both eyes. Once again there was no difference between the controls and the T group, but the NT group was significantly worse than either of the other two groups ($p < 0.001$). Failures on both acuity tests were not necessarily in one eye, as would be expected from strabismic or anisotropic amblyopia.

Bilateral acuity deficits, which do not fit with conventional ideas of amblyopia as a competitive process, were common. .

Comparison of Control, Offered Treatment, and Not Offered Treatment Groups. A total of 8.8% (6 of 68) of the OT group became strabismic compared to 23.2% (13 of 56) of the NOT group (significant on χ-square test, $p < 0.05$). The controls showed a significantly lower level of strabismus (2 of 123) than the OT group ($p < 0.05$) and the NOT group ($p < 0.001$).

A total of 16.4% (9 of 55) of the OT group compared to 33.9% (20 of 59) of the NOT group failed the single optotype test at 4 years (significant at the 0.05% level). The controls were just significantly better than the OT group on single letters ($p < 0.05$) and much better than the NOT group ($p < 0.001$).

A total of 36.4% (20 of 55) of the OT group compared to 69.6% (39 of 56) of the NOT group failed to reach the 4-year-old pass criterion on the Cambridge Crowding Cards (significant difference $p = 0.001$). The controls, however, did significantly better than both the OT group and the NOT group ($p = 0.001$) on the Crowding Cards.

MERIDIONAL AMBLYOPIA

One possibility is that early astigmatism is a contributory cause in some cases (as children with large astigmatisms were more likely to appear in the hyperopic group than among the controls). Meridional amblyopia—reduced acuity in one meridian—has been demonstrated in astigmatic adults (Mitchell et al., 1973) and is presumed to be a consequence of differential

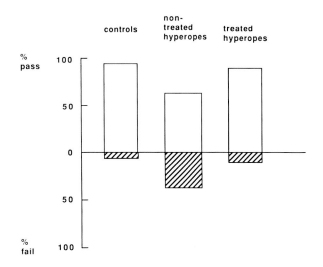

FIG. 21-6. Outcome of screen groups: pass/failure rates for acuity using the single letter matching test.

image blur caused by marked astigmatism during an early critical period.

Recognition of letter targets could be impaired by poor acuity in any meridian. Grating stimuli were used to test for meridional amblyopia in a subset of the NOT group. We used an automated FPL procedure (Atkinson et al., 1982; Atkinson and Braddick, 1982) with acuity estimated for different orientations of gratings. We used a statistically reliable reduced staircase procedure (Atkinson et al., 1986a,b) and compared acuity in the two major meridians. The children were tested at 4 years wearing a full astigmatic correction at the time of testing. If a reliable difference of more than 0.67 octave was found between acuity in the two major meridians, we deemed the child "meridionally amblyopic." We also looked at reduction in astigmatism over the course of the first 3 years in the same children and divided the group into those who were persistently astigmatic (> 1 D) after 2 years of age and those who had lost their astigmatism by 2 years. As can be seen in Figure 21-8 there is a strong relation between those showing meridional amblyopia and those with persistent astigmatism. We also compared our measures of meridional amblyopia with the child's failure on the acuity test at 4 years (Fig. 21-9). Children who failed the acuity tests tended also to show meridional amblyopia. There is a significant group, however, who failed the letter test but were not deemed to be meridional amblyopes. Our conclusion to date would be that although meridional amblyopia probably contributes to poor preschool acuity in the uncorrected hyperopic group, it is not the only cause.

So why do many of our children who had been infant hyperopes and had not worn correcting spectacles fail the Cambridge Crowding Cards test? It appears that there is no one single cause. Some are indeed truly amblyopic at 4 years, and it remains to be seen if treatment at this stage can alleviate this condition in this group. Some of the children who had been hyperopic during

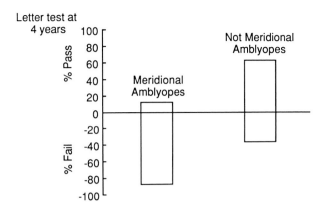

FIG. 21-9. Meridional amblyopia and letter acuity of 4-year-olds who had been infant hyperopes.

infancy appeared to fail the crowded acuity task because they failed to understand the task of matching only one letter in the center of the array. Their behavior was often rather like that of a younger child or Down syndrome child: They would have no difficulty with single letter matching but when presented with the crowded cards became confused and lost attention. We suspect that the development of some of these children is generally delayed, and that it is not specific to the visual domain. However, we did not build into our outcome protocol nonvisual indicators of development and so cannot present substantial evidence for this idea. One suggestive piece of evidence for this general delay is presented in Figure 21-10. A subset of certain groups has been followed up to 5 years. From Figure 21-10 we can see that a substantial number of the failures at 4 years in the NT group pass at the 4-year-old level when they are 5 years old. It is as though they are still 1 year behind in acuity development. Whether this delay persists into the early school years we do not know, but we are attempting to retest as many of the children as possible from all groups at school age, to try and answer this question.

ACCOMMODATIVE ABILITY IN CHILDREN WITH REFRACTIVE ERRORS

Some information about the infants' accommodative behavior can be obtained from the photorefractive testing without cycloplegia, which was carried out at each follow-up examination, while the infant was looking at a target close to the camera at 75 cm distance (Braddick et al., 1988). Whereas the control subjects generally focus close to the camera and sometimes slightly in front of it, a significant proportion of the hyperopic infants maintain a more distant position of focus. This finding implies that, at least in some cases under test conditions, infant hyperopes are not overaccommodating to the full

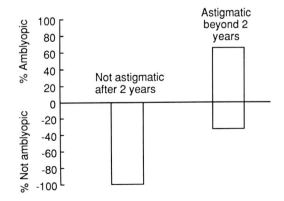

FIG. 21-8. Astigmatism and meridional amblyopia in 4-year-olds who had been infant hyperopes.

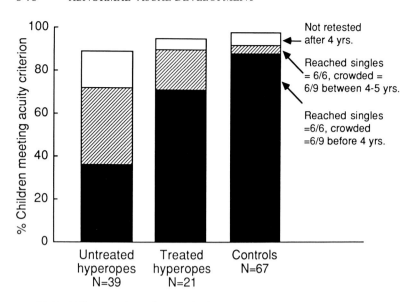

FIG. 21-10. Follow-up of visual acuity development at 4 and 5 years.

extent necessary to achieve maximally clear vision. This increase in accommodative lag in hyperopic infants has been confirmed by Bobier et al. (1988). Bobier also found that whereas the accommodative lag increases for emmetropic infants when they view near targets (30–40 cm), some hyperopic infants show a decreased lag and may even overaccommodate at these distances. It appears, then, that the accommodative behavior of hyperopes may be more complicated than would be expected from a simple account of failing to meet excessive accommodative demands.

SUMMARY AND CONCLUSIONS

The complex set of data we have outlined has indicated a number of relations among the variables of visual development over the first years of life, although most of the causal mechanisms involved are still unclear. We briefly summarize these relations.

A high level of hyperopia under cycloplegia at around 6 months is a strong predictor of later visual problems, including relatively poor preschool acuity. A likely mechanism is deprivation amblyopia due to image blur, but the contributions of blur due to spherical hyperopia and that due to astigmatism have not yet been distinguished. Strabismus is also predictively linked to hyperopia during infancy. This relation is often explained in terms of the hypothesis of accommodative esotropia, but this hypothesis leaves a good deal more to be explained. The extent to which the developmental visual problems of hyperopes can be alleviated by spectacle correction suggests that the optical effects of hyperopia play a causal role. We suspect, however, that hyperopia may

be correlated with much more general developmental variables, going beyond purely visual performance.

Refraction is not constant over the preschool years, particularly for the hyperopic group. The possibility exists in our studies that changes in refraction may be under some control by visual processing, but it is certainly not proved. Changes in astigmatism seem difficult to explain in this way; they show asymmetries that seem more likely to be an expression of a maturational process.

Normal, binocular, pattern vision is the result of an interplay of three factors: (1) optical, in the image formation of the eye; (2) sensorineural, in the processing of that image and interaction of the images of the two eyes; and (3) muscular, in both the active adjustment of accommodation and the control of eye movements. The balance of these mechanisms is delicate, and the plasticity of the developing system is not always adequate to the task of maintaining it. A fuller understanding of this developmental interaction will not only enhance our grasp of the general principles of how complex neural systems develop; it will also improve our chances of intervening effectively to maintain the balance when it is perturbed.

Acknowledgments. This work is supported by the Medical Research Council of Great Britain and by a grant from the East Anglia Regional Health Authority. Dr. David Allen, Shirley Anker, Bill Bobier, Jackie Day, Kim Durden, Carol Evans, Dr. Fiona Griffith, Ann MacIntyre, Dr. Michael Mair, Elizabeth Pimm-Smith, Claire Towler, and John Wattam-Bell have assisted in carrying out the screening and follow-up. I thank Mr. P. G. Watson, Consultant Ophthalmologist, and members of the Department of Community Health, Cambridge Health Authority, for their support, and many general practitioners and health visitors for their cooperation. Dr. Sue Atkinson, Dr. Oliver

Braddick, and I jointly designed the study, and Dr. Sue Atkinson administered a parallel screening program in Bristol. For an earlier, but extended, discussion of these issues, see Atkinson and Braddick (1988).

REFERENCES

ANGI, M. R. (1991). Results of photorefractometric screening for ambloyogenic deficits in children aged 20 months. In *Transactions of the 3rd Meeting of the Child Vision Research Society, Rotterdam.*

ANKER, S., ATKINSON, J., BOBIER, W., TRICKLEBANK, J., AND WATTAM-BELL, J. (1991). *Abstracts of the 7th International Orthoptic Congress, Nuremberg.*

ATKINSON, J. (1985). Assessment of vision in infants and young children. In S. HAREL AND N. J. ANASTASIOW (eds). *The At-Risk Infant: Psycho/Socio/Medical Aspects.* Baltimore: Paul H. Brookes Publishing.

ATKINSON, J., AND BRADDICK, O. J. (1982). Assessment of visual acuity in infancy and early childhood. *Acta Ophthalmol. Suppl. (Copenh.)* 157, 18–26.

ATKINSON, J., AND BRADDICK, O. J. (1983a). The use of isotropic photorefraction for vision screening in infants. *Acta Ophthalmol. Suppl. (Copenhh.)* 157, 36–45.

ATKINSON, J., AND BRADDICK, O. J. (1983b). Vision screening and photorefraction: the relation of refractive errors to strabismus and amblyopia. *Behav. Brain Res.* 10, 71–80.

ATKINSON, J., AND BRADDICK, O. (1988). Infant precursors of later visual disorders: correlation or causality? In A. YONAS (ed.). *20th Minnesota Symposium on Child Psychology.* Hillsdale, NJ: Erlbaum, pp. 35–65.

ATKINSON, J., AND VAN HOF-VAN DUIN, J. (in press). Assessment of normal and abnormal development during the first years of life. In A. FIELDER AND M. BAX (eds.). *Management of Visual Handicap in Childhood.* MacKeith Press.

ATKINSON, J., ANKER, S., EVANS, C., AND MCINTYRE, A. (1987a). The Cambridge Crowding Cards for preschool visual acuity testing. In *Transactions of the 6th International Orthoptic Congress, Harrogate, England.*

ATKINSON, J., BRADDICK, O. J., AND FRENCH, J. (1980). Infant astigmatism: its disappearance with age. *Vision Res.* 20, 891–893.

ATKINSON, J., BRADDICK, O. J., AND PIMM-SMITH, E. (1982). "Preferential looking" for monocular and binocular acuity testing of infants. *Br. J. Ophthalmol.* 66, 264–268.

ATKINSON, J., BRADDICK, O. J., AYLING, L., PIMM-SMITH, E., HOWLAND, H. C., AND INGRAM, R. M. (1981). Isotropic photorefraction: a new method for refractive testing of infants. *Doc. Ophthalmol. Proc. Ser.* 30, 217–223.

ATKINSON, J., BRADDICK, O. J., DURDEN, K., WATSON, P. G., AND ATKINSON, S. (1984). Screening for refractive errors in 6–9 month old infants by photorefraction. *Br. J. Ophthalmol.* 68, 105–112.

ATKINSON, J., BRADDICK, O., WATTAM-BELL, J., DURDEN, K., BOBIER, W., POINTER, J., AND ATKINSON, S. (1987b). Photorefractive screening of infants and effects of refractive correction. *Invest. Ophthalmol. Vis. Sci.* 28 (suppl.), 399.

ATKINSON, J., GARDNER, N., TRICKLEBANK, J., AND ANKER, S. (1989). Atkinson Battery of Child Development for Examining Functional Vision (ABCDEFV). *Ophthalmic Physiol. Opt.* 9.

ATKINSON, J., PIMM-SMITH, E., EVANS, C., HARDING, G., AND BRADDICK, O. J. (1986a). Visual crowding in young children. *Doc. Ophthalmol. Proc. Ser.* 45, 210–213.

ATKINSON, J., SMITH, J., ANKER, S., WATTAM-BELL, J., BRADDICK, O. J., AND MOORE, A. T. (1991). Binocularity and amblyopia before and after early strabismus surgery. *Invest. Ophthalmol. Vis. Sci.* 32, 820.

ATKINSON, J., WATTAM-BELL, J., PIMM-SMITH, E., EVANS, C., AND

BRADDICK, O. J. (1986b). Comparison of rapid procedures in forced choice preferential looking for estimating acuity in infants and young children. *Doc. Ophthalmol. Proc. Ser.* 45, 192–200.

BANKS, M. S. (1980a). Infant refraction and accommodation. *Int. Ophthalmol. Clin.* 20, 205–232.

BANKS, M. S. (1980b). The development of visual accommodation during early infancy. *Child Dev.* 51, 646–666.

BANKS, M. S., ASLIN, R. N., AND LETSON, R. D. (1975). Sensitive period for the development of human binocular vision. *Science* 190, 675–677.

BAX, M. C. O., AND WHITMORE, K. (1990). Health for all children [book review]. *Arch. Dis. Child.* 65, 141–142.

BEARDSELL, R. (1989). Orthoptic visual screening at 3½ years by Huntingdon Health Authority. *Br. Orthoptic J.* 46, 7–13.

BELLUGI U., ET AL. (in press). Language, cognition and brain organization in a neurodevelopmental disorder. In M. GUNNAR AND C. NELSON (eds.). *Developmental Behavioural Neuroscience.* Hillsdale, NJ: Erlbaum.

BLAKEMORE, C. (1978). Maturation and modification in the developing visual system. In R. HELD, H. W. LEIBOWITZ, AND H. L. TEUBER (eds.). *Handbook of Sensory Physiology. Vol. VIII. Perception.* Heidelberg: Springer.

BOOTHE, R. G., DOBSON, V., AND TELLER, D. Y. (1985). Postnatal development of vision in human and nonhuman primates. *Annu. Rev. Neurosci.* 8, 495–545.

BRADDICK, O. J., AND ATKINSON, J. (1983). Photorefractive techniques: application in testing infants and young children. In *Transactions of the British College of Ophthalmic Opticians (Optometrists) 1st International Congress.* Vol. 2, pp. 26–34.

BRADDICK, O. J., ATKINSON, J., FRENCH, J., AND HOWLAND, H. C. (1979). A photorefractive study of infant accommodation. *Vision Res.* 19, 1319–1330.

BRADDICK, O. J., ATKINSON, J., WATTAM-BELL, J., ANKER, S., AND NORRIS, V. (1988). Videorefractive screening of accommodative performance in infants. *Invest. Ophthalmol. Vis. Sci.* 29 (suppl.), 60.

CASTANERA DE MOLINA, A., MUNOZ, L. G., AND CASTANERA, A. S. (1989). El metodo de fotorrefraccion coaxial isotropica (VPR-1) en la deteccion precoz de la ambliopia. Presented at the X Congreso de la Sociedad Espanola de Estrabologia, Madrid.

COURT, D. (1975). *Report of the Committee on the Child Health Services.* London: HMSO.

DOBSON, V. (1991). Posterior pole status and grating acuity at 12 months following cryotherapy for retinopathy of prematurity. In *Transactions of the 3rd Meeting of the Child Vision Research Society, Rotterdam.*

EHRLICH, M. I., REINECKE, R. D., AND SIMONS, K. (1983). Preschool vision screening for amblyopia and strabismus: programs, methods, guidelines, 1983. *Surv. Ophthalmol.* 28(3), 145–163.

HALL, D. B. M. (ED.) (1989). *Health for All Children (Report of the Joint Working Party on Child Health Surveillance).* Oxford: Oxford University Press.

HILTON, A. F., AND STANLEY, J. C. (1972). Pitfalls in testing children's vision by the Sheridan Gardiner single optotype method. *Br. J. Ophthalmol.* 56, 135–139.

HOLLAND, W. W., AND STEWART, S. S. (1990). *Screening in Health Care.* Nuffield: Nuffield Provincial Hospitals Trust.

HOOD, B., AND ATKINSON, J. (1990). Sensory visual loss and cognitive deficits in the selective attentional system of normal infants and neurologically impaired children. *Dev. Med. Child Neurol.* 32, 1067–1077.

HOWLAND, H. C. (1991). Advances in instrumentation for biometry of infant refractive error. *Invest. Ophthalmol. Vis. Sci.* 32(4) (suppl.), xii.

HOWLAND, H. C., ATKINSON, J., BRADDICK, O., AND FRENCH, J. (1978). Infant astigmatism measured by photorefraction. *Science* 202, 331–333.

HOWLAND, H. C., BRADDICK, O. J., ATKINSON, J., AND HOWLAND, B. (1983). Optics of photorefraction: orthogonal and isotropic methods. *J. Opt. Soc. Am.* 73, 1701–1708.

HUBEL, D. H., AND WIESEL, T. N. (1965). Binocular interaction in striate cortex of kittens reared with artificial squint. *J. Neurophysiol.* 28, 1041–1059.

HYVARINEN, L. (1988). Vision and eye screening in Finland: an overview. Presented at the Joint Meeting of the American Orthoptic Council and the American Association of Certified Orthoptists, Dallas.

INGRAM, R. M. (1979). Refraction as a means of predicting squint and amblyopia in preschool siblings of children known to have these defects. *Br. J. Ophthalmol.* 63, 238–242.

INGRAM, R. M., ET AL. (1985). A first attempt to prevent squint and amblyopia by spectacle correction of abnormal refractions from age 1 year. *Br. J. Ophthalmol.* 69, 851–853.

INGRAM, R. M., TRAYNAR, M. J., WALKER, C., AND WILSON, J. M. (1979). Screening for refractive errors at age 1 year: a pilot study. *Br. J. Ophthalmol.* 63, 243–250.

JACOBSON, S. G., MOHINDRA, I., AND HELD, R. (1982). Visual acuity in infants with ocular diseases. *Am. J. Ophthalmol.* 93, 198–209.

McCLELLAN, A. V. (1977). Area vision screening. *Br. Orthoptic J.* 34(26), 2833.

MILES, F. A., AND JUDGE, S. J. (1982). In G. LENNERSTRAND, D. S. ZEE, AND E. KELLER (eds.). *Functional Basis of Ocular Motility Disorders.* Oxford: Pergamon Press.

MITCHELL, D. E. (1981). Sensitive periods in visual development. In R. N. ASLIN, J. R. ALBERTS, AND M. R. PETERSON (eds.). *The Development of Perception. Vol. 2. The Visual System.* Orlando, FL: Academic Press.

MITCHELL, D. E., FREEMAN, R. D., MILLODOT, M., AND HAEGERSTROM, G. (1973). Meridional amblyopia: evidence for modification of the human visual system by early visual experience. *Vision Res.* 13, 535–558.

MOHINDRA, I., HELD, R., GWIAZDA, J., AND BRILL, S. (1978). Astigmatism in infants. *Science* 202, 329–331.

ROYAL NATIONAL INSTITUTE FOR THE BLIND (1990). *New Directions: Towards a Better Future for Multihandicapped Visually Impaired Children and Young People.* RNIB.

SCOTTISH HOME AND HEALTH DEPARTMENT (1991). *Scottish Low Birthweight Study.* Social Paediatric and Obstetric Research Unit, University of Glasgow.

SHERIDAN, M. D. (1976). Manual for the STYCAR vision tests. Slough: NFER Publishing.

SOMOV, E. E. (1989). The videorefractometry for the children of different age on the device of Clement Clarke International Ltd (London). Presented at the Plenary Meeting of the Leningrad Scientific Medical Society of Ophthalmologists.

TAYLOR, D., AND RICE, N. S. C. (1982). Congenital cataract, a cause of preventable child blindness. *Arch. Dis. Child.* 57, 165–167.

VAN DER LEM, G. J., ET AL. (eds.) (1990). Early detection of vision, hearing, and language disorders in childhood. In *Final Report of Workshop Sponsored by Commission of the European Communities, Concerted Action Committee on Health Service Research.*

VON NOORDEN, G. K. (1974). Factors involved in the production of amblyopia. *Br. J. Ophthalmol.* 58, 158–175.

WATTAM-BELL, J., BRADDICK, O., ATKINSON, J., AND DAY, J. (1987). Measures of infant binocularity in a group at risk for strabismus. *Clin. Vis. Sci.* 1, 327–336.

22 | Detection and treatment of congenital esotropia

STEVEN M. ARCHER

Although not a new topic, a chapter devoted to congenital esotropia must be prefaced with some discussion of its definition. It is a relatively common entity that is easy to recognize clinically when the presentation is typical; in the spectrum of childhood esotropias, however, it is not always easy to decide whether a given case falls into the category of congenital esotropia. After exclusion of better defined entities (Duane syndrome, abducens palsy, accommodative esotropia, esotropia associated with global neurological disease) the most important factor in the diagnosis of congenital esotropia has traditionally been the age of onset. In the original use of the term congenital esotropia (Costenbader, 1950), an onset of the deviation before 6 months of age was an essential part of the definition. The term infantile esotropia was subsequently introduced for esotropia with an onset before 12 months of age (Costenbader, 1961). This usage may have originally been intended to denote a broad diagnostic category that included other entities as well; however, the term has subsequently been used synonymously with congenital esotropia to reflect uncertainty about the actual age of onset in this group of patients. To avoid becoming bogged down in semantics, the historical term congenital esotropia is retained for the purposes of this discussion. However, the onset of congenital esotropia and its relation to the normal development of ocular alignment has implications beyond any controversy over the correctness of the terminology.

Developmental considerations suggest another basis for the definition of congenital esotropia (Romano, 1971). If binocular cooperation normally develops after 4 months, infants with an onset of esotropia prior to this age would not have an opportunity to experience normal binocular vision. Therefore Romano's definition of congenital esotropia was "the presence of a constant esodeviation at 4 months of age." The age of onset that can be properly attributed to congenital esotropia and its relation to the normal development of ocular alignment are explored in this section.

DETECTION OF CONGENITAL ESOTROPIA

Because the hallmark sign of congenital esotropia is readily appreciated by direct observation, detection is largely a question of examining an infant at the right time and correctly interpreting any esotropia that may be found. If the ocular deviation of congenital esotropia is present at birth, the newborn nursery would be an ideal place for detecting this condition. Essentially all babies are available for examination as they pass through the nursery, and a neonatal diagnosis may be optimal in terms of treatment options. Absence of esotropia at birth would make detection efforts more complicated. If congenital esotropia is an acquired condition, cases could be detected only as the deviation develops. On the other hand, if the term "congenital esotropia" is technically correct and the as yet unidentified underlying defect is an innate condition that manifests only at a later stage of development, it may still be possible to find a means of detecting this defect before the esotropia develops.

Parents of infants with congenital esotropia often give a history of the eyes crossing since birth. The fact that esotropia is rarely if ever documented during the neonatal period is not necessarily inconsistent with the parents' observations because ophthalmologists do not routinely examine otherwise healthy neonates, and those with esotropia are generally not referred until long after the deviation is first noted. The picture is further confused by the fact that visual behavior in neonates is difficult to evaluate and tends not to be scrutinized closely by parents or physicians.

Screening Neonates for Esotropia

In an initial attempt to detect congenital esotropia during the neonatal period, 1219 neonates were examined in a newborn nursery; not a single case of esotropia was identified (Nixon et al., 1985). Given the reported 1%

incidence of congenital esotropia (Graham, 1974; Friedman et al., 1980), it was argued statistically that there should have been at least one patient who would develop congenital esotropia in a sample of this size. It was concluded that congenital esotropia cannot be detected during the neonatal period. This conclusion remained suspect, however, because there was no follow-up to confirm the inclusion of congenital esotropia patients and to allow direct correlation of the neonatal motility findings with the eventual diagnosis of congenital esotropia. Moreover, there was reason to suspect that the incidence of congenital esotropia in the study population was significantly lower than might be expected from the previously published incidence figures. Perhaps the most important contribution of this study was the demonstration that in most neonates sufficient visual behavior can be elicited for a meaningful (although gross) ocular motility examination.

The initial conclusion of Nixon and coworkers was supported by two subsequent studies that were specifically designed to correlate neonatal motility findings with the eventual diagnosis of congenital esotropia (Friedrich and de Decker, 1987; Archer et al., 1989). Friedrich and de Decker examined 1024 neonates and obtained follow-up examinations on about 180 of them. Sufficient follow-up for the confirmation of any diagnoses of congenital esotropia was difficult to obtain; however, none of the infants suspected of having congenital esotropia was esotropic as a neonate. One infant had neonatal esotropia that resolved at 2 months of age. Ten others first developed esotropia at 1–3 months of age; four of them were not available for follow-up, and in the remainder the disorder resolved spontaneously.

In the study by Archer and coworkers (1989), 3316 neonates were examined. Follow-up to an age of at least 4 months was obtained for 582 of these infants; and three cases of congenital esotropia were identified in this cohort. As neonates, one of these infants was grossly orthotropic, one had a small exotropia, and one was orthotropic with a small exotropia noted on a subsequent examination at 2 months of age; none had esotropia as neonates. This study established definitively that esotropia during the neonatal period is not necessarily a prerequisite for the diagnosis of congenital esotropia. Because there was nothing to distinguish the ocular motility of the three congenital esotropia patients from normal neonates, it appears that in most cases there is no basis for the detection of congenital esotropia during the neonatal period. These data, however, do not exclude the possible existence of a minor subset of congenital esotropia patients who have esotropia at birth.

A small number (0.7%) of neonates in this study had transient esodeviations. Most were unimpressive, small, intermittent deviations, but two had larger, more constant esotropias that would have been called congenital esotropia if the subsequent course had been consistent with this diagnosis. All neonatal esodeviations resolved by 2 months of age. It is possible that neonatal esotropia is associated with an increased risk of persistent esodeviation; however, the spontaneous resolution of the esodeviation in all three patients in both this study and the Friedrich and de Decker study suggests that neonatal esotropia is an incidental finding. If so, some of the occasionally convincing anecdotal reports of congenital esotropia dating from birth could be explained as the rare infant with a neonatal esodeviation who happens to develop congenital esotropia, unrelated to the neonatal alignment.

The findings from these infant studies make detection of congenital esotropia a complicated problem. It would be helpful if one could examine infants of a specific age and be certain of detecting most cases of congenital esotropia early in the course of the disorder; these studies, however, seem to show an ill-defined age of onset that is generally not at birth. On the other hand, when esotropia is observed in an infant, there appears to be no way of knowing with certainty whether it is a case of congenital esotropia and not just a benign transient phenomenon. Is there an age at which most congenital esotropia cases can be detected and yet be distinguished from transient neonatal esotropia? Insights and perhaps even an answer to this question may be provided by comparing the course of congenital esotropia with the development of ocular alignment in normal infants.

Orthotropization of Normal Infants

Although esotropia was rarely seen in these studies of neonatal alignment, good ocular alignment was hardly the rule. Exotropia was at least as prevalent as orthotropia (Nixon et al., 1985; Friedrich and de Decker, 1987; Sondhi et al., 1988; Archer et al., 1989). This observation had previously been made in sleeping neonates (Réthy, 1969) and in photographic studies of infant alignment (Ling, 1942; Salapatek and Kessen, 1966; Wickelgren, 1967, 1969) but was discounted as an artifact due to a large angle κ (Slater and Findlay, 1972) or a Bell's phenomenon in drowsy infants. Further studies sidestepped the problems inherent in using the center of the pupil to judge the direction of gaze for an individual eye by looking at the relative change in alignment between the two eyes at various fixation distances (Slater and Findlay, 1975; Aslin, 1977). It was found that infants make more or less appropriate relative changes in vergence angle for fixation of objects at various distances. It has thus been concluded that the infant's eyes must be aligned if the infant makes changes in vergence position for the presumed purpose of maintaining ocular alignment.

All these data show is that infants have an accommodative convergence/accommodation (AC/A) ratio; they do not support any conclusion about the ocular alignment. As an illustration, imagine performing the same tests on a (not at all unusual) congenital esotropia patient with a 30 Δ deviation at both 6 meters and 30 cm fixation distances. Although the patient has made a change in vergence position to maintain the same vergence relative to the fixation target at the two fixation distances, all that can be concluded is that the AC/A ratio is relatively normal. It would be erroneous to conclude on this basis that the eyes were aligned. Although a significant positive angle κ is frequently present and needs to be accounted for, it does not appear to account fully for the ocular divergence seen in the previous photographic studies (Salapatek et al., 1972). It has been our experience that, when not actively attending, neonates often assume a symmetrically divergent eye position that could be mistaken for fixation with a large angle κ. In the current generation of studies (Nixon et al., 1985; Friedrich and de Decker, 1987; Sondhi et al., 1988; Archer et al., 1989) the data are controlled for inattention and fixation someplace other than the intended target because the examiner interactively verifies refixation behavior on his or her face before judging the ocular alignment. Motility findings were reported as indeterminate in any infant for whom refixation behavior could not be confirmed. In these studies, neonatal exotropia appears to be a real finding because the fixating eye can be identified interactively, and its line of sight and consequently the angle κ can be judged. An infant was not designated exodeviated unless the ocular divergence was larger than could be accounted for by the magnitude of the angle κ. A large angle κ also cannot account for the spontaneous alternation of fixation, the intermittence of the deviation, and day-to-day variability of the exodeviation that were frequently observed during the course of these studies. Cover testing, the clinical gold standard for judging ocular alignment, is not subject to error due to the angle κ. Unfortunately, cover testing cannot be carried out on neonates because they behave poorly when one eye is occluded, usually by assuming a divergent position with the unoccluded eye and ceasing to exhibit refixation behavior. However, the true nature of the exotropia could be confirmed by cover testing on some of the older infants (usually 2 months or older).

Neonatal ocular alignment is not consistently orthotropic because, unlike the closed-loop vergence system of an adult, which maintains registration of the two retinal images, the sensory limb of the vergence loop in neonates is, if at all, only loosely coupled to motor vergence activity. In addition to the high prevalence of ocular deviations (mostly exotropia), the variability of alignment and absence of a prism vergence response

(Aslin, 1977) support the concept that young infants do not have a closed-loop vergence system. At some point an infant must make the transition from the loosely coupled vergence system of a neonate to the closed-loop vergence system of an adult, resulting in stable orthotropia. It may occur as a result of maturation of the neural pathways through which the sensory cortex exerts control over the motor vergence centers in the brainstem, or it may simply reflect increased sensory appreciation of binocular disparity and diplopia. There is no reason to expect it to occur at the same age in each infant; indeed, the ages at which the onset of orthotropia occurs in a cohort of infants can be reasonably well described by a normal distribution curve.

Figure 22-1A shows how the reported data for the percent of orthotropic infants at various ages (Archer et al., 1989) can be approximated by a cumulative normal distribution function. The equation used in this weighted least-squares fit is

Infants appearing to be orthotropic at a given age

$$= C + (100 - C) * CDF [(Age - M)/S]$$

where M = mean onset age; S = standard deviation of the onset age; CDF = cumulative normal distribution function representing the sum of all infants who have made the transition to a closed-loop vergence system prior to a given age; C = a fixed percentage (21.2%) of the remaining infants without a closed-loop vergence system who, by chance, happen to be close enough to straight to be called orthotropic by the gross examination technique. Figure 22-1B shows the normal distribution with the same mean and standard deviation used to fit the curve in Figure 22-1A. With these cross-sectional data, this curve represents the rate at which the fraction of orthotropic infants in the population is increasing. By inference, one can think of it as the distribution of ages at which individual infants make the transition to a closed-loop vergence system. In this model the mean age for this transition is 2.7 months, and the standard deviation is 1.2 months.

Onset of Congenital Esotropia

The age of transition to a closed-loop vergence system is a point of special significance for the diagnosis of congenital esotropia. As alluded to earlier, if an infant's onset of esotropia occurs after closure of the vergence loop, there would be an opportunity for normal binocular sensory experience during the interval between these two events. Such an infant might have a better prognosis than that usually associated with congenital esotropia. On the other hand, esotropia prior to the age at which closure of the vergence loop would normally occur is of questionable significance. It cannot be regarded as

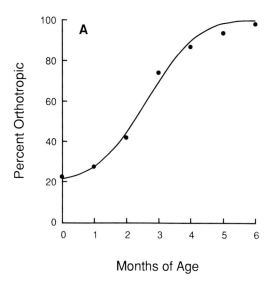

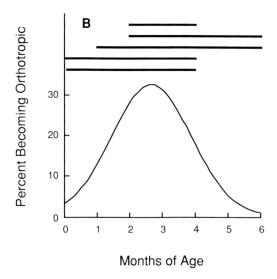

FIG. 22-1. (A) Percent of apparently orthotropic infants at various ages. Points represent actual data (Archer et al., 1989). Curve is the weighted least-squares fit of cumulative normal distribution function to these data. (B) Normal distribution for age of onset of orthotropia derived from above cumulative normal distribution function. Horizontal bars are possible onset age ranges for all infants known to the author who were examined prior to the onset of esotropia and later diagnosed as having congenital esotropia.

an anomalous binocular sensory experience because normal infants do not have their eyes aligned at this time either; moreover, the esotropia may subsequently resolve if and when closure of the vergence loop occurs, as it did in the three documented cases of significant esotropia in neonates. Because of these difficulties of interpreting esotropia before and after closure of the vergence loop, detection of congenital esotropia is ideally based on the ocular alignment at the exact age that closure of the vergence loop should be occurring.

The age of the expected transition to a closed-loop vergence system may be more than just a theoretically clean point at which to detect congenital esotropia. An etiological significance has been suggested (Archer et al., 1989). It was hypothesized that the pathological deviation of congenital esotropia is a result of the attempt to close a defective vergence loop. Further speculation placed the defect in the coupling between the sensory and motor portions of the vergence loop, as the motor output (full abduction and normal AC/A ratio) and sensory input (documented stereopsis, at least early in the course of congenital esotropia) (Archer et al., 1986; Rogers et al., 1986; Birch et al., 1990) portions of the loop appear to be comparatively intact. The ocular alignment of a neonate who eventually develops congenital esotropia is indistinguishable from that of a normal neonate because the defective portion of the vergence loop is not in use by either infant during the neonatal period. It is only later, when the infant with congenital esotropia attempts to make the transition to a closed-loop vergence system, that the defect in this portion of the vergence loop becomes evident and a large, manifest strabismus develops. Nonrefractive accommo-

dative esotropia might provide an analogous example where an abnormal coupling constant (the AC/A ratio in this case) between normal accommodation and vergence systems result in esotropia when the infant's development reaches a point that demands active use of these systems.

The conception of this vergence loop defect hypothesis originated with the observation that infants with congenital esotropia apparently develop esotropia at about the same age that normal infants (including those who had esotropia as a neonate) are becoming orthotropic. This relation between the development of normal ocular alignment and the onset of the deviation in congenital esotropia is now explored in more detail. The exact onset of esotropia in any individual case of congenital esotropia is difficult to establish, and it may evolve gradually over a period of several weeks. There are several infants, however—four reported cases (Archer and Helveston, 1989; Archer et al., 1989) and one from the author's current practice—who have had documented motility examinations prior to the onset of esotropia and were subsequently diagnosed as having congenital esotropia. This finding restricts the possible age ranges for the onset of esotropia in these infants, which are plotted as the horizontal bars in the upper portion of Figure 22-1B. Although the range for each infant is broad, the ages at which these ranges overlap coincides with the peak of the normal curve shown in the lower portion of Figure 22-1B. Empirically then, the distribution for the age of onset of the pathological deviation in congenital esotropia is grossly homologous to the distribution for the age of transition to a closed-loop vergence system in normal infants. The two distributions should, of course, be identical if the hypothesis regarding the deviation of congenital esotropia as the result of the attempt to close a defective vergence loop is correct.

Recognizing the relation between the onset of the deviation in congenital esotropia and the onset of orthotropia in normal infants is, in itself, of little practical value, as the age at which these events occur shows some variation and cannot be known in an individual infant except in retrospect. However, a model such as the one developed here can provide a useful statistical handle on a number of issues pertaining to the detection of congenital esotropia. The percent of infants with congenital esotropia who will manifest their esotropia at a given age can be predicted from this model. For example, more than 99% of all cases of congenital esotropia should be detected by a program in which infants are screened at 6 months of age. Although there is no reason to believe that an onset before 6 months of age has any nosological significance, it appears that Constenbader's original definition of congenital esotropia has a certain practical aptness. Statistical inferences about individual infants can also be made. For example, there is slightly less than a 15% likelihood that a 4-month-old infant with esotropia has yet to attempt closure of the vergence loop and could therefore still have resolution of the esotropia. Ironically, the diagnosis of congenital esotropia is probably more certain in such an infant if the esotropia is known to have developed subsequently rather than having been present at birth.

TREATMENT OF CONGENITAL ESOTROPIA

The standard treatment for congenital esotropia is surgical. Other modes of therapy such as orthoptic exercises, segmental occlusion, and plus lenses for low hyperopia have been advocated; reports of these treatments, however, have tended to be either philosophical or anecdotal. None of these methods has gained wide acceptance because of this lack of rigorously documented efficacy. Although having become the standard of care, most aspects of surgical treatment either remain controversial or are the object of continued refinement efforts. There can be a number of secondary or independent contributory problems associated with congenital esotropia such as A and V patterns, inferior oblique overaction, dissociated vertical deviation, latent nystagmus with or without a compensatory head posture, hyperopia with an accommodative component of esotropia, and amblyopia. When present, these factors may also require surgical or nonsurgical treatment; however, the following discussion is limited to treatment of the horizontal strabismus that is the hallmark feature of congenital esotropia.

Motor Alignment

For treatment of congenital esotropia, there is general agreement that perfect alignment, bifoveal fixation, is seldom obtained (Parks, 1984). However, a subnormal form of binocular vision referred to as monofixation syndrome can be achieved with some regularity and is considered an optimal result (Parks, 1975). Because a residual deviation of 8 Δ or less is compatible with the development of monofixation syndrome (Parks, 1969), realignment of the eyes to within 8 or 10 Δ of straight has become the generally accepted definition of a surgical success. This definition of a motor success is the one used in the following discussion.

Historically, surgery for congenital esotropia has been fairly conservative with an emphasis on avoiding overcorrections. The number of muscles operated on and the amount of surgery performed on each muscle was limited; as a result, satisfactory alignment was not often achieved with a single procedure. Correction of esotropia was regarded as a staged treatment (Sugar, 1952) in which the options left open for a second procedure were an important consideration when planning the initial surgery (Arnoult et al., 1976). More recently, concern has shifted away from whether satisfactory alignment can be achieved at all and emphasis placed on achieving satisfactory alignment with a minimum number of procedures, preferably one. There is no disadvantage to more aggressive surgery for congenital esotropia if an effective means for dealing with overcorrections exists. The worst outcome, a reoperation with its associated expense and risk of repeat anesthesia, is the usual outcome with more conservative surgery. Optimizing the success rate for the initial procedure also makes sense in terms of providing any possible sensory benefit from ocular alignment as quickly as possible.

Specifics of Surgical Approach. The traditional surgical treatment of congenital esotropia has consisted in (1) recession of the medial rectus muscle and resection of the lateral rectus muscle of one eye, or (2) recession of the medial recti of both eyes. Comparison of these two procedures generally demonstrated a similarly low success rate when either was performed as the initial procedure (Miles and Burian, 1967; Arnoult et al., 1976; Zak and Morin, 1984; Bartley et al., 1985), but no consistent advantage of one over the other was found. As discussed below, improvements in the bimedial recession have led to increased satisfaction with this technique; however, no study has demonstrated any inherent advantage of bimedial recession, and it is possible that similar results could also be obtained with larger recess-resect procedures. Perhaps because of the tissue-sparing aesthetics of a recession procedure, as much as any other reason, bimedial recession is currently the two-muscle procedure favored by most strabismus surgeons.

A significant improvement in the initial success rate with a two-muscle procedure was reported after several modifications to the usual bimedial recession technique. An 85.7% success rate was obtained when bimedial recession was performed with recession of the overlying conjunctiva and a simple system of grading the recession in three increments based on the distance from the limbus rather than the original insertion of the muscle (Helveston et al., 1983). Subsequent studies confirmed the success rate for this regimen of recessing the medial rectus to a specified distance from the limbus (Kushner and Morton, 1984), at least for moderate deviations (Richler and Barsoum-Homsy, 1989); however, it was not clear which factors contributed to the higher success rate. Although there is some evidence that recession of the overlying conjunctiva can enhance the effect of a medial rectus recession (Willshaw et al., 1986; Kushner and Morton, 1987), the success rate did not appear to suffer from elimination of this portion of the regimen (Kushner and Morton, 1984).

The remaining question is why recession from the limbus produced better results. The rationale for measuring the recession from the limbus was that it reduced the variability of the reattachment site. The medial rectus insertion is variable and often significantly closer to the limbus than the 5.5 mm that is usually assumed (Goldstein, 1969; Helveston et al., 1978; Apt, 1980; Barsoum-Homsy, 1981). It results in great variability of the reattachment site if a recession is measured from the original insertion. The muscle may inadvertently be left further anterior or posterior to the equator of the globe than might have been intended (Rogers and Bremer, 1985). Additionally, the original insertion site can shift during the course of the procedure (Kushner et al., 1987; Keech et al., 1990), which introduces more variability to the reattachment site for a recession measured from the insertion. However, had the recessions measured from the limbus in these studies been measured from the insertion, they would have been relatively large compared to what was customary at the time. It is therefore conceivable that using the limbus as a reference point is not, of itself, responsible for the high success rate, and that the same results could have been obtained by performing larger recessions measured from the insertion (Greenwald, 1984; Saunders, 1984). Analysis of this possibility showed that the response to bimedial recession is better correlated with the recession distance from the original insertion and that the distance from the limbus is not an independent predictor of surgical response (Kushner et al., 1989b). Thus it appears that the most rational point from which to measure a recession is the original insertion if artifacts due to intraoperative manipulation can be minimized. This point is consistent with the view that the major effect of a recession is due to alteration of the muscle's length-tension curve rather than alteration of the relation of its insertion to the center of rotation of the globe (Biesner, 1971; Kushner and Vrabec, 1987).

Surgical Dose-Response Curve. In an effort to refine the appropriate amount of surgery for a given preoperative deviation, the relation between the amount of correction obtained with a bimedial recession and the size of the recession has been analyzed in the context of a dose-response curve (Mims et al., 1985; Kushner and Morton, 1987), a concept borrowed from the field of pharmacology. Titrating the "dose" of surgery to the preoperative deviation is hardly new to the field of strabismology; however, computerized curve-fitting of retrospective data has recently permitted more detailed guidelines to be generated. A prospective study (Mims and Wood, 1989) showed an 85% success rate when bimedial recessions were graded according to such a retrospectively generated curve; however, this result does not necessarily validate either the dose-response concept in general or any specific curve in particular for the reasons discussed below.

When the size of the recession is a function of the preoperative deviation, it is not possible to determine the extent to which each of these variables is an independent predictor of the surgical effect. To illustrate with an extreme example, suppose the response to surgery (regardless of the amount) is related only to the size of the original deviation. As outrageous as it sounds, it is not a new concept and has been supported by data from one study in which the response to surgery was highly correlated with the preoperative deviation despite the fact that all patients were treated with the same 6 mm medial rectus recessions (Scobee, 1951). It has also been found in more recent work that the preoperative deviation is strongly correlated with the amount of correction obtained per millimeter of recession (Kushner and Morton, 1987). If the response to surgery is a function of the preoperative deviation, any hypothetical dose-response curve will appear to show a tight dose-response relation because the amount of surgery performed is correlated with the preoperative deviation, the factor to which the surgical response is correlated. This scenario cannot be entirely correct because large medial rectus recessions have certainly led to markedly improved success rates; however, if the relation between the size of recession and the amount of correction is as strong as generally believed, it becomes difficult to explain how two completely different prescriptions for the amount of recession—one with only three gross gradations (Helveston et al., 1983) and the other with recessions specified to within 0.1 mm for each 1 Δ increment in preoperative deviation (Mims et al., 1985)—

could have comparably high success rates. It appears that enough surgery must be done to bring the patient within striking range of orthotropia; but having made this statement, the exact amount of surgery within this range may not be critical.

Uniform and Selective Surgery. Although the overall success rate in surgery for congenital esotropia has improved, correction of the largest deviations with a single procedure has remained problematical. There are two basic ways in which the surgical effect can be increased to deal with these large deviations. One is to increase the amount of surgery performed on each muscle, and the other is to increase the number of muscles operated on. Claims of increased success rates with the latter approach (Fisher et al., 1968; Goldstein, 1974; Foster et al., 1976) preceded the current use of larger bimedial recessions. Operating on two, three, or four muscles at the initial surgery, depending on the size of the preoperative deviation, has been termed the *selective approach*. Using a two-muscle procedure as the initial surgery, regardless of the preoperative deviation, has been termed the *uniform approach*. Advocates of the selective approach point to better initial success rates for large deviations (Lee and Dyer, 1983; Scott et al., 1986). However, large bimedial recessions, on the order of 7 mm, can also produce high success rates in large deviations, apparently without crippling adduction (Hess and Calhoun, 1979; Edwards et al., 1984; Skov and Mazow, 1985; Szmyd et al., 1985; Nelson et al., 1987). It appears that initially satisfactory alignment can be obtained in most cases with one procedure by either the uniform or the selective approach. All else being equal, the technically easier operation on fewer muscles with the associated shorter operating time should favor the uniform approach. However, the subsequent risk of deteriorating alignment, particularly the development of secondary exotropia, may not be equal with these two approaches. If long-term studies eventually show a significant advantage in this regard for one approach or the other, it will certainly be the most important factor when choosing between them.

Long-Term Results. Up to this point, the high success rates described with an initial procedure (80+%) have reflected relatively short-term outcome results after only a few months or a few years. Because the pathogenesis of congenital esotropia is fundamentally unknown, surgical treatment is necessarily directed at its secondary manifestations rather than the underlying defect itself. Although reasonably good ocular alignment can be obtained in the short run, recurrent strabismus should occur frequently if the original defect that prevented proper closure of the vergence loop and the normal development of orthotropia remains. It is not surprising,

then, that an initially good surgical result is not necessarily stable over time (Hiles et al., 1980; Lunder et al., 1985). The development of dissociated vertical deviation and inferior oblique overaction may require secondary surgery for cosmetic reasons. Accommodative esotropia frequently develops and requires spectacle or miotic therapy (Freeley et al., 1983; Nirenberg and Mazow, 1985; Baker and DeYoung-Smith, 1988).

The most striking late complication in patients who initially appeared to be treated successfully for congenital esotropia is the development of a large secondary exotropia. Most strabismus surgeons have anecdotal experience with this problem, and it has been reported with some regularity in long-term studies of congenital esotropia. The possible magnitude of the problem, however, has not been appreciated until recently. In a study of congenital esotropia patients (patients with other neurological disease were specifically excluded) who were aligned to within 10 Δ at 6 weeks and 6 months postoperatively, the prevalence of secondary exotropia was 11% at 3 years and 25% at 6 years (Caputo et al., 1990). Only about half of the patients initially included in this study had follow-up at 6 years, so it is possible that the increase in the percent of patients with secondary exotropia between 3 and 6 years of follow-up may have been inflated by inadvertent selection for those who continued to have problems. Within the smaller 6-year follow-up group, however, the actual number of patients with exotropia is larger, so the increase in the percent of patients with exotropia cannot be entirely explained as a selection artifact.

It has been suggested that, if monofixation syndrome develops, the vergence amplitudes found in this condition should ensure stable long-term alignment (Parks, 1969). This contention was supported by one study (Botet et al., 1981) in which congenital esotropia patients with an initially good surgical result were recalled for examination years later. All patients with evidence of monofixation syndrome at that time had also retained good alignment. It was concluded that monofixation is a permanent condition that reduces the chances of needing further surgery; however, the data do not necessarily support this conclusion (Arthur et al., 1989). The manner in which the data were collected makes the association between monofixation and long-term horizontal ocular alignment tautological. At the time of recall, patients could not have been diagnosed as having monofixation syndrome if they did not have good horizontal alignment. The number of patients who previously had monofixation syndrome but lost it and developed a significant postoperative deviation prior to the time of recall cannot be ascertained from these data. It is significant, however, that only 26% of these patients still had monofixation syndrome at the time of recall, suggesting that there may have been some attrition. Other studies are in agreement that monofixation syndrome is not necessarily retained throughout life and does not guarantee stable long-term alignment (Hiles et al., 1980; Lunder et al., 1985; Robb and Rodier, 1987). Longitudinal study of patients with initially good alignment shows that progressively more patients lose their ocular alignment with the passage of time, although it occurs at a less rapid rate in patients who have monofixation syndrome than in those who do not (Arthur et al., 1989). It is an ongoing process; and because this study did not find a postoperative interval at which the deterioration rate drops to zero, it is possible that patients remain at risk for deterioration of their ocular alignment for the remainder of their lives.

Other Refinements. Two other systems of refining the amount of surgery have been proposed. The first involves using the axial length as a factor when adjusting the amount of surgery to be performed (Gillies and Hughes, 1984; Kushner et al., 1989a). The second involves using the ocular deviation under anesthesia in various ways to adjust the amount of surgery intraoperatively (Apt and Isenberg, 1977; Bedrossian, 1983; Lingua et al., 1983, 1986; Romano, 1985; Romano and Gabriel, 1985; Romano et al., 1988; Mims and Wood, 1989). None of these adjustments has been employed prospectively with appropriate controls on a large enough number of patients to verify its usefulness; the adjustments thus remain controversial without widespread acceptance. In general, it is not clear that the potential benefits of additional minor refinements to the amount of surgery are likely to justify the effort. Despite differences between them, most current surgical schedules are converging to the same 80 + % initial success rate. It may be time to entertain the possibility that failure of success rates to go significantly beyond this point and the suboptimal sensory results are not due to subtle errors in the amount of surgery but, rather, reflect a fundamental limitation of a treatment modality that does not directly address the underlying pathophysiology of congenital esotropia.

Sensory Results

The sensory outcome of congenital esotropia treatment is an issue that is closely linked to the question of the optimal age for surgery. It is generally agreed that normal binocular function with normal stereopsis rarely if ever results after treatment of congenital esotropia (Ing et al., 1966). Reported cases with normal stereopsis (40 seconds on the Titmus test) are so rare that there is some question as to whether they have the same pathology as the bulk of congenital esotropia patients (Parks, 1984). Indeed it is possible, particularly in cases where surgery was performed before 6 months of age (van

Selm, 1988), that the infant is in the tail of the normal distribution in Figure 22-1B and has yet to pass through the transition to a closed-loop vergence system. Such a patient may not have had congenital esotropia but, rather, a transient esotropia that would have resolved spontaneously even if surgery had not been performed.

Interpretation of Sensory Testing. Although normal binocular function is not an expected outcome of congenital esotropia treatment, lesser degrees of binocular cooperation may be found. They are referred to as subnormal binocular vision (von Noorden, 1984), microtropia (Helveston and von Noorden, 1967), or monofixation syndrome (Parks, 1969). In studies addressing binocular function in congenital esotropia, a normal response on the Worth 4-dot test at one-third meter is used as evidence of peripheral fusion, and any response on the Titmus stereotest is reported as "gross stereopsis." Both of these findings in the setting of a manifest deviation of 8 Δ or less is used as evidence for diagnosis of monofixation syndrome. It has been pointed out, however, that a "fusion" response on the Worth 4-dot test and "gross stereopsis" are not necessarily proof of fusion, as both can also be found in the setting of manifest strabismus with anomalous retinal correspondence (von Noorden, 1984).

The Worth 4-dot test is questionable as a test of sensory fusion, as it contains no fusible features (von Noorden, 1984). The only portion of the stimulus that is visible to both eyes is the white dot, which is usually perceived with color rivalry. Normal subjects seldom report a yellow dot, the response that occurs with color fusion of a red and a green dot. A "fusion" response on the Worth 4-dot test means only that the retinal correspondence matches the alignment (abnormal retinal correspondence if there is a manifest deviation and normal retinal correspondence if there is not), and that if any central scotoma is present it is smaller than 6 degrees. The greatest value of the Worth 4-dot test is that a "fusion" response correlates with the presence of vergence amplitudes (Parks, 1969).

It would be easy to conclude from the literature that treated congenital esotropia patients frequently have stereopsis; however, these reports are all based on the Titmus test, which is notorious for its nonstereoscopic artifacts (Simons and Reinecke, 1974; Cooper and Warshowsky, 1977; Clarke and Noel, 1990). Often reports of stereopsis on the Titmus test are verified by reversing the test booklet or Polaroid glasses; but even when care is taken to ask for a response without suggesting what the answer should be, artifactual responses still occur (Archer, 1988). Moreover, congenital esotropia patients may in fact have depth perception (Henson and Williams, 1980; Campos et al., 1987), properly termed *bathopsis*. It may occur on the basis of a number of cues: perspective, motion parallax, parallax resulting from the image shift that occurs when alternating fixation between the two eyes (Archer, 1988), and perhaps even binocular disparity. *Stereopsis*, which literally means "seeing solid" (Walls, 1963), is a different matter. Stereopsis is a distinctive sensation that is qualitatively different from anything that can be experienced monocularly. Random-dot stereograms uniquely elicit this sensation in isolation from the context of monocular cues with which it is normally commingled. Comparison of stereotests invariably shows that esotropia patients perform better on the Titmus test than on a random-dot test of stereopsis (Brenneisen et al., 1975; Frisby et al., 1975; Okuda et al., 1977; Cooper et al., 1979; Marsh et al., 1980; Lin and Jeng, 1984; Clarke and Noel, 1990). Typically, even congenital esotropia patients who pass the Titmus test at a fairly small disparity fail to perform on a random-dot test at any disparity. In fact, it is claimed that no congenital esotropia patient with normal stereopsis on a random-dot test has ever been reported (von Noorden, 1990).

Benefits of Early Surgery. Despite these reservations about the meaning of the tests employed, a surprisingly consistent picture has emerged from studies of the sensory outcome in congenital esotropia. Animal studies have shown that anomalous binocular sensory experience early in life, during a "critical period" of development (Yinon, 1976; Berman and Murphy, 1981) can result in loss of behavioral evidence of stereopsis (Crawford et al., 1983) and electrophysiological evidence of cortical binocularity (Hubel and Wiesel, 1965; Yinon and Auerbach, 1975; Crawford and von Noorden, 1979a,b, 1980; Bennett et al., 1980; Crawford et al., 1984; Cynader et al., 1984; Kalil et al., 1984; Chino et al., 1988). Extension of this concept to congenital esotropia in humans suggests that the binocular sensory deficits these patients experience may be secondary to the presence of strabismus during their critical period. If so, patients who are surgically realigned early in their lives should have less anomalous binocular experience during their critical period and a better sensory outcome than those who undergo surgery later.

With rare exception (von Noorden et al., 1972), most studies relating the age of surgical alignment to the sensory outcome show that favorable results are more likely if alignment is achieved before 2 years of age (Ing et al., 1966; Taylor, 1967, 1972; Fisher et al., 1968; Uemura et al., 1973; Foster et al., 1976; Botet et al., 1981; Ing, 1981, 1983a,b; Zak and Morin, 1982; Bateman et al., 1983; Deller, 1988; Teller et al., 1988; von Noorden, 1988). Some of these studies claim to show evidence of binocularity in 90–100% of such patients; however, other studies that were more critical in their application and interpretation of sensory tests indicate

a range of 20–30% (Pratt-Johnson and Tillson, 1983; von Noorden, 1988). One puzzling feature of these studies is that among children whose eyes were aligned before 2 years of age there does not appear to be a significant advantage to being aligned during the early, rather than the latter portion of this time range (Fisher et al., 1968; Foster et al., 1976; Ing, 1983b). In the context of minimizing anomalous experience during the critical period, one would expect that younger should always be better. In any event, it is generally accepted that there is no additional risk in performing surgery as early as 6 months of age so long as the patient can be adequately examined; the conventional recommendation is currently to perform surgery between 6 months and 2 years of age.

New Frontiers

Surgery Before 6 Months. The logical extension of the critical period concept is to perform surgery at an even younger age. Despite the increasing number of infant eyes aligned as early as 6 months of age, the optimum sensory outcome remains the monofixation syndrome. One possible explanation is that the anomalous sensory experience resulting from esotropia has already caused permanent damage by 6 months. This idea is supported by animal studies showing that irreversible loss of cortical binocularity can occur with brief periods of artificial strabismus (Crawford and von Noorden, 1979b). The critical period for binocularity could conceivably begin as early as the time of transition to a closed-loop vergence system. If so, delaying surgery until 6 months of age would permit, on the average, 3.3 months of anomalous sensory experience.

Several objections to earlier surgery may be raised. First, it has been pointed out that if medial rectus recession is performed before 6 months of age, normal growth of the eye may place the equator anterior to the new insertion of the muscle (Swan and Wilkins, 1984), which may lead to crippling of adduction and a high incidence of secondary exotropia. Second, there is concern that surgery before 6 months may include some infants whose esotropia would have resolved spontaneously (Friedrich and de Decker, 1987; Archer et al., 1989). The percent of infants with esotropia at a given age who are potentially normal can be estimated from the normal distribution shown in Figure 22-1. There are also reports of a few patients (without neurological damage) whose esotropia spontaneously resolved well beyond the time of expected vergence loop closure (Clarke and Noel, 1982; Robb and Rodier, 1987); of course these cases pose a problem for surgery performed after 6 months as well. However, many of these patients develop the same constellation of secondary motility problems that are found in congenital esotropia (inferior oblique overaction, dissociated vertical deviation, and latent nystagmus) and probably have the same sensory outcome as well. Figure 22-2 shows the Brückner test of a 13-month-old patient who had photographically documented early-onset esotropia that improved to a small intermittent esotropia. Note that although his alignment was fairly good, he did not fixate bifoveally. Later, his esotropia became more constant; it did not improve with echothiophate iodide, and surgery was performed. Despite reduction to a 6–8 Δ esophoria, he subsequently developed inferior oblique overaction and dissociated vertical deviation. If the benefits of earlier surgical alignment can be proved, it appears that these unusual patients stand to benefit as much as those with a more typical course of congenital esotropia.

The fact that the underlying pathology in congenital esotropia is unknown poses a theoretical problem for the concept of earlier surgery. If surgery does not correct the underlying defect, why should stable and precise alignment compatible with the development of bifoveal fixation be any more likely after surgery than it was at the time esotropia first developed? A possible answer to this question is that, if the offending portion of the vergence loop is only delayed and not completely aberrant, early surgery may afford a second chance at loop closure after that portion of the loop has matured but before there has been significant sensory damage from anomalous binocular experience. One series of congenital esotropia patients operated on before 6 months of age appears to show favorable sensory results (Gale, 1972), and in a second series there is not yet enough follow-up for conclusions (Helveston et al., 1990). Early surgery did not always eliminate the need for reoperations in either series.

Botulinum Toxin. Botulinum toxin chemodenervation has been introduced as an alternative to incisional surgery for treatment of strabismus (Scott, 1981). Certain properties of botulinum treatment make it a particularly interesting alternative for the management of congenital esotropia. Botulinum toxin is a paralytic agent that causes presynaptic interference with acetylcholine release at the neuromuscular junction (Kelly et al., 1979). When botulinum toxin is injected into a medial rectus muscle, it can correct esotropia by producing a temporary medial rectus palsy. An interesting and unexpected finding in congenital esotropia patients treated with botulinum toxin is that they develop a face turn (Magoon, 1984; Magoon and Scott, 1987). The face turn has been construed as evidence of fusion because of its similarity to the face turn seen with Duane syndrome, a nonconcomitant cause of esotropia in infants that is usually associated with normal stereopsis.

Like conventional surgical management, botulinum does not treat the underlying defect of congenital esotropia; it is possible, however, that botulinum treatment bypasses the defective portion of the vergence loop by taking control away from the vergence centers in the

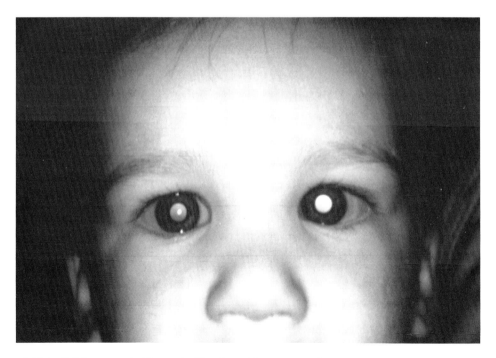

FIG. 22-2. Brückner test of a 13-month-old patient with spontaneously improving intermittent esotropia. Cycloplegic refraction was + 1.00 D in both eyes. Dark red reflex indicates the fixating right eye.

brainstem and allowing the sensory system to control ocular alignment through the neck muscles. As such, botulinum could potentially produce improved sensory results, which cannot be obtained with conventional surgery. Unfortunately, though, once the botulinum has worn off one is again left with the same vergence loop defect that caused the esotropia in the first place. Prolonged maintenance of fusion might be possible (but tedious) with repeated injections of botulinum; however, given this circumstance it would be preferable to find a longer-acting paralytic agent such as cadmium (Breinin et al., 1985).

Published studies dealing with botulinum use in children (Scott, 1987; Magoon, 1989b; Scott et al., 1989, 1990) have demonstrated its safety and efficacy in producing long-term reduction of the strabismic deviation, although multiple injections are often needed to produce satisfactory results (Magoon and Scott, 1987; Magoon, 1989a). As yet, no sensory outcomes from these series have been reported. The only other series in which botulinum-treated congenital esotropia patients are discussed as a specific group (Biglan et al., 1989) included only 12 congenital esotropia patients, and the development of a face turn was not mentioned; the average age of these patients was 6.5 years, however, which may be too old to expect any residual binocular function. This study pointed out that, in addition to the frequent need for reinjection, the prolonged period of misalignment and the occasionally severe blepharoptosis after injection are counterproductive when attempting rapid establishment of ocular alignment to minimize damage from anomalous sensory experience and promote the development of normal binocular function.

Botulinum may have special value in the context of surgery before 6 months of age, as discussed in the previous section. If all that is needed is a period of protection from anomalous binocular experience while some portion of the vergence loop gets a chance to mature, botulinum might be the ideal agent. Its use could be considered even in infants as young as 2−4 months (Scott et al., 1990) because the mechanical effect of botulinum, unlike medial rectus recession, is temporary. Even if intervention during this age range leads to inadvertent treatment of an occasional infant whose problem could have still resolved spontaneously, the botulinum effect eventually wears off and, hopefully, no harm has been done. The possibility of treating any infant unnecessarily is not a matter to be dismissed cavalierly. This type of tradeoff between unnecessary treatment and better outcome is not foreign to the practice of medicine. An analogy might be the removal of a certain number of normal appendices in order to be certain of adequately treating all cases of appendicitis.

Of course, the benefit of esotropia treatment in the 2- to 4-month age range would have to be established in ethically designed controlled studies before any risk of unnecessary intervention would be acceptable.

Another possible use of botulinum in congenital esotropia might be as an adjunct to conventional surgery. Here, one might hope to exploit the advantages of both treatment modalities by intraoperatively injecting a single medial rectus with a comparatively small dose of botulinum at the time of bimedial recession. Because the basic alignment is due to the bimedial recession, this combined procedure should share the high initial success rate of conventional surgery. The contribution of the botulinum is to provide a postoperative period of nonconcomitance during which a face turn can be used to fine-tune the alignment and obtain bifoveal fixation. It is, in effect, a postoperative period of orthoptic fusion exercise. A congenital esotropia patient with a bifoveal result after combined treatment is pictured in the Brückner test photographs shown in Figure 22-3. It is not known at this time whether this postoperative period of binocular experience will prove to be beneficial in regard to the long-term alignment or sensory outcome.

SUMMARY

Detection of congenital esotropia is largely a question of differentiating it from benign transient forms of neonatal strabismus on the one hand and later acquired forms of esotropia on the other. An understanding of the relation between the onset of the deviation in congenital esotropia and the normal orthotropization process may be helpful for providing a statistical approach to making these differentiations and for selecting an optimal age at which to perform screening examinations. With the current focus on intervention at progressively earlier ages, issues regarding the detection and treatment of congenital esotropia have become increasingly intertwined.

Conventional surgical management of congenital esotropia is a well-evolved treatment modality. Considering that it is directed only at a secondary manifestation of the unknown underlying defect, the motor and sensory results are remarkably good; however, subnormal binocular vision is still the best outcome that can be expected. Studies have shown that congenital esotropia patients may have the potential for true stereopsis, at least early in their course (Archer et al., 1986; Rogers et al., 1986; Birch et al., 1990). Any significant new advances in treatment that permit congenital esotropia patients to realize this potential will probably have to come from some new direction in which the underlying pathology is better addressed.

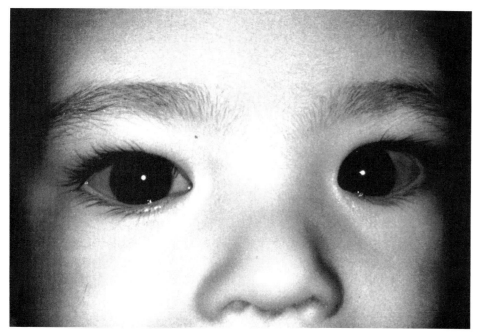

A

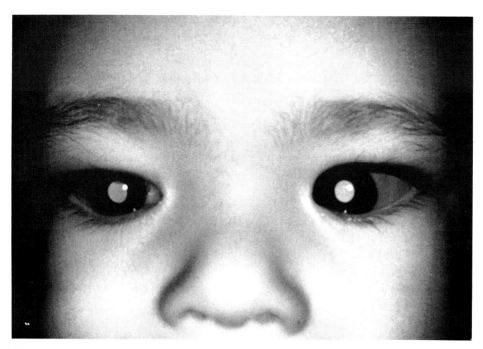

B

FIG. 22-3. Brückner test of a 7-month-old congenital esotropia patient treated with a combination of bimedial recession and botulinum toxin injection of the right medial rectus. (A) Subtle face turn has developed 10 days postoperatively that results in bifoveal fixation, indicated by equally dark fundus reflexes. (B) Off-axis photograph shows expected brightness for nonfixating eyes. This method controls for the possibility that the equal fundus reflexes in (A) were due to neither eye fixating.

360

REFERENCES

APT, L. (1980). An anatomical reevaluation of rectus muscle insertions. *Trans. Am. Ophthalmol. Soc.* 78, 365–375.

APT, L., AND ISENBERG, S. (1977). Eye position of strabismus patients under general anesthesia. *Am. J. Ophthalmol.* 84, 574–579.

ARCHER, S. M. (1988). Stereotest artifacts and the strabismus patient. *Graefes Arch. Clin. Exp. Ophthalmol.* 226, 313–316.

ARCHER, S. M., AND HELVESTON, E. M. (1989). Strabismus and eye movement disorders. In S. J. ISENBERG (eds.). *The Eye in Infancy.* Chicago: Year Book, pp. 215–237.

ARCHER, S. M., HELVESTON, E. M., MILLER, K. K., AND ELLIS, F. D. (1986). Stereopsis in normal infants and infants with congenital esotropia. *Am. J. Ophthalmol.* 101, 591–596.

ARCHER, S. M., SONDHI, N., AND HELVESTON, E. M. (1989). Strabismus in infancy. *Ophthalmology* 96, 133–137.

ARNOULT, J. B., YESHURUN, O., AND MAZOW, M. L. (1976). Comparative study of the surgical management of congenital esotropia of 50 prism diopters or less. *J. Pediatr. Ophthalmol.* 13, 129–131.

ARTHUR, B. W., SMITH, J. T., AND SCOTT, W. E. (1989). Long-term stability of alignment in the monofixation syndrome. *J. Pediatr. Ophthalmol. Strabismus* 26, 224–231 [erratum appears in *J. Pediatr. Ophthalmol. Strabismus* 27(1):following 55, 1990].

ASLIN, R. N. (1977). Development of binocular fixation in human infants. *J. Exp. Child Psychol.* 23, 133–150.

BAKER, J. D., AND DEYOUNG-SMITH, M. (1988). Accommodative esotropia following surgical correction of congenital esotropia, frequency and characteristics. *Graefes Arch. Clin. Exp. Ophthalmol.* 226, 175–177.

BARSOUM-HOMSY, M. (1981). Medial rectus insertion site in congenital esotropia. *Can. J. Ophthalmol.* 16, 181–186.

BARTLEY, G. B., DYER, J. A., AND ILSTRUP, D. M. (1985). Characteristics of recession-resection and bimedial recession for childhood esotropia. *Arch. Ophthalmol.* 103, 190–195.

BATEMAN, J. B., PARKS, M. M., AND WHEELER, N. (1983). Discriminant analysis of congenital esotropia surgery: predictor variables for short- and long-term outcomes. *Ophthalmology* 90, 1146–1153.

BEDROSSIAN, R. H. (1983). Adjusting adjustable eye muscle sutures in anesthetized patients. *Ann. Ophthalmol.* 15, 800–804.

BENNETT, M. J., SMITH III, E. L., HARWERTH, R. S., AND CRAWFORD, M. L. (1980). Ocular dominance, eye alignment and visual acuity in kittens reared with an optically induced squint. *Brain Res.* 193, 33–45.

BERMAN, N., AND MURPHY, E. H. (1981). The critical period for alteration in cortical binocularity resulting from divergent and convergent strabismus. *Brain Res.* 254, 181–202.

BIESNER, D. H. (1971). Reduction of ocular torque by medial rectus recession. *Arch. Ophthalmol.* 85, 13–17.

BIGLAN, A. W., BURNSTINE, R. A., ROGERS, G. L., AND SAUNDERS, R. A. (1989). Management of strabismus with botulinum A toxin. *Ophthalmology* 96, 935–943.

BIRCH, E. E., STAGER, D. R., BERRY, P., AND EVERETT, M. E. (1990). Prospective assessment of acuity and stereopsis in amblyopic infantile esotropes following early surgery. *Invest. Ophthalmol. Vis. Sci.* 31, 758–765.

BOTET, R. V., CALHOUN, J. H., AND HARLEY, R. D. (1981). Development of monofixation syndrome in congenital esotropia. *J. Pediatr. Ophthalmol. Strabismus* 18, 49–51.

BREININ, G. M., SADOVNIKOFF, N., PFEFFER, R., DAVIDOWITZ, J., AND CHIARANDINI, D. J. (1985). Cadmium reduces extraocular muscle contractility in vitro and in vivo. *Invest. Ophthalmol. Vis. Sci.* 26, 1639–1642.

BRENNEISEN, D., DE SAUNIERS, E., AND CHEVELERAUD, J. P. (1975). Importance of the random stereogram test in evaluation of strabismus with a small angle of anomaly. *J. Fr. Orthoptics* 7, 131–134.

CAMPOS, E. C., ALDROVANDI, E., AND BOLZANI, R. (1987). Distance judgement in concomitant strabismus with anomalous retinal correspondence. *Doc. Ophthalmol.* 67, 229–235.

CAPUTO, A. R., GUO, S., WAGNER, R. S., AND PICCIANO, M. V. (1990). Preferred postoperative alignment after congenital esotropia surgery. *Ann. Ophthalmol.* 22, 269–272.

CHINO, Y. M., RIDDER III, W. H., AND CZORA, E. P. (1988). Effects of convergent strabismus on spatio-temporal response properties of neurons in cat area 18. *Exp. Brain Res.* 72, 264–278.

CLARKE, W. N., AND NOEL, L. P. (1982). Vanishing infantile esotropia. *Can. J. Ophthalmol.* 17, 100–102.

CLARKE, W. N., AND NOEL, L. P. (1990). Stereoacuity testing in the monofixation syndrome. *J. Pediatr. Ophthalmol. Strabismus* 27, 161–163.

COOPER, J., AND WARSHOWSKY, J. (1977). Lateral displacement as a response cue in the Titmus stereo test. *Am. J. Optom. Physiol. Opt.* 54, 537–541.

COOPER, J., FELDMAN, J., AND MEDLIN, D. (1979). Comparing stereoscopic performance of children using the Titmus, TNO, and Randot stereo tests. *J. Am. Optom. Assoc.* 50, 821–825.

COSTENBADER, F. D. (1950). The management of convergent strabismus. In J. H. ALLEN (ed.). *Strabismus Ophthalmic Symposium.* St. Louis: Mosby, pp. 343.

COSTENBADER, F. D. (1961). Infantile esotropia. *Trans. Am. Ophthalmol. Soc.* 59, 397–429.

CRAWFORD, M. L., AND VON NOORDEN, G. K. (1979a). Concomitant strabismus and cortical eye dominance in young rhesus monkeys. *Eye* 99, 369–374.

CRAWFORD, M. L., AND VON NOORDEN, G. K. (1979b). The effects of short-term experimental strabismus on the visual system in *Macaca mulatta. Invest. Ophthalmol. Vis. Sci.* 18, 496–505.

CRAWFORD, M. L., AND VON NOORDEN, G. K. (1980). Optically induced concomitant strabismus in monkeys. *Invest. Ophthalmol. Vis. Sci.* 19, 1105–1109.

CRAWFORD, M. L., AND VON NOORDEN, G. K., MEHARG, L. S., RHODES, J. W., HARWERTH, R. S., SMITH III, E. L., AND MILLER, D. D. (1983). Binocular neurons and binocular function in monkeys and children. *Invest. Ophthalmol. Vis. Sci.* 24, 491–495.

CRAWFORD, M. L. J., SMITH III, E. L., HARWERTH, R. S., AND VON NOORDEN, G. K. (1984). Stereoblind monkeys have few binocular neurons. *Invest. Ophthalmol. Vis. Sci.* 25, 779–781.

CYNADER, M., GARDNER, J. C., AND MUSTARI, M. (1984). Effects of neonatally induced strabismus on binocular responses in cat area 18. *Exp. Brain Res.* 53, 384–399.

DELLER, M. (1988). Why should surgery for early-onset strabismus be postponed? *Br. J. Ophthalmol.* 72, 110–115.

EDWARDS, W. C., HESS, J. B., LOWERY, B., AND LOWERY, R. D. (1984). Surgical correction of large-angle esotropia. Part II. *J. Ocular Ther. Surg.* 2, 10–12.

FISHER, N. F., FLOM, M. C., AND JAMPOLSKY, A. (1968). Early surgery of congenital esotropia. *Am. J. Ophthalmol.* 65, 439–443.

FOSTER, R. S., PAUL, T. O., AND JAMPOLSKY, A. (1976). Management of infantile esotropia. *Am. J. Ophthalmol.* 82, 291–299.

FREELEY, D. A., NELSON, L. B., AND CALHOUN, J. H. (1983). Recurrent esotropia following early successful surgical correction of congenital esotropia. *J. Pediatr. Ophthalmol. Strabismus* 20, 68–71.

FRIEDMAN, Z., NEUMANN, E., HYAMS, S. W., AND PELEG, B. (1980). Ophthalmic screening of 38,000 children age 1 to 1½ years, in child welfare clinics. *J. Pediatr. Ophthalmol. Strabismus* 17, 261–267.

FRIEDRICH, D., AND DE DECKER, W. (1987). Prospective study of the development of strabismus during the first 6 months of life. In M. LENK-SCHÄFER (ed.). *Orthoptic Horizons.* Harrogate, UK: LIPS, pp. 21–28.

FRISBY, J. P., MEIN, J., SAYE, A., AND STANWORTH, A. (1975). Use of random-dot stereograms in the clinical assessment of strabismic patients. *Br. J. Ophthalmol.* 59, 545–552.

GALE, D. (1972). The surgical management of estropia in infancy. *Trans. Ophthalmol. Soc. UK* 92, 675–683.

GILLIES, W. E., AND HUGHES, A. (1984). Results in 50 cases of strabismus after graduated surgery designed by A scan ultrasonography. *Br. J. Ophthalmol.* 1984, 790–795.

GOLDSTEIN, J. H. (1969). Strabismus and the insertion of the horizontal rectus muscles. *Am. J. Ophthalmol.* 68, 695–698.

GOLDSTEIN, J. H. (1974). Large angle esotropia. *Ann. Ophthalmol.* 6, 1025–1027.

GRAHAM, P. A. (1974). Epidemiology of strabismus. *Br. J. Ophthalmol.* 58, 224–231.

GREENWALD, M. J. (1984). A randomized comparison of surgical procedures for infantile esotropia [letter]. *Am. J. Ophthalmol.* 98, 642–643.

HELVESTON, E. M., AND VON NOORDEN, G. K. (1967). Microtropia: a newly defined entity. *Arch. Ophthalmol.* 78, 272–281.

HELVESTON, E. M., ELLIS, F. D., PLAGER, D. A., AND MILLER, K. K. (1990). Early surgery for essential infantile esotropia. *J. Pediatr. Ophthalmol. Strabismus* 27, 115–118, discussion on p. 119.

HELVESTON, E. M., ELLIS, F. D., SCHOTT, J., MITCHELSON, J., WEBER, J. C., TAUBE, S., AND MILLER, K. (1983). Surgical treatment of congenital esotropia. *Am. J. Ophthalmol.* 96, 218–228.

HELVESTON, E. M., PATTERSON, J. H., ELLIS, F. D., AND WEBER, J. C. (1978). En-bloc recession of the medial recti for concomitant esotropia. In: *Symposium on Strabismus. Transactions of the New Orleans Academy of Ophthalmology*. St. Louis: Mosby, pp. 230–243).

HENSON, D. B., AND WILLIAMS, D. E. (1980). Depth perception in strabismus. *Br. J. Ophthalmol.* 64, 349–353.

HESS, J. B., AND CALHOUN, J. H. (1979). A new rationale for the management of large angle esotropia. *J. Pediatr. Ophthalmol. Strabismus* 16, 345–348.

HILES, D. A., WATSON, B. A., AND BIGLAN, A. W. (1980). Characteristics of infantile esotropia following early bimedial rectus recession. *Arch. Ophthalmol.* 98, 697–703.

HUBEL, D. H., AND WIESEL, T. N. (1965). Binocular interaction in striate cortex of kittens reared with artificial squint. *J. Neurophysiol.* 28, 1041–1059.

ING, M. R. (1981). Early surgical alignment for congenital esotropia. *Trans. Am. Ophthalmol. Soc.* 79, 625–663.

ING, M. R. (1983a). Early surgical alignment for congenital esotropia. *Ophthalmology* 90, 132–135.

ING, M. R. (1983b). Early surgical alignment for congenital esotropia. *J. Pediatr. Ophthalmol. Strabismus* 20, 11–18.

ING, M., COSTENBADER, F. D., PARKS, M. M., AND ALBERT, D. G. (1966). Early surgery for congenital esotropia. *Am. J. Ophthalmol.* 61, 1419–1427.

KALIL, R. E., SPEAR, P. D., AND LANGSETMO, A. (1984). Response properties of striate cortex neurons in cats raised with divergent or convergent strabismus. *J. Neurophysiol.* 52, 514–537.

KEECH, R. V., SCOTT, W. E., AND BAKER, J. D. (1990). The medial rectus muscle insertion site in infantile esotropia. *Am. J. Ophthalmol.* 109, 79–84.

KELLY, R. B., DEUTSCH, J. W., CARLSON, S. S., AND WAGNER, J. A. (1979). Biochemistry of neurotransmitter release. *Annu. Rev. Neurosci.* 2, 399–446.

KUSHNER, B. J., AND MORTON, G. V. (1984). A randomized comparison of surgical procedures for infantile esotropia. *Am. J. Ophthalmol.* 98, 50–61.

KUSHNER, B. J., AND MORTON, G. V. (1987). The effect of surgical technique and amount, patient age, abduction quality and deviation magnitude on surgical success rates in infantile esotropia. *Binocular Vision* 2, 25–40.

KUSHNER, B. J., AND VRABEC, M. (1987). Theoretical effects of surgery on length tension relationships in extraocular muscles. *J. Pediatr. Ophthalmol. Strabismus* 24, 126–131.

KUSHNER, B. J., LUCCHESE, N. J., AND MORTON, G. V. (1989a). The influence of axial length on the response to strabismus surgery. *Arch. Ophthalmol.* 107, 1616–1618.

KUSHNER, B. J., LUCCHESE, N. J., AND MORTON, G. V. (1989b). Should recessions of the medial recti be graded from the limbus or the insertion? *Arch. Ophthalmol.* 107, 1755–1758.

KUSHNER, B. J., PRESLAN, M. W., AND VRABEC, M. (1987). Artifacts of measuring during strabismus surgery. *J. Pediatr. Ophthalmol. Strabismus* 24, 159–164.

LEE, D. A., AND DYER, J. A. (1983). Bilateral medial rectus muscle recession and lateral rectus muscle resection in the treatment of congenital esotropia. *Am. J. Ophthalmol.* 95, 528–535.

LIN, L. L. K., AND JENG, S. (1984). Disparity in stereotests. In R. D. REINECKE (eds.). *Strabismus II*. Orlando, FL: Grune & Stratton, pp. 541–546.

LING, B-C. (1942). A genetic study of sustained visual fixation and associated behavior in the human infant from birth to six months. *J. Genet. Psychol.* 61, 227–277.

LINGUA, R. W., AZEN, S., SZIRTH, B., EDELMAN, P., AND WALONKER, F. (1983). Succinylcholine as a predictor in strabismus surgery. *J. Pediatr. Ophthalmol. Strabismus* 20, 145–148.

LINGUA, R. W., AZEN, S. P., WALONKER, F., LEVIN, L., AND BAKER, S. (1986). A comparison of the succinylcholine induced ocular position and the postoperative alignment in strabismus. *J. Pediatr. Ophthalmol. Strabismus* 23, 69–73.

LUNDER, D., MAZOW, M. L., AND JENKINS, P. F. (1985). Stability of surgical alignment in early onset esotropia. *Am. Orthoptic J.* 35, 75–80.

MAGOON, E. H. (1984). Botulinum toxin chemo-denervation for strabismus in infants and children. *J. Pediatr. Ophthalmol. Strabismus* 21, 110–113.

MAGOON, E. H. (1989a). Botulin therapy in pediatric ophthalmology. *Int. Ophthalmol. Clin.* 29, 30–32.

MAGOON, E. H. (1989b). Chemodenervation of strabismic children. *Ophthalmology* 96, 931–934.

MAGOON, E., AND SCOTT, A. B. (1987). Botulinum toxin chemodenervation in infants and children: an alternative to incisional strabismus surgery. *J. Pediatr.* 110, 719–722.

MARSH, W. R., RAWLINGS, S. C., AND MUMMA, J. V. (1980). Evaluation of clinical stereoacuity tests. *Ophthalmology* 87, 1265–1272.

MILES, D. R., AND BURIAN, H. M. (1967). Computer statistical analysis of symmetrical and asymmetrical surgery in esotropia. *Trans. Am. Acad. Ophthalmol. Otol.* 71, 290–302.

MIMS III, J. L., AND WOOD, R. C. (1989). Verification and refinement of surgical guidelines for infantile esotropia: a prospective study of 40 cases. *Binoc. Vision* 4, 7–14.

MIMS III, J. L., TREFF, G., KINCAID, M., SCHAFFER, B., AND WOOD, R. (1985). Quantitative surgical guidelines for bimedial recession for infantile esotropia. *Binoc. Vision* 1, 7–14.

NELSON, L. B., CALHOUN, J. H., SIMON, J. W., WILSON, T., AND HARLEY, R. D. (1987). Surgical management of large angle congenital esotropia. *Br. J. Ophthalmol.* 71, 380–383.

NIRENBERG, N., AND MAZOW, M. (1985). The frequency and correction of accommodative esotropia following surgical correction of congenital esotropia. *Binoc. Vision* 1, 71–76.

NIXON, R. B., HELVESTON, E. M., MILLER, K., ARCHER, S. M., AND ELLIS, F. D. (1985). Incidence of strabismus in neonates. *Am. J. Ophthalmol.* 100, 798–801.

OKUDA, F. C., APT, L., AND WANTER, B. S. (1977). Evaluation of the TNO-random-dot stereogram test. *Am. Orthoptic J.* 27, 124–130.

PARKS, M. M. (1969). The monofixation syndrome. *Trans. Am. Ophthalmol. Soc.* 67, 609–657.

PARKS, M. M. (1975). Monofixation syndrome: a frequent end stage of strabismus surgery. *Trans. Am. Acad. Ophthalmol. Otolaryngol.* 79, 733–735.

PARKS, M. M. (1984). Congenital esotropia with a bifixation result: report of a case. *Doc. Ophthalmol.* 58, 109–114.

PRATT-JOHNSON, J. A., AND TILLSON, G. (1983). Sensory results following treatment of infantile esotropia. *Can. J. Ophthalmol.* 18, 175–177.

RÉTHY, I. (1969). Development of the simultaneous fixation from the divergent anatomic eye-position of the neonate. *J. Pediatr. Ophthalmol.* 6, 92–96.

RICHLER, M., AND BARSOUM-HOMSY, M. (1989). Bimedial rectus recession measured from the limbus for congenital esotropia. *Can. J. Ophthalmol.* 24, 304–307.

ROBB, R. M., AND RODIER, D. W. (1987). The variable clinical characteristics and course of early infantile esotropia. *J. Pediatr. Ophthalmol. Strabismus* 24, 276–281.

ROGERS, G. L., AND BREMER, D. L. (1985). Reference points for recessions [letter]. *Binoc. Vision* 1, 65.

ROGERS, G. L., BREMER, D. L., LEGUIRE, L. E., AND FELLOWS, R. R. (1986). Clinical assessment of visual function in the young child: a prospective study of binocular vision. *J. Pediatr. Ophthalmol. Strabismus* 23, 233–235.

ROMANO, P. E. (1971). Congenital esotropia: definition, course, and management. *J. Pediatr. Ophthalmol.* 8, 88–92.

ROMANO, P. E. (1985). Classification into three stages of intra-operative adjustments of eye muscle surgery performed under general anesthesia. *Binoc. Vision* 1, 233–236.

ROMANO, P., AND GABRIEL, L. (1985). Intraoperative adjustment of eye muscle surgery: correction based on eye position during general anesthesia. *Arch. Ophthalmol.* 103, 351–353.

ROMANO, P. E., GABRIEL, L., BENNETT, W. L., AND SNYDER, B. M. (1988). Stage I intraoperative adjustment of eye muscle surgery under general anesthesia: consideration of graduated adjustment. *Graefes Arch. Clin. Exp. Ophthalmol.* 226, 235–240.

SALAPATEK, P., AND KESSEN, W. (1966). Visual scanning of triangles by the human newborn. *Exp. Child. Psychol.* 3, 155–167.

SALAPATEK, P., HAITH, M., MAURER, D., AND KESSEN, W. (1972). Error in the corneal-reflection technique: a note on Slater and Findlay. *J. Exp. Child Psychol.* 14, 493–499.

SAUNDERS, R. A. (1984). A randomized comparison of surgical procedures for infantile esotropia [letter]. *Am. J. Ophthalmol.* 98, 643–645.

SCOBEE, R. G. (1951). Esotropia: incidence, etiology and results of therapy. *Am. J. Ophthalmol.* 34, 817–833.

SCOTT, A. B. (1981). Botulinum toxin injection of eye muscles to correct strabismus. *Trans. Am. Ophthalmol. Soc.* 79, 734–770.

SCOTT, A. B. (1987). Botulinum injection treatment of congenital esotropia. In M. LENK-SCHÄFER (ed.). *Orthoptic Horizons.* Harrogate, UK: LIPS, pp. 21–28.

SCOTT, A. B., MAGOON, E. H., McNEER, K. W., AND STAGER, D. R. (1989). Botulinum treatment of strabismus in children. *Trans. Am. Ophthalmol. Soc.* 87, 174–180.

SCOTT, A. B., MAGOON, E. H., McNEER, K. W., AND STAGER, D. R. (1990). Botulinum treatment of childhood strabismus. *Ophthalmology* 97, 1434–1438.

SCOTT, W. E., REESE, P. D., HIRSH, C. R., AND FLABETICH, C. A. (1986). Surgery for large-angle congenital esotropia: two vs three and four horizontal muscles. *Arch. Ophthalmol.* 104, 374–377.

SIMONS, K., AND REINECKE, R. D. (1974). A reconsideration of amblyopia screening and stereopsis. *Am. J. Ophthalmol.* 78, 707–713.

SKOV, C. M. B., AND MAZOW, M. L. (1985). The surgical effect on esotropia of greater than 5 mm recessions. *Am. Orthoptic J.* 35, 71–74.

SLATER, A. M., AND FINDLAY, J. M. (1972). The measurement of fixation position in the newborn baby. *J. Exp. Child Psychol.* 14, 349–364.

SLATER, A. M., AND FINDLAY, J. M. (1975). Binocular fixation in the newborn baby. *J. Exp. Child Psychol.* 20, 248–273.

SMITH III, E. L., BENNETT, M. J., HARWERTH, R. S., AND CRAWFORD, M. L. (1979). Binocularity in kittens reared with optically induced squint. *Science* 204, 875–877.

SONDHI, N., ARCHER, S. M., AND HELVESTON, E. M. (1988). Development of normal ocular alignment. *J. Pediatr. Ophthalmol. Strabismus* 25, 210–211.

SUGAR, H. S. (1952). An evaluation of results in the use of measured recessions and resections in the correction of horizontal concomitant strabismus. *Am. J. Ophthalmol.* 35, 959–967.

SWAN, K. C., AND WILKINS, J. H. (1984). Extraocular muscle surgery in early infancy—anatomical factors. *J. Pediatr. Ophthalmol. Strabismus* 21, 44–49.

SZMYD, S. M., NELSON, L. B., CALHOUN, J. H., AND SPRATT, C. (1985). Large bimedial rectus recessions in congenital esotropia. *Br. J. Ophthalmol.* 69, 271–274.

TAYLOR, D. M. (1967). Congenital strabismus: the common sense approach. *Arch. Ophthalmol.* 77, 478–484.

TAYLOR, D. M. (1972). Is congenital esotropia functionally curable? *Trans. Am. Ophthalmol. Soc.* 70, 529–576.

TELLER, J., SAVIR, H., YELIN, N., COHEN, R., LEVIAV, A., AND ELSTIN, R. (1988). Late results of surgery for congenital esotropia. *Metab. Pediatr. Syst. Ophthalmol.* 11, 156–159.

UEMURA, Y. (1973). Surgical correction of infantile esotropia. *Jpn. J. Ophthalmol.* 17, 50–59.

VAN SELM, J. L. (1988). Primary infantile-onset esotropia—20 years later. *Graefes Arch. Clin. Exp. Ophthalmol.* 226, 122–125.

VON NOORDEN, G. K. (1984). Infantile esotropia: a continuing riddle. *Am. Orthoptic J.* 34, 52–62.

VON NOORDEN, G. K. (1988). A reassessment of infantile esotropia: XLIV Edward Jackson memorial lecture. *Am. J. Ophthalmol.* 105, 1–10.

VON NOORDEN, G. K. (1990). *Binocular Vision and Ocular Motility.* 4th Ed. St. Louis: Mosby, p. 303.

VON NOORDEN, G. K., ISAZA, A., AND PARKS, M. E. (1972). Surgical treatment of congenital esotropia. *Trans. Am. Acad. Ophthalmol. Otolaryngol.* 76, 1465–1478.

WALLS, G. L. (1963). *The Vertebrate Eye and Its Adaptive Radiation.* New York: Hafner, p. 315.

WICKELGREN, L. W. (1967). Convergence in the human newborn. *J. Exp. Child Psychol.* 5, 74–85.

WICKELGREN, L. W. (1969). The ocular response of human newborns to intermittent visual movement. *J. Exp. Child Psychol.* 8, 469–482.

WILLSHAW, H. E., MASHHOUDI, N., AND POWELL, S. (1986). Augmented medial rectus recession in the management of esotropia. *Br. J. Ophthalmol.* 70, 840–843.

YINON, U. (1976). Age dependence of the effect of squint on cells in kittens' visual cortex. *Exp. Brain Res.* 26, 151–157.

YINON, U., AND AUERBACH, E. (1975). The ocular dominance of cortical neurons in cats developed with divergent and convergent squint. *Vision Res.* 15, 1251–1256.

ZAK, T. A., AND MORIN, J. D. (1982). Early surgery for infantile esotropia: results and influence of age upon results. *Can. J. Ophthalmol.* 17, 213–218.

ZAK, T. A., AND MORIN, J. D. (1984). Early surgery of infantile esotropia: a comparison of surgical procedures. *J. Ocular Ther. Surg.* 3, 67–70.

23 | Motion sensitivity and the origins of infantile strabismus

LAWRENCE TYCHSEN

The visual experience made possible by eye alignment early in life plays an important role in development of the visual cortex. Most studies devoted to this topic have described the effects of experimentally induced strabismus on cortical development in animals (for reviews see Movshon and Van Sluyters, 1981; Wiesel, 1982; Boothe et al., 1985b). The major finding emerging from these studies is that strabismus causes a permanent loss of binocularity in the response of cells in the primary visual area (Hubel and Wiesel, 1965; Crawford and von Noorden, 1979; Van Sluyters and Levitt, 1980; Wiesel, 1982). Analogous losses of binocularity are evident in humans who had strabismus early in life, as measured by deficits in the perception of depth using binocular cues (stereopsis) (Birch and Stager, 1985; Mohindra, 1985; Dobson and Sebris, 1989) and deficits in interocular transfer (Movshon et al., 1972).

In addition to producing permanent losses of binocularity, both experimental and natural strabismus in animals and natural strabismus in humans have been shown to cause a permanent deficit in pursuit and optokinetic eye movement (Cynader and Harris, 1980; Schor and Levi, 1980; Tychsen et al., 1985; Walton and Lisberger, 1989; Tychsen et al., 1991a). The deficit is evident as a bias favoring stimuli that move in a nasal direction under conditions of monocular viewing. The directional deficit is qualitatively similar to that observed in all healthy young infants (Atkinson, 1979; Atkinson and Braddick, 1981; Naegele and Held, 1982; Demer and von Noorden, 1988) before onset of binocular vision. For this reason, it can be used as a marker of arrested binocular development when it persists beyond the first months of life.

The assumptions on which most studies of natural strabismus are based are (1) that the visual cortex has little to do with eye alignment; and (2) that eye alignment in normal humans and in animals is established at birth. Working from these premises, natural strabismus with onset during infancy has been viewed by and large as an ill-defined congenital problem of the ocular muscles analogous to experimental strabismus produced by surgical weakening of eye muscles in animals.

With experimental strabismus, the absence of normal ocular alignment during the critical period causes a secondary maldevelopment of neurons mediating stereopsis and pursuit eye movement.

The cause of the ocular motor signs of naturally occurring infantile strabismus are unknown, and converging lines of evidence now suggest that maldevelopment of the visual pathways mediating eye movement and motion processing may be the primary deficit. Implicit in this paradigm is the notion that eye alignment is immature and unstable at birth, and that normal eye alignment is the result of an active visual process that takes place during the critical period of the first months of life. Viewed from this vantage point, strabismus is not a congenital muscle problem but, rather, a problem of visually guided motor learning.

ONSET OF EYE ALIGNMENT DURING THE FIRST YEAR OF LIFE

More than 75% of all strabismic children are esotropic (the visual axes are deviated nasally), and more than 90% of strabismus that develops during the first year of life manifests as an initial esotropia (Tychsen, 1991). Esotropic infants typically have large angles of deviation but normal visual acuity and minimal refractive errors in each eye (Costenbader, 1961; Birch and Stager, 1985; Dickey et al., 1991). They fixate monocularly at any given moment and often alternate viewing with the right or left eye. Onset of the esotropia is rare before the fourth postnatal month (Nixon et al., 1985; Archer et al., 1989; Tychsen, 1991).

The normal position of the visual axes in most healthy infants over the first four postnatal months is one of moderate divergent misalignment. Figure 23-1 is based on the data of Archer et al. (1989), plotting vergence alignment of the eyes of 3316 healthy infants examined serially over the first 9 months of life. Onset of eye alignment occurred sometime between postnatal months 2 and 6 for most of the infants, as shown by the interval

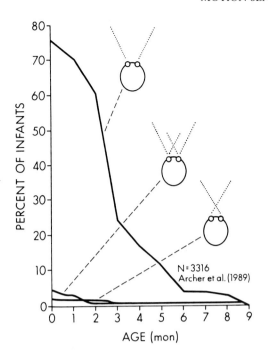

FIG. 23-1. Eye misalignment in 3316 normal term human infants as a function of postnatal age. Most infants had transient divergent misalignment during the neonatal period. A smaller proportion varied between divergent and convergent or were predominantly convergent. Decreasing proportions along the y-axis with time indicating that the onset of eye alignment in most infants was established by age 3–5 months. None of the infants who had early convergent misalignment developed infantile esotropia. (Replotted from the data of Archer et al., 1989.)

disparity signals are the two classes of signal principally responsible for establishing eye alignment. According to this model, the nasally directed bias of pursuit when viewing with each eye provides a chronic visual signal driving the eyes from a position of divergence to a position of more normal eye alignment. At the same time, the emerging sensitivity to binocular disparity provides a negative feedback signal that helps calibrate vergence neutrons within an envelope of approximate alignment (orthophoria). Eye alignment in this schema is an active visual process that takes place during the first 6 months of life. Alignment depends on motion and disparity signals of the correct magnitude being presented to vergence neurons at the appropriate time. If the motion bias is too great or the disparity signal too weak, the system is driven to esotropic strabismus.

The visual motion mechanism is appealing because it can parsimoniously account for a number of otherwise unrelated phenomena: (1) time of onset, direction, and magnitude of the strabismus; (2) other ocular motor signs that accompany the strabismus, e.g., latent fixation nystagmus and pursuit asymmetry; (3) associated motion misperceptions; and (4) recurrence of the strabismus despite optimal, initial, surgical correction.

METHODS THAT PROBE MOTION PATHWAYS OF THE VISUAL CORTEX

The direction of the asymmetry of smooth pursuit that is seen in subjects who have onset of strabismus during infancy and normal visual acuity in each eye is determined by the eye doing the viewing (Fig. 23-2). Pursuit of sinusoidal target motion is normal when the target moves nasally with respect to the viewing eye, and pursuit is weak when the target moves temporally with respect to the viewing eye. The direction of the deficit reverses instantaneously when the viewing eye is changed, and the deficit is much less apparent when the subject is allowed to view binocularly (Fig. 23-3). The directional asymmetry of pursuit is present transiently in healthy infants before the onset of binocularity and persists permanently if normal binocularity fails to develop during infancy.

The bias in pursuit implies an arrest of development of the motion pathway in visual cortex, as the motion pathway of the cortex provides the signals driving pursuit (for review see Lisberger et al., 1987). We were able to test this hypothesis by taking advantage of experimental methods that use pursuit eye movements and judgments of target velocity to probe the motion pathway (Lisberger and Westbrook, 1985; McKee and Welch, 1985; Tychsen and Lisberger, 1986b). A key advantage

along the x-axis corresponding to the portion of the upper curve having the steepest negative slope.

During months 0–3, normal infants display, in addition to unstable eye alignment, other signs of immature binocularity (for review see Boothe et al., 1985a). Normal infants fail to display compensatory vergence movements in response to prism-induced horizontal image disparity (Aslin, 1977), and they fail to show binocular summation of visually evoked potentials (VEPs) or sensitivity to stereoscopic targets (Braddick and Atkinson, 1983; Birch and Stager, 1985; Gwiazda et al., 1989).

POSSIBLE VISUAL SIGNALS GUIDING EYE ALIGNMENT

Given these observations, one may ask what visual signals the infant ocular motor system uses to establish normal alignment from a neonatal state of ocular divergence and absent binocularity. In the sections that follow it is postulated that visual motion and visual

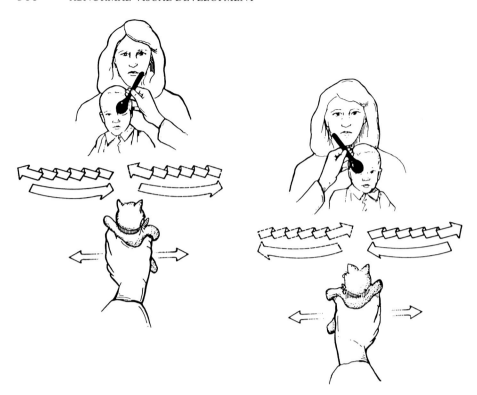

FIG. 23-2. Asymmetry of horizontal smooth pursuit evident during monocular viewing. When a handheld toy is moved from temporal to nasal before the fixating eye, pursuit is smooth. Pursuit is absent or cogwheel when the target moves in a nasal to temporal direction. The movements of the two eyes are conjugate, and the direction of the asymmetry reverses instantaneously with a change of fixating eye, so the direction of robust pursuit is always for nasally directed targets in the visual field. The asymmetry is seen best by moving the target at a brisk pace. The asymmetry indicates immaturity of motion processing connections in visual cortex.

of these methods was that they permitted placement of the stimulus probe anywhere in the visual field so a retinotopic map of visual motion processing could be constructed noninvasively. As shown in the pursuit initiation trial of Figure 23-4, a ramp of probe motion was used to evoke transient eye acceleration. By systematically altering the location, direction, speed, size, and contrast of the stimulus, transient eye acceleration was used to infer tuning properties of motion neurons in the cortex. The tuning properties measured in normal adult humans proved to be remarkably similar to the tuning properties measured by extracellular recordings in monkey visual area MT (Maunsell and Van Essen, 1983a; Lisberger and Westbrook, 1985; Tychsen and Lisberger, 1986a).

Using the evoked pursuit method, we then compared the processing of visual motion signals in normal versus strabismic humans (Tychsen and Lisberger, 1986b). The strabismic humans proved to have two major abnormalities of their visual motion pathway: one a directional bias, and the other a topographical distortion.

NASOTEMPORAL BIASES OF MOTION PROCESSING IN STRABISMUS

The nasotemporal biases of pursuit that we found in strabismic humans can be appreciated more easily when compared side by side with the performance of normal subjects. Figure 23-5 (left panels) is typical of the pursuit response of normal humans and monkeys when viewing monocularly (Tychsen and Lisberger, 1986a). When a ramp motion stimulus is delivered to different locations in the visual field, the evoked eye acceleration (plotted along the y-axis in the lower panels) is equal for nasally directed and temporally directed target motion. Each half visual field shows a centripetal bias for stimulus motion toward the vertical meridian. (The centripetal bias is independent of eye position in the orbit and is therefore a property of visual rather than motor pathways.) When combined, the two half visual fields show remarkable symmetry, so the whole visual field has no nasotemporal bias.

In marked contrast, a nasotemporal bias across the

Both Eyes Tracking

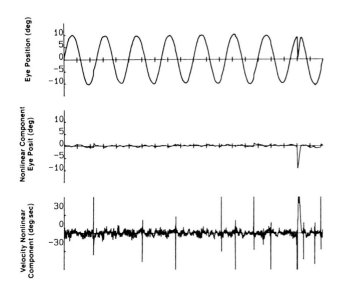

Right Eye Tracking

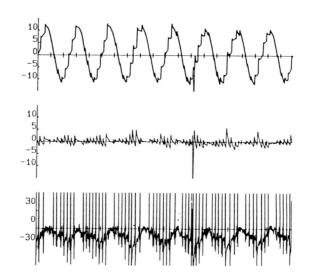

FIG. 23-3. Nasal bias of horizontal smooth pursuit in an adult human who had arrested development of motion processing during the critical period and normal visual acuity in both eyes. The target (a spot subtending 6 arc minutes) moved sinusoidally at 0.4 Hz, 20 degrees peak to peak. (A) Pursuit was normal and symmetrical under conditions of binocular viewing. (B) Pursuit was asymmetrical when viewing monocularly, showing normal gain when target motion was nasally directed (leftward for the right eye), but low gain with saccadic intrusions when target motion was temporally directed. The mirror image was seen when viewing monocularly with the left eye (not shown). Top tracing of each pair is eye position. Middle tracing is the nonlinear component of eye position, computed by comparing eye position to target position on a millisecond time scale. Bottom tracing was computed by comparing target velocity to eye velocity. Right is upward. Eye position (digitized at 1 kHz) was recorded using the magnetic search coil technique.

visual field typifies the response of the strabismic human (Tychsen and Lisberger, 1986b). Nasally directed stimulus motion evokes much greater eye acceleration than temporally directed motion, as shown by the difference in the height of the curves plotted in Figure 23-5 (right panels). That the directional bias is visual is supported by (1) the finding that each eye achieves vigorous temporally directed eye acceleration when the other eye is viewing, (2) the demonstration of directional biases in the judgment of stimulus velocity independent of pursuit, and (3) the absence of a directional bias when eye rotations are evoked by head rotation in total darkness (Tychsen et al., 1985; Tychsen and Lisberger, 1986b).

When the experimental task is to judge stimulus velocity but not pursue (McKee and Welch, 1985), nasally directed stimulus motion is perceived as being faster than temporally directed motion. The perceptual bias persists even when the nasally directed stimulus is presented to the naive subject at a speed that is actually 40% *slower* than the temporally directed stimulus (Fig. 23-6). Viewing with a given eye, the magnitude of the bias in velocity perception correlates with the magnitude of the bias in pursuit acceleration (Tychsen and Lisberger, 1986b).

Although it would be possible to argue from these results that strabismic humans have two deficits—one in the cerebral pathways responsible for velocity perception and one in the cerebral pathways that subserve pursuit—the correspondence between the perceptual and pursuit biases argues for a more parsimonious interpretation; namely, that the deficit is in a general visual motion pathway that provides signals for both perception and pursuit. This conclusion is justified by the findings that correlated deficits in pursuit and velocity judgment are produced in normal monkeys by lesions of the MT area (Newsome et al., 1985; Newsome and Pare, 1988).

NASAL MOTION BIAS AND INTERRUPTIONS OF BINOCULARITY DURING THE CRITICAL PERIOD

That humans who had strabismus during infancy should have these biases of motion processing is compatible with the notion that the pathways mediating motion processing are immature at birth and develop normally only if the animal develops normal binocularity. Binocularity in the form of stereopsis and motion processing appear to develop in parallel during similar critical periods. Healthy human and monkey infants lack

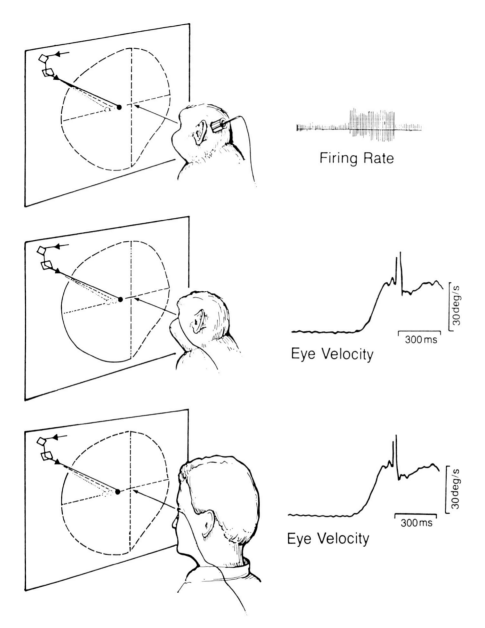

FIG. 23-4. Motion sensitivity as measured by excitation of visual motion neuron or initiation of pursuit eye movement. Response is evoked by a brief ramp of target motion in the left visual hemifield. Each trial begins by having the subject steadily fixate a spot target at zero eccentricity in the visual field under conditions of monocular viewing (the left eye in this case). After a random interval, the fixation spot disappears and a rightward moving spot appears at an eccentric position. (Top) Increase in firing rate of a motion neuron in extrastriate cortex whose receptive field is traversed by the moving spot. (Middle) After a latency period of about 100 ms, rightward pursuit (smooth eye velocity) is initiated. To maintain foveation, eye velocity eventually stabilizes at target velocity, which in the trials shown was 30 degrees/ second. Abrupt upward deflection indicates a saccade. Upward direction indicates rightward movement. (Bottom) Pursuit initiation in the normal human is remarkably similar to that recorded in the macaque monkey (Tychsen and Lisberger, 1986a).

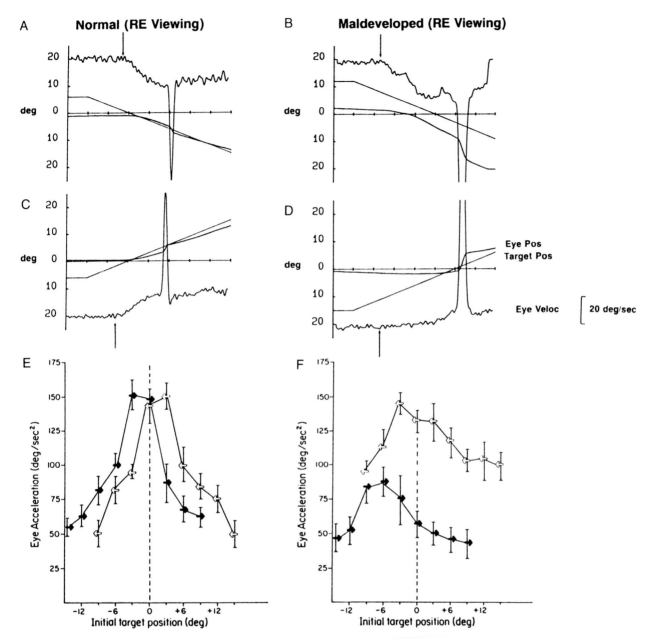

FIG. 23-5. Trials of nasally directed versus temporally directed horizontal pursuit initiation in a normal subject (A, B, C) compared to a subject who had a nasal bias of motion processing (D, E, F). In both cases the subjects viewed monocularly with the right eye. (A) The trial begins by having the subject fixate a stationary spot at zero eccentricity, while a second spot is visible but stationary at 6 degrees eccentric along the horizontal meridian in the right hemifield. The 0 degree spot disappears, and 100 ms later the eccentric spot begins a ramp of leftward motion at 30 degrees/second. After a latency period of about 125 ms (arrow), the subject initiates leftward pursuit and eventually foveates the target. Raw data tracings of target position, eye position, and eye velocity are shown for each trial. (B) Eccentric spot begins a ramp of rightward motion from a position 6 degrees eccentric along the horizontal meridian in the left hemifield. (C) Plots of mean smooth eye acceleration ± SEM for nasally versus temporally

directed target motion at eccentricities of 0–15 degrees in the left and right hemifields. Note the mirror-image symmetry of nasally directed (white arrows) versus temporally directed (black arrows) pursuit in this normal subject. (D, E) Pursuit initiation is normal for nasally directed target motion but weak for temporally directed target motion. (F) Nasal bias of pursuit initiation is evident as higher smooth eye accelerations in response to nasally directed targets in either hemifield. The topography of the response is distorted compared with that of the normal subject in (C). (A, B, D, E) Upward direction indicates rightward. Eye position was recorded using infrared oculography. Each symbol plotted in (C) and (F) is a mean of 10 trials for eccentricity and direction of motion drawn from one experimental session. Within a session, trials were randomized for direction and eccentricity.

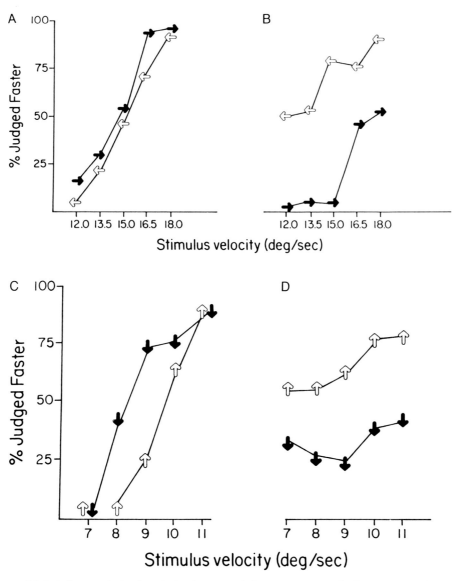

FIG. 23-6. Judgment of stimulus velocity during steady fixation, in a normal subject versus a subject who had maldeveloped motion processing. Viewing was monocular through the right eye. Stimulus was a white rectangle (6 minutes wide by 10 minutes high) that moved horizontally or vertically across the fovea in individual trials of ramp motion (the paradigm of McKee and Welch, 1985). Target speed and direction for any given trial was randomized from 12 to 18 degrees/second with a mean of 15 degrees/second. The subject's task was to judge whether an individual trial was "faster" or "slower" than a subjective mean of all of the trials seen up to that point in the session. Responses are plotted as the percent judged faster at each stimulus velocity; nasally directed stimulus motion (white arrows) versus temporally directed motion (black arrows). (A) The normal subject judges nasally versus temporally directed targets to be moving at the same speeds. Higher velocities of stimulus motion are judged to be "faster" than slower velocities. (B) The subject with maldeveloped motion processing consistently judges nasally directed stimuli to be moving "faster" than temporally directed stimuli, despite the fact that the stimuli were actually moving at the same speed. (C, D) Analogous biases occur for vertical stimulus motion. The normal subject judges upward-directed stimuli to be moving at approximately the same speed as downward stimuli, but the subject with maldeveloped motion processing consistently judges upward-directed stimuli to be moving "faster." The vertical bias verifies that the horizontal bias is not merely an adaptation to latent fixation nystagmus. The vertical bias of velocity perception is accompanied by an upward bias of vertical smooth pursuit. The vertical bias may provide a mechanism for dissociated vertical deviation observed in these subjects. (For a discussion of this topic see Tychsen, 1991, 1992.)

signs of normal binocular function and have biases in visual tracking similar to those seen in strabismic subjects (Atkinson, 1979; Atkinson and Braddick, 1981; Naegele and Held, 1982; Demer and von Noorden, 1988). When viewing monocularly, small field and large field optokinetic stimuli elicit normal tracking only when the direction of stimulus motion is nasal. This nasotemporal bias disappears by about 6 months of age if signs of normal binocularity appear.

The pursuit asymmetry is also apparent in humans (Atkinson, 1979; Schor and Levi, 1980; Maurer et al., 1983; Lewis et al., 1989) and monkeys (Sparks et al., 1986) who have infantile-onset, unilateral amblyopia. The critical factor causing maldeveloped motion processing in these cases appears to be disruption of binocularity during the critical period and not the deprivation itself. Onset of amblyopia after infancy is not associated with pursuit asymmetries (Tychsen et al., 1985).

Nonprimates who have been monocularly deprived (van Hof-van Duin, 1978; Hoffmann, 1979) or who have had their visual cortex removed (Wood et al., 1973), show analogous tracking biases. They retain the ability to track nasally directed optokinetic targets but show no response to temporally directed targets. Hoffman hypothesized that temporally directed tracking in these animals was lost because it involved an indirect, ontogenetically and phylogenetically more recent cortical pathway that was easily disrupted by deprivation (Hoffman, 1979). Nasally directed tracking was retained because it involved only direct subcortical inputs from retina to brainstem pretectum, which were resistant to deprivation.

Is it valid to use Hoffman's hypothesis to explain the nasally directed bias of pursuit in strabismic or amblyopic humans? The answer is yes and no. There is ample evidence to support the argument that, in the human infant, visual cortex neurons mediating temporally directed motion processing develop later, are fewer in number, and are more susceptible to deprivation (for review see Tychsen, 1992). Thus extending this part of Hoffman's hypothesis to the human appears to be reasonable. However, extending the second part of the hypothesis—that one direction of motion processing is mediated by subcortical pathways and the other by cortical pathways—is less valid for several reasons.

First, the nasotemporal motion asymmetry in human infant is present at the level of striate cortex in that evoked potentials recorded over the occipital lobes in very young human infants show responses biased for nasally directed motion (Norcia et al., 1989, 1990; Hamer et al., 1990). Second, humans who have nasally directed biases in pursuit have correlative biases in velocity perception (Tychsen and Lisberger, 1986b; Tychsen, 1989).

It would be difficult to explain velocity perception biases on the basis of subcortical pathways. Third, subcortical inputs for optokinetic tracking in nonprimates cannot be equated with inputs for motion processing and foveal pursuit in the human and monkey. Nonprimates lack well developed foveas or smooth pursuit. Primates have well developed foveas and exquisite pursuit, and they show profound, permanent deficits in pursuit after loss of visual cortex (Zee et al., 1987; Tusa et al., 1988; Tychsen et al., 1988). Moreover, the deficits in strabismic humans are most pronounced for the initiation of pursuit (Tychsen and Lisberger, 1986b), and recordings from pretectal nuclei (nucleus of the optic tract) in the monkey indicate that the subcortical pathway in primates is not involved in initiation or maintenance of pursuit (Kato et al., 1986; Mustari and Fuchs, 1990).

NASOTEMPORAL INPUTS TO THE PRIMARY VISUAL CORTEX: EXAMPLE OF NASAL DOMINANCE

The appearance of binocularity with the disappearance of the nasal motion bias compels a closer look at nasotemporal development of the primary visual cortex, as the primary visual cortex is a major component in the motion pathway. In cats and monkeys, geniculostriate input from the nasal hemiretina to each area V1 is initially stronger than that from the temporal hemiretina (Rodieck, 1979; LeVay et al., 1980; Movshon and Van Sluyters, 1981; Stone, 1983; Segal et al., 1991; Tychsen and Burkhalter, unpublished data). "Stronger" in this context means that the nasal input is established earlier, drives a greater number of primary visual area neurons, and has less tendency to regress as development proceeds. As shown in Figure 23-7, normal human infants have an analogous bias in that cell density measurements of magnocellular lamina 1 in the lateral geniculate nucleus exceed density measurements in lamina 2 by an average of 7% (lamina 1 receives input from the nasal retina of the contralateral eye, and lamina 2 from the temporal retina of the ipsilateral eye) (Segal et al., 1991). Normal human infants preferentially attend to visual targets in the temporal field (Mohn and van Hof-van Duin, 1985), and it is well established that the corresponding region of the nasal retina in normal infants is more mature at birth (Nissenkom, 1990).

Neuroanatomically, the development of ocular dominance columns in area V1 is remarkably similar in cats, Old World monkeys, and humans (Hendrickson, 1985). In V1 of normal adult monkey, dominance columns driven by the nasal hemiretina are 7–10% wider than columns driven by the temporal hemiretina (LeVay et al., 1975; Tychsen and Burkhalter, unpublished data). Neurophysiologically, strabismus in cats and monkeys causes a loss of binocularity in the response of the cells

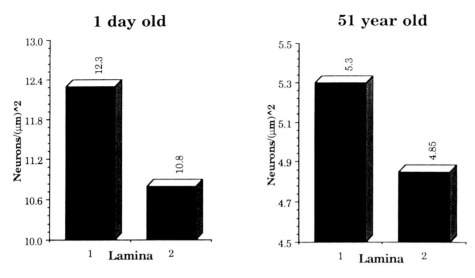

FIG. 23-7. Nasal bias in density of neurons in lamina 1 versus lamina 2 of the human lateral geniculate nucleus. Lamina 1 receives input from the contralateral nasal hemiretina; lamina 2 from the ipsilateral temporal hemiretina. Equivalent biases are apparent in total number of neurons (the product of laminar volume and neuron density). Cell counts and laminar areas were digitized from Nissl-stained 40-μm sections using a camera lucida method (Segal et al., 1991).

that comprise these columns. The result is two populations of monocularly driven cells, each column driven by either a nasal or a temporal hemiretina. In strabismic and amblyopic animals, a consistent nasal bias develops, evident as a greater number of units in the cell population driven by the nasal retina of the contralateral eye (Wiesel and Hubel, 1963; Sherman et al., 1974; Shatz et al., 1977; Singer, 1978; LeVay et al., 1980; Moushon and Van Sluyters, 1981; von Grunau and Rauschecker, 1983; Kalil et al., 1984). Humans presumably have a loss of binocularity in homologous cell populations, as those who had strabismus during infancy continue to display deficits in the perception of depth using binocular cues, even if surgery is performed to realign the eyes (Birch and Stager, 1985; Mohindra, 1985; Archer et al., 1986; Birch et al., 1990). It is therefore reasonable to argue that the primary visual cortex of strabismic humans contains a similar nasal bias.

This nasal hemiretinal bias cannot, however, explain the bias for nasally directed motion processing in the immature visual pathway. The principal reason it cannot is seen in the lower right panel of Figure 23-5, which shows that the bias favoring nasally directed motion is not restricted to the temporal visual field but extends beyond the vertical meridian, well into the nasal field, i.e., onto the temporal hemiretina. As developed in more detail later in the chapter, the evidence suggests that dominance of the nasal hemiretina and dominance of nasally directed motion processing early in life represent two types of nasal dominance and are not related as chicken-and-egg. The anatomical bias reflects the num-

ber and weight of inputs from the lateral geniculate nucleus (LGN) to lamina 4cα of area V1. The motion bias may merely reflect the ordering of early monocular connections between adjacent temporal field neuron pairs and nasal field neuron pairs from lamina 4cα to 4b of V1.

TOPOGRAPHICAL DISTORTIONS OF THE MOTION PATHWAY IN STRABISMUS

Callosal axons normally interdigitate a narrow strip of the nasal and temporal visual fields at the vertical meridian (Hubel and Wiesel, 1967; Shatz et al., 1977; Tusa et al., 1978; Dehay et al., 1986; Bourdet and Van Sluyters, 1989). Neuroanatomically, it is represented by the callosal efferent zone at the border of area V1 and V2.

Immature neurons in this area send axon collaterals to several targets in area V1 of the opposite hemisphere (Lund et al., 1978; Innocenti and Frost, 1979; Berman and Payne, 1983, Innocenti and Clarke, 1984; Innocenti et al., 1985). It was initially reported that the representation of the vertical meridian in area V1 of kittens made artificially strabismic was two to five times as broad as normal, implying that pruning of abnormal connections occurred only in animals that developed normal binocularity. However, Van Sluyters and coworkers have now shown, using more extensive sampling techniques, that the callosal distribution in strabismic cats is, if anything, narrower than that in normal adult cats (Bourdet and Van Sluyters, 1989).

Development of visual field topography is mentioned here because strabismic humans have distortions in the topography of the visual field for motion processing (Tychsen and Lisberger, 1986b), and any comprehensive model of visual motion development must offer some explanation for the distortions. The distortions are so systematic that it seems reasonable to argue that heterotopic callosal connections could be responsible. The abnormal connections need not involve the V1–V2 border. Conceivably, the abnormal topography could be based on projections from V1 to V3–MT. In area MT of normal monkeys, extensive regions of the peripheral visual fields are connected by callosal inputs (Maunsell and Van Essen, 1987), and receptive fields are several times larger than those found in area V1.

The greatest topographical distortions occur in strabismic humans who have pronounced nasally directed biases of pursuit. The most pronounced nasally directed biases of pursuit occur in subjects who have the largest angles of strabismus, so the three variables (topography, pursuit bias, strabismus) vary systematically. Comparing normal (Fig. 23-8, top) to mildly, moderately, and severely strabismic humans (Fig. 23-8, middle and bottom), the covariation of these variables presents a consistent picture.

The subject of Figure 23-8 (top) has a moderate angle of strabismus and a mild nasotemporal bias (quantified as the difference between peak eye acceleration for nasally directed versus temporally directed target motion). The subject shows little if any shift in the normal location of the peaks of the curves with respect to the vertical meridian of the visual field. The peaks are sharp. The subject (Fig. 23-8, bottom), however, has a severe strabismus and a marked nasally directed bias. Compared to normal, the location of the peaks is markedly shifted, and the peaks are broadened.

It would be difficult to explain the topographical abnormality of this subject (Fig. 23-8, bottom) as deprivation of the nasal visual field by the nose: (1) in several subjects, stimuli located in the nasal field evoked the *most vigorous* response; (2) the topographical distortion is within the central 15 degrees of the visual field, whereas the nose blocks stimuli in the human visual field only at eccentricities of 50 degrees or more; and (3) the subject has normal visual acuity, so viewing alternates between the eyes, which are fully mobile in the orbits. It would also be difficult to ascribe the topographical distortion to an albino-like abnormality of the optic chiasm, in which retinal ganglion cells normally projecting to the ipsilateral LGN decussate inappropriately to project to the contralateral LGN (Guillery, 1979, 1986; Leventhal et al., 1985). Humans with classical infantile esotropia lack the funduscopic abnormalities, acuity deficits, and pendular nystagmus seen in albinos and do not show the abnormal lateralization

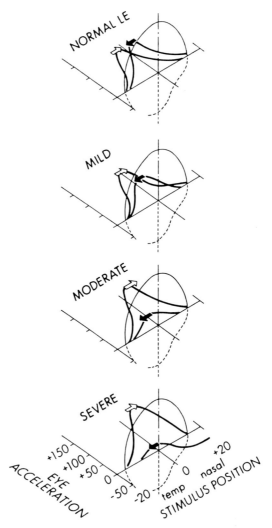

FIG. 23-8. Covariation of magnitude of strabismus, bias favoring nasally directed motion processing for pursuit, and distortion of normal topography of motion processing, viewing monocularly using the left eye. A normal human is shown at the top of the figure, and three humans with infantile-onset esotropia are shown below (angle of strabismus during infancy was smallest for subject "mild" and largest for subject "severe"). Motion processing was measured as average smooth eye acceleration (y-axis) evoked by moving spots placed at different locations across the central 30 degrees of the horizontal visual field (x-axis). Curve under the white arrow indicates eye acceleration to nasally directed spots and the curve under the black arrow to temporally directed spots. Eye acceleration for temporally directed spots beyond 5–10 degrees eccentric evoked wrong-way (negative eye acceleration) pursuit in subjects who had the most severe nasal biases. Each subject had strabismus surgery during childhood and at the time of eye movement recording had cosmetically inapparent, residual angles of strabismus. (Data redrawn from Tychsen and Lisberger, 1986b.)

of the VEP that typifies albinism (Apkarian et al., 1984; Hoyt and Caltrider, 1984).

The topographical distortion of the "motion field" shown in Figures 23-5 and 23-8 was quantified by computing a topographical median for each curve relating eye acceleration to stimulus position across the visual field. The topographical median was the location in the field that divided the integrated area under the curve into two equal parts. For normal subjects, the topographical median fell within a narrow 2- to 3-degree strip around the position of fixation. Strabismic subjects, however, had topographical medians falling as much as 5–6 degrees away from the normal position (Tychsen and Lisberger, 1986b). As depicted in Figure 23-9, the net effect of convolving the topographical distortion onto the directional bias is that an abnormally large region of each monocular vision field is preferentially sensitive to nasally directed motion.

CODEVELOPMENT OF MOTION PROCESSING, STEREOPSIS, AND EYE ALIGNMENT

Stereopsis, visual motion processing, and eye alignment codevelop during similar critical periods: normal human and monkey infants are born stereoblind; they

have nasal biases for pursuit and optokinetic nystagmus (OKN) eye movement; and they display unstable eye alignment (Day and Norcia, 1990; Tychsen, 1991). Stereopsis, symmetrical nasotemporal pursuit, and normal eye alignment emerge together at age 3–5 months. The available evidence indicates that development of these three binocular functions shows interdependency: Normal binocularity depends on development of each, and interrupting development of any one function appears to interrupt development of the others.

A logical place to begin thinking about the neural conjunction of this development is at lamina 4 of striate cortex. The first order neurons of lamina 4c in monkey are known to be strictly segregated in nasal versus temporal columns (Hubel and Wiesel, 1972, 1977; LeVay et al., 1975) with a neonatal bias favoring nasal inputs (Segal et al., 1991). Motion-sensitive cells of 4cα are necessary to provide monocularly segregated signals for opponent motion (looming)(cf. Tychsen, 1992). As shown in Figure 23-10, these neurons converge on binocular neurons of lamina 4b (Hubel et al., 1977), which play a major role in disparity sensitivity and motion processing (Van Essen, 1985; Hawken et al., 1988; Poggio et al., 1988). The binocular neurons of lamina 4b provide the major projection to extrastriate area MT (Lund et al., 1975; Maunsell and Van Essen, 1983a), which is in turn known to provide a major signal driving eye movements (Newsome et al., 1985; Lisberger et al., 1987).

Following this line of reasoning, normal development

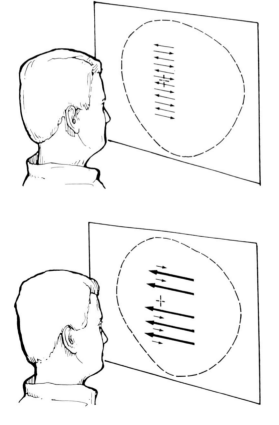

FIG. 23-9. Symmetry of motion sensitivity in a normal human (top) and asymmetry in a strabismic human (bottom) viewing monocularly with the right eye. Figure is a conceptual simplification of the data of Figures 23-5, 23-6, and 23-8. The size of the arrows represents the motion sensitivity: the strength of pursuit initiation to moving targets or judgment of target velocity for nasally directed versus temporally directed target motion.

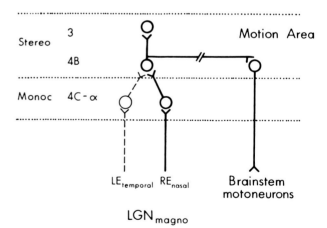

FIG. 23-10. Inputs and intrinsic-extrinsic connections of motion-pathway neurons in visual cortex of the newborn primate. Neurons from LGN laminae 1 and 2 provide input to monocular direction-selective neurons of lamina 4Cα in area V1. These monocular cells converge on first binocular neurons in the magnocellular pathway, lamina 4B. Neurons of 4B provide major extrinsic projection to visual areas V3–MT. These areas in turn provide signals to pursuit and vergence premotor neurons. Not shown: extrinsic projection of 4C or monocular 4B neurons to V3–MT for opponent motion (looming cells).

of disparity sensitivity, symmetrical development of motion processing, and unbiased signals for pursuit and vergence would require normal development of 4b and 4b-like neurons in striate cortex. The critical factor in this development would be anatomically balanced and physiologically synchronous nasal and temporal axon input to 4cα and 4b, which, stated another way, would be simultaneous, equal right eye and left eye input. Any one of a number of postulated perturbations (e.g., monocular deprivation, artificial strabismus, striate cortex hypoxia, or genetic influences on axon sprouting) could retard symmetrical nasotemporal input to 4b neurons. The retarded development would be manifested chiefly as a prolonged bias favoring nasally directed motion.

VICIOUS CYCLE: VISUAL MOTION PATHWAY IN IMMATURITY AND ESOTROPIA

The established paradigm that strabismus causes maldevelopment of the visual cortex and the paradigm presented here that maldevelopment of the visual cortex causes strabismus are not mutually exclusive but may, in fact, work together in a vicious cycle (Fig. 23-11).

The vicious cycle incorporates the old paradigm, "strabismus causes maldevelopment of the visual cortex," into a new paradigm, "maldevelopment of the visual cortex can also cause strabismus."

The vicious cycle would ensue once the nasally directed bias of the immature motion pathways produced the initial strabismus. The strabismus would confound the development of disparity sensitivity in visual area V1 (and the projection to disparity neurons in V2–V3) through the mechanism of image uncorrelation. Image uncorrelation would also further retard the maturation of motion neurons preferring temporally directed motion by a high-pass filter mechanism discussed later in the chapter. Lack of temporally directed motion processing would deprive the immature visual cortex of a means to oppose the esotropic drive. The notion of the vicious cycle is attractive because the motion bias in human and monkey infants (Atkinson, 1979; Atkinson and Braddick, 1981; Naegele and Held, 1982) is apparent months before the development of natural strabismus (Nixon et al., 1985), and yet artificial strabismus is an effective way to make the motion bias persist permanently (Cynader and Harris, 1980; Walton and Lisberger, 1989). Monocular deprivation is in many cases also effective, as the image uncorrelation accom-

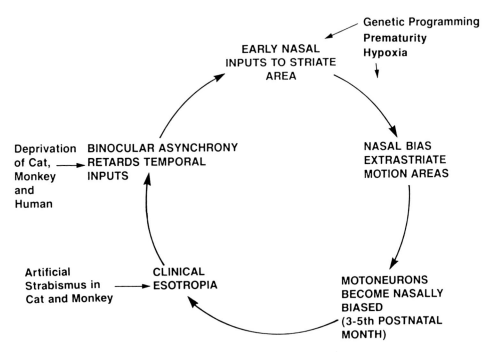

FIG. 23-11. Vicious cycle in which nasal biases of motion processing precipitate eye misalignment, and eye misalignment disrupts development of binocularity, further aggravating the motion bias. The nasal bias of motion processing is both cause and effect. Top right: Inborn and environmental insults to the visual pathways delay development, which prevents resolution of the nasal bias in the primary visual area, eventually biasing development of MT, and, in turn, vergence motoneurons. Lower left: Artificial strabismus produces a nasal bias by causing image uncorrelation. The uncorrelation causes asynchrony and, via Hebbian mechanisms, failure to develop binocularity. If severe and of early onset, amblyopia (monocular deprivation) produces the same result.

panying amblyopia disrupts binocularity. This idea is supported by the finding that monocularly deprived animals (Vital-Durand et al., 1974; van Hof-van Duin, 1978; Sparks et al., 1986) and humans (Schor and Levi, 1980; Maurer et al., 1983; Lewis et al., 1989) have nasal tracking biases analogous to the nondeprived strabismic subjects. Monocularly deprived monkeys often develop esotropia (Quick et al., 1989); and monocularity deprived humans develop esotropia and nasally directed fixation nystagmus (Helveston et al., 1985; Metz, 1985; Seabar, 1991).

ESOTROPIA AS A MOTOR ADAPTATION TO A VISUAL BIAS

The time of onset and the direction of the strabismus provide support for the notion that the esotropia is a motor adaptation to a visual bias. First, the motor pathways are unbiased at birth, as indicated by the symmetry of smooth eye movements evoked by head rotations in the dark (Ornitz et al., 1979; Finocchio et al., 1990). Second, in infants who develop strabismus, the esotropia is not apparent at birth and typically does not appear until 3 months of age or later (Nixon et al., 1985; Archer et al., 1989). Third, ocular motor adaptation to visual motion inputs is well documented in adult monkeys and humans (Gauthier and Robinson, 1975; Gonshor and Melvill Jones, 1976; Collewijn et al., 1981; Miles and Lisberger, 1981). Asymmetrical motion has been produced by wearing magnifying, minifying, or reversing-prism lenses or by exposure to a scene that always moves in one direction. Vergence can be adapted to produce a convergence bias that persists for hours in normal viewing conditions (Collewijn et al., 1981; Oohira et al., 1989); and pursuit pathways can be adapted to produce a nystagmus that persists for hours in total darkness (Miles, 1976). Fourth, vergence and pursuit adaptations would be expected to be more pronounced were the visual stimulation applied during a labile period of early ocular motor development. Fifth, the notion that development of vergence is guided by binocular disparity is supported by the finding that infant monkeys, reared under conditions of alternating monocular viewing, fail to develop stable vergence eye movements and remain stereoblind (Tychsen et al., 1991a). Finally, the direction of the visual motion bias and the direction of the strabismus coincide in more than 90% of cases of human infantile strabismus. The remaining cases appear to involve additional nonvisual factors (infants who develop early-onset constant exotropia tend to have major structural anomalies of the eye or brain) (Tychsen, 1991).

GENETIC AND ENVIRONMENTAL FACTORS THAT MAY RETARD MOTION PATHWAY DEVELOPMENT AND PROMOTE ESOTROPIA

Implicit in the adaptation paradigm is the notion that the ocular motor signs of strabismus develop only if the visual motion bias persists at a given magnitude for a given interval during the first months of life (Fig. 23-12). The threshold magnitude and interval producing strabismus could be altered by a number of genetic and environmental factors.

As for genetic factors, in the study reported by Tychsen and Lisberger in 1986 the strabismic subject who had the most severe motion processing bias had two siblings with infantile strabismus (Tychsen and Lisberger, 1986a). Nonstrabismic kindred in pedigrees of infantile strabismus have been found who manifest nasally directed biases of pursuit and velocity perception not present in the normal population (Tychsen, 1989), and large-scale studies have documented that approximately 20–30% of children born to a strabismic parent do themselves develop strabismus (Cross, 1975; Spivey, 1980; Judisch, 1985; Hakim et al., 1989).

As for environmental factors, the prevalence of strabismus and amblyopia is substantially higher in low-birth-weight, premature infants (Kitchen et al., 1979; Hoyt, 1980; Kushner, 1982; Manning et al., 1982; van Hof-van Duin et al., 1989) and in infants who suffer perinatal hypoxia (Kitchen et al., 1979; Groenendaal et al., 1989). Infants born weighing less than 1500 g have a prevalence of amblyopia and strabismus seven times that of normal-weight, term infants (Kitchen et al., 1979). Infants born weighing less than 2500 g have a prevalence of strabismus four times that of normal-weight infants (Hoyt, 1980). The risk of strabismus increases roughly 4% for each 100-g decrease in birth weight under 5 pounds (Hakim et al., 1989).

The increased risk of strabismus in these infants is most likely due to maldevelopment of binocular connections in visual cortex. The occipital lobes in newborns are especially vulnerable to damage from hypoxia (Tychsen and Hoyt, 1985; Volpe, 1987). Premature infants frequently suffer ischemic injury to the optic radiations near the occipital trigone. Term infants are prone to hypotensive injury to the dorsal motion processing area of extrastriate cortex, as this area represents the watershed zone for all three major cerebral vessels. Striate cortex in humans has the highest neuron/glia ratio of the entire cerebrum (Bailey and von Bonin, 1951; Huttenlocher et al., 1982; Huttenlocher, 1984) and the highest regional cerebral consumption of glucose (Phelps et al., 1981).

Maternal smoking, drug, or alcohol abuse are associated with increases in amblyopia or strabismus risk

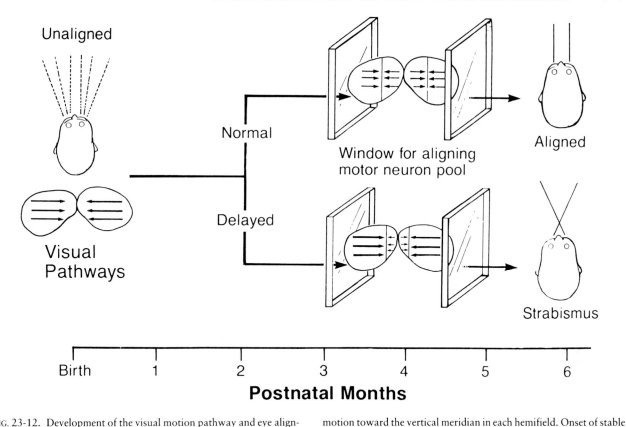

FIG. 23-12. Development of the visual motion pathway and eye alignment during the first 6 months of life. Left: At birth, motion sensitivity when viewing monocularly with either eye is heavily weighted in favor of nasally directed motion. The directional bias is present across the visual field and is not hemiretinal. Eye alignment during the first months of life is unstable, varying between exo-deviated and eso-deviated. Middle: About 98% of infants (normal) outgrow the nasal bias and develop symmetrical motion sensitivity. A small centripetal bias is apparent in the motion pathways, favoring horizontal stimulus motion toward the vertical meridian in each hemifield. Onset of stable eye alignment occurs in most infants within a developmental window spanning the third to fifth month postnatally. Approximately 2% of infants (about 1% of whom were born at term and another 1% who were premature or from complicated pregnancies) suffer developmental delay of the visual motion pathway and enter the alignment "window" with signals strongly biased for nasally directed motion. Many of these infants begin to manifest the constellation of ocular motion findings that typify infantile strabismus.

equivalent to those seen with prematurity or hypoxia (Rantakallio et al., 1978; Miller et al., 1981; Hakim et al., 1989).

SCHEMATIC FOR THE TOPOGRAPHICAL ABNORMALITIES OF NASALLY BIASED MOTION PROCESSING

The available data suggest that the maturation of ocular dominance and cortical topography influence development of motion processing. These data were used to build the flow diagram of motion pathway maldevelopment shown in Figure 23-13, which is based on inferences drawn from psychophysical, neurophysiological, and neuroanatomical studies of normal and strabismic humans and monkeys. Its validity rests on the assumption that the motion pathways of adult strabismic humans represent early, immature stages in the development of a normal motion pathway.

A nasally directed moving stimulus in the monocular vision field of the right eye (left edge of the figure) evokes a response in magnocellular neurons of motion streams in both the ipsilateral and contralateral hemisphere. The visual inputs are conveyed to the hemispheres via ipsilateral LGN lamina 2 and contralateral LGN lamina 1, through monocular neurons in V1 lamina 4cα, to disparity and direction selective neurons in laminae 4B and 6. The contralateral projection is more robust than the ipsilateral as depicted by the bold symbology. Callosal transfer of motion inputs is accomplished by efferents arising from supragranular layers as well as lamina 4. A major interhemispheric transfer occurs from ipsilateral 4 to contralateral MT.

Weak centripetal biases for the population of motion-sensitive neurons have been found in areas V1 and MT of the normal monkey (Maunsell and Van Essen, 1983b; Albright et al., 1984). The centripetal directional bias can be accounted for by simple cortical magnification factors without invoking elaborate circuitry; for ex-

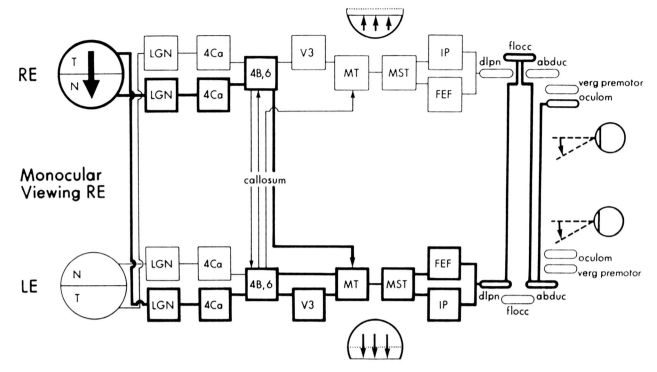

FIG. 23-13. Topographical abnormalities of nasally directed motion processing under conditions of monocular viewing with the right eye. For explanation, see text. RE = right eye; LE = left eye; black arrows = stimulus motion in visual field; T = temporal hemifield; N = nasal hemifield; LGN = dorsal lateral geniculate nucleus; 4Cα = LGN recipient lamina of area V1 (striate cortex), input is monocular from either the nasal of temporal hemifield; 4B, 6 = laminae of area V1 containing a large number of directionally selective binocular neurons that provide extrinsic projection to areas V3–MT; callosum = corpus callosum; MT = middle temporal visual area; MST = medial superior temporal visual area, contiguous with MT; IP = intraparietal sulcus area; FEF = frontal eye field; dlpn = dorsolateral pontine nucleus; flocc = cerebellar flocculus; abduc = abducens nucleus; verg premotor = near response cells dorsolateral to midbrain oculomotor complex; oculom = oculomotor complex; motion bias causes smooth, conjugate eye movement to the left.

ample, the preferred direction of motion for most of the cells in each cerebral hemisphere is that of a stimulus that moves from a more eccentric to a more central position along the horizontal meridian.

The centripetal bias convolved on the transfer of inputs from ipsilateral V1 to heterotopic receptive fields in contralateral MT produces a weak nasally directed bias of motion sensitivity that extends across the vertical meridian of the hemifield (shown as a broadened representation of the vertical meridian in the retinotopical map of area MT in the left hemisphere). The retinotopical map of directional sensitivity in area MT contralateral to the viewing eye is here depicted as being similar to the topographical map of motion sensitivity plotted from the pursuit data of strabismic humans (Tychsen and Lisberger, 1986b).

Signal flow proceeds from area MT to MST, an area known to be involved in visual control of ipsilateral conjugate smooth pursuit eye movement in primates (Dursteler et al., 1987; Komatsu and Wurtz, 1988; Newsome et al., 1988). Projections from MST, VIP, and FEF descend to ipsilateral DLPN and other pontine premotor nuclei (Tusa et al., 1988).

The combined output of areas MT in the ipsilateral and contralateral hemispheres yields a weak bias for nasally directed motion at all loci except those in the eccentric nasal hemifield. The eccentric nasal field retains a weak centripetal bias for temporally directed motion. Note that the combination is not strictly a hemiretinal model but, rather, a schematic of motion processing across a larger portion of the monocular visual field. The schematic is attractive because it depicts only known connections and is one way of accounting for the topographical abnormalities of motion processing documented in strabismic humans.

The serious weakness of the schematic of Figure 23-13 is that it fails to account in a straightforward way for the strong bias favoring nasally directed motion in each eye. The biases favoring centripetal motion in area MT of normal animals are mild, and even if exaggerated it would be difficult to account for the marked biases of the strabismic subject on this basis. Also, imputing the bias to MT would be difficult in neonates, as it is reasonable to assume that areas such as MT that receive projections from V1 are not fully operational near birth. Both of these weaknesses are eliminated if one assumes that the bias involves a simple mechanism early in the motion pathway, e.g., at lamina $4c\alpha$ and 4b of V1, the first level at which directional selectivity is known to be present in the visual system of primates.

MOVEMENT DETECTOR MODEL FOR NASALLY DIRECTED BIAS[1]

Such a mechanism is depicted in the signal processing diagram of Figures 23-14 and 23-15. The diagram uses components drawn from standard models of movement detection (Reichardt, 1961; Barlow and Levick, 1965; Wyatt and Daw, 1975; Torre and Poggio, 1978). For the sake of clarity the units are depicted as Reichardt-type motion detectors.[2] The simplest unit for asymmetrical movement detection is shown in Figure 23-14A. A pair of receptors is connected in such a way that when the left-hand receptor is excited by a spot of light its output is sent through two temporal filters: H, a high-pass or fast filter; and L, a low-pass filter that delays the signal a small amount. When the spot of light is moving in the preferred rightward direction it excites the rightward receptor and coincidence (or multiplicative nonlinear interaction) takes place, allowing a signal to pass. Movement in the null direction does not produce coincidence of signals, as there is no equivalent delay line for movement to the left. The asymmetrical movement detector can be converted to a symmetrical detector by adding a low-pass filter (L) for leftward motion (Fig. 23-14B). The spacing of receptors or the amount of filter delay determines the image velocities to which the detector responds.

Figure 23-14C shows an asymmetrical movement detector that has two low-pass temporal filters: L_1 and L_2. If L_1 had a short delay and L_2 a longer delay, they would provide detection of high and low image velocities, respectively. This mechanism is applied in the signal flow diagram of Figure 23-15, which depicts a preference for nasally directed image motion in each eye under conditions of monocular viewing. Viewing with the left eye, the preferred direction of motion is rightward (nasally directed motion); and viewing with the right eye, the preferred direction is leftward.[3] The temporal filters L_1 and L_2 for the preferred direction are here depicted as present at birth. The L_1 filters have longer time delays than the L_2 filters and so pass signals for lower image velocities. To produce asymmetrical movement detection it is assumed that the L_1 and L_2 filters are not fully functional for the nonpreferred direction at birth. The monocular preference for nasally directed motion in healthy infants and in strabismic infants and adults is most apparent at higher image velocities (or higher temporal frequencies of stimulation). This point is depicted in the figure as a dashed line indicating weak flow through the L_2 filters in the direction of temporally directed motion. With proper maturation the dashed line would be replaced by a solid line indicating unimpeded flow.

Binocular connections are depicted as the dashed lines feeding from the output of each detector to an "AND" gate in the opposite detector. Under conditions of binocular viewing the AND gate would receive input from the L_2 filter of its own receptor and input from the opposite eyes detector, allowing higher-frequency signals to pass. After several months of normal development the AND gate would be replaced by a solid line, converting the asymmetrical detector to a symmetrical detector and making the binocular signal superfluous. The receptors depicted are adjacent pairs of receptors, e.g., two receptors on the left temporal hemiretina and two receptors on the right nasal hemiretina providing input to the left LGN and the left area V1. The four receptors feed into adjacent dominance columns representing corresponding points in the right visual hemifield. The dashed binocular connections could be horizontal axons in lamina 4B, the stria of Gennari.

The asymmetry favoring nasally directed motion under conditions of monocular viewing is most striking at higher image velocities and higher frequencies of image flicker, in both normal young infants and adults whose strabismus had its onset during infancy (for review see Tychsen, 1982). The asymmetry at high velocities or frequencies is demonstrable by testing monocular pursuit or OKN, by measuring the amplitude of the motion-elicited VEP, and by flicker-induced nystagmus. These observations indicate that low-frequency filters are functioning for temporally directed motion detection at or near birth. The high-frequency filters mature much later, and their maturation requires binocular interaction. For this reason, the movement detectors of Figure 23-15 are depicted as containing two types of delay filter, a lower frequency filter operational at birth (the solid line) and a higher frequency filter that is not operational until several months after birth and that requires synchronous binocular input (the dashed line and the AND gate).

The primacy of nasally directed motion detection appears to be an example of an early structural asymmetry

---

1. The idea that someone should begin to modify existing models of asymmetrical motion detection to account for binocular motion development arose from conversations with A. M. Norcia.

2. Equivalent Adelson and Bergen-type detectors can be substituted by taking the sums and differences of the output of the filter pairs, squaring each of them, and adding them together as quadrature pairs (Adelson and Bergen, 1985). Spatial filters can be substituted for the receptor symbols used here.

3. Motion is shown for target motion in the visual field. For the sake of clarity the direction of image motion on the retina is not reversed, as occurs with the image inversion produced by the optics of the eye.

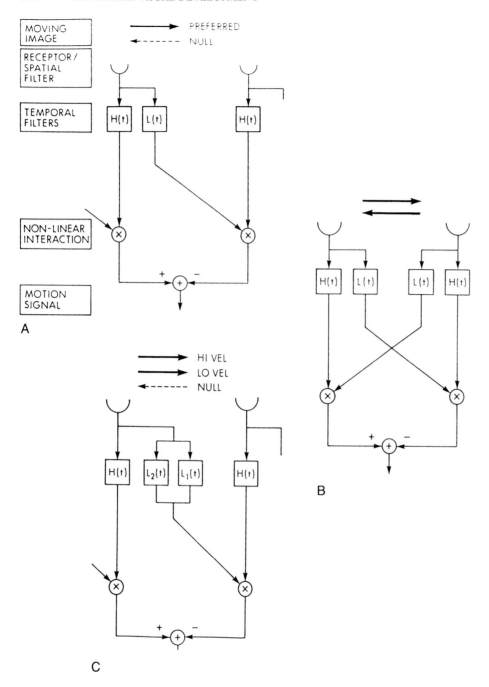

FIG. 23-14. Movement-detector model for the nasally directed bias. For description, see text. Arrows = direction of image motion; H(t) = high pass temporal frequency filter, or neuron; L(t) = low pass filter producing a small delay; $L_1(t)$ = low pass filter with higher cutoff (less delay) than $L_2(t)$; $L_2(t)$ = low pass filter with lower cutoff (more delay) than $L_1(t)$.

that is overcome by development of activity-dependent symmetrical connections. One might expect the structural asymmetry to "reemerge" in normal adults if the activity-dependent connections were severely perturbed. An example may be the motion-detection asymmetries that have been documented in adult humans who have chronically elevated intraocular pressure. The pressure is known to cause selective loss of large-caliber

magnocellular neurons (i.e., the first-order temporal frequency filters). These adults show a progressive bias favoring detection of nasally directed motion, with gradual loss of temporally directed motion sensitivity (Silverman et al., 1990). Random dropout of filters would impair overall signal detection in the motion system but would disproportionately impair more recently developed, fragile motion detectors having narrower tolerances.

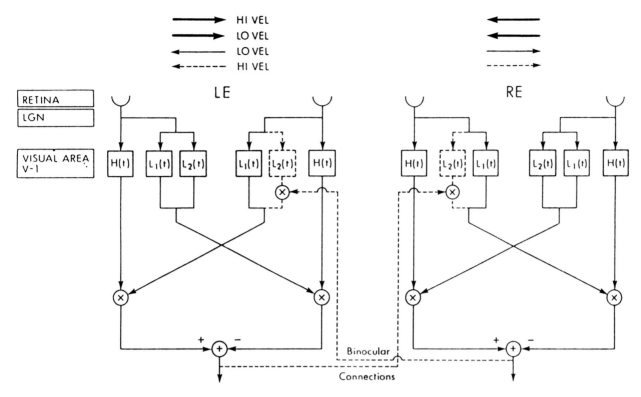

FIG. 23-15. Movement-detector model showing detector modules for both eyes in visual area V1 of the left cerebral hemisphere. The receptors shown at the top of the figure are adjacent receptive fields in the two eyes, e.g., adjacent ganglion cells on the left tremporal retina and right nasal retina. They convey their signals through a high-pass and two kinds of low-pass temporal frequency filters, the $L_2(t)$ filters producing more delay than the $L_1(t)$ filters. The $L_2(t)$ filter and its connections for temporally directed motion are not present at birth (dashed lines) but develop postnatally and require binocular interaction [input to an "and" gate shown as a multiplicative summing junction underneath $L_2(t)$]. When fully mature, the binocular interaction is superfluous, and motion detection is symmetrical for nasally directed versus temporally directed images (the dashed line would become solid). The binocular connections could be collateral axons of lamina 4B between adjacent dominance columns, representing corresponding regions in the right visual field.

BINOCULAR MOTION PROCESSING INPUTS TO VERGENCE

Figure 23-16 shows the model of Figure 23-13 under conditions of binocular input. The retinotopical map of area MT in each hemisphere is biased for nasally direction motion (an exaggeration of the centripetal bias observed in the MT population of the normal macaque) and is expanded to include a region of the ipsilateral hemifield. As noted above, it could occur because of two factors in the V1 to MT projection: (1) conveyance of a strong signal to ipsilateral MT from the nasally biased motion neurons of V1 that receive input from the nasal retina; and (2) a projection to contralateral MT from the motion neurons that receive input from the temporal retina. Independent of the mechanism for the MT bias, the notion of an MT bias itself would be difficult to contest, given the magnitude of the biases in pursuit and correlative biases in velocity perception that have been documented in strabismic humans. In Figure 23-15, summation of the output from the two areas MT (binocular counterphase motion) evokes a response appropriate for crossed disparity motion, namely convergence.

The model is appealing because it is consistent with current notions of the visual signals necessary to drive vergence to moving targets. It assumes that vergence signals arise from combination of signals used to drive simpler conjugate eye movements (in-phase binocular motion). Counterphase frontoparallel motion (i.e., looming) evokes the perception of increasing near disparity and evokes convergence eye movements in humans (Tyler, 1983; Regan et al., 1986). Recordings from area MST in behaving monkeys have shown that these cells encode both pursuit and vergence signals (Gnadt and Mays, 1989), and recordings from premotor vergence neurons (near response neurons) in behaving monkeys have shown that vergence and versional eye movement signals sum algebraically (Mays and Porter, 1984; Mays et al., 1986).

Figure 23-17 depicts the vergence promotor neuron pool as a cross-linked matrix driven by disparity and motion signals [analogous to the accommodative-vergence models of Semmlow and Hung (1983) and

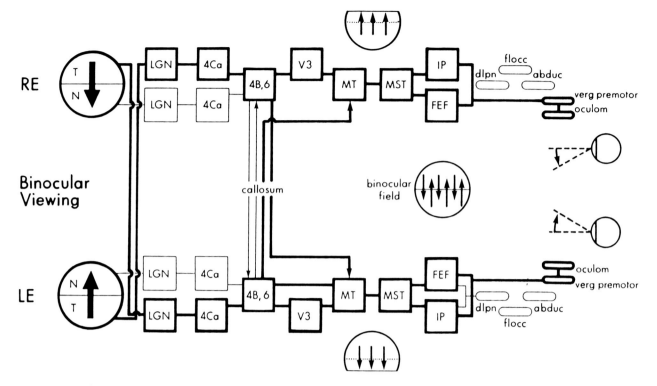

FIG. 23-16. Nasally directed biases of motion processing under conditions of binocular viewing. The nasal bias of motion processing in the visual pathway of each hemisphere leads to a combined bias favoring convergence (nasally directed motion in each eye, or opponent motion signally image movement toward the head). The ocular motor response is a bias toward convergence. Strong disparity signals would need to counteract the biased motion signals to maintain eye alignment. For explanation of abbreviations see Figure 23-13.

Hain and Zee (1989)]. Disparity and motion pathways drive individual vergence neurons with unequal weight. The vergence pool is calibrated by negative feedback loops. Failure to develop robust disparity sensitivity and temporally directed motion sensitivity allows the system to run open loop.

EXPERIMENTS NECESSARY TO VALIDATE THE MODEL

The model in its current state is acceptable as a first approximation, given that its inferences are based on known connections and properties of motion neurons in the primate. Major gaps are apparent, however, and several critical experiments are necessary to confirm or refute important assumptions. Falsification of the model should be attempted by neurophysiological and neuroanatomical experimentation at several specific levels of the motion pathway of the strabismic monkey.

The naturally occurring infantile esotropia of the monkey provides an ideal opportunity for such study (Kiorpes and Boothe, 1981; Boothe et al., 1985b; Kiorpes et al., 1985). One advantage of studying monkeys is that they, like humans, possess a well developed fovea centralis and smooth pursuit. The functional organization of motion processing is highly similar in the mon-

key and human (Tychsen and Lisberger, 1986b; for review see Lisberger et al., 1987). The monkey visual system is sensitive to fine binocular disparities (Poggio and Fischer, 1977; Poggio et al., 1988) and displays robust vergence (Mays and Porter, 1984; Judge and Cumming, 1986).

Preliminary ocular motor recordings have been obtained from naturally strabismic monkeys who have normal visual acuity in both eyes. These animals exhibit the constellation of eye movement signs seen in strabismic humans (Matsumoto et al., 1991). Recordings have documented latent fixation nystagmus, dissociated vertical deviation, and directional asymmetry of horizontal smooth pursuit. Further training and more detailed recordings are required to determine if these animals have the topographical distortion of pursuit initiation and the asymmetry of velocity perception detectable in strabismic humans.

Extracellular recordings are planned for lamina 4 of visual area V1 in these animals. The cells in lamina 4 are of major interest for several reasons: (1) they are segregated into nasotemporal columns more conspicuously than cells in other laminae of V1; (2) they send and receive callosal visual axons; (3) they are both disparity and direction selective; and (4) they are the source of the major projection into visual area MT (Ungerlei-

Unstable Eye Alignment

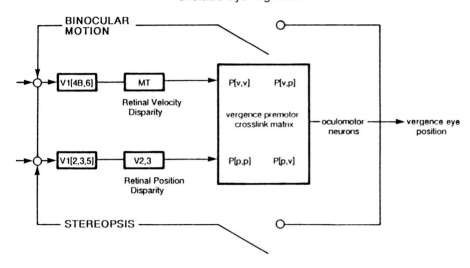

Stable Eye Alignment

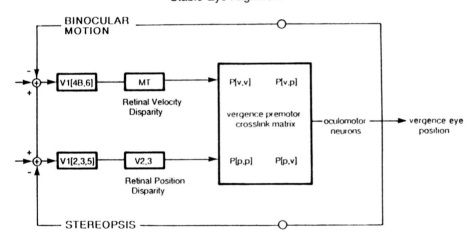

FIG. 23-17. Vergence premotor neuron pool as a crosslink matrix driven by motion and disparity inputs. Before age 3–5 months, image disparity and binocular motion feedback loops are open, and motion input is nasally biased. At age 3–5 months, binocular motion and stereopsis emerge, and eye alignment is stable. P = premotor neuron; v,v = neuron driven exclusively by image velocity (motion) inputs; v,p = neuron driven predominantly by iamge velocity with some image position (disparity) inputs; p,p = neurons driven exclusively by disparity inputs; p,v = neuron driven predominantly by disparity inputs with some image velocity inputs.

der and Mishkin, 1979; Maunsell and Van Essen, 1983b; Hawken et al., 1988). The combination of recording and injection of neuroanatomical tracers should be able to determine if a larger number of lamina 4 neurons are driven by input from the contralateral eye; a tracer study should also reveal if lamina 4 callosal efferents interconnect heteroptic locations in the two hemispheres. The cell populations of visual area MT should be similarly studied. Seventy-nine percent of the MT cells in normal monkeys are driven binocularly, and no attempt has been made to determine the binocular responsiveness of these cells in strabismic animals or to

test the directional selectivity in MT of normal or strabismic animals under conditions of monocular viewing (Maunsell and Van Essen, 1983b; Van Essen, personal communication). Similar recordings from MST cells should be attempted to determine if cell population biases exist that favor nasally directed stimulus or eye motion.

As for behavioral study, efforts should be made to produce esotropia by rearing conditions that deprive animals of disparity and motion channel inputs. A small body of numerical data is currently available describing the tuning properties of these channels as a function of postnatal age (Mohn, 1989; Norcia et al., 1990). Better psychophysical estimates of the spatiotemporal properties of the channels will allow quantitative definition of the way in which motion inputs and disparity inputs could influence vergence, e.g.:

$$(N/T_{re} + N/T_{le} + D_u) - (D_c) = 0 = Error_{verg}$$

where N/T = a nasotemporal motion asymmetry index when viewing monocularly with the right eye (re) or left eye (le); D_c = sensitivity to crossed disparities; and D_u = sensitivity to uncrossed disparities. The equation states that subjects who failed to develop sensitivity to temporally directed motion when viewing with either eye (N/T ratios > 1.0) could maintain eye alignment if they developed sufficient sensitivity to uncrossed disparities (large value of D_u).

HISTORICAL NOTIONS OF THE CAUSE OF INFANTILE STRABISMUS

Up to this point in the discussion of visual processing and the possible mechanism of infantile esotropia I have made little effort to place recent data into the context of historical schools of thought on the origins of strabismus. In this final section I briefly outline historical hypotheses.

To help clarify thinking I have attempted to bring each hypothesis into a modern frame of reference by assigning it to anatomical components of known pathways. In some cases it is an arbitrary assignment for several reasons. First, there is the problem of translating what the author has said into current physiological terms; data on motion and form streams in the visual cortex were unavailable before the 1980s. Second, there is a problem of specificity regarding whether the authors were limiting their hypotheses to typical esotropia with onset during infancy (e.g., excluding discussion of the esotropia associated with large hyperopic refractive errors). Third, there is the problem caused by clinical uses of the term "fusion." By "fusion," did the authors mean the blending of images from the two eyes to form the percept of a single object in depth, or did they mean vergence movements undertaken to align the visual axis of each eye on a stimulus?

Historical hypotheses regarding the mechanism of infantile esotropia suffer from two general weaknesses. As noted above, the first is lack of anatomical or physiological specificity. To say that esotropia is caused by an excess of tonic convergence is a meaningless tautology, as it does not explain the origin of the excess. A second general weakness is a lack of comprehensiveness: a failure to account for the timing, constellation of ocular motor signs, perceptual deficits, and predicted response to treatment. Although it might be reasonable to postulate that the esotropia itself is due to a primary myopathy of the eye muscles, it cannot account for sudden emergence of the esotropia 3 months after birth, for nystagmus and conjugate asymmetries of pursuit, for deficits in motion processing, or for the high prevalence in infants who suffer delayed development of cerebral cortex.

Nature Versus Nurture

Perhaps the clearest point of departure for a discussion of opposing views on the cause of infantile strabismus can be drawn along the "nature-nurture" axis (Figure 23-18). Worth (1903) was a strong proponent of an inborn irreversible defect of fusion. Although he did not specify exactly what he meant by fusion or a location in the central nervous system for the congenital defect, it is reasonable to interpret his language as a defect of disparity sensitive neurons in the primary visual area. Crones' (1973) "nature" hypothesis is similar to that of Worth. Crone argued for a primary dysfunction in the development of binocular sensitivity based on the following findings in infantile esotropia: absence of gross optical or orbital abnormalities that would impede binocularity or eye alignment; the disappointing rate of restoration of normal binocularity despite early therapy; and the ability of many individuals to develop excellent binocularity despite impediments such as congenital extraocular muscle fibrosis or palsy.

The leading proponent of the "nurture" hypothesis was Chavasse (1939). Chavasse contended that everything necessary for normal binocular fusion had been present in strabismic individuals at birth, but that the development of fusion postnatally was impeded by abnormalities of optical input (e.g., monocular cataract) or muscular output (e.g., a cranial nerve palsy). The argument is couched in the terminology of Pavlovian reflexes, binocular vision being a reflex conditioned during the early postnatal period. A key point in Chavasse's argument was that normal binocularity could still be learned by the strabismic subject if the input or output impediments were removed by early therapy. Thus the cause and the cure of infantile strabismus could be largely localized to the end-organ itself.

Costenbader (1961) and Parks (1975), as advocates of early intervention, subscribed to the outline of the "nurture" hypothesis. Parks described a binocular fixation conditioned reflex much like that noted by Chavasse.[4]

---

4. For other interpretations of the Worth–Chavasse controversy the reader is referred to an article by Day and Norcia (1990) and von Noorden's text (1990).

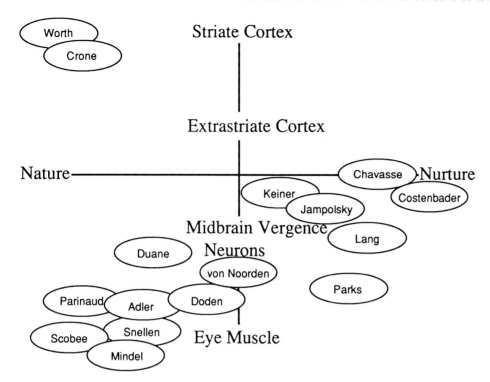

FIG. 23-18. Historical notions of the cause of infantile strabismus arrayed along prenatal versus postnatal and visual pathway versus motor pathway axes. See text for discussion. Early authors appear behind more recent authors. The list of authors is not exhaustive but includes almost all those who proposed a mechanism for infantile esotropia in their writings. Excluded are those who did not address specifically the topic of nonrefractive infantile esotropia.

Visual Pathways Versus Motor Pathways

Opposing viewpoints on the origins of infantile esotropia are also arrayed along a visuomotor axis. Worth and Crone, arguing for a congenital deficit in binocularity, can be positioned at the visual cortex end of this axis. Most other hypotheses fall into a vague middle ground between visual cortex and muscle. Snellen (1913), Scobee (1948), and Mindel et al. (1980, 1983) defined the muscle end of the axis.

Keiner (1956) postulated a defect of cortical binocularity compounded by direct subcortical "light tonus" inputs (Keiner, 1956). Keiner claimed that, at birth, illumination of the temporal retina drove the eyes nasalward. Keiner's writing repeatedly touched on the topics of unstable infant vergence, a vague nasally directed bias, and what can be interpreted as a defect of disparity sensitivity. Keiner firmly believed that esotropia developed postnatally: "All children are born with a potentiality to squint and an almost total dissociation of the two eyes. Congenital squint does not exist; strabismus cannot occur until the light stimulus is able—in connection with the stage of development of the reflex paths—to produce a motor effect" (Keiner, 1951). Jampolsky's (1978) "bilateral monocular esotropia" hy-pothesis was thematically related to the thinking of Keiner (Jampolsky, 1978). "I offer the hypothesis that very early neonatal visual influences may be responsible for motor misalignment and anomalous motor development. Light stimulus in the premature insufficiently developed eyes (with yet incompletely resolved media diffusors in the vitreous and lens) fulfills the essential overall diffusion stimulus criterion—the chain of exaggerated monocular and binocular dominances with altered muscle tonus." According to this model, the diffuse light excites a primitive brainstem motor reflex, driven by the nasal hemiretinas, which evokes bilateral monocular adduction movements. Lang's (1984) hypothesis similarly cited subcortical light inputs as the mechanism for infantile esotropia. The subcortical inputs cause "fixation on the nasal side of both foveae, and the eyes assume a convergent position. Only with development does fixation return to the fovea, but it has a tendency to slide over to the nasal retinal half." Lang postulated that delay in myelination of the optic nerves may be a factor, as may "difficulty in coordination between ocular and vestibular influences."

The notion of a primary defect of vergence motoneurons, "excessive tonic convergence," has attracted the largest number of proponents. Duane (1897) ascribed the esotropia to an excess of subcortical "convergent tonus" unopposed by cortical influences. Parinaud (1899) and Adler (1945) pointed to a primary anomaly of convergence innervation that produced, over time, secondary changes in the medial rectus muscle attachments. Parks (1975) noted that the mechanism for excessive convergence was unknown. von Noorden (1988) proposed that "a delay in the development or a permanent defect of motor . . . vergences in a sensorially normal infant causes esotropia during the vulnerable first three months of visual immaturity under the influence of factors that destabilize the oculomotor equilibrium." These factors are "uncorrected hypermetropia and anisometropia already mentioned by Worth, excessive tonic convergence, an abnormally high AC/A ratio, or anomalies of the neural integrators for vergence movements. . . ."

Doden and Adams (1957) implicated an unspecified lower brainstem vestibuloocular mechanism for esotropia, based on the observation that strabismus was highly associated with fixation nystagmus. Snellen (1913) believed the primary defect to be partial muscle paralysis. Similarly, Scobee (1948) argued that infantile esotropia was caused by inborn defects of the extraocular muscles and their tendinous attachments. Mindel appears to share some of the views of both Snellen and Scobee (Mindel et al., 1980, 1983). Mindel postulated that the cause of esotropia is a relative excess of en grappe acetylcholine receptors on the medial rectus muscles. A secondary increase in such receptors would be expected following chronic excitation of the muscles from any cause. Mindel et al. implied a primary excess.[5]

Acknowledgments. My interpretation of different schools of thought on strabismus causality has been greatly aided by conversations with many participants in the workshop Anthony Norcia and I conducted on form and motion pathway development at the 1988 and 1990 meetings of the Association for Pediatric Ophthalmology and Stra-

---

5. Those seeking broader perspectives on the origins of strabismus are referred to three important monographs: Keiner's *New Viewpoints on the Origin of Squint* (1951); Jampolsky's "Unequal Visual Inputs and Strabismus Management: A Comparison of Human and Animal Strabismus" (1978); and Flynn's *Strabismus: A Neurodevelopmental Approach* (1991). The first chapter of Keiner's book is a review of hypotheses to midcentury, followed by a series of observations from his own patient cases and speculation on the importance of the "monocular adduction reflexes." Jampolsky's work is a single, lengthy chapter, but it is so full of ideas that it is considered a monograph by students of strabismus. Highlights are speculations on the importance of nasotemporal asymmetries and his now famous cautions regarding the invalidity of extrapolating findings in amblyopic and strabismic cats to a discussion of humans. Flynn's book provides a bird's-eye view of the phenomenon of childhood strabismus. He reviewed human embryology and neonatology, encouraging neuroscientists to study strabismus as a fascinating growth disorder of the cerebral hemispheres.

bismus. I am indebted especially to Anthony Norcia for helpful criticisms and to Andreas Burkhalter, Stephen Lisberger, Ronald Boothe, Nigel Daw, and Fran Mizen. Several students helped in data analysis: Robert MacDonald (supported by the March of Dimes), Bertram Matsumoto, and William Segal. Eileen McGowan provided valuable technical assistance. This work was supported by a Career Development Award from Research to Prevent Blindness; by the Knight's Templar Eye Research Foundation; by Biomedical Research Support Grant 54329A from Washington University School of Medicine; and by LDIR 77552420 from the USAF School of Aerospace Medicine.

REFERENCES

ADELSON, E. H., AND BERGEN, J. R. (1985). Spatiotemporal energy models for the perception of motion. *J. Opt. Soc. Am. [A]* 2, 284–299.

ADLER, F. (1945). Pathologic physiology of convergent strabismus: motor aspects of the non-accommodative type. *Arch. Ophthalmol.* 33, 362.

ALBRIGHT, T., DESIMONE, R., AND GROSS, C. (1984). Columnar organization of directionally selective cells in visual area MT of the macaque. *N. Neurophys.* 51(1), 16–31.

APKARIAN, P, REITS, D., AND SPEKREIJSE, H. (1984). Component specificity in albino VEP asymmetry: maturation of the visual pathway anomaly. *Exp. Brain Res.* 53, 285–294.

ARCHER, S., HELVESTON, E., MILLER, K., AND ELLIS, F. D. (1986). Stereopsis in normal infants and infants with congenital esotropia. *Am. J. Ophthalmol.* 101, 591–596.

ARCHER, S. M., SONDHI, N., AND HELVESTON, E. M. (1989). Strabismus in infancy. *Ophthalmology* 96, 133–137.

ASLIN, R. N. (1977). Development of binocular fixation in human infants. In *Eye Movements: Cognition and Visual Perception.* Hillsdale, NJ: Erlbaum, pp. 31–51.

ATKINSON, J. (1979). Development of optokinetic nystagmus in the human infant and monkey infant: an analogue to development in kittens. In R. D. FREEMAN (eds.). *Developmental Neurobiology of Vision.* New York: Plenum, pp. 277–287.

ATKINSON, J., AND BRADDICK, O. (1981). Development of optokinetic nystagmus in the human infant and monkey infant. In D. F. FISHER, R. A. MONTY, AND J. W. SENDERS (eds.). *Eye Movements: Cognition and Visual Perception.* Hillsdale, NJ: Erlbaum, pp. 53–64.

BAILEY, P., AND VON BONIN, G. (1951). *The Isocortex of Man.* Urbana: University of Illinois Press.

BARLOW, H. B., AND LEVICK, W. R. (1965). The mechanism of directionally selective units in rabbit's retina. *J. Physiol. (Lond.)* 178, 477–504.

BERMAN, N. E., AND PAYNE, B. R. (1983). Alterations in connections of the corpus callosum following convergent and divergent strabismus. *Brain Res.* 274, 201–212.

BIRCH, E. E., AND STAGER, D. R. (1985). Monocular acuity and stereopsis in infantile esotropia. *Invest. Ophthalmol. Vis. Sci.* 26, 1624–1630.

BIRCH, E. E., STAGER, D. R., BERRY, P., AND EVERETT, M. E. (1990). Prospective assessment of acuity and stereopsis in amblyopic infantile esotropes following early surgery. *Invest. Ophthalmol. Vis. Sci.* 31, 758–765.

BOOTHE, R. G., DOBSON, V., AND TELLER, D. Y. (1985a). Postnatal development of vision in human and nonhuman primates. *Annu. Rev. Neurosci.* 8, 495–546.

BOOTHE, R. G., KIORPES, L., AND CARLSON, M. R. (1985b). Studies of strabismus and amblyopia in infant monkeys. *J. Pediatr. Ophthalmol. Strabismus* 22, 206–212.

BOURDET, C., AND VAN SLUYTERS, R. C. (1989). Visual callosal development in strabismic cats. *Soc. Neurosci. Abstr.* 15, 1338.

BRADDICK, O., AND ATKINSON, J. (1983). The development of binocular function in infancy. *Acta. Ophthalmol. Suppl. 157 (Copenh.)* 62, 27–35.

CHAVASSE (1939).

COLLEWIJN, H., MARTINS, A., AND STEINMAN, R. (1981). Natural retinal image motion: origin and change. *Ann. N.Y. Acad. Sci.* 374, 312–329.

COSTENBADER, F. D. (1961). Infantile esotropia. *Trans. Am. Ophthalmol. Soc.* 59, 397–429.

CRAWFORD, M. L. J., AND VON NOORDEN, G. K. (1979). The effects of short-term experimental strabismus on the visual system in *Macaca mulatta*. *Invest. Ophthalmol. Vis. Sci.* 18, 496–505.

CRONES (1973).

CROSS, H. E. (1975). The heritability of strabismus. *Am. Orthoptic J.* 25, 11–17.

CYNADER, M., AND HARRIS, L. (1980). Eye movement in strabismic cats. *Nature* 286, 64–65.

DAY, S. H., AND NORCIA, A. M. (1990). Infantile esotropia and the developing visual system. *Pediatr. Ophthalmol.* 3, 281–287.

DEHAY, C., KENNEDY, H., AND BULLIER, J. (1986). Callosal connectivity of area V1 and V2 in the newborn monkey. *J. Comp. Neurol.* 254, 20–33.

DEMER, J. L., AND VON NOORDEN, G. K. (1988). Optokinetic asymmetry in esotropia. *J. Pediatr. Ophthalmol. Strabismus* 25, 286–292.

DICKEY, C. F., METZ, H. S., STEWART, S. A., AND SCOTT, W. E. (1991). The diagnosis of amblyopia in cross-fixation. *J. Pediatr. Ophthalmol. Strabismus* 28, 171–176.

DOBSON, V., AND SEBRIS, S. L. (1989). Longitudinal study of acuity and stereopsis in infants with or at-risk for esotropia. *Invest. Ophthalmol. Vis. Sci.* 30, 1146–1158.

DODEN, W., AND ADAMS, W. (1957). Elektronystagmographische Ergebnisse der Prufung des optischvestigularen Systems bei Schielenden. *Ber. Zusammenkrunft Dtsch. Ophthalmol. Ges.* 60, 316–317.

DUANE, A. (1897). *A New Classification of the Motor Anomalies of the Eye*. New York: J. H. Vaio.

DURSTELER, M., WURTZ, R., AND NEWSOM, W. (1987). Directional pursuit deficits following lesions of the foveal representation within the superior temporal sulcus of the macque monkey. *J. Neurophysiol.* 57, 1262–1287.

FINOCCHIO, D. V., PRESTON, K. L., AND FUCHS, A. F. (1990). A quantitative analysis of the development of the vestibulo-ocular reflex and visual-vesibular interactions in human infants. *Invest. Ophthalmol. Vis. Sci.* 19(suppl.), 83.

FLYNN, J. T. (1991). *Strabismus: A Neurodevelopmental Approach*. New York: Springer-Verlag.

GAUTHIER, G., AND ROBINSON, D. (1975). Adaptation of the human vestibulo-ocular reflex to magnifying lenses. *Brain Res.* 92, 331–335.

GNADT, J., AND MAYS, L. (1989). Posterior parietal cortex, the oculomotor near response and spatial coding in 3-D space. *Soc. Neurosci. Abstr.* 15, 786.

GONSHOR, A., AND MELVILL JONES, G. (1976). Extreme vestibulo-ocular adaptation induced by prolonged optical reversal of vision. *J. Physiol. (Lond.)* 256, 381–414.

GROENENDAAL, F., VAN HOF-VAN DUIN, J., ET AL. (1989). Effects of perinatal hypoxia on visual development during the first year of (corrected) age. *Early Hum. Dev.* 20, 267–279.

GUILLERY, R. (1979). Normal and abnormal visual pathways. *Trans. Ophthalmol. Soc. UK* 99, 352.

GUILLERY, R. (1986). Neural abnormalities of albinos. *TINS* 9, 364–367.

GWIAZDA, J., BAUER JR., J. A., AND HELD, R. (1989). Binocular function in human infants: correlation of stereoptic and fusion-rivalry discriminations. *J. Pediatr. Ophthalmol. Strabismus* 26, 128–132.

HAIN, T. C., AND ZEE, D. S. (1989). Vergence. *Bull. Soc. Belge Ophthalmol.* 237, 145–161.

HAKIM, R., TIELSCH, J., CANNER, J., AND GUYTON, D. (1989). Prenatal and fetal risk factors for childhood strabismus. *Invest. Ophthalmol. Vis. Sci.* 30, 107.

HAMER, R. D., NORCIA, A. M., OREL-BIXLER, D., AND HOYT, C. S. (1990). Cortical responses to nasalward and temporalward motion are asymmetric in early but not late-onset strabismus. *Invest. Ophthalmol. Vis. Sci.* 31(suppl.), 289.

HAWKEN, M. J., PARKER, A. J., AND LUND, J. S. (1988). Laminar organization and contrast sensitivity of direction-selective cells in the striate cortex of the old world monkey. *J. Neurosci.* 8, 3541–3548.

HELVESTON, E. M., PINCHOFF, B., ELLIS, F. D., AND MILLER, K. (1985). Unilateral esotropia after enucleation in infancy. *Am. J. Ophthalmol.* 100, 96–99.

HENDRICKSON, A. E. (1985). Dots, stripes and columns in monkey visual cortex. *Trends Neurosci.* 406–410.

HOFFMANN, K. (1979). Optokinetic nystagmus and single-cell responses in the nucleus tractus opticus after early monocular deprivation in the cat. In R. D. FREEMAN (ed.). *Developmental Neurobiology of Vision*. New York: Plenum, pp. 63–72.

HOYT, C. (1980). The long-term visual effects of short-term binocular occlusion of at-risk neonates. *Arch. Ophthalmol.* 98, 1967–1970.

HOYT, C., AND CALTRIDER, N. (1984). Hemispheric visually-evoked responses in congenital esotropia. *J. Pediatr. Ophthalmol. Strabismus* 21, 19–21.

HUBEL, D. H., AND WIESEL, T. N. (1965). Binocular interaction in striate cortex of kittens reared with artificial squint. *J. Neurophysiol.* 28, 1041–1059.

HUBEL, D. H., AND WIESEL, T. N. (1967). Cortical and callosal connections concerned with the vertical meridian of visual field in the cat. *J. Neurophysiol.* 30, 1561–1573.

HUBEL, D. H., AND WIESEL, T. N. (1972). Laminar and columnar distribution of geniculocortical fibers in macaque monkeys. *J. Comp. Neurol.* 146, 421–450.

HUBEL, D. H., AND WIESEL, T. N. (1977). Ferrier lecture: functional architecture of macaque monkey visual cortex. *Proc. R. Soc. Lond. [Biol.]* 198, 1–59.

HUBEL, D., WIESEL, T., AND LEVAY, S. (1977). Plasticity of ocular dominance columns in monkey striate cortex. *Philos. Trans. R. Soc. Lond. [Biol.]* 278, 377–409.

HUTTENLOCHER, P. R. (1984). Synapse elimination and plasticity in developing human cerebral cortex. *Am. J. Ment. Defic.* 88, 488–496.

HUTTENLOCHER, P., DE COURTEN, C., GAREY, L., AND VAN DER LOOS, H. (1982). Synaptogenesis in human visual cortex: evidence for synapse elimination during normal development. *Neurosci. Lett.* 33, 247–252.

INNOCENTI, G., AND CLARKE, S. (1984). The organization of immature callosal connections. *J. Comp. Neurol.* 230, 287–309.

INNOCENTI, G. M., AND FROST, D. O. (1979). Effects of visual experience on the maturation of the efferent system to the corpus callosum. *Nature* 280, 231–234.

INNOCENTI, G., FROST, D., AND ILLES, J. (1985). Maturation of visual callosal connections in visually deprived kittens: a challenging critical period. *J. Neurosci.* 5, 255–267.

JAMPOLSKY, A. (1978). Unequal visual inputs and strabismus management: a comparison of human and animal strabismus. In E. M. HELVESTON, A. JAMPOLSKY, P. KNAPP, K. W. MCNEER, M. M. PARKS, R. D. REINECKE, W. E. SCOTT, AND G. K. VON NOORDEN (eds.). *Symposium on Strabismus: Transactions of the New Orleans Academy of Ophthalmology*. St. Louis: Mosby, pp. 358–492.

JUDGE, S. J., AND CUMMING, B. G. (1986). Neurons in the monkey midbrain with activity related to vergence eye movement and accommodation. *J. Neurophysiol.* 55, 915–929.

JUDISCH, G. F. (1985). Basis of inheritance. In T. D. DUANE AND E. A. JAEGER (eds.). *Biomedical Foundations of Ophthalmology*. Philadelphia: Harper & Row.

KALIL, R. E., SPEAR, P. D., AND LANGSETMO, A. (1984). Response properties of striate cortex neurons in cats raised with divergent or convergent strabismus. *J. Neurol.* 52, 514–536.

KATO, I., HARADA, K., HASEGAWA, T., AND IKARASHI, T. (1986). Role of the nucleus of the optic tract in monkeys in relation to optokinetic nystagmus. *Brain Res.* 364, 12–22.

KEINER, G. B. J. (1951). *New Viewpoints on the Origin of Squint: A Clinical and Statistical Study on Its Nature, Cause and Therapy*. The Hague: Martinus Nijhoff.

KEINER, G. B. J. (1956). Physiology and pathology of the optomotor reflexes. *Am. J. Ophthalmol.* 42, 233–249.

KIORPES, L., AND BOOTHE, R. G. (1981). Naturally occurring strabismus in monkeys (*Macaca nemestrina*). *Invest. Ophthalmol. Vis. Sci.* 20, 257–263.

KIORPES, L., BOOTHE, R., CARLSON, M., AND ALF, D. (1985). Frequency of naturally occurring strabismus in monkeys. *J. Pediatr. Ophthalmol. Strabismus* 22, 60–64.

KITCHEN, W., RICKARDS, A., RYAN, M. M., MCDOUGALL, A. B., BILLSON, F. A., ET AL. (1979). A longitudinal study of very low-birthweight infants. II. Results of controlled trial of intensive care and incidence of handicaps. *Dev. Med. Child Neurol.* 21, 582–589.

KOMATSU, H., AND WURTZ, R. (1988). Relation of cortical areas MT and MST to pursuit eye movements. III. Interaction with full-field visual stimulation. *J. Neurophysiol.* 60, 621–644.

KUSHNER, B. J. (1982). Strabismus and amblyopia associated with regressed retinopathy of prematurity. *Arch. Ophthalmol.* 100, 256–261.

LANG, J. (1984). *Strabismus* (G. W. Cibis, trans.). Thorofare, NJ: Slack.

LEVAY, S., HUBEL, D., AND WIESEL, T. (1975). The pattern of ocular dominance columns in macaque visual cortex revealed by a reduced silver stain. *J. Comp. Neurol.* 159, 559–576.

LEVAY, S., WIESEL, T., AND HUBEL, D. (1980). The development of ocular dominance columns in normal and visually-deprived monkeys. *J. Comp. Neurol.* 191, 1–51.

LEVENTHAL, A., VITEK, D., AND CREEL, D. (1985). Abnormal visual pathways in normally pigmented cats that are heterozygous for albinism. *Science* 229, 1395–1396.

LEWIS, T. L., MAURER, D., AND BRENT, H. P. (1989). Optokinetic nystagmus in normal and visually deprived children: implications for cortical development. *Can. J. Psychol.* 43(2), 121–140.

LISBERGER, S. G., AND WESTBROOK, L. E. (1985). Properties of visual inputs that initiate horizontal smooth pursuit eye movements in monkeys. *J. Neurosci.* 5, 1662–1673.

LISBERGER, S. G., MORRIS, E. J., AND TYCHSEN, L. (1987). Visual motion processing and sensory-motor integration for smooth pursuit eye movements. *Annu. Rev. Neurosci.* 10, 97–129.

LUND, J., LUND, R., HENDRICKSON, A., BUNT, A., AND FUCHS, A. (1975). The origin of efferent pathways from the primary visual cortex, area 17, of the macaque monkey as shown by retrograde transport of horseradish peroxidase. *J. Comp. Neurol.* 164, 287–304.

LUND, R., MITCHELL, D., AND HENRY, G. (1978). Squint-induced modification of callosal connections in cats. *Brain Res.* 144, 169–172.

MANNING, K., FULTON, A., HANSEN, R., MAYER, D., ET AL. (1982). Preferential looking vision testing: application to evaluation of high-risk, prematurely born infants and children. *J. Pediatr. Ophthalmol. Strabismus* 19, 286–293.

MATSUMOTO, B., MACDONALD, R., AND TYCHSEN, L. (1991). Constellation of ocular motor findings in naturally-strabismic macaque: animal model for human infantile strabismus. *Invest. Ophthalmol. Vis. Sci.* 32(suppl.), 820.

MAUNSELL, J. H. R., AND VAN ESSEN, D. C. (1983a). The connections of the middle temporal visual area (MT) and their relationship to a cortical hierarchy in the macaque monkey. *J. Neurosci.* 3, 2563–2586.

MAUNSELL, J. H. R., AND VAN ESSEN, D. C. (1983b). Functional properties of neurons in middle temporal visual area of the macaque monkey. I. Selectivity for stimulus direction, speed, and orientation. *J. Neurophysiol.* 49, 1127–1147.

MAUNSELL, J. H. R., AND VAN ESSEN, D. C. (1987). Topographic organization of the middle temporal visual area in the macaque monkey: representational biases and the relationship to callosal connections and myeloarchitectonic boundaries. *J. Comp. Neurol.* 266, 535–555.

MAURER, D., LEWIS, T. L., AND BRENT, H. P. (1983). Peripheral vision and optokinetic nystagmus in children with unilateral congenital cataract. *Behav. Brain Res.* 10, 151–161.

MAYS, L. E., AND PORTER, J. D. (1984). Neural control of vergence eye movements: activity of abducens and oculomotor neurons. *J. Neurophysiol.* 52, 743–761.

MAYS, L. E., PORTER, J. D., GAMLIN, P. D. R., AND TELLO, C. A. (1986). Neural control of vergence eye movements: neurons encoding vergence velocity. *J. Neurophysiol.* 56, 1007–1021.

MCKEE, S. P., AND WELCH, L. (1985). Sequential recruitment in the discrimination of velocity. *J. Opt. Soc. Am. [A]* 2, 243–251.

METZ, H. S. (1985). Unilateral esotropia after enucleation in infancy. *Am. J. Ophthalmol.* 859–860.

MILES, F. (1976). Effects of a continuously moving environment on the rhesus monkey's ocular stability in the dark. *Soc. Neurosci. Abstr.* 2, 273.

MILES, F. A., AND LISBERGER, S. G. (1981). Plasticity in the vestibulo-ocular reflex: a new hyothesis. *Annu. Rev. Neurosci.* 4, 273–299.

MILLER, M., ISRAEL, J., AND CUTTONE, J. (1981). Fetal alcohol syndrome. *J. Pediatr. Ophthalmol. Strabismus* 18, 6–15.

MINDEL, J., RAAB, E., EISENKRAFT, J., AND TEUTSCH, G. (1980). Succinyldicholine-induced return of the eyes to the basic deviation: a motion picture study. *Ophthalmology* 12, 1288–1295.

MINDEL, J. S., EISENKRAFT, J. B., RAAB, E. L., AND TEUTSCH, G. (1983). Succinyldicholine and the basic ocular deviation. *Am. J. Ophthalmol.* 95, 315–326.

MOHINDRA, I. (1985). Development of acuity and stereopsis in infants with esotropia. *Ophthalmology* 92, 691–697.

MOHN, G. (1989). The development of binocular and monocular optokinetic nystagmus in human infants. *Invest. Ophthalmol. Vis. Sci.* 30(suppl.), 49.

MOHN, G., AND VAN HOF-VAN DUIN, J. (1985). The development of the binocular and monocular visual field in fullterm and preterm human infants. *Invest. Ophthalmol. Vis. Sci.* 26(suppl.), 137.

MOVSHON, J. A., AND VAN SLUYTERS, R. C. (1981). Visual neural development. *Annu. Rev. Psychol.* 32, 477–522.

MOVSHON, J. A., CHAMBERS, B. E. I., AND BLAKEMORE, C. (1972). Interocular transfer in normal humans, and those who lack stereopsis. *Perception* 1, 483–490.

MUSTARI, M. J., AND FUCHS, A. F. (1990). Discharge patterns of neurons in the pretectal nucleus of the optic tract (NOT) in the behaving primate. *J. Neurophysiol.* 64, 77–90.

NAEGELE, J. R., AND HELD, R. (1982). The postnatal development of monocular optokinetic nystagmus in infants. *Vision Res.* 22, 341–346.

NEWSOME, W. T., AND PARE, E. B. (1988). A selective impairment of motion perception following lesions of the middle temporal visual area MT. *J. Neurosci.* 8, 2201–2211.

NEWSOME, W., WURTZ, R., AND KOMATSU, H. (1988). Relation of cortical areas MT and MST to pursuit eye movements. II. Differentiation of retinal from extraretinal inputs. *J. Neurophysiol.* 60, 604–620.

NEWSOME, W. T., WURTZ, R. H., DURSTELER, M., AND MIKAMI, A. (1985). Deficits in visual motion processing following ibotenic acid lesions of the middle temporal visual area of the macaque monkey. *J. Neurosci.* 5, 825–840.

NISSENKOM, I. (1990). Nasal vs. temporal preretinal vasoproliferation in retinopathy of prematurity. *Surv. Ophthalmol.* 34, 474–475.

NIXON, R. B., HELVESTON, E. M., MILLER, K., ARCHER, S. M., AND ELLIS, F. D. (1985). Incidence of strabismus in neonates. *Am. J. Ophthalmol.* 100, 798–801.

NORCIA, A. M., HAMER, R. D., AND OREL-BIXLER, D. (1990). Temporal tuning of the motion VEP in infants. *Invest. Ophthalmol. Vis. Sci.* 31(suppl.), 10.

NORCIA, A. M., HUMPHREY, R., GARCIA, H., AND HOLMES, A. (1989). Anomalous motion VEPS in infants and in infantile esotropia. *Invest. Ophthalmol. Vis. Sci.* 30(suppl.), 327.

OOHIRA, A., ZEE, D., AND DAS, S. (1989). Disconjugate ocular motor adaptation in rhesus monkeys. *Invest. Ophthalmol. Vis. Sci.* 30(suppl.), 183.

ORNITZ, E., ATWELL, C., AND WALTER, D. (1979). The maturation of the vestibular nystagmus in infancy and childhood. *Acta Otolaryngol. (Stockh.)* 88, 244–256.

PARINAUD, H. (1899). *Le Strabisme et Son Traitement*. Paris: Gaston Doin & Cie.

PARKS, M. (1975). *Ocular Motility and Strabismus*. Hagerstown: Harper & Row.

PHELPS, M., MAZZIOTTA, J., KUHL, D., NUWER, M., PACKWOOD, J., METTER, M., AND ENGEL, J. (1981). Tomographic mapping of human cerebral metabolism: visual stimulation and deprivation. *Neurology* 31, 517–529.

POGGIO, G. F., AND FISCHER, B. (1977). Binocular interaction and depth sensitivity in striate and prestriate cortex of behaving rhesus monkey. *J. Neuropysiol.* 40, 1392–1405.

POGGIO, G. F., GONZALEZ, F., AND KRAUSE, F. (1988). Stereoscopic mechanisms on monkey visual cortex: binocular correlation and disparity selectivity. *J. Neurosci.* 8, 4531–4550.

QUICK, M. W., TIGGES, M., GAMMON, J. A., AND BOOTHE, R. G. (1989). Early abnormal visual experience induces strabismus in infant monkeys. *Invest. Ophthalmol. Vis. Sci.* 30, 1012–1017.

RANTAKALLIO, P., KRAUSE, U., AND KRAUSE, K. (1978). The use of the ophthalmological services during the preschool age, ocular findings and family background. *J. Pediatr. Ophthalmol. Strabismus* 15, 253–258.

REGAN, D., ERKELENS, C. J., AND COLLEWIJN, H. (1986). Visual field defects for vergence eye movements and for stereomotion perception. *Invest. Ophthalmol. Vis. Sci.* 27, 806–819.

REICHARDT, W. (1961). Autocorrelation: a principle for the evaluation of sensory information by the central nervous system. In W. A. ROSENBLITH (ed.). *Sensory Communication*. Cambridge, MA: MIT Press, pp. 303–317.

RODIECK, R. W. (1979). Visual pathways. *Annu. Rev. Neurosci.* 2, 193–225.

SCHOR, C., AND LEVI, D. (1980). Disturbances of small-field horizontal and vertical optokinetic nystagmus in amblyopia. *Invest. Ophthalmol. Vis. Sci.* 19, 668–683.

SCOBEE, R. (1948). Anatomic factors in the etiology of heterotropia. *Am. J. Ophthalmol.* 31, 781.

SEABAR, J. (1991). Amblyopia in monocular aphakia. In *American Association of Certified Orthopists*. Anaheim, CA: AACO.

SEGAL, W., MACDONALD, R., BURKHALTER, A., AND TYCHSEN, L. (1991). Topographic variation of magnocellular neurons in normal human lateral geniculate nucleus: temporal and lower field visual biases. *Invest. Ophthalmol. Vis. Sci.* 32(suppl.), 1116.

SEMMLOW, J. L., AND HUNG, G. K. (1983). The near response: theories of control. In C. M. SCHOR AND K. J. CIUFFREDA (eds.).

Vergence Eye Movements: Basic and Clinical Aspects. Boston: Butterworths, pp. 175–195.

SHATZ, C. J., LINDSTROM, S. H., AND WIESEL, T. N. (1977). The distribution of afferents representing the right and left eyes in the cat's visual cortex. *Brain Res.* 131, 103–116.

SHERMAN, S. M., GUILLERY, R. W., KAAS, J. H., AND SANDERSON, K. J. (1974). Behavioral, electrophysiological and morphological studies of binocular competition in the development of the geniculo-cortical pathway of cats. *J. Comp. Neurol.* 158, 1–18.

SILVERMAN, S. E., TRICK, G. L., AND HART, W. M. (1990). Motion perception is abnormal in primary open-angle glaucoma and ocular hypertension. *Invest. Ophthalmol. Vis. Sci.* 31, 722–729.

SINGER, W. (1978). The effects of monocular deprivation on cat parastriate cortex: asymmetry between crossed and uncrossed pathways. *Brain Res.* 157, 351–355.

SNELLEN, H. (1913). Die Ursache des Strabismus convergens concomitans. *Arch. Ophthalmol.* 24, 433.

SPARKS, D., MAYS, L., GURSKI, M., AND HICKEY, T. (1986). Long and short-term monocular deprivation in the rhesus monkey: effects on visual fields and optokinetic nystagmus. *J. Neurosci.* 6, 1771–1780.

SPIVEY, B. (1980). Strabismus: factors in anticipating its occurrence. *Aust. J. Ophthalmol.* 8, 5–9.

STONE, J. (1983). *Parallel Processing in the Visual System*. Oxford: Plenum.

TORRE, V., AND POGGIO, T. (1978). A synaptic mechanism possibly underlying directional selectivity to motion. *Proc. R. Soc. Lond. [Biol.]* 202, 409–416.

TUSA, R. J., HERDMAN, S. J., AND MISHKIN, M. (1988). Ocular motor deficits in retinotopic and craniotopic space in monkeys with unilateral striate and corpus callosum lesions. *Soc. Neurosci. Abstr.* 14, 796.

TUSA, R. J., PALMER, L. A., AND ROSENQUIST, A. C. (1978). The retinotopic organization of area 17 (striate cortex) in the cat. *J. Comp. Neurol.* 177, 213–236.

TYCHSEN, L. (1989). Primary maldevelopment of visual motion pathway in humans. *Invest. Ophthalmol. Vis. Sci.* 30(suppl.), 302.

TYCHSEN, L. (1991). Pediatric ocular motility disorders of neuro-ophthalmic significance. In W. T. SHULTS (ed.). *Ophthalmology Clinics of North America*. Philadelphia: Saunders, pp. 615–643.

TYCHSEN, L. (1992). Binocular vision. In W. H. HART (ed.). *Adler's Physiology of the Eye: Clinical Applications*. St. Louis: Mosby.

TYCHSEN, L., AND HOYT, W. F. (1985). Occipital lobe dysplasia. *Arch. Ophthalmol.* 103, 680–682.

TYCHSEN, L., AND LISBERGER, S. G. (1986a). Visual motion processing for the initiation of smooth-pursuit eye movements in humans. *J. Neurophysiol.* 56, 953–968.

TYCHSEN, L., AND LISBERGER, S. G. (1986b). Maldevelopment of visual motion processing in humans who had strabismus with onset in infancy. *J. Neurosci.* 6, 2495–2508.

TYCHSEN, L., HURTIG, R. R., AND SCOTT, W. E. (1985). Pursuit is impaired but the vestibulo-ocular reflex is normal in infantile strabismus. *Arch. Ophthalmol.* 103, 536–539.

TYCHSEN, L., QUICK, M., AND BOOTHE, R. G. (1991a). Alternating monocular input from birth causes stereoblindness, motion processing asymmetries, and strabismus in infant macaque. *Invest. Ophthalmol. Vis. Sci.* 32(suppl.), 1044.

TYCHSEN, L., RIZZO, M., HURTIG, R. R., STEVENS, R. W., AND ENGELKEN, E. J. (1988). Visual motion processing in humans after loss of striate cortex. *Soc. Neurosci. Abstr.* 14, 796.

TYLER, C. W. (1983). Sensory processing of binocular disparity. In C. M. SCHOR AND K. J. CUIFFREDA (eds.). *Vergence Eye Movements: Basic and Clinic Aspects*. Boston: Butterworths, pp. 199–296.

UNGERLEIDER, L. G., AND MISHKIN, M. (1979). The striate projection zone in the superior temporal sulcus of *Macaca mulatta*: location and topographic organization. *J. Comp. Neurol.* 188, 347–366.

VAN ESSEN, D. C. (1985). Functional organization of primate visual cortex. In A. PETERS AND E. JONES (eds.). *Cerebral Cortex.* New York: Plenum, pp. 259–329.

VAN HOF-VAN DUIN, J. (1978). Direction-preference of optokinetic responses in monocularly tested normal kittens and light-deprived cats. *Arch. Ital. Biol.* 116, 471–477.

VAN HOF-VAN DUIN, J., EVENHUIS-VAN LAUNEN, A., ET AL. (1989). Effects of very low birth weight (VLBW) on visual development during the first year term. *Early Hum. Dev.* 20, 255–266.

VAN SLUYTERS, R. C., AND LEVITT, F. B. (1980). Experimental strabismus in the kitten. *J. Neurophysiol.* 43, 686–699.

VITAL-DURAND, F., PUTKONEN, P. T. S., AND JEANNEROD, M. (1974). Motion detection and optokinetic responses in dark-reared kittens. *Vision Res.* 14, 141.

VOLPE, J. J. (1987). Hypoxic-ischemic encephalopathy: neuropathology and pathogenesis. In J. VOLPE (ed.). *Neurology of the Newborn.* Philadelphia: Saunders, pp. 209–235.

VON GRUNAU, M. W., AND RAUSCHECKER, J. P. (1983). Natural strabismus in non-Siamese cats: lack of binocularity in the striate cortex. *Exp. Brain Res.* 52, 307–310.

VON NOORDEN, G. K. (1988). Current concepts of infantile esotropia: XLIV Edward Jackson memorial lecture. *Am. J. Ophthalmol.* 105, 1–10.

VON NOORDEN, G. K. (1990). *Binocular Vision and Ocular Motility.* St. Louis: Mosby.

WALTON, P., AND LISBERGER, S. G. (1989). Binocular misalignment in infancy causes directional asymmetries in pursuit. *Invest. Ophthalmol. Vis. Sci.* 30(suppl.), 304.

WIESEL, T. N. (1982). Postnasal development of the visual cortex and the influence of environment. *Nature* 299, 583.

WIESEL, T. N., AND HUBEL, D. N. (1963). Single-cell responses in striate cortex of kittens deprived of vision in one eye. *J. Neurol.* 26, 1003–1017.

WOOD, C., SPEAR, P., AND BRAUN, J. (1973). Direction-specific deficits in horizontal optokinetic nystagmus following removal of visual cortex in the cat. *Brain Res.* 60, 231–237.

WORTH (1903).

WYATT, H., AND DAW, N. (1975). Directionally sensitive ganglion cells in the rabbit retina: specificity for stimulus direction, size, and speed. *J. Neurophysiol.* 38, 613–626.

ZEE, D., TUSA, R., HERDMAN, S., AND BUTLER, P. (1987). Effects of occipital lobectomy upon eye movements in primate. *J. Neurophysiol.* 58, 883.

24 | Amblyopia: A consequence of abnormal visual development

DENNIS M. LEVI AND ANDREW CARKEET

Amblyopia, a disorder of spatial vision, is almost always associated with the presence of strabismus, anisometropia, or form deprivation *early in life* (Ciuffreda et al., 1990). If the same disorders (i.e., strabismus, anisometropia, or form deprivation) occur late in life, amblyopia does not develop. The powerful notion of amblyopia as a developmental disorder was first articulated by Worth (1903), who formulated the theory that the reduced vision of the amblyopic eye represented arrested sensory development. Specifically, Worth suggested that the presence of a "sensory obstacle" (e.g., unilateral strabismus) arrested the development of visual acuity ("amblyopia of arrest"), so the patient's acuity remained at the level achieved at the time of onset of strabismus. In this view, the depth of amblyopia is a direct function of the age of onset of the "sensory obstacle." Worth further suggested that if amblyopia of arrest were allowed to persist, "amblyopia of extinction" could occur as a result of binocular inhibition. In Worth's view, only this "extra" loss of sensory function (i.e., the amblyopia of extinction) could be recovered by treatment. Although the latter notion appears to be untenable in the light of present knowledge, the ideas of Worth (1903) have had a powerful influence on both clinicians and basic scientists. Thus many of our currently held concepts of amblyopia, such as plasticity, sensitive periods, and abnormal binocular interaction, were described almost a century ago.

In this chapter we examine the notion of amblyopia as a developmental disorder of spatial vision. We begin by sketching out the nature of the deficit in strabismic and anisometropic amblyopia and then ask whether the amblyopic visual system may be considered to be immature (i.e., arrested development) or, put another way: Is the infant visual system a good model for understanding amblyopia? In particular, we examine a developmental hypothesis that might account for the differences in performance between strabismic and anisometropic amblyopes. Finally, we ask if the normal (adult) retinal periphery offers a reasonable model for understanding the spatial vision of amblyopes and infants.

VISUAL FUNCTION IN AMBLYOPIA

In clinical practice, the defining characteristic of amblyopia is reduced visual acuity in an otherwise healthy, properly corrected eye. Amblyopia is generally accompanied by *strabismus* (a turned eye), *anisometropia* (unequal refractive error), or both (strabismus and anisometropia) in approximately equal proportions (Flom and Neumaier, 1966; Ciuffreda et al., 1990), and these "sensory obstacles" are widely presumed to be the cause of the visual loss. In psychophysical studies, amblyopes demonstrate many, various, and often curious visual losses (for a detailed review see Levi, 1991). An attempt is made throughout to compare and, where possible, contrast the performance of strabismic and anisometropic amblyopes (other categories of amblyopes, e.g., stimulus deprivation, which are rare, receive only cursory consideration in this chapter). This task is easier said than done, as many studies have not paid attention to distinctions that may exist between amblyopias associated with different presumptive etiologies. Moreover, even studies that have attempted to make distinctions are confronted with two potential sources of ambiguity: (1) difficulty of clinical diagnosis (e.g., failure to discover microstrabismus in a patient with anisometropia); and, perhaps more critical, (2) the difficulty of ascertaining an accurate and complete history of the development of the amblyopia and its associated conditions. Despite these difficulties, there is strong evidence that strabismic and anisometropic amblyopia differ in their psychophysical performance. We argue that these differences may be understood by considering the time course of development of form perception and by the nature of the "sensory obstacles" represented by strabismus and anisometropia.

"Light Sense"

The earliest psychophysical studies of amblyopia were concerned with the integrity of basic processes in the amblyopic visual system. Specifically, early workers were interested in learning about the status of rod and cone mechanisms in the amblyopic eye. More than a century ago, Bjerrum (1884) noted that there was essentially no difference in the "light sense" between the amblyopic and nonamblyopic eye. In their classic study, Wald and Burian (1944) measured dark adaptation and spectral sensitivity curves in a group of amblyopes. Their results showed essentially identical dark adaptation curves in the two eyes and normal scotopic and photopic spectral sensitivity, both centrally and peripherally. These findings have been widely accepted; and although several investigators have noted slightly elevated cone thresholds in amblyopic eyes (e.g., Oppel and Kranke, 1958), these losses were found in only some observers and were small in magnitude. The conclusion drawn by Wald and Burian, now widely accepted, was that the basic retinal sensory mechanisms (rods, cones, and photopigments) are intact and normal in the amblyopic visual system. Wald and Burian argued further that amblyopia represents a dissociation between the "light sense" and the "form sense."

Luminance Increment Thresholds. Both strabismic and anisometropic amblyopes show elevated luminance increment thresholds for small targets (Miller, 1955; Grosvenor, 1957) and increased spatial summation (Flynn, 1967). The increment threshold task requires the observer to detect a target (e.g., a bar, slit, or spot) superimposed on a homogeneous background. Thus the task is actually contrast discrimination. Although Miller, Grosvenor, and Flynn all interpreted their results in terms of altered retinal receptive field characteristics (i.e., increased receptive field size or reduced lateral inhibition), this explanation does not seem tenable in light of more recent studies. A more plausible alternative explanation does not depend on alterations in either the size or the shape of retinal receptive fields but, rather, is based on the spatial frequency specific loss of contrast sensitivity of the amblyopic eye (Levi and Harwerth, 1982).

Stiles-Crawford Effect. Enoch (1957, 1967) was the first to suggest that the amblyopia could be a consequence of a specific retinal receptor abnormality, i.e., "receptor amblyopia." Enoch's suggestion came from his studies of the Stiles-Crawford effect of the first type in amblyopic eyes. His results showed that amblyopes may have slightly distorted Stiles-Crawford functions. Enoch hypothesized that tilting, or "malorientation," of the retinal receptors could lead to both the abnormal Stiles-Crawford functions and the reduced central visual acuity characteristic of amblyopes. This conclusion has been questioned on a number of grounds. First, marked malorientation of the receptors would produce only a minor reduction in acuity (Campbell and Gregory, 1960). Second, undetected eccentric fixation in an amblyopic

eye could mimic malorientation of the retinal receptors (Marshall and Flom, 1970). More recently, Bedell (1980) has reconsidered the question of photoreceptor misalignment in amblyopic eyes. Bedell noted that all of the amblyopic eye peaks were clustered within a subregion of the pupil, as occurs in normal eyes. His results clearly demonstrated that the reduced vision of amblyopes cannot be attributed to disturbances in the physical or optical properties, or in the malorientation of the retinal receptors.

Color Vision. Harwerth and Levi (1978), using flicker photometry, corroborated the earlier report of Wald and Burian (1944) that photopic (as well as scotopic) spectral sensitivity are essentially normal in the amblyopic eye. Although the cone color mechanisms have not been studied in detail psychophysically in the amblyopic visual system, it is likely that they are normal. Thus Francois and Verriest (1967) have found that the color vision of amblyopes is essentially normal except for a few severe cases of strabismic amblyopia (visual acuity worse than 20/200). These deficits are similar to those found in normal peripheral vision, as are many other aspects of visual performance in strabismic amblyopes.

Amblyopes do, however, demonstrate anomalies in their increment threshold spectral sensitivity functions (Harwerth and Levi, 1977). Increment threshold spectral sensitivity is measured by superimposing the test spot on a bright, uniform, white background, so the observer's task is to distinguish the test spot from the background. Experiments using sinusoidal gratings (Bradley et al., 1986) showed that the contrast sensitivity of the amblyopic eye is similarly reduced for chromatic and achromatic gratings, suggesting that the reduction in increment threshold spectral sensitivity in the amblyopic eye can be understood in terms of its reduced spatial contrast sensitivity.

Temporal Processing in the Amblyopic Visual System

Although amblyopia is typically characterized as an anomaly of spatial vision, a large number of studies have addressed the question of temporal processing in amblyopia. Several aspects of the temporal processing of amblyopic eyes are discussed in this section.

Temporal Resolution. Many early studies were concerned with the critical fusion frequency (CFF) of the amblyopic eye, i.e., the highest flicker rate at which an intermittent stimulus appears to just flicker. The results of these studies are somewhat contradictory. For example, Feinberg (1956) found a significant and consistent reduction in the CFF of his subjects. Alpern et al. (1960) found rather smaller losses, and Miles (1949) found the CFF to be superior in the amblyopic eye of about half of his sample. Thus CFF is sometimes but not always reduced in amblyopic eyes, and the losses are generally small. This finding is not really surprising, considering that the stimuli used for measuring CFF generally have a lot of low spatial frequency information. Although CFF represents one limit of temporal resolution, it is in many respects analogous to the measurement of visual acuity in the spatial domain.

Temporal Contrast Sensitivity. A more complete description of temporal processing may be obtained by measuring the temporal contrast sensitivity function (de Lange function), i.e., 1/ the threshold contrast needed to detect temporal variations in a uniform field over a wide range of temporal frequencies (de Lange, 1958). Because the stimulus is temporally modulated about a constant mean luminance level, adaptation level is easily controlled.

The temporal contrast sensitivity of amblyopic eyes also shows considerable between-subject variation. For example, substantial losses in the temporal contrast sensitivity function of the amblyopic eye, particularly at low temporal frequencies, were observed in some studies (e.g., Spekreijse et al., 1972; Wesson and Loop, 1982), whereas little or no loss was evident in other studies. For example, Manny and Levi (1982a) found small losses in about half of their population. These losses were most prominent at low temporal frequencies and were found to depend on both the adaptation level (they normalize at low luminance levels) and the field size.

Bradley and Freeman (1985) have addressed the question of field size in more detail by reanalyzing data from seven studies of flicker sensitivity as a function of the stimulus field size. Their analysis clearly show an inverse relation between the stimulus size and the observed deficits. Small deficits in CFF and temporal contrast sensitivity were found with large stimuli (e.g., Manny and Levi, 1982a), and large deficits in CFF (e.g., Feinberg, 1956) or temporal contrast sensitivity (Wesson and Loop, 1982) were found with small targets. This analysis makes it clear that much of the deficit in "temporal" processing of amblyopes revealed by uniform field flicker studies are a consequence of the spatial parameters of the stimulus.

Summary. The results of the psychophysical studies reviewed above suggest that (1) the basic retinal receptor processes (rods and cones) of the amblyopic eye are essentially normal. In fact, there is little hard evidence for any primary retinal abnormality in the amblyopic eye. (2) Wald and Burian in 1944 concluded that amblyopia is an anomaly of the "form sense" rather than the "light sense." However, as was pointed out by Hecht and Mintz (1939), this distinction is specious. Rather, it may be more appropriate to describe the threshold

abnormalities of strabismic and anisometropic amblyopes in terms of reduced contrast sensitivity for high spatial frequencies (i.e., fine detail). In the next section, this conclusion is developed further, and we argue that amblyopia may be regarded as a developmental anomaly involving primarily those cortical mechanisms involved in form and shape perception. (3) Amblyopes show abnormalities in spatiotemporal processing that can be largely understood in terms of the reduced spatial contrast sensitivity of the amblyopic eye. Thus amblyopes show either small or no losses for large uniform fields or low spatial frequency gratings flickering rapidly. Amblyopes do show reduced sensitivity for small fields and for high spatial frequencies, however, and these losses are most pronounced at low temporal frequencies (Schor and Levi, 1980; Manny and Levi, 1982b; Bradley and Freeman, 1985). Whether this temporal dependence is a result of abnormal eye movements or a selective loss of slow mechanisms is still a matter of controversy. In addition, amblyopes show normal velocity discrimination for high velocities but poor velocity discrimination for slow velocities (Steinman et al., 1988), a finding that may bear on their reduced ability to track slowly drifting targets.

Spatial Vision in Amblyopia

Visual Acuity. Reduced visual acuity is the defining feature of amblyopia. Surprisingly, the distribution of Snellen acuities provides some interesting insights into the differential effects of anisometropia and strabismus. For both anisometropic and strabismic amblyopes, the most frequently encountered acuities fall between 1.5 and 3.0 minutes (20/30–20/60), whereas the preponderance of poorer Snellen acuities are found in strabismic amblyopes (Levi, 1990).

Spatial Contrast Sensitivity. Amblyopia is generally defined by a decrease in visual acuity; however, visual acuity represents only one limit of visual capacity, i.e., the smallest high contrast stimuli that can be resolved. Most objects in everyday vision are larger than this limit, but many have lower contrast. In fact, the ability to perceive spatial detail is determined to a great extent by one's ability to discern contrast, i.e., differences in brightness of adjacent areas. It is interesting to note that neurons in primary visual cortex are indifferent to variations in luminance (e.g., Shapley, 1986). Changes in adaptation level are handled by retinal gain control mechanisms (e.g., Green, 1986). Abnormal contrast functions have long been implicated in the amblyopic eye. The studies of Miller (1955), Grosvenor (1957), and Flynn (1967) suggested that amblyopes have difficulty detecting contrast variations in small stimuli. Lawwill and Burian (1966) measured the contrast required by each eye of amblyopes to read letters of varying size. They found that, at photopic luminance levels, amblyopic eyes required considerably higher contrast to detect the letters than did the fellow eyes.

The use of sine-wave gratings to measure contrast sensitivity in amblyopic eyes has a particular advantage. By using an extended stimulus, it is possible to ensure that the target is imaged on the fovea, even in amblyopes with eccentric fixation. Using this approach, it is now well established that strabismic and anisometropic amblyopia result in marked losses of threshold contrast sensitivity (Gstalder and Green, 1971; Hess and Howell, 1977; Hilz et al., 1977; Levi and Harwerth, 1977; Thomas, 1978; Bradley and Freeman, 1981; Selby and Woodehouse, 1981). The reduced contrast sensitivity found in most amblyopic eyes is most marked at high spatial frequencies, with a smaller or no loss at low spatial frequencies. Hess and Howell (1977) argued for two categories of loss in strabismics, i.e., high spatial frequency only, or both high and low spatial frequencies. It now appears likely that there are at least two sources that can contribute to the low spatial frequency losses they and other workers observed: (1) the use of small fields (Katz et al., 1984); and (2) relative image magnification effects associated with anisometropia (Bradley and Freeman, 1981). Katz et al. (1984) found that in amblyopic observers the magnitude of the loss of contrast sensitivity at low spatial frequencies depends on the size of the stimulus field. With large fields little or no loss was evident, whereas with small fields there were substantial reductions in contrast sensitivity in the amblyopic eye at low spatial frequencies. This low spatial frequency loss with small fields may be related to edge effects, which extend over long distances in the amblyopic eye. In any event, the loss of contrast sensitivity is always greatest at high spatial frequencies.

The loss of contrast sensitivity at high spatial frequencies increases with the severity of the amblyopia (Levi, 1988). The high spatial frequency cutoff (i.e., the highest spatial frequency that can be detected with 100% contrast) provides a measure of the resolution capacity of the eye. With normal foveal vision, the cutoff is around 40–50 cycles/degree (cpd), i.e., equivalent to normal Snellen acuity levels of about 20/15. In amblyopic eyes the cutoff is also highly correlated with Snellen acuity. Correlation coefficients are often on the order of 0.9; however, high correlations do not imply perfect correspondence. Gstalder and Green (1971) first pointed out that the grating acuity of strabismic amblyopes was much better than their Snellen acuity. This finding has been confirmed by a number of investigators (Hess et al., 1978; Levi and Klein, 1982a,b; Selenow et al., 1986); and Hess and colleagues (1978) have reported on several strabismic amblyopes who showed abnormal Snellen acuity and almost normal contrast sensitivity.

Despite the failure of the contrast sensitivity function (CSF) to provide a complete account of the visual losses of strabismic amblyopes, it does provide a number of important insights into the functioning of the amblyopic visual system. First, the results outlined above stress the spatial frequency-dependent nature of the losses that occur in amblyopia. These losses occur primarily at high spatial frequencies, so it is not surprising that studies using large stimuli (e.g., spots or slits) failed to find significant loss of function. Second, because of the steep slope of the high spatial frequency limb of the CSF a small reduction in acuity is reflected by a large loss in contrast sensitivity. Thus measurements in the contrast domain (vertical axis of the CSF) are inherently more sensitive than those in the acuity domain (horizontal axis). Third, and perhaps most importantly, the reduced contrast sensitivity of the amblyopic eye does not result from optical factors (Fankhauser and Rohler, 1967; Hess and Smith, 1977; Levi and Harwerth, 1977) or unsteady fixational eye movements (Higgins et al., 1982). Nor is it a result of eccentric fixation, as it occurs when the grating is sufficiently large to encompass the fovea. Thus the reduced CSF of the amblyopic eye represents a neural loss in foveal function.

"Spatial Sense"

Although clinicians generally consider spatial vision in terms of Snellen acuity, with a limiting acuity of about 20/20 (i.e., critical detail of about 1 minute), the visual system is capable of making much finer spatial discriminations. For example, relative position can be judged with an accuracy of 3–6 arc seconds or better (Westheimer, 1975). These low spatial thresholds are 5–10 times finer than either the cutoff spatial frequency or the intercone spacing. For this reason, Westheimer (1975) coined the term "hyperacuity" to describe a variety of tasks that involve sensing the direction of spatial offset of a line or point relative to a reference. Hyperacuity, or positional acuity, has been the focus of much research and modeling for both normal and anomalous vision. There are several reasons. First, it is of basic interest to understand how the visual system achieves this high degree of accuracy. Second, several lines of evidence suggest that performance on hyperacuity tasks reflects cortical processing (Levi et al., 1985; McKee and Levi, 1987). Third, it seems likely that the mechanisms underlying hyperacuity have the more general task of form and shape analysis (Marr, 1982). Thus studying hyperacuity may provide a "window" to the operation of the cortical mechanisms of form perception. Not surprisingly, with amblyopia, which is considered to be an abnormality of the "form" sense, hyperacuity is markedly degraded. With hyperacuity tasks, several lines of evidence suggest that the losses of strabismic and anisometropic amblyopes are fundamentally different. In particular, Levi and Klein (1982a,b, 1983, 1985, 1990b) have shown that in *anisometropic* amblyopes, grating acuity (or resolution) and positional acuity are similarly affected by the amblyopic process. However, *strabismic* amblyopes show greater losses in the accuracy of positional acuity than for grating resolution. Figure 24-1 plots the resolution/Vernier acuity (R/V) ratio for a group of normal and amblyopic observers. For normal foveal vision and for anisometropic amblyopes the resolution thresholds/Vernier thresholds (R/V) ratio is approximately 7.5:1.0 (in other words, Vernier acuity is about 7.5 times finer than resolution). However, the R/V ratio of strabismic amblyopes and those with both strabismus and anisometropia is considerably poorer, even approaching 1:1. This result is similar to the decoupling of Snellen acuity and grating acuity in strabismic amblyopes described in the section on contrast sensitivity. Levi and Klein (1982b) showed that the reduced positional acuity of amblyopes could not be accounted for on the basis of eccentric fixation or faulty eye movements and thus represents a neural deficit(s) in the amblyopic visual system. Although the differences in performance between strabismic and anisometropic amblyopes may represent fundamentally different neural deficits, we examine the possibility that the different pattern of losses of strabismic and anisometropic amblyopes represent differential effects of development.

VISUAL FUNCTION IN INFANTS

There is now a great deal of insight into the development of visual mechanisms and sensitivities. One concept is that different visual functions may emerge at different times and develop at different rates. For example, the rod system appears to be functional during early infancy (Powers et al., 1981; Werner, 1982; Teller and Bornstein 1986; Fulton, 1988; Brown, 1990; see also Chapter 13). Whereas rods and rhodopsin are functional early, postreceptoral mechanisms may mature later, as dark-adapted spatial summation areas of infants are considerably enlarged compared to those of adults (Hamer and Schneck, 1984). Most of the investigations of cone-mediated vision have focused on the development of mechanisms of color vision, visual acuity, and contrast sensitivity. It is now reasonably well established that by 2–3 months of life infants must have three functioning cone types. The question of when each of these three types functions normally is less clear. Infants less than 1 month old fail to make chromatic discriminations; however, what remains unclear is whether these failures reflect immature cones, postreceptoral mechanisms (Teller and Bornstein, 1986; Teller and Movshon, 1986), or lack of attention. Uniform field flicker sensitivity appears to be adult-like by 3 months of age (Regal, 1981), whereas acuity and contrast sensitivity for high spatial frequencies develop slowly and may not reach adult levels until several years of age (see below).

Spatial Vision: Acuity, Contrast Sensitivity, Hyperacuity

Much effort has focused on the development of spatial vision in human infants, and it seems of particular relevance to the development of amblyopia. Almost all recent studies suggest that grating acuity develops rapidly within the first year of life and then continues to develop more slowly, reaching adult levels near age 3–6 years (Dobson and Teller, 1978; Mayer and Dobson, 1982; Teller and Movshon, 1986; Gwiazda, 1987; Carkeet et al., 1990). Studies show that visually evoked potential (VEP) acuity approaches 20 cpd by the end of the first year of life (Norcia and Tyler, 1985), considerably earlier than behavioral (forced-choice preferential looking, or FPL) techniques suggest. The discrepant estimates of these techniques have not been resolved (Dobson and Teller, 1978; Teller and Movshon, 1986), but the VEP data of Norcia and Tyler may be considered to provide a lower boundary on the spatial resolution of the afferent visual pathway, up to striate cortex. Interestingly, Wilson's (1988) analysis of acuity and cone spacing in the infant retina suggests that VEP acuity at age 1 month is consistent with lim-

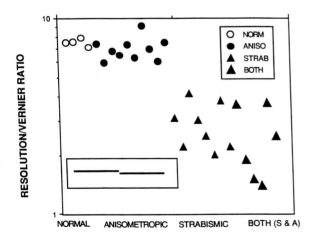

FIG. 24-1. Ratio of resolution to Vernier acuity for a group of normal and amblyopic observers. The abutting Vernier stimuli are defined in the inset, and experimental details were given by Levi and Klein (1985). With normal foveal vision (○) and in anisometropic amblyopes (●), the R/V ratio is approximately 7.5:1.0 (in other words, Vernier acuity is about 7.5 times finer than resolution). However, the R/V ratio of strabismic amblyopes (medium ▲) and those with both strabismus and anisometropic (larger ▲) is considerably poorer, even approaching 1:1.

itations imposed by cone sampling, whereas FPL acuity is considerably lower. The highest spatial frequency mechanisms (those responsible for acuities approaching 60 cpd in adults) continue to develop well beyond the first year of life (de Vreis-Khoe and Spekreijse, 1982).

Studies of the development of contrast sensitivity in infants are sparse, but the emerging picture suggests that peak contrast sensitivity increases, and the peak of the CSF shifts toward higher spatial frequencies with age. Low spatial frequency sensitivity develops much more rapidly than high spatial frequency sensitivity. Thus peak contrast sensitivity may reach adult levels as early as about 9 weeks of age, whereas sensitivity at higher spatial frequencies continues to develop dramatically; and there remains a roughly 20-fold difference in the contrast sensitivity of adults and that of 8-month-olds (Norcia et al., 1990). There remains some debate about the shape of the infant CSF (Banks and Salapatek, 1976; Movshon and Kiorpes, 1988). Much of the developmental change in visual resolution and contrast sensitivity can be understood on the basis of developmental changes in the retina and cortex. For example, the growth of foveal cone outer segments causes an increase in mechanism sensitivity, whereas migration of foveal cones produces a change in spatial scale and a progressive shift of mechanism tuning toward higher spatial frequencies (Wilson, 1988). Development of cortical inhibition is thought to contribute significantly to the development of bandpass spatial frequency and orientation tuning. From the perspective of amblyopia, it is relevant to note that sensitivity to different spatial frequencies develops at different rates, with low frequencies reaching adult levels of sensitivity sooner than high spatial frequencies. Thus the CSF progressively shifts upward (higher sensitivity) and to the right (higher spatial frequencies) with age (Boothe et al., 1985). The poor spatial and good temporal resolution of 1-month-olds suggests that mechanisms tuned to lower spatial frequencies and higher temporal frequencies mature earliest. Because sensitivity to high spatial frequencies develops last, it may not be surprising that amblyopia, which develops early in life, primarily influences the sensitivity of high spatial frequency mechanisms, and that sensitivity to large uniform fields (low spatial frequencies) modulated at high temporal frequencies is reasonably intact. It would be interesting to determine if the degree of loss at low spatial frequencies present in some amblyopes is closely related to the age of onset of the amblyopia.

Because amblyopia is well characterized by a reduced resolution and a loss of precision in making spatial localization judgments, we focus in this section on the development of resolution and Vernier acuity. Figure 24-2 shows the development of Vernier acuity and grating acuity. The data for ages below 2 years are from

the studies of Shimojo et al. (1984), Shimojo and Held (1987), and Manny and Klein (1984). Also shown are VEP estimates of grating acuity from Norcia et al. (1990). The data for ages from 3 years and older are from our laboratory (Carkeet et al., 1990). The early development of Vernier acuity appears to be somewhat delayed compared to resolution. In fact, Shimojo and coworkers (1984, 1987) suggested that Vernier acuity is initially worse than grating acuity and then dramatically improves (relative to grating acuity) between about 2 and 8 months. At 8 months Vernier acuity was about twice as good as grating acuity. The Vernier acuity of very young infants remains controversial, so we have placed a question mark on that part of the curve. Shimojo and Held (1987) interpreted their results on the basis of undersampling in young infants, and the rapid development of cortical organization; however, there are alternative explanations. For example, poor Vernier acuity of the youngest infants may reflect the effects of crowding or stimulus spatial frequency, as the stimulus was a repetitive grating, and crowding effects may be extensive in infants (Mohn et al., 1989; Skoczenski and Aslin, 1989). Moreover, Manny and Klein (1984) suggested that Vernier acuity and grating acuity developed in parallel between birth and 6 months, with Vernier acuity being about twice as good as grating acuity at all ages. Whereas Manny and Klein's estimates of Vernier acuity were similar to those of Shimojo et al. (1984), their grating acuities were low, perhaps due to the small fields used. The discrepancies in the results may also be due, at least in part, to the different stimuli utilized by the two laboratories; however, it is interesting to note that data from monkeys (Kiorpes and Movshon, 1988, 1989) parallel the Shimojo and Held data closely (when the 4:1 rule for equating monkey and human ages is applied).

The attainment of adult levels of hyperacuity—which is 6–10 times better than grating acuity—is delayed compared to resolution. Our own studies (Carkeet et al., 1990) suggest that resolution reaches half its maximal adult value at age 2 years, whereas Vernier reaches half its adult maximum value at age 4; and our results and those of Gwiazda (1987) suggest that Vernier acuity may reach adult levels only near age 10. The critical point is that Vernier acuity and grating acuity reach adult levels of performance at different ages. Thus the resolution/Vernier acuity ratio varies during development. For example, in monkeys the ratio is 0.5:1.0 at 2 weeks of age, almost 1:1 by 12 weeks, 2:1 at 20 weeks, and 4:1 at 70 weeks.

In Figure 24-3 are the R/V ratios, calculated from the paired resolution and Vernier data of Figure 24-2 (i.e., we omitted the Manny and Klein, 1985, data because there were no direct resolution comparison data). The small circles represent data from Manny and Klein (1984),

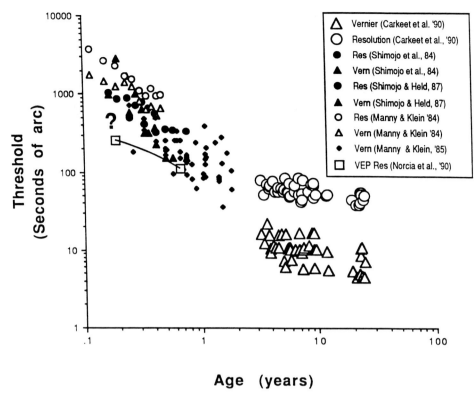

FIG. 24-2. Development of Vernier acuity and grating acuity. The data for ages below 2 years are from the studies of Shimojo et al. (1984), Shimojo and Held (1987), and Manny and Klein (1984, 1985). □ = VEP estimates of grating acuity from Norcia et al. (1990). ♦ = three alternative tracking data of Manny and Klein (1985). The data for ages 3 years and older are from our laboratory (Carkeet et al., 1990). Res = resolution; Vern = Vernier.

the small open squares data from Shimojo et al. (1984), and the solid squares data from Shimojo and Held (1987). As indicated by the question mark, the "true" R/V ratio of young infants (< 6 months) is in serious question; however, it appears that by 6 months the ratio is approaching 2:1, and it may be underestimated by the data of Shimojo et al. (shown by the three squares at ages 0.5–0.7 years) because of equipment limitations.

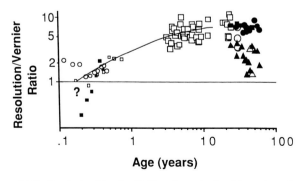

FIG. 24-3. Resolution/Vernier (R/V) ratios, calculated from the paired resolution and Vernier data of Figure 24-2. Also shown here are the R/V ratios of the adult amblyopes shown in Figure 24-1, plus several amblyopes tested with the same three alternative forced-choice procedure as the young children in Figure 24-2.

Our data suggest that the ratio is between 3:1 and 5:1 (roughly half the adult level) by age 4.

It is interesting to speculate why Vernier acuity has slow, late development, reaching adult levels considerably later than resolution. If we consider that Vernier acuity is limited by the precision with which the brain "knows" the position of each afferent, it is perhaps not surprising that intrinsic positional uncertainty can reach adult levels only after retinal development is complete. The primary postnatal changes in the retina concern differentiation of the macular region (Boothe et al., 1985). After birth, foveal receptor density and cone outer segment length both increase, as foveal cones become thinner and more elongated. There is a dramatic migration of ganglion cells and inner nuclear layers from the foveal region as the foveal pit develops during the first 4 months of life, and it is not until about 4 years of age that the fovea is fully adult-like (Youdelis and Hendricksen, 1986). From birth to beyond 4 years of age, cone density increases in the central region owing to both migration of receptors and decreases in their dimensions. Both of these factors result in finer cone sampling (by decreasing the distance between neighboring cones). It is likely that alterations in cone spacing and the light-gathering properties of the cones during early development contribute

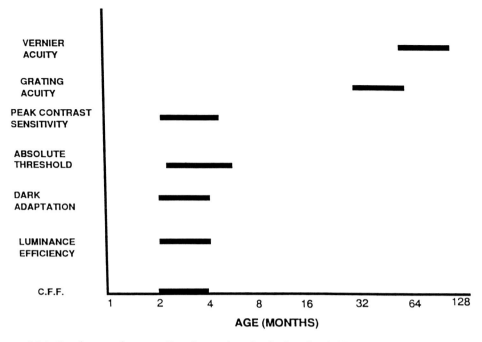

FIG. 24-4. Developmental cartoon. Functions such as the absolute threshold, CFF, and sensitivity to low spatial frequencies develop rapidly, whereas grating acuity and Vernier acuity develop much later. Each bar represents the range of ages over which adult-like performance is achieved (estimated from studies cited in the text plus several reviews [Teller and Movshon, 1986; Brown, 1990; Van Sluyters et al., 1990]).

a great deal to the improvements in acuity and contrast sensitivity during the first months of life. The massive migration of retinal cells and the alterations in the size of retina and eyeball (along with changes in interpupillary distance) may necessitate the plasticity of cortical connections early in life. It seems reasonable to speculate that the brain cannot "know" the positions of foveal cones with high levels of precision until after these changes in the retina are complete. Interestingly, the peripheral retina appears to develop much more rapidly than the fovea (Youdelis and Hendricksen, 1986).

Summary

One of the most interesting aspects of visual development is that different structures and functions develop at different rates. Figure 24-4 summarizes this development, showing that functions such as the absolute threshold, CFF, and sensitivity to low spatial frequencies develop rapidly, whereas grating acuity and Vernier acuity develop much later. Each bar in Figure 24-4 represents the range of ages over which adult-like performance is achieved.

SUSCEPTIBILITY TO ABNORMAL VISUAL INPUT: "DETROIT MODEL"

The presence of amblyopia is always associated with an early history of a "sensory obstacle": binocular mis-registration (strabismus) or image degradation (high refractive error, anisometropia, cataract, ptosis, or lid closure consequent to treatment). The severity of the amblyopia appears to be associated with the degree of imbalance between the two eyes (e.g., dense unilateral cataract results in severe loss) and to the age at which the amblyogenic factor occurred. Precisely how these factors interact is not yet known. Clinicians are well aware that amblyopia does not develop after age 6–8 years of age (Worth, 1903; von Noorden, 1981), suggesting that there is a "sensitive period" for its development; however, in humans with naturally occurring amblyopia, the age of onset of the amblyogenic condition(s) are difficult to ascertain, and the effects of intervention combine to make it difficult to obtain a clear picture of the "natural history" of amblyopia development. Thus much of our current understanding of the development of amblyopia accrues from animal studies (for a review see Boothe et al., 1985) and from retrospective studies of clinical records (e.g., von Noorden, 1981). Technological improvements in infant testing are also beginning to provide more direct data on the development of naturally occurring amblyopia in humans (Mohindra et al., 1979; Jacobson et al., 1981; Birch, 1983; Maurer et al., 1983) and monkeys (Kiorpes and Boothe, 1981; Kiorpes et al., 1984, 1989). All of these studies provide strong evidence that there is a sensitive period for the development of amblyopia.

Consider the hypothesis that structures and functions that develop earliest are most robust to the effects of abnormal visual input, whereas those that develop more slowly seem most susceptible. We think of this situation as the biological analog of the "last hired, first fired" philosophy; a sort of "Detroit model." This notion suggests that different structures, or functions may be susceptible to the effects of visual deprivation at different times during development. There is now clear evidence from anatomical and physiological studies that the sensitive period in layer IVc (the input layer) of the cortex of monkeys is considerably shorter than that of other layers (LeVay et al., 1980). The behavioral studies of lid-sutured monkeys by Harwerth et al. (1987, 1990) provided strong evidence that different psychophysical functions are affected by lid suture at different times. For example, these authors found that early lid suture (at age 3–6 months) had a marked influence on scotopic and photopic spectral sensitivity, and that it essentially abolished pattern and binocular vision. A later onset of deprivation (up to about 25 months) had no influence on spectral sensitivity but resulted in reduced contrast sensitivity at high spatial frequencies and reduced binocular summation. Lid suture beyond 25 months had no effect on contrast sensitivity but still disrupted binocular functioning. There are several points worth noting. First, to extrapolate these results to monocular pattern deprivation in humans, the 1:4 rule should be applied (i.e., 1 monkey year is equivalent to about 4 human years). Second, the effects of deprivation seem to be the "mirror image" of the developmental sequence. Thus, as noted above, different visual functions (and presumably their underlying anatomical and physiological structures) develop at different rates. Those that develop earliest seem most robust to the influences of pattern deprivation, whereas those that develop last are most at risk and remain susceptible for the longest time.

Although the upper limit for susceptibility of excitatory binocular interactions is not yet certain, it appears to be later than that for acuity or contrast sensitivity in monkeys and may extend to at least 7–8 years (and possibly more) in humans. Psychophysical studies of interocular transfer in humans with a history of strabismus (Banks et al., 1975; Hohmann and Creutzfeldt, 1975) have provided an indirect estimate of the period of susceptibility of binocular connections. The results of both studies suggested that binocular connections are highly vulnerable during the first 18 months of life and remain susceptible to the effects of strabismus until at least age 7 years.

DOES THE INFANT VISUAL SYSTEM PROVIDE A REASONABLE MODEL FOR AMBLYOPIA?

The preceding brief description of the visual capacities of infants provides at least a qualitative sense that many aspects of the abnormal visual functions of amblyopes

may be understood on the basis of abnormal development, due to either arrest or extinction. Thus the amblyopic visual system resembles in many respects the immature visual system. Both show normal or near-normal receptoral functions (light sense); relatively normal function at low spatial frequencies; near normal CFF (Regal, 1981); reduced acuity and contrast sensitivity, particularly at high spatial frequencies; and reduced hyperacuity. In this section, we focus on the development of resolution and Vernier acuity and the losses of these two functions in amblyopes.

As noted above, strabismic and anisometropic amblyopes show different relative losses of grating and Vernier acuity (Fig. 24-1), which raises the intriguing question of whether strabismus and anisometropia exert their effects on the developing visual nervous system at different times during development (discussed further below) or in different manners. In Figure 24-3, the large filled symbols represent the data from Figure 24-1 using conventional abutting line Vernier acuity (Levi and Klein, 1985) (the points have been scattered randomly along the horizontal axis between 20 and 50 years of age). The squares represent data for normal observers, circles for anisometropic amblyopes, and the triangles for strabismic amblyopes. Also shown are data of three anisometropic (open circles) and three strabismic (open triangles) amblyopes using the identical three-alternative forced choice method (Carkeet et al., 1990) as was used to gather the children's data (open squares). It is of special interest to note that for the anisometropes the R/V ratio is similar to that of normal adults and within the range of R/V ratios achieved beyond 3 years of age. In contrast, many of the strabismic amblyopes show a much lower ratio, similar to the level of performance achieved below the age of 1 year.

We have estimated the "effective" age of each of our adult amblyopes by fitting (by eye) a line to the children's data and interpolating the age corresponding to each amblyopes R/V ratio. Figure 24-5 shows the "ef-

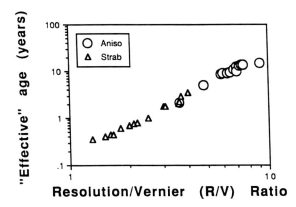

FIG. 24-5. "Effective" age (i.e., the age corresponding to each amblyope's R/V ratio) is plotted as a function of the R/V ratio of each amblyope from Figure 24-4.

fective" age plotted against the R/V ratio of each amblyope. The results, although preliminary, are interesting. The spatial vision of strabismic amblyopes, as characterized by the R/V ratio, is continuously distributed between effective ages of about 4 months and 4 years. The visual system of anisometropic amblyopes, on the whole, appears more developed using their amblyopic R/V ratios as an index. Effective ages for anisometropic amblyopes are distributed between 4 years and adulthood, showing only slight overlap with effective ages for strabismic amblyopes. Thus we hypothesize that strabismic amblyopia develops early in life, whereas anisometropic amblyopia develops later (when the R/V ratio is adult-like). We wish to point out some caveats. First, when constructing the "effective age" plot, it should be kept in mind that there is almost no reliable paired resolution and Vernier data between the ages of 1 and 3 years, and that much of the data in infants may be suspect (because of possible "crowding" or spatial frequency effects or because of the use of target motion); thus we have not attempted to make a more quantitative analysis. Second, there remains a question about whether the apparent distinctions between strabismic and anisometropic amblyopes could be simply based on the depth of amblyopia. We do not believe that this situation is the case. If two amblyopes, one strabismic and the other anisometropic, are matched for resolution, the strabismic invariably demonstrates a greater loss of Vernier acuity (Levi and Klein, 1982a,b, 1985) (Fig. 24-6). Third, although much of the limitation in performance of infants can be ascribed to immaturity of the retina (Banks and Bennett, 1988; see also Chapter 6), the limitations in performance of amblyopes are almost certainly cortical (von Noorden, 1977; Hess and Baker, 1984; Hendrickson et al., 1987; Movshon et al., 1987).

Fourth, Figure 24-5 is, in fact a kind of "gedanken" plot (i.e., given the greater loss of Vernier than grating acuity of strabismic amblyopes and the late development of the R/V ratio, it could not have come out any other way) and in no way proves that strabismic amblyopia develops earlier than anisometropic amblyopia. Nonetheless, Figure 24-5 is consistent with our tentative hypothesis that the visual system of *strabismic* amblyopes shares many features with the vision of older infants and young toddlers (i.e., that strabismic amblyopes are like infants who somewhere along the line took a wrong "turn"). The "light sense" is basically intact, and peak contrast sensitivity is normal or near-normal. On the other hand, sensitivity to high spatial frequencies is reduced, and the R/V ratio is well below that found in normal adults. These losses in strabismic amblyopes are thought to be primarily restricted to the central visual field (Hess and Pointer, 1985; Kolia and Levi, 1989). In contrast, the visual system of the anisometropic amblyope appears to be more closely approximated by a normal (mature) visual system that has been blurred (Levi and Klein, 1990a,b).

It is important to note that, although the qualitative similarity between strabismic amblyopia and infant vision is striking, the "effective age" hypothesis is probably an oversimplification. This point can be seen by considering the absolute performance of infants and amblyopes. Figure 24-6A replots all the "paired" resolution and Vernier data from Figure 24-2. [We have omitted the Manny and Klein (1985) Vernier data, as there are no paired resolution measures.] The resolution and Vernier thresholds of the two adult amblyopes, one strabismic and the other anisometropic, were measured using the identical three-alternative forced choice procedure that was used to obtain the children's data. This

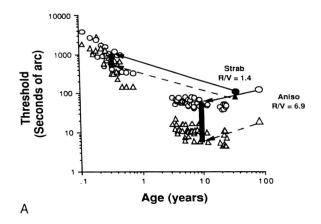

A

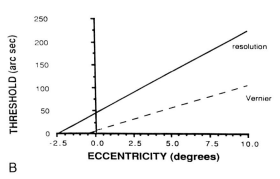

B

FIG. 24-6. (A) Replot of all the "paired" resolution (small circles) and Vernier acuity (small triangles) data from Figure 24-2. The large circles and triangles are the resolution and Vernier thresholds of a strabismic amblyope (filled symbols) and an anisometropic amblyope (open symbols). The vertical bars show the effective ages of the two amblyopes. The length of the bars corresponds to the R/V ratio, and the horizontal position of the bars corresponds to the effective age (i.e., the age with the same R/V ratio). (B) Linear variation in resolution and Vernier acuity with eccentricity.

plot makes it possible to compare not only the R/V ratios, shown by the vertical distance between the resolution and Vernier thresholds, but the absolute performance levels. Several points are noteworthy. First, these two amblyopes have similar resolution thresholds but different R/V ratios. The anisometrope has a ratio of 6.9:1.0, whereas the strabismic has a ratio of 1.4:1.0. As noted above, this finding argues that the differences between strabismic and anisometropic amblyopes are not simply a consequence of the severity of amblyopia. Second, there is not good correspondence between the "effective age" of these amblyopes and their absolute level of performance. First consider the strabismic amblyope. His 1.4:1.0 R/V ratio represents an effective age of about 0.2–0.3 years. Note that his resolution is considerably better than that of a 0.2 to 0.3-year-old, at least as measured by FPL techniques. Note that this strabismic observer's resolution is better than that of an infant with the same R/V ratio, as shown by the upward slope of the diagonal arrow. One should remember that infant performance is probably closer to that of adult strabismic amblyopia than our analysis predicts because FPL procedures underestimate performance.[1] However, this strabismic amblyope's resolution is still about twofold better than VEP acuity at 0.2–0.3 years. What does this finding imply? Suppose our strabismics have had some sort of "sensory obstacle" that impairs their ability to extract displacement information from cortical filters (perhaps due to undersampling or high degrees of positional uncertainty) and fixes their R/V ratio at that of a given age. The upper pass limit of their visual filters may continue to improve despite this "obstacle." One might not expect the overall resolution performance to improve to normal adult levels because of increased pooling. In addition, developmental scale changes at the fovea and increasing axial length might act as factors that passively improve a strabismic amblyopic child's overall performance to that of a strabismic amblyopic adult. The main point, however, is that although the strabismic amblyopic adult's R/V ratio is similar to that of an infant or toddler the absolute level of performance may be better.

Now consider the anisometrope. This observer has an R/V ratio of 6.9:1.0, similar to that of an adult, and her "effective age is represented by the vertical bar, at approximately 10 years old. Note that her resolution is worse than that of an adult (or 10-year-old). Anisometropic amblyopes apparently suffer injuries (obsta-

cles) that are selective for higher spatial frequencies, but in other respects the processes that integrate the information from cortical filters into position information are unimpeded. Thus the vision of anisometropic amblyopes may be better represented as a spatial scale change than as an immature visual system. On this basis one would predict an adult or near-adult R/V ratio.[2]

"NATURAL HISTORY" OF AMBLYOPIA DEVELOPMENT

Several lines of evidence suggest that the period of susceptibility to deprivation does not begin at birth, which has raised interesting debates regarding when treatment should begin. For example, Hubel and Wiesel (1970) reported that the period of susceptibility in monocularly deprived kittens began abruptly at about 4 weeks of age. In humans, neither congenital cataract nor congenital esotropia produce a loss of acuity prior to 2 months of age (Mohindra et al., 1979; Taylor et al., 1979; Maurer et al., 1983). It appears that the onset of amblyopia may not begin before the normal development of binocular interaction in striate cortex (Held, 1984). This notion receives further support from the findings of Harwerth et al. (personal communication) that a prior period of prism rearing that severely disrupts binocular neurons "protects" monkeys from the harmful effects of monocular lid suture. Moreover, there is frequently a period of uninterrupted continued parallel acuity development in the two eyes following the onset of experimental strabismus. It can also be seen in the development of resolution in monkeys with experimental strabismus (Kiorpes et al., 1989), providing some support for the notion that the development of amblyopia involves binocular competition and suppression (von Noorden, 1977).

Our hypothesis, as outlined above, is that strabismus and anisometropia exert their influence on the developing visual nervous system at different times during development. Note that we do not wish to imply that visual development is necessarily simply arrested at different times. For example, several studies (e.g., Mohindra et al., 1979) have suggested that there may also be extinction of function as a consequence of strabismus. It seems plausible, however, that amblyopia of extinction (as well as amblyopia of arrest) may be more severe early in life than later. The key point we raise here is that strabismus and anisometropia might produce amblyopia at different times during development.

---

1. One advantage of using the R/V ratio, rather than the absolute levels, is that to the extent that nonsensory factors influence the absolute performance they should have similar effects on resolution and Vernier acuity, leaving the ratio as a good estimate of sensory development.

2. Some models might predict a small additional loss of Vernier acuity on the basis that the more narrowly tuned higher frequency filters yield relatively better spatial sensitivity than broadly tuned lower frequency filters (e.g., Wilson, 1988).

Why? Consider the effect of a constant unilateral strabismus. Binocular cortical neurons with foveal representation receive signals that on average are uncorrelated. Thus a competitive developmental process dependent on the average signal strength from each eye (e.g., Wiesel, 1982) would result in neurons driven by one eye or the other, but not both. Decorrelation of the foveal images could have an influence immediately, as sensitivity to binocular correlation is adult-like by 3–4 months of age (Braddick et al., 1980; Petrig et al., 1983). As Wilson (1991) pointed out, if one eye has a competitive advantage, there would be a significant loss of cells driven by the deviating eye that results in spatial undersampling and irregularity. A competitive advantage could result from one eye being out of focus (anisometropia) or from small differences in the time of arrival at the lateral geniculate nucleus (LGN) or cortex, of afferents from the two eyes (Keiner, 1951). One interesting and important question is why some (most) strabismics do not develop amblyopia, whereas others do. Strabismic amblyopia is reported to occur in 35–50% of children with strabismus (Ciuffreda et al., 1990), which suggests a kind of threshold of competitive advantage (otherwise we might all develop amblyopia, as there are presumably small differences in binocular input in most normal infants, but they do not cascade to amblyopia). Once this threshold is overstepped, amblyopia develops. The competitive threshold presumably diminishes as we get older. Several factors appear to be important in determining the development of strabismic amblyopia: the type of strabismus (more frequent in constant esotropia); the presence of high refractive error or a refractive imbalance; and age of onset (amblyopia is more likely to develop with early-onset strabismus than with the later-onset variety). The difficulty is to determine the relative weighting of each of these factors and the possibility of other factors that have not yet been determined. Interestingly, Kiorpes et al. (1989) found that in monkeys with experimental strabismus those with the *earliest* onset were most likely to develop amblyopia.

With anisometropia, the signals from the two eyes are positively correlated; however, if the image of one eye is blurred, and thus of lower contrast, its signal is somewhat weaker. Thus cortical neurons driven through the defocused eye would have a lower sensitivity, particularly for high spatial frequencies, as they are affected most by blur (Levi and Klein, 1985, 1990a,b; Wilson 1991). Consider, for example, an anisometrope whose one eye has a high hyperopic refractive error. The retinal image is blurred, thereby reducing high spatial frequencies in the retinal image. However, because high spatial frequency sensitivity does not develop until late, this blur does not influence neural processing until it exceeds the "neural" blurring of the image by the developing visual nervous system. It is only at this stage that monocular defocus is likely to result in a binocular neural imbalance. Although little is known about the development of anisometropia, it seems at least plausible that anisometropic amblyopia may have its onset considerably later than amblyopia associated with strabismus. Interestingly, meridional amblyopia (associated with high degrees of astigmatism early in life), does not develop during the first year of life and perhaps not until age 3 (Mohindra et al., 1979; Teller et al., 1982). Note that for both strabismic and anisometropic amblyopia, the mechanism is the same (i.e., binocular competition); it is the period of susceptibility to, and the consequences of the two conditions that are different.

It is worth noting that presently little is known about the development of anisometropia, and the literature is conflicting as to its prevalence (Flom and Bedell, 1985; Almeder et al., 1990; Laird, 1990). However, several points are now becoming clear. First, refractive error and the emmetropization process do not seem to be so tightly linked in the two eyes early in life as previously thought (Abrahamsson et al., 1990a,b). Consequently, anisometropia present at an early age may not be persistent (Abrahamsson et al., 1990a,b; Almeder et al., 1990). Second, there appears to be a subgroup of young children whose anisometropia persists (Abrahamsson et al., 1990a,b); and perhaps it is these children, exposed to continuous unilateral blur, who develop amblyopia. For example, Abrahamsson et al. (1990a,b) found that 14 of 33 patients who were anisometropic at age 1 year remained anisometropic at age 4 years, and 25% of these patients developed amblyopia. Interestingly, those patients whose anisometropia did not persist showed no increased risk of amblyopia. This finding suggests that the development of anisometropic amblyopia may require a prolonged period of continuous unilateral blur. We do know that there is a significant proportion of amblyopes, perhaps as many as one-third (Flom and Bedell, 1985), who present with anisometropia and no strabismus. These anisometropic amblyopes demonstrate different psychophysical losses from strabismic amblyopes, have different clinical characteristics (Ciuffreda et al., 1990), and have different prognosis with treatment (Kivlin and Flynn, 1981).

In summary, it is our hypothesis that although strabismic and anisometropic amblyopia share a common neural mechanism (i.e., binocular competition) it is the period of susceptibility to, and the consequences of the two conditions for *cortical* processing that differ. In the next section, we ask whether the (adult) retinal periphery may offer a reasonable model for the spatial vision of amblyopes and infants and perhaps provide some additional insights into the nature of the reduced spatial vision.

Spatial Vision in the Periphery

The normal adult fovea is remarkably adept at discerning and recognizing shapes and patterns. A great deal of the neural machinery of the human fovea seems to be dedicated to the task of pattern recognition. A central question in vision science is how pattern discrimination varies with eccentricity. Almost 140 years ago, Aubert and Foerster (1857) demonstrated that visual acuity declines in an orderly fashion with eccentricity. Aubert and Foerster's important observation has been often repeated and extended to numerous tasks over the years (e.g., Weymouth, 1958; Levi et al., 1985). Weymouth (1958) was perhaps the first to recognize that for a wide range of pattern discrimination tasks (including visual acuity), visual performance varies *approximately linearly* with eccentricity, as do many of the anatomical and physiological functions thought to constrain performance. Figure 24-6B illustrates the nature of the linear variation in both structure and function with eccentricity. Plotted here are resolution (grating acuity) and Vernier acuity as a function of eccentricity. Note that for the fovea the values for resolution and Vernier acuity are 45 arc second and 6 arc second, similar to the adult foveal performances shown in Figure 24-2. Both the resolution and the Vernier thresholds (Th) increase with eccentricity according to:

$$Th = Th_f(1 + ECC/E_2)$$

where Th_f = foveal value; ECC = eccentricity of the stimulus; and E_2 = eccentricity at which the foveal value is doubled. E_2 is a scale free factor, shown graphically as the x-axis intercept in Figure 24-1, that captures the rate at which structure and function vary with eccentricity. Note that the two lines in Figure 24-6B each have a different value of E_2. A variety of studies suggest that, within the central 10 degrees, resolution has an E_2 values of about 1.5–4.0 degrees, with a mean value of approximately 2.5 degrees (Levi et al., 1985; Levi and Klein, 1990a,b; Wilson et al., 1990). Much of the variation in the reported E_2 values may reflect meridional differences in sensitivity. Although the optimal position acuity is precise in the fovea, it declines more rapidly with eccentricity than does resolution or contrast sensitivity. Thus tasks such as Vernier acuity (Westheimer, 1982; Levi et al., 1985), bisection (Klein and Levi, 1987; Yap et al., 1987), and spatial interval discrimination (Yap et al., 1989; Levi and Klein, 1990a) show a precipitous decline with eccentricity, with E_2 values between 0.3 and 0.9 degrees (see also Wilson et al., 1990). It has been suggested (Levi et al., 1985; Levi and Klein, 1990a) that the rapid decline of position acuity in peripheral vision reflects the high degree of intrinsic spatial uncertainty, which increases in the periphery in proportion to the inverse cortical magnifi-

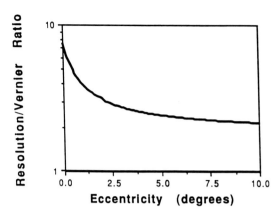

FIG. 24-7. One consequence of the differential decline of resolution and position acuity with eccentricity (Fig. 24-6B) is that the R/V ratio varies with eccentricity from 7.5:1.0 in the fovea to around 2:1 at 10 degrees.

cation factor [M^{-1}, i.e., the number of degrees of visual space per millimeter of cortex (Dow et al., 1981)]. One consequence of the differential decline of resolution and position acuity with eccentricity is that the R/V ratio varies with eccentricity, as illustrated in Figure 24-7, where the ratio declines from 7.5:1.0 in the fovea to around 2:1 at 10 degrees.

"Effective" Eccentricity

We have estimated the "effective" eccentricity of each of our adult amblyopes by interpolating to the eccentricity corresponding to each amblyope's R/V ratio in a manner analogous to that used to construct the "effective" age plot (Fig. 24-3). Figure 24-8 shows the "effective" eccentricity plotted against the R/V ratio of each amblyope. The triangles represent the data of the strabismic amblyopes and the circles those of the anisometropic amblyopes. The results are interesting. The anisometropic amblyopes show effective eccentricities close to 0 degrees (i.e., their R/V ratios are similar to the normal fovea) whereas the strabismic amblyopes have effective eccentricities from about 1 degree to at least 20 degrees.[3]

In Figure 24-9, the dotted line plots effective eccentricity as a function of age. Note that the spatial vision of infants and young toddlers (characterized by the R/V ratio) is similar to that of the periphery. The decrease in effective eccentricity with age is precipitous; for example, at around 7 months of age the R/V ratio is similar to that found at 20 degrees eccentricity; at 9 months it is equivalent to an eccentricity of 10 degrees;

---

3. We have not calculated effective eccentricities beyond 20 degrees because we are uncertain as to whether the linear relations for resolution and Vernier acuity are maintained beyond 20 degrees.

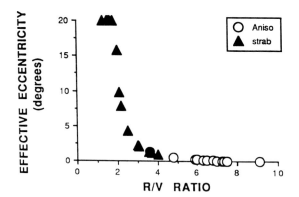

FIG. 24-8. "Effective" eccentricity plotted against the R/V ratio of each amblyope.

and at 1 year it is equal to an effective eccentricity of about 4 degrees. Note that we have not tried to define the effective eccentricity for younger infants because of the uncertainty with *both* the infant data and the peripheral data. It is worth noting that projections of the linear eccentricity functions described above to eccentricities as large as 90 degrees always yield R/V ratios greater than unity.

The qualitative and quantitative similarity between the spatial vision of strabismic amblyopes and the normal periphery has been well documented elsewhere (e.g., Flynn, 1967; Levi and Klein, 1985, 1990b). Our present analysis suggests that infant spatial vision may also be qualitatively similar to that at the periphery (but see Brown, 1990). Of course many of the same caveats that pertain to the issue of effective age pertain also to effective eccentricity. Moreover, our analysis leads to the suspicion that R/V ratios less than 1:1 (as seen in the infant data of Shimojo and Held, 1987) might reflect other limitations (e.g., stimulus limitations such as "crowding effects," rather than visual system constraints).

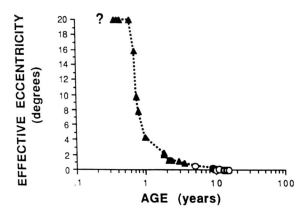

FIG. 24-9. Effective eccentricity versus age (dotted line). The symbols are the adult amblyopes' data from Figure 24-8.

To summarize, the analyses here suggest that spatial vision in infants, strabismic amblyopes, and the normal periphery are remarkably similar. What is the connection between these three visual systems? One hypothesis is that infants and strabismic amblyopes effectively have a central scotoma and therefore use a more sensitive peripheral locus to make their spatial judgments. In the case of infants, this might occur because peripheral retinal development precedes foveal development (see Chapter 17). In strabismus, it may be a consequence of binocular competition or suppression (or both). At least in strabismic amblyopes, this hypothesis seems unlikely, because using repetitive targets that are imaged on the fovea does not improve their performance (e.g., Levi and Klein, 1982a,b). The alternative hypothesis (which we prefer) is that both infant and adult strabismic amblyopic foveae are similar to the normal periphery. Banks and colleagues (e.g., Sekuler et al., 1990; see also Chapter 6) have been examining the optical and retinal constraints on spatial vision in infants and in the normal periphery using an "ideal discriminator" approach. Their work suggests that "front end" (retinal) constraints lead to reduced quantal efficiency in the periphery and in infants. To the extent that performance is quantum limited, their modeling suggests that both the infant and the peripheral visual system may have low R/V ratios. Presumably these "front end" constraints are also reflected in the cortex. These optical and retinal constraints, however, do not extend to strabismic amblyopes, whose abnormalities appear to be cortical (see Chapter 18). Our hypothesis, which unifies the reduced spatial vision of infants, strabismic amblyopes, and the periphery, is that each of these three visual systems is uncertain about the positions of the retinal afferents carrying the signals to the brain, perhaps due to sparse and irregular sampling in the cortex. This hypothesis is illustrated in Figure 24-10. All current models of spatial vision are based on the general notion that any point in space is sampled by an array of receptive fields of different sizes (spatial scales), so each row represents a different mechanism center size (smallest at the top; note that we do not intend to imply that there are only three mechanism sizes). For each mechanism size, the spacing is regular and is equal to approximately 0.5σ, where σ = the standard deviation of receptive field center. Note that as the receptive field size increases (from top to bottom in Figure 24-10), the spacing also increases proportionally. Although little is known about how cortical mechanisms in the human visual system sample the image, the spacing shown here would provide adequate spatial sampling.

The righthand panel of the figure illustrates our hypothesis for the three degraded visual systems (periphery, infancy, and strabismic amblyopia) as outlined above. Note that the largest mechanisms are similar to those

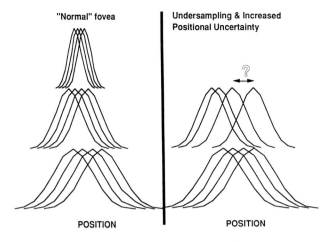

"Normal" fovea   Undersampling & Increased Positional Uncertainty

POSITION   POSITION

FIG. 24-10. Cortical sampling. (Left) "Normal" adult fovea. Each row illustrates the excitatory centers of four overlapped receptive fields, with receptive field center size increasing from top to bottom. Each receptive field is regularly spaced, with the separation between neighbors equal to approximately 0.5σ (where σ is the standard deviation of receptive field center). (Right) Our hypothesis for the three degraded visual systems (periphery, infancy, and strabismic amblyopia) as described in the text.

of the normal adult fovea; however, the figure differs from normal in three ways: (1) The smallest mechanisms are eliminated. This absence of small (high spatial frequency) mechanisms implies that there is increased pooling or neural blur, as occurs in the normal periphery, in amblyopes (both strabismic and anisometropic) (e.g., Levi and Klein, 1990a,b; Wilson, 1991) and presumably in infants (Wilson, 1988). (2) The smallest (highest spatial frequency) remaining mechanisms are undersampled. (3) The spacing is irregular. In contrast to the normal (adult) fovea (middle row, lefthand panel), the mean spacing has been increased, on average, twofold (the mean spacing has been increased from 0.5σ to σ); however, the spacing between neighboring mechanisms is jittered. The question mark is intended to illustrate the uncertainty in the positions of neighboring cortical mechanisms (i.e., the positional uncertainty).

Wilson (1991) has shown that a model of this sort can quantitatively account for the degraded spatial vision of the normal periphery and strabismic amblyopes. In the periphery, there is now clear evidence for spatial undersampling at the retina (e.g., Coletta and Williams, 1987). Moreover, the standard deviation of cone separation increases more rapidly than actual cone separation (Hirsch and Miller, 1987; Hirsch and Curcio, 1989); and Wilson (1991) has suggested that the increase in uncertainty of the position of peripheral cones may limit peripheral positional acuity. We argue here that the uncertainty (or jitter) in the positions of peripheral cones is reflected in the cortex. Similar arguments may account for the high positional uncertainty in the developing visual system. Although there is no

evidence one way or the other on the question of undersampling in the infant visual system, it seems likely that there is a high degree of positional uncertainty in the developing retina. As discussed earlier, the massive migration of retinal cells and the alterations in the size of the retina and eyeball (along with changes in interpupillary distance) may necessitate the plasticity of cortical connections early in life. Thus the brain probably cannot "know" precisely the positions of foveal cones with high levels of precision until after these (and many other) changes in the retina are complete. Finally, if as we speculated earlier there is an early "sensory obstacle" to normal visual development early in life, the cortices of strabismic amblyopes may never develop precise knowledge of the positions of the foveal cones.

SUMMARY

We have examined the notion of amblyopia as a developmental disorder of spatial vision. We considered two models for the amblyopic visual system: the infant visual system and the normal (adult) retinal periphery. Our analysis suggests that there is a good deal of similarity between the spatial vision of *strabismic* amblyopes and that of both the immature and peripheral visual systems.

Acknowledgments. This work was supported by a grant from the National Eye Institute, RO1EY 01728. We are grateful to Ruth Manny for providing us with three tons of infant data and for helpful comments on an early draft of the manuscript. We also thank Marty Banks, Ron Harwerth, Stan Klein, Steve Morse, Sarah Waugh, and Bruce Wick for their thoughtful comments.

REFERENCES

ABRAHAMSSON, M., ANDERSSON, A. K., AND SJOSTRAND, J. (1990a). A longitudinal study of a population based sample of astigmatic children. I. Refraction and amblyopia. *Acta Ophthalmol.* (*Copenh.*) 68, 428–434.

ABRAHAMSSON, M., FABIAN, G., AND SJOSTRAND, J. (1990b). A longitudinal study of a population based sample of astigmatic children. II. The changeability of anisometropia. *Acta Ophthalmol.* (*Copenh.*) 68, 435–440.

ALMEDER, L. M., PECK, L. B., AND HOWLAND, H. C. (1990). Prevalence of anisometropia in volunteer laboratory and school screening populations. *Invest. Ophthalmol. Vis. Sci.* 31, 2448–2455.

ALPERN, M., FLITMAN, D. B., AND JOSEPH, R. H. (1960). Centrally fixed flicker thresholds in amblyopia. *Am. J. Ophthalmol.* 49, 1194–1202.

AUBERT, H., AND FOERSTER, R. (1857). Beitraege zur Kenntnisse der indirecten Sehens. *Graefes Arch. Ophthalmol.* 3, 1–37.

BANKS, M. S., AND SALAPATEK, P. (1976). Contrast sensitivity function of the infant visual system. *Vision Res.* 16, 867–869.

BANKS, M. S., AND BENNETT, P. J. (1988). Optical and photoreceptor immaturities limit the spatial and chromatic vision of human neonates. *J. Opt. Soc. Am.* [A] 5, 2059–2079.

BANKS, M. S., ASLIN, R. N., AND LETSON, R. D. (1975). Sensitive period for the development of human binocular vision. *Science* 190, 675–677.

BEDELL, H. E. (1980). Central and peripheral retinal photoreceptor orientation in amblyopic eyes as assessed by the psychophysical Stiles-Crawford effect. *Invest. Ophthalmol. Vis. Sci.* 19, 49–59.

BIRCH, E. E. (1983). Assessment of binocular function during infancy. *Ophthalmic Paediatr. Genet.* 2, 43–50.

BJERRUM, J. (1884). Untersuchungen uber den Lichtsinn und den Raumsinn bei verschiedenen Augenkrankheiten. *Arch. Ophthalmol.* 30, 201.

BOOTHE, R. G., DOBSON, V., AND TELLER, D. Y. (1985). Postnatal development of vision in human and non-human primates. *Annu. Rev. Neurosci.* 8, 495–545.

BRADDICK, O., ATKINSON, J., JULESZ, B., KROPFL, W., BODIS-WOLNER, I., AND RAAB, E. (1980). Cortical binocularity in infants. *Nature* 288, 363–365.

BRADLEY, A., AND FREEMAN, R. D. (1981). Contrast sensitivity in anisometropic amblyopia. *Invest. Ophthalmol. Vis. Sci.* 21, 467–476.

BRADLEY, A., AND FREEMAN, R. D. (1985). Temporal sensitivity in amblyopia: an explanation of conflicting reports. *Vision Res.* 25, 39–46.

BRADLEY, A., DAHLMAN, C., SWITKES, E., AND DE VALOIS, K. (1986). A comparison of color and luminance discrimination in amblyopia. *Invest. Ophthalmol. Vis. Sci.* 27, 1404–1409.

BROWN, A. M. (1990). Development of visual sensitivity to light and color vision in human infants: a critical review. *Vision Res.* 30, 1159–1188.

CAMPBELL, F. W., AND GREGORY, A. H. (1960). The spatial resolving power of the human retina with oblique incidence [letter to the editor]. *J. Opt. Soc. Am.* 50, 831.

CARKEET, A., LEVI, D. M., AND MANNY, R. E. (1990). Development of Vernier and resolution after age 3. *Invest. Ophthalmol. Vis. Sci.* 31 (suppl.), 9.

CIUFFREDA, K. J., LEVI, D. M., AND SELENOW, A. (1990). *Amblyopia: Basic and Clinical Aspects*. Stoneham, MA: Butterworth-Heinemann.

COLETTA, N. J., AND WILLIAMS, D. R. (1987). Psychophysical estimate of extrafoveal cone spacing. *J. Opt. Soc. Am. [A]* 4, 1503–1513.

DE LANGE, H. (1958). Research into the dynamic nature of the human fovea-cortex systems with intermittent and modulated light. I. Attenuation characteristics with white and colored light. *J. Opt. Soc. Am.* 48, 777–784.

DE VRIES-KHOE, L., AND SPEKREIJSE, H. (1982). Maturation of luminance and pattern EPs in man. *Doc. Ophthalmol. Proc. Ser.* 31, 461–475.

DOBSON, V., AND TELLER, D. Y. (1978). Visual acuity in human infants: a review and comparison of behavioral and electrophysiological studies. *Vision Res.* 18, 1469–1483.

DOW, B. M., SNYDER, R. G., VAUTIN, R. G., AND BAUER, R. (1981). Magnification factor and receptive field size in foveal striate cortex of the monkey. *Exp. Brain Res.* 44, 213–228.

ENOCH, J. M. (1957). Amblyopia and the Stiles-Crawford effect. *Am. J. Optom. Arch. Am. Acad. Optom.* 34, 298–309.

ENOCH, J. M. (1967). The current status of receptor amblyopia. *Doc. Ophthalmol.* 23, 130–148.

FANKHAUSER, F., AND ROHLER, R. (1967). The physical stimulus, the quality of the retinal image and foveal brightness discrimination in one amblyopic and two normal eyes. *Doc. Ophthalmol.* 23, 149–184.

FEINBERG, I. (1956). Critical flicker frequency in amblyopia ex anopsia. *Am. J. Ophthalmol.* 42, 473–481.

FLOM, M. C., AND NEUMAIER, R. W. (1966). Prevalence of amblyopia. *Public Health Rep.* 81, 329–341.

FLOM, M. C., AND BEDELL, H. E. (1985). Identifying amblyopia using associated conditions, acuity, and nonacuity features. *Am. J. Optom. Physiol. Opt.* 62, 153–160.

FLYNN, J. T. (1967). Spatial summation in amblyopia. *Arch. Ophthalmol.* 78, 470–474.

FOX, R., ASLIN, R. N., SHEA, S. L., AND DUMAIS, S. T. (1980). Stereopsis in human infants. *Science* 207, 323–324.

FRANCOIS, J., AND VERRIEST, G. (1967). La discrimination chromatique dans l'amblyopie strabique. *Doc. Ophthalmol.* 23, 318.

FULTON, A. B. (1988). The development of scotopic retinal function in human infants. *Doc. Ophthalmol.* 69, 101–109.

GREEN, D. G. (1986). The search for the site of visual adaptation. *Vision Res.* 26, 1417–1429.

GROSVENOR, T. (1957). The effects of duration and background luminance upon the brightness discrimination of an amblyope. *Am. J. Optom. Physiol. Opt.* 34, 634–663.

GSTALDER, R. J., AND GREEN, D. G. (1971). Laser interferometric acuity in amblyopia. *J. Pediatr. Ophthalmol.* 8, 251–256.

GWIAZDA, J. (1987). Development of grating and Vernier acuity in the detection of amblyopia in human infants. In *Orthoptic Horizons: Transactions of the Sixth International Orthoptic Congress*, Harrowgate, UK.

HAMER, R. D., AND SCHNECK, M. E. (1984). Spatial summation in dark-adapted human infants. *Vision Res.* 24, 77–85.

HARWERTH, R. S., AND LEVI, D. M. (1977). Increment threshold sensitivity in anisometropic amblyopia. *Vision Res.* 17, 585–590.

HARWERTH, R. S., AND LEVI, D. M. (1978). A sensory mechanism for amblyopia: psychophysical studies. *Am. J. Optom. Physiol. Opt.* 55, 151–162.

HARWERTH, R. S., SMITH III, E. L., DUNCAN, G. C., CRAWFORD, M. L. J., AND VON NOORDEN, G. K. (1987). Multiple sensitive periods in the development of the primate visual system. *Science* 232, 235–238.

HARWERTH, R. S., SMITH III, E. L., DUNCAN, G. C., CRAWFORD, M. L. J., AND VON NOORDEN, G. K. (1990). Behavioral studies of the sensitive periods of development of visual functions in monkeys. *Behav. Brain Res.* 41, 179–198.

HECHT, S., AND MINTZ, E. U. (1939). The visibility of single lines of various illuminations and the retinal basis of visual resolution. *J. Gen. Physiol.* 22, 593–612.

HELD, R. (1984). Binocular vision . . . behavioral and neuronal development. In J. MEHLER AND R. FOX (eds.). *Neonate Cognition: Beyond the Blooming, Buzzing Confusion*. Hillsdale, NJ: Erlbaum.

HENDRICKSON, A., MOVSHON, J. A., BOOTHE, R. G., EGGERS, H., GIZZI, M., AND KIORPES, L. (1987). Effects of early unilateral blur on the macaque's visual system. II. Anatomical observations. *J. Neurosci.* 7, 1327–1339.

HESS, R. F., AND BAKER, C. L. (1984). Assessment of retinal function in severely amblyopic individuals. *Vision Res.* 24, 1367–1376.

HESS, R. F., AND HOWELL, E. R. (1977). The threshold contrast sensitivity function in strabismic amblyopia: evidence for a two-type classification. *Vision Res.* 17, 1049–1055.

HESS, R. F., AND POINTER, J. S. (1985). Differences in the neural basis of human amblyopias: the distribution of the anomaly across the visual field. *Vision Res.* 25, 1577–1594.

HESS, R. F., AND SMITH, G. (1977). Do optical aberrations contribute to visual loss in strabismic amblyopia? *Am. J. Optom. Physiol. Opt.* 54, 627–633.

HESS, R. F., CAMPBELL, F. W., AND GREENHALGH, T. (1978). On the nature of the neural abnormality in human amblyopia: neural aberrations and neural sensitivity loss. *Pflugers Arch. Ges. Physiol.* 377, 201–207.

HIGGENS, K. E., DAUGMANN, J. G., AND MANSFIELD, J. W. (1982). Amblyopic contrast sensitivity: insensitivity to unsteady fixation. *Invest. Ophthalmol. Vis. Sci.* 23, 113–120.

HILZ, R., RENTSCHLER, I., AND BRETTEL, H. (1977). Myopia and strabismic amblyopia: substantial differences in human visual development. *Exp. Brain Res.* 30, 445–446.

HIRSCH, J., AND CURCIO, C. A. (1989). The spatial resolution capacity of human foveal retina. *Vision Res.* 29, 1095–1101.

HIRSCH, J., AND MILLER, W. H. (1987). Does cone positional disorder limit resolution. *J. Opt. Soc. Am. [A]* 4, 1481–1492.

HOHMANN, A., AND CREUTZFELDT, O. D. (1975). Squint and the development of binocularity in humans. *Nature* 254, 613–614.

HUBEL, D. H., AND WIESEL, T. N. (1970). The period of susceptibility to the physiological effects of unilateral eye closure in kittens. *J. Physiol. (Lond.)* 206, 419–436.

JACOBSON, S. G., MOHINDRA, I., AND HELD, R. (1981). Age of onset of amblyopia in infants with esotropia. *Ophthalmol. Proc. Ser.* 30, 210–216.

KATZ, L. M., LEVI, D. M., AND BEDELL, H. E. (1984). Central and peripheral contrast sensitivity in amblyopia with varying field size. *Doc. Ophthalmol.* 58, 351–373.

KEINER, G. B. J. (1951). *New Viewpoints on the Origin of Squint.* The Hague: Martinus Nijhoff.

KIORPES, L., AND BOOTHE, R. G. (1981). Naturally occurring strabismus in monkeys (*Macaca nemestrina*). *Invest. Ophthalmol. Vis. Sci.* 20, 257–263.

KIORPES, L., AND MOVSHON, J. A. (1988). Development of vernier and grating acuity in strabismic monkeys. *Invest. Ophthal. Visual Sci.* 29 (suppl.), 9.

KIORPES, L., AND MOVSHON, J. A. (1989). Differential-development of two visual functions in primates. *Proc. Natl. Acad. Sci. USA* 86, 8998–9001.

KIORPES, L., BOOTHE, R. G., AND CARLSON, M. R. (1984). Acuity development in surgically strabismic monkeys. *Invest. Ophthalmol. Vis. Sci.* 25 (suppl.), 216.

KIORPES, L., CARLSON, M. R., ALFI, D., AND BOOTHE, R. G. (1989). Development of visual acuity in experimentally strabismic monkeys. *Clin. Vis. Sci.* 4, 95–106.

KIVLIN, J. D., AND FLYNN, J. T. (1981). Therapy of anisometropic amblyopia. *J. Pediatr. Ophthalmol.* 18, 47–56.

KLEIN, S. A., AND LEVI, D. M. (1987). The position sense of the peripheral retina. *J. Opt. Soc. Am. [A]* 4, 1544–1553.

KOLIA, F., AND LEVI, D. M. (1989). Distribution of the loss in position acuity and resolution across the visual field of amblyopes. *Invest. Ophthalmol. Vis. Sci.* 30 (suppl.), 303.

LAIRD, K. (1990). Anisometropia. In T. GROSVENOR AND M. C. FLOM (eds.). *Refractive Anomalies.* Stoneham, MA: Butterworth-Heinemann.

LAWWILL, T., AND BURIAN, H. M. (1966). Luminance, contrast function and visual acuity in functional amblyopia. *Am. J. Ophthalmol.* 62, 511–520.

LEVAY, S., WIESEL, T. N., AND HUBEL, D. H. (1980). The development of ocular dominance columns in normal and visually deprived monkeys. *J. Comp. Neurol.* 191, 1–5.

LEVI, D. M. (1988). The "spatial grain" of the amblyopic visual system. *Am. J. Optom. Physiol. Opt.* 65, 767–786.

LEVI, D. M. (1990). Visual acuity in strabismic and anisometropic amblyopia: a tale of two syndromes. *Ophthalmol. Clin. North Am.* 3, 289–301.

LEVI, D. M. (1991). Spatial vision in amblyopia. In J. CRONLY-DILLON (ed.). *Vision and Visual Dysfunction.* Vol. 10B. New York: Macmillan.

LEVI, D. M., AND HARWERTH, R. S. (1977). Spatio-temporal interactions in anisometropic and strabismic amblyopia. *Invest. Ophthalmol. Vis. Sci.* 16, 90–95.

LEVI, D. M., AND HARWERTH, R. S. (1982). Psychophysical mechanisms in humans with amblyopia. *Am. J. Optom. Physiol. Opt.* 59, 936–951.

LEVI, D. M., AND KLEIN, S. A. (1982a). Hyperacuity and amblyopia. *Nature* 298, 268–270.

LEVI, D. M., AND KLEIN, S. A. (1982b). Differences in vernier discrimination for gratings between strabismic and anisometric amblyopes. *Invest. Ophthalmol. Vis. Sci.* 23, 398–407.

LEVI, D. M., AND KLEIN, S. A. (1983). Spatial localization in normal and amblyopic vision. *Vision Res.* 23, 1005–1017.

LEVI, D. M., AND KLEIN, S. A. (1985). Vernier acuity, crowding and amblyopia. *Vision Res.* 25, 979–991.

LEVI, D. M., AND KLEIN, S. A. (1990a). Equivalent intrinsic blur in spatial vision. *Vision Res.* 30, 1971–1993.

LEVI, D. M., AND KLEIN, S. A. (1990b). Equivalent intrinsic blur in amblyopia. *Vision Res.* 30, 1995–2022.

LEVI, D. M., KLEIN, S. A., AND AITSEBAOMO, A. P. (1985). Vernier acuity, crowding and cortical magnification. *Vision Res.* 25, 963–977.

MANNY, R. E., AND KLEIN, S. A. (1984). The development of vernier acuity in infants. *Curr. Eye Res.* 3, 453–462.

MANNY, R. E., AND KLEIN, S. A. (1985). A three alternative tracking paradigm to measure vernier acuity of older infants. *Vision Res.* 25, 1245–1252.

MANNY, R. E., AND LEVI, D. M. (1982a). Psychophysical investigations of the temporal modulation sensitivity function in amblyopia: uniform field flicker. *Invest. Ophthalmol. Vis. Sci.* 22, 515–524.

MANNY, R. E., AND LEVI, D. M. (1982b). Psychophysical investigations of the temporal modulation function in amblyopia: spatiotemporal interactions. *Invest. Ophthalmol. Vis. Sci.* 22, 525–534.

MARR, D. (1982). *Vision.* San Francisco: W. H. Freeman.

MARSHALL, R. L., AND FLOM, M. C. (1970). Amblyopia, eccentric fixation, and the Stiles-Crawford effect. *Am. J. Optom. Arch. Am. Acad. Optom.* 42, 81–90.

MAURER, D., LEWIS, T. L., AND TYTLA, M. E. (1983). Contrast sensitivity in cases of unilateral congenital cataract. *Invest. Ophthalmol. Vis. Sci.* 24 (suppl.), 21.

MAYER, D. L., AND DOBSON, V. (1982). Visual acuity development in infants and young children, as assessed by operant preferential looking. *Vision Res.* 22, 1141–1152.

MCKEE, S. P., AND LEVI, D. M. (1987). Dichoptic hyperacuity: the precision of nonius alignment. *J. Opt. Soc. Am. [A]* 4, 1104–1108.

MILES, W. P. (1949). Flicker fusion frequency in amblyopia ex anopsia. *Am. J. Ophthalmol.* 32, 225–231.

MILLER II, E. F. (1955). The nature and cause of impaired visual acuity in amblyopia. *Am. J. Optom. Arch. Am. Acad. Optom.* 32, 10–28.

MOHINDRA, I., JACOBSON, S. G., THOMAS, J., AND HELD, R. (1979). Development of amblyopia in infants. *Trans. Ophthalmol. Soc. UK* 99, 344–346.

MOHN, G., VAN NIEUWENHUIZEN, O., AND FAHLE, M. (1989). Vernier acuity and "crowding" in human infants. In *Perception 18, 12th ECVP Abstracts*, p. 490.

MOVSHON, J. A., AND KIORPES, L. (1988). Analysis of the development of spatial contrast sensitivity in monkey and human infants. *J. Opt. Soc. Am. [A]* 5, 2166–2172.

MOVSHON, J. A., EGGERS, H. M., GIZZI, M. S., HENDRICKSON, A., KIORPES, L., AND BOOTHE, R. G. (1987). Effects of early unilateral blur on the macaque's visual system. III. Physiological observations. *J. Neurosci.* 7, 1340–1351.

NORCIA, A. M., AND TYLER, C. W. (1985). Spatial frequency sweep VEP: visual acuity during the first year of life. *Vision Res.* 25, 1399–1408.

NORCIA, A. M., TYLER, C. W., AND HAMER, R. D. (1990). Development of contrast sensitivity in the human infant. *Vision Res.* 30, 1475–1486.

OPPEL, O. (1960). Uber unsere gegenwartigen Vorstellungen vom Wesen der funktionellen Schwachsichtigkeit. *Klin. Monatsbl. Augenheilkd.* 136, 1–20.

OPPEL, O., AND KRANKE, D. (1958). Vergleichende Untersuchunger uber das Verhalten der Dunkeladaption normaler und schielamblyopen Augen. *Graefes Arch. Ophthalmol.* 159, 486–501.

PETRIG, B., JULESZ, B., KROPFL, W., BAUMGARTNER, G., AND ANLIKER, M. (1983). Development of stereopsis and cortical binocularity in human infants: electrophysiological evidence. *Science* 213, 1402–1405.

POWERS, M. K., SCHNECK, M., AND TELLER, D. Y. (1981). Spectral sensitivity of human infants at absolute visual threshold. *Vision Res.* 21, 1005–1016.

REGAL, D. M. (1981). Development of critical flicker frequency in human infants. *Vision Res.* 21, 549–555.

SCHOR, C. M., AND LEVI, D. M. (1980). Direction selectivity for perceived motion in strabismic and anisometric amblyopia. *Invest. Ophthalmol. Vis. Sci.* 19, 1094–1104.

SEKULER, A. B., BANKS, M. S., AND ANDERSON, S. J. (1990). Receptor pooling and peripheral spatial vision. *Invest. Ophthalmol. Vis. Sci.* 31 (suppl.), 495.

SELBY, S. A., AND WOODHOUSE, J. M. (1981). The spatial frequency dependence of interocular transfer in amblyopes. *Vision Res.* 21, 1401–1408.

SELENOW, A., CIUFFREDA, K. J., MOZLIN, R., AND RUMPF, D. (1986). Prognostic value of laser interferometric visual acuity in amblyopia therapy. *Invest. Ophthalmol. Vis. Sci.* 27, 273–277.

SHAPLEY, R. M. (1986). The importance of contrast for the activity of single neurons, the VEP and perception. *Vision Res.* 26, 45–61.

SHIMOJO, S., AND HELD, R. (1987). Vernier acuity is less than grating acuity in 2- and 3-month-olds. *Vision Res.* 27, 77–86.

SHIMOJO, S., BIRCH, E. E., GWIAZDA, J., AND HELD, R. (1984). Development of vernier acuity in infants. *Vision Res.* 24, 721–724.

SKOCZENSKI, A. M., AND ASLIN, R. N. (1989). Spatiotemporal influences on Vernier acuity in human infants. *Invest. Ophthalmol. Vis. Sci.* 30 (suppl.), 312.

SPEKREIJSE, H., KHOE, L. H., AND VAN DER TWEEL, L. H. (1972). A case of amblyopia, electrophysiology and psychophysics of luminance and contrast. In G. B. ARDEN (ed.). *The Visual System: Proceedings 9th ISCERG Symposium.* New York: Plenum, pp. 141–156.

STEINMAN, S. B., LEVI, D. M., AND MCKEE, S. P. (1988). Discrimination of time and velocity in the amblyopic visual system. *Clin. Vis. Sci.* 2, 265–276.

TAYLOR, D. M., VAEGAN, MORRIS, J. A., ROGERS, J. E., AND WARLAND, J. (1979) Amblyopia in bilateral infantile and juvenile cataract. *Trans. Ophthalmol. Soc. UK* 99, 170–175.

TELLER, D. Y., AND BORNSTEIN, M. H. (1986). Infant color vision and color perception. In P. SALAPATEK AND L. B. COHEN (eds.). *Handbook of Infant Perception.* Orlando, FL: Academic Press.

TELLER, D. Y., AND MOVSHON, J. A. (1986). Visual development. *Vision Res.* 26, 1483–1506.

TELLER, D. Y., ALLEN, J. L., REGAL, D. M., AND MAYER, D. L. (1982). Astigmatism and acuity in two primate infants. *Invest. Ophthalmol. Vis. Sci.* 17, 344–349.

THOMAS, J. (1978). Normal and amblyopic contrast sensitivity functions in central and peripheral retinae. *Invest. Ophthalmol. Vis. Sci.* 17, 746–753.

THOMAS, J. P. (1986). Spatial vision then and now. *Vision Res.* 26, 1523–1532.

VAN SLUYTERS, R. C., ATKINSON, J., BANKS, M. S., HELD, R. M., HOFFMANN, K. P., AND SHATZ, C. (1990). The development of vision and visual perception. In L. SPILLMAN AND J. WERNER (eds.). *The Neurophysiological Foundations of Visual Perception.* Orlando, FL: Academic Press.

VON NOORDEN, G. K. (1977). Mechanisms of amblyopia. *Adv. Ophthalmol.* 34, 92–115.

VON NOORDEN, G. K. (1981). New clinical aspects of stimulus deprivation amblyopia. *Am. J. Ophthalmol.* 92, 416–421.

WALD, G., AND BURIAN, H. M. (1944). The dissociation of form vision and light perception in strabismic amblyopia. *Am. J. Ophthalmol.* 27, 950–963.

WERNER, J. S. (1982). Development of scotopic sensitivity and the absorption spectrum of the human ocular media. *J. Opt. Soc. Am.* 72, 247–258.

WESSON, M. D., AND LOOP, M. S. (1982). Temporal contrast sensitivity in amblyopia. *Invest. Ophthalmol. Vis. Sci.* 22, 98–102.

WESTHEIMER, G. (1975). Visual acuity and hyperacuity. *Invest. Ophthalmol.* 14, 570–572.

WESTHEIMER, G. (1982). The spatial gain of the perifoveal visual field. *Vision Res.* 22, 157–162.

WEYMOUTH, F. W. (1958). Visual sensory units and the minimal angle of resolution. *Am. J. Ophthalmol.* 46, 102–113.

WIESEL, T. N. (1982). Postnatal development of the visual cortex and the influence of environment. *Nature* 299, 583–591.

WILSON, H. R. (1988). Development of spatiotemporal mechanisms in the human infant. *Vision Res.* 28, 611–628.

WILSON, H. R. (1991). Model of peripheral and amblyopic hyperacuity. *Vision Res.* 31, 967–982.

WILSON, H. R., LEVI, D. M., DE VALOIS, R., MAFFEI, L., AND ROVAMO, J. (1990). The perception of form: retina to striate cortex. In L. SPILLMAN AND J. WERNER (eds.). *The Neurophysiological Foundations of Visual Perception.* Orlando, FL: Academic Press.

WORTH, C. A. (1903). *Squint: Its Causes, Pathology and Treatment.* Philadelphia: Blakiston.

YAP, Y. L., LEVI, D. M., AND KLEIN, S. A. (1987). Peripheral hyperacuity: 3-dot spatial interval scales to a single factor from 0 to 10 deg. *J. Opt. Soc. Am. [A]* 4, 1554–1561.

YAP, Y. L., LEVI, D. M., AND KLEIN, S. A. (1989). Peripheral position acuity: retinal and cortical constraints on 2-dot spatial interval discrimination under photopic and scotopic conditions. *Vision Res.* 29, 789–802.

YOUDELIS, C., AND HENDRICKSEN, A. (1986). A qualitative and quantitative analysis of the human fovea during development. *Vision Res.* 26, 847–855.

25 | Stereoscopic neurontropy and the origins of amblyopia and strabismus

KURT SIMONS

The probabilistic nature of physiological dysfunction is surely nowhere better illustrated than in the complex of sensorimotor disorders classified clinically as strabismus and amblyopia. Even as "obvious" a condition as infantile esotropia turns out to be a taxonomically blurry collage of symptoms that represent a whole subfamily of sensorimotor dysfunction (see discussions in von Noorden, 1988a,b). The diversity of variables involved is illustrated in the equivalent diversity of outcomes seen over the natural (i.e., untreated) history of strabismus, ranging from variability of deviation to outright change in sign, such as from eso- to exo-deviated (Fletcher, 1971; Moore, 1971; Burian, 1972; Keiner, 1978; Folk, 1979; Clark and Noel, 1982; Robb and Rodier, 1987; Quick et al., 1990). Furthermore, the distinction between the statically defined symptom of misalignment (strabismus) and the dynamically defined symptom of nystagmus may be useful taxonomically but misleading etiologically, as illustrated by the co-occurrence of various forms of nystagmus with strabismus and by developing evidence of a dynamic deficit (motion processing) being at least partially responsible for the static (strabismus) deficit (see Chapters 23 and 26). Similarly, the cause-and-effect relation between strabismus (or strabismus-nystagmus) and amblyopia may be bidirectional, rather than the unidirectional vector indicated by the traditional term "strabismus amblyopia," as illustrated by evidence of sensory deficits giving rise to strabismus or nystagmus in animal models (reviewed by Quick et al., 1989; Tusa et al., 1991) and human patients (von Noorden, 1990, pp. 313, 336, 435ff).

The present chapter considers some nontraditional risk factors possibly contributing to the onset of the amblyopia-nystagmus-strabismus complex. They include proposals that: (1) the key concept in understanding amblyopia and strabismus onset is that visual function and development involves a reciprocally inhibitory relation between monocular vision in each eye and the integrated global stereopsis of binocular vision; (2) risk factors for amblyopia may include (a) a "micro" form of the retinotopic neural miswiring to the cortex in albino heterozygotes similar to that seen in gross form in homozygous albinos, (b) a developmentally transient cone matrix malformation from birth-stress-related retinal microdetachments exacerbated by poststress phagocytosis or short-wavelength-light photic insult, or (c) stereopsis neural time-encoding defects; (3) the cortical origin of amblyopia lies in the global stereopsis mechanism and specifically that mechanism's sensitivity to excessive discrepancies in retinotopic mapping to the cortex between the two eyes, possibly involving the "cone position known" (Hirsch and Miller, 1987) retinal matrix distortion-compensation systems; (4) strabismus risk factors include (a) fusion or optomotor deficits from albino heterozygote neural miswiring to the midbrain or to cerebral, midbrain, or cerebellar hydraulic insult from birth trauma, (b) deficient fusion or asynchrony in developmental onset of fusion and stereopsis, possibly due to corpus callosum-based mechanisms, (c) abnormal fovea-to-disc distance; (5) the relation between the two eyes' nasal and temporal hemiretinas influences the direction of strabismus deviation, and the associated signed stereopsis disparity mechanism may partially explain the difficulty of treating the accommodative component in esotropia; and (6) maternal birth posture may affect birth trauma incidence. A stereoscopic "neurontropy" (Julesz and Tyler, 1976) process is proposed to explain amblyopiagenesis, and new detection and therapeutic approaches are proposed to improve binocular prognosis in early strabismus and amblyopia.

VISUAL DEVELOPMENT: BIOCULARITY TO BINOCULAR STEREOPSIS

Before considering developmental aberrations, it is useful to review the physiological developmental context that sets the stage for them, in the form of a refinement of the traditional idea of visual ontogeny recapitulating phylogeny (Duke-Elder, 1958). The idea is based on there being a developmental parallel to the shift from the nonoverlapping panoramic visual field of lower species, such as the rabbit (Figure 25-1), to the overlapped,

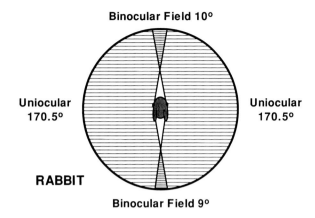

FIG. 25-1. Monocular and binocular visual fields of the rabbit. (Adapted from Duke-Elder, 1958.)

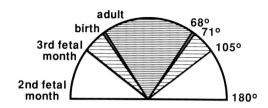

FIG. 25-3. Plot of the angular relation of orbital axes in humans from the second fetal month to adulthood. (Adapted from Duke-Elder and Cook, 1963.)

stereopsis-capable binocular field of the adult primate (Figure 25-2). An anterior visual axes rotation with ascent up the phylogenetic scale is recapitulated in every human fetus in the form of the swing forward in orbital alignment that takes place between early fetal life and birth, with a final asymptote extending postnatally (Figure 25-3).

From Fusion to Coarse and Fine Global Stereopsis

We consider the hypothesis that the infant begins postnatal development in a state of alternating bi-monocular, or "bi-ocular," vision in lieu of binocular fusion. Thus most neonates have slightly more diverged orbital axes (Figure 25-3) and relatively less sensitive nasal visual fields monocularly (see Chapter 7) than adults and adopt an exotropic vergence posture, many with motor indications of alternating fixation as well (Archer and Helveston, 1989; see also Chapter 22). When binocular fusion has its onset, it apparently begins with a quasi-binocularity in the form of non-eye-selective monocular

visual field superposition, which appears to be followed by a crude level of fusion (see Chapters 12, 13, and 15) that seems almost depth-indifferent, or "pyknostereoscopic" (Tyler, 1983, 1990) and results in initially poor control of vergence (see Chapter 3). This depth insensitivity is enhanced by the infant's small interorbital, and resulting interpupillary, stereo base distance (Zimmerman et al., 1929; Aslin and Dumais, 1980).

The infant thus appears to begin life with an alternation-based bi-ocular view of the world and with only crude spatial resolution, or "grain" (Table 25-1). It is useful to reflect on the adaptive reason for this situation. Although it has a fetal history of lateral eye placement, at birth the infant has frontal eye placement, open eyes,

TABLE 25-1. *The visual development spectrum.*

Postnatal visual development onset	Adult vision
Small orbital stereo base	Large orbital stereo base
Coarser cone/RF "grain," "area centralis"	Fine cone/RF grain, fovea
Wide acceptance angle COS/CIS	Narrow acceptance angle COS/CIS
Small, homogeneous retina/ monocular VF	Large, central vs. peripheral-differentiated retina/ monocular VF
Alternating monocular VF	Fused binocular VF
Alternate fixation	Stereopsis
Midbrain predominance	Cortical predominance
High callosal axon count, no myelin	Low callosal axon count, high myelin
Nasal hemiretina dominant	Temporal/nasal balance
Robust OKAN	Weak or absent OKAN
Large + angle κ	Small angle κ
Large interval of Sturm astigmatism	Small interval of Sturm
Large depth of focus	Small depth of focus
Often hyperopic	Nominally emmetropic
No accommodation	Accommodation
Reduced CSF	Normal CSF
3:1 Ratio cone/RF density for nasal/temporal retina periphery	3:1 Ratio cone/RF density for nasal/temporal retina periphery
Exo-deviation tonus	Exo-deviation tonus

Sources: Curcio and Hendrickson (1991); Duke-Elder (1963); Aslin and Dumais (1980); LaMantia and Rakic (1990); Chapters 1, 3, 7, 13, 14, 22, 26; Powers and Dobson (1982); Schor (1983); Schor et al. (1983b); Westall and Schor (1985).

RF = receptive field; VF = visual field; COS = cone outer segment; CIS = cone inner segment; OKAN = optokinetic afternystagmus; CSF = contrast sensitivity function; + = positive.

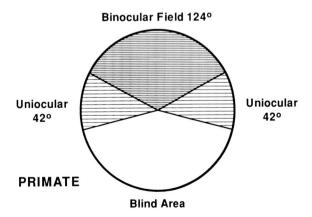

FIG. 25-2. Monocular and binocular visual fields of a primate. (Adapted from Duke-Elder, 1958.)

and an at least crudely functional monocular visual capacity. Why then does it not develop globally integrated binocular vision until 3–4 months postnatally? Levi and Carakeet note that robustness in the face of abnormal visual input appears to be a key characteristic of visual functions with onset earlier, rather than later, in development (see Chapter 24). Binocular vision is particularly neuronally fragile and thus easier to disrupt than monocular vision (Timney, 1983, 1990; Crawford et al., 1991), and so by this logic would be expected to have its onset later than the more neurally robust monocular function. The computational task confronting global stereoscopic interocular matching is daunting even in the anatomically stable adult. In the infant, during rapid early neural development, ongoing stereoscopic matching that incorporates the necessary multidimensional calibration changes in the complex set of changes in the binocular substrate (Table 25-1) and the vagaries of visual experience may thus be a computational problem to adaptively avoid. Instead, the infant apparently first alternates, which does not interfere with initial development of monocular vision, via "equal time" in the alternation that allows development of both monocular pathways. The rate of change in the substrate apparently has decreased in rate terms by 3–4 months of age to the extent that binocular vision is computationally feasible and safe from the neural disruptive hazards of the developmental structural asynchronies of normal, if not abnormal, development. However, there remains the potential for abandonment of the global stereopsis computational struggle at some stage of developmental "arrest" (Chavasse, 1939; Worth, 1903) due to genetic, pathological or experiential obstacle. The results of such abandonment are binocularly regressive, influenced by the (in Linksz's words) "continuous undercurrent of monocular vision (panoramic vision) in spite of all the provisions of binocularity. . . . They are all later grafts, later mappings on a basically panoramic-pyramidal setup of eyes and brain" (quoted in Jampolsky, 1978, p. 379). Thus the baseline form of "arrest" is to halt development at the starting point, alternation, seen in infants with the earliest and most profound binocular deficits, such as that typically associated with early-onset esotropia (or exotropia) (von Noorden, 1990, p. 314). Whether the primitive alternation state should also represent the goal of treatment for amblyopia patients is discussed later in the chapter.

If we assume that, as with monocular visual development (see Chapters 24 and 32), stereoscopic development parallels the functional change across the retina from peripheral to foveal vision, it suggests a shift with development from coarse to fine stereopsis (Table 25-2). In other words, it implies a shift from a stereopsis that is initially sensitive to coarse disparities, perhaps only motion-based, to the fine stereopsis of visual adult-

TABLE 25-2. *Classes of stereopsis.*

Global	Local
Fovea dominant	Periphery dominant
Fine	Coarse
Small disparity	Large disparity
On-horopter	Off-horopter
Static, position-sensitive	Motion-sensitive
LGB parvocellular routing	LGB magnocellular routing

Adapted from Tyler (1990).
LGB = lateral geniculate body.

hood. As noted above, the genesis of stereopsis function appears to be a relatively depth-insensitive "pyknostereoscopic" state that then develops more precise depth localization capabilities. During the developmental transition, small disparity thresholds are worse than those of adults (Simons, 1981a; Heron et al., 1985),[1] but large disparity fusion capacity is better than that of the adult (Dowd et al., 1980). In other words, in keeping with Tyler's concept of a "larval" state unique to early development (see Chapter 16), there may be an initial stereopsis status in which the infant or child sees in a way the adult cannot. Specifically, it seems reasonable to propose that the child has a stereoscopic system based on what would be a combination of opposites in the adult (Table 25-2), being both relatively coarse disparity-sensitive and yet global, in keeping with the pyknostereoscopic idea. The adaptive advantage of coarse global stereopsis is that it is tolerant of mismatches (Parker and Yang, 1989), as suggested by the reduced stereopsis sensitivity, particularly for low spatial frequency stimuli, at off- than on-horopter loci (Badcock and Schor 1985). In sum, such a coarse global stereopsis appears to be relatively robust, tolerant of interocular

---

1. Fox et al. (1986) questioned if in fact stereoacuity shows development between 3–5 years of age and adulthood. Using a Howard-Dolman apparatus, they demonstrated better stereoacuity thresholds in children of this age than was obtained on the Titmus Circles test. This result, however, is simply another demonstration of the variability of absolute stereoacuity thresholds found between tests (e.g., Simons, 1981a; Heron et al., 1985). Comparison of the Fox et al.'s child versus adult thresholds on the Howard-Dolman test indicates the same approximately 2:1 within-test threshold difference that is found between these two age groups on other stereo tests, even when "motivated" methodology such as theirs is used (Heron et al., 1985). Birch and Hale (1989) found a threshold plateau of stereoacuity at 36 months of age, but it coincided with the smallest test disparity available and so may have constituted a ceiling effect. Ciner et al. (1991) attributed the threshold improvement at these ages to a reduction in response variability. Such variability is an inescapable reality of testing young children, as attested to by Ciner et al.'s test–retest correlation of only $r = .62$, and is the reason for reliance on population sample-based estimates of threshold in this age group. On a group basis, Ciner et al.'s results too support a conclusion of continuing development in the 3- to 5-year-old age period. Indeed, the relatively constant standard error extending from their 30- to 35-month-old to 60- to 65-month-old age groups (Ciner et al., 1991, Fig. 3) makes the case for continuing stereoacuity development over this age range particularly convincing.

mismatches in a way that later fine-structure adult global stereopsis (Table 25-2) is not. This coarse—and developmentally transient—form appears to be responsible for the transient stereopsis found in infant and toddler esotropes (Birch and Stager, 1985; Mohindra et al., 1985; Archer et al., 1986; Stager and Birch, 1986; Birch et al., 1990; Atkinson et al., 1991).

There seems reason to conclude, then, that the underlying tendency toward bi-ocular vision translates, in a binocularly wired cortex, into suppression or amblyopia when, and to the extent that, there is an obstacle to normal development of the merged monocularity of fusion and stereopsis. In adaptive fashion, these dysfunctions appear to arrest disturbed central binocular visual development at the infantile bi-ocular level, leaving what may be innate, crude residual binocular vision at the periphery (e.g., Sireteanu and Fronius, 1982; Sireteanu 1982) but either bi-ocular "time-sharing" alternation or bilateral (see Chapter 21) or unilateral amblyopia centrally.

Development of Binocular Optomotor Alignment

In motor terms, the strength of the atavistic bi-monocular-tropic "undercurrent" is seen in the fact that, with the exception of the esotropia of infancy and childhood, decrement of oculomotor control typically results in a divergent "exotropic" eye position. Thus the eyes assume a divergent posture under anesthesia, even in the case of esotropes, and postmortem (Jampolsky, 1978; von Noorden, 1990, p. 305); and most visually "normal" adults are exophoric (von Noorden, 1990). Furthermore, as noted above, some human (Moore, 1971; Burian, 1972; Keiner, 1978; Folk, 1979; Clarke and Noel, 1982; Robb and Rodier, 1987) and naturally strabismic monkey (Quick et al., 1990) esotropes exhibit spontaneous reductions, resolutions, or even reversals of their deviation over time, i.e., become relatively more exo-deviated. More dramatically, there are patients who appear to have a true genetic "fusion defect" (Worth, 1903) absence of retinal correspondence that results not simply in bi-ocularity but in exotropic, nonoverlapped monocular visual field vision (von Noorden, 1990, p. 330). Walls (1962) reported one such patient who "could drive a milk truck down the street and be watching where he was going with one eye while reading the house numbers with the other, without the least confusion." Patients with hyperteliorism from craniofacial dysostoces, which produces an interocular stereo base exaggerated beyond what the binocular vision system can fuse, typically become exotropic as well (Lloyd, 1975; Miller and Pruzansky, 1981; von Noorden, 1990, p. 323). Finally, with the milder and more pervasive condition of intermittent

exotropia, where there is often suppression of distance viewing, Fletcher (1971) noted that,

> This visual pattern, using one eye while looking in the distance, and both eyes when viewing near objects, resembles the visual pattern of a large group of lower animals. The horse surveys his surroundings with one eye at a time but uses both eyes when eating. This type of strabismus could well be a throwback to a former sub-primate visual pattern.

Apparently to achieve the motor alignment basis for the phylogenetic/ontogenetic ascent from bi-ocular to normal binocular vision, the infant is provided with a relatively crude but powerful subcortically mediated tool to counter his or her exotropic vergence tonus: a monocular-based sensitivity to nasalward stimulus motion and relative insensitivity to temporalward stimulus motion (see reviews in Chapters 5, 23, and 26) characterized clinically as an adduction reflex (Keiner, 1951; Jampolsky, 1978; von Noorden, 1990, p. 136). The strength of this nasalward bias is sufficient that the optokinetic after-nystagmus exhibited in the dark following optokinetic nystagmus (OKN) stimulation in young infants always has a nasalward slow phase, whether the preceding OKN stimulus was in the nasalward or temporalward direction (Schor et al., 1983b). This response asymmetry is based on dominance of output of the cortical and subcortical projections of the temporal hemiretina (THR) by that of the nasal hemiretina (NHR), which is phylogenetically older and more mature at birth than the THR (Westall and Schor, 1985; see also Chapters 7 and 23) and has a cone density in the periphery three times that of the THR (Packer et al., 1990). The nasalward motion bias is an NHR bias (Westall and Schor, 1985). A similar response asymmetry is seen in afoveate animals (Howard and Gonzalez, 1987) and an exaggerated form with amblyopia (Westall and Schor, 1985) and in premature infants (see Chapter 26). The NHR dominance extends interocularly as well, as illustrated even in normal visual adults, where in a rivalry task the NHR of either eye dominates the THR of the contralateral eye (Fahle, 1987).

It appears that developmental onset of the nasalward motion sensitivity sets up a primal tug-of-war between the NHR's "esotonic" adduction-vergence and the original exotropic tonus (see Chapters 7 and 23). The onset and refinement of function of cortically mediated binocular vision, and specifically of the interocularly integrative process of fusion, apparently becomes the arbitrator of the resulting vergence alignment. For instance, binocularly presented optokinetic stimuli produce the highest slow-phase tracking gain when located at the horopter, with far lower gain or outright lack of response at a binocularly disparate (i.e., off-horopter) depth locus (Howard and Gonzalez, 1987). The task of successfully achieving the delicate balance of precise bifix-ation necessary to achieve high resolution stereoacuity in the presence of this exotropic/esotonic conflict is a formidable one, especially when the balance must be maintained over a long course of development, with multiple changing substrates (Table 25-1) and neurally open to influence by the vagaries of visual experience.

BINOCULAR VERSUS MONOCULAR VISION IN DEVELOPMENT

The development from bi-ocularity to full stereoscopic vision appears to involve not simply a progression but a classic agonist-antagonist reciprocal relation between the two ends of the recapitulation spectrum involved. That is, we propose here (not originally, see Tyler, 1983) that (bi)monocular vision does not simply coexist with binocular vision but in fact stands in a mutually inhib-itory reciprocal relation with it.

General Experimental Evidence

On the motor side, Rashbass and Westheimer (1961) suggested three decades ago that conjugate and vergence eye movements are controlled by independent mecha-nisms. During that same era, Riggs and Niehl (1960) demonstrated that a target moved closer to a subject along the line of sight of one eye does not initially result in the most fixationally efficient solution, of a mon-ocular refixation of the contralateral eye, resulting in an interocularly asymmetric vergence posture change. Instead, there is initially a binocular vergence response that misaligns the ipsilateral eye, followed by a conju-gate (i.e., again, both eyes involved) corrective saccade to at last bring both eyes into alignment with the target. What appears to be illustrated in the present context is that when a target is fusible binocular control is par-amount, even when that control is paradoxically inef-ficient. More recently there has been demonstration of default of binocular to monocular control of fixation when stereo targets are moved beyond fusion threshold due to misalignment extent or velocity: When random dot stereo targets are dichoptically pulled apart in tem-poralward motion until fusion is lost, the visual axes drop back to, for the stimulus, an overconverged po-sition (Hyson et al., 1983). Reversal of motion to bring the targets back into fusible alignment results initially in binocular-fusional-inappropriate, but (bi)monocular-fixation-logical, further "convergence"–actually bi-monocular adduction (Hyson et al., 1983). When the targets are aligned enough to re-fuse, that refusion is preceded by a pair of abducting saccades that cancel the vergence error, i.e., motions, again, of a bi-mon-

ocular fixation (not vergence) type (Hyson et al., 1983). Similarly, random dot targets pulled apart at a too rapid speed to maintain fusion result in the default of bilat-erally symmetrical vergence tracking to accurate mon-ocular tracking by one eye and the assignment of the retinal disparity "slip" entirely to the tracking error of the other eye, which is also partially sensorially sup-pressed (Erkelens and Collewijn, 1985). In other words, this fixation behavior too is in keeping with the idea of independent monocular and binocular fixation mech-anisms, with a default to bi-monocular precedence when fusion is lost.

On the sensory side, monocular Vernier acuity is greatly reduced by fusion of the monocular Vernier image into a stereo pair (McKee et al., 1990), and there is greater lag (i.e., lower gain) for (monocular-mediated) pursuit tracking of random dot stereogram targets than of equivalent monocularly visible targets in both infants (Shea, 1986) and adults (Julesz and Oswald, 1979; Archer et al., 1986). Again, the predominance of fused binoc-ular vision in normal circumstances is demonstrated (see Neurontropy Model of Mapping Distortion Origins, below, for other examples). On the other hand, a variety of evidence suggests that retinal rivalry is the default outcome when stereoscopic binocular correspondence cannot be established (Blake, 1989; Blake et al., 1991), i.e., that monocular function dominance—in this case alternating monocular dominance—arises to inhibit bi-nocular function in reciprocal fashion when binocular-ity is disrupted. Under appropriate conditions, equi-dominance of monocular *and* binocular vision can be demonstrated, such as the simultaneous perception of fusion or stereopsis and (bi-monocular-based) diplopia in normal subjects (Boman and Kertesz, 1985a; Wolfe, 1986). An equivalent phenomenon is seen in strabismic patients who experience diplopia with small centrally located stimuli for which they cannot initiate (binocu-larly controlled) vergence movements in response (Bo-man and Kertesz, 1985b). Mildly amblyopic patients viewing motion-in-depth stimuli (oscillating squares) are also reported who see neither (normal binocular) mo-tion-in-depth nor (monocular component) lateral mo-tion but, rather, diagonal motion at a vectorial position intermediate between motion-in-depth and lateral mo-tion (Mohn et al., 1986).

Vernier acuity has been found to deteriorate more with eccentricity than stereoacuity (Schor and Badcock, 1985). Vernier acuity is already a sub-cone-matrix-res-olution "hyper" acuity (Westheimer, 1987), suggesting that there is a further level of "hyper"-ness that supports stereoacuity and that is beyond the resolution of the monocular Vernier component, i.e., again, that two sys-tems are involved. The "superhyper" aspect of stereop-sis is suggested in demonstrations of stereopsis from target structure features too subtle to be detected monocularly [Julesz and Spivack, 1967 (but see Nishihara and Poggio, 1982); Julesz and Oswald, 1979].

Finally, demonstration that sensory and motor monocular versus binocular interactions are coordinated, and on a binocular visual field locus-by-locus basis, is found in studies that investigated stereomotion detection using small targets at different locations around the visual field (Richards and Regan, 1973; Regan et al., 1986). Although normal eyes were used, a surprisingly large proportion of the binocular fields were found to be defective in detecting this localized stereomotion. Lateral motion was perceived, however, accompanied by normal conjugate eye tracking movements at these loci, again demonstrating operation of monocular vision in default of binocular vision.

Developmental Evidence

Many neonates who, as noted above, appear exodeviated fix with one eye and then adduct the exodeviated eye into appropriate "vergence" alignment (Archer and Helveston, 1989). This behavior stands in contrast to the adult normal (binocular) behavior of the Riggs and Niehl (1960) study reviewed above. Instead of an "inefficient" bi-ocular vergence followed by a bi-ocular conjugate corrective saccade, in the young infant there appears to be an efficient (and apparently monocular) adduction of each eye independently. Again, in the absence of normal binocularity, in this case due to immaturity, monocular vision is transcendent.

There appears to be no correlation between dark vergence and dark focus resting state points in infants (Aslin et al., 1982), and these two points are at different fixation distances in adults (Owens and Leibowitz, 1980). Furthermore, accommodation and convergence in infants have been found to correlate with target distance but not with each other (Widdershein et al., 1990). Although the linkage between accommodation and convergence in infants is not well understood (see Chapter 3), these findings appear compatible with the idea of accommodation being controlled by a system at least partially independent of that controlling vergence, i.e., another example of monocular versus binocular control.

Clinical Evidence

Much of the symptomatology of strabismus can be interpreted as, and perhaps is causally related to, a reciprocal battle for predominance of binocular and monocular vision. This idea is attested to by the fundamental tool for strabismus diagnosis, the *cover test*, which compares fixation and motility status under binocular versus monocular viewing conditions. The differences under these two viewing conditions clearly demonstrate that the fixational zero point is different between the conditions of monocular vision (cover present) and simultaneous binocular and monocular viewing conditions (no cover present). The influence of the binocular-monocular reciprocal battle for predominance is also seen sensorially in the existence of amblyopia and suppression in the first place, which demonstrate both the existence of the two systems and the primacy of one (binocular/interocular) over the other (monocular). The predominance contest is also seen in such forms as the binocular condition of anomalous retinal correspondence (ARC) and monocular eccentric fixation, both of which seem due to the result of being influenced during visual development by the reciprocal system, especially in the case of unharmonious ARC or paradoxic eccentric fixation, i.e., opposite laterality for a deviation from what would be expected, such as temporal eccentricity in esotropia (von Noorden, 1990, p. 224). Thus eccentric fixation is not correlated with visual acuity (von Noorden, 1990, p. 222), as would be expected if it had a purely monocular origin. Furthermore, eccentric fixation can develop in an occluded eye in nonstrabismic patients (von Noorden, 1990, p. 212), an outcome difficult to explain on the basis of (occluded) monocular processes, as is the converse case of eccentric fixation in the monocular acuity-defined "normal" eye of strabismic amblyopes (Kandel et al., 1977, 1980). The presence of ARC in most patients with eccentric fixation (von Noorden, 1990, p. 226) suggests that, in fact, these two conditions may be reciprocally related.

Other measures illustrate the variety and complexity of the *modus vivendi* of binocular and monocular vision arrived at under conditions of subnormal binocularity. When strabismic patients are presented with the asymmetrical vergence task of Riggs and Niehl's experiment, like young infants they reverse the normal order of events in so-called accommodative vergence: A saccade is initially used to fixate the sound eye on the target followed by an asymmetrical vergence movement to properly align the two eyes (Ciuffreda and Kenyon, 1983; Boman and Kertesz, 1985b). In other words, saccade-driving monocular function takes precedence in lieu of the (disparity-based) binocular precedence of normal vision. Similarly, visual acuity of both the amblyopic or suppressing and the nominally sound eye of amblyopes may be reduced under dichoptic (vectographic) testing conditions compared to standard unilateral testing (Awaya and von Noorden, 1972; Morgan et al., 1972). In other words, although there is monocular system predominance in the better eye, it remains influenced by the binocular system, a point also illustrated by the variety of sensory and motor defects in the better eye of both human amblyopes (Kandel et al., 1980; Bedell et al., 1985; Mac Cana et al., 1986; Leguire et al., 1990; see

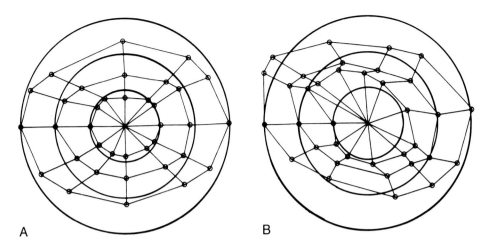

FIG. 25-4. Spatial distortion maps from the normal (A) and amblyopic (B) eyes of an amblyope. From circle construction task, using 4-, 8-, and 12-degree circles, with reference loci indicated by circles. (Reprinted from *Vision Research*, Volume 31, W-L. Lagrèze and R. Sireteanu, "Two-dimensional spatial distortions in human strabismic amblyopia," pp. 1271–1288, Copyright 1991, with permission from Pergamon Press Ltd., Headington Hall, Oxford OX3 OBW, UK.)

also Chapter 26) and in naturally occurring strabismic monkeys (Kiorpes and Boothe, 1981). That active interocular inhibition and not simply rupture is involved in this process is demonstrated by patients and primate models who regain vision in an amblyopic eye during postdevelopmental life when vision is lost in the sound eye (Tommila, 1964; Harwerth et al., 1986; Tierney, 1989). Finally, there are two components of amblyopia—one based on "abnormal binocular interaction" and one on visual deprivation (Mitchell and Timney, 1984; von Noorden, 1990)—that suggest operation of binocular and monocular mechanisms, respectively. [Whether a third form, anisometropic amblyopia, is a cause or effect of its associated refractive error is at this point unclear (von Noorden, 1990, p. 211; see also Chapter 1), but it seems likely to be a vectorial result of a combination of the other two forms rather than an etiological distinct third class of amblyopia].

Final evidence of the possible significance of monocular function in strabismus is found in two unusual reports: Infants and children with an enucleated or congenitally blind eye have been reported to exhibit "esotropia" in the remaining eye in the form of face turn while fixating and nystagmus symptoms often characteristic of esotropia (Helveston et al., 1985; Kushner, 1985). Clearly, only monocular processes are involved. In another study, a penlight was projected into one eye of strabismic patients in an otherwise dark room (Mitsui et al., 1979). With exophoria it caused the opposite eye to abduct, and with hyperdeviations it caused the opposite eye to hyperdeviate—both results that would be expected from cover test responses.[2] With esophoria

or esotropia, however, the *illuminated* eye adducted, a finding difficult to explain by other than a monocular process, as the contralateral eye received no stimulation. This response had originally been reported in strabismic infants by Keiner (1951) but was not previously replicated (von Noorden, 1990, p. 137).

RISK FACTORS FOR SPATIAL MAPPING DISTORTIONS IN STRABISMIC AMBLYOPIA

It has been known for years that some amblyopes report visual anomalies beyond simply acuity loss, specifically spatial distortions and abnormal spatial directionalization (Pugh, 1958, 1962; Hess et al., 1978). More recent research indicates that these anomalies (Figure 25-4) occur with strabismic amblyopia and are due to spatial localization errors or distortions in retinotopic mapping to the visual cortex (Bedell and Flom, 1983; Fronius and Sireteanu, 1989; Lagrèze and Sireteanu, 1991). Although primarily reported as a foveal effect, some studies indicate that the spatial mapping errors involved are found as far as 7 degrees in the periphery. So characteristic of strabismic amblyopia do these mapping errors appear to be that one investigator has proposed that the term "amblyopia," meaning "blunted sight," should be replaced by the term "tarachopia," from the Greek for confused or jumbled sight (Hess, 1982). Other investigators have proposed that the distortions should be incorporated in the basic clinical differential diagnosis of amblyopia, as they distinguish strabismic amblyopia from nonamblyopic reduced vision, e.g., due to refractive error or immaturity, in a way the traditional visual acuity criterion cannot (Flom and Bedell, 1983).

---

2. Illumination of either eye in exotropia produced no movement.

Albino Heterozygote Retinocortical Pathway Localized Misrouting

Strabismus has a hereditary component (Aurrell and Norsell, 1990; von Noorden, 1990, p. 144ff), as illustrated by such findings as common characteristics of strabismus in twins reared apart (Knobloch et al., 1985). However, the specific physiological mechanisms involved remain a matter of debate. I here consider the possibility that a subtle version of the retinocortical pathway misrouting seen in oculocutaneous and ocular albinism is one such mechanism, resulting in either a static positional retinotopic mapping distortion or incompatibly interleaved out-of-phase projections to the lateral motion or motion-in-depth sensitive binocular cells of the primary visual cortex (Poggio and Talbot, 1981).

What makes the albinotic mapping error of initial interest here is that the defect involves the visual field of the temporal hemiretina (THR), that, as noted earlier, is fundamentally involved in strabismic maldevelopment. The proportion of fibers from the THR that project to the same side of the brain, or are uncrossed, is normally related to the degree that a species' eyes are frontally placed and so capable of binocular vision, with more frontal placement associated with a greater proportion of uncrossed fibers (Kinnear et al., 1985). In the albino, there is a phylogenetic atavism, with some THR fibers near the midline routed inappropriately to the contralateral side of the cortex, in reversed mirror image form of the normal projection. That is, the projections are in proper retinotopic order but are sent to the wrong side of the brain (Kinner et al., 1985; Guillery, 1986, 1990). There is also evidence of similar misprojection to the midbrain (Dräger, 1985a; Creel et al., 1990). The result of this misrouting is an interocular mapping conflict that degrades binocular function in albinos, who typically lack central stereopsis, are often strabismic, and may exhibit reversed OKN (Kinnear et al., 1985; Guo et al., 1989; Creel et al., 1990).

Although many albinos are strabismic, evoked potential studies have demonstrated that geniculocortical misrouting on the scale of that present in albinos does not occur in normally pigmented strabismus patients (McCormack, 1975; Hoyt and Caltrider, 1984). However, the relatively gross evoked potential measurement does not exclude the possibility of more localized mapping errors of the albino type in normally pigmented strabismus patients.

Evidence compatible with the idea that "micro" misrouting errors may exist is found in the studies of Sireteanu and colleagues of localized motion-in-depth responses in strabismic and amblyopic patients (Sireteanu et al., 1981; Sireteanu, 1982; Mohn et al., 1986). The stimulus used was a dichoptically presented pair of small

(2.5 degrees on a side) squares moving laterally in opposite directions to create an appearance, to normal binocular vision, of motion in depth directly toward or away from the observer. This stimulus was presented at a variety of loci within a ± 40 degrees horizontal and ± 20 degrees vertical visual field. The noteworthy finding here was perception by some patients of motion-in-depth bias skewed laterally left or right (rather than orthogonal to the observer) at different parts of the field. For instance, one nonstrabismic amblyope saw the square moving toward the right between 20 and 40 degrees in the left visual field at the vertical midline and between 0 to 20 degrees in the right field but toward the left at the interleaved at 0–20 degrees in the left field and 20–40 degrees in the right field (Fig. 25-5). This kind of response is compatible with the idea of interleaved patches of normal and abnormal misrouting or of misrouting of opposite motion-sensitive directional polarity. Dräger has proposed that the misrouting in albinism results in a 180-degree reversal in directional selectivity of adjacent projections, forming the basis for the inverted following movements of albinism (Dräger, 1985a). Many of the cortical neurons most sensitive to positional disparity are also sensitive to lateral motion (Poggio and Talbot, 1981), so opposite directional selectivity of such interdigitated projections would presumably interfere with global stereoscopic integration of the positioned disparity for such a cell ensemble.

Albinism is variable in expression, with some patients difficult to distinguish from normal subjects (Kinnear et al., 1985; Creel et al., 1990). Some even have central stereopsis (Apkarian and Reites, 1989; Guo et al., 1989). Such variation suggests that there is a normally distributed continuum, rather than a discrete genetic distinc-

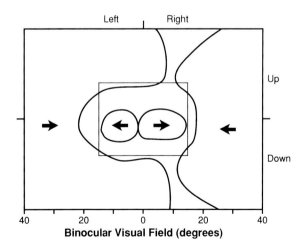

FIG. 25-5. Motion sensitivity discrepancies at different loci in the binocular visual field of an amblyope in response to a motion-in-depth target. Arrows indicate the direction of the perceived lateral motion. (Adapted from Mohn et al., 1986.)

tion, between the misrouting of albinism and the routing of normal pigmentation. Leventhal et al. (1985) found normally pigmented cats that were heterozygous for a recessive allele for tyrosine-negative albinism that had misrouting similar to that of homozygous albinos and that showed a relatively low proportion of binocular cells, also like the full albinos, although none of the heterozygotes were strabismic. Leventhal et al. pointed out that heterozygotes for the different classes of albinism in humans may comprise 1–2% or more of the population and suggest that this heterozygote status may be responsible for reduced binocularity in this sector of the population. Guillery has proposed that the known incidence of albino misrouting may represent only the "tip of the iceberg" of this disorder and that a wider population may have lesser degrees of misrouting (Guillery, 1972, cited in Regan, 1988). The heterozygote prevalence figure of Leventhal et al. is similar to that for strabismus (Simons and Reinecke, 1978), which is not proof of a connection but certainly a necessary prerequisite for establishing that such a connection may exist. Evidence of idiosyncratic localized variations of stereoscopic sensitivity across the visual field of normals (Richards and Regan, 1973; Regan et al., 1986) and localization irregularities across the horopter in normals (Bourdy, 1973; Bedell and Flom, 1983); would also be in keeping with smaller amounts of misrouting at the "normal" end of a misrouting population distribution. [Qualitatively similar horopter irregularities, but with much larger standard deviations of localization, can be demonstrated in strabismus patients (Bagolini and Capobianco, 1965; Reading, 1985).]

Fetal melanin pigment appears fundamental to the albino misrouting and specifically that found in the retinal pigment epithelium (RPE), which is the first melanin formed anywhere in the body during fetal development (Guillery, 1986). The size of the misrouted component is related to the severity of the RPE melanin abnormality (Guillery, 1990). The misrouting process in neurogenesis is not well understood, but the RPE melanin anomaly localization suggests that the misrouting begins with the retinal projection to the lateral geniculate nucleus (Guillery, 1986). In mice, reduced melanin has been found explicitly to affect only those projections involved in binocular vision, and it has been suggested that melanin has a role in establishing the line of decussation (Balkema and Dräger, 1990).

If melanin is critical to the misrouting defect, another place to look for insight into its influence would be in populations with melanin differences not of albino origin. In fact, one of the more dramatic and as yet unexplained epidemiological findings with regard to strabismus is that there appears to be a higher incidence of esotropia among caucasians than noncaucasians (Mann,

1966; Cass, 1973, 1976; Wyatt and Boyd, 1973[3]; Ing and Pang, 1974; Chiapella et al., 1984; Johnson et al., 1984; Adler-Grinberg, 1986; Kikudie et al., 1988; von Noorden, 1990, p. 325; Bruce et al., 1991) and a greater incidence of esotropia among caucasians and exotropia among Afro-Americans in the United States (James Tielsch, Dana Center for International Ophthalmology, Wilmer Institute, personal communication). In many cases, noncaucasians exhibit no strabismus prevalence at all (Mann, 1966; Wick and Crane, 1976). One report found virtually no "accommodative strabismus" among various tribes of Indians and Eskimos living in the Canadian Northwest Territories except when there had been intermarriage with caucasians (Cass, 1976). In one tribe that had in general avoided intermarriage, the only concomitant, apparently esotropic patient in the tribe had a white father. When acquired strabismus did occur it was a sequela of unilateral visual impairment from trauma or other disease. [Another relatively isolated Eskimo group near Hudson Bay in Canada was found to contain cases of strabismus, however, but eight of nine of the patients were eso- or exotropic alternators (Woodruff and Samek, 1976), i.e., without amblyopia.]

There is evidence that refractive status has a racial component, with noncaucasians typically exhibiting a reduced degree of myopia compared to caucasians, except in the case of Asians, particularly in the case of native peoples living in their original habitats (Mann, 1966; Cass, 1973, 1976; Curtin, 1985). It raises the question of whether the refractive and strabismus racial components are causally related, i.e., whether the strabismus is a secondary effect of a racially determined refractive error or whether it has a racial genetic component independent of refractive status. One large study of a mostly Eskimo and Native American population found no difference in myopia prevalence between the study population and urban Western population samples despite the presence of the typical divergent strabismus preponderance in the Eskimo and Native American (Wyatt and Boyd, 1973). Another study found a 14:1 divergent/convergent strabismus ratio in a sample of Native American children despite a preponderance of the hyperopia that would be expected to be associated with esotropia (Wick and Crane, 1976). A third study's Eskimo sample, mentioned above, contained eight of nine individuals with alternating convergent or divergent strabismus, but all had "no or minimal" refractive error and only one of the nine "could be termed an accommodative esotrope" (Woodruff and Samek, 1976).

---

3. This large study ($n = 4,450$) found a 1.6:1.0 ratio of divergent to convergent squint prevalence despite including 499 (11%) caucasians in the sample.

The latter findings support the hypothesis of independence, or perhaps a final common pathway, in the strabismus and refractive error etiologies, rather than a causal link. In keeping with this hypothesis is evidence suggesting that anisometropia may be a consequence rather than a cause of amblyopia (see Chapter 1) and a growing body of evidence that refraction is plastic in a manner similar to early neural development (see Chapter 2). There is also a report of unequal refractive emmetropization or myopization between the two eyes of patients ($n = 329$) with unilateral but not alternating esotropia, the nonfixing eye development lagging behind that of the fixing eye in the unilateral cases (Leffertstra, 1977). This finding too suggests a visual basis for refractive development either independent, or a result rather than a cause, of strabismus. Finally, there is evidence that with-the-rule astigmatism is typical in Oriental infants, in contrast to the hyperopic against-the-rule typical of caucasian infants (Thorn et al., 1987). Because early with-the-rule astigmatism has been found to substantially increase, not decrease, the risk factor for amblyopia, at least for caucasians (Sjöstrand and Abrahamsson, 1990), and excessive astigmatism in any axis to increase the risk of both strabismus and amblyopia (Ingram et al., 1986), a refractive error causal basis of strabismus appears not to be supported. Some other racial difference factor must be responsible.

In summary, then, there is at least circumstantial evidence suggesting that albino-like misrouting of neural projections from the retina during fetal development may occur more widely in reduced form than previously thought as a result of a genetically influenced modulation of melanin formation (or breakdown) (Guillery, 1986) in the fetal RPE. The racial differences data suggest that this defect is specifically a precursor of esotropia, though strabismic albinos may be eso- or exotropic (Kinnear et al., 1985).

The Question of Retinal Origins

In work mainly from the 1950s, Pugh (1954, 1958, 1962) and Enoch (1957, 1959a,b), in a classic example of *zeitgeist*, independently proposed and provided data in support of the idea that amblyopia had its origin in morphological anomalies of the photoreceptors of the central retina. Pugh, whose only instrumentation was the "orthoptoscope," a clinical haploscope of her own design that presaged contemporary instruments (Editorial, 1972), performed a meticulous and exhaustive series of studies of sensory and motor function in amblyopes that in some respects have never been either equaled or adequately explained by later literature in the area. Using observations that were extensively replicated in the same patients over months and even years in some cases, she obtained detailed phenomenological

reports from her amblyopes, together with associated quantitative measurements, that stand in some contrast to the point, line, and grating thresholds used to characterize amblyopia in many of the contemporary studies of this condition.

Most noteworthy of Pugh's findings in the present context were her amblyopic subjects' detailed reports and measurements of perceived image distortions. White-on-black letters were reported as being seen, across their extent, in several "shades of grey" (Pugh, 1958). Black-on-white letters appeared " 'jagged,' 'dragged,' 'smudged,' or 'rubbed' " or "faded away so that there was no clear end to the horizontal bars of the E, F and the T" (Pugh, 1958) and "extra fragments of the target's image appeared to one side of the main image" (Pugh, 1962). Rows of letters "appeared to run together 'as if a fold occurs to run one letter into the other' " (Pugh, 1958). The overall effect was "outside the usual visual experience of the normal eye; descriptive terms such as 'iridescent,' 'dragged,' 'unreal,' 'splintered,' even 'not in the same plane,' suggested the . . . quality of pattern disturbance. The effect was quite unlike that of suppression, the [optotype] letter sometimes appearing to have more than less" (Pugh, 1958). The direction along which this distortion was scaled was correlated with the direction of deviation and eye involved. Thus the image appeared to be "dragged" toward the right, with the left-edge contours clear, for a right amblyopic eye, or toward the left, with right-edge contours clear, for a left amblyopic eye, or with an equivalent gradient opposite to a vertical deviation, or with a vectorial sum direction for combined horizontal and vertical deviations.

It is not difficult when rereading Pugh's reports to see the intuitive appeal of a retinal origin explanation for amblyopia, as the reported distortions would be compatible with degradation of the normally highly ordered foveal cone matrix. Enoch's originally reported Stiles-Crawford anomalies in amblyopes appeared to give explicit evidence of a retinal origin as well (Enoch, 1957, 1959a,b).

Although the reality of the spatial distortions of at least strabismic amblyopia have been more fully documented during the decades since these early reports, at levels ranging from the phenomenological (Hess et al., 1978; Bradley et al., 1985; Haase, 1988), to visual field mapping (Sireteanu and Fronius, 1982; Flom and Bedell, 1983), to small receptive field anomalies (reviewed by Levi, 1988; Levi and Klein, 1990; Wilson, 1991), the retinal origin idea has lost favor. A cortical locus is now routinely assumed, arising from deprivation or secondary to the rivalry of strabismic misalignment (e.g., Levi et al., 1987; Wilson, 1991). There is a variety of evidence bearing on the retina involvement issue, but virtually all of it is inconclusive:

1. Administration of levodopa has been found to improve acuity and contrast sensitivity in adult amblyopes and to reduce the size of the associated suppression scotoma (Gottlob and Stangler-Zuschrott, 1990; Leguire et al., 1991); and, conversely, dopaminergic blockage in nonamblyopes reduces the high spatial frequency response (and enhances medium and low spatial frequency response) (Harris et al., 1990). Because dopamine is known to be a neurotransmitter in the amacrine and interplexiform cells of the retina and has been found to be reduced in concentration by visual deprivation in infant monkeys (Iuvone et al., 1989), the levodopa effect may argue for a retinal defect. Evidence in the rat suggests that dopamine acts on the horizontal cells to reduce the size of the receptive field (Hankins and Ikeda, 1991), which would explain the importance of dopamine's presence for increasing visual resolution. However, there are also dopaminergic neurons in the cortex and midbrain (Gottlob and Stangler-Zuschrott, 1990; Witkovsky and Dearry, 1991).

2. Fluorescein angiography (Romano and Bird, 1980) and conventional electroretinography (ERG) (Hess and Baker, 1984; Hess et al., 1985) of amblyopes cannot be distinguished from that of normals, arguing against retinal involvement. However, a new type of pattern ERG recording measures both luminance response and lateral interaction within the retina (Sutter and Tran, 1991). Anomalies in both components were found in an amblyopic eye (Brown and Sutter, 1991), but only one eye was measured, and it was grossly amblyopic and so perhaps not representative.

3. Enoch's original report of Stiles-Crawford anomalies in amblyopes (Enoch, 1959a,b) supported the idea of retinal involvement, but his results were not replicated in a larger amblyope sample (Bedell, 1980). Both studies are open to the question of how meaningful a Stiles-Crawford measurement can be taken with the reduced visual acuity of amblyopia, however.

4. The pupillary light reflex has been assumed to be a measure of retinal function, as its neural control pathway branches out at the pregeniculate level and so has been thought to be controlled by local, pregeniculate mechanisms, a conclusion reinforced by evidence of a decrement in the response in patients with macular disease (reviewed by Portnoy et al., 1983). A variety of studies have found at least subtle afferent defects in pupillary responses in some amblyopic eyes, with the detection rate roughly proportional to the sensitivity of the method used (Harms, 1938; Trimarchi et al., 1976; Greenwald and Folk, 1983; Portnoy et al., 1983; Kase et al., 1984; Firth, 1990), suggesting not simply a history but an extant retinal disorder in these visual adults. The deficit is specifically localized to the central retina, as stimulation in the periphery exhibits no difference between amblyopic and normal eyes (Harms, 1938; Tri-

marchi et al., 1976). The degree of deficit has not been found to correlate with the level of visual acuity (Greenwald and Folk, 1983; Portnoy et al., 1983; Kase et al., 1984), which might be due to postretinal cortical processing. More difficult to explain on a retinal basis are reports of normalization of pupillary response in some cases of successfully treated amblyopia (Greenwald and Folk, 1983; Kase et al., 1984; Firth, 1990), as occlusion of the contralateral eye would have no effect on a truly locally determined ipsilateral pupillary response. Whether this response improvement is due to modulation of retinal inhibition by postretinal processes (Brenner et al., 1969; Trimarchi et al., 1976; Firth, 1991) or other causes, it means that the pupillary data cannot be interpreted as clearly supporting or contradicting a retinal origin of amblyopia. There is also evidence of pupillary defect in the eyes, with better acuity in patients with interocular differences in function due to retinal or optic nerve dysfunction and, conversely, no difference in pupillary function between eyes in patients with interocular differences due to various ocular media and retinal dysfunctions (Bullock, 1990).

A final difficulty when interpreting this body of research is that it has been done on adults and thus depends on the implicit assumption that any amblyopiagenic retinal morphological anomalies are still present. If in fact such anomalies are developmentally transient (Simons, cited in Enoch et al., 1973) as a result of healing or retinal maturational processes, measurement in the adult may be unproductive or misleading. There appear never to have been histological studies of any human strabismic amblyope retinas—infant or adult—that would throw light on this matter.

If we assume, however, that the retinotopic mapping distortions of amblyopia have a retinal origin, the question arises of just what physiological forces might give rise to them. As is discussed in detail later in the Chapter, orderliness of the retinal geometry and its mapping to the cortex, especially in terms of bilateral congruency, may be critical to achieving normal global stereopsis development. To the extent this is true, forces interfering with such orderliness become potential amblyopiagenic factors. There appear to be several possible sources of such factors, which may interact.

Retinal Structure Maturation and Globe Growth. The retina is in a state of multidimensional morphological and ultrastructural flux during development, not simply during infancy but stretching well into early childhood. This flux affects both cone packing geometry and the optical microenvironment of cone (and rod) inner and outer segments and appears open to both developmental variability and to insult. The size of the rod-free zone decreases, and its cone density increases with the thinning of the foveal cones with maturation (Curcio and

Hendrickson, 1991; see also Chapter 17). In the parafovea and periphery, there is a three-layer cellular lateral movement with development, illustrated in Figure 25-6. Initially, there is a centrifugal movement of inner nuclear and ganglion cells out from the area of the fovea, as well as of the cells of the retinal pigment epithelium (RPE) (Hendrickson and Yuodelis, 1984; Robb, 1985; Curcio and Hendrickson, 1991; see also Chapter 17). Starting about the same time but extending much later, there is centripetal movement of the cones and rods sandwiched between these two other layers. Nor is it simply a question of transposed laminar motion (if motion of three nonhomogeneous cellular sheets of different radii and changing cellular morphology moving inside a maturationally expanding eye globe can be said to be simple): The inner retinal layers move proportionally farther to hollow out the foveal pit. Meanwhile, individual cone morphology is changing profoundly in both the orthogonal and parallel dimensions. The cone outer segment elongates sevenfold between birth and 15 months, and by 14-fold between birth and adulthood (Curcio and Hendrickson, 1991).

Eye globe growth itself has both "radial" (out from the posterior pole) and "tangential" (orthogonal to radial) components, with radial growth greater at any given retinal locus and more rapid during early development (Packer et al., 1990). Although this globe expansion is confined to the peripheral rather than the central retina, it seems possible that it may have traction effects on more central cellular translocation. Finally, the different elasticity of the retina and choroid, as well as the difference between the choroid and sclera (Blank et al., 1975; Enoch, 1981), create a viscoelastic source of force vector influence on movement of the various layers, particularly if there are local differences in interlayer adhesion. It has been suggested that this latter elastic variability may provide part of the substrate of cone phototropism (Blank et al., 1975; Enoch, 1981).

There thus appears to be a substrate basis for considerable idiosyncratic variation in the homogeneity of photoreceptor placement during visual development. The opposite motion vector of the inner retina and RPE layers surrounding the photoreceptor layer, the differential motion between the inner retina and photoreceptor layer responsible for excavation of the foveal pit, and the globe expansion and retina-versus-choroid elasticity differences (Fig. 25-6) create shear and rotational stresses affecting cone placement with several degrees of freedom; and it seems unlikely that these stresses would be identical in both eyes. Transposition among cones resulting from these processes would present a particular departure from homogeneity (discussed below). Rod intrusion would abet such transposition, as cones tend to develop a round profile on the sides where they abut rods, in lieu of the more transposition-resistant polygonal shape of abutment to other cones (Curcio et al., 1990). Localized irregularities in globe growth would add another potentially rotary force vector to cone placement. As discussed later in the Chapter, there are retinal distention effects of efforts to accommodation in adults (Blank et al., 1975; Enoch, 1975), even if the lens is not changing shape (Enoch, 1981); to the extent accommodation is active in infants, a similar result would be expected, which would add a further rotary force vector, and there is extraocular muscle torsional stress as well.

Evidence of the possibility of a population distribution of the amount of transretinal cone movement with development is suggested by the subnormal amount apparent in albinos (Wilson et al., 1988) and possibly monochromats (Glickstein and Heath, 1975) on the one hand. At the other extreme is the subject with the supranormal stereoacuity and reduced night vision (Efron and Wolfe, 1966) that would be expected if the extent of cone movement was supranormal, expanding the size of the rod-free area beyond the central foveal bouquet.

Further evidence of idiosyncratic developmental variability in the cone matrix of normal adult central retina is found in a report of greater packing geometry disorder in the foveal center than at the edge of the rod-free zone of one adult normal retina (Curcio and Hendrickson, 1991). Some degree of disordered geometry in the normal parafovea (i.e., 1.5–14.0 degrees eccentricity) of both center-to-center and rotational positional disorder appears near-universal, for instance as demonstrated by the two-dimensional visual noise appearance of fine gratings viewed by it (Colleta and Williams, 1987; Hirsch and Miller, 1987). Furthermore, the standard deviation of cone separation increases more rapidly with eccentricity than cone separation itself (Hirsch and Miller, 1987; Hirsch and Curcio, 1989).

We can thus see, in the multidimensional ultrastructure transformation of postnatal retinal development,

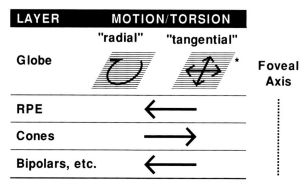

FIG. 25-6. Summary of lateral and rotational directional forces on photoreceptor matrix during early development. See text for details.

a possible physiological basis for interocular differences in retinal homology, even in normals. Indeed, there is evidence of some degree of interocular difference in adult human foveal cone density distribution (Curcio et al., 1990). The functional significance of this variability appears confirmed at the monocular level by variability among normals in Stiles-Crawford effect sensitivity profiles (Enoch and Bedell, 1981) and binocularly by microvariations among normals of the horopter at the fovea (Bourdy, 1973).

Birth Trauma.   *Retinal Hemorrhages?* The idea that amblyopia might have a retinal origin in the perinatal hydraulic stress on the retina of the cranial and ocular globe compression-decompression sequence during the birth process also dates to the 1950s. Burian, commenting on one of Enoch's reports, suggested the specific mechanism of perinatal retinal hemorrhages (RHs) (Burian, 1959). Such hemorrhages have been found in many studies to have an incidence as high as one-third or more of all neonates (see von Barsewisch's monumental 1979 study and review of earlier studies; see also Richter, 1976; Besio et al., 1979; Egge et al., 1980; Bist et al., 1989). It seems clear, however, that the RHs themselves are not amblyopiagenic. Most occur in the retinal periphery, not the macula; and most follow-up studies have found no difference in strabismus or amblyopia incidence between children with and without a history of them (Richter, 1976; von Barsewisch, 1979; Gillebo et al., 1987). It should be noted, however, that there are reports of such sequelae in these children: Microstrabismus and amblyopia have been reported in long-term follow-up of a few cases of RH (Schenk and Stangler-Zuschrott, 1974; Lowes et al., 1976; Gillebo et al., 1987), as well as reduced fusional amplitudes in otherwise visually normal children (Stangler-Zuschrott, 1978). There is also a report of a primate with a history of RH developing esotropia (Quick et al., 1990).

Nonetheless, it seems unlikely that RHs constitute an amblyopic risk factor. In fact, a case could be made that they evolved specifically to serve as a hydraulic "safety valve," rupturing the integrity of the retinal vasculature to allow distribution via the ocular media of vascular-based hydraulic stress throughout the eye globe's inner surface (Simons, cited in Enoch, 1981). Such hemorrhages have been found to arise in a variety of other contexts, from head trauma and intracranial hemorrhage (von Barsewisch, 1979) to pneumoencephalography (Mosely and Pilling, 1976) and high altitude mountain climbing (Vogt et al., 1978), where they may also be adaptively intended to protect cone matrix integrity. By this logic, it seems possible that it is the infants who do *not* exhibit RHs who are most at risk for retinal structural insult from birth trauma (Simons, cited in Enoch, 1981).

Retinal Microdetachments. Although retinal hemorrhages have been extensively studied (von Barsewisch, 1979), there has been little consideration in the literature of the specific mechanics of how hydraulic force may be applied to the retina by the dynamics of head and eye globe compression and decompression during birth. Data from such better-documented conditions as hydrocephalus effects on the eye are of questionable value because they do not involve the diversity of forces at work in the perinatal case. Something like an adaptation of a balloon model of globe growth (Mastronarde et al., 1984) is needed to elucidate the compression-decompression force and phase relations of hydraulic interchange between two spheres, the soft perinatal skull and soft infant eye globe (contained within the larger sphere), and so open to direct force asymmetry. At the same time, the two spheres are hydraulically connected by two sets of vasculature (arterial and venous) and by cerebrospinal fluid (CSF) contained in the optic nerve sheath, which are themselves contained within the two spheres. Once the amniotic sac is ruptured, ending the hydraulic force equilibrium of fetal life, the retina is in principle at hydraulic risk for every stage from labor contractions and initial entry into the birth canal to at least full emergence of the head. Infants who bypass this process via cesarean section delivery thus have a much lower incidence of RH than do those with standard deliveries (Bergen and Margolis, 1976; Besio et al., 1979; von Barsewisch, 1979).

If we take the incidence of RH as an index of hydraulic stress on the retina, however, some specific characteristics of the hydraulic force generation are suggested. Although the many variables associated with delivery indicate caution when drawing conclusions in this area, it is of interest that breech presentation results in both reduced incidence and severity of RH (von Barsewisch, 1979, p. 85). Furthermore, a study using a pressure transducer positioned between the fetal head and wall of the birth canal found no correlation between fetal head compression and RH appearance (Svenningsen et al., 1988). These findings suggest a further degree of complexity in the form of thoracic compression involvement. In this context, it is of interest to note that, although the early literature is conflicting on the point (von Barsewisch, 1979), some studies have reported that, relative to spontaneous delivery, RH incidence is increased through use of vacuum extraction and decreased by forceps-aided delivery (Egge et al., 1980, 1981; O'Leary et al., 1986), although the amount of vacuum extraction force was not correlated with RH incidence (Svenningsen et al., 1987). There is also reduced RH incidence in preterm infants and no difference in the latter group in terms of spontaneous versus forceps delivery (Maltau et al., 1984). Vacuum extraction exacerbates the pressure differential of the thoracic "push" of spontaneous delivery and forceps delivery reduces it; and the smaller thoracic diameter of the preterm infant presumably fits less tightly in the birth canal—findings that appear to be compatible with thoracic involvement in the RH onset.

If we assume a hydraulic column connecting the thorax with the head by means of a complex of body fluid and tissue (i.e., not just vasculature) via the neck, birth involves a complex sequence of alternating positive and negative pressures on the retina, beginning with head and eye, followed by thoracic compression at entry into the birth canal, and concluding with cranial and globe release, followed by thoracic release at expulsion from the birth outlet. The possible end result appears to be a flexing of the retina from the interaction of these sequential compressions and releases. One specific sequela of such a compression/decompression/flexing sequence, especially from CSF involvement, could be a distributed set of retinal "micro" detachments, from localized separations of the photoreceptor and RPE or RPE and choroid layers. Such localized separations would, under this hypothesis, involve no bleeding or other ophthalmoscopically apparent sign, especially if the separation paralleled that seen in more massive form in the serous macular detachments of the congenital morning glory and optic pit syndromes (Irvine et al., 1986; Sadun, 1989). Most notable would be the possibility of a centrifugal forced flow of CSF through the (immature) lamina cribrosa similar to that implicated in some theories of the pathogenesis of these latter syndromes in which there is evidence of absent or incompletely developed lamina cribrosa (Irvine et al., 1986).

Hayreh (1964) inserted balloons into the monkey skull at different locations and inflated the balloon with liquid (to simulate tumor growth effects on optic disc edema). RHs resulted from balloon inflation at cerebellar, but not cranial, sites. There is simulation evidence derived from human neonate cadavers that birth stress may have a distorting effect on the cerebellum (Issel et al., 1977). The retinal hemorrhages found in the Hayreh study were on the same side of the disc as the edematous changes, "generally after some violent straining on the part of the animal" (Hayreh, 1964). The combination of elevated CSF pressure (from the balloon inflation) and this straining appears to comprise a relevant model for the microdetachment effect proposed here.

It has been reported that even momentary separation of the retina from the RPE causes realignment of the RPE apical surface into a flattened sheet, with the apical processes assuming an orientation perpendicular to that surface (Iwasaki et al., 1990). The short, thick structure of the infant cone (see Chapter 17) and the fact that the RPE is the last element to mature in the retina (Borwein, 1981) suggest that the interdigitation of the infant

cone matrix with its RPE microvilli does not have the depth or extent that is the case in the adult retina. This supposition in turn suggests that the infant retina may be more prone than that of the adult to RPE-flattening separation, such as from birth trauma. Furthermore, the high metabolic demand of photoreceptors, the fact that cone discs are open to the extracellular space and that these discs are more easily disrupted than rod discs (Borwein, 1981), and the reactivity of the RPE to retinal injury (Gass, 1989) suggest that early localized trauma might have relatively far-reaching morphological effects.

Of particular note here is a study that hydraulically induced very small localized retinal detachments in the macula of adult monkeys by saline microinjection (Guèrin et al., 1989). The authors qualified the findings' applicability to adult human retinal detachment—the focus of their study—as their experimental detachments were rapidly produced, did not involve large retinal tears or breaks, involved virtually no intraretinal bleeding, and were small enough to allow substantial recovery (at the ophthalmoscopic level) within a relatively brief period (1 week). These very features, however, make their model pertinent here, where a hydraulically produced, small, localized detachment is the mechanism of interest. Guèrin et al. found that their "minidetachment" caused persistent abnormal cone outer segment alignment and disc stacking, as well as RPE proliferation in areas where there was a lack of outer segment regeneration, typically outside the macula but in one case in the fovea. Outer segment regeneration underlying areas of proliferation was poor. [Small focal congenital RPE lesions in humans are in some cases accompanied by amblyopia (Gass, 1989).] With adult human retinal detachment there is also evidence of protracted and incomplete morphological recovery, possibly due to either dilution of a trophic factor resulting from the increased subretinal space or release of some factor that interferes with disc assembly (Kaplan et al., 1990).

A further ramification is suggested by the finding in the monkey model study of phagocyte appearance in the subretinal space following the minidetachment, from both the RPE and blood-borne monocytes (Guèrin et al., 1989). There is evidence that macrophages may digest intact photoreceptor material as well as debris by generating oxidizing free radicals (Tso, 1989). Thus introduction of these macrophages could in principle set in motion a domino-like train of destructive events, as the presence of their free radicals opens up opportunity for photooxidative damage, and there is evidence in cases of adult retinal detachment that once present in the subretinal space the macrophages may remain there for years (Tso, 1989).

Another aspect to note here with regard to adult retinal detachments is that reattachments are frequently attended by micropsia or metamorphopsia (Ameniya et al., 1983; Sjöstrand and Anderson, 1986), i.e., a clearly retina-based phenomenon resembling the spatial distortions seen with strabismic amblyopia. The micropsia/metamorphopsia effects have been attributed to photoreceptor separation as the result of subclinical levels of macular edema (Sjöstrand and Anderson, 1986). More complex effects of retinal distortion on photoreceptor orientation have been demonstrated by Stiles-Crawford effect variations in patients with various retinally localized pathologies (Fankhauser et al., 1961; Fitzgerald et al., 1980; Bedell et al., 1981; Hamer et al., 1986; Yasuma et al., 1986). Here again, the possibility of inter-eye, corresponding point, retinal mapping differences are introduced. On the other hand, there is also evidence of photoreceptor orientation being maintained in adults in the presence of serous retinal detachment (Fitzgerald et al., 1980).

A final possible source of insult from birth trauma might be an effect involving early vascular development. The Michaelson hypothesis is that no intraretinal vasculature develops when the retinal structure can be oxygenated by vasculature being directly within a radius of 140 μm (Burns et al., 1986) and, presumably, intact. Adjacency of the choriocapillaris within this radius of the photoreceptors provides the basis for development of the foveal avascular zone. Separation or rupture of the integrity of the choriocapillaris/Bruch's membrane/RPE sandwich due to birth stress could perhaps cause violation of this limit or interfere with the oxygen exchange itself.

Phototoxic Insult

It has become apparent that the traditional characterization of light hazard to the eye, based simply on thermal burn threshold considerations, is inadequate. It now appears that there is a complex relation between the spectral content and intensity of incident light and the eye's absorptive, visual transduction, and reparative responses to that light (Cronly-Dillon et al., 1986; Waxler and Hitchins, 1986; Mainster, 1987; Tso, 1989; Vos et al., 1990). There appears to be, in a word, a multivariate interaction reminiscent of the aerospace concept of a performance "envelope," rather than a single threshold, needed to characterize the boundary between safe and hazardous light input to the eye. The main basis of need for this expanded concept derives from the findings of the last two decades that radiation at the blue (< 500 nm) end of the spectrum, including the near-ultraviolet, induces damage by photochemical means at energy levels that are as much as orders of magnitude below that required to cause thermal damage from longer-wavelength light. Evidence of damage from blue or ultraviolet light has been found for an expanding list of

biochemical component and physiological sites in the retina, including the visual pigments, Müller cells, RPE, intraretinal vitamin A, cytochrome C oxidase, the DNA structure of the photoreceptor nucleus, and blood components in the choriocapillaris (Berler, 1989; Tso, 1989; Borges et al., 1990; Gottsch et al., 1990; Pautler et al., 1990; Vos et al., 1990).

The retinas of infants and young children are particularly exposed to blue light and near-ultraviolet radiation, as their ocular media is far more transmissive of these spectra than is that of adults (Werner, 1982; Hansen and Fulton, 1989). For instance, there is 75–85% lenticular transmission of UV-A (320–400 nm) radiation up to 8 years of age versus 5–10% transmission at age 25 or older (Lerman, 1984). Infants' protective blue-absorbing carotenoid macular pigment level may be three or four times lower than that of adults (Bone et al., 1988) and is four times as transmissive of UV-A radiation as it is of blue light as well (Handelman et al., 1991). The carotenoids in adults are densest over the macula (Snodderly et al., 1984), and their photoprotective significance is suggested by the inverse correlation of carotenoid macular distribution with the areal configuration of "bulls-eye" maculopathies (Weiter et al., 1988). Infant rhodopsin levels are also about one-third that of the adult (Fulton et al., 1991), which limits rhodopsin's threat as a photosensitizer (Vos et al., 1990) but also limits its role in blue light absorption. Infants with lighter irides have larger pupils (Roarty and Keltner, 1990), and both transmit more blue light. The premature's pupil is both large and fixed (Isenberg et al., 1990).

Thus what constitutes safe short-wavelength light and UV-A intensity for the adult retina may be hazardous for the infant or young child. The retinal irradiance for preterm infants in neonatal units lit by "everyday" fluorescent light may exceed levels shown to cause cone damage in (adult) monkeys (Robinson and Fielder, in press). Whether the neonate human's photoreceptor regenerative capacity can compensate to the extent that the neonate rat's does (Malik et al., 1986) is unknown. However, melanin formation in the retina is not complete in the newborn (Mund and Rodrigues, 1979) and may continue at a low level even into adult life (Boulton et al., 1990). The melanogenesis process may represent a significant phototoxic threat: Not only is there less photoprotective (Dràger, 1985b; Young, 1988) melanin present as a result, but dopa, a melanin precursor, acts synergistically with oxygen to damage or suppress proliferation of RPE and vascular endothelial cells, particularly in blue light (Akeo et al., 1989; Dorey et al., 1990). Blue light also maximizes photooxidant production by an erythrocytic blood component, protoporphyrin IX (PPIX), that could interfere with the neonate's vascular endothelium development as well (Gottsch et al., 1990). Either the melanogenesis or PPIX mechanism may have some bearing on the question of whether neonatal nursery fluorescent light, which radiates more than 25% of its power below 500 nm (Kaufman and Haynes, 1981), constitutes a risk factor in retinopathy of prematurity (ROP) (Glass et al., 1985; Stobie, 1985; Hommura et al., 1988; Ackerman et al., 1989. Seiberth et al., 1991; Fielder et al., in press). This situation would be particularly the case if the eye's defensive antioxidant enzymes are not fully developed before birth (Katz and Robison, 1988; Naash et al., 1988).

Although the possible implications of phototoxicity in the infant for late-life age-related macular degeneration has been considered (Simons, in press), its amblyopiagenic potential apparently has not. It is of interest to note that otherwise normal individuals with a history of prematurity tend to have slightly lower visual acuity than do term controls (Sebris et al., 1984; Snir et al., 1988; Cats and Tan, 1989; Burgess and Johnson, 1991), as do infants with regressed ROP who are nominally free of amblyopia or neurological deficit (Birch and Spenser, 1991; Katsumi et al., 1991). Although potentially attributable to a variety of factors, it seems possible, in view of the particularly low level of pigmentation and large pupil of the premature infant, that these acuity deficits might have originated in a mild phototoxically induced amblyopia.

It should be noted that, whereas any phototoxic insult would be delivered equally to both eyes, the interocular competition aspect of neural development would convert it to a unilateral amblyopia, although initially bilateral amblyopia may be more prevalent than traditionally realized (see Chapter 21).

It has been suggested that the photoreceptor axons, or fibers of Henle, may act as fiberoptic waveguides that channel blue light from the axon pedicle at their anterior end to the fovea (Mainster, 1988). This hypothesis is based on the assumption that the refractive index of the Henle fiber is greater than that of the surrounding lucent Müller cell "cladding" and that the pedicle expansion of the fiber funnels light to the fiber in a manner similar to that of the cone inner segment (Mainster, 1988). This condition provides a potential source of increased foveal irradiance of greater cross-sectional area than the fovea itself. The optical characteristics of this waveguide functionality would be particularly efficient for wavelengths below 460 nm (Mainster, 1988), which would be significant for the infant as the highest concentration of protective carotenoid pigment in the adult is found in the Henle fibers (Snodderly et al., 1984), and this protection, as noted above, is largely lacking in the infant. In sum, this waveguide capability might provide a means of optically bypassing even the low level of foveal carotenoid protection in the infant. The kind of extraaxonal edema that might result from birth trauma and that is known to

be induced in Müller cells by light exposure (Berler, 1989) would increase the axon's fiberoptic efficiency still further, as water and plasma have even lower refractive indices than Müller cytoplasm (Mainster, 1987). The increased efficiency might be offset by microbends, optical inhomogeneities, or fiber thickness variations (Mainster, 1987) that might also arise from the trauma but that would simply distribute the photic insult to other intraretinal structures.

Light Scatter, Autofluorescence, and Cone Phototropism. There is an appreciable degree of stray alight arising from cone capture inefficiency in even normal adult retinas, with it being estimated, for instance, that at least half of incident light passes through more than one cone prior to capture (Chen and Makous, 1989). For infants, it seems clear that the amount of stray light is appreciably greater, in view of the clarity of the infant ocular media (Hansen and Fulton, 1989), the infant cone quantal catch inefficiency (Banks and Bennett, 1988; see also Chapters 6 and 32), and subadult levels of rhodopsin and retinal pigmentation (Mund and Rodriguez, 1979; Fulton et al., 1991). Futhermore, like the peripheral cones of adults (Miller and Snyder, 1973), it seems likely that the undeveloped infant cone radiates as well as collects incident light. Even the normal infant retina, in a word, is a prime candidate for susceptibility to scatter. It seems possible that birth-stress-related retinal trauma would increase that susceptibility by the following mechanism: The refractive index difference between the cone outer segment and its interphotoreceptor matrix cladding is not large in even adult normal eyes (Horowitz, 1981), and small changes in refractive index of photopigments have appreciable effects on photoreceptor absorption spectra as well (Snyder and Richmond, 1972). Thus relatively subtle local edematous or choroidal-vascular-compromise-based metabolic anomalies induced by birth trauma or phototoxicity could have significant scatter-increasing effects through affecting refractive indices of the outer segment, interphotoreceptor matrix cladding, or photopigment regeneration. This condition would in turn degrade outer segment waveguide quality and increase scatter.

An initial effect of increased scatter is to increase the phototoxic effect of incident light, as light not absorbed otherwise in the eye is available to photooxidative chemistry. There is, however, also another potential effect: Development of normal high resolution foveal vision depends not simply on high packing density of cones but also on precise optical localization of the light acceptance apertures of individual cones (Enoch and Tobey, 1981). The inner and outer segment optical waveguide characteristics, in conjunction with the light-absorption capabilities of the adjacent retinal pigment epithelium, are fundamental to achieving this precision

(Enoch and Bedell, 1981; Enoch and Tobey, 1981), with an adaptive phototropic mechanism apparently operative in cone alignment to optimize it (Enoch, 1981). Interference with the optical integrity of this system from increased light scatter causes reduced capability of optical localization from the point of view of a retinotopic cortical mapping output even if the cone matrix itself is structurally normal. From the point of view of that mapping, there is no difference between positional variance from loss of cone outer and inner segment integrity due to cone matrix malformation and poor localization due to high levels of scatter. This problem is illustrated in the contrast sensitivity losses associated with increased scatter in the retinas of albinos (Abadi et al., 1990).

Optical localization has still further ramifications. If we assume that during early development foveal cones are phototropic in the same way, if not to the same extent, as adult cones (Enoch, 1981), excessive optical scatter introduces correspondingly increased positional "noise" into the phototropic orientation input. Patients with retinitis pigmentosa who develop shortened and thickened cone inner and outer segments (Flannery et al., 1989) reminiscent of that of the infant (Curcio and Hendrickson, 1991; see also Chapter 17) appear to have an abnormally enlarged acceptance angle of individual cones, as demonstrated by a reduced degree of Stiles-Crawford effect directionality (Bailey et al., 1991) and abnormally large positional errors on a bisection task (Turano, 1991). Assuming the infant's cone acceptance angle is similarly enlarged, and taken together with the infant's low foveal cone density (Curcio and Hendrickson, 1991), low visual acuity and stereoacuity (see Chapter 13), and hence low receptive field resolution, there seems reason to conclude that infant cone phototropism is more tolerant of positional noise than the visual adult. As the cones elongate with development (see Chapter 17) and each cone seeks adaptively to minimize scatter via optimum phototropic alignment under the optical circumstances of its particular retinal locus, a high degree of optical scatter would result in a positionally "noisy" optical input similar in retinal mapping result to the positional input of Enoch's original amblyopic "general malorientation" hypothesis (Enoch, 1959a,b).[4] As discussed later in the chapter, the visual results of any such positional variance appear to be magnified by the interocular corresponding point comparison of stereoscopic vision.

---

4. In fact, there is evidence of some degree of physical "general malorientation" or "splaying" (Hamer et al., 1986) in normal adult parafovea (Colletta and Williams, 1987; Hirsch and Miller, 1987), and that cones in normal adult fovea are arranged in several commonly aligned groups (Enoch and Bedell, 1981), suggesting that there may be cone position as well as optical basis for mapping noise.

A final source of scatter would occur if the optical integrity of the cone fiberoptic characteristics either remain compromised from early birth trauma insult or are degraded by the phagocytic or phototoxic sequelae of such insult. This source would be from optical coupling or "crosstalk" between adjacent cone outer or inner segments (Enoch, 1967; Horowitz, 1981), as such coupling capability is increased with increasing fiber length and decreasing fiberoptic interfiber distance and core diameter (Mainster, 1987). The latter description neatly characterizes the developing foveal cone matrix, with its thinning and elongating cones (Curcio and Hendrickson, 1991; see also Chapter 17).

Stereopsis Time Encoding Defects and "Temporal Amblyopia"

There is evidence of spatial- and motion-based stereopsis subsystems (Tyler, 1990) and evidence of deficits in both systems in the presence of strabismus (Schor et al., 1983a; Kitaoji and Toyama, 1987). Even in normal eyes there are localized but visual-field-wide discrepancies between the spatial- and motion-based stereoscopic field maps (Richards and Regan, 1973; Regan et al., 1986). The highly idiosyncratic nature of these discrepancies suggests a developmental origin and, by extrapolation, the possibility of even larger discrepancies.

Amblyopic temporal processing losses are generally considered to be most significant at low temporal frequencies (see Chapter 24). It has been proposed that the motion-processing deficits in amblyopia are a function of the amblyope's spatial-processing deficit and specifically of the absence of small-receptive field velocity reference (Steinman et al., 1988). We explore here the possibility of a direct temporal coding deficit in amblyopia, as suggested by findings of delayed reaction time to (nonmoving) light flash onset in the central fields of amblyopes. Of particular interest in view of the discussion of hemiretinal differences later in the chapter is the finding that these reaction-time measures show a greater deficit in the nasal than the temporal hemiretina of the esotropic amblyope (Chelazzi et al., 1988).

A variety of evidence suggests that stereopsis is neurally encoded by interocular differences in time of arrival at the cortex of neural input from corresponding points in the two eyes, most familiarly seen in the Pulfrich phenomenon (see review in Carney et al., 1989), and there is evidence of other forms of neural transmission time-based stereopsis encoding as well (Bower, 1966; Lee, 1970; Harker, 1973). There is evidence in the cat that this time encoding is directly confounded with positional disparity encoding in the individual binocular cortical cell (Carney et al., 1989).

The significance in the present context of the temporal encoding aspect of stereopsis is suggested by patients with interocularly asymmetrical transmission-slowing demyelination of the optic nerve, typically due to optic neuritis. Some of these patients have been reported to exhibit a spontaneous Pulfrich effect, that is, a Pulfrich effect without the normally required neutral density filter before one eye. Indeed, in these cases, the effect was abolished by placing a neutral density filter over the normal eye (Frisen et al., 1973; Heron and Dutton, 1989). It thus seems likely that the reduced stereoacuity of such patients is due to this timing deficit, especially as the stereoacuity deficit is disproportionate to visual acuity loss (Friedman et al., 1985; Newman et al., 1991) and may continue after the condition is nominally, in visual acuity terms, resolved (Fleishman et al., 1987). [In one report, patients with the spontaneous Pulfrich effect had normal visual acuity in both eyes (Frisen et al., 1973).]

A variety of evidence has demonstrated a delay in retinocortical transmission time in amblyopic eyes (Chelazzi et al., 1988; von Noorden, 1990, p. 236ff) and there is a report of a spontaneous Pulfrich effect in three cases of anisometropic amblyopia (Tredici and von Noorden, 1984). These effects, however, are found in visual adults and so may be confounded with cortical components of amblyopia.

One origin of precortical timing deficits in amblyopia could be interocular differences in rates of myelination of the optic nerves or more central structures, originally proposed by Keiner (1951), as optic nerve myelination is not complete until at least 1 month after birth and perhaps as long as 2 years postnatally (reviewed by Nakayama, 1972; Atkinson, 1984). As is discussed later, a relatively small unilateral deficit may be magnified in effect as a result of binocular interaction. However, our focus here is on possible retinal origins of amblyopia. In that context, the question from a (mal)developmental point of view is whether timing deficits could have a birth-stress-related or phototoxic origin. In fact, there is evidence of transmission delays in a variety of retinal disorders and particularly in serous retinal detachment (Hofeldt et al., 1985) and central serous choroidopathy (Sherman et al., 1986). This delay was accompanied by the spontaneous Pulfrich effect in four patients with serous detachment, with one of the four exhibiting a visual acuity of 20/20 in both eyes and another with a reduction in the affected eye to only 20/30. The spontaneous Pulfrich effect and abnormal evoked potential latency both reverted to normal with resolution of the retinopathy in these patients (Hofeldt et al., 1985).

Electrophysiological studies suggest the origin of the delay in serous retinal detachment to lie in a disturbance of the interface between the photoreceptors and RPE (Papakostopoulos et al., 1984). In view of the possible involvement of dopaminergic processes in amblyopia, it may also be significant that there is a retinal-level response latency found in dopamine-depleted rats (Dyer et al., 1981), suggesting interference with dopamine generation metabolism as a possible site of birth trauma or phototoxic insult.

Temporal stereo encoding would exhibit two types of defect: (1) creation of latency differences between eyes of corresponding points; and (b) temporal phase reversals between adjacent binocular loci as a result of transposition of cone or receptive fields, so a stimulus passing from locus A to locus B in one eye passes from corresponding loci B′ and A′ in the contralateral eye. This latter effect might be expected as a sequela of albino heterozygote misrouting (discussed earlier). Either form of temporal deficit could interact with spatial mapping disorders in a complex way in terms of the resulting retinocortical mapping because, again, the spatial and temporal stereo inputs appear to be confounded at the cortical cell level (Carney et al., 1989). Again, there are localized but visual-field-wide discrepancies between static and motion-based stereoscopic field maps even in normal subjects (Richards and Regan, 1973; Regan et al., 1986), and more exaggerated versions of these discrepancies are seen in strabismic and amblyopic patients (Sireteanu et al., 1981; Sireteanu, 1982; Mohn et al., 1986).

OPTOMOTOR AND FUSION DEFECTS

Albino Heterozygote Optomotor Miswiring

As noted above, there is evidence that the albino misrouting may extend to the midbrain as well as the cortex (Creel et al., 1990). If the micro-misrouting hypothesis is correct, a more localized midbrain as well as cortical misrouting may be present with strabismus. It could conceivably affect midbrain binocular fusion, though that fusion is crude (Schor, 1983). The extensive evidence of motion-processing anomalies in strabismic infants and adults (Norcia et al., 1991; see also Chapters 23 and 26) makes it more likely, however, that such misrouting would cause localized phase reversals between adjacent receptive fields in motion sensing (Dräger, 1985a), with a consequent decrement in oculomotor control.

Birth Trauma-Based Defects

Strabismus is often associated with brain damage of traumatic or malformation origin (von Noorden, 1990, pp. 142ff, 305, 433). It seems likely that this damage is due to insult to the fusion rather than fine stereo mechanism, as illustrated by the finding of loss of fusion but continued functionality of stereopsis during momentary eye alignment in some adults with posttraumatic fusion deficiency (von Noorden, 1990, p. 433). The evidence is conflicting as to whether birth trauma is associated with increased strabismus incidence, except as part of the symptomatology associated with severe problems such as cerebral palsy or significant anoxia (Billings, 1969; Aichmair, 1975; Ellingham et al., 1976; McBride et al., 1979; Ham et al., 1984; von Noorden, 1990, p. 143). Scobee (1951) reported an inverse relation between duration of labor and age of heterotropia onset in a large ($n = 524$) patient group. Another study found a significantly higher strabismus incidence with breech deliveries than with normal vertex deliveries, as well as significantly poorer stereopsis in the postbreech delivery population; but it suggested that prenatal motor deficiencies may be responsible for failure of the fetus to assume the vertex position as well as the strabismus (McBride et al., 1979). This study found no difference in strabismus incidence between an elective cesarean delivery sample and the vaginal delivery sample, although the cesarean group had a lower mean gestational age (38.4 versus 39.4 weeks) and higher rate of jaundice (33% versus 20%) than the remainder of the sample, and reasons for the cesarean decision are not reported, making conclusions difficult to draw. A report of one group of Eskimos in northwestern Canada, who typically do not develop strabismus, observed that:

> At parturition, the Eskimo squats to deliver her baby, and another woman gets behind her and puts a knee in her back, squeezing her stomach hard, sometimes to the point of causing involution of the uterus. Where birth is difficult, the Shaman (Medicine Man) sometimes danced on the stomach. Birth trauma, therefore, was frequent in Eskimos, and there were cases of congenital strabismus, with no evidence of a family history. [Cass, 1976, p. 379]

A key question here is whether, as in the case of retinal hemorrhages the hydraulic trauma of even routine deliveries or other less obvious birth-related factors such as subtle anoxic damage (Kervick, 1986) are sufficient to cause subcortical or cortical damage that in turn constitutes a risk factor for strabismus. Such births might appear normal to standard obstetrical diagnostic indicators and so be difficult to distinguish epidemiologically from nonstrabismogenic births. There is evidence from birth process simulation on fresh neonate cadavers that the hydraulic pressure involved in even standard deliveries can cause a variety of effects on the brain, including cerebral distortions, vascular elongation and venous blood congestion, and displacement and kinking of the brainstem (Issel et al., 1977).

Although birthing histories were not reported, it is of interest to note here a report of gait and posture control anomalies found in otherwise healthy children with convergent but not divergent strabismus, suggesting the presence of brainstem anomalies in the eso- but not the exo-deviated group (Odenrick et al., 1984; Sandstedt et al., 1986). At the same time, there was a correlation between fusional amplitude and postural control in the exo- but not the eso-deviated children, leading to a hypothesis of vision-related cerebral involvement in the origin of exo-deviations, rather than a brainstem origin of eso-deviations (Sandstedt et al., 1986). The study of birthing variables that found breech-presenting children to have a higher incidence of strabismus also found them to perform significantly worse than normal subjects on walking balance and eye-hand tracking tasks (McBride et al., 1979).

NEURONTROPY MODEL OF MAPPING DISTORTION ORIGINS

Neurontropy and the Binocular Deficit Cascade

How might such relatively subtle anomalies as the albino heterozygote micro-misrouting or cone matrix distortion mechanisms cascade into a substantial enough deficit to contribute significantly to amblyopia or suppression? The general concept we consider is that cortex-based comparison of the two eyes' noncongruent images causes a greater stereopsis decrement than might be predicted from the image quality decrement of either eye alone. The resulting compromise of binocular cortical function is then proposed to both induce amblyopia and compromise the cortical dominance of subcortical binocular vision, contributing in turn to strabismic misalignment. The details of what might be referred to as the "binocular deficit cascade" are as follows.

We have already reviewed evidence in support of the concept of a binocular versus monocular vision reciprocal relation. Within binocular vision, there is also evidence of two mechanisms, global and local stereopsis. *Local stereopsis* is that which processes disparity in one part of the visual field without reference to other loci. *Global stereopsis* is that which involves interaction between multiple loci (Tyler, 1990).[5] This distinction is in practice somewhat arbitrary in that there is evidence of intrastimulus interaction in almost any multielement stimulus configuration (e.g., Kumar and Glaser, 1991), so that only a single point may fully satisfy the definition of "local." We here adopt the convention of using "local" to refer to small-area stereo matching and "global" to refer to matching of more binocular field-wide extent.

---

5. Global stereopsis should not be confused with *cyclopean stereopsis*, which refers to stereo image features invisible to monocular vision (Tyler, 1990).

There is evidence of global and local processing at the monocular form processing as well as binocular stereoscopic level (Julesz and Schumer, 1981; Williams and Sekuler, 1984; Burr et al., 1986; DeValois and DeValois, 1988; Fendrich et al., 1990; Tyler, 1990) with global function possibly localized in the lateral geniculate nucleus (LGN) parvocellular-mediated "P system" and local function in the magnocellular "M system" (Tyler, 1990). There is also, presumably, interaction between the binocular–monocular and global–local dyads. For instance, adding global monocular information in the form of connecting lines between the test and reference lines markedly increases threshold on a local stereopsis-mediated stereoacuity task (Westheimer, 1979; McKee, 1983) or overrides conflicting local stereopsis-mediated surface perception (Stevens and Brookes, 1988). On the other hand, (monocular local) Vernier acuity is greatly reduced by fusion of the monocular Vernier target into a (binocularly local) stereo pair (McKee et al., 1990). More subtly, subjective contours, a clear case of purely global monocular perception, have been found able to cause perceived organizational shifts in global stereoscopic form perception (Ramachandran and Cavanaugh, 1985). Finally, there is evidence that the spatial frequency tuning of global stereopsis processing is different from that underlying global form discrimination (Yang and Blake, 1991).

Interaction between the binocular–monocular and

global–local dyads seems to follow a scale in the stages of amblyopic deterioration of function I have characterized as the Neurontropy Predominance Scale, outlined in Figure 25-7. The fundamental thrust of this deterioration is characterized by extrapolation of Tyler and Julesz's concept of "neurontropy," a stereo equivalent of entropy in which the stereo system is biased toward orderly fusion, with fusion being a more efficient process than the alternative state of rivalry (Julesz and Tyler, 1976; Tyler and Julesz, 1976). Once there is a loss of fusional order, in the form of interocular decorrelation, return to that order is difficult, in keeping with the second law of thermodynamics. Julesz and Tyler applied the term "catabolism" to this relative irreversibility, from the term for degenerate metabolism in physiology.

Julesz and Tyler applied the neurontropy concept to the question of the relation of fusion and rivalry, concluding that these functions are mediated by separate mechanisms. This specific question remains controversial (Wolfe, 1986; Blake, 1989; Blake et al., 1991; Yang and Blake, 1991). Under the hypothesis presented here, the neurontropy concept is applied more broadly. I am suggesting that unified global stereoscopic perception fragments neurontropically, in the presence of retinotopic image mapping distortion "noise," into a lesser or greater plurality of its local stereopsis component parts. This action represents a decline from the normal

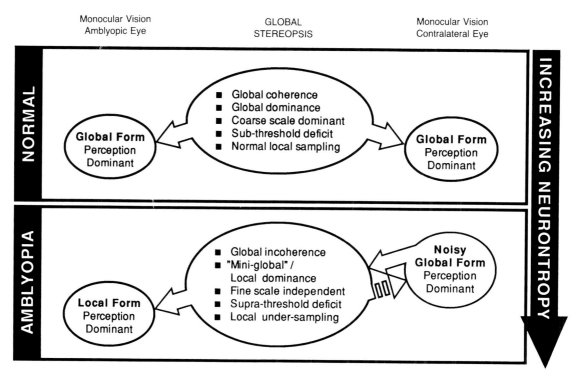

FIG. 25-7. Neurontropy Predominance Scale in normal (upper tier) and amblyopic (lower tier) vision. Horizontal arrows indicate direction of predominance. See text for details.

constraint of coarse-on-fine spatial scales in fusion (Wilson et al., 1991) to a condition of greater fine-scale independence and global disjunction among fine scales at different visual field loci (Fig. 25-7).

A prediction of the neurontropy scale would be that global stereopsis, at the highest predominance level in ordering the binocular percept, must necessarily be less adaptive than the local stereopsis mechanisms it modulates and integrates. In fact, local stereopsis has been reported to adapt to the disparity inversion of eye-transposing prisms within 2 days, whereas global stereopsis shows no sign of so adapting after a week of prismatically induced experience (Shimojo and Nakajima, 1981). Another illustration of the neurontropy scale occurs with the milder degrees of amblyopia, where normal stereopsis function is decremented to the extent that global stereopsis random dot stereogram targets can no longer be perceived, but local stereopsis targets (i.e., with monocularly visible contours) can still be discriminated (Simons, 1981b; Rutstein and Eskridge, 1984).

Global processing, as a field-wide process, would also seem by definition a low frequency mechanism. In fact, there is evidence of global stereopsis function being based primarily on channels with spatial frequencies centered on 3 and 5 cycles/degree (cpd) (Schor et al., 1984; Yang and Blake, 1991). A corollary of this assumption is that the higher energy high spatial frequencies necessary for resolving spatial detail can constitute a threat to the coherence of global processing if they contain interocularly nonhomologous global disparity information. The global stereopsis sensitivity to this threat is indicated in the finding that targets containing higher spatial frequency harmonics, which have less threshold-increasing matching ambiguity than fundamental-only gratings (Legge and Gu, 1989), provide lower stereoacuity thresholds than do targets of equal contrast at the fundamental, but at the same time have lower fusion limits than equivalent targets containing only the fundamental (Schor et al., 1989). High spatial frequency global (random dot) stereograms are more sensitive than low spatial frequency stereograms to disruptions by masking noise (Yang and Blake, 1991) and do not support global stereopsis (Mowforth et al., 1981). Similarly, at the monocular level, the suprathreshold presence of a higher spatial frequency or spatial frequency harmonic has been found to force perception of a pattern at the local rather than the global processing level, with the reverse case, global form perception dominant, obtaining when low pass filtering removes the harmonic or low spatial frequencies are dominant (Burr et al., 1986; Fendrich et al., 1990). The coarse-on-fine scaling basis proposed for global binocular function (Wilson et al., 1991) seems likely to be directed toward constraining these higher frequency mechanisms to preserve the global percept, compatible with detailed stereoscopic and monocular form discrimination.

Like the global–local characterization, the neurontropy scale is a continuum. For instance, modeling experiments have documented a breakdown of unified global stereopsis under dissociating conditions into patch-like "miniglobal" regions (Blake et al., 1991; Wilson et al., 1991), suggesting that there can be multiple coarse-on-fine scale hierarchies operating in parallel in different parts of the binocular visual field (Wilson et al., 1991). This situation appears to constitute a variant on Tyler's "pyknostereopsis" and "diastereopsis" classifications (Tyler, 1983, 1990) that might be categorized, from an overall binocular field point of view, as "polystereopsis," comprised of an assembly of "miniglobal" regions. In terms of global stereo versus global monocular predominance, the continuous nature of the neurontropy scale is illustrated by demonstration of the result of incremental increase of rivalry-inducing noise in one eye's image of a random texture stereogram. At low noise levels, the global stereo figure is seen simultaneously with the (monocular) global rivalry-inducing texture (Blake et al., 1991); at higher levels of noise, when stereopsis is impaired the texture associated with the stereo (in contrast to rivalry-inducing) target remains monocularly visible (Yang and Blake, 1991). There is evidence in the cat of a continuum, rather than generically different classes, of disparity-sensitive cells (LeVay and Voight, 1988) and preliminary evidence of a stereo neural processing mechanism based on multiple spatial frequency scale phase-disparity sensitivity (Freeman and Ohzawa, 1990).

Because by definition the binocular field would not fragment from an integrated global status into the assembly of "miniglobal" regions if those regions could be coordinated from a depth-matching point of view, the "patches" in the miniglobal collage must stand in antagonistic relation to each other. This relation may take the form of stereo "repulsion" (Westheimer, 1986; Westheimer and Levi, 1987; Stevenson et al., 1991). In cascade-like fashion, the degree of this repulsion sets in train a deterioration of global binocular function to a level of amblyopia or suppression adequate to adaptively conceal the level of resulting neurontropic chaos[6] from perception under normal viewing conditions.

An objectively measurable demonstration of the neurontropy scale was reported in a study noted earlier of

---

6. This situation in fact seems to fit the description of Walls' vivid caveat on the phylogenetic development of binocular vision, that "unless the monocular images were automatically kept upon corresponding spots (within the leeway provided by Panum's areas), the stereoscopic image would break up into a horrid, uninterpretable diplopic mess and all advantage of binocularity would be lost" (Walls, 1962).

the tracking of the two eyes in response to a random dot stereo image as the two half-images were moved laterally in opposite directions (Erkelens and Collewijn, 1985). At low target speeds fusion remained intact, and both eyes tracked symmetrically; that is, binocular predominance was intact. As target speed was increased, so long as fusion was maintained there was increasing phase lag, but the two eyes continued to track symmetrically. When target speed reached the point where fusion was lost, binocular tracking congruence was lost as well. Specifically, as the neurontropy scale would predict, one eye tracked accurately and the combined disparity tracking error, or interocular phase lag, of *both* eyes was assigned to the contralateral eye and its vision partially suppressed. In other words, the loss of binocular predominance resulted in not independent bilateral symmetry but monocular predominance of one eye, indicated by its tracking dominance, to achieve optimum performance and amblyopia-like degradation of contralateral eye visual and motor performance to absorb the resulting variance between the two eyes' images. An equivalent demonstration in actual amblyopia is seen when such a patient attempts to fixate a small target in a dark room. Both eyes show the small jerk nystagmus while fixating that is characteristic of amblyopia (Schor, 1983), indicating the binocular basis of the condition, but with greater nystagmus amplitude (i.e., fixational variance) in the amblyopic eye, indicating the interocular predominance of the better eye.

Binocular Catabolism, Amblyopiagenesis, and Anomalous Retinal Correspondence

Interocular competition for synaptic representation at the binocular cells of the visual cortex is fundamental to primate visual development (Mitchell and Timney, 1984) and appears responsible for the adaptive mechanism that maintains better vision in one eye in strabismic amblyopia, at the price of reduced binocular function as well as monocular function in the amblyopic eye. In terms of the neurontropy precedence mechanism, this competition appears to result in such cases in the global form perception of monocular processes of the better eye achieving a higher level of function through the arrest of maturational development at a lower level on the scale of both the amblyopic eye and binocular global stereopsis. In short, it appears that normal binocular global predominance in cortical neural coordination is displaced by that of the monocular global mechanism of the better eye (Fig. 25-7).

That the binocular global mechanism remains the inhibitory global mediator of the interocular competition process, however, is seen under haploscopic testing conditions that allow measurement of acuity (i.e., monocular form perception) in each eye simultaneously but

independently. The result in many cases of amblyopia is either reduction of *both* eyes' acuity compared to unilaterally determined thresholds or a reduction of the better eye's acuity and improvement of the amblyopic eye's acuity (Awaya and von Noorden, 1972; Morgan et al., 1972). The binocular/interocular influence is also seen indirectly in other high spatial frequency monocular form processing defects in the better eye of both human amblyopes (Kandel et al., 1980; Bedell et al., 1985; Mac Cana et al., 1986; Leguire et al., 1990), and naturally occurring strabismic monkeys (Kiorpes and Boothe, 1981), as well as in the improvement of vision in an amblyopic eye in visual adults that occurs when vision in the sound eye is lost (Tommila, 1964; Harwerth et al., 1986; Tierney, 1989). There is also evidence that amblyopia in infants (Day et al., 1988) and young children (see Chapter 21) may be bilateral more frequently than traditionally thought, as it is in the naturally strabismic monkey (Kiorpes, 1989).

A stereogram-based modeling experiment (Simons, submitted), summarized below, demonstrated that bilaterally symmetrical variance distributions of stereogram pixel positional "jitter," modeling image mapping distortion, was less disruptive of stereopsis function than when the combined interocular jitter variance was asymmetrically assigned to the image of only one eye. In terms of the model, it demonstrated that inversion of the global stereopsis and better-eye monocular predominance, to improve global monocular form processing integrity of the better eye in the presence of increased disparity "noise" at the price of increased monocular positional noise in the contralateral eye, is more disruptive of stereopsis than when global stereopsis predominance is maintained in the form of equal noise assignment to both eyes.

There is evidence that mapping distortion resulting from cone matrix irregularities in the fovea are compensated for by mapping of the retinal locus of individual cones to the cortex (reviewed by Costaridou et al., 1990; Curcio and Hendrickson, 1991). This "cone position known" (Hirsch and Miller, 1987) system has been specified to date only for monocular vision (Costaridou et al., 1990; Curcio and Hendrickson, 1991). In a binocular system, especially one in which neural development environment involves interocular competition (Mitchell and Timney, 1984), a problem arises if the retinal remapping of this monocular image disorder compensation process for one eye conflicts (via the homologous comparison between eyes of stereopsis) with the disorder compensation remapping of the contralateral eye. Is there such a conflict, or is the cone-position-known system binocularly based?

I propose that, in keeping with the binocular versus monocular theme of early development, there is a conflict between an innately defined neural basis for the homologous stereoscopic comparison between the two eyes and the experientially calibrated monocular "cone position known" distortion compensation system. The literature on artificially induced amblyopia makes clear that monocular vision can be modified on the basis of experience (Mitchell and Timney, 1984; Crawford et al., 1989, Harwerth et al., 1989; Mitchell, 1991), as especially demonstrated by the remodification experiments such as reverse occlusion. Evidence for the traditional assumption of an innate basis for stereoscopic retinotopic mapping (Linksz, 1952) is not as clear-cut but is circumstantially suggestive. Binocular, and particularly stereoscopic, vision can be inhibited (i.e., via suppression) or neurally ruptured (Linksz, 1952; Freeman and Tsumoto, 1983; Timney, 1983, 1990; Crawford et al., 1991; Harwerth et al., 1991). Furthermore, there is a greater decrement in performance on vertical than horizontal gratings in monkeys raised with surgically induced strabismus (Harwerth et al., 1989) and greater loss of vertically than horizontally tuned neurons in cats raised with optically induced strabismus (Chino et al., 1991), as would be expected if horizontal disparity-sensing mechanisms are responsible for the rupture. However, as Sireteanu and Fronius note in their review of the question, the findings from animal compensation experiments support the existence of a significant mapping compensation capability only in the vertical direction, i.e., that horizontal mapping is indeed immutable (Sireteanu and Fronius, 1989).

In humans it appears difficult to explain the abrupt onset and rapid initial stereoacuity improvement in infants by other than an innately wired mechanism, especially as this change is coincident with an uninterrupted gradual development of monocular acuity (see Chapter 13). However, the critical question is what interpretation is to be given to "anomalous" retinal correspondence (ARC), which appears to show a plasticity of stereoscopic inter-eye homology. We suggest below (step 4) that in fact ARC represents the attempt by the (crippled) global stereopsis mechanism to integrate a variety of disjunct local, or "miniglobal," regions of the binocular field that cannot be integrated into a coherent global whole. The result is an uneasy collage of these localized "patches" that change—and thus give the appearance that correspondence status itself changes—as a function of both the visual system status and testing conditions. What is significant here is that such a theory is compatible with the existence of innate binocular retinotopic wiring of the primary visual cortex for horizontal disparity, with the global "ARC" shifts due to the operation of more central processing, such as in area 18 of the cortex. Demonstrations of change of ARC angle in different gaze positions, instantaneous change of angle under various testing conditions, and rapid postoperative adjustment of the angle (von Noorden, 1990, pp. 259, 260) also argue against a long-term neural wiring change basis of ARC and for simply a (global) reorganization of innately wired retinotopic representations.

We consider the hypothesis, then, that amblyopiagenesis proceeds by the following sequence.

Step 1. *Interocular mapping homology discrepancy detection and arrest of binocular receptive field refinement.* There appears to be reason to think that, at its developmental onset, stereopsis may be characterized as a coarse global mechanism. As the binocular receptive field (Ferster, 1981) resolution improves with development, however, the model predicts that homologous matching will be impeded when that resolution reaches the detection threshold of a given level of interocular retinotopic mapping distortion discrepancy. This discrepancy is illustrated in the interocular vectorial subtraction of the image maps of the two eyes of an amblyope (Fig. 25-8). As noted earlier, the higher density resulting from the developmentally improved resolution "grain" increases the (horopteral) sensitivity to mismatches (Badcock and Schor, 1985; Parker and Yang, 1989). Thus stereopsis sensitivity to rivalrous noise is inversely proportional to spatial frequency (Blake et al., 1991; Yang and Blake, 1991), in this case with the spatial frequency increase due to maturation. Furthermore, the nonlinearity of the neurontropy transfer characteristic (Tyler and Julesz, 1976, Fig. 5) predicts that relatively small amounts of interocular decorrelation (e.g., 10%) can seriously disrupt stereopsis, as the reader can see by viewing Figure 8.1-2 of Julesz (1971).[7] This sensitivity is presumably the result of the multiplying effects of what has been characterized as disparity "recruiting" (Kertesz, 1983a), "cooperativity" (Julesz, 1971; Julesz and Chang, 1976), or "pooling" (Westheimer and Levi, 1987; Parker and Yang, 1989), or, alternatively, its rivalry zone complement (Mueller and Blake, 1990). Instead of normal cooperativity/recruiting/pooling, the interocular mapping distortion positional "noise" appears to result in disrecruiting/cooperativity/pooling that reduces stereoscopic depth localization accuracy in an adaptive attempt to maintain global stereopsis to the extent possible in the presence of the matching noise.

The developmental result of this attempt to maintain intact global stereopsis is "arrest" (Chavasse, 1939) of maturational improvement of binocular receptive field resolution at an "undersampled" (Levi et al., 1987; Levi, 1988) level that hence limits development of ster-

---

7. This sensitivity also applies for the "diffrequency" (Tyler, 1990) stereopsis mechanism based on fusing targets of two spatial frequencies. This form of stereopsis is lost when the two targets differ in frequency by more than 25% (Halpern et al., 1987).

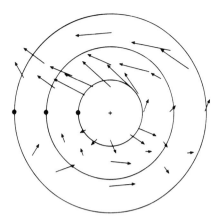

FIG. 25-8. Vector subtraction plot of the interocular positional discrepancies between the monocular maps of the amblyope illustrated in Figure 25-4. (Reprinted from *Vision Research*, Volume 31, W-L. Lagrèze and R. Sireteanu, "Two-dimensional spatial distortions in human strabismic amblyopia," pp. 1271–1288, Copyright 1991, with permission from Pergamon Press Ltd., Headington Hall, Oxford OX3 OBW, UK.)

eoscopic spatial frequency response at an abnormally "pyknosteroscopic" stage. (If there is trauma or pathology that introduces positional noise during the sensitive period, there may be an outright reversal of development, causing reenlargement of the binocular receptive field.)

Step 2. *Mapping distortion interocular reassignment.* The global stereopsis system assigns the combined interocular positional variance resulting from the difference between the two eyes' maps to the eye with the greater amount of mapping distortion, i.e., the eye requiring the greatest degree of distortion compensation. This assignment to what becomes the amblyopic eye takes the form of inhibition by the global stereoscopic mechanism of the disorder compensation mechanism in that eye, illustrated in our simulation (Fig. 25-6). That this interocular competition-based process is both fundamental to binocular development and based on predominance of an innate binocular mechanism over a plastic monocular mechanism is suggested by two findings: Cats that are fitted bilaterally with a prism during early development (Chino et al., 1991) and monkeys raised with full bilateral deprivation (Harwerth et al., 1991) nonetheless show interocularly asymmetrical losses of spatial resolution and contrast sensitivity. The reassignment process is also illustrated by amblyopic patient reports that the visual distortion seen monocularly in their amblyopic eye increases when the better eye is opened (Sireteanu and Fronius, 1982). Another illustration, as noted above, is that the visual acuity of the amblyopic (or sound) eyes in some amblyopes is further reduced under dichoptic testing conditions from what it is with standard unilateral testing (Awaya and von Noorden, 1972; Morgan et al., 1972). On the motor

side, also as noted above, greater nystagmus amplitude "variance" may be seen when the amblyopic eye is fixating than when the better eye is (Schor, 1983).

Step 3. *Arrest of amblyopic eye monocular receptive field refinement.* The binocular receptive field arrest at a field-undersampled level also halts the normal shrinkage with development of the monocular receptive field, or "cortical processing module" (Levi, 1988) grain, at an undersampled level as well, the localized "positional uncertainty" (Levi, 1988; Levi and Klein, 1990) of amblyopia. Here the undersampling is particularly reminiscent of that found in the normal peripheral field, where cone angular position is less predictable than at the fovea (Hirsch and Miller, 1987) and where there may be neural mapping errors as well (Hess and Watt, 1990). Undersampling has been demonstrated to provide an effective compensation for such distortion in monocular vision (see Wilson, 1991, Fig. 10).

It should be noted that many strabismus children do not develop amblyopia but, instead, alternate fixation and exhibit suppression (von Noorden, 1990). Others exhibit a combination of suppression and amblyopia (Dickey et al., 1991). In terms of the present hypothesis, it appears that the alternator has a more complete, presumably innate, "fusion defect" (Worth, 1903) that precludes establishment of even coarse global stereopsis to begin with, although more localized "miniglobal" stereopsis may be possible.

Step 4. *Global stereopsis and monocular form processing conversion to disjunct "miniglobal"/local "patches."* Even with normal vision there is some degree of spatial mapping distortion across the visual field (e.g., Bedell and Flom, 1983; Hess and Watt, 1990), but the "global-tropic" coarse-on-fine scale mechanism is able to integrate a field-wide global stereopsis percept. With the amblyopiagenic condition of significant interocular mapping discrepancies, I propose that this integration is successful only at a more localized level, in the form of multiple "patches" that can be stereoscopically matched with homologous patches contralaterally in "miniglobal" fashion, but not at a field-wide global stereopsis level. This effect has been modeled in ambiguous and rivalrous stereograms, where a patch-like breakup of the global image is observed (Parker and Yang, 1989; Blake et al., 1991), and there is evidence of parallel operation of multiple parallel coarse-on-fine processes operating in different parts of the visual field (Wilson et al., 1991). In the amblyope, in whom I propose that this condition follows some degree of visual development, and possibly in the alternator, where it may be innate, the result is variations in retinal correspondence across the visual field (Mohn et al., 1986; Fronius and Sireteanu, 1989; Sireteanu and Fronius, 1989). This state of disjunct "miniglobal"/local stereopsis-mediated patches of correspondence and noncorrespondent rivalry across the visual field seems likely to underlie the group of symptoms associated with the term "anomalous" retinal correspondence.

"Anomalous" retinal correspondence has been clinically notorious for its variability as to both presence and size, varying not simply idiopathically across patients but for a given patient for different tests or visual field loci or across time (Jennings, 1985; Sireteanu and Fronius, 1989; von Noorden, 1990). The variability appears to be simply explained, however, by a binocular visual field comprised of a shifting collage of local stereopsis and rivalry patches, with ARC status a function of the most globally stable binocular visual field organization possible under the reigning visual system status—and diagnostic test condition—constraints. For instance, coarser, more dissociative tests such as the after-image method indicate a smaller angle or lack of ARC anomaly than do less-dissociating tests such as the Bagolini striated lenses (von Noorden, 1990, pp. 252ff), as would be expected if low spatial frequency coarse stereo function were relatively unaffected by localized higher spatial frequency patch disjunction. Similarly, ARC tends to be harmonious (angle of anomaly matches angle of strabismic deviation) in the periphery or to less-localized testing, and unharmonious (noncongruent angles) in central vision and for more localized testing (Sireteanu and Fronius, 1989) that pinpoints "patch" correspondence differences. In sum, under our hypothesis, "ARC" is in fact "DGS," or Disjunct Global Stereopsis.

It seems possible that a similar breakdown of the global process to a miniglobal/local process is responsible at the monocular level for decoupling grating acuity from letter or Vernier acuity in many patients with amblyopia, with grating thresholds much nearer normal than that of the other two acuity tests (see Chapter 24). Visual acuity on the redundant "full-field E" target is also less affected by amblyopia than linear Snellen acuity (Walsh et al., 1984). We may speculate that the redundancy of the grating and "full-field E" targets makes them able to be processed by more local monocular form processing mechanisms than the nonredundant Snellen or Vernier stimuli. If we assume, again, that local monocular form processing mechanisms remain functional to a larger extent than the global mechanisms in amblyopia (Fig. 25-7), the improved performance on the local task compared to the global task is explained.

Step 5. *Binocular catabolism/monocular predominance.* The breakdown of global into disjunct miniglobal/local stereopsis patches comprises the condition of binocular "catabolism" (Julesz and Tyler, 1976; Tyler and Julesz, 1976). A fundamental property of binocular neurontropy is that stereopsis acts like a (leaky) neural diode, responding only to conditions of positive interocular image correlation but failing to function in the presence of either a lack of such correlation or the presence of negative correlation (Julesz and Tyler, 1976; Tyler and Julesz, 1976). Thus, as noted in step 1, a relatively small amount of interocular homologous mapping discrepancy can produce significant stereoscopic degradation. Global monocular form perception in the better eye is thus placed at a competitive neurontropy predominance advantage. This condition comprises amblyopia, the state in which, again, monocular global form processing in the better eye functions at a level of organization competitive with or higher than that of stereoscopic or contralateral eye monocular form processing global function (Fig. 25-7).

Step 6. *The catabolism loop.* Julesz and Miller (1975) originally reported that a given spatial frequency's stereopsis masking noise could affect other channels only if the channels involved were no more than 2.0 octaves of spatial frequency apart. More recent studies have suggested that this value may be smaller if other factors such as noise energy are taken into account (Wilson et al., 1991; Yang and Blake, 1991). The range question is significant here as it bears on the question of how great an amblyopiagenic effect from the "masking" noise a given degree of interocular mapping discrepancy may have, especially if that degree is relatively subtle. Our simulation experiment suggests that, when the mapping distortion is asymmetrically assigned between eyes, the effect is magnified relative to bilaterally symmetrical presentation. Furthermore, the effect would presumably be magnified still further in the chronic "presentation" of such noise in the developmental context, especially if there is a loop-like degenerative (i.e., neurontropic catabolism) interaction with developing optomotor vergence control.

Farther down the neurontropy scale into amblyopia, the only remaining binocular function is motion-based local stereopsis, illustrated by findings that such stereopsis is better preserved (e.g., present at larger angles of deviation) in strabismic subjects than is static, position stereopsis (Sireteanu et al., 1981; Sireteanu, 1982; Schor et al., 1983a; Kitaoji and Toyama, 1987). As with static ARC, there is disjunct local variability across the visual field of this residual motion-based stereo sensitivity (Sireteanu et al., 1981; Sireteanu, 1982; Mohn et al., 1986).

Neurontropy Precedence Illustration: Photophobia

Operation of the neurontropy precedence mechanism appears to be demonstrated in photophobia, most clinically familiar in intermittent exotropia (Wiggins and von Noorden, 1990). In fact, the greater tolerance for high luminance in monocular vision—typically via monocular eye closure—than in binocular vision is

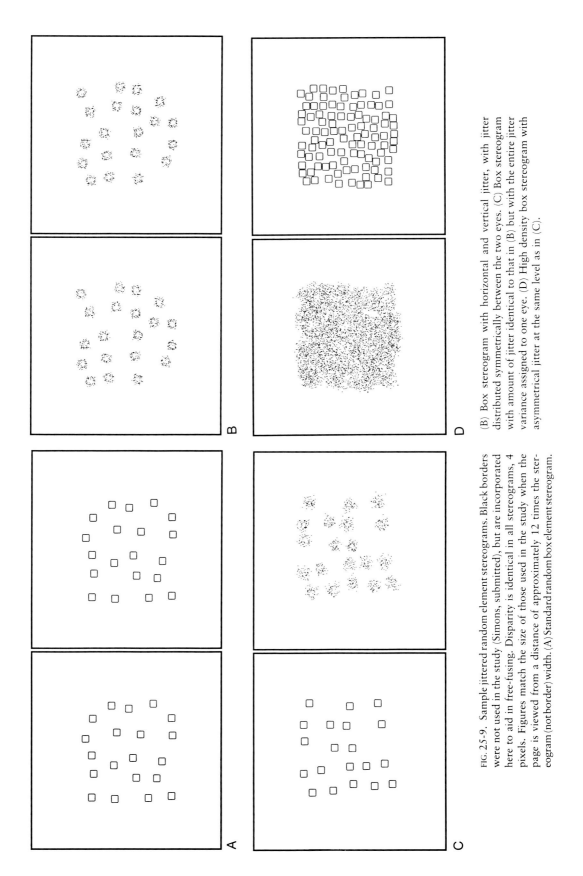

FIG. 25-9. Sample jittered random element stereograms. Black borders were not used in the study (Simons, submitted), but are incorporated here to aid in free-fusing. Disparity is identical in all stereograms, 4 pixels. Figures match the size of those used in the study when the page is viewed from a distance of approximately 12 times the stereogram (not border) width. (A) Standard random box element stereogram. (B) Box stereogram with horizontal and vertical jitter, with jitter distributed symmetrically between the two eyes. (C) Box stereogram with amount of jitter identical to that in (B) but with the entire jitter variance assigned to one eye. (D) High density box stereogram with asymmetrical jitter at the same level as in (C).

characteristic of normals and patients with other forms of strabismus as well. A binocular interaction is obviously responsible for the effect, and that it is not simply a binocular summation effect is illustrated by evidence in normals that the photophobic aversion is specifically associated with the presence of binocular fusion and relieved (i.e., luminance tolerance threshold increased) by loss of fusion (Mathis and Bourassa, 1968). On the other hand, that it is the stereopsis rather than the fusion system that is involved is suggested by the lack of effect of luminance level on fusional vergence amplitudes (Wiggins and von Noorden, 1990). The magnitude of the Stiles-Crawford effect increases at the fovea at high luminance in normal subjects (Enoch and Bedell, 1981), suggesting that these high luminance conditions exaggerate the sensitivity to interocular mapping distortion discrepancies beyond that to which the global stereopsis sytem had been adapted at normal luminance levels. The result is aversion and eye closure in normals, an analog of clinical suppression or amblyopia. The intermittent exotrope, whose fusion status clearly is subnormal, as evidenced by his exo-deviation, does the eye closure at lower luminance levels than normals. In the absence of such closure (or, more typically, transiently prior to eye closure), some of these patients are even driven to decompensate into a constant exotropia (Eustace et al., 1973; Wiggins and von Noorden, 1990), presumably due to the same mechanism. Significantly, the eye closure is more likely to occur in the intermittent exotrope with normal than abnormal retinal correspondence (Wang and Chryssanthou, 1988). Finally, that this effect may have larger significance is suggested by studies and anecdotal evidence indicating a higher prevalence of exotropia (in Caucasians) at latitudes and times of year with greater sun exposure (Berg, 1982; Editorial, 1990a). In other words, inadequate image mapping distortion compensation appears to create a risk factor for exotropia.

Jittered Stereogram Simulation

To explicitly simulate the effects of cone misalignment on stereopsis, a new type of stereogram was devised, the Jittered Random Element Stereogram (JRES) (Simons, submitted). The JRES has the unique property of allowing manipulation of individual monocular receptive field-equivalent loci, in the form of pixels, at the local stereopsis level while exhibiting the monocular artifact-free random pattern of the standard random element stereogram (Fig. 25-9). The manipulation takes the form of pixel static positional displacement, or "jitter," according to a binomial approximation to a Guassian distribution. To fully model mapping distortion, the JRES allows jitter in the horizontal or vertical axis (Fig. 25-9). Using more- and less-localized measures of

perceived depth position, serving as measures of "local" and "global" stereopsis function, the following findings were observed: (1) The amount of jitter positional variance was inversely related to accuracy of depth localization. (2) Jitter-induced stereopsis decrement reduced the congruence of perceived direction of disparity between the local and global measures (e.g., the JRES stereo figure perceived in crossed disparity on the local measure and in uncrossed disparity on the global measure), modeling the ARC "miniglobal" breakdown effect. (3) At higher levels of jitter variance, there was a loss of depth percept and, in some cases, a perception of disparity sign reversal, i.e., a crossed disparity target being perceived as uncrossed, also in keeping with the proposed ARC mechanism. (4) Jitter variance asymmetrically assigned to one eye (Fig. 25-9C) caused appreciably greater local and global stereopsis decrement than jitter distributed symmetrically between eyes (Fig. 25-9B), an explicit model of amblyopiagenesis. (5) Increasing stereogram density (Fig. 25-9D), modeling the effect of the increasing visual sampling density of development increased the amount of stereopsis-decrementing effect of a given amount of jitter, especially in the interocularly asymmetric distribution condition. (6) Jitter in the horizontal axis caused greater stereopsis decrement than in the vertical axis. (7) Above a threshold minimum, the proportion of pixels jittered caused greater stereopsis decrement than a variance-equivalent jittering of fewer pixels. The last finding is of interest because it indicates that the individually small but widely distributed mapping distortions such as that resulting from the hypothesized heterozygote micromis-routing or birth trauma/photic insult process could in fact have a disproportionately large stereopsis-decrementing effect.

FUSION VERSUS STEREOPSIS IN STRABISMOGENESIS

Jampolsky (1978) has suggested, and illustrated with clinical examples, that interocular asymmetry of any combination of central and peripheral visual field loss can cause strabismus, whereas symmetrical loss may not. Other clinical (von Noorden, 1990, p. 313) and animal model (reviewed in Quick et al., 1989) findings also demonstrate that interocular asymmetries of visual input cause strabismus. Boman and Kertesz (1985a), in a modeling experiment with normal adult subjects using artificial central or annular scotomas, found fusion response and interocular alignment anomalies to result from various symmetrical and asymmetrical combinations of both types of scotoma. Thus it appears that compromise of function of almost any combination of central and peripheral vision may create an amblyopia or strabismus risk factor.

Neurontropic Amblyopiagenesis and Subcortical Disinhibition

One result of the stereopsis neurontropic catabolism process described above might be degradation of the binocularity-based cortical projection to the midbrain. Midbrain binocularity deficits have been implicated as the origin of monocular OKN asymmetries and possibly esotropia (see Chapters 5, 23, and 26). Although it was previously thought that deficits in the midbrain's own (crude) binocularity were primarily responsible for these dysfunctions (Schor, 1983; Westall and Schor, 1985; see also Chapter 26), other studies have suggested a more dominant role of cortical input—or its lack—into this process (van Hof-van Duin and Mohn, 1986; see also Chapter 26). Thus amblyopic defects in cortically mediated stereopsis in humans may cascade into a larger effect on oculomotor alignment control than previously thought. The vergence-sustaining fusional response mechanism appears to be narrowly tuned for disparity (Jones and Stephens, 1989), and modeling experiments on adult normals with stabilized image-based scotomatic stimuli demonstrate a reduced degree of vergence response (Boman and Kertesz, 1985a).

Fusion/Stereopsis Developmental Asynchrony and the Corpus Callosum

Infant esotropia is virtually never present at birth but has a postnatal onset, following the same type of initial exo-deviation seen in normal subjects (Archer and Helveston, 1989; see also Chapter 22), a sequence also seen in naturally esotropic cats (Schoppman and Hoffman, 1985) and monkeys exposed to alternating (Tyschen et al., 1991) as well as unilateral (Quick et al., 1989) deprivation. These findings suggest a maturation-related process rather than connatally present condition. The idea of absent or delayed development of fusion as a cause of strabismus dates back to at least the work of Worth (1903) and Keiner (1951) and has been promulgated most recently by von Noorden (1988b, 1990).[8] Of particular interest in this respect are demonstrations of stereopsis, including global random dot stereopsis, in esotropic infants, either transiently pre- or postoperatively or for a more extended period, when alignment deficits are compensated for by prism correction (Birch and Stager, 1985; Mohindra et al., 1985; Archer et al., 1986; Stager and Birch, 1986; Birch et al., 1990; Atkinson et al., 1991). [A study that did not use prisms failed to replicate this finding (Dobson and Sebris, 1989).] These findings suggest onset of coarse global stereopsis in the absence of or prior to the development of adequate coarse fusional control of interocular alignment at the level needed to support such stereopsis. In fact, there is evidence of "late starters" on a visually evoked potential (VEP)-based binocular fusion measure exhibiting an appreciably higher level of strabismus incidence in a prospective study than the general population or a group of infants with earlier fusion onset (Wattam-Bell et al., 1987). The independence of fusion and stereopsis in development is also suggested by findings in older patients of lack of correlation between stereoacuity and fusional vergence amplitudes in small-angle esotropia, including monofixators (Parks, 1971; Pratt-Johnson and Barlow, 1975; Hiles et al., 1980; Ing, 1983). For instance, one study reported a postoperative esotropia patient with only a 12 prism diopter fusional vergence amplitude and a 400 arc-second stereoacuity threshold and another with 27 prism diopter amplitude but no measurable stereoacuity (Pratt-Johnson and Tillson, 1983); in yet another study, patients were orthophoric but had no central fusion (Pratt-Johnson, 1973).

When considering physiological substrates that might underlie a fusion-stereopsis onset asynchrony, the corpus callosum is of interest, in view of Bishop and Henry's (1971) proposal that it may mediate coarse stereopsis function, if we add the qualification that this mediation may be developmentally transient. Though there is support for such a hypothesis, the literature needs careful interpretation (see review by Timney et al., 1985). For instance, sectioning the callosum in adult cat or monkey has no effect on stereopsis function, though it does have such an effect in humans, as does callosal agenesis (Timney et al., 1985; Fisher, 1986).[9] The difference may be due to the lower species' naso-temporal overlap, the lack of which appears unique to humans (Lines and Milner, 1983; Lines, 1984; Fendrich and Gazzaniga, 1989). Of particular significance in the present context, however, is evidence that the callosum appears to have its greatest influence on binocular vision during the early postnatal period (Elberger, 1989, 1990). It is not surprising in view of the fact that, in terms of axon count, the callosum presence is more dominant immediately postnatally than it ever is again. In keeping with what has been characterized as "negative" neural development effects (Blakemore, 1988) that involve neural elimination rather than growth, there is elimination of 70% of callosal axons during the first 4 months of postnatal life in the primate (LaMantia and

---

8. Delayed maturation of temporalward motion processing has also been proposed as responsible for strabismus-linked monocular OKN asymmetry (see Chapter 5).

9. A study that reports normal stereo function in callosal agenesis in human patients (Ettlinger et al., 1974) used a stereo task with potential monocular artifacts, including motion parallax.

Rakic, 1990). That normal binocular visual function is required for this decline to take place is indicated by findings in the cat that induced strabismus or deprivation leaves axons more widely spread than in normal cortex, suggesting a visual experience-dependent competition between callosal and intracortical axons during early development (Innocenti et al., 1985). Early callosal-mediated interocular integration appears to be required for later achievement of high spatial frequency visual acuity function of individual cortical neurons (Elberger, 1989, 1990).

It seems possible, then, that a hypernormal-for-date level of development of the monocular substrate of visual acuity (i.e., the inverse case from callosum sectioning) could competitively eliminate too much of the callosal axonal wiring, producing subnormal binocular fusion. The reduction of interhemispheric transfer would be particularly disruptive if global stereopsis is localized in only one cerebral hemisphere (the right), as suggested by studies of patients with unilateral brain disease (Hamsher, 1978; see also Rothstein and Sacks, 1972). More subtle binocular deficits, involving temporal aspects of function, might result from delays or interocular asynchronies in callosal axon myelination, which is normally most intense during the period following axon elimination (LaMantia and Rakic, 1990), as originally proposed by Keiner (1951).

Unlike virtually all other visual function, binocular summation as measured by evoked potential reaches a peak during infancy and then declines (reviewed in Leguire et al., 1991). In terms of physiological substrate, it suggests pre-axon-elimination callosal involvement, although other substrates must also be involved as summation during early infancy begins at a low level, presumably due to the bi-ocularity of early infant vision.

Hemiretina and Disparity Sign Biases

The demonstration in normal adults of visual field-wide small but distinct stereoanomalies of both position and motion stereopsis on both sensory and vergence measures (Richards, 1970a, 1971a; Richards and Regan, 1973; Jones, 1977, 1983; Patterson and Fox, 1984; Regan et al., 1986) on the one hand, and demonstration of related patterns of residual stereopsis in strabismus patients (Sireteanu et al., 1981; Sireteanu 1982; Schor et al., 1983a; Mohn et al., 1986; Kitaoji and Toyama, 1987), on the other, suggests the possibility of defects in disparity detector pools due to genetic (Richards, 1970a, 1971a) or experiental factors. Esophoric patients have been reported to exhibit better stereoacuities on uncrossed (UC) disparity on a local stereopsis test and exophores better crossed (C) disparity (Shippman and Cohen, 1983), in keeping with the concept of C disparity deficit giving rise to eso-deviations and UC dis-

parity to exo-deviations. [The fact that some esophores were found selectivity unable to discriminate any C disparity targets and some exophores unable to resolve any UC targets suggests that a true disparity pool functionality difference is reflected in this finding, despite the use of nominally relative (Blakemore, 1970) rather than absolute signed disparity stereo test stimuli.] Parents of eso-deviated propositi have also been found to exhibit poorer C disparity than parents of exo-deviated or randomly selected propositi (UC disparity was not tested) (Smith et al., 1972).

It is not generally correct to identify C and UC disparity with the temporal hemiretina (THR) and nasal (NHR) hemiretina, respectively, except near the fovea (Tyler, 1983). However, the "area centralis"-like nature of infant central retina, with its large cone diameters and consequent low receptive field density, combined with the absolutely smaller infant retina and visual field, may make the C-THR and UC-NHR congruence more of a reality in the infant than is the case in the adult. To the extent this point is true, the initial dominance of NHR function suggests a basis for an eso-deviation bias, as NHR dominance in stereoscopic terms would represent a UC dominance or, reciprocally, a C deficit, i.e., a condition conducive to eso-deviation. It seems possible that avoidance of such deviation is the reason normal infants appear to develop C disparity before UC disparity (Reuss, 1981; see also Chapter 13), although ultimately UC disparity develops more in young children (Kitao, 1960; Simons, 1975). By this logic, adequate C function depends on THR function being established adequately at the onset of binocular function. In fact, as noted earlier, it appears to be the THR that is the locus of subcortically mediated deficits in early-onset esotropia (Westall and Schor, 1985; see also Chapters 23 and 26) as well as the locus of functional deficit for at least some types of cortically mediated psychophysical tasks in the presence of intermediate levels of amblyopia (reviewed by Chelazzi et al., 1988; Sireteanu and Fronius, 1990).

Panum's area for UC detection increases with accommodation in normal adults, whereas C detection may decrease or increase to a plateau (Richards, 1971b). There is also greater tolerance of binocular rivalry at near (Richards, 1970b). A temporal aspect of neural coding may be involved in the latter mechanism, as increased convergence has also been found to increase fusion frequency of dichoptic image alternation (Guttmann and Spatz, 1985) and decrease critical flicker frequency (Harvey, 1970). There may be at least a partial monocular receptive field "zooming" basis for these mechanisms (Richards, 1968), as near fixation improves unilaterally determined visual acuity in some amblyopes (von Noorden and Helveston, 1970; von Noorden, 1990, p. 219). If the mechanism involved in these effects is present in infants, those with UC dominance or a C deficit would have a stimulus to accommodation independent of any hyperopia, i.e., the need to increase Panum's area and so improve fusion.

There is also evidence that flexing of the globe during accommodation causes a nasally directed tilt or, more precisely, shearing over of the photoreceptors located in the NHR between the disc and the posterior pole as a result (apparently) of elasticity differences between the retina and choroid (Blank and Enoch, 1973; Blank et al., 1975; Enoch, 1975). This effect, which results in monocular spatial distortions and a shift in the Stiles-Crawford function peak, would presumably be maximized during the accommodative response to the hyperopia found in many infants (see Chapter 1). In disparity terms, the nasal shear would displace that portion of the stereo match set localized along the fovea-disc axis in a UC direction, which in turn would create a stereoscopic mapping distortion relative to non-sheared adjacent retinal regions.

There are thus two additional mechanisms involved in infant accommodation and vergence in addition to the basic response to defocus and diplopia: (1) the Panum enlargement; and (2) induction of a UC disparity bias along the fovea-disc axis. The interaction of all four mechanisms over the course of the anatomical and morphological changes of ocular development may explain the complexity of the accommodative component in esotropia. For instance, some accommodative esotropes deteriorate to the nonaccommodative form, whereas others do not despite sharing similar characteristics such as the AC/A ratio (Raab and Spierer, 1986; Ludwig et al., 1988; von Noorden, 1990), whereas others with nonaccommodative esotropia that is apparently successfully aligned early in life develop an accommodative component (Baker and De Young-Smith, 1988).

Interpupillary Distance, Fovea-Disc Distance, and Angle κ

Interocular separation, typically measured as interpupillary distance, increases by a factor of 1.6 postnatally, from about 4.0 cm in the infant to 6.5 cm in the adult (Zimmerman et al., 1929; Aslin and Dumais, 1980). This growth has the effect of increasing the stereo base, i.e., the angular disparity between two points a fixed z-axis distance apart. Maintaining depth-gauging accuracy during this period seems to be one of the major adaptive justifications for neural plasticity (Mitchell and Timney, 1984), suggested by the finding that the waning of the sensitive period in the cat coincides with completion of the developmental change in interpupillary distance (Timney, 1990).

There seems to be need of a stable geometric anatomical reference to base stereopsis calibration during

development, and a likely candidate is the position of the fovea at the eye's posterior pole, which remains constant throughout life (Packer et al., 1990). One source of interocular alignment error, then, would be displacement of that reference, such as the pseudoexotropia that arises from the macula being dragged temporally in those with ROP (Hunter and Mukai, 1992). There is evidence suggesting an abnormal temporal displacement of the area centralis in naturally microesotropic cats (Schoppmann and Hoffman, 1985; Distler and Hoffmann, 1991) and that angle κ in esotropia may have a similar origin (Scott and Mash, 1973). Subnormal interpupillary distance has been reported to be associated with esophoria (and hyperopia) in humans and supernormal interpupillary distance with exophoria (and myopia) (Ditmars, 1966); there is also evidence of a correlation between the peak of an apparently compensatory (monocular) Stiles-Crawford effect and the direction of phoria, a temporally biased peak in the eyes of esophoric subjects and a nasally biased peak in exophores (Bourdy, 1970).

CONCLUSIONS: CLINICAL AND RESEARCH IMPLICATIONS

Maternal Birth Posture

The possibility that birth-related cerebral, midbrain, cerebellar, or retinal insult may be a risk factor for strabismus and amblyopia suggests a reconsideration of contemporary obstetrical technique. One obvious candidate for such reconsideration is maternal birth posture. Use of the supine posture is a relatively recent innovation of Western culture, rather than the vertical birth posture in the form of squatting or other variants used in most other times and cultures (Naroll et al., 1961; Russell, 1982). In view of the stark threats of morbidity and mortality facing mother and infant in settings lacking modern obstetrical care, there has been fundamental incentive to devise the most efficient delivery method possible (Russell, 1982).

Vertical posture has, to begin with, the basic mechanical/hydraulic advantage over the supine position of making gravity's action on the fetus an ally rather than an obstacle to be overcome by increased contractive effort on the part of the mother. Of note here is the fact that the expulsive effort in supine deliveries has, necessarily, a forced lateral fetal motion component completely absent from vertical deliveries. Furthermore, the supine position has the negative consequence of maternal hypotension in some cases, apparently due to venous compression by the uterus on the inferior vena cava (Ellington et al., 1991), with fetal asphyxia in some cases as well (Humphrey et al., 1973). Simply tilting the mother laterally out of the supine position appears to have beneficial hemodynamic effects (Humphrey et al., 1973; Johnstone et al., 1987; Ellington et al., 1991). Vertical posture or an approximation to it seems to increase the transverse and anteroposterior diameters of the birth outlet and the sagittal diameter of the birth inlet (Russell, 1982; Lilford et al., 1989) and has been reported to increase maternal capillary oxygen tension and decrease capillary carbon dioxide tension (Ang et al., 1969), reduce the duration of labor (Lu, 1974; Gardosi et al., 1989a), increase the regularity of uterine contractions (Lu, 1974), and reduce the need for forceps (Gardosi et al., 1989a,b), among other effects (Gardosi et al., 1989a,b; Stewart and Spiby, 1989; Editorial, 1990b). An important distinction appears to be that a vertical posture assumed by means of a birth chair reduces much of the effectiveness of the posture (Crowley et al., 1991) owing to the changed weight distribution of sitting compared to kneeling or squatting (Gardosi et al., 1989a). [Use of a "birth cushion" has been reported effective in terms of aiding the mother to maintain upright posture while providing obstetrical access (Brown, 1989; Gardosi, 1989; Gardosi et al., 1989a; Gupta et al., 1989; Samra et al., 1989).] There is even some evidence suggesting that not simply a vertical posture but ambulation during at least the first stage of labor is beneficial, e.g., shortening labor (Lupe and Gross, 1986; Roberts, 1989).

There appear to have been no eye-morbidity-related studies of neonates in regard to birth posture outcome. Of particular interest in the present context would be a study of retinal hemorrhage incidence as a measure of hydraulic stress on the retina and a longer-term follow-up case-controlled study comparing strabismus incidence in supine versus, for instance, cushion-aided squat deliveries.

Recapitulation in Strabismus and Amblyopia Treatment

Strabismus and amblyopia are not *deus ex machina* dysfunctions; they arise as adaptive reactions to a set of abnormal ocular sensorimotor conditions. Therapeutically riding roughshod over the adaptive state that has given rise to them may thus exacerbate rather than relieve the sensorimotor dysfunction. Certainly there must be food for thought in the fact that, on the one hand, no infant begins life esotropic (Archer and Helveston, 1989; see also Chapter 22) and, on the other, that "subnormal binocular vision" (von Noorden, 1988a,b, 1990) is the best achievable binocular vision outcome by current surgery-oriented treatment techniques—and for only a minority of patients (Dobson and Sebris, 1989; Birch et al., 1990). Futhermore, long-term follow-up data indicate instability or deterioration of interocular alignment in some successfully treated

strabismic infants such as a patient achieving a stereoacuity of 40 arc seconds at the age of 8 years subsequently developing dissociated vertical deviation and losing his level of stereoacuity (Hiles et al., 1980).

A key question, highlighted by current studies of early refractive correction for strabismus and amblyopia prophylaxis (Ingram et al., 1990, 1991; see also Chapter 21) is whether early nonsurgical intervention can produce better binocular results. One theme of any such approach appears to be the need to bring the infant's visual status into congruence with normal-for-date status in the bi-ocular to global stereopsis development process. It may even be useful to consider reducing visual performance temporarily to that of an earlier ontogenetic state and recapitulating the normal development sequence.

One critical need in the strabismic infant is to improve fusional capacity. We noted earlier that fixation at near increases both the Panum's area for UC disparity and the tolerance of binocular rivalry (Richards, 1970b, 1971b), both antiesotropic compensations. This mechanism may partially explain the nystagmus "compensation" or "blockage" form of convergent strabismus (von Noorden, 1990, p. 438). That is, whether the mechanism is based on a monocular receptive field "zoom" increase (Richards, 1968) or binocular Panum increase (Richards, 1971b), near viewing may reduce the nystagmus through reduced spatial frequency sensitivity rather than simply dampening the nystagmus through mechanical constriction of muscle action. The implication is that creating conditions that stimulate convergence or accommodation, rather than relieving them, may aid the infant in such cases.

Refraction. The hyperopia of many infants (see Chapters 1 and 3) stimulates accommodation and convergence, and the question arises as to whether this too is a Panum's area-enlarging, "fusion-tropic" mechanism. The against-the-rule astigmatism (i.e., hyperopic in the vertical axis) of many (caucasian) infants (see Chapter 1) preferentially favors resolution of lateral-disparity-stimulating contours, suggesting a refractive "stereo-tropic" vector as well. It is of interest in this regard that there is less reduction of against-the-rule astigmatism with development in such infants than is the case for with-the-rule astigmatism (see Chapter 21).[10] Thus fusion effects and not simply ametropia may need to be taken into account when determining an appropriate correction. Failure to consider this aspect may explain the unpre-

---

10. There is also evidence of an unusually high incidence of substantial with-the-rule astigmatism of corneal origin in albinos (Dickinson and Abadi, 1984) and correlated horizontal grating acuity deficits (Bedell and Loshin, 1991), suggesting a melanin-associated genetic basis for astigmatism development.

dictable combination of efficacy and failure found to result from early fitting of partial corrections in reducing strabismus and amblyopia incidence (Ingram et al., 1990, 1991; see also Chapter 21) as well as the other traditional problems when predicting treatment outcome in the accommodative component of esotropia. The correction may create a developmental asynchrony-like condition in which monocular acuity and hence monocular predominance (Figure 25-7) is refractively improved beyond what the stereopsis or fusion system can integrate or control binocularly at that developmental stage or if there are abnormalities in either of those systems. The result would be to exacerbate rather than relieve a condition of amblyopiagenic rivalry. For instance, presenting large-disparity high spatial frequency stereograms that an (adult) subject cannot fuse causes the vergence system to go into unstable oscillation (Mowforth et al., 1981), suggesting a model of strabismus or nystagmus. Similarly, correcting against-the-rule astigmatism, at least in caucasian infants (Thorn et al., 1987), may be removing a needed stereotropic capacity, in keeping with demonstrations of significant increase of relative risk of amblyopia (again in caucasians, apparently) in with-the-rule astigmatism (Sjöstrand and Abrahamsson, 1990).

One possible implication that becomes apparent here is that, as noted above, instead of attempting to maximize all aspects of visual and motor function simultaneously, thereby in effect contravening the adaptive strabismic state, deliberate retardation of one function while the other(s) developmentally "catches up" in recapitulation fashion is sometimes appropriate. Thus bilateral contrast reduction via optical fogging may be called for to retard monocular acuity maturation and maintain sloppy but functional ocular alignment until a delayed fusion substrate development becomes appropriately functionally synchronous. Similarly, deliberately creating a condition of myopic against-the-rule astigmatism to enhance disparity-stimulating vertical contour resolution at near might be called for in infants with a disparity-sensing deficit, or, conversely, myopic with-the-rule astigmatism to degrade such contours to retard stereoscopic development into synchrony with delayed fusion/vergence development.

One implication of this reasoning is that further investigation may be warranted into devising extended-wear contact lenses practical for routine use with infants. The hyperopic or cylindrical corrections that are required to correct significant infant ametropia, when used in a spectacle format, replace the ametropic blur in the periphery with blur from optical aberration that may interfere with fusion and hence fusional control of alignment, as illustrated clinically (Jampolsky, 1978) and in modeling experiments using stabilized annular (i.e., peripheral) scotomas (Boman and Kertesz, 1985a).

Occlusion. Question has periodically been raised about the threat of occlusion treatment of amblyopia to the development of binocular vision (Hubel and Wiesel, 1963; Wiesel and Hubel, 1963; Jampolsky, 1978; Simons and Reinecke, 1978; Schor, 1983; Harwerth et al., 1991). The great neural vulnerability of binocular vision to irreversible rupture, compared to monocular vision's relative robustness (Timney, 1983, 1990; Crawford et al., 1989, 1991; Harwerth et al., 1989, 1991; Mitchell, 1991), binocularity's particular sensibility to conditions of interocular imbalance, and patching's potential for causing strabismus or increasing a preexisting angle of deviation in both animal models (reviewed by Quick et al., 1989) and human patients (von Noorden, 1990, p. 469; Holbach et al., 1991), suggest that the monocular acuity-maximization priority used to justify occlusion may work against stereopsis achievement, maintenance, or improvement. Alternating occlusion to some extent between eyes is used clinically to prevent occlusion amblyopia (von Noorden, 1990, p. 468). However, animal studies indicate alternating occlusion causes as great binocular deficit as unilateral occlusion (Mitchell and Timney, 1984; Tyschen et al., 1991), unless, that is, the occlusion is alternated every 500 ms or less (Altmann et al., 1987).

The "neurontropy" model implies that sound eye occlusion improves the amblyopic eye's vision by overriding the binocular predominance mechanism and allowing the consequently disinhibited amblyopic eye to move up the neurontropy scale and make full use of its monocular cone-position-known image disorder-compensation mechanism (Hirsch and Miller, 1987).[11] However, this situation may be achieved at the price of moving the amblyope phylogenetically backward from binocularity toward the more primitive condition of interocularly independent pools of monocular neurons in the central visual field, similar to those normally found in the temporal crescents. [That the connections are inhibited and not ruptured is demonstrated in amblyopic patients whose vision is improved with administration of levodopa and by amblyopes and primate models that regain vision in an amblyopic eye in postdevelopmental life when vision is lost in the sound eye (Tommilla, 1964; Harwerth et al., 1986; Tierney, 1989).] This point is illustrated by the converse case in a monkey model: If binocularity is ruptured by optically induced strabismus prior to occlusion onset, most of the deleterious monocular effects of occlusion are prevented (Smith et al., 1991).

The neurontropy model also predicts that the amount of improvement possible in the amblyopic eye is a func-

---

11. Flom and Bedell (1983) proposed, similarly, that patching results in remapping of visual space but on the basis of error feedback to saccadic eye movements.

tion of the extent to which that eye's disinhibited mapping distortion compensation mechanism is able to effect mapping correction in its monocular global form processing (Fig. 25-7). To the extent that the mapping distortion variance exceeds the available compensation capacity, the model predicts that the eye will remain amblyopic in true "organic" (von Noorden, 1990) amblyopia style despite occlusion treatment. There seems to be some support for this idea in the long-term follow-up evidence that amblyopic patients whose disorder compensation mechanism is adequate to allow achievement of normal or near-normal acuity from occlusion treatment are more likely to maintain their improvement than are patients unable to achieve such acuity levels (Scott and Dickey, 1988), presumably because the distortion compensation limits are exceeded.

The problem with patching from a retinotopic mapping point of view is that animal experiments indicate that deprivation results in expansion of the cortical dominance columns of the nondeprived eye at the expense of the cortical area occupied by those of the deprived eye (Wiesel, 1982). Thus patching appears to introduce a further interocular mapping distortion discrepancy at the cortical level in addition to that originally causing the amblyopic adaptive response. This effect seems particularly well modeled in reverse-sutured cats, whose original occlusion-induced mapping distortion is presumably counterdistorted by the reverse occlusion. In fact, mapping position-sensitive Vernier acuity (Levi et al., 1987) is relatively more reduced than grating acuity in these cats, to the extent that the Vernier threshold in some cases becomes a "hypoacuity," i.e., absolutely worse than grating acuity (Murphy and Mitchell, 1991). The mapping modification of occlusion is also illustrated in the Siamese cat, which has innate temporal hemiretina interocular mapping discrepancies. These discrepancies are eliminated by occlusion, allowing normal function to develop in the temporal hemiretina of the nondeprived eye (Guillery and Casagrande, 1974). Indeed, if the albino heterozygote hypothesis of amblyopia origin is correct, this Siamese model may directly illustrate the basis of the improvement of vision from patching.

In addition to reduction of binocular function itself, another binocular implication of occlusion-induced mapping distortion is suggested by the familiar clinical finding of recurrence of amblyopia at the end of a regimen of patching treatment, i.e., when binocular stimulation is resumed (von Noorden, 1990, p. 469). This effect is seen in the animal model in the finding that visual improvement obtained in a reverse-occluded eye may be lost when that eye is exposed to binocular viewing conditions, with the vision of the other eye often reduced as well (Mitchell, 1991; Murphy and Mitchell, 1991). This rule applies even when the reverse depri-

vation is interleaved with initial deprivation via occlusion alternated on a daily basis (Mitchell, 1991). This effect is reminiscent of the acuity reductions in both the sound and amblyopic eyes often demonstrable in human amblyopes under haploscopic viewing conditions (Awaya and von Noorden, 1972; Morgan et al., 1972).

An alternative to the monocular vision-maximizing occlusion approach would be to make binocular vision the initial priority for treatment and reduce the image quality in a graded manner in one or both eyes sufficient to reestablish crude binocular function. Then image quality would be titrated back up to at least an approximation to normal-for-date levels of binocular and monocular vision in recapitulation-like fashion. This approach would not undo a genetically determined mapping distortion, but it might produce a better binocular result than occlusion. Such an approach does not seem to have received extensive clinical consideration. At present, creating such interocular image quality asymmetry is typically thought of as a postocclusion acuity maintenance technique using fogging filters, with the sound eye fogged to an acuity level below that of the postocclusion amblyopic eye (von Noorden, 1990), although there have been occasional anecdotal reports of use of such filters to improve amblyopic stereopsis function (e.g., Rubin, 1965). Yet it seems possible that the efficacy of the "penalization" treatment of amblyopia (von Noorden, 1990, p. 471) may result from creating just such a compensatory image quality asymmetry. That is, penalization creates a condition of graded interocular relative blur that at some point in the anteroposterior axis (i.,e., z-axis) may allow fusion. Unfortunately, there apparently remain sufficient conflicting rivalrous stereo matches at other binocular visual field lateral and z-axis locations, so the results of penalization may be equivocal. The neurontropy model suggests that nonrefractive compensatory graded vision reduction works more effectively in this respect, specifically by invoking the stereo "repulsion" mechanism (Westheimer, 1986; Levi and Westheimer, 1987; Stevenson et al., 1991) in off-horopter mismatch-tolerant fusional space (Yang and Blake, 1991). The reader can model this treatment by squinting at the amblyopia-modeling stereograms of Figure 25-9 or viewing them through two or three layers of a contrast-reducing plastic sandwich bag (Simons, 1984). Neutral density filter-modulated compensation for "temporal amblyopia" stereo time-encoding anomalies may also be required (Wesson, 1983).

Surgery. As in the case of the glasses and patching, so surgically compromised muscle function may present the (by definition) already compromised strabismic sensorimotor system with a new condition that is as much challenge as solution. Indeed, if in fact a maturational delay of fusion is responsible for the strabismus, the surgery may turn out to be a permanent "solution" to what was a temporary developmental problem, with, as in the case of patching, binocular dysfunction-exacerbating sequelae. Results ranging from postsurgical susceptibility to amblyopia induced in previously cross-fixing eyes (Hoyt et al., 1984), to consecutive exotropia, to less obvious confounding variables that muscle surgery may introduce into the infant or child's oculomotor gain calibration process (Aslin, 1988) suggest caution when drawing conclusions as to the true binocular visual efficacy of early surgery.

A second question here is of the utility of the alternative concept of fitting prism as compensatory for nonparetic strabismus, an issue that has long been controversial (von Noorden, 1990, p. 460ff). Wearing of such prisms during testing has been demonstrated to aid stereo function in pre- and postoperative esotropic infants and toddlers (Birch and Stager, 1985; Mohindra et al., 1985; Stager and Birch, 1986; Birch et al., 1990). [A study that did not use the prisms failed to replicate this finding (Dobson and Sebris, 1989).][12] Long-term compensatory prism wearing prior to surgery has been found to improve binocular function in some older children with acquired esotropia (Prism Adaptation Study Research Group, 1990) and optically similar treatment with wide-angle fusional stimulation to have some fusion-improving efficacy even in adult strabismics (Kertesz, 1982, 1983b).

Photoprotection for Strabismus and Amblyopia

The use of photoreceptive filters for prophylaxis against photic insult effects in age-related macular degeneration and ROP has been suggested (Glass et al., 1985; Mainster, 1987; Young, 1988; Gottsch et al., 1990; Simons, in press). To the extent that phototoxicity is a risk factor for strabismus and amblyopia, it may be useful to consider such filters for prophylaxis here as well. Infant ametropia may provide some protection against photic insult by preventing focused illumination on the retina. If the ametropia is corrected, again perhaps use of photoprotective corrections should be considered.

Early Screening and Esotropia Prophylaxis

Evidence that esotropia has a postnatal onset (Archer and Helveston, 1989; see also Chapter 22) suggests the possibility of not simply early corrective intervention but perhaps outright prophylaxis, as does evidence of

reduction of strabismus incidence resulting from early refractive correction (Ingram et al., 1991a,b; see also Chapter 21). Prophylaxis by definition requires new methods of detection of not simply manifest deviation but of developmental precursors to such deviation. Refractive precursors have received considerable attention. Other measures might also be of use. An indexed ratio standard comparing performance on a binocular fusion test (see Chapters 12, 13, and 15) and monocular OKN asymmetry (see Chapters 23 and 26), for instance, might serve to quantify the relative early status of the binocular and monocular vision systems in prestereocapable young infants (i.e., under 3 months of age), with a substandard ratio constituting an early flag for incipient strabismus.

If the birth-stress-based retinal microdetachment theory is valid, techniques for early detection of cone matrix malformation such as those used for objective determination of the Stiles-Crawford effect (van Blokland, 1986) may have screening potential. Such measures, as well as other instrumented means of objectively quantifying infant ocular scatter or retinal densitometry (Kilbride et al., 1989), may provide more information about the phototoxicity hazard in infant eyes and constitute a potential screening modality.

Binocular Heredity

In view of strabismus being by definition a binocular dysfunction, and in view of it having a certain, if poorly defined, genetic component (Aurrell and Norsell, 1990; von Noorden, 1990, p. 144ff), there seems reason to consider renewed study of the binocular vision components of heredity in light of contemporary knowledge of binocular vision to determine if more explicit hereditary risk factors can be specified. More investigation of the binocular capabilities of albino heterozygotes seems to be a potentially fruitful line of inquiry. There is also evidence of a lack of binocular cells in congenitally strabismic cats (Hoffmann and Schoppmann, 1984). In humans, families of propositi with "low binocularity" without deviation (Richter, 1976) or with microtropia (Cantolino and von Noorden, 1969) or large angle eso- or exotropia (Niederecker et al., 1972; Smith et al., 1972; Mash et al., 1975) have been found to have reduced horizontal fusional vergence amplitudes and reduced stereoacuity on local stereopsis (monocularly visible target contour) stereotests (Wirt or Titmus circles). However, there appear to be as yet no studies of heritability patterns of signed disparity stereoacuity, although genetic defects in these mechanisms have been hypothesized (Richards, 1971a, 1975); nor are there heritability studies of global (e.g., random dot) stereopsis, signed or relative, or vertical fusional vergence amplitudes. Vertical fusional vergence amplitude seems to be of in-

---

12. A study of residual stereopsis in adult strabismic patients also utilized compensatory prism (Schor et al., 1983a).

terest for several reasons: (1) the high incidence of vertical anomalies, including dissociated vertical deviation, oblique overactions, and rotary nystagmus (which has a vertical component), in early esotropia (von Noorden, 1990); (2) the vertical amplitude's normally small size relative to horizontal amplitudes (Kertesz, 1983a) and the corresponding relative small size of the vertical dimension of Panum's area (Tyler, 1983) and hence relatively greater susceptibility to degradation from a given degree of function loss than in the horizontal dimension (Nielsen and Poggio, 1984), potentially giving rise in turn to a horizontal deviation (Burian, 1950); (3) the reduction of vertical fusional vergence amplitudes by larger horizontal disparities (Boman and Kertesz, 1983), meaning that genetically reduced amplitudes could magnify the degradative effect on stereoscopic function of retinotopic mapping distortion; and (4) conversely, the association of abnormally large vertical amplitudes and dissociated vertical deviation in early-onset esotropia (von Noorden, 1990).

Finally, in view of the possible significance of birthing variables to strabismus and amblyopia onset suggested in this chapter, further study of these variables is suggested, perhaps including instrumented deliveries (Svenningsen et al., 1987). It also may be appropriate to consider nonvisual hereditary variables, such as maternal pelvic diameter versus infant head and trunk diameter.

Acknowledgments. The author gratefully acknowledges comments received on earlier versions of this manuscript by Richard Aslin, Ph.D., Eileen Birch, Ph.D., Anne Fulton, M.D., David L. Guyton, M.D., and David Hunter, M.D., Ph.D.

REFERENCES

ABADI, R. V., AND PASCAL, E. (1991). Visual resolution in human albinism. *Vision Res.* 31, 1445–1448.

ABADI, R. V., DICKINSON, C. M., PASCAL, E., PAPAS, E. (1990). Retinal image quality in albinos: a review. *Ophthalmic Pediatr. Genet.* 11, 171–176.

ACKERMAN, B., SHERWORIT, E., AND WILLIAMS, J. (1989). Reduced incidental light exposure: effect on the development of retinopathy of prematurity in low birth weight infants. *Pediatrics* 83, 958–962.

ADLER-GRINBERG, D. (1986). Need for eye and vision care in an under-served population: refractive errors and other ocular anomalies in the Sioux. *Am. J. Optom. Physiol. Opt.* 63, 553–558.

AICHMAIR, H. (1975). Risk factors inducing the formation of concomitant squint. *Klin. Monatsbl. Augenheilkd.* 167, 311–313.

AKEO, K., EBENSTEIN, D. B., AND DOREY, C. K. (1989). Dopa and oxygen inhibit proliferation of retinal pigment epithelial cells, fibroblasts and endothelial cells in vitro. *Exp. Eye Res.* 49, 335–346.

ALTMANN, L., LUHMANN, H. J., GREUEL, J. M., AND SINGER, W. (1987). Functional and neuronal binocularity in kittens raised with rapidly alternating monocular occlusion. *J. Neurophysiol.* 58, 965–980.

AMENIYA, T., IIDA, Y., AND YOSHIDA, H. (1983). Subjective and objective disturbances in reattached retina after surgery for retinal detachment, with special reference to visual acuity and metamorphopsia. *Ophthalmologica* 186, 25–30.

ANG, C. K., TAN, T. H., WALTERS, W. A., WOOD, C. (1969). Postural influence on maternal capillary oxygen and carbon dioxide tension. *BMJ* 4, 201.

APKARIAN, P., AND REITES, D. (1989). Global stereopsis in human albinos. *Vision Res.* 29, 1359–1370.

ARCHER, S. M., AND HELVESTON, E. M. (1989). Strabismus and eye movement disorders. In S. J. ISENBERG (ed.). *The Eye in Infancy.* Chicago: Year Book Medical Publishers.

ARCHER, S. M., HELVESTON, E. M., MILLER, K. K., AND ELLIS, F. (1986). Stereopsis in normal infants and infants with congenital esotropia. *Am. J. Ophthalmol.* 101, 591.

ASLIN, R. N. (1988). Anatomical constraints on oculomotor development: implications for infant perception. In A. YONAS (ed.). *Perceptual Development in Infancy.* Hillsdale, NJ: Erlbaum.

ASLIN, R., AND DUMAIS, S. (1980). Binocular vision in infants, a review and theoretical framework. *Adv. Child Dev.* 15, 53.

ASLIN, R. N., DOBSON, V., AND JACKSON, R. W. (1982). Dark vergence and dark focus in human infants. *Invest. Ophthalmol. Vis. Sci.* 22 (suppl.), 105.

ATKINSON, J. (1984). Human visual development over the first 6 months of life: a review and a hypothesis. *Hum. Neurobiol.* 3, 61–74.

ATKINSON, J., SMITH, J., ANKER, S., WATTAM-BELL, J., BRADDICK, O., AND MOORE, T. (1991). Binocularity and amblyopia before and after early strabismus surgery. *Invest. Ophthalmol. Vis. Sci.* 32 (suppl.), 820.

AURRELL, E., AND NORRSELL, K. (1990). A longitudinal study of children with a family history of strabismus. *Br. J. Ophthalmol.* 74, 589–594.

AWAYA, S., AND VON NOORDEN, G. K. (1972). Visual acuity of amblyopic eyes under monocular and binocular conditions. *J. Pediatr. Ophthalmol.* 9, 8–13.

BADCOCK, D. R., AND SCHOR, C. M. (1985). Depth-increment detection function for individual spatial channels. *J. Opt. Soc. Am. [A]* 2, 1211–1215.

BAGOLINI, B., AND CAPOBIANCO, N. M. (1965). Subjective space in comitant squint. *Am. J. Ophthalmol.* 59, 430–442.

BAILEY, J. E., LAKSHMINARAYANAN, V., AND ENOCH, J. M. (1991). The Stiles-Crawford function in an aphakic subject with retinitis pigmentosa. *Clin. Vis. Sci.* 6, 165–170.

BAKER, J. D., AND DE YOUNG-SMITH, M. (1988). Accommodative esotropia following surgical correction of congenital esotropia, frequency and characteristics. *Graefes Arch. Clin. Exp. Ophthalmol.* 226, 175–177.

BALKEMA, G. W., AND DRÄGER, U. C. (1990). Origins of uncrossed retinofugal projections in normal and hypopigmented mice. *Vis. Neurosci.* 4, 595–604.

BANKS, M. S., AND BENNETT, P. J. (1988). Optical and photoreceptor immaturities limit the spatial and chromatic vision of human neonates. *J. Opt. Soc. Am. [A]* 5, 2059–2079.

BEDELL, H. E. (1980). Central and peripheral retinal photoreceptor orientation in amblyopic eyes as assessed by the psychophysical Stiles-Crawford function. *Invest. Ophthalmol. Vis. Sci.* 19, 49–59.

BEDELL, H. E., AND FLOM, M. C. (1983). Normal and abnormal space perception. *Am. J. Optom. Physiol. Opt.* 60, 426–435.

BEDELL, H. E., AND LOSHIN, D. S. (1991). Interrelations between measures of visual acuity and parameters of eye movement in congenital nystagmus. *Invest. Ophthalmol. Vis. Sci.* 32, 416–421.

BEDELL, H. E., ENOCH, J. M., AND FITZGERALD, C. R. (1981). Photoreceptor orientation: a graded disturbance bordering a region of choroidal atrophy. *Arch. Ophthalmol.* 99, 1841.

BEDELL, H. S., FLOM, M. C., AND BARBEITO, R. (1985). Spatial aberrations and acuity in strabismus and amblyopia. *Invest. Ophthalmol. Vis. Sci.* 26, 909–916.

BERG, P. H. (1982). Effect of light intensity on the prevalence of exotropia in strabismus populations. *Br. Orthoptic J.* 39, 55–56.

BERGEN, R., AND MARGOLIS, S. (1976). Retinal hemorrhages in the newborn. *Ann. Ophthalmol.* 8, 53–56.

BERLER, D. K. (1989). Müller cell alterations from long-term ambient fluorescent light exposure in monkeys: light and electron microscopic fluorescein and lipofuscin study. *Trans. Am. Ophthalmol. Soc.* 87, 553–576.

BESIO, R., CABALLERO, C., MEERHOFF, E., AND SCHWARZ, R. (1979). Neonatal retinal hemorrhages and influence of perinatal factors. *Am. J. Ophthalmol.* 87, 74–76.

BILLINGS, E. L. (1969). Traumatic and anoxic births: follow-up examination of 478 babies. *Med. J. Aust.* 2, 1146–1151.

BIRCH, E., GWIAZDA, J., AND HELD, R. (1982). Stereoacuity development for crossed and crossed disparities in human infants. *Vision Res.* 22, 507.

BIRCH, E. E., AND HALE, L. A. (1989). Operant assessment of stereoacuity. *Clin. Vis. Sci.* 4, 295–300.

BIRCH, D. G., AND SANDBERG, M. A. (1982). Psychophysical studies of cone optical bandwidth in patients with retinitis pigmentosa. *Vision Res.* 22, 1113–1118.

BIRCH, E. E., AND STAGER, D. R. (1985). Monocular acuity and stereopsis in infantile esotropia. *Invest. Ophthalmol. Vis. Sci.* 26, 1624.

BIRCH, E., AND SPENCER, R. (1991). Visual outcome in infants with cicatricial retinopathy of prematurity. *Invest. Ophthamol. Vis. Sci.* 32, 410–415.

BIRCH, E. E., SHIMOJO, S., AND HELD, R. (1985). Preferential-looking assessment of fusion and stereopsis in infants aged 1 to 6 months. *Invest. Ophthalmol. Vis. Sci.* 26, 366–370.

BIRCH, E. E., STAGER, D. R., BERRY, P., AND EVERETT, M. E. (1990). Prospective assessment of acuity and stereopsis in amblyopic infantile esotropes following early surgery. *Invest. Ophthalmol. Vis. Sci.* 31, 758–765.

BISHOP, P. O., AND HENRY, G. H. (1971). Spatial vision. *Annu. Rev. Psychol.* 22, 119–160.

BIST, H. K., SINGH, M., SATSANGI, S. K., ET AL. (1989). Retinal hemorrhages in newborn—fetal causative factors. *Indian Pediatr.* 26, 558–565.

BLAKE, R. (1989). A neural theory of binocular rivalry. *Psychol. Rev.* 96, 145–167.

BLAKE, R., YANG, Y., AND WILSON, H. R. (1991). On the coexistance of stereopsis and binocular rivalry. *Vision Res.* 31, 1191–1203.

BLAKEMORE, C. (1970). The range and scope of binocular depth discrimination in man. *J. Physiol. (Lond.)* 211, 599.

BLAKEMORE, C. (1988). The sensitive periods in the monkey's visual cortex. In G. LENNERSTRAND, G. K. VON NOORDEN, E. C. CAMPOS (eds.). *Strabismus and Amblyopia. Experimental Basis for Advances in Clinical Management.* New York: Plenum.

BLANK, K., AND ENOCH, J. M. (1973). Monocular spatial distortions induced by marked accommodation. *Science* 182, 392–395.

BLANK, K., PROVINE, R. R., AND ENOCH, J. M. (1975). Shift in the peak of the photopic Stiles-Crawford function with marked accommodation. *Vision Res.* 15, 499–507.

BOMAN, D. K., AND KERTESZ, A. E. (1983). Interaction between horizontal and vertical fusional responses. *Percept. Psychophys.* 33, 565.

BOMAN, D. K., AND KERTESZ, A. E. (1985a). Horizontal fusional responses to stimuli containing artificial scotomas. *Invest. Ophthalmol. Vis. Sci.* 26, 1051–1056.

BOMAN, D. K., AND KERTESZ, A. E. (1985b). Fusional responses of strabismics to foveal and extrafoveal stimulation. *Invest. Ophthalmol. Vis. Sci.* 26, 1731–1739.

BONE, R. A., LANDRUM, J. T., FERNANDEZ, L., AND TARSIS, S. L. (1988). Analysis of the macular pigment by HPLC retinal distribution and age study. *Invest. Ophthalmol. Vis. Sci.* 29, 843–849.

BORGES, J., ZONG-LI, L., AND TSO, M. O. M. (1990). Effects of repeated photic exposures on the monkey macula. *Arch Ophthalmol.* 108, 727–733.

BORWEIN, B. (1981). The retinal receptor: a description. In J. M. ENOCH AND F. L. TOBEY JR. (eds.). *Vertebrate Photoreceptor Optics.* New York: Springer-Verlag.

BOULTON, M., DOCCHIO, F., DAYHAW-BARKER, P., RAMPONI, R., AND CUBEDDU, R. (1990). Age-related changes in the morphology, absorption and fluorescence of melanosomes and lipofuscin granules of the retinal pigment epithelium. *Vision Res.* 30, 1291–1230.

BOURDY, C. (1970). Effet Stiles-Crawford, et fixation. *Vision Res.* 10, 859–874.

BOURDY, C. (1973). Etude des variations des disparite's re'tiniennes autour du point de fixation par le me'thode du Vernier binoculaire dans la re'gion fove'le. *Vision Res.* 13, 149–160.

BOWER, T. G. B. (1966). Stereopsis by binocular delay. *Nature* 248, 363–364.

BRADLEY, A., AND FREEMAN, R. D. (1985). Is reduced vernier acuity in amblyopia due to position, contrast or fixation deficits? *Vision Res.* 25, 55–66.

BRADLEY, A., FREEMAN, R. D., AND APPLEGATE, A. R. (1985). Is amblyopia spatial frequency or retinal locus specific? *Vision Res.* 25, 47–54.

BRENNER, R. L., CHARLES, S. T., AND FLYNN, J. T. (1969). Pupillary responses in rivalry and amblyopia. *Arch. Ophthalmol.* 82, 23–29.

BROWN, B., AND SUTTER, E. E. (1991). Pattern ERG in amblyopia: a case report and demonstration of a new technique. Paper presented at the Annual Meeting, American Academy of Optometry.

BROWN, S. J. (1989). Squatting in the second stage of labor [letter to the editor]. *Lancet* 2, 750.

BRUCE, A., HURST, M. A., ABBOTT, H., AND HARRISON, H. (1991). The incidence of refractive error and anomalies of binocular vision in infants. *Br. Orthopt. J.* 48, 32–35.

BULLOCK, J. D. (1990). Relative afferent pupillary defect in the "better" eye. *J. Clin. Neuro. Ophthalmol.* 10, 45–51.

BURGESS, P., AND JOHNSON, A. (1991). Ocular defects in infants of extremely low birth weight and gestational age. *Br. J. Ophthalmol.* 75, 84–86.

BURIAN, H. M. (1950). Etiology of heterophoria and heterotropia. In J. Y. ALLEN (ed.). *Strabismus Ophthalmic Symposium.* St. Louis: Mosby.

BURIAN, H. (1959). Discussion. *Am. J. Ophthalmol.* 48, 273–274.

BURIAN, H. M. (1972). Hypermetropia and esotropia. *J. Pediatr. Ophthalmol.* 9, 135.

BURNS, M. S., BELLHORN, R. W., KORTE, G. E., AND HERIOT, W. J. (1986). Plasticity of the retinal vasculature. *Prog. Retinal Res.* 5, 254–307.

BURR, D. C., MORRONE, M. C., AND ROSS, J. (1986). Local and global visual processing. *Vision Res.* 26, 749–757.

CANTOLINO, S. J., AND VON NOORDEN, G. K. (1969). Heredity in microtropia. *Arch. Ophthalmol.* 753.

CARNEY, T., PARADISO, M. A., AND FREEMAN, R. D. (1989). A physiological correlate of the Pulfrich effect in cortical neurons of the cat. *Vision Res.* 29, 1555–1565.

CASS, E. (1973). A decade of northern ophthalmology. *Can. J. Ophthalmol.* 8, 210–217.

CASS, E. (1976). Types of strabismus occurring among Indians and Eskimos of the Northwest Territories. In R. J. SHEPHARD AND S. ITOH (eds.). *Circumpolar Health Proceedings of the 3rd International Symposium.* Toronto: University of Toronto Press.

CATS, B. P., AND TAN, K. E. (1989). Prematures with and without regressed retinopathy of prematurity, comparison of long-term (6–10 years) ophthalmological morbidity. *J. Pediatr. Ophthalmol. Strabismus* 26, 271–275.

CHAVASSE, B. F. (1939). *Worth's Squint or the Binocular Reflexes and the Treatment of Strabismus.* Philadelphia, Blakiston.

CHELAZZI, L., MARZI, C. A., PANOZZO, G., PASQUALINI, N., TASSINARI, G., AND TOMAZZOLI, A. (1988). Hemiretinal differences in speed of light detection in esotropic amblyopes. *Vision Res.* 28, 95–104.

CHEN, B., AND MAKOUS, W. (1989). Light capture by human cones. *J. Physiol. (Lond.)* 414, 89–109.

CHIAPELLA, A. P., ROSENTHAL, A. R., EDWARDS, C., TANNER, J., FIELDER, A. R. (1984). Use of computers in ophthalmology: Leicester computer ophthalmology index. *Trans. Ophthalmol. Soc. UK* 104, 106.

CHINO, Y. M., SMITH, E. L., WADA, H., RIDDER, W. H., LANGSTON, A. L., AND LESHER, G. A. (1991). Disruption of binocularly correlated signals alters the postnatal development of spatial properties in cat striate cortical neurons. *J. Neurophysiol.* 65,841–859.

CINER, E. B., SHCNEL-KLITSCH, E., AND SCHEIMAN, M. (1991). Stereoacuity development in young children. *Optom. Vis. Sci.* 68, 533–536.

CIUFFREDA, K. J., AND KENYON, R. V. (1983). Accommodative vergence and accommodation in normals, amblyopes and strabismics. In C. M. SCHOR AND K. J. CIUFFREDA (eds.). *Vergence Eye Movements: Basic and Clinical Aspects.* London: Butterworths.

CLARKE, W. N., AND NOEL, L. P. (1982). Vanishing infantile esotropia. *Can. J. Ophthalmol.* 17, 100.

COLLETTA, N. J., AND WILLIAMS, D. R. (1987). Psychophysical estimate of extrafoveal cone spacing. *J. Opt. Soc. Am. [A]* 4, 1503.

COSTARIDOU, L., SPYROS, S., HIRSCH, J., AND ORPHANOUDAKIS, S. (1990). Image reconstruction based on human and monkey cone mosaics. *J. Vis. Comm. Image Rep.* 1, 137–152.

CRAWFORD, M. L. J., DE FABER, J-T., HARWERTH, R. S., AND VON NOORDEN, G. K. (1989). The effects of reverse monocular deprivation in monkeys. II. Electrophysiological and anatomical studies. *Exp. Brain Res.* 74, 338–347.

CRAWFORD, M. L. J., PESCH, T. W., VON NOORDEN, G. K., HARWERTH, R. S., AND SMITH, E. L. (1991). Bilateral form deprivation in monkeys: Electrophysiologic and anatomic consequences. *Invest. Ophthalmol. Vis. Sci.* 32, 2328–2336.

CREEL, D. J., SUMMERS, C. G., AND KING, R. A. (1990). Visual anomalies associated with albinism. *Ophthalmic Pediatr. Genet.* 11, 193–200.

CRONLY-DILLON, J., ROSEN, E. S., AND MARSHALL, J. (eds.) (1986). *Hazards of Light.* London: Pergamon.

CROWLEY, P., ELBOURNE, D., ASHURST, H., GARCIA, J., MURPHY, D., AND DUIGNAN, N. (1991). Delivery in an obstetric birth chair, a randomized controlled trial. *Br. J. Obstet. Gynaecol.* 98, 667–674.

CURCIO, C. A., AND HENDRICKSON, A. E. (1991). Organization and development of the primate photoreceptor mosaic. *Prog. Retinal Res.* 10, 89–120.

CURCIO, C. A., SLOAN, K. R., CALINA, R. E., AND HENDRICKSON, A. E. (1990). Human photoreceptor topography. *J. Comp. Neurol.* 292, 497–523.

CURCIO, C. A., SLOAN, K. R., PACKER, O., HENDRICKSON, A. E., AND KALINA, R. E. (1987). Distribution of cones in human and monkey retina: individual variability and radial asymmetry. *Science* 236, 579–582.

CURTIN, B. J. (1985). *The Myopias. Basic Science and Clinical Management.* Philadelphia: Harper and Row.

DAY, S. H., OREL-BIXLER, D. A., AND NORCIA, A. M. (1988). Abnormal acuity development in infantile esotropia. *Invest. Ophthalmol. Vis. Sci.* 29, 327–329.

DEVALOIS, R. L., AND DEVALOIS, K. K. (1988). *Spatial Vision.* New York: Oxford University Press.

DICKEY, D. F., METZ, H. S., STEWART, S. A., AND SCOTT, W. E. (1991). The diagnosis of amblyopia in cross-fixation. *J. Pediatr. Ophthalmol. Strabismus* 28, 171–175.

DICKINSON, C. M., AND ABADI, R. V. (1984). Corneal topography of humans with congenital nystagmus. *Ophthalmol. Physiol. Opt.* 4, 3–13.

DISTLER, C., AND HOFFMANN, K-P. (1991). Depth perception and cortical physiology in normal and innate microstrabismic cats. *Vis. Neurosci.* 6, 25–41.

DITMARS, D. (1966). Relationship between refractive error, phoria, and interpupillary distance in 500 patients. *J. Am. Optom. Assoc.* 37, 361.

DOBSON, V., AND SEBRIS, S. L. (1989). Longitudinal study of acuity and stereopsis in infants with or at-risk for esotropia. *Invest. Ophthalmol. Vis. Sci.* 30, 1146–1158.

DOREY, C. K., DELORI, F. C., AND AKEO, K. (1990). Growth of cultured RPE and endothelial cells is inhibited by blue light but not green or red light. *Curr. Eye Res.* 9, 549–558.

DOWD, J. M., CLIFTON, R. K., ANDERSON, D. R., AND EICHELMAN, W. H. (1980). Children perceive large-disparity random-dot stereograms more readily than adults. *J. Exp. Child Psychol.* 29, 1.

DRÄGER, U. C. (1985a). Albinism and visual pathways. *N. Engl. J. Med.* 314, 1636–1638.

DRÄGER, U. C. (1985b). Calcium binding in pigmented and albino eyes. *Proc. Natl. Acad. Sci. USA* 73, 6716–6720.

DUKE-ELDER, A. (1958). The eye in evolution. In S. DUKE-ELDER (ed.). *System of Ophthalmology.* Vol. I. St. Louis: Mosby.

DUKE-ELDER, S., AND COOK, C. (1963). Normal and abnormal development. Part 1. Embryology. In S. DUKE-ELDER (ed.). *System of Ophthalmology.* Vol. III. St. Louis: Mosby.

DYER, R. S., HOWELL, W. E., AND MACPHAIL, R. C. (1981). Dopamine depletion slows retinal transmission. *Exp. Neurol.* 71, 326.

Editorial (1972). MARY AGNES PUGH, MRCS, LRCP, 1900–1972. *Br. J. Ophthalmol.* 56, 382.

Editorial (1990a). The relationship between light and exotropia. *Binoc. Vis. Q.* 5, 11–12.

EDITORIAL (1990b). Stand and deliver. *Lancet* 335, 761–762.

EFRON, R., AND WOLFE, E. (1966). An unusual form of night-blindness associated with increased stereoscopic acuity. *Vision Res.* 6, 717–724.

EGGE, K., LYNG, G., AND MALTAU, J. M. (1980). Retinal haemorrhages in the newborn. *Acta Ophthalmol. (Copenh.)* 58, 231–236.

EGGE, K., LYNG, G., AND MALTAU, J. M. (1981). Effect of instrumental delivery on the frequency and severity of retinal hemorrhages in the newborn. *Acta Obstet. Gynecol. Scand.* 60, 153.

ELBERGER, A. J. (1989). Binocularity and single cell acuity are related in striate cortex of corpus callosum sectioned and normal cats. *Exp. Brain Res.* 77, 213–216.

ELBERGER, A. J. (1990). Spatial frequency threshold of single striate cortical cells in neonatal corpus callosum sectioned cats. *Exp. Brain Res.* 82, 617–627.

ELLINGHAM, T. R., SILVA, P. A., AND BUCKFIELD, P. M. (1976). Neonatal at risk factors, visual defects and the preschool child: a report from the Queen Mary Hospital multidisciplinary child development study. *N.Z. Med. J.* 83, 74–77

ELLINGTON, C., KATZ, V. L., WATSON, W. J., AND SPIELMAN, F. (1991). The effect of lateral tilt on maternal and fetal hemodynamic variables. *Obstet. Gynecol.* 77, 201–203.

ENOCH, J. M. (1957). Amblyopia and the Stiles-Crawford effect. *Am. J. Optom.* 34, 298–308.

ENOCH, J. M. (1959a). Further studies on the relationship between amblyopia and the Stiles-Crawford effect. *Am. J. Optom.* 36, 111–128.

ENOCH, J. M. (1959b). Receptor amblyopia. *Am. J. Ophthalmol.* 48, 262–273.

ENOCH, J. M. (1967). The current status of receptor amblyopia. *Doc. Ophthalmol.* 23, 130–148.

ENOCH, J. M. (1975). Marked accommodation, retinal stretch, monocular space perception and retinal receptor orientation. *Am. J. Optom. Physiol. Opt.* 52, 376.

ENOCH, J. M. (1981). Retinal receptor orientation and photoreceptor optics. In J. M. ENOCH AND F. L. TOBEY JR. (eds.). *Vertebrate Photoreceptor Optics*. New York: Springer-Verlag.

ENOCH, J. M., AND BEDELL, H. E. (1981). The Stiles-Crawford effects. In J. M. ENOCH AND F. L. TOBEY JR. (eds.). *Vertebrate Photoreceptor Optics*. New York: Springer-Verlag.

ENOCH, J. M., AND TOBEY, JR., F. L. (1981). Waveguide properties of retinal receptors: techniques and observations. In J. M. ENOCH AND F. L. TOBEY JR. (eds.). *Vertebrate Photoreceptor Optics*. New York: Springer-Verlag.

ENOCH, J. M., VAN LOO, J. A., AND OKUN, E. (1973). Realignment of photoreceptors disturbed in orientation secondary to retinal detachment. *Invest. Ophthalmol. Vis. Sci.* 12, 849–853.

ERKELENS, C. J., AND COLLEWIJN, H. (1985). Eye movements and stereopsis during dichoptic viewing of moving random dot stereograms. *Vision Res.* 25, 1689–1700.

ETTLINGER, G., BLAKEMORE, C. B., MILNER, A. D., AND WILSON, J. (1974). Agenesis of the corpus callosum: a further behavioural investigation. *Brain* 97, 225–234.

EUSTACE, P., WESSON, M. E., AND DRURY, D. J. (1973). The effect of illumination on intermittent divergent squint of the divergent excess type. *Trans. Ophthalmol. Soc. UK* 93, 559.

FAHLE, M. (1987). Naso-temporal asymmetry of binocular inhibition. *Invest. Ophthalmol. Vis. Sci.* 28, 1016–1017.

FANKHAUSER, F., ENOCH, J., AND CIBIS, P. (1961). Receptor orientation in retinal pathology. *Am. J. Ophthalmol.* 52, 767–783.

FENDRICH, R., AND GAZZANIGA, M. S. (1989). Evidence of foveal splitting in a commissurotomy patient. *Neuropsychologia* 27, 273–281.

FENDRICH, R., REUTER-LORENZ, P. A., AND HUGHES, H. C. (1990). A loss of global precedence with stimuli devoid of low spatial frequencies. *Invest. Ophthalmol. Vis. Sci.* 31 (suppl.), 324.

FERSTER, D. (1981). A comparison of binocular depth mechanisms in areas 17 and 18 of the cat visual cortex. *J. Physiol. (Lond.)* 311, 623–655.

FIELDER, A. R., ROBINSON, J., SHAW, D. E., NG, Y. K., AND MOSELEY, M. J. (in press). Light and retinopathy of prematurity, does retinal location offer a clue? *Pediatrics* 89, 648–653.

FIRTH, A. Y. (1990). Pupillary responses in amblyopia. *Br. J. Ophthalmol.* 74, 676–680.

FISHER, N. F. (1986). The optic chiasm and the corpus callosum: their relationship to binocular vision in humans. *J. Pediatr. Ophthalmol. Strabismus* 23, 126–131.

FITZGERALD, C. R., ENOCH, J. M., BIRCH, D. G., BENEDETTO, M. D., TEMME, L. A., AND DAWSON, W. W. (1980). Anomalous pigment epithelial photoreceptor relationships and receptor orientation. *Invest. Ophthalmol. Vis. Sci.* 19, 956.

FLANNERY, J. G., FARBER, D. B., BIRD, A. C., AND BOK, D. (1989). Degenerative changes in a retina affected with autosomal dominant retinitis pigmentosa. *Invest. Ophthalmol. Vis. Sci.* 30, 191–211.

FLEISHMAN, J. A., BECK, R. W., LINORES, O. A., AND KLEIN, J. W. (1987). Deficits in visual function after recovery from optic neuritis. *Ophthalmology* 94, 1029–1035.

FLETCHER, M. C. (1971). Natural history of idiopathic strabismus. In *Symposium on Strabismus. Transactions of the New Orleans Academy of Ophthalmology*. St. Louis: Mosby.

FLOM, M. C., AND BEDELL, H. E. (1983). Identifying amblyopia using associated conditions, acuity, and nonacuity features. *Am. J. Optom. Physiol. Opt.* 62, 153–160.

FOLK, E. (1979). Intermittent congenital esotropia. *Ophthalmology* 86, 2107.

FOX, R., PATTERSON, R., AND FRANCIS, E. L. (1986). Stereoacuity in young children. *Invest. Ophthalmol. Vis. Sci.* 27, 598.

FREEMAN, R. D., AND OHZAWA, I. (1990). On the neurophysiological organization of binocular vision. *Vision Res.* 30, 1661–1676.

FREEMAN, R. D., AND TSUMOTO, T. (1983). An electrophysiological comparison of convergent and divergent strabismus in the cat: electrical and visual activation of single cortical cells. *J. Neurophysiol.* 49, 238–253.

FRIEDMAN, J. R., KOSMORSKY, G. S., AND BURDE, R. M. (1985). Stereoacuity in patients with optic nerve disease. *Arch. Ophthalmol.* 103, 37–38.

FRISEN, L., HOYT, W. F., BIRD, A. C., AND WEALE, R. A. (1973). Diagnostic uses of the Pulfrich phenomenon. *Lancet* 2, 385.

FRONIUS, M., AND SIRETEANU, R. (1989). Monocular geometry is selectively distorted in the central visual field of strabismic amblyopes. *Invest. Ophthalmol. Vis. Sci.* 30, 2034–2044.

FULTON, A. B., DODGE, J., HANSEN, R. M., SCHREMSER, J-L., AND WILLIAMS, T. P. (1991). The quantity of rhodopsin in young human eyes. *Curr. Eye Res.* 10, 977–982.

GARDOSI, J. (1989). Squatting in the second stage of labor [letter to the editor]. *Lancet* 2, 750.

GARDOSI, J., HUTSON, N., AND B-LYNCH, C. (1989a). Randomised, controlled trial of squatting in the second stage of labor. *Lancet* 2, 74–77.

GARDOSI, J., SYLVESTER, S., AND B-LYNCH, C. (1989b). Alternative positions in the second stage of labor, a randomized controlled trial. *Br. J. Obstet. Gynaecol.* 96, 1290–1296.

GASS, J. D. M. (1989). Focal congenital anomalies of retinal pigment epithelium. *Eye* 3, 1–18.

GILLEBO, K., BOSTAD, R., OFTEDAL, G., RYE, H. H., AND EGGE, K. (1987). Perinatal retinal haemorrhages and development. *Acta Paediatr. Scand.* 76, 745–750.

GLASS, P., AVERY, G. B., KOLINJAVADI, N., ET AL. (1985). Effect of bright light in the hospital nursery on the incidence of prematurity. *N. Engl. J. Med.* 313, 401–404.

GLICKSTEIN, M., AND HEATH, G. G. (1975). Receptors in the monochromat eye. *Vision Res.* 15, 633–636.

GOTTLOB, I., AND STANGLER-ZUSCHROTT, E. (1990). Effects of levodopa on contrast sensitivity and scotomas in human amblyopia. *Invest. Ophthalmol. Vis. Sci.* 31, 776–780.

GOTTSCH, J. D., POU, S., BYNOE, L. A., AND ROSEN, G. M. (1990). Hematogenous photosensitization: a mechanism for the development of age-related macular degeneration. *Invest. Ophthalmol. Vis. Sci.* 31, 1674–1682.

GREENWALD, M. J., AND FOLK, E. R. (1983). Afferent pupillary defects in amblyopia. *J. Pediatr. Ophthalmol. Strabismus* 20, 63–67.

GREGOR, Z., AND JOFFE, L. (1981). Senile macular changes in the black African. *Br. J. Ophthalmol.* 13, 1053–1056.

GUÈRIN, C. J., ANDERSON, D. H., FARISS, R. N., AND FISHER, S. K. (1989). Retinal reattachment of the primate macula: photoreceptor recovery after short-term detachment. *Invest. Ophthalmol. Vis. Sci.* 30, 1708–1725.

GUILLERY, R. W. (1986). Neural abnormalities of albinos. *Trends Neurosci.* 8, 364–367.

GUILLERY, R. W. (1990). Normal and abnormal visual field maps in albinos. *Ophthalmic. Paediatr. Genet.* 11, 177–183.

GUILLERY, R. W., AND CASAGRANDE, V. A. (1974). Studies of the modifiability of the visual pathways in midwestern Siamese cats. *J. Comp. Neurol.* 174, 15–46.

GUO, S., REINECKE, R. D., FENDICK, M., AND CALHOUN, J. H. (1989). Visual pathway abnormalities in albinism and infantile nystagmus: VECPs and stereoacuity measurements. *J. Pediatr. Ophthalmol. Strabismus* 26, 97–104.

GUPTA, J. K., LEAL, C. B., JOHNSON, N., AND LILFORD, R. J. (1989). Squatting in second stage of labor [letter to the editor]. *Lancet* 2, 561–562.

GUTTMANN, J., AND SPATZ, H-C. (1985). Frequency of fusion and loss of fusion, and binocular depth perception with alternating stimulus presentation. *Perception* 14, 5–12.

HAASE, W. (1988). Amblyopia: clinical aspects. In G. LENNER-STRAND, G. K. VON NOORDEN, AND E. C. CAMPOS (eds.). *Strabismus and Amblyopia. Experimental Basis for Advances in Clinical Management.* New York: Plenum.

HALPERN, D. L., PATTERSON, R., AND BLAKE, R. (1987). What causes stereoscopic tilt from spatial frequency disparity. *Vision Res.* 27, 1619–1630.

HAM, O., PUENTES, F., CABRERA, F., HAMEDO, D., DIAZ, T., SILVA, M. L., AND CLARAMUNT, M. (1984). Etiology of early strabismus. In R. D. REINECKE (ed.). *Strabismus.* Vol. II. Orlando, FL: Grune & Stratton.

HAMER, R. D., LAKSHMINARAYANAN, V., ENOCH, J. M., AND O'DONNELL, J. J. (1986). Selective adaptation of the Stiles-Crawford function in a patient with gyrate atrophy. *Clin. Vis. Sci.* 1, 103–106.

HAMPTON, D. R., AND KERTESZ, A. (1985). The extent of Panum's area and the human cortical magnification factor. *Perception* 12, 162–165.

HAMSHER, D. (1978). Stereopsis and unilateral brain disease. *Invest. Ophthalmol. Vis. Sci.* 17, 340–343.

HANDELMAN, G. J., DRATZ, E. A., REAY, C. C., AND VAN KUJIK, J. G. M. (1988). Carotenoids in the human macula and whole retina. *Invest. Ophthalmol. Vis. Sci.* 29, 850–855.

HANDELMAN, G. J., SNODDERLY, D. M., KRINSKY, N. I., RUSSETT, M. D., AND ADLER, A. J. (1991). Biological control of primate macular pigment. *Invest. Ophthalmol. Vis. Sci.* 32, 257–267.

HANKINS, M. W., AND IKEDA, H. (1991). The role of dopaminergic pathways at the outer plexiform layer of the mammalian retina. *Clin. Vis. Sci.* 6, 87–93.

HANSEN, R. M., AND FULTON, A. B. (1989). Psychophysical estimates of ocular media density of human infants. *Vision Res.* 29, 687–690.

HARKER, G. S. (1973). The Mach-Dvorak phenomenon and binocular fusion of moving stimuli. *Vision Res.* 13, 1041–1058.

HARMS, H. (1938). Ort und Wesen der Bildhemmung bei Scheilended. *Graefes Arch. Klin. Exp. Ophthalmol.* 138, 149–210.

HARRIS, J. P., CALVERT, J. E., LEENDERTZ, J. A., AND PHILLIPSON, T. (1990). The influence of dopamine on spatial vision. *Eye* 4, 806–812.

HARVEY, L. O. (1970). Critical flicker frequency as a function of viewing distance, stimulus size and luminance. *Vision Res.* 10, 65–78.

HARWERTH, R. S., AND SMITH, E. L. (1983). Oblique effects, vertical effects and meridional amblyopia in monkeys. *Exp. Brain Res.* 53, 142–150.

HARWERTH, R. S., SMITH, E. L., DUNCAN, G. C., CRAWFORD, M. L. J., AND VON NOORDEN, G. K. (1986). Effects of enucleation of the fixating eye on strabismic amblyopia in monkeys. *Invest. Ophthalmol. Vis. Sci.* 27, 246–254.

HARWERTH, R. S., SMITH, E. L., PAUL, A. D., CRAWFORD, M. L. J., AND VON NOORDEN, G. K. (1989). The effects of reverse monocular deprivation in monkeys. I. Psychophysical experiments. *Exp. Brain Res.* 74, 327–337.

HARWERTH, R. S., SMITH, E. L., PAUL, A. D., CRAWFORD, M. L. J., AND VON NOORDEN, G. K. (1991). Functional effects of bilateral form deprivation in monkeys. *Invest. Ophthalmol. Vis. Sci.* 32, 2311–2327.

HAYREH, S. S. (1964). Pathogenesis of oedema of the optic disc (papilloedema). *Br. J. Ophthalmol.* 48, 522–543.

HELVESTON, E. M., AND VON NOORDEN, G. K. (1967). Microtropia, a newly defined entity. *Arch. Ophthalmol.* 78, 272.

HELVESTON, E. M., PICHOFF, B., ELLIS, F. D., AND MILLER, K. (1985). Unilateral esotropia after enucleation in infancy. *Am. J. Ophthalmol.* 11, 96–99.

HENDRICKSON, A. E., AND YUODELIS, C. (1984). The morphological development of the human fovea. *Ophthalmology* 91, 603–612.

HERON, G., AND DUTTON, G. N. (1989). The Pulfich phenomenon and its alleviation with a neutral density filter. *Br. J. Ophthalmol.* 73, 1004–1008.

HERON, G., DHOLAKIA, S., COLLINS, D. E., AND MCLAUGHLIN, M. (1985). Stereoscopic thresholds in children and adults. *Am. J. Optom. Physiol. Opt.* 62, 505.

HESS, R. F. (1982). Developmental sensory impairment, amblyopia or tarachopia? *Hum. Neurobiol.* 1, 17–29.

HESS, R. F., AND BAKER, C. L. (1984). Assessment of retinal function in severely amblyopic individuals. *Vision Res.* 24, 1367–1376.

HESS, R. F., AND WATT, R. J. (1990). Regional distribution of the mechanisms that underlie spatial localization. *Vision Res.* 30, 1021–1030.

HESS, R. F., BAKER, C. L., VERHOEVE, J. N., KEESEY, U. T., AND FRANCE, T. D. (1985). The pattern evoked electroretinogram: its variability in normals and its relationship to amblyopia. *Invest. Ophthalmol. Vis. Sci.* 26, 1610–1623.

HESS, R. F., CAMPBELL, F. W., AND GREENHALGH, T. (1978). On the nature of the neural abnormality in human amblyopia: neural aberrations and neural sensitivity loss. *Pflugers Arch.* 377, 201–207.

HILES, D. A., WATSON, B. A., AND BIGLAN, A. W. (1980). Characteristics of infantile esotropia following early bimedial rectus recession. *Arch. Ophthalmol.* 98, 697–703.

HIRSCH, J., AND CURCIO, C. A. (1989). The spatial resolution capacity of the human fovea. *Vision Res.* 29, 2095–1101.

HIRSCH, J., AND MILLER, W. H. (1987). Does cone positional disorder limit resolution? *J. Opt. Soc. Am.* [A] 4, 1481–1492.

HOFELDT, A. J., LEAVITT, J., AND BEHRENS, M. M. (1985). Pulfrich stereo-illusion phenomenon in serous sensory retinal detachment of the macula. *Am. J. Ophthalmol.* 100, 576–580.

HOFFMANN, K. P., AND SCHOPPMANN, A. (1984). Shortage of binocular cells in area 17 of visual cortex in cats with congenital strabismus. *Exp. Brain Res.* 55, 470–482.

HOLBACH, H. T., VON NOORDEN, G. K., AND AVILLA, C. M. (1991). Changes in esotropia after occlusion therapy in patients with strabismic amblyopia. *J. Pediatr. Ophthalmol. Strabismus* 28, 6–9.

HOMMURA, S., USUKI, Y., TAKEI, K., SEKIU, Y., FUKUDA, Y., TERAUCHI, M. (1988). Ophthalmic care of very low birthweight infants: report 4, clinical studies of the influence of light on the incidence of ROP. *Acta Soc. Ophthalmol. Jpn.* 92, 456–461.

HOROWITZ, B. R. (1981). Theoretical considerations of the retinal receptor as a waveguide. In J. M. ENOCH AND F. L. TOBEY JR. (eds.). *Vertebrate Photoreceptor Optics.* New York: Springer-Verlag.

HOWARD, I. P., AND GONZALEZ, E. G. (1987). Human optokinetic nystagmus in response to moving binocularly disparate stimuli. *Vision Res.* 27, 1807–1816.

HOYT, C. S., AND CALTRIDER, N. (1984). Hemispheric visually-evoked responses in congenital esotropia. *J. Pediatr. Ophthalmol. Strabismus* 21, 19.

HOYT, C. S., JASTRZEBSKI, G. B., AND MARG, E. (1984). Amblyopia and congenital esotropia: visually evoked potential measurements. *Arch. Ophthalmol.* 102, 58–61.

HUBEL, D. H., AND WIESEL, T. N. (1963). Receptive fields of cells in striate cortex of very young, visually inexperienced kittens. *J. Neurophysiol.* 26, 994–1002.

HUMPHREY, M., HOUNSLOW, D., MORGAN, S., AND WOOD, C. (1973). The influence of maternal posture at birth on the fetus. *J. Obstet. Gynaecol. Br. Commonw.* 80, 1075–1080.

HUNTER, D. G., AND MUKAI, S. (1992). Retinopathy of prematurity: pathogenesis, diagnosis and treatment. *Int. Ophthalmol. Clin.* 32, 163–184.

HYSON, M. T., JULESZ, B., AND FENDER, D. H. (1983). Eye movements and neural remapping during fusion of misaligned random-dot stereograms. *J. Opt. Soc. Am.* 73, 1665–1673.

ING, M. (1981). Early surgical alignment for congenital esotropia. *Trans. Am. Ophthalmol. Soc.* 79, 625–663.

ING, M. R., AND PANG. S. W. L. (1974). The racial distribution of strabismus—a statistical study. *Hawaii Med. J.* 33, 22–23.

INGRAM, R. M., ARNOLD, P. E., DALLY, S., AND LUCAS, J. (1990). Results of a randomised trial of treating abnormal hypermetropia from the age of 6 months. *Br. J. Ophthalmol.* 74, 158–159.

INGRAM, R. M., ARNOLD, P. E., DALLY, S., AND LUCAS, J. (1991). Emmetropisation, sauint, and reduced visual acuity after treatment. *Br. J. Ophthalmol.* 75, 414–416.

INGRAM, R. M., WALKER, C., WILSON, J. M., ARNOLD, P. E., AND DALLY, S. (1986). Prediction of amblyopia and squint by means of refraction at age 1 year. *Br. J. Ophthalmol.* 70, 12–15.

INNOCENTI, G. M., FROST, D. O., AND ILLES, J. (1985). Maturation of visual callosal connections in visual deprived kittens, a challenging critical period. *J. Neurosci.* 5, 255–267.

IRVINE, A. R., CRAWFORD, J. B., AND SULLIVAN, J. H. (1986). The pathogenesis of retinal detachment with morning glory disc and optic pit. *Retina* 6, 146–150.

ISENBERG, S. J., MOLARTE, A., AND VASQUEZ, M. (1990). The fixed and dilated pupils of premature neonates. *Am. J. Ophthalmol.* 110, 168–171.

ISSEL, von E. P., NEUMÄKER, K-J., NEUMÄKER, M., LOETZKE, H-H., KUNZ, G., AND WILCKE, G. (1977). Significance of model studies for explanation of the pathogenesis of mechanical induced birth trauma. *Zentralbl. Gynaekol.* 99, 9–16.

IUVONE, P. M., TIGGES, M., FERNANDES, A., ET AL. (1989). Dopamine synthesis and metabolism in rhesus monkey retina, development, aging, and the effects of monocular visual deprivation. *Vis. Neurosci.* 2, 465–471.

IAWASAKI, M., RAYBORN, M. E., TAWARA, A., AND HOLLYFIELD, J. G. (1990). Topography of the apical surface of the RPE: loss of cisternal invaginations following retinal separation. *Invest. Ophthalmol. Vis. Sci.* 31, 151.

JAMPOLSKY, A. (1978). Unequal visual inputs and strabismus management, a comparison of human and animal strabismus. In *Symposium on Strabismus. Transactions of the New Orleans Academy of Ophthalmology.* St. Louis: Mosby.

JENNINGS, J. A. M. (1985). Anomalous retinal correspondence—a review. *Ophthalmic Physiol. Opt.* 5, 357–368.

JOHNSON, G. J., GREEN, J. S., PATERSON, G. D., AND PERKINS, E. S. (1984). Survey of ophthalmic conditions in a Labrador community. II. Ocular disease. *Can. J. Ophthalmol.* 19, 224–233.

JOHNSTONE, F. D., ABOELMAGD, M. S., AND HAROUNY, A. K. (1987). Maternal posture in second stage and fetal acid base status. *Br. J. Obstet. Gynaecol.* 94, 753–757.

JONAS, J. B., MARDIN, C. Y., SCHLÖTZER-SCHREHARDT, U., AND NAUMANN, G. O. H. (1991). Morphometry of the human lamina cribrosa surface. *Invest. Ophthalmol. Vis. Sci.* 32, 401–405.

JONES, R. (1977). Anomalies of disparity detection in the human visual system. *J. Physiol. (Lond.)* 264, 621.

JONES, R. (1983). Horizontal disparity vergence. In C. M. SCHOR AND K. J. CIUFFREDA (eds.). *Vergence Eye Movements. Basic and Clinical Aspects.* Boston: Butterworths.

JONES, R., AND STEPHENS, G. L. (1989). Horizontal fusional amplitudes: evidence for disparity tuning. *Invest. Ophthalmol. Vis. Sci.* 30, 1638–1642.

JULESZ, B. (1971). *Foundations of Cyclopean Perception.* Chicago: University of Chicago Press.

JULESZ, B., AND CHANG, J. J. (1976). Interaction between pools of binocular disparity detectors tuned to different disparities. *Biol. Cybern.* 22, 107–119.

JULESZ, B., AND OSWALD, H-P. (1979). Binocular utilization of monocular cues that are undetectable monocularly. *Perception* 7, 315–322.

JULESZ, B. AND SCHUMER, R. A. (1981). Early visual perception. *Ann. Rev. Psychol.* 32, 575–627.

JULESZ, B., AND SPIVACK, G. J. (1967). Stereopsis based on vernier clues alone. *Science* 157, 563–565.

JULESZ, B., AND TYLER, C. W. (1976). Neurontropy, an entropy-like measure of neural correlation, in binocular fusion and rivalry. *Biol. Cybern.* 23, 25–32.

KANDEL, G. L., GRATTAN, P. E., AND BEDELL, H. E. (1977). Monocular fixation and acuity in amblyopic and normal eyes. *Am. J. Optom. Physiol. Opt.* 54, 598.

KANDEL, G. L., GRATTAN, P. E., AND BEDELL, H. E. (1980). Are the dominant eyes of amblyopes normal? *Am. J. Optom. Physiol. Opt.* 57, 1.

KAPLAN, M. W., IWATA, R. T., AND STERRETT, C. B. (1990). Retinal detachment prevents normal assembly of disk membranes in vitro. *Invest. Ophthalmol. Vis. Sci.* 31, 1–8.

KASE, M., NAGATA, R., YASHIDA, A., AND HANADA, I. (1984). Pupillary light reflex in amblyopia. *Invest. Ophthalmol. Vis. Sci.* 25, 467–471.

KATSUMI, O., MEHTA, M. C., MATSUI, Y., TETSUKA, H., AND HIROSE, T. (1991). Development of vision in retinopathy of prematurity. *Arch. Ophthalmol.* 109, 1394–1398.

KATZ, M. L., AND ROBISON, JR., W. G. (1988). Autooxidative damage to the retina: potential role in retinopathy of prematurity. *Birth Defects* 24, 237–248.

KAUFMAN, J. E., AND HAYNES, H. (eds.) (1981). *IES Lighting Handbook. Application Volume.* New York: Illuminating Engineering Society of North America.

KEINER, E. C. J. F. (1978). Spontaneous recovery in microstrabismus. *Ophthalmologica* 177, 280.

KEINER, G. B. J. (1951). *New Viewpoints on the Origin of Squint.* The Hague: Martinus Nijhoff.

KERTESZ, A. E. (1982). The effectiveness of wide-angle fusional stimulation in the treatment of convergence insufficiency. *Invest. Ophthalmol. Vis. Sci.* 22, 690–693.

KERTESZ, A. E. (1983a). Vertical and cylofusional disparity vergence. In C. M. SCHOR AND K. J. CIUFFREDA (eds.). *Vergence Eye Movements. Basic and Clinical Aspects.* London: Butterworths.

KERTESZ, A. E. (1983b). The effectiveness of wide-angle fusional stimulation in strabismus. *Am. Orthoptic J.* 33, 83–90.

KERVICK, G. (1986). The importance of birth history in the aetiology of strabismus. *Br. Orthoptic J.* 43, 68–71.

KIKUDI, A., MAERTENS, K., AND KAYEMBE, L. (1988). Strabismus and heterophoria, the situation in Zaire. *J. Fr. Ophthalmol.* 11, 765–768.

KILBRIDE, P. E., ALEXANDEER, K. R., FISHMAN, M., AND FISHMAN, G. A. (1989). Human macular pigment assessed by imaging fundus reflectometry. *Vision Res.* 29, 663–674.

KINNEAR, P. E., JAY, B., AND WITKOP, C. J. (1985). Albinism. *Surv. Ophthalmol.* 30, 75–101.

KIORPES, L. (1989). The development of spatial resolution and contrast sensitivity in naturally strabismic monkey. *Clin. Vis. Sci.* 4, 279–294.

KIORPES, L., AND BOOTHE, R. G. (1981). Naturally occurring strabismus in monkeys (*Macca menstrina*). *Invest. Ophthalmol. Vis. Sci.* 20, 257–262.

KITAO, H. (1960). Studies on the development of the depth perception for near and distant object in the childhood. *Jpn. J. Ophthalmol.* 4, 67.

KITAOJI, H., AND TOYAMA, K. (1987). Preservation of position and motion stereopsis in strabismic subjects. *Invest. Ophthalmol. Vis. Sci.* 28, 1260–1267.

KNOBLOCH, W. H., LEAVENWORTH, N. M., BOUCHARD, T. J., AND ECKERT, E. D. (1985). Eye findings in twins reared apart. *Ophthalmic Paediatr. Genet.* 5, 59–66.

KUMAR, T., AND GLASER, D. G. (1991). Influence of remote objects on local depth perception. *Vision Res.* 31, 1687–1700.

KUSHNER, B. (1985). Unilateral esotropia after enucleation in infancy [letter to the editor]. *Am. J. Ophthamol.* 11, 744–745.

LAGRÈZE, W-D., AND SIRETEANU, R. (1991). Two-dimensional spatial distortions in human strabismic amblyopia. *Vision Res.* 31, 1271–1288.

LAMANTIA, A-S., AND RAKIC, P. (1990). Axon overproduction and elimination in the corpus callosum of the developing rhesus monkey. *J. Neurosci.* 10, 2156–2175.

LEE, D. N. (1970). A stroboscopic stereophenomenon. *Vision Res.* 10, 587–594.

LEFFERTSTRA, L. J. (1977). [A comparative study of the differences in the evolution of refraction in the two eyes in patients with convergent strabismus.] *Klin. Monatsbl. Augenheilkd.* 170, 74–79.

LEGGE, G. E., AND GU, Y. (1989). Stereopsis and contrast. *Vision Res.* 29, 989–1004.

LEGUIRE, L. E., ROGERS, G. L., AND BREMER, D. L. (1990). Amblyopia: the normal eye is not normal. *J. Pediatr. Ophthamol. Strabismus* 27, 32–38.

LEGUIRE, L. E., ROGERS, G. L., BREMER, D. L., WILSON, P., AND WALI, N. (1991). Levadopa treatment for childhood amblyopia. *Invest. Ophthalmol. Vis. Sci.* 32 (suppl.), 820.

LERMAN, S. (1984). Biophysical aspects of corneal and lenticular transparency. *Curr. Eye Res.* 3, 3–13.

LEVAY, S., AND VOIGT, T. (1988). Ocular dominance and disparity coding in cat visual cortex. *Vis. Neurosci.* 1, 395–414.

LEVANTHAL, A. G., VITEK, D. J., AND CREEL, D. J. (1985). Abnormal pathways in normally pigmented cats that are heterozygous for albinism. *Science* 229, 1395–1397.

LEVI, D. M. (1988). The spatial grain of the amblyopic visual system. *Am. J. Optom. Physiol. Opt.* 10. 767–786.

LEVI, D. M., AND KLEIN, S. A. (1990). Equivalent intrinsic blur in amblyopia. *Vision Res.* 30, 1995–2022.

LEVI, D. M., KLEIN, S. A., AND YAP, Y. L. (1987). Positional uncertainty in peripheral and amblyopic vision. *Vision Res.* 27, 581–598.

LILFORD, R. J., GLANVILLE, J. N., GUPTA, J. K., SHRESTHA, R., AND JOHNSON, N. (1989). The action of squatting in the early postnatal period marginally increases pelvic dimensions. *Br. J. Obstet. Gynaecol.* 96, 964–966.

LINES, C. R. (1984). Nasotemporal overlap investigated in a case of agenesis of the corpus callosum. *Neuropsychologia* 22, 85–90.

LINES, C. R., AND MILNER, A. D. (1983). Nasotemporal overlap in the human retina investigated by means of a simple reaction time to lateralized light flash. *Exp. Brain Res.* 50, 166–172.

LINKSZ, A. (1952). *Physiology of the eye. Vol. 2. Vision.* Orlando, FL: Grune and Stratton.

LLOYD, L. A. (1975). Craniofacial reconstruction, ocular management of orbital hyperteleorism. *Trans. Am. Ophthalmol. Soc.* 73, 123, 140.

LOWES, M., EHLERS, N., AND JENSEN, I. K. (1976). Visual functions after perinatal macular haemhorrage. *Acta Ophthalmol. (Copenh.)* 54, 227–232.

LU, Y. C. (1974). Effects of an upright position during labor. *Am. J. Nurs.* 74, 2202–2205.

LUDWIG, I. H., PARKS, M. M., GETSON, P. R., AND KAMMERMAN, L. A. (1988). Rate of deterioration in accommodative esotropia correlated to the AC/A relationship. *J. Pediatr. Ophthalmol. Strabismus* 25, 8–12.

LUPE, P. J., AND GROSS, T. L. (1986). Maternal upright posture and mobility in labor—a review. *Obstet. Gynecol.* 67, 727–734.

MAC CANA, F., CUTHBERT, A., AND LOVEGROVE, W. (1986). Contrast and phase processing in amblyopia. *Vision Res.* 26, 781–789.

MAINSTER, M. A. (1987). Light and macular degeneration, a biophysical and clinical perspective. *Eye* 1, 304–310.

MAINSTER, M. A. (1988). Henle fibers may direct light toward the center of the fovea. *Laser Light Ophthalmol.* 2, 79–86.

MALIK, S., COHEN, D., MEYER, E., AND PERLMAN, I. (1986). Light damage in the developing retina of the albino rat: an electroretinographic study. *Invest. Ophthalmol. Vis. Sci.* 27, 164–167.

MALTAU, J. M., EGGE, K., AND MOE, N. (1984). Retinal hemorrhages in the preterm neonate: a prospective randomized study comparing the occurrence of hemorrhages after spontaneous versus forceps delivery. *Acta. Obstet. Gynecol. Scand.* 63, 219–221.

MANN, I. (1966). *Culture, Race, Climate and Eye Disease. An Introduction to the Study of Geographical Ophthalmology.* Springfield, IL: Charles C. Thomas.

MASH, A. J., HEGMANN, J. P., AND SPIVEY, B. E. (1975). Genetic analysis of vergence measures in populations with varying incidences of strabismus. *Am. J. Ophthalmol.* 79, 978.

MASTRONARDE, D. N., THIBEAULT, M. A., AND DUBIN, M. W. (1984). Non-uniform postnatal growth of the cat retina. *J. Comp. Neurol.* 228, 598–608.

MATHIS, W., AND BOURASSA, C. M. (1968). Fusion and nonfusion as factors in aversion to high luminance. *Vision Res.* 8, 1501.

MCBRIDE, W. G., BLACK, B. P., BROWN, C. J., DOLBY, R. M., MURRAY, A. D., AND THOMAS, D. B. (1979). Method of delivery and developmental outcome at five years of age. *Med. J. Aust.* 1, 301–304.

MCCORMACK, E. L. (1975). Electrophysiologic evidence for normal optic nerve projections in normally pigmented squinters. *Invest. Ophthalmol. Vis. Sci.* 14, 931.

MCKEE, S. M. (1983). The spatial requirements for fine stereoacuity. *Vision Res.* 23, 191–198.

MCKEE, S. M., LEVI, D. M., AND BOWNE, S. F. (1990). The imprecision of stereopsis. *Vision Res.* 30, 1763.

MILLER, M., AND PRUZANSKY, S. (1981). Craniofacial anomalies. In G. A. PEYMAN, D. R. SANDERS, AND M. F. GOLDBERG (eds.). *Principles and Practice of Ophthalmology.* Philadelphia: Saunders.

MILLER, W. H., AND SNYDER, A. W. (1973). Optical function of human peripheral cones. *Vision Res.* 13, 2185–2194.

MITCHELL, D. E. (1970). Properties of stimuli eliciting vergence eye movements and stereopsis. *Vision Res.* 10, 145.

MITCHELL, D. E. (1991). The long-term effectiveness of different regimens of occlusion on recovery from early monocular deprivation in kittens. *Philos. Trans. R. Soc. Lond. [Biol.]* 333, 51–79.

MITCHELL, D. E., AND TIMNEY, B. (1984). Postnatal development of function in the mammalian visual system. In S. R. GEIGER (ed.). *Handbook of Physiology. Vol. III. The Nervous System.* Bethesda: American Physiological Society.

MITSUI, Y., HIRAI, K., AKAZAWA, K., AND MASUDA, K. (1979). The sensorimotor reflex and the strabismus. *Jpn. J. Ophthalmol.* 23, 227–256.

MOHINDRA, I., ZWAAN, J., HELD, R., BRILL, S., AND ZWAAN, F. (1985). Development of acuity and stereopsis in infants with esotropia. *Ophthalmology* 92, 691.

MOHN, G., SIRETEANU, R., AND VAN HOF-VAN DUIN, J. (1986). The relation of monocular optokinetic nystagmus to peripheral binocular interactions. *Invest. Ophthalmol. Vis. Sci.* 27, 565–573.

MOORE, S. (1971). The natural course of esotropia. *Am. Orthoptic J.* 21, 80.

MORGAN, R. A., BUDD, G. E., AND BOYD, T. A. S. (1972). Vectographic suppression studies in strabismus patients. In J. MEIN, J. J. M. BIERLAAGH, AND T. E. A. BRUMMELKAMP-DONS (eds.). *Orthoptics, Proceedings of the Second International Orthoptics Congress.* Amsterdam: Excerpta Medica.

MOSELEY, I. F., AND PILLING, J. B. (1976). Intraocular haemorrhage as a complication of pneumoencephalography. *J. Neurol. Neurosurg. Psychiatry* 39, 375–380.

MOSELEY, M. J., AND FIELDER, A. R. (1988). Light toxicity and the neonatal eye. *Clin. Vis. Sci.* 3, 75–82.

MOWFORTH, P., MAYHEW, J. E. W., AND FRISBY, J. P. (1981). Vergence eye movements made in response to spatial-frequency-filtered random dot stereograms. *Perception* 10, 299.

MUELLER, T. J., AND BLAKE, R. (1990). Estimating the size of a zone of suppression for binocular rivalry. *Invest. Ophthalmol. Vis. Sci.* 31 (suppl.), 525.

MUND, M. L., AND RODRIGUES, M. M. (1979). Embryology of the human retinal pigment epithelium. In K. M. ZINN AND M. J. MARMOR (eds.). *The Retinal Pigment Epithelium.* Cambridge, MA: Harvard University Press.

MURPHY, K. M., AND MITCHELL, D. E. (1991). Vernier acuity of normal and visually deprived cats. *Vision Res.* 31, 253–266.

NAASH, M. I., NIELSEN, J. C., AND ANDERSON, R. E. (1988). Regional distribution of glutathione and peroxidase and glutathione-S-transferase in adult and premature human retinas. *Invest. Ophthalmol. Vis. Sci.* 29, 149–152.

NAKAYAMA, K. (1972). Studies on the myelization of the human optic nerve. *Jpn. J. Ophthalmol.* 11, 132–140.

NAROLL, F., NARROLL, R., AND HOWARD, F. H. (1971). Position of women in childbirth. *Am. J. Obstet. Gynecol.* 82, 943–954.

NEWMAN, N. J., WOLFE, J. M., STEWART, M. I., AND LESSELL, S. (1991). Binocular visual function in patients with a history of monocular optic neuritis. *Clin. Vis. Sci.* 6, 95–108.

NIEDERECKER, O., MASH, A. J., AND SPIVEY, B. E. (1972). Horizontal fusional amplitudes and versions. *Arch. Ophthalmol.* 87, 283.

NIELSEN, K. R. K., AND POGGIO, T. (1984). Vertical image registration in stereopsis. *Vision Res.* 24, 1133.

NISHIHARA, H. K., AND POGGIO, T. (1982). Hidden cues in random-line stereograms. *Nature* 300, 347–349.

NORCIA, A. M., GARCIA, H., HUMPHRY, R., HOLMES, A., HAMER, R. D., AND OREL-BIXLER, D. (1991). Anomalous motion of VEPs in infants and infantile esotropia. *Invest. Ophthalmol. Vis. Sci.* 32, 436–439.

ODENRICK, P., STANDSTEDT, P., AND LENNERSTRAND, G. (1984). Postural sway and gait of children with convergent strabismus. *Dev. Med. Child Neurol.* 26, 495–499.

O'LEARY, J. A., FERRELL, R. E., AND RANDOLPH, C. R. (1986). Retinal hemorrhage and vacuum extraction delivery. *J. Perinat. Med.* 14, 197–199.

OWENS, D. A., AND LEIBOWITZ, H. W. (1980). Accommodation, convergence and distance perception in low illumination. *Am. J. Optom. Physiol. Opt.* 57, 540.

PACKER, O., HENDRICKSON, A. E., AND CURCIO, C. A. (1990). Developmental redistribution of photoreceptors across the *Macca nemestrina* (pigtail macaque) retina. *J. Comp. Neurol.* 298, 472.

PAPAKOSTOPOULOS, D., HART, D., COOPER, R., AND NATSIKOS, V. (1984). Combined electrophysiological assessment of the visual system in central serous retinopathy. *Electroencephalogr. Clin. Neurophysiol.* 59, 77.

PARKER, A. J., AND YANG, Y. (1989). Spatial properties of disparity pooling in human stereo vision. *Vision Res.* 29, 1525.

PARKS, M. M. (1971). The monofixation syndrome. In *Symposium on Strabismus. Transactions of the New Orleans Academy of Ophthalmology.* St. Louis: C. V. Mosby.

PATTERSON, R., AND FOX, R. (1984). The effect of testing method on steroanomaly. *Vision Res.* 24, 403–408.

PAUTLER, E. L., MORITA, M., AND BEEZLEY, D. (1990). Hemoprotein(s) mediate blue light damage in the retinal pigment epithelium. *Photochem. Photobiol.* 51, 599–605.

POGGIO, G. F., AND TALBOT, W. H. (1981). Mechanisms of static and dynamic stereopsis in foveal cortex of the rhesus monkey. *Vision Res.* 315, 469–492.

PORTNOY, J. Z., THOMPSON, H. S., LENNARSON, L., AND CORBETT, J. J. (1983). Pupillary defects in amblyopia. *Am. J. Ophthalmol.* 96, 609–614.

POWERS, M. K., AND DOBSON, V. (1982). Effect of focus on visual acuity of human infants. *Vision Res.* 22, 521.

PRATT-JOHNSON, J. A. (1973). Binocular function and acquired esotropia. *Am. J. Orthop.* 23, 52.

PRATT-JOHNSON, J. A., AND BARLOW, J. M. (1975). Stereoacuity and fusional amplitude in foveal suppression. *Can. J. Ophthalmol.* 10, 56.

PRATT-JOHNSON, J. A., AND TILLSON, G. (1983). Sensory results following treatment of infantile esotropia. *Can. J. Ophthalmol.* 18, 175.

PRISM ADAPTATION STUDY RESEARCH GROUP (1990 Efficacy of prism adaptation in the surgical management of esotropia. *Arch. Ophthalmol.* 108, 1248–1256.

PUGH, M. (1954). Foveal vision in amblyopia. *Br. J. Ophthalmol.* 38, 321–331.

PUGH, M. (1958). Visual distortion in amblyopia. *Br. J. Ophthalmol.* 42, 449–460.

PUGH, M. (1962). Amblyopia and the retina. *Br. J. Ophthalmol.* 46, 193–211.

QUICK, M., EGGERS, M., AND BOOTHE, R. (1990). Convergence errors in normal and naturally strabismic monkeys. *Invest. Ophthalmol. Vis. Sci.* 31 (suppl.), 83.

QUICK, M. W., TIGGES, M., GAMMON, J. A., AND BOOTHE, R. G. (1989). Early abnormal visual experience induces strabismus in infant monkeys. *Invest. Ophthalmol. Vis. Sci.* 30, 1012–1017.

RAAB, E. L., AND SPIERER, A. (1986). Persisting accommodative esotropia. *Arch. Ophthalmol.* 104, 1777.

RAMACHANDRAN, V., AND CAVANAUGH, P. (1985). Subjective contours capture stereopsis. *Nature* 317, 527–529.

RASHBASS, C., AND WESTHEIMER, G. (1961). Independence of conjugate and disjunctive eye movements. *J. Physiol. (Lond.)* 159, 361–364.

READING, R. W. (1985). Determinations of the horopter in esotropia. *Doc. Ophthalmol.* 61, 175–181.

REGAN, D. (1988). *Human Brain Electrophysiology. Evoked Potentials and Evoked Magnetic Fields in Science and Medicine.* New York: Elsevier.

REGAN, D., ERKELENS, C. J., AND COLLEWIJN, H. (1986). Visual field defects for vergence eye movements and for stereomotion perception. *Invest. Ophthalmol. Vis. Sci.* 27, 806–819.

REUSS, J. L. (1981). Human stereopsis, detection and development. PhD thesis, Northwestern University.

RICHARDS, W. (1968). Spatial remapping in the primate visual system. *Kybernetik* 4, 146–156.

RICHARDS, W. (1970a). Stereopsis and stereoblindness. *Exp. Brain Res.* 10, 380–388.

RICHARDS, W. (1970b). Oculomotor effects upon binocular rivalry. *Psychol. Forsch.* 33, 136–154.

RICHARDS, W. (1971a). Anomalous stereoscopic depth perception. *J. Opt. Soc. Am.* 61, 410.

RICHARDS, W. (1971b). Independence of Panum's near and far limits. *Am. J. Optom. Physiol. Opt.* 48, 103.

RICHARDS, W. (1975). Stereoblindness and fixation disparity. Paper presented at Annual Meeting, American Academy of Optometry, Columbus, Ohio, December 14, 1975 (abstract in *Am. J. Optom. Physiol. Opt.* 52, 716A).

RICHARDS, W., AND REGAN, D. (1973). A stereo field map with implications for disparity processing. *Invest. Ophthalmol. Vis. Sci.* 12, 904–909.

RICHTER, S. (1976). [The significance of retinal hemorrhages in newborns.] *Padiatr. Grenzgebiete* 15, 103–107.

RIGGS, A. L., AND NIEHL, E. W. (1960). Eye movements recorded during convergence and divergence. *J. Opt. Soc. Am.* 50, 913–920.

ROARTY, J. D., AND KELTNER, J. L. (1990). Normal pupil size and anisocoria in newborn infants. *Arch. Ophthalmol.* 108, 94–95.

ROBB, R. M. (1985). Regional changes in retinal pigment epithelial cell density during ocular development. *Invest. Ophthalmol. Vis. Sci.* 26, 614.

ROBB, R. M., AND RODIER, D. W. (1987). The variable clinical characteristics and course of early infantile esotropia. *J. Pediatr. Ophthalmol. Strabismus* 24, 276.

ROBERTS, J. (1989). Maternal position in the first stage of labour. In I. CHALMERS, M. ENKIN, AND M. J. N. KEIRSE (eds.). *Effective Care in Pregnancy and Childbirth.* Oxford: Oxford University Press.

ROBINSON, J., AND FIELDER, A. R. (1990). Pupillary diameter and reaction to light in preterm neonates. *Arch. Dis. Child.* 65, 35–38.

ROBINSON, J., AND FIELDER, A. R. (1991). Spectral characteristics of the neonatal unit lighting. *Invest. Ophthalmol. Vis. Sci.* 32 (suppl.), 1146.

ROBINSON, J., AND FIELDER, A. R. (1992). Light and the neonatal eye. *Behav. Brain Res.* 49, 51–55.

ROMANO, O. P. E., AND BIRD, J. J. (1980). Fluorescein retinal angiographic studies of functional amblyopia. *J. Pediatr. Ophthalmol. Strabismus* 17, 318–319.

ROTHSTEIN, T. B., AND SACKS, J. G. (1972). Defective stereopsis in lesions of the parietal lobe. *Am. J. Ophthalmol.* 73, 281.

RUBIN, W. (1965). Reverse prism and calibrated occlusion in the treatment of small-angle deviations. *Am. J. Ophthalmol.* 59, 271–277.

RUSSELL, J. G. B. (1982). The rationale of primitive delivery positions. *Br. J. Obstet. Gynaecol.* 89, 712–715.

RUTSTEIN, R. P., AND ESKRIDGE, J. B. (1984). Stereopsis in small-angle strabismus. *Am. J. Optom. Physiol. Opt.* 61, 491.

SADUN, A. A. (1989). Optic disc pits and associated serous macular detachment. In. S. J. RYAN (ed.). *Retina*, Vol. 2. St. Louis: C. V. Mosby.

SAMRA, J. S., TANG, L. C., AND OBHRAI, M. S. (1989). Squatting in the second stage of labor [letter to the editor]. *Lancet* 2, 1150–1151.

SANDSTEDT, P., ODENRICK, P., AND LENNERSTRAND, G. (1986). Gait and postural control in children with divergent strabismus. *Binocular Vision* 1, 141–146.

SCHENK, H., AND STANGLER-ZUSCHROTT, E. (1974). [Sequelae of central retinal hemorrhages in the newborn in regard to visual acuity and muscle equilibrium.] *Klin. Monatsbl. Augenheilkd.* 165, 867–870.

SCHOPPMAN, A., AND HOFFMAN, K-P. (1985). The development of eye alignment in normal and naturally strabismic kittens. *Invest. Ophthalmol. Vis. Sci.* 26, 3350–3358.

SCHOR, C. (1983). Subcortical binocular suppression affects the development of latent and optokinetic nystagmus. *Am. J. Optom. Physiol. Opt.* 60, 481–502.

SCHOR, C. M., AND BADCOCK, D. R. (1985). A comparison of stereo and vernier acuity within spatial channels as a function of distance from fixation. *Vision Res.* 25, 1113.

SCHOR, C., BRIDGEMAN, B., AND TYLER, C. W. (1983a). Spatial characteristics of static and dynamic stereoacuity in strabismus. *Invest. Ophthalmol. Vis. Sci.* 24, 1572–1579.

SCHOR, C., HECKMAN, T., AND TYLER, C. W. (1989). Binocular fusion limits are independent of contrast, luminance gradient and component phases. *Vision Res.* 29, 821–835.

SCHOR, C., NARAYAN, V., AND WESTALL, C. (1983b). Postnatal development of optokinetic afternystagmus in human infants. *Vision Res.* 23, 1643–1648.

SCHOR, C., WOOD, I., AND OGAWA, J. (1984). Spatial tuning of static and dynamic local stereopsis. *Vision Res.* 24, 573–578.

SCOBEE, R. G. (1951). Esotropia. *Am. J. Ophthalmol.* 34, 817.

SCOTT, W. E., AND DICKEY, C. F. (1988). Stability of visual acuity in amblyopic patients after visual maturity. *Graefes Arch. Clin. Exp. Ophthalmol.* 226, 154–157.

SCOTT, W. E., AND MASH, A. J. (1973). Kappa angle measures of strabismic and non-strabismic individuals. *Arch. Ophthalmol.* 89, 18.

SEBRIS, S. L., DOBSON, V. L., AND HARTMAN, E. E. (1984). Assessment and prediction of visual acuity in 3- to 4-year-old children born prior to term. *Hum. Neurobiol.* 3, 87–92.

SEIBERTH, B., LINDERKAMP, O., KNORZ, M. C., AND LIESENHOFF, H. (1991). The effect of bright light on the incidence of retinopathy of prematurity: a controlled clinical trial. *Ophthalmology* 98 (suppl.), 120–121.

SHEA, S. L. (1986). Quantitative measurements of infant eye movements to dynamic random element stereograms. *Invest. Ophthalmol.* 27 (suppl.), 152.

SHERMAN, J., BASS, S. J., NOBLE, K. G., NATH, S., AND SATIJA, V. (1986). Visual evoked potential (VEP) delays in central serous choroidopathy. *Invest. Ophthalmol. Vis. Sci.* 27, 214–221.

SHIMOJO, S., AND NAKAJIMA, Y. (1981). Adaptation to the reversal of binocular depth cues: effects of wearing left-right reversing spectacles on stereoscopic depth perception. *Perception* 10, 391–402.

SHIPPMAN, S., AND COHEN, K. R. (1983). Relationship of heterophoria to stereopsis. *Arch. Ophthalmol.* 101, 609.

SIMONS, K. (1975). The development of stereopsis in children. Thesis, Harvard University.

SIMONS, K. (1981a). Stereoacuity norms in young children. *Arch. Ophthalmol.* 99, 439–445.

SIMONS, K. (1981b). A comparison of the Frisby, Random Dot E, TNO and Randot Circles stereotests in screening and office use. *Arch. Ophthalmol.* 99, 446.

SIMONS, K. (1984). Effects on stereopsis of monocular versus binocular degradation of image contrast. *Invest. Ophthalmol. Vis. Sci.* 25, 987–989.

SIMONS, K. (submitted). The effects of monocular and binocular spatial distortion on stereopsis.

SIMONS, K. (in press). Artificial light and early-life exposure in age-related macular degeneration and in cataractogenic phototoxicity [letter]. *Arch. Ophthalmol.*

SIMONS, K., AND REINECKE, R. D. (1978). Amblyopia screening and stereopsis. In *Symposium on Strabismus Transactions of the New Orleans Academy of Ophthalmology.* St. Louis: Mosby.

SIRETEANU, R. (1982). Binocular vision in strabismic humans with alternating fixation. *Vision Res.* 22, 889–909.

SIRETEANU, R., AND FRONIUS, M. (1982). Naso-temporal asymmetries in human amblyopia: consequence of long-term interocular suppression. *Vision Res.* 21, 1055–1063.

SIRETEANU, R., AND FRONIUS, M. (1989). Different patterns of retinal correspondence in the central and peripheral fields of strabismics. *Invest. Ophthalmol. Vis. Sci.* 30, 2023–2033.

SIRETEANU, R., AND FRONIUS, M. (1990). Human amblyopia, structure of the visual field. *Exp. Brain Res.* 79, 603–614.

SIRETEANU, R., FRONIUS, M., AND SINGER, W. (1981). Binocular interaction in the peripheral visual field of humans with strabismic and anisometropic amblyopia. *Vision Res.* 21, 1065.

SJÖSTRAND, J., AND ABRAHAMSSON, M. (1990). Risk factors in amblyopia. *Eye* 4, 787–793.

SJÖSTRAND, J., AND ANDERSON, C. (1986). Micropsia and metamorphopsia in the re-attached macula following retinal detachment. *Acta Ophthalmol. (Copenh.)* 64, 425–432.

SMITH, D., GRUTZNER, P., COLENBRANDER, A., HEGMANN, J. P., AND SPIVEY, B. (1972). Selected ophthalmologic and orthoptic measurements in families. *Arch. Ophthalmol.* 87, 278–282.

SMITH, E. L., HARWERTH, R. S., SIDEROV, J., WINGARD, M., CRAWFORD, M. L. J., AND VON NOORDEN, G. K. (1991). Prior strabismus protects young monkeys from the effects of monocular deprivation. *Invest. Ophthalmol. Vis. Sci.* (s)32, 1239.

SNIR, M., NISSENKORN, I., SHERF, I., COHEN S., AND SIRA, I. B. (1988). Visual acuity, strabismus and amblyopia in premature babies without retinopathy of prematurity. *Ann. Ophthalmol.* 20, 256–258.

SNODDERLY, D. M., AURAN, J. D., AND DELORI, F. C. (1984). The macular pigment. II. Spatial distribution in primate retinas. *Invest. Ophthalmol. Vis. Sci.* 25, 674–685.

SNODDERLY, D. M., HANDELMAN, G. J., AND ADLER, A. J. (1991). Distribution of individual macular pigment carotenoids in central retina of macaque and squirrel monkeys. *Invest. Ophthalmol. Vis. Sci.* 32, 268–279.

SNYDER, A. W., AND RICHMOND, P. (1972). Effect of anomalous dispersion on visual photoreceptors. *J. Opt. Soc. Am.* 62, 1278–1283.

STAGER, D. R., AND BIRCH, E. E. (1986). Preferential-looking acuity and stereopsis in infantile esotropia. *J. Pediatr. Ophthalmol. Strabismus* 23, 160.

STANGLER-ZUSCHROTT, E. (1978). [Disturbances of fusion after extensive retinal hemorrhaeges in newborn infants.] *Klin. Monastbl. Augenheilkd.* 172, 209–212.

STEINMAN, S. B., LEVI, D. M., AND MCKEE, S. P. (1988). Discrimination of time and velocity in the amblyopic visual system. *Clin. Vis. Sci.* 2, 265–272.

STEVENS, K. A., AND BROOKES, A. (1988). Integrating stereopsis with monocular interpretations of planar surfaces. *Vision Res.* 28, 371–386.

STEVENSON, S. B., CORMACK, L. K., AND SCHOR, C. M. (1991). Depth attraction and repulsion in random dot stereograms. *Vision Res.* 31, 805–813.

STEWART, P., AND SPIBY, H. (1989). Posture in labour. *Br. J. Obstet. Gynaecol.* 96, 1258–1260.

STOBIE, P. E. (1985). Bright light and retinopathy of prematurity [letter to the editor]. *N. Engl. J. Med.* 314, 448–449.

SUTTER, E. E., AND TRAN, D. (1991). Identification of pattern ERG components by means of their field topography. *Invest. Ophthalmol. Vis. Sci.* 32 (suppl.), 929.

SVENNINGSEN, L., LINDEMANN, R., EIDAL, K., AND JENSEN, Ø. (1987). Neonatal retinal hemorrhages and neurobehavior related to tractive force in vacuum extraction. *Acta Obstet. Gynecol. Scand.* 66, 165–169.

SVENNINGSEN, L., LINDEMANN, R., AND EIDAL, K. (1988). Measurements of fetal head compression during bearing down and their relationship to the condition of the newborn. *Acta Obstet. Gynecol. Scand.* 67, 129–133.

THORN, F., HELD, R, AND FANG. L. (1987). Orthogonal astigmatic axes in Chinese and Caucasian infants. *Invest. Ophthalmol. Vis. Sci.* 28, 191–194.

TIERNEY, D. W. (1989). Vision recovery in amblyopia after contralateral subretinal hemorrhage. *J. Am. Optom. Assoc.* 60, 281–283.

TIMNEY, B. (1983). The effects of early and late monocular deprivation on binocular depth perception in cats. *Dev. Brain Res.* 7, 235.

TIMNEY, B. (1990). Effects of brief monocular deprivation on binocular depth perception in the cat. *Vis. Neurosci.* 5, 273–280.

TIMNEY, B., ELBERGER, A. J., AND VANDEWATER, M. L. (1985). Binocular depth perception in the cat following early corpus callosum section. *Exp. Brain Res.* 60, 19–26.

TOMMILA, V. (1964). Treatment of amblyopia in loss of vision in the other eye. *Acta Ophthalmol. (Copenh.)* 42, 489–494.

TREDICI, T. D., AND VON NOORDEN, G. K. (1984). The Pulfrich effect in anisometropic amblyopia and strabismus. *Am. J. Ophthalmol.* 98, 499–503.

TRIMARCHI, F., CASALI, G., FRANCHINI, F., AND GILARDI, E. (1976). Pupillographic responses in patients with untreated amblyopia. In S.

MOORE, J. MEIN, AND L. STOCKBRIDGE (eds.). *Orthoptics: Past, Present, Future.* Chicago: Year Book Medical Publishers.

TSO, M. O. M. (1989). Experiments on visual cells by naute and man: in search of treatment for photoreceptor degeneration; Friedenwald lecture. *Invest. Ophthalmol. Vis. Sci.* 30, 2430–2454.

TURANO, K. (1991). Bisection judgment in patients with retinitis pigmentosa. *Clin. Vis. Sci.* 6, 119–130.

TUSA, R. J., REPKA, M. S., SMITH, C. B, AND HERDMAN, S. J. (1991). Early visual deprivation results in permanent strabismus and nystagmus in monkeys. *Invest. Ophthalmol. Vis. Sci.* 32, 134–141.

TYLER, C. W. (1983). Sensory processing of binocular disparity. In C. M. SCHOR AND K. J. CIUFFREDA (eds.). *Vergence Eye Movements. Basic and Clinical Aspects.* Boston: Butterworths.

TYLER, C. W. (1990). A stereoscopic view of visual processing streams. *Vision Res.* 30, 1877–1895.

TYLER, C. W., AND JULESZ, B. (1976). The neural transfer characteristic (neurontropy) for binocular stochastic stimulation. *Biol. Cybern.* 23, 33–37.

TYSCHEN, L., QUICK, M., AND BOOTHE, R. G. (1991). Alternating monocular input from birth causes stereoblindness, motion processing asymmetries and strabismus in infant macaque. *Invest. Ophthalmol. Vis. Sci.* 32 (suppl.), 1044.

VAN BLOKLAND, G. J. (1986). Directionality and alignment of the foveal receptors assessed with light scattered from the human fundus in vivos. *Vision Res.* 26, 495–500.

VAN HOF-VAN DUIN, J., AND MOHN, G. (1986). Monocular and binocular optokinetic nystagmus in humans with defective stereopsis. *Invest. Ophthalmol. Vis. Sci.* 27, 574–583.

VOGT, C., GREITE, J-H., AND HESS, J. (1978). [High altitude retinal hemorrhages in mountain climbers.] *Klin. Monatsbl. Augenheilkd.* 172, 770–775.

VON BARSEWISCH, B. (1979). *Perinatal Retinal Haemorrhages: Morphology, Aetiology and Significance.* New York: Springer-Verlag.

VON NOORDEN, G. K. (1988a). Reassessment of infantile esotropia. *Am. J. Ophthalmol.* 105, 1.

VON NOORDEN, G. K. (1988b). Current concepts of infantile esotropia. *Eye* 2, 343–357.

VON NOORDEN, G. K. (1990). *Binocular Vision and Ocular Motility.* 4th Ed. St. Louis: Mosby.

VON NOORDEN, G. K., AND FRANK, J. W. (1976). Relationship between amblyopia and the angle of strabismus. *Am. Orthop. J.* 26, 31.

VON NOORDEN, G. K., AND HELVESTON, E. M. (1970). Influence of eye position on fixation behavior and visual acuity. *Am. J. Ophthalmol.* 70, 199–204.

VOS, J. J., KREMERS, J. J. M., AND VAN NOOREN, D. (1990). The two-pigment model for retinal light damage and its consequence for occupational safety. *Laser Light Ophthalmol.* 3, 251–260.

WALLS, G. L. (1962). The evolutionary history of eye movements. *Vision Res.* 2, 69–80.

WALSH, P. M., HARRIS, M. J., ROBINS, D., FINE, S. L., AND GUYTON, P. L. (1984). "Full field" visual acuity in patients with impaired fixation. *Invest. Ophthalmol. Vis. Sci.* 25 (suppl.), 310.

WANG, F. M., AND CHRYSSANTHOU, G. (1988). Monocular eye closure in intermittent exotropia. *Arch. Ophthalmol.* 106, 941.

WATTAM-BELL, J., BRADDICK, O., ATKINSON, J., AND DAY, J. (1987). Measures of infant binocularity in a group at risk for strabismus. *Clin. Vis. Sci.* 1, 327–336.

WAXLER, M., AND HITCHINS, V. M. (eds.). (1986). *Optical Radiation and Visual Health.* Boca Raton, FL: CRC Press.

WEITER, J. J., DELORI, F., AND DOREY, C. K. (1988). Central sparing in annular macular degeneration. *Am. J. Ophthalmol.* 106, 286–292.

WERNER, J. S. (1982). Development of scotopic sensitivity and the absorption spectrum of the human ocular media. *J. Opt. Soc. Am.* 72, 247–258.

WESSON, M. D. (1983). Use of light intensity reduction for amblyopia therapy. *Am. J. Optom. Physiol. Opt.* 60, 112–117.

WESTALL, C. N., AND SCHOR, C. M. (1985). Asymmetries of optokinetic nystagmus in amblyopia: the effect of selected retinal stimulation. *Vision Res.* 25, 1431–1438.

WESTHEIMER, G. (1979). Cooperative neural processes involved in stereoscopic acuity. *Exp. Brain Res.* 36, 585–597.

WESTHEIMER, G. (1986). Spatial interaction in the domain of disparity signals in human stereoscopic vision. *J. Physiol. (Lond.)* 370, 619–629.

WESTHEIMER, G. (1987). Visual acuity and hyperacuity, resolution, localization, form. *Am. J. Optom. Physiol. Opt.* 64, 567–574.

WESTHEIMER, G., AND LEVI, D. M. (1987). Depth attraction and repulsion of disparate foveal stimuli. *Vision Res.* 27, 1361–1368.

WICK, B., AND CRANE, S. (1976). A vision profile of American Indian children. *Am. J. Optom. Physiol. Opt.* 53, 34–40.

WIDDERSHEIM, K. P., PECK, L. B., AND HOWLAND, H. (1990). Studies of accommodation and convergence in infants and young children. *Invest. Ophthalmol. Vis. Sci.* 31, 82.

WIESEL, T. N. (1982). Postnatal development of the visual cortex and the influence of environment. *Nature* 299, 583–591.

WIESEL, T. N., AND HUBEL, D. H. (1963). Effects of visual deprivation on morphology and physiology of cells in the cat's lateral geniculate body. *J. Neurophysiol.* 26, 978–993.

WIGGINS, R. E., AND VON NOORDEN, G. K. (1990). Monocular eye closure in sunlight. *J. Pediatr. Ophthalmol. Strabismus* 27, 16.

WILLIAMS, D. R., AND COLETTA, N. J. (1987). Cone spacing and the visual resolution limit. *J. Opt. Soc. Am. [A]* 4, 1514.

WILLIAMS, D. W., AND SEKULER, R. (1984). Coherent global motion percepts from stochastic local motions. *Vision Res.* 24, 55–62.

WILSON, H. R. (1991). Model of peripheral and amblyopic hyperacuity. *Vision Res.* 31, 967–982.

WILSON, H. R., BLAKE, R., AND HALPERN, L. H. (1991). Coarse spatial scales constrain the range of binocular vision on fine scales. *J. Opt. Soc. Am. [A]* 8, 229–236.

WILSON, H. R., METS, B., NAGY, S. E., AND KRESSEL, A. B. (1988). Albino spatial vision as an instance of arrested visual development. *Vision Res.* 28, 979–990.

WITKOVSKY, P., AND DEARRY, A. (1991). Functional properties of dopamine in the vertebrate retina. *Prog. Retinal Res.* 11, 247–289.

WOLFE, J. (1986). Stereopsis and binocular rivalry. *Psychol. Rev.* 93, 269–282.

WOO, G. C., AND SILLANPAA, V. (1979). Absolute stereoscopic thresholds as measured by crossed and uncrossed disparities. *Am. J. Optom. Physiol. Opt.* 56, 350.

WOODRUFF, M. E., AND SAMEK, M. J. (1976). The refractive status of Belcher Island Eskimos. *Can. J. Public Health* 67, 314–319.

WORTH, C. (1903). *Squint, Its Causes, Pathology, and Treatment.* London: Baillière, Tindall & Cox.

WYATT, H. T., AND BOYD, T. A. S. (1973). Strabismus and strabismic amblyopia in northern Canada. *Can. J. Ophthalmol.* 8, 244–251.

YANG, Y., AND BLAKE, R. (1991). Spatial frequency tuning of human stereopsis. *Vision Res.* 31, 1177.

YASUMA, T., DAMER, R. D., LAKSHMINARAYANAN, V., ENOCH, J. M., AND O'DONNELL, J. J. (1986). Retinal receptor alignment and directional sensitivity in a gyrate atrophy patient. *Clin Vis. Sci.* 1, 93–102.

YOUNG, R. D. (1988). Solar radiation and age-related macular degeneration. *Surv. Ophthalmol.* 32, 252–269.

YUODELIS, C., AND HENDRICKSON, A. (1986). A qualitative and quantitative analysis of the human fovea during development. *Vision Res.* 26, 847–855.

ZIMMERMAN, A. A., ARMSTRONG, E. L., AND SCAMMON, R. E. (1929). The change in position of the eyeballs during fetal life. *Anat. Rec.* 59, 109.

26 | Visual outcomes after infantile cataract

DAPHNE MAURER AND TERRI L. LEWIS

Children treated for congenital cataract afford an opportunity to study the effects of experience on visual development. A cataract is an opacity in the lens of the eye that scatters light and blurs the images on the retina. Treatment requires surgical removal of the cataract and renders the eye aphakic (without a natural lens). The aphakic eye is then fitted with an optical correction to focus visual input, although this correction focuses input perfectly at only one distance. In unilateral cases, ophthalmologists recommend patching the fellow eye part of the time during infancy and childhood in order to encourage use of the previously deprived eye.

For many visual functions, the effect of deprivation from cataract depends on whether the deprivation was unilateral or bilateral. The abnormalities following binocular deprivation indicate that deprivation per se interferes with normal visual development. The greater abnormalities following monocular deprivation indicate that, in addition, the deprived eye is disadvantaged by its inability to compete with the fellow "normal" eye for connections within the nervous system. Patching presumably promotes recovery by reducing that competition. The effect of deprivation from cataract also depends on how long the deprivation lasted. For many visual functions, the deficits are worse when the cataract was present from birth and when treatment (surgery and contact lens fitting) was late. The pattern of influence, however, varies for different visual functions. Because of these differences, we have organized this chapter by visual functions. In each case we summarize the basic findings and analyze the effects of the type of deprivation (monocular or binocular) and its duration.

We introduce two types of literature in an effort to understand why deprivation has such diverse effects. First, we describe the normal pattern of development for each visual function. We do so to examine if there is a relation between the influence of deprivation on the development of a visual function and the level of development of that function at birth, subsequent qualitative changes in it, if any, and subsequent quantitative changes. Second, we describe the effect of similar deprivation in cats and monkeys on the development of visual behavior and its electrophysiological and ana-

tomical underpinnings. In most of these studies, one or both of the animal's eyes were sutured shut so only diffuse light could reach the retina. This form of deprivation is analogous to that caused by a dense, central cataract.

Most of the results come from our own studies of 89 children treated for unilateral congenital cataract and 161 eyes of 84 children treated for bilateral congenital cataracts. All cataracts had been diagnosed during the first eye examination, which was always before 6 months of age. All the cataracts were judged by an ophthalmologist to interfere seriously with central vision because: (1) the eye would not fixate or follow a light source; (2) the cataract completely blocked the ophthalmologist's view of the fundus; (3) it prevented a red reflex from being reflected from the retina; or (4) it looked dense and central. Eyes with additional serious problems likely to interfere with vision (e.g., glaucoma, detached retina) were excluded. Children with the common associated abnormalities of strabismus (misaligned eyes), nystagmus (repetitive jerky eye movements), and microcornea or microphthalmos (an unusually small eye) were included. The data from eyes with persistent hyperplastic primary vitreous (PHPV) were analyzed separately or excluded except in cases where the results were the same for those with and without PHPV (i.e., the symmetry of optokinetic nystagmus and vision in the fellow eye of children treated for unilateral congenital cataract).

Because the age at the time of referral varied, the age at which the child had surgery to remove the cataract and was first given an optical correction also varied (between 35 days and 15 years, although in most cases it was between 1 and 7 months). This variation allows us to assess the effects of the duration of deprivation, which had always begun before 6 months of age. We can also compare the effects of monocular versus binocular deprivation by contrasting children who were treated at the same age for a cataract in one versus both eyes. Although in unilateral cases the parents were instructed to patch the fellow eye 50% of the waking time throughout early childhood, compliance varied. This variation allows us to evaluate the effect of different amounts of patching following monocular deprivation.

454

For all tests included in the final analyses, aphakic eye(s) were corrected optically for the testing distance.

To monitor compliance with the prescribed patching regimen as accurately as possible, we questioned parents during each visit. We phrased our questions to make it easy for a parent to admit to little or no patching (e.g., "Is he still giving you a fight about patching?" or "Would you say that you have been patching about 15 minutes a day?"). We also observed whether the parent's report was consistent with how easily he or she was able to patch the child for our visual tests, and we questioned the parents again if we doubted their initial estimates. Although parents were instructed to patch the fellow eye 50% of the waking time, we treated a patient as compliant despite occasional lapses during an illness or short periods without a contact lens so long as the occlusion averaged at least 40% of the waking time.

GRATING ACUITY

Because many of the children treated for congenital cataract are too young to read a conventional letter chart, researchers have used nonverbal techniques to monitor the development of grating acuity, that is, the smallest stripes the eye can resolve. Three techniques have been developed: preferential looking (see Chapter 20), optokinetic nystagmus, and visually evoked potentials. The rationale in each case is that the child makes some response if, and only if, he or she can resolve the patterning in the stimulus. The smallest pattern eliciting a response provides a measure of grating acuity. We have confined our discussion to studies based on preferential looking and optokinetic nystagmus, the two techniques we have used ourselves.

Preferential Looking

Method. Preferential looking (PL) takes advantage of the fact that young infants look longer at a patterned stimulus than at a plain gray field (Fantz et al., 1962). After about 6–12 months of age, the preference must be strengthened by rewarding the child for looking at, or pointing toward, the stripes (Mayer and Dobson, 1980, 1982; Birch et al., 1983). Typically, black-and-white stripes are paired with a plain gray stimulus, and the size of stripe is varied across trials. An observer, blind to the side on which the stripes appear, guesses their location based on the child's response. Either a staircase or the method of constant stimuli is used to determine the smallest stripes the observer can locate correctly. A more subjective version of this test, commonly called Acuity Cards, has been introduced (McDonald et al., 1985; Teller et al., 1986).

The literature contains a number of case reports on the grating acuity of children treated for congenital cataract (Jacobson et al., 1981, 1982; Rogers et al., 1981; Mohindra et al., 1983; Catalano et al., 1987) and systematic reports from two laboratories on unilateral cases (Birch et al., 1986; Birch and Stager, 1988; Mayer et al., 1989). This literature is difficult to summarize because some studies include (1) patients with other serious problems likely to interfere with visual development, e.g., case 4 with retinal detachment reported by Jacobson et al. (1981) and 5 of 16 patients with persistent hyperplastic primary vitreous reported by Birch et al. (1986); (2) patients in whom the cataract was apparently not dense, e.g., case 3 of Jacobson et al. (1981) and case C, left eye, of Mohindra et al. (1983); and (3) patients in whom the cataract may not have been congenital because it was not diagnosed until late during the first year of life, e.g., case 2 of Catalano et al. (1987).

There are also methodological problems in some of these studies. Rogers et al. (1981) developed their own testing procedure, which appears to reach a ceiling at 13 weeks, yet six of their seven patients were tested after 13 weeks of age. The tests also appear to have been binocular. The staircase used by Jacobson and his colleagues (Jacobson et al., 1981, 1982; Mohindra et al., 1983) has been criticized (Banks et al., 1982; Teller et al., 1982), but their confirmation of many of the results by the method of constant stimuli suggests that the overall picture they described is correct. Catalano et al. (1987) have no normative data before 3 months or after 18 months of age to which to compare their four patients, and between these ages there were only 39 control children divided among five ages. Mayer et al. (1989) used a staircase to determine grating acuity for the first half of their patients; but for the second half, they used an Acuity Card procedure in which the observer's expectation of poor results in some cases could have biased the results.

In the summary below, we have ignored these methodological concerns but restricted our coverage to monocular tests of children treated for dense cataracts diagnosed before 6 months of age.

Previous Studies: Bilateral Cases. The literature contains reports of five eyes from three children treated for bilateral congenital cataracts (in the sixth eye, the cataract was not dense) (Jacobson et al., 1981, 1982; Mohindra et al., 1983). In every test during the first year of life, grating acuity was within normal limits, except when the eye was covered by a secondary membrane or immediately following a period of being patched full-time. There are no reports (other than our own, which are summarized below) of development after the first year or of the effects of the duration of deprivation.

Previous Studies: Unilateral Cases. It is unclear whether the grating acuity of the deprived eye immediately after surgery and contact lens fitting is abnormal (Mayer et al., 1989) or within normal limits (Jacobson et al., 1981; Birch et al., 1986; Catalano et al., 1987; Birch and Stager, 1988). Nonetheless, all published reports agree that the grating acuity of the deprived eye improves during the first year and is generally within normal limits, except after periods when the contact lens has been lost (Jacobson et al., 1981; Birch et al., 1986; Catalano et al., 1987; Birch and Stager, 1988; Mayer et al., 1989). In most of these patients the period of deprivation was short, and the normal eye was patched at least 50% of the waking time. The amount of patching appears to be important because the interocular difference in grating acuity at 1 year of age correlates significantly with the mean number of hours per week that the fellow eye was patched after contact lens fitting (Mayer et al., 1989).

Although the grating acuity of children treated for unilateral congenital cataract typically continues to improve after the first year of life, it does not keep pace with the improvement shown by normal children and hence falls below normal limits (Birch et al., 1986; Birch and Stager, 1988; Mayer et al., 1989). This result is found even in patients without PHPV (Mayer et al., 1989), and even when treatment occurred within 6 weeks of birth and was followed by extensive patching (Birch et al., 1986). There are no reports of the effect on the acuity of the aphakic eye of the extent of patching or the duration of deprivation, but the interocular difference in grating acuity at 3 years of age (but not at 2 years) correlates significantly with the amount of previous patching (Mayer et al., 1989). [Mayer et al. (1989) reported no effect of the child's age at surgery on interocular differences in grating acuity at 1, 2, and 3 years of age. Because the children were not fitted with a contact lens immediately after surgery and they typically required a +30 diopter (D) correction, a better indicator of the duration of deprivation would have been the age when the eye was first given an optical correction.]

The fellow eyes of children treated for unilateral congenital cataract generally show normal grating acuity throughout the first 5 years of life (Jacobson et al., 1981; Birch et al., 1986; Catalano et al., 1987; Birch and Stager, 1988). The graphs of Mayer et al. (1989), however, indicated that the acuity of the fellow eye was above normal limits at 12 months and below normal limits at both 24 and 36 months. The low values are not likely to be related to patching, as patching was even more aggressive for the patients reported by Birch (Birch et al., 1986; Birch and Stager, 1988) and their fellow eyes showed no such acuity deficit.

Our Studies. We have been using preferential looking (PL) to monitor the development of grating acuity in 44 children treated for unilateral congenital cataract without PHPV, 16 children treated for unilateral congenital cataract with PHPV, and 92 eyes from 51 children treated for bilateral congenital cataracts (the remaining 10 eyes have additional abnormalities). Details of the patients followed with PL are given in Table 26-1. All testing was monocular, and in each case aphakic eyes were corrected optically for the testing distance. Because developmental delay can influence adversely the performance on tests of grating acuity (Wyngaarden et al., 1991), we excluded from our analyses of both PL acuity and optokinetic nystagmus acuity the data for 13 children, all treated for bilateral congenital cataracts, whose scores on standardized cognitive tests were more than 2 standard deviations (SD) below the normal mean.

In our version of PL (Lewis and Maurer, 1986), the child sits 50 cm from a panel with 10-degree portholes to the left and right of a central observation hole. (If it is necessary to create stripes smaller than 1 minute, the child is moved back to 100 cm.) Black-and-white stripes are presented through one porthole, and a plain gray through the other porthole. The gray is one of four luminances that bracket the luminance of the stripes. (Because we have found that the gray necessary for a perfect match is different for the fovea and the peripheral retina, we do not attempt an exact match but, instead, "jitter" the luminance of the gray.) We begin with wide stripes (66 minutes wide) and train the child first to look toward the stripes by projecting a colored picture onto a screen beside them whenever the child makes an appropriate response. After training, the observer must guess the location of the stripes solely on the basis of the child's behavior. During the testing phase, we use a modification of Taylor and Creelman's (1967) PEST staircase to "zero in" on the narrowest size of stripe the child/observer can locate accurately 75% of the time. When comparing these acuity values to those from normal children, we adjusted the age of the six children who were born before 37 weeks' ges-

TABLE 26-1. *Subjects who contributed to the data on preferential looking.*

Group	Age of first optical correction (months)		
	No.	Median	Range
Unilateral congenital cataract without PHPV	44	4.7	1.2–16.1
Unilateral congenital cataract with PHPV	16	3.4	1.2–10.5
Bilateral congenital cataract	92 Eyes from 51 children	4.6	1.3–18.0

tation for the number of weeks of prematurity because improvements in acuity measured by PL are related more tightly to postconceptional age than to postnatal age (reviewed by Dobson, 1990).

Table 26-2 indicates that more than 75% of the tests attempted with children treated for congenital cataract were completed successfully. The exceptions were mainly incomplete tests because the child would not cooperate until the end of the staircase. The procedural errors were tests during which the eye was not corrected for the testing distance.

Bilateral Cases. Figure 26-1 shows the median acuity at six testing ages for eyes treated for bilateral congenital cataracts plotted against the values obtained from 168 normal children (24–57 per age). The number of deprived eyes at each age varied from 41 eyes at 24 and 30 months to 55 eyes at 36 months, with each eye, on average, contributing data during three age periods. Although the median acuity was below the normal median at all ages, it was within normal limits through 18 months of age. Moreover, even at 24 months of age, 60% of the eyes with treatment (surgery and contact lens fitting) before 3 months of age had PL acuity values within normal limits. The median acuity of the group as a whole improved between 24 and 36 months but not sufficiently to keep pace with normal children. Figure 26-2 indicates that by 30 months fewer than 25% of these eyes had normal PL acuity.

Table 26-3 shows the Pearson correlation between PL acuity and the duration of deprivation in eyes treated

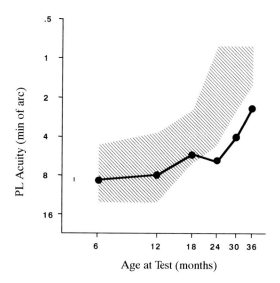

FIG. 26-1. Acuity measured by preferential looking as a function of the age of testing in children treated for bilateral congenital cataracts. Each point represents the median acuity for that age. Shaded area represents the range of values obtained from 95% of the normative sample.

for bilateral congenital cataract. For these analyses, we included one eye per child at each age, grating acuity was converted to a $\log_2$ scale, and duration of deprivation was defined as the time from birth until the first optical correction after surgery. There was a significant correlation only for tests at 12 months of age: At that age, better grating acuity was associated with shorter deprivation.

Unilateral Cases. Figure 26-3 shows the median acuity at six testing ages of eyes treated for unilateral congenital cataract plotted against our normative data (Lewis

TABLE 26-2. *Testing success with preferential looking.*

Age (months)	No. of tests Attempted	No. of tests Successful	Percent of tests Successful	Percent of tests Unsuccessful Incomplete	Percent of tests Unsuccessful Procedural error
Unilateral congenital cataract without PHPV					
6	25	19	76	20	4
12	33	26	79	21	—
18	26	22	85	15	—
24	22	16	73	27	—
30	27	23	85	4	11
36	21	20	95	5	—
Unilateral congenital cataract with PHPV					
6	11	9	82	9	9
12	9	9	100	—	—
18	12	10	83	17	—
24	11	8	73	18	9
30	9	7	78	22	—
36	7	7	100	—	—
Bilateral congenital cataract					
6	47	42	89	2	9
12	51	44	86	4	10
18	63	50	79	8	13
24	54	41	76	11	13
30	46	41	89	9	2
36	61	55	90	5	2

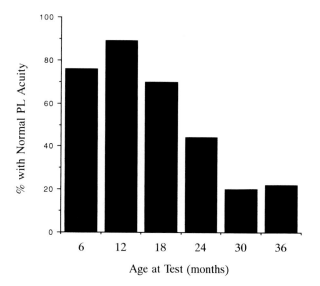

FIG. 26-2. Percent of eyes with normal preferential looking acuity at six test ages for children treated for bilateral congenital cataracts.

TABLE 26-3. *Correlation between PL acuity and duration of deprivation.*

Testing age (months)	Bilateral congenital cataract		Unilateral congenital cataract without PHPV	
	No.	Correlation[a]	No.	Correlation[a]
6	25	.03	19	.42*
12	28	.54***	26	−.07
18	30	−.09	22	.19
24	25	.23	16	.60**
30	25	.04	23	−.14
36	33	.17	20	−.10

[a]*$p < 0.05$ (one-tailed); **$p < 0.01$; ***$p < 0.001$.

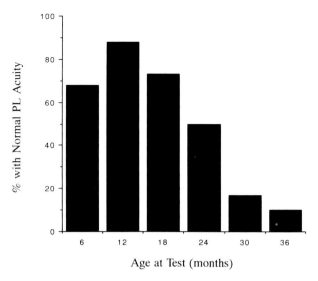

FIG. 26-4. Percent of eyes with normal preferential looking acuity at six test ages for deprived eyes without PHPV from children who had been treated for unilateral congenital cataract.

and Maurer, 1986). For eyes without PHPV, the number of cases ranged from 16 at 24 months to 26 at 12 months. For eyes with PHPV, the number ranged from 7 cases at 30 and 36 months to 10 cases at 18 months. In both groups, each eye contributed, on average, to three age periods. Eyes with and without PHPV showed a similar pattern: median acuity within (or nearly within) normal limits through 24 months of age and then little change, so median acuity fell increasingly below normal (Figs. 26-4 and 26-5).

Table 26-3 indicates that in eyes without PHPV better grating acuity was associated with shorter deprivation at 6 and 24 months of age, but there was no significant correlation at 12, 18, 30, or 36 months. (There were not sufficient data to perform correlations for eyes with PHPV.)

In eyes without PHPV, there was a significant correlation ($r = 0.43$; $n = 26$; $p < 0.025$; one-tailed) between PL acuity at 12 months (converted to $\log_2$) and the mean number of hours each day that the fellow eye

had been patched since contact lens fitting. That is, PL acuity improved as patching increased. Because patching success may be negatively correlated with the duration of deprivation, we calculated the correlation separately for eyes treated before versus after 3 months of age. The correlation between PL acuity at 12 months and the amount of patching was significant for the eight eyes treated before 3 months ($r = 0.79$; $p < 0.01$) but not for the 18 eyes treated later ($r = 0.30$; $p > 0.05$). The correlations were not significant for tests at 24 months or 36 months, although there were too few eyes

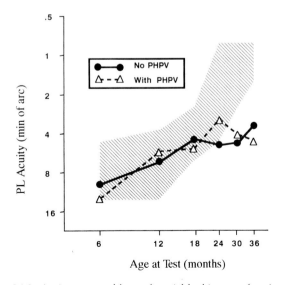

FIG. 26-3. Acuity measured by preferential looking as a function of age of testing in the deprived eyes of children treated for unilateral congenital cataract with or without persistent hyperplastic primary vitreous (PHPV). Other details as in Figure 26-1.

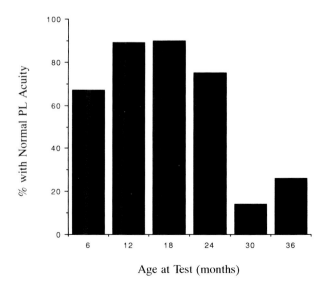

FIG. 26-5. Percent of deprived eyes with normal preferential looking acuity at six ages for deprived eyes with PHPV from children who had been treated for unilateral congenital cataract.

with early treatment for a separate analysis. (There were also too few cases to evaluate the effects of patching in eyes with PHPV.)

The pattern of results for children treated for unilateral cataract is similar to that reported above for children treated for bilateral cataracts. The two groups had similar durations of deprivation (Table 26-1); the PL acuity of both developed within normal limits during the first 18 months and fell increasingly below normal after 2 years (compare Figures 26-1 and 26-3). This similarity is surprising given the much greater deficits in later linear letter acuity in unilateral cases than in bilateral cases (see below).

Optokinetic Nystagmus

Method. Optokinetic nystagmus (OKN) can be used to measure grating acuity by progressively reducing the size of the stripe until it no longer elicits OKN. Other than our own report (Maurer et al., 1989b), there are only two published case reports based on OKN (Enoch and Rabinowicz, 1976; Enoch et al., 1979). Enoch and colleagues used an OKN drum to measure the acuity of two infants treated for unilateral congenital cataract during the first (Enoch and Rabinowicz, 1976) and sixth (Enoch et al., 1979) months of life. For tests of one patient (Enoch and Rabinowicz, 1976), the stripes were made smaller by moving the drum farther from the child. As the authors acknowledged, this method makes the results difficult to interpret because (1) the aphakic eye could not change its focus with the testing distance and (2) the child appeared not to pay attention to the drum beyond 1.2 meters. In both patients, Enoch and his colleagues found improvement in the acuity of the aphakic eye during the 3–4 months after optical correction, with the aphakic eye always performing more poorly than the fellow eye.

Our Studies. In our version of the OKN test (Lewis et al., 1990a), the baby has one eye patched and is seated 50 cm (or, to create the smallest stripes, 100 cm) from a large rear projection screen (84 × 84 degrees when viewed from 50 cm). Vertical black-and-white stripes move across the screen at 13 degrees/second (or 6.5 degrees/second from 100 cm) for 7 seconds at a time in the direction from the temporal field toward the nasal field of the unpatched eye. Movement is limited to this direction because normal young infants and children with eye problems often show OKN only for stripes moving in this direction (see Symmetry of OKN, below). Observers watch the child's eye movements through peepholes beside the screen and determine the smallest stripes eliciting OKN. They also make sure that they can differentiate nystagmus elicited by the stripes from

any spontaneous nystagmus seen on control trials during which no stimulus is projected. In cases where the child has to be moved back to 100 cm to create smaller stripes, we also show the child large stripes from that distance to verify that OKN can still be elicited despite the reduction in field size and velocity. Note that the smallest stripes we can create in this setup are 6 minutes wide when viewed from 100 cm, and hence the range of values cuts off at this value. Note also that, with a constant velocity, increases in spatial frequency simultaneously increase the temporal frequency of luminance changes on the retina. Hence our OKN thresholds may be limited by either temporal or spatial resolution.

Our OKN test can be completed by virtually all normal children within a short time, and the results are reliable for both normal children and children treated for cataracts (Maurer et al., 1989b; Lewis et al., 1990a). It is difficult to test children treated for cataracts, however, primarily because many have a spontaneous or latent nystagmus that cannot be differentiated from nystagmus elicited by the stripes. This problem occurred for about half the attempts to test children treated for unilateral congenital cataract and for most of the attempts to test children treated for bilateral congenital cataracts (Table 26-4). Because there were so few successful tests, we report the average pattern of development of OKN acuity for ages with at least five data points, but we do not correlate it with the duration of deprivation or with the amount of patching. The average eye in these series was tested successfully at two ages with a range from one to five. Table 26-5 lists the characteristics of the children included.

There are no published reports on the effects of prematurity on the development of OKN acuity. Because PL acuity is so closely tied to postconceptional age, however, we corrected for prematurity the age of the three children born before 37 weeks' gestation.

Bilateral Cases. The number of eyes tested ranged from 6 eyes at 6 months to 11 eyes at 24 months (there were too few tests to report at 18 months). Figure 26-6 shows the median OKN acuity from children treated for congenital cataracts plotted against the range at five ages seen in 24–30 children per age without eye problems (Lewis et al., 1990a). The treated eyes fell at the bottom of the normal range at 6 months and then improved slightly but still fell outside the normal range at all other ages. Figure 26-7 indicates that by 36 months no eye showed OKN acuity within normal limits.

Unilateral Cases. The data for children treated for unilateral congenital cataract without PHPV are plotted in Figure 26-8. The number of data points ranges from 9 points at 6 and 18 months to 14 points at 12 months. (There were too few data points to report for children treated for unilateral congenital cataract with PHPV.) Figures 26-8 and 26-9 indicate that the OKN acuity of

TABLE 26-4. *Testing success with OKN.*

Age (months)	No. of tests		Percent of tests			
				Unsuccessful		
	Attempted	Successful	Successful	Too much nystagmus	Could not elicit OKN	Procedural error
Unilateral congenital cataract without PHPV						
6	22	9	41	50	4	4
12	29	14	48	45		7
18	22	9	41	59		
24	26	12	46	46		8
36	20	11	55	40		5
Unilateral congenital cataract with PHPV						
6	11	6	55	27		18
12	13	5	38	54	8	
18	9	4	44	56		
24	8	2	50	50		
36	3	1	33	67		
Bilateral congenital cataract						
6	62	6	9	84		6
12	65	9	14	77	3	6
18	63	3	5	90		5
24	58	11	19	76	2	3
36	57	8	14	86		

TABLE 26-5. *Subjects who contributed to the data on OKN acuity.*[a]

Group	No.	Age of first optical correction (months)	
		Median	Range
Unilateral congenital cataract without PHPV	27	4.8	1.3–16.1
Bilateral congenital cataract	21 Eyes from 15 children	4.2	1.3–17.9

[a]Includes only ages at which there were at least five data points.

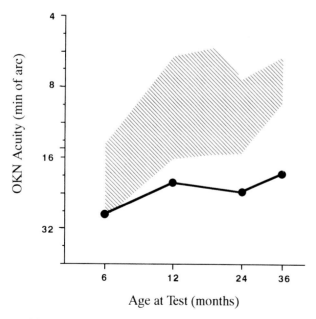

FIG. 26-6. Acuity measured by optokinetic nystagmus (OKN) as a function of the age of testing in children treated for bilateral congenital cataracts. Each point represents the median acuity for that age. Shaded area represents the range of values obtained from 95% of the normative sample.

unilateral cases fell outside the normal range at all ages, with no normal values at 12, 18, or 36 months.

Comparison of Figures 26-6 and 26-8 and of Figures 26-7 and 26-9 indicates that the OKN acuity of unilateral cases was slightly worse than that of bilateral cases. It is the same pattern we found with later linear acuity (see below) but differs from the pattern we found with PL acuity, where unilateral cases performed just as well as bilateral cases.

The eyes that could be tested with OKN may represent the eyes with the best prognosis: They showed steady enough fixation to complete the test successfully. Despite this biased selection, OKN acuity was outside the normal range during the first 1–2 years, whereas PL acuity was normal. This difference is emphasized by

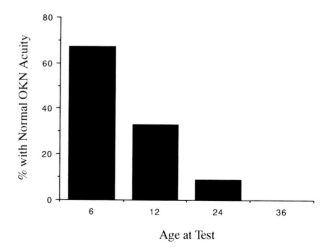

FIG. 26-7. Percent of eyes with normal OKN acuity at four test ages for children treated for bilateral congenital cataracts.

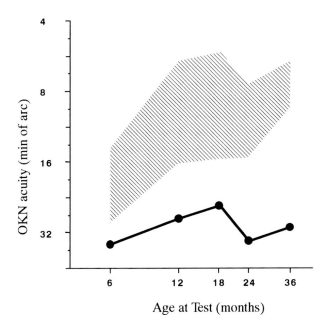

FIG. 26-8. OKN acuity as a function of the age of testing in the deprived eyes of children treated for unilateral congenital cataract without PHPV. Other details as in Figure 26-6.

TABLE 26-6. *Agreement between PL and OKN on whether the acuity of an eye was normal or abnormal.*

Testing age (months)	No.	% Agreement
6	12	58
12	22	23
18	10	20
24	17	41
36	19	95

Table 26-6, which compares eyes tested at the same age by the two techniques: Agreement was good at 36 months of age, at which point both techniques indicated that the acuity of most eyes was below normal limits; but agreement was poor before that age because in most instances OKN acuity was abnormal whereas PL acuity was within normal limits.

Synthesis and Conclusions

Our results indicate that children treated for unilateral or bilateral congenital cataracts have PL acuities within the normal range during early infancy but later fail to keep pace with normal children. In unilateral cases, this pattern seems not to depend on whether the eye also had PHPV. However, the pattern does vary with the duration of deprivation and, in unilateral cases, with the extent to which the fellow eye was patched. These patterns are similar to those shown by aphakic monkeys (deprived by having the natural lens removed) tested with Acuity Cards (O'Dell et al., 1989). In contrast to the results from PL, we found that OKN acuity shows little improvement with age and falls outside the normal range virtually throughout early childhood. Like our results from normal children, the different patterns of results for the two tests suggest that our versions of OKN and PL measure different aspects of vision and may tap different neural circuits.

One possible reason for the different patterns is that PL is an insensitive test of visual acuity, at least during early infancy. First, children treated for congenital cataract rarely develop 20/20 linear acuity. Yet measurements with our version of PL yielded acuity values that were within normal limits for most children during the first 1–2 years. This pattern is consistent with previous reports using a variety of other versions of PL (Jacobson et al., 1981; Birch et al., 1986; Catalano et al., 1987; Birch and Stager, 1988; Mayer et al., 1989). Second, the linear acuity of eyes treated for unilateral congenital cataract is usually worse than that of eyes treated for bilateral congenital cataract (see below), especially if there has been little patching in the unilateral cases. Yet there was no difference in PL acuity between unilateral and bilateral cases, even though our sample included children who received little patching. Third, the PL acuity of esotropic children is usually normal in both eyes during early infancy (Birch and Stager, 1985; Stager and Birch, 1986) and even the first 2 years of life (Dobson and Sebris, 1989), and the relative acuity of their two eyes often does not agree with fixation preference (Stager and Birch, 1986). It is tempting to conclude that either (1) PL acuity is not a sensitive measure during infancy; or (2) it takes several years for deficits in PL acuity to develop, longer than it takes for fixation preferences to emerge in strabismic amblyopes or for OKN acuity deficits to emerge in deprivation amblyopes.

Correlational evidence argues against the first hypothesis that PL is an insensitive measure during early

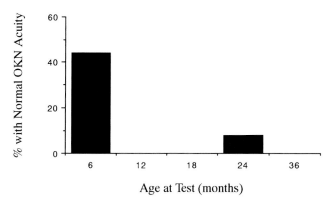

FIG. 26-9. Percent of eyes with normal OKN acuity at five test ages for deprived eyes without PHPV from children who had been treated for unilateral congenital cataract.

infancy. Even though most of the eyes we studied had normal PL acuity during the first 1–2 years of life, variables known to influence later linear acuity were correlated significantly with PL acuity at several points during the first 2 years: In unilateral cases, the duration of deprivation influenced the results at 6 and 24 months, and the duration of patching influenced the results at 12 months. Moreover, in children treated for bilateral congenital cataracts with a stable prognosis (i.e., no intervening complications), there is a significant correlation between PL acuity at 12 months and later linear letter acuity (Maurer et al., 1989a). (Because intervening patching affects the outcome in unilateral cases, we did not calculate a similar correlation for that group). Such correlations suggest that PL measurements during infancy are sensitive to differences among cases that affect their long-term prognosis. Moreover, Birch and Hale (1988) have shown that PL assessments based on differences in acuity between the two eyes are a more sensitive measure of amblyopia than assessments based on the comparison of each eye's performance to the normal range.

The second possibility is that PL acuity measures a different aspect of vision than does OKN acuity, an aspect that is not degraded severely during infancy by a period of deprivation, the resulting aphakia, or other abnormalities such as strabismus. Limitations on the acuity of children treated for cataracts are likely to occur at the level of the cortex. In the monkey, retinal ganglion cells are apparently unaffected by deprivation, provided the deprivation did not extend from birth past 2 years of age (reviewed by Boothe et al., 1985). In contrast, after binocular deprivation, many cells in the striate cortex are unresponsive, and others respond sluggishly and unreliably with ill-defined or broadly tuned receptive fields (reviewed by Movshon and Van Sluyters, 1981; Boothe et al., 1985; but see Crawford et al., 1991). As in the striate cortex of the infant monkey, no cells respond to fine stripes (Blakemore, 1988). Similar changes occur after monocular deprivation in cortical cells driven by the deprived eye, which are scarce (Blakemore, 1988). Moreover, lesions of the monkey's striate cortex drastically reduce contrast sensitivity for all stripe sizes (Pasik and Pasik, 1982).

Much of the limitation on the PL acuity of normal infants can be accounted for by immaturities in the density and shape of photoreceptors in the macula (Banks and Bennett, 1988). It is possible that during early infancy such retinal immaturities are more limiting than are the developing cortical abnormalities in children treated for cataract. Hence the PL acuity of deprived eyes is no worse than that of normal eyes. With increasing age, retinal immaturity ceases to limit the acuity of normal children, and the acuity of eyes treated for congenital cataract falls increasingly behind because of cortical abnormalities.

Although Banks and Bennett (1988) analyzed the effect of immature macular photoreceptors on infants' acuity, several lines of evidence suggest that peripheral photoreceptors (and their projections) are likely to be more important for PL acuity. First, the striped fields used for PL testing are large (10 degrees in our version). When older amblyopic children are tested with smaller striped fields, their PL results are poorer and correspond more closely to their recognition acuities (Mayer, 1986). Second, infants with no anatomical fovea because of oculocutaneous albinism show surprisingly little deficit in PL acuity—much less deficit than is shown by infants with general retinal degeneration (Mayer et al., 1985). Anatomical data from the monkey indicate that the near peripheral retina takes many years to mature (Packer et al., 1990). If it is also the case in humans, the cortical limitations on the acuity of children treated for cataracts might not become apparent until immaturities in the peripheral retina are no longer limiting normal PL acuity. This hypothesis is strengthened by our finding that children treated for congenital cataract have abnormally small visual fields (Bowering et al., 1989) and lower than normal sensitivity to both light and contrast throughout the visual field (Bowering et al., 1991; Tytla et al., 1991). It suggests that the peripheral retina or its projections do not develop normally in children treated for congenital cataract.

Paradoxically, OKN acuity is more likely to be affected by the central retina and its projections than by the peripheral retina. On the one hand, reducing a field of moving stripes to an area as small as a 5-degree strip over the central retina has little effect on the gain of OKN, and masking a part of the stimulus falling on the near periphery has no effect (van Die and Collewijn, 1982, 1986). Similarly, an area of moving stripes just 10 × 20 degrees is as effective at driving OKN as an area of 10 × 65 degrees so long as the edges of the moving stimulus are blurred (Howard and Ohmi, 1984). On the other hand, occluding even the central 5 degrees of the stimulus dramatically lowers the gain of OKN (van Die and Collewijn, 1986) and does so over a range of velocities (Howard and Ohmi, 1984). The deleterious effects of central occlusion are not due entirely to the effects of sharp vertical edges on the masks (Howard and Ohmi, 1984; van Die and Collewijn, 1986; Murasugi et al., 1989). Similarly, patients with a central scotoma show lower OKN gain in the affected eye than in their fellow normal eye over a wide range of velocities (van Die and Collewijn, 1986). Together these findings indicate that the central retina plays a larger role than the peripheral retina in driving OKN. It is interesting that at least by 7 years of age children treated for congenital cataract show less than normal visual sensitivity throughout the visual field, but the losses are greatest in the center of the field (Bowering et al., 1991)—the part of the field that has the greatest influence on OKN.

In summary, OKN acuity and PL acuity show a different pattern of development in normal infants. It might be because the two tests differ in the extent to which they are influenced by central versus peripheral vision. It is tempting to speculate that in children treated for congenital cataract OKN acuity shows deficits at an early age because it is influenced strongly by the central retina and its projections, which do not develop normally. PL acuity may not show deficits during infancy because it is influenced strongly by the peripheral retina and its projections, which are not damaged as seriously by deprivation or because the cortical deficits in children treated for cataract are not manifest until the immaturity of the peripheral retina no longer limits the PL acuity of normal infants.

Alternatively (and not mutually exclusively), the poor OKN acuity of children treated for congenital cataract may be caused by abnormal cortical influence on the midbrain. As we discuss later in the chapter, deprived eyes show little if any OKN to stripes moving from the nasal field toward the temporal field. This asymmetrical OKN seemingly reflects a failure of cortical pathways to influence OKN (Hoffmann, 1989) or abnormal development within those cortical pathways (Norcia et al., 1991a,b). In the normal adult cat, the cortex is not necessary for OKN to stripes moving temporally to nasally, but in the normal adult monkey and human there is evidence for greater cortical influence over OKN in general (see Symmetry of OKN, below). Thus during normal development, temporal-to-nasal OKN may improve because of changes in the visual cortex. Because of cortical deficits, the OKN acuity of children treated for cataracts may show no such improvement.

LINEAR LETTER ACUITY

By linear letter acuity we mean acuity as measured by tests that require the child to recognize or match letters arranged in rows (e.g., Snellen chart, Bailey-Lovie chart, linear versions of the Sheridan Gardiner test, or linear E game). We do not include single letter tests such as the Sheridan Gardiner singles, or the single tumbling Es that require the child to recognize a letter presented in isolation because children with eye problems often do well when their acuity is measured with single letters but do poorly when it is measured with rows of letters (reviewed by Birch, 1989; Mohn and van Hof-van Duin, 1990). Nor do we include tests with single letters surrounded by crowding bars because we have found that at least some of these tests also overestimate linear letter acuity (unpublished results).

Numerous studies have shown that children treated for congenital cataract have poor linear acuity in the affected eyes despite suitable optical correction (reviewed by Maurer et al., 1989b; see also Lewis et al., 1986; Robb et al., 1987; Birch and Stager, 1988; Drummond et al., 1989). The results are more promising for patients who were treated during early infancy and, in unilateral cases, who received extensive patching of the fellow eye. For example, Birch and Stager (1988; see also Everett et al., 1989) reported a median acuity of 20/60 for children who had surgery for a unilateral congenital cataract before 2 months of age and a median acuity of counting fingers for those who underwent later surgery. Patching appears also to be important: The results were significantly better for the nine children who complied with the patching regimen and contact lens wear throughout early childhood, all of whom had had surgery before 5 months of age, than for the 10 children with poorer compliance, who were treated at a variety of ages. Similarly, Drummond et al. (1989; see also Scott et al., 1989) reported linear acuities of 20/60 or better for their six patients who received their first optical correction before 17 weeks of age and who patched the fellow eye aggressively, in contrast to acuities of 20/200 or worse for the three patients who received later treatment and less patching. (We have omitted the results for two patients with secondary glaucoma and for patients not tested with a linear letter chart.) Robb et al. (1987) found that 5 of their 12 patients treated for a unilateral congenital cataract during the first 6 months of life had a Snellen E acuity of at least 20/70, although in this sample the acuity was not correlated with age of surgery and the data were not analyzed in terms of compliance with patching. Scattered reports of 17 children who were treated for bilateral congenital cataracts during early infancy suggest that in bilateral cases a good outcome can be achieved after early treatment: In 6 of the 33 tested eyes, vision was 20/100 or better (reviewed by Maurer et al., 1989b).

These studies suggest that children visually deprived from birth by dense cataracts can at least sometimes achieve good visual acuity when the period of deprivation is short. However, a number of problems make these studies difficult to interpret (reviewed by Maurer et al., 1989b). Many studies have not described the density of the cataract, the age at which it was first noted, the age at which the deprivation ended because the aphakic eye was given a suitable optical correction, and in unilateral cases the extent to which the fellow eye was patched (Hiles and Wallar, 1977; Francois, 1979, 1984; Pratt-Johnson and Tillson, 1981; Robb et al., 1987; Birch and Stager, 1988). Some samples included eyes with PHPV or posterior lenticonus, which may alter the prognosis (Birch and Stager, 1988; Everett et al., 1989), whereas other studies restricted their sample to eyes without these additional abnormalities (Robb et al., 1987; Drummond et al., 1989). Moreover, no previous study, other than previous reports of our own (Brent et al., 1986; Maurer et al., 1989b), has compared unilateral cases to bilateral cases or examined the influence of the duration of deprivation in bilateral cases.

Our Studies

We have examined the linear letter acuity of 34 children treated for unilateral congenital cataract without PHPV, 7 children treated for unilateral congenital cataract with PHPV, and 64 eyes from 36 children treated for bilateral congenital cataracts (Table 26-7). Figures 26-10 to 26-12 show the linear letter acuity for each group, plotted as a function of the duration of deprivation. Each value represents the median of all tests of an eye; the average value is based on six tests with a range of 1–36 tests. All of the children were at least 3 years old at the time of the test.

Among unilateral cases without PHPV, the four children who had 5 months or less of deprivation and whose fellow eye was patched at least 40% of the waking time throughout early childhood achieved a linear letter acuity in the deprived eye of between 20/40 and 20/80 (Table 26-8). The results were much worse for the remaining 30 children, who received later treatment or less extensive patching, with one-third of the values no better than counting fingers. Results for the 7 eyes with PHPV also ranged from 20/200 to counting fingers. (There were no children in this group whose fellow eye was patched extensively.) The eyes treated for bilateral congenital cataracts achieved a median acuity of 20/77 when deprivation ended at or before 5 months of age. However, bilateral cases did much better than unilateral cases when deprivation ended later, with only 3 of 64 values as poor as counting fingers.

To evaluate statistically the effect of the duration of deprivation over the whole range of values, we calculated the Pearson correlation between the duration of deprivation and the denominator of the linear acuity value (converted to $\log_2$). For these analyses we included only one eye from each child treated for bilateral congenital cataracts. The correlation was significant for unilateral cases without PHPV ($r = 0.37$; $p < 0.025$; one-tailed) but not for the other two groups. To com-

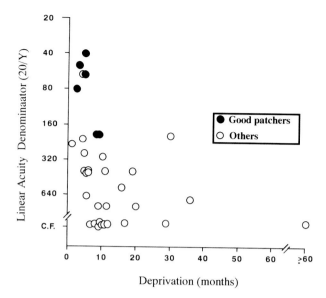

FIG. 26-10. Linear letter acuity as a function of the duration of deprivation for children treated for unilateral congenital cataract without PHPV whose good eye was (●) or was not (○) patched 40–50% of the waking time throughout early childhood. The ordinate represents the denominator of the Snellen fraction (20/Y). C.F. = counting fingers.

pare the linear acuity of unilateral versus bilateral cases, we performed a t-test using the 34 unilateral cases and one eye from each of 36 bilateral cases. The linear acuity of the unilateral cases was significantly worse, despite the fact that in these samples the mean duration of deprivation was one month shorter in the unilateral sample [$t(68) = 4.92$; $p < 0.0001$].

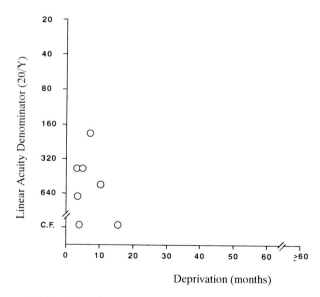

FIG. 26-11. Linear letter acuity in deprived eyes with PHPV from children treated for unilateral congenital cataract. Other details as in Figure 26-10.

TABLE 26-7. *Subjects who contributed to data on linear acuity.*

| Group | No. | Age of first optical correction (months) | |
		Median	Range
Unilateral congenital cataract without PHPV	34	8.8	1.3–72.8
Unilateral congenital cataract with PHPV	7	5.1	3.3–15.3
Bilateral congenital cataract	64 Eyes from 36 children	6.1	1.3–82.3

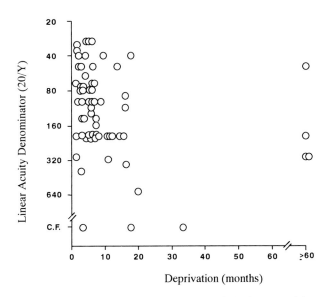

FIG. 26-12. Linear letter acuity as a function of the duration of deprivation in children treated for bilateral congenital cataracts.

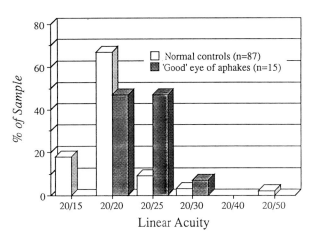

FIG. 26-13. Frequency histogram of linear letter acuities for the good eyes of 6- and 7-year-olds who had been treated for unilateral congenital cataract (dark bars) and for the right eyes of normal age-mates (white bars).

To evaluate the linear acuity of the fellow eyes in children treated for unilateral congenital cataract, we compared the linear letter acuity in the fellow eye of 15 children aged 6–7 years to that of 87 age-matched controls (Lewis et al., 1989b). All of the fellow eyes were ophthalmologically normal with minimal refractive error (< 2 D of spherical error and 1 D of cylindrical error). As Figure 26-13 indicates, the frequency of acuity of at least 20/20 was significantly lower in the patients ($\chi^2 = 9.3$; $p < 0.01$). There was no relation between the percent of time the good eye had been patched and its linear letter acuity (Fig. 26-14). For this analysis, patching represents a weighted mean of the percent of time the fellow eye had been patched from birth until 5 years of age.

Synthesis and Conclusions

Our results indicate that the linear letter acuity of eyes treated for congenital cataract is worse following monocular deprivation than following binocular deprivation; and at least in unilateral cases, it is worse following long periods of deprivation than following shorter periods. As in previous studies (Pratt-Johnson and Tillson,

1981; Robb et al., 1987; Birch and Stager, 1988; Drummond et al., 1989), our results indicate that good linear acuity can be achieved even in unilateral cases if the deprivation is short *and* if the fellow eye is patched at least 40% of the waking time throughout early childhood. This finding is reminiscent of our results for PL acuity (see above) in which the extent of patching was correlated with PL acuity at 12 months in children treated for unilateral congenital cataract with short deprivation. Also like the results of Mayer et al. (1989) for PL acuity in unilateral cases (see earlier in the chapter), the linear acuity of the fellow eye was good but statistically less than that of age-matched controls.

In bilateral congenital cases, any effect of the duration of deprivation must be subtle: Despite considerable variation in the age at treatment, we found no significant difference in the linear letter acuity of eyes with more or less than 5 months of deprivation and no significant correlation between the duration of deprivation and linear letter acuity. The contrasting results in unilateral and bilateral congenital cases imply that the nervous system is considerably more resilient when it must cope only with deprivation and not also with unfair competition between the two eyes for synaptic connections. The results from unilateral cases indicate that such unfair competition can also be mitigated by patching.

TABLE 26-8. *Linear acuity.*

Group	Deprivation ≤ 5 months and good patching in unilateral cases			Deprivation > 5 months and/or poor patching in unilateral cases		
	No.	Median	Range	No.	Median	Range
Unilateral congenital cataract without PHPV	4	20/55	20/40–20/80	30	20/600	20/60–CF
Unilateral congenital cataract with PHPV	—			7	20/550	20/200–CF
Bilateral congenital cataract	22	20/77	20/30–CF	42	20/180	20/30–CF

CF = counting fingers.

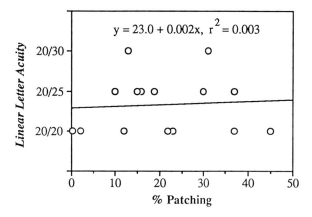

FIG. 26-14. Scatter plot showing the relation between linear letter acuity and the percent of time the good eye had been patched between birth and 5 years of age. Each point represents the results from the good eye of one child treated for unilateral congenital cataract. The solid line plots the regression equation.

Moreover, it can even lead to subtle deficits in the non-deprived eye.

Parallel results have been reported for animals deprived by lid suture, which were allowed to recover and then tested for grating acuity. Adult cats and monkeys that had been visually deprived for a period after birth usually show poor acuity in the previously deprived eye(s). As in humans, the longer monocular deprivation lasts after birth, the poorer the acuity (Mitchell and Timney, 1982; Smith and Holdeter, 1985; Harwerth et al., 1989). Following binocular deprivation, at least in monkeys, the duration of deprivation does not have an obvious effect (Harwerth et al., 1991). Also as in humans, animals that had been deprived monocularly had much poorer acuity in the formerly deprived eye than in either eye of animals that had been deprived binocularly (Smith, 1981; Harwerth et al., 1991). However, following monocular deprivation, as in humans, the reduced acuity of the formerly deprived eye can be improved by reverse occlusion (i.e., by shutting the fellow eye after the deprived eye is opened) (Harwerth et al., 1989; Mitchell, 1991). After short-term monocular deprivation from birth in cats or corrected aphakia from early infancy in monkeys, the best results for both eyes are achieved by occluding the fellow eye 50–75% of the time (Wilson et al., 1991; Mitchell, 1991). The overall pattern of results from cats and monkeys suggests that, as in humans, deprivation per se and competition between a deprived and nondeprived eye interfere with the development of visual resolution.

CONTRAST SENSITIVITY

Unlike acuity, which provides a measure only of the smallest stimulus the eye can resolve, contrast sensitivity provides a measure of the eye's sensitivity across a wide

range of spatial frequencies. Figure 26-15 illustrates the contrast sensitivity function of typical normal adults. The abscissa represents spatial frequency ranging from wide (0.33 cycles/degree, or cpd) stripes to narrow (20 cpd) stripes. The ordinate represents contrast sensitivity, the reciprocal of the minimum contrast necessary to detect a grating. Extrapolation of the right half of the function to the abscissa provides an estimate of grating acuity, the finest stripes the eye can resolve at 100% contrast. As shown in Figure 26-15, adults are less sensitive to wide or narrow stripes than to stripes of medium width.

Other than our own work (Tytla et al., 1988), little is known about the contrast sensitivity of patients treated for congenital cataract. The results differ for the only two patients who had had a unilateral cataract diagnosed during early infancy and an ophthalmologically normal fellow eye [patient C.T. reported by Manny and Levi (1982) and patient R.C. reported by Hess et al., (1981)]. Both suffered long-term deprivation (13–16 years) because they wore no optical correction after surgery until the time of the contrast sensitivity test. Patient C.T. could detect the pattern in 1-cpd stripes (the only width tested) only at high contrast and could not detect movement or flicker across a wide range of temporal frequencies (Manny and Levi, 1982). Patient R.C. could detect no pattern in even wider stripes (0.05–

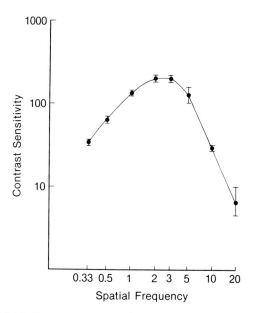

FIG. 26-15. Contrast sensitivity plotted as a function of spatial frequency for normal adults tested in our apparatus. Curve illustrates the reciprocal of the threshold contrast at various spatial frequencies, with higher values on the ordinate representing greater sensitivity. Curve shows mean and standard error for five adults. (From Maurer, D., Lewis, T. L., and Brent, H. P. (1988b). The effects of deprivation on human visual development: studies of children treated for cataracts. In F. J. Morrison, C. Lord, and D. P. Keating (eds.). *Applied Developmental Psychology. Vol. 3. Psychological Development in Infancy.* San Diego: Academic Press. By permission.)

1.00 cpd) but could detect flicker up to 10 Hz if the stripes were of high contrast (Hess et al., 1981). Eight patients born with dense bilateral cataracts who had suffered 9–30 months of deprivation had a much more favorable outcome (Kocher and Perenin, 1983; Mioche and Perenin, 1986). Nonetheless, most showed deficits in contrast sensitivity at all spatial frequencies, deficits that increased with increasing spatial frequency.

Our Results

Unilateral Cases. We measured the contrast sensitivity of a larger group of patients, including many who received more prompt and successful treatment than in previous studies (Tytla et al., 1988). To examine the effects of monocular deprivation, we tested 10 children aged 4–12 years who were treated for unilateral congenital cataract. The aphakic eye had first been fitted with a contact lens at ages ranging from 3 to 29 months; patching ranged from excellent (50% of the waking time throughout early childhood) to poor (occasional, or 1 hour per week). For comparison, we tested the right eyes of 20 normal children aged 4–12 years and three children treated for traumatic cataract who had been deprived for 5–7 months beginning after age 5 years.

Results from the traumatic cases were essentially normal, indicating that surgery for cataract and the subsequent aphakia (with suitable optical correction) do not in themselves alter contrast sensitivity. Figure 26-16 shows the loss in contrast sensitivity relative to the normal control group for the deprived eye of each of the 10 children treated for unilateral congenital cataract. Each point shows, for a particular spatial frequency and rate of flicker, the log of the ratio relating sensitivity in the deprived eye to mean sensitivity in the normal sample. Thus ordinate values of zero represent no difference from the average normal eye. Negative values signify less sensitivity than in normal eyes. Values outside the dashed lines are beyond the normal 99% confidence interval.

Across all 10 eyes treated for unilateral congenital cataract, there were two obvious trends. First, for stationary gratings (0 Hz, Fig. 26-16), sensitivity loss increased with increasing spatial frequency. Second, for all but the coarsest stripes, the extent of the loss decreased as the flicker rate increased from 0–1 Hz and from 1–8 Hz.

Of all the patients treated for unilateral congenital cataract shown in Figure 26-16, David and Janine showed the least loss in contrast sensitivity. Only these two patients had had early treatment (first optical correction at 3 and 5 months, respectively) and had had the fellow eye patched close to 50% of the waking time throughout early childhood. Both have good linear letter acuity in the aphakic eye (20/50 and 20/40, respectively), and

both show some evidence of fusion and stereopsis. In contrast, Sandra, Krista, and Kim had much poorer results despite early treatment (first optical correction by 6 months of age). They had had the fellow eye patched less than 25% of the time throughout early childhood. All had poor linear letter acuity in the aphakic eye (20/200–20/600) with no evidence of fusion or stereopsis. Together, these results indicate that nearly normal contrast sensitivity can be achieved in cases of unilateral congenital cataract if the treatment is prompt and if the fellow eye is patched regularly.

Casual inspection of the results from the fellow eye of patients treated for unilateral congenital cataract initially suggested normal contrast sensitivity (Tytla et al., 1989). A more detailed analysis, however, revealed subtle deficits (Lewis et al., 1989b). Figure 26-17 shows the contrast sensitivity of the fellow eyes of each of nine patients treated for unilateral congenital cataract compared to the normal control group. (Kim's data were excluded because her fellow eye had a significant astigmatism of 2.50 D.) Contrast sensitivity was within normal limits at low and medium spatial frequencies but was significantly below normal at 10 and 20 cpd. Further analyses indicated no relation between the extent of the deficit in the fellow eye and the extent to which it had been patched. Like our results from linear letter acuity, reduced contrast sensitivity in the fellow eye of children treated for unilateral congenital cataract suggests that deprivation amblyopia may affect both eyes. Others have reached similar conclusions for strabismic and anisometropic amblyopia (Levi and Klein, 1985; Leguire et al., 1990).

Bilateral Cases. To examine the effects of binocular deprivation, we tested 13 eyes of eight children, aged 4–9 years, who were treated for bilateral congenital cataracts. The aphakic eyes had first been fitted with contact lenses (or, in two cases, with glasses) at ages ranging from 5 to 18 months. Figure 26-18 shows the loss in contrast sensitivity, relative to the normal control group, for each of the 13 eyes tested. As in unilateral cases, the loss in sensitivity for stationary gratings increased with increasing spatial frequency. When the gratings were flickered, however, all but one patient (Terri) showed no systematic change in the slope or extent of the loss function. Thus the loss in sensitivity in eyes treated for bilateral congenital cataracts is a constant ratio of normal sensitivity regardless of flicker frequency. This finding agrees with previous data from patients treated for bilateral congenital cataracts (Mioche and Perenin, 1986) but is in marked contrast to that from our patients treated for unilateral congenital cataract.

A comparison of Figures 26-16 and 26-18 indicates that after comparable periods of deprivation bilateral cases showed less deficit in contrast sensitivity than did

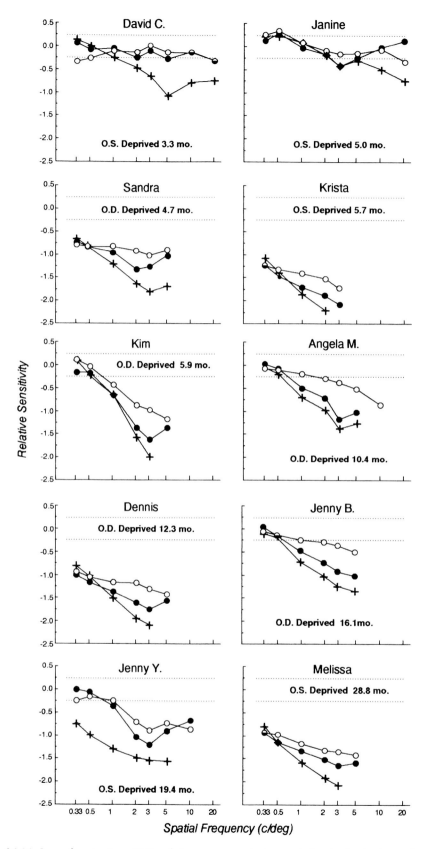

FIG. 26-16. Loss of contrast sensitivity relative to age-matched controls for the deprived eye of each of 10 children treated for unilateral congenital cataract. Each point shows the log of the ratio relating sensitivity in the deprived eye to mean sensitivity in the normal sample for gratings of a particular spatial frequency that were static (0 Hz) (+), or flickering at 1 Hz (●) or 8 Hz (○). Values outside the dashed lines are beyond the normal 99% confidence interval. (From Tytla et al., 1988. By permission.)

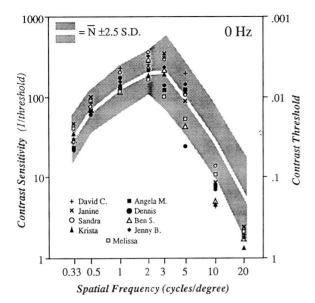

FIG. 26-17. Contrast sensitivity for the good eyes of children treated for unilateral congenital cataract tested with static gratings (0 Hz). Each point represents the result for one eye. The shaded area defines the normal range (99% confidence interval) about the mean sensitivity (white curve) derived from 28 visually normal children.

unilateral cases. Compared to unilateral cases, there was a wider range of spatial frequencies over which responses were normal or nearly normal. (Exceptions are David C. and Janine, whose unique visual histories were discussed above.) Furthermore, no child treated for bilateral congenital cataracts had losses exceeding 1.5 log units, whereas 5 of the 10 unilateral cases had losses of 2 log units or more.

Our eight patients treated for dense bilateral congenital cataracts exhibited considerably higher contrast sensitivity than did the eight reported by Mioche and Perenin (1986). The most likely reason is that, despite similar ages of surgery, their patients endured much longer periods of uncorrected aphakia (mean 7.4 months versus 2.3 months) after removal of the cataracts.

Peripheral Contrast Sensitivity. In addition to measuring contrast sensitivity in the central visual field, we measured it at 10, 20, and 30 degrees in the temporal and nasal visual fields (Tytla et al., 1991). We tested the deprived eye of six children treated for unilateral congenital cataract (mean duration of deprivation 8.0 months, range 4.7–16.1 months) and one eye of each of five children treated for bilateral congenital cataracts (mean duration of deprivation 10.8 months, range 7.0–16.4 months), all of whom had sufficiently steady fixation to produce reliable results in the periphery.

In age-matched normal controls (*n* = 12), sensitivity to high spatial frequencies showed the typical decline with eccentricity. Three children who had incurred a

traumatic cataract after 6 years of age showed subtle losses at high frequencies that were constant across eccentricities relative to normal.

For the bilaterally deprived children, the loss was much more severe but was fairly constant compared to the normal controls regardless of eccentricity. However, unlike normal controls and bilaterally deprived children, the deprived eye of children treated for unilateral congenital cataract showed no consistent decrease in sensitivity in the periphery compared to the center of the field so the amount of loss decreased with eccentricity. These results paralleled our findings with flicker: Children treated for bilateral congenital cataracts showed a constant loss compared to normal regardless of flicker rate, but the deprived eye in unilateral cases showed less loss at all but the lowest spatial frequencies with increasing rates of flicker up to 8 Hz (the highest frequency tested) (Tytla et al., 1988). In addition, eyes treated for unilateral congenital cataract differed from all other groups in showing less sensitivity to high spatial frequencies in the nasal visual field than to those at comparable locations in the temporal visual field.

Of the six children treated for unilateral congenital cataract whose contrast sensitivity was tested in the periphery, only Janine had had early treatment and had had the fellow eye patched regularly throughout early childhood (see above for details). Only her contrast sensitivity was within normal limits at all peripheral locations. These encouraging results suggest that at least some of the deficits common in children treated for unilateral congenital cataract can be ameliorated by prompt treatment and regular patching of the fellow eye.

Our findings for bilateral cases agree with those of Mioche and Perenin (1986), who tested peripheral contrast sensitivity out to 20 degrees. However, our finding of a different pattern of results for monocular versus binocular deprivation again indicates that the two types of deprivation have different effects on the developing nervous system.

Comparison to Normal Infants

Like grating acuity, contrast sensitivity has been measured in human infants using PL, visually evoked potentials (VEPs), and OKN (e.g., Atkinson et al., 1977; Pirchio et al., 1978; Hainline et al., 1986). The three methods yield similar results when the same stimuli are used in the same infant (Atkinson and Braddick, 1989). Young babies require more contrast than do adults to respond to any spatial frequency, have reduced grating acuity, and are most sensitive to the coarsest stripes tested (reviewed by Banks, 1982–1983). By 3 months, the curve has an adult shape, but sensitivity to coarse stripes is relatively more mature than sensitivity to fine

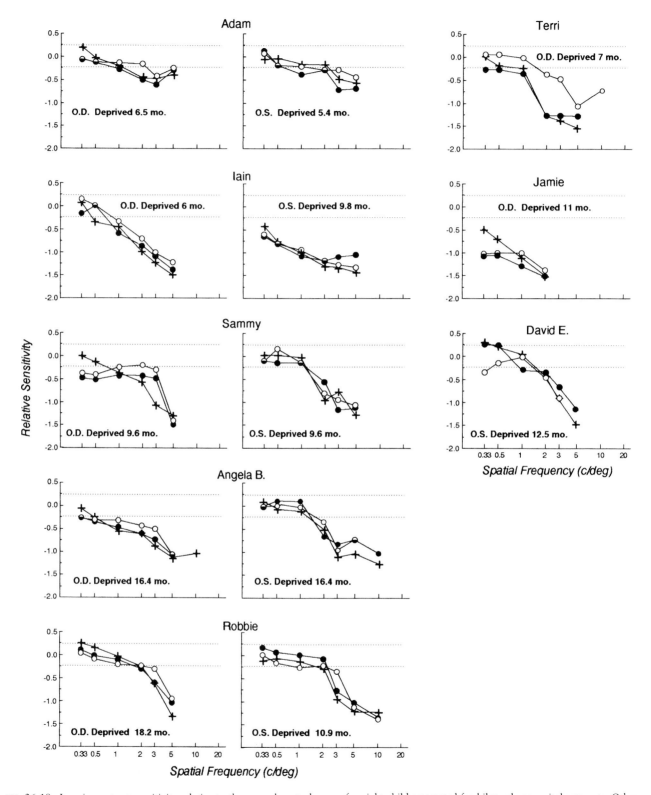

FIG. 26-18. Loss in contrast sensitivity relative to the normal control group for eight children treated for bilateral congenital cataracts. Other details as in Figure 26-16. (From Tytla et al., 1988. By permission.)

stripes (Norcia et al., 1990; reviewed by Banks, 1982–1983). At 8 months, sensitivity is still at least 1.0 octave below adult values at all spatial frequencies (Norcia et al., 1990; reviewed by Banks, 1982–1983); the age at which it is fully adult-like is not clear from the literature (Derefeldt et al., 1979; Beazley et al., 1980; Atkinson et al., 1981; Bradley and Freeman, 1982; Abramov et al., 1984).

There appears to be a relation between the developmental time course in normal infants and the type of loss in unilateral cases. First, in unilateral cases, the extent of the loss decreased as flicker rate increased up to 8 Hz (the highest frequency tested) for all but the coarsest gratings; but in bilateral cases, the extent of the loss was a constant ratio of normal sensitivity at all spatial frequencies, regardless of flicker frequency. Better acuity for stripes modulating in this range compared to stationary stripes is typical of normal young infants but not of adults (Sokol et al., 1988, 1992). Moreover, adult-like responses to flicker develop earlier for coarse gratings (to which even unilateral cases showed the adult-like pattern) than for finer gratings (to which unilateral cases showed the infant-like pattern) (Swanson and Birch, 1990). Second, only in unilateral cases did the extent of the loss decrease with increasing eccentricity relative to normals. This finding reflects the fact that with increasing eccentricity their sensitivity did not decline consistently, as it does in normals. Young normal infants also show little decline in sensitivity with increasing eccentricity in that their grating acuity is similar at 10 and 30 degrees in the periphery (Maurer et al., 1986; see also Chapter 7). Third, only in unilateral cases was sensitivity compromised more in the nasal visual field than in the temporal visual field. Normal young infants, unlike adults, have especially poor sensitivity in the nasal visual field (Lewis et al., 1985a; reviewed by Maurer and Lewis, 1991; Lewis and Maurer, 1992; see also Chapter 7). Together these results indicate that vision in children treated for unilateral congenital cataract resembles an earlier phase of development than does vision in children treated for bilateral congenital cataracts.

Comparison with Animal Studies

Early visual deprivation interferes with the development of contrast sensitivity in both cats and monkeys. In cats, suturing the lids of one or both eyes at the age of 1.5–16.0 months profoundly reduces later contrast sensitivity (Lehmkuhle et al., 1982; Mitchell and Murphy, 1984; Mitchell, 1988). There is a suggestion that monocular deprivation produces greater losses than binocular deprivation (Lehmkuhle et al., 1982), although this conclusion is tentative as the two groups of cats also differed regarding the periods of deprivation and recovery. Slight recovery of vision in monocularly deprived cats can occur after extended periods of binocular visual input (Mitchell et al., 1977). After short-term monocular deprivation, however, both eyes can achieve equal and normal contrast sensitivity only if the fellow eye is occluded 50–70% of the time (Mitchell, 1991). Thus some of the original loss is caused by suppression of the deprived eye by the nondeprived eye. Our data point to a strong parallel between cats and humans in terms of the effects of reverse occlusion after monocular deprivation. The sensitivities of patients Janine and David C., both of whom had received close to 50% occlusion throughout childhood, far surpassed those of Sandra and Krista, who had received little occlusion after comparable deprivation.

Monkeys also show profound losses of contrast sensitivity following 2–12 weeks of monocular deprivation beginning at the age of 1 month, losses that increase with spatial frequency (Harwerth et al., 1989). The losses following binocular deprivation are much less profound (Harwerth et al., 1991). When losses do occur, the pattern of sensitivity in the deprived eye(s) resembles that found in normal infant monkeys (Boothe et al., 1988) in much the same way as the overall sensitivity shown by our congenital cases resembles that of human infants (reviewed by Banks, 1982–1983). In the monocularly deprived monkey, some recovery is seen after several months of reverse occlusion (or by producing a lesion on the central retina of the nondeprived eye), even after 10–12 months of deprivation from birth (Hendrickson et al., 1977). Nearly normal contrast sensitivity can be achieved if deprivation lasted no more than 1 month and was followed by reverse occlusion (Harwerth et al., 1989). Unlike the cat, however, binocular visual input alone after early monocular deprivation effects no recovery (Blakemore et al., 1981; Harwerth et al., 1981) likely because monocular deprivation produces larger refractive errors in monkeys than in cats (reviewed by Harwerth et al., 1989). The fact that in the monkey reverse occlusion can effect some recovery after up to 1 year of monocular deprivation raises the possibility that in humans also some of the deficit following longer-term monocular deprivation might be reversible by patching. We have been unable to test this hypothesis because none of the children in our sample followed the prescribed patching regimen after long-term monocular deprivation from birth.

Synthesis and Conclusions

The results from contrast sensitivity complement the findings from linear letter acuity. Both show that visual deprivation during infancy affects the development of visual sensitivity, with the effect being more severe in unilateral cases than in bilateral cases. After long deprivation ($\geq$ 5 months), the deprived eyes of children treated for unilateral congenital cataract have poor acuity and substantial losses in contrast sensitivity at all spatial frequencies. Their deficits show an infant-like variation with increasing eccentricity, different rates of flicker, and location (i.e., especially poor sensitivity in the nasal visual field). In contrast, also after long deprivation, children treated for bilateral congenital cataracts have less severely reduced acuity and less severe losses in contrast sensitivity. Their deficits show an adult-like pattern of variation with increasing eccentricity, different rates of flicker, and location (i.e., comparable losses in the temporal and nasal visual fields). Nevertheless, even in unilateral cases, good visual sensitivity can be attained, provided the deprivation was short and the normal eye was patched regularly after the deprivation.

FUSION AND STEREOPSIS

In the dozens of studies on the visual acuity of children treated for congenital cataract (see above), there is little evidence of fusion or stereopsis. Children treated for unilateral congenital cataract have shown no evidence of fusion or stereopsis even after optimal treatment (e.g., Beller et al., 1981). Only if the cataract developed late (estimates of the age conflict, varying from 3 to 12 years) is there evidence of binocular function (Davies and Tarbuck, 1977; Frank and France, 1977; Vaegan and Taylor, 1979; Beller et al., 1981; Yamamoto et al., 1983). Among children treated for bilateral congenital cataracts, there are only a few scattered reports of fusion (2 of 16 cases studied by Davies and Tarbuck, 1977)

or stereopsis (1 of 23 cases studied by Taylor et al., 1979).

Most children treated for congenital cataract have strabismus (e.g., Beller et al., 1981; Gelbart et al., 1982), and many have profound amblyopia (reviewed by Maurer et al., 1989b; see also above). Consequently, they may fail clinical tests of stereovision, such as the Titmus or the Randot test, not because they have no stereopsis but because they cannot see the small test stimuli or the test stimuli do not fall on corresponding retinal points. We investigated that possibility by using a custom-made set of large stereograms that were easily visible to the amblyopic eye and by presenting them in a synoptophore to permit alignment on corresponding points on the two hemiretinas (Tytla et al., in press).

The stimuli were nine pairs of slides with crossed disparity ranging from 14 to 3600 arc seconds in 1.0-octave increments. Each pair contained five wide (2 degree) vertical bars of high contrast (94%), of which two or three were in crossed disparity (Fig. 26-19). Each pair also contained a stimulus for verifying alignment and for detecting suppression. We aligned the stimuli in the synoptophore and then decreased disparity from the largest value until the child could no longer identify which bars appeared "in front."

Figure 26-20 shows stereoacuity on our test (TLMB) plotted against clinical stereoacuity as measured by the Randot or the Titmus test. Normal controls (n = 25, aged 4–16 years) had values close to the unity line, a finding that suggests our test and the clinical stereotests measure similar functions. Seven children who had incurred a traumatic cataract after 6 years of age all dem-

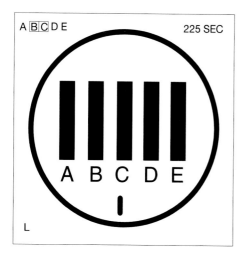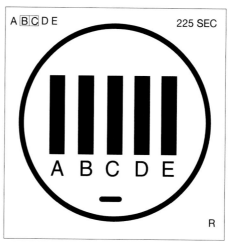

FIG. 26-19. Example of a stereo-pair used to test amblyopic children. Only the circle and its contents are visible when viewed in the synoptophore. The lines below the letter C intersect when the stereo-pairs are fused. The bars above the letters B and C are displaced nasalward (crossed disparity) and when fused appear to be closer to the observer than the rest of the display, all elements of which are in perfect register (zero disparity) and lie on the horopter. (From Tytla et al., in press. By permission.)

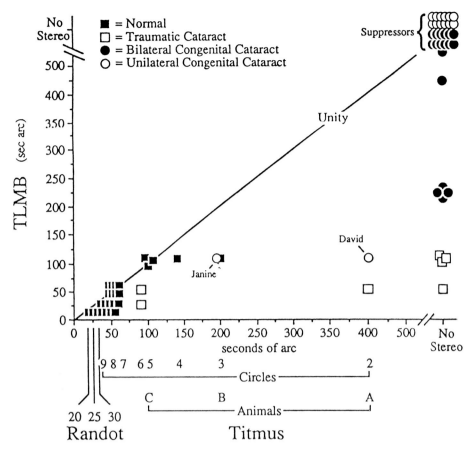

FIG. 26-20. Stereoacuity on our test (TLMB) versus stereoacuity on the Titmus and Randot stereotests for each subject. The diagonal line of unity slope represents no difference between TLMB and clinical stereoacuities. (From Tytla et al., in press. By permission.)

onstrated good stereoacuity on our test, even though the four with strabismus showed no stereovision on the clinical tests (Fig. 26-20).

Of the 32 children tested who had been treated for congenital cataract, 25 (78%) showed suppression on all tests of stereovision. These 25 children had endured relatively long periods of deprivation (4.7–19.4 months for the unilateral cases and 9.6–18.0 months for the bilateral cases) and, in unilateral cases, did not follow the prescribed patching regimen. The remaining seven patients (two unilateral and five bilateral cases) had measurable stereopsis on our test. Only the two treated for unilateral cataract showed any evidence of stereopsis on clinical tests. These seven patients treated for congenital cataract and with measurable TLMB stereoacuity are among those with the shortest deprivation and the best spatial vision. The two treated for unilateral cataract were also the only ones to comply with the 50% patching regimen throughout early childhood.

Two control conditions indicated that extraneous cues did not permit correct performance on the test. First, to evaluate monocular extraneous cues, we tested the normal controls monocularly; they performed randomly. Second, to evaluate nonstereoscopic cues that might be used by a patient with simultaneous vision (diplopia) rather than true binocular fusion, we retested one of the children treated for unilateral congenital cataract (Janine) with the bars oriented in their normal vertical position and again with the bars oriented horizontally. When the bars are oriented horizontally, the disparity is vertical and hence should not support true stereopsis. With the vertical bars, Janine replicated her previous result of 112 arc seconds of stereoacuity. In contrast, with the horizontal bars, she failed even the largest disparity. These control results rule out explanations other than stereovision in patients with positive results on our test.

Most of the children treated for congenital cataract had no measurable stereopsis. This finding is consistent with the fact that cats and monkeys that had been deprived by lid suture show both a loss of neurons tuned to binocular disparity and few cortical cells that respond to input from both eyes (Crawford et al., 1989, 1991; reviewed by Blakemore and Vital-Durand, 1981; Movshon and Van Sluyters, 1981; Boothe et al., 1985).

Like most children treated for congenital cataract, normal young infants show no evidence of fusion or stereopsis until about 3 months of age (e.g., Birch et al., 1985). Then there is a dramatic improvement over the next few months, and stereoacuity is nearly adult-like by 5 months (Held et al., 1980; reviewed in Chapter 13). The results of our study suggest that visual deprivation during this period usually disrupts binocular function.

By compensating for amblyopia and strabismus, however, stereopsis can be demonstrated in some children treated for congenital cataract. The seven children with positive TLMB stereovision do not necessarily appreciate stereopsis during everyday life. Nonetheless, the presence of stereopsis in these children implies the existence of some binocular cortical neurons such as those found in cats with bilateral deprivation, short unilateral deprivation, or distributed reverse occlusion after unilateral deprivation (e.g., Watkins et al., 1978; Crewther et al., 1983; Malach et al., 1984a; Freeman and Ohzawa, 1988).

SYMMETRY OF OKN

Cats visually deprived by lid suture during early infancy show asymmetrical OKN when tested as adults: OKN is elicited easily when a patterned stimulus moves from the temporal visual field toward the nasal visual field but not when it moves in the opposite direction (van Hof-van Duin, 1976, 1978, 1979; Harris et al., 1980; Hoffmann, 1981, 1983; Malach et al., 1984b). Moreover, this asymmetry is usually present in the previously deprived eye and the nondeprived eye (van Hof-van Duin, 1976, 1979; Hoffmann, 1981, 1983; Malach 1984b; but see Malach et al., 1981; Markner and Hoffmann, 1985). As is described later, the asymmetry appears to reflect abnormalities in the visual cortex or its input to the midbrain.

Only one study has looked for asymmetrical OKN in visually deprived monkeys tested monocularly (Sparks et al., 1986). After 1–2 weeks of monocular deprivation from the second week of life, OKN was asymmetrical in the deprived eye; but after 18–26 months of monocular deprivation, no OKN could be elicited from the deprived eye in most monkeys. Unfortunately, because of an equipment failure, Sparks et al. (1986) could not measure accurately the symmetry of OKN in the nondeprived eye of monkeys after long-term monocular deprivation, but it appeared to be grossly normal.

Like visually deprived cats and monkeys, normal young human infants show asymmetrical OKN. Estimates of the age at which their OKN becomes symmetrical have ranged from 3 months (Atkinson, 1979; Atkinson and Braddick, 1981; van Hof-van Duin and Mohn, 1984,

1985, 1986b; Lewis et al., 1992) to 5–6 months (Naegele and Held, 1982, 1983; Roy et al., 1989). All these studies, however, used wide stripes or large random dots. If spatial frequency is varied, even 12-month-olds require much larger stripes (or lower temporal frequencies) to show OKN for nasal-to-temporal motion than for temporal-to-nasal motion (Lewis et al., 1991), although the size of the asymmetry is not nearly as large as it is in 3-month-olds (Lewis et al., 1990b).

Other than our own work (Maurer et al., 1983; Lewis et al., 1985b, 1986, 1989a), there have been few published reports on the symmetry of OKN in children treated for congenital cataract. Schor and Levi (1980) found asymmetrical OKN in the nondeprived eyes of two children treated for unilateral congenital cataract. In contrast, Atkinson and Braddick (1981) found symmetrical OKN in the deprived eye of a 6-month-old treated for unilateral cataract, and Naegele and Held (1983) found symmetrical OKN in the nondeprived eye of a 1-year-old who still had a cataract in the other eye. In neither case, however, is there any indication that the cataract was dense from birth.

Our Studies

To examine more thoroughly the effect of deprivation on the symmetry of OKN in humans, we tested a large number of children with steady fixation who had been treated for cataracts in one or both eyes (Lewis et al., 1989a). The age at which deprivation began and its duration varied widely across patients. Subjects faced an 84 × 84 degree rear projection screen entirely filled with black-and-white vertical stripes (contrast 91%; space average luminance 39.2 candelas/m²) moving horizontally at 13 degrees/second. All subjects were tested with stripes 50 minutes wide unless wider stripes were required to elicit OKN for temporal-to-nasal motion. Each subject was given 39 seven-second trials: 15 trials with stripes moving from the temporal field toward the nasal field, 15 trials with stripes moving from the nasal field toward the temporal field, and 9 control trials with a plain gray field. An observer, who was unaware of the type of trial, watched the child's unpatched eye through a peephole beside the screen and reported whether OKN had occurred. Children who showed OKN on control trials (i.e., had a spontaneous nystagmus) were eliminated from the study.

For each child, we used χ^2 tests to compare the frequency of trials on which OKN was judged to occur when stripes moved temporally to nasally versus nasally to temporally. A significant difference for the two directions indicates asymmetrical OKN.

Children treated for unilateral congenital cataract showed OKN on most trials when stripes moved temporally to nasally but on few trials when stripes moved nasally to temporally. The asymmetry was significant in every deprived eye ($n = 15$) and in every fellow eye ($n = 23$) tested. The magnitude of the asymmetry was not related to the duration of deprivation (ranging from 3 to 16 months), the patching regimen (ranging from excellent to poor compliance), or linear letter acuity (ranging from 20/40 to counting fingers): Children who had good linear acuity in the aphakic eye after early treatment with aggressive patching of the fellow eye had asymmetries as large as those who had poor linear acuity after later treatment with little or no patching of the fellow eye.

Asymmetrical OKN cannot be attributed to unequal refractive errors between eyes in children treated for unilateral congenital cataract because anisometropes with 5.0–17.5 D of myopia in one eye and a normal fellow eye showed asymmetrical OKN in only 2 of the 22 myopic eyes tested and in none of the 17 fellow eyes tested. Nor can asymmetrical OKN be attributed to aphakia per se because children who had had a normal early history and then incurred a cataract sometime after 2.5 years of age showed asymmetrical OKN in none of the aphakic eyes ($n = 14$) or fellow eyes ($n = 10$) tested despite deprivation lasting up to 17 months. These results indicate that monocular deprivation from birth results in asymmetrical OKN, whereas similar deprivation after age 2.5 does not. Unfortunately, our sample of monocular cases did not include children who incurred a cataract after birth but before age 2.5. Thus we cannot pinpoint a sensitive period for the development of asymmetrical OKN.

Like eyes in the unilateral congenital group, eyes in the bilateral congenital group showed OKN more frequently when stripes moved from the temporal field toward the nasal field than when they moved in the opposite direction. There was a significant asymmetry in 8 of the 10 individual eyes tested. The size of the asymmetry was similar to that following monocular deprivation from birth. Eyes treated for bilateral developmental cataracts had mixed results: There was a significant asymmetry in 3 of the 20 individual eyes. For this group, however, the age at which a dense cataract was first detected varied from 7.5 months to 10 years, and the asymmetry was shown only by eyes that developed dense cataracts before 18 months of age.

Figure 26-21 suggests that there is no effect of the duration of binocular deprivation on the symmetry of OKN. Nine of the eleven eyes that had congenital cataracts or that had developmental cataracts diagnosed before 12 months of age showed asymmetrical OKN regardless of the duration of deprivation. Moreover, the size of the asymmetry (not shown in Figure 26-21) was as large after 5–6 months of deprivation as after 12 months or more of deprivation. In contrast, none of the 14 eyes that developed dense cataracts after 18 months

of age showed asymmetrical OKN, even though six of the eyes that developed cataracts after 2.5 years were deprived for more than 5 months.

In summary, we found that the timing of deprivation, but not its duration, is important for determining whether OKN is asymmetrical. Moreover, we found no differences between monocular and binocular deprivation: After early monocular or binocular deprivation, whatever its duration, OKN was asymmetrical; whereas after late deprivation, whatever its duration, OKN was symmetrical. These conclusions, however, must be limited to the particular variation in our sample of the duration and timing of deprivation and to the particular method we used to measure the symmetry of OKN. For example, a more sensitive measure (e.g., Lewis et al., 1990b) might reveal differences in the size of the asymmetry for monocular versus binocular deprivation.

Factors other than early pattern deprivation per se might have contributed to the asymmetries we observed: Asymmetrical OKN has been reported in subjects with amblyopia from other causes, with esotropia, or with reduced stereopsis for whatever reason (e.g., Schor and Levi, 1980; Atkinson and Braddick, 1981; Mohn et al., 1986; van Hof-van Duin and Mohn, 1986a). In our study, however, none of these factors was more common in children who showed an asymmetry than in children who did not.

Mechanisms Underlying Asymmetrical OKN

The nucleus of the optic tract (NOT) in the pretectum and the related dorsal terminal nucleus (DTN) in the accessory optic tract are a scattered group of cells in the midbrain that play an important role in the mediation of OKN in the cat and monkey (reviewed in Hoffmann et al., 1988; Simpson et al., 1988). The NOT-DTN cells are the main link between sensory input from the retina and the motor output of OKN through the brainstem (Hoffmann, 1986; Hoffmann and Distler, 1989). The left NOT-DTN is activated maximally by large patterns moving from right to left, and the right NOT-DTN is activated maximally by large patterns moving from left to right (e.g., Hoffmann and Schoppmann, 1981; Hoffmann et al., 1988). There are at least three pathways that project to each NOT-DTN: two from the contralateral eye and one from the ipsilateral eye (Hoffmann, 1986, 1989). These pathways are illustrated in Figure 26-22 for the right eye of the adult cat and monkey.

There are three important similarities between cats and monkeys in the mediation of OKN (Harris et al., 1980; Montarolo et al., 1981; Hoffmann, 1982; Williams and Chalupa, 1983; Strong et al., 1984; Kato et al., 1986; Zee et al., 1986, 1987; Simpson et al., 1988). First, the direct pathway from the retina through the

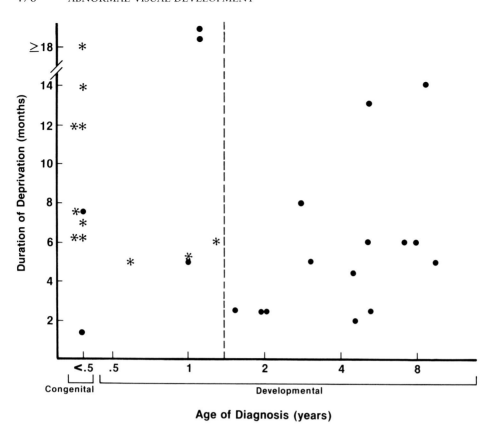

FIG. 26-21. Asymmetry of OKN in children treated for bilateral congenital or developmental cataracts as a function of (1) the age of diagnosis of a dense cataract and (2) the duration of deprivation. Each point represents the results for one eye. Asterisks indicate that the asymmetry was significant and the dots that it was not. The vertical dashed line separates eyes that had cataracts diagnosed before and after 18 months of age. (Adapted from Lewis, T. L., Maurer, D., and Brent, H. P. (1985b). Optokinetic nystagmus in children treated for bilateral cataracts. In R. Groner, G. W. McConkie, and C. Menz (eds.). *Eye Movements and Human Information Processing*. Amsterdam: North Holland. By permission.)

contralateral NOT-DTN is sufficient to mediate OKN when patterns move from the temporal visual field toward the nasal visual field, especially when movement is slow. Second, the indirect pathway from the retina through the ipsilateral lateral geniculate nucleus and visual cortex to the ipsilateral NOT-DTN is necessary for consistent OKN when stripes move from the nasal visual field toward the temporal visual field. Finally, although there is also a direct retinal projection to the ipsilateral NOT-DTN (not shown in Fig. 26-22), it is much smaller than the contralateral projection, and its contribution to OKN is minimal. Nonetheless, important differences do exist between species. In the cat all NOT-DTN cells receive input directly from the retina, whereas in the monkey only 30% do so; conversely, only 40% of NOT-DTN cells receive cortical input in the cat, but all do so in the monkey (Hoffmann et al., 1988). These differences suggest greater cortical influence on the OKN of monkeys than of cats.

Hoffmann (1989) hypothesized that in cats, monkeys, and humans, OKN early in life is mediated entirely by subcortical projections to NOT-DTN, which develop in the absence of visual experience. The cortical projections to NOT-DTN develop later and depend on normal binocular visual experience. After the cortical projections are established, the subcortical projections lose influence over NOT-DTN cells. This reduction in subcortical influence occurs to a small extent in cats, to a greater extent in monkeys, and almost completely in humans. In all three species, however, any abnormality that interferes with cortical input to the midbrain, such as pattern deprivation or strabismus during early infancy, leaves OKN mediated by subcortical pathways and asymmetrical.

Although the findings of asymmetrical OKN in cats, monkeys, and humans tested early in life or after early pattern deprivation are consistent with Hoffmann's (1989) hypothesis that under these conditions OKN is

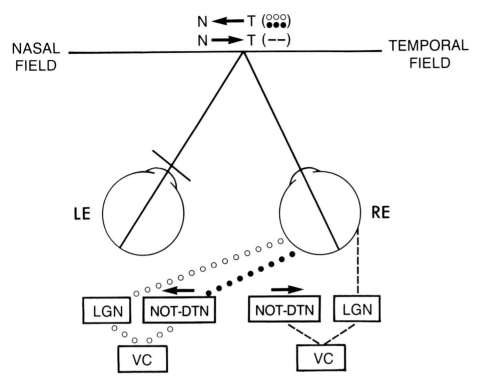

FIG. 26-22. Pathways projecting from the right eye (RE) to the nucleus of the optic tract and dorsal terminal nucleus (NOT-DTN) in the midbrain of the normal cat and monkey. LE = left eye; LGN = lateral geniculate nucleus; VC = visual cortex. (Adapted from Lewis, T. L., Maurer, D., and Brent, H. P. (1985b). Optokinetic nystagmus in children treated for bilateral cataracts. In R. Groner, G. W. McConkie, and C. Menz (eds.). *Eye Movements and Human Information Processing*. Amsterdam: North Holland. By permission.)

mediated by subcortical pathways in all three species, there is an alternative explanation for humans. Psychophysical studies by Harris and colleagues that compared monocular and binocular responses to plaids indicate, as Hoffmann (1989) predicted, that subcortical pathways are involved in the OKN of normal adult cats but apparently not in the OKN of normal adult humans (Harris and Smith, 1990; Harris et al., 1991; Smith and Harris, 1991). Other studies using evoked potentials, however, have revealed asymmetries in the *cortical* response to motion in normal young infants and in infants with abnormal binocular experience early in life caused by strabismus (Norcia et al., 1991a,b; see also the model of development proposed by Tychsen in Chapter 23). Thus in children treated for congenital cataract, OKN is asymmetrical either because the cortical pathways mediating OKN are nonfunctional and the subcortical pathways favor temporal-to-nasal motion (Hoffmann, 1989) or because OKN is mediated entirely by cortical pathways that respond asymmetrically to motion (Norcia et al., 1991a,b). At this point it is impossible to choose between the two hypotheses, but both agree that asymmetrical OKN in humans is caused by immaturities or abnormalities in cortical input to the midbrain.

GENERAL DISCUSSION

Our studies of children treated for dense, central cataracts indicate that visual deprivation affects the development of vision in humans: They show deficits in grating acuity, linear letter acuity, contrast sensitivity, stereopsis, and the symmetry of OKN. All of these deficits point to abnormalities in the visual cortex. As summarized in earlier sections of this chapter, visual deprivation in monkeys reduces the resolution of cells in the visual cortex, and cortical lesions reduce the monkey's sensitivity to contrast at all spatial frequencies. Visual deprivation results in a loss of neurons tuned to binocular disparity and alters the distribution of ocular dominance columns in the monkey's visual cortex, so fewer cells can be driven by both eyes. The asymmetrical OKN shown by children treated for cataracts is what would be expected if there is no (or an abnormal) influence of the visual cortex over the midbrain.

Nevertheless, children treated for cataract show some abilities dependent on the cortex. For example, all of the children we tested could read large letters of high contrast at some distance or at least distinguish the number of fingers held up in front of them. This finding implies at least some rudimentary ability to discriminate among shapes, which we have confirmed in a systematic test designed to eliminate extraneous cues (Maurer et al., 1989b): Children treated for cataracts made virtually no errors. Such good performance likely depends on some cortical pathway because extensive cortical lesions abolish the monkey's ability to discriminate among shapes (e.g., Schilder et al., 1972).

The pattern of results we obtained also suggests that deprivation has different effects on different cortical projections. The symmetry of OKN showed one pattern: OKN was asymmetrical in children treated for congenital cataract regardless of the duration of deprivation, whether it was monocular or binocular, or, in unilateral cases, the extent to which the fellow eye was patched, provided the deprivation began during the first 1–3 years of life. Linear letter acuity and contrast sensitivity in the central visual field showed a second pattern: Although all eyes showed deficits, the deficits were worse in unilateral cases than in bilateral cases, and in unilateral cases after long deprivation than after short deprivation, unless there had been extensive patching of the fellow eye. In unilateral cases variations in contrast sensitivity as a function of flicker rate and eccentricity resembled those of infants, whereas in bilateral cases variations in contrast sensitivity resembled those of adults. The pattern of results for stereopsis was similar to that for linear letter acuity and contrast sensitivity: All eyes showed deficits, but some stereopsis was achieved after short-term binocular deprivation and after short-term monocular deprivation, provided the fellow eye had been patched extensively. As with linear letter acuity and contrast sensitivity, without extensive patching stereodeficits were more pronounced after monocular deprivation than after binocular deprivation: Patients treated for unilateral cataract who had had little patching demonstrated no stereopsis, whereas some of those treated for bilateral cataracts did. As noted above, the discrimination of shape showed a still different pattern: no evidence of abnormality even following monocular deprivation of long duration.

We speculated previously (Maurer et al., 1989b) that the different patterns of deficit shown in children treated for cataract can be related to the maturity of the function at birth and to its subsequent rate of development. (Levi and Carkeet present similar hypotheses about strabismic and anisometropic amblyopes in Chapter 24.) Most of the results reported in this chapter support that speculation. OKN is asymmetrical during early infancy, but nasal-to-temporal OKN improves markedly between 2 and 3 months of age, so that by 3–5 months there is little evidence of asymmetry when the stimuli include large elements, as they did in our tests of deprived eyes. Grating acuity and contrast sensitivity are immature at birth and take several years to develop

fully. In contrast, even newborns can discriminate between shapes. These different developmental patterns likely reflect different underlying cortical mechanisms, which mature at different rates and are differentially affected by deprivation. Our results for OKN acuity can also be understood within this framework: They were probably influenced by both the mechanisms underlying the development of visual resolution *and* those underlying the development of symmetrical OKN, i.e., the development of mature cortical influence over OKN.

The results for stereopsis and PL acuity, however, indicate that the relation between the normal developmental pattern and the effects of deprivation are more complex. As summarized above, the pattern of deficits in stereopsis was similar to the pattern of deficits in linear letter acuity and contrast sensitivity. Yet these visual functions have different developmental patterns. On the one hand, there is no evidence of stereopsis at birth, but stereopsis emerges and then develops rapidly during early infancy. On the other hand, even newborns can detect large stripes of high contrast, and contrast sensitivity improves gradually over many years. Thus two visual functions with different courses in normal development can show the same pattern of deficits after deprivation.

Our results for PL acuity also deviate from the pattern we would have predicted from the normal developmental pattern. Like contrast sensitivity and OKN acuity, PL acuity improves gradually over several years. Unlike the OKN acuity of deprived infants and the later contrast sensitivity of children treated for congenital cataract, however, PL acuity was within normal limits during the first 1.5–2.0 years, and the results following monocular and binocular deprivation did not differ. We hypothesized that PL acuity may reflect mainly the development of the peripheral retina and its projections. It would be fruitful to reexamine the relation between the normal developmental pattern and the effects of deprivation when more data become available regarding the normal development of peripheral visual resolution and the effects of deprivation thereon.

A further complication is that how one characterizes a developmental pattern may depend on the parameters of the study. For example, our characterization of the developmental pattern for stereopsis is based on the fact that stereoacuity improves dramatically during the few months after stereopsis first emerges. It takes many years, however, for stereoacuity to reach adult levels (Gwiazda et al., 1989b; reviewed by Gwiazda et al., 1989a; see also Chapter 13). Similarly, OKN becomes symmetrical between 3 and 5 months of age for patterns containing large elements, a finding that suggests a qualitative change; but OKN asymmetry for small stripes changes more gradually and is still present at 12 months of age (Lewis et al., 1991).

Whatever the relation to normal human development, our data make clear that there are multiple sensitive periods during which the human visual system can be affected adversely by deprivation. The data also indicate that there are at least two mechanisms by which deprivation can cause deficits: deprivation per se and competition between the eyes. Some deficits appear to result from deprivation per se: For PL acuity, OKN acuity, linear letter acuity, contrast sensitivity, stereopsis, and the symmetry of OKN, there were deficits in *both* eyes following binocular deprivation. In some circumstances, unfair competition between the eyes for cortical synapses appears to increase the deficit caused by deprivation. Such competition would occur in every unilateral case and, to a lesser extent, in bilateral cases in which one eye has worse acuity or is suppressed. Such competition could be reduced in unilateral cases by extensive patching of the fellow eye. We found evidence of competitive effects for OKN acuity, linear letter acuity, contrast sensitivity, and stereopsis. For each of these areas, the deficits were worse after monocular deprivation than after binocular deprivation unless the monocular deprivation was followed by extensive patching of the fellow eye. The competition appears to leave vision in monocular cases more like the vision of normal human infants: Like normal human infants, children treated for unilateral congenital cataract who did not follow the prescribed patching regimen showed poor visual resolution and contrast sensitivity, no evidence of stereopsis, better visual resolution for flickering than for stationary stripes, poorer sensitivity in the nasal than in the temporal visual field, and little decline in visual resolution with eccentricity. Of course, these generalizations should be limited to the particular tests we used and the particular variation in our sample. For example, a more sensitive test might reveal a difference between unilateral and bilateral cases in the symmetry of OKN or reveal deficits in the ability to discriminate among shapes.

The data from our studies of children treated for cataracts fit well with the results from cats and monkeys that had been deprived by lid suture (reviewed by Movshon and Van Sluyters, 1981; Boothe et al., 1985; Blakemore, 1988; Mitchell, 1991). As in the children we studied, their visual acuity and contrast sensitivity are degraded, with the deficit worse after monocular than after binocular deprivation unless short-term monocular deprivation was followed by occlusion of the fellow eye at least 50% of the time. The results for the symmetry of OKN and the discrimination of shape also parallel those from cats and monkeys, although they have not been studied as extensively: Long-term early monocular or binocular deprivation leads to asymmetrical OKN but has relatively little effect on the discrimination of large shapes of high contrast. Moreover,

in both cats and monkeys, visual deprivation interferes with the development of cells in the visual cortex during a series of critical periods shortly after birth. During at least some of those critical periods, longer deprivation has more deleterious effects than shorter deprivation, monocular deprivation has more deleterious effects than binocular deprivation, and some of the effects can be mitigated by subsequent normal experience, especially if, after monocular deprivation, the previously open eye is occluded. Thus the principles governing the effects of visual deprivation that emerge from behavioral, anatomical, and electrophysiological studies of cats and monkeys are the same as the principles that our results suggest govern the effects in humans. The similar results after lid suture in cats and monkeys and after treatment for congenital cataract in humans allow us to use information about the accompanying physiological changes in the cat or monkey to hypothesize about the physiological effects of deprivation in humans.

Like visually deprived monkeys (Quick et al., 1989), children treated for congenital cataract usually develop strabismus. Thus some of the deficits we observed could result from the secondary strabismus rather than from the original deprivation. Strabismic amblyopes show deficits in visual abilities that are abnormal in our patients: reduced visual resolution, reduced stereopsis, and asymmetrical OKN (reviewed by Boothe et al., 1985; see also Atkinson and Braddick, 1981; Birch and Stager, 1985). We cannot discount the possibility that the secondary strabismus underlies the deficits in stereopsis and in asymmetrical OKN seen in children treated for congenital cataract. In fact, when Malach and Van Sluyters (1989) compared recovery from 2 days of monocular deprivation in kittens with and without strabismus induced at the end of the deprivation, they found that the strabismus interfered with the recovery of normal ocular dominance. However, secondary strabismus seems not to account for the deficits we observed in visual resolution. First, the deficits in visual resolution shown by children treated for congenital cataract are much larger than those found in strabismic amblyopes (e.g., Hess and Howell, 1977; Levi and Harwerth, 1977). Second, the deficits were as large in children who developed exotropia secondary to the congenital cataract as in the children who developed esotropia. Yet exotropia on its own has a much smaller effect on visual resolution than does esotropia (e.g., Burian and von Noorden, 1985). Third, strabismus was equally common among the unilateral and bilateral cases; yet these groups had distinctly different patterns of deficit, with the patients who had a unilateral cataract exhibiting a greater loss than those affected bilaterally. Fourth, in cats, strabismus following short-term monocular deprivation does not interfere with the recovery of the deprived eye's ability to drive cortical neurons (Malach and Van Sluyters, 1989). Nor does it increase the deficits in grating acuity, contrast sensitivity, and Vernier acuity caused by the original deprivation (Mitchell, 1991). Thus it appears that deprivation has a more profound effect on the development of visual resolution than does secondary strabismus.

A second factor, nystagmus, also cannot account entirely for the deficits shown by children treated for congenital cataract. Nystagmus was present in its latent or manifest form in many, but not all, bilateral cases and in some unilateral cases. Nystagmus conceivably might blur high frequency gratings oriented orthogonally to the direction of the nystagmus and reduce grating acuity, letter acuity, contrast sensitivity, and stereopsis. It cannot, however, account for the profound loss in contrast sensitivity that some children showed at low spatial frequencies. Nor can it account for the differences between bilateral and unilateral cases, as those treated for bilateral cataracts tended to have nystagmus of greater amplitude but showed better visual resolution and better stereopsis than did those treated for unilateral cataract (except for PL acuity, where there was no difference between unilateral and bilateral cases). Moreover, it cannot account for the asymmetrical OKN to large stripes of high contrast shown by patients without a spontaneous nystagmus.

Third, the deficits might have been caused not entirely by the initial deprivation induced by cataract but also by the continued though mild deprivation caused by the child's inability to accommodate after cataract surgery. The degree of deprivation would depend on the focal length of the aphakic correction and on the child's viewing preferences throughout the remainder of the sensitive period. We do not know if intermittent unclear images are sufficient to produce amblyopia, but they cannot account for the different patterns of deficits for different visual functions. (Note that aphakia at the time of testing does not account for the deficits because all eyes were corrected for the testing distance and we found essentially normal results in the aphakic eyes of children treated for traumatic cataract.)

In unilateral cases, or bilateral cases fitted with two contact lenses of different focal length, aphakia would be compounded by *aniseikonia*, that is, different image sizes on the two retinas. Aniseikonia might lead to additional competition between the eyes. Like the effect of aphakia, this possibility is difficult to evaluate, but it is unlikely to account for all of the deficits we observed or the different patterns of deficits for different visual functions. Moreover, anisometropes, who also suffer from aniseikonia, show no evidence of asymmetrical OKN, a finding which suggests that aniseikonia is not a major contributor to the asymmetrical OKN of children treated for congenital cataract.

Our results not only have theoretical relevance for understanding the effects of visual deprivation on human visual development, they also have clinical relevance to the treatment of children with eye disorders. They indicate that children born with dense cataracts can achieve essentially normal vision in many areas provided the treatment is prompt and, in unilateral cases, followed by regular patching of the normal eye. Prompt treatment includes not only surgery but also fitting the then aphakic eye with a contact lens so that some focused patterned input reaches the retina. So far, no child in our sample who was born with dense cataracts has achieved completely normal vision: In every case, there has been reduced linear letter acuity, a loss of sensitivity to high spatial frequencies, reduced peripheral sensitivity to light, and reduced stereopsis. It is possible that with treatment at birth some or all of these aspects of vision also would be normal. Alternatively, it is possible that even with such early treatment, some aspects of vision would be abnormal because of the continuing, though mild, form of deprivation caused by the inability of an aphakic eye to change its focus or because the development of a cataract is associated with permanent neural deficits regardless of the timing of treatment.

Acknowledgments. We thank Dr. Henry Brent, the director of the Contact Lens Clinic at The Hospital for Sick Children in Toronto, for his skilled treatment of the patients, his many years of advice, and his comment on an earlier draft of this chapter. We thank Dr. J. Donald Morin, Ophthalmologist-in-Chief at The Hospital for Sick Children, for his encouragement and support. We also thank our many research assistants who helped to collect and analyze the data. Special thanks go to the patients at The Hospital for Sick Children and to the normal subjects for volunteering their time. We appreciate the helpful suggestions on an earlier draft of this manuscript from Robert Hess, Milan Tytla, and other participants at the meeting in Irvine.

This research was supported by grants from the National Eye Institute (NIH EY0-3475), from the Ontario Ministry of Health (PR 928), from the Medical Research Council of Canada (8894 and 1475C) and from the National Foundation March of Dimes (1251).

REFERENCES

ABRAMOV, I., HAINLINE, L., TURKEL, J., LEMERISE, E., SMITH, H., GORDON, J., AND PETRY, S. (1984). Rocket-ship psychophysics: assessing visual functioning in young children. *Invest. Ophthalmol. Vis. Sci.* 25, 1307–1315.

ATKINSON, J. (1979). Development of optokinetic nystagmus in the human infant and monkey infant: an analogue to development in kittens. In R. D. FREEMAN (ed.). *Developmental Neurobiology of Vision.* New York: Plenum, pp. 277–287.

ATKINSON, J., AND BRADDICK, O. (1981). Development of optokinetic nystagmus in infants: an indicator of cortical binocularity? In D. G. FISHER, R. A. MONTY, AND J. W. SENDERS (eds.). *Eye Movements: Cognition and Visual Perception.* Hillsdale, NJ: Erlbaum, pp. 53–64.

ATKINSON, J., AND BRADDICK, O. (1989). Newborn contrast sensitivity measures: do VEP, OKN, & FPL reveal differential development of cortical and subcortical streams? [Abstract]. *Invest. Ophthalmol. Vis. Sci.* 30 (suppl.), 311.

ATKINSON, J., BRADDICK, O., AND MOAR, K. (1977). Contrast sensitivity of the human infant for moving and static patterns. *Vision Res.* 17, 1045–1047.

ATKINSON, J., FRENCH, J., AND BRADDICK, O. (1981). Contrast sensitivity function of preschool children. *Br. J. Ophthalmol.* 65, 525–529.

BANKS, M. (1982–1983). The development of spatial and temporal contrast sensitivity. *Curr. Eye Res.* 2, 191–198.

BANKS, M. S., AND BENNETT, P. J. (1988). Optical and photoreceptor immaturities limit the spatial and chromatic vision of human neonates. *J. Opt. Soc. Am.* 5, 2059–2079.

BANKS, M. S., STEPHENS, B. R., AND DANNEMILLER, J. L. (1982). A failure to observe negative preference in infant acuity testing. *Vision Res.* 22, 1025–1032.

BEAZLEY, L., ILLINGWORTH, D., JAHN, A., AND GREER, D. (1980). Contrast sensitivity in children and adults. *Br. J. Ophthalmol.* 64, 863–866.

BELLER, R., HOYT, C. S., MARG, E., AND ODOM, J. V. (1981). Congenital monocular cataracts: good visual function with neonatal surgery. *Am. J. Ophthalmol.* 91, 559–567.

BIRCH, E. E. (1989). Visual acuity testing in infants and young children. *Ophthalmol. Clin. North Am.* 2, 369–389.

BIRCH, E. E., AND HALE, L. A. (1988). Criteria for monocular acuity deficit in infancy and early childhood. *Invest. Ophthalmol. Vis. Sci.* 29, 636–643.

BIRCH, E. E., AND STAGER, D. R. (1985). Monocular acuity and stereopsis in infantile esotropia. *Invest. Ophthalmol. Vis. Sci.* 26, 1624–1630.

BIRCH, E. E., AND STAGER, D. R. (1988). Prevalence of good visual acuity following surgery for congenital unilateral cataract. *Arch. Ophthalmol.* 106, 40–43.

BIRCH, E. E., GWIAZDA, J., BAUER, J. A., NAEGELE, J., AND HELD, R. (1983). Visual acuity and its meridional variations in children aged 7–60 months. *Vision Res.* 23, 1019–1024.

BIRCH, E. E., SHIMOJO, S., AND HELD, R. (1985). Preferential-looking assessment of fusion and stereopsis in infants aged 1–6 months. *Invest. Ophthalmol. Vis. Sci.* 26, 366–370.

BIRCH, E. E., STAGER, D. R., AND WRIGHT, W. W. (1986). Grating acuity development after early surgery for congenital unilateral cataract. *Arch. Ophthalmol.* 104, 1783–1787.

BLAKEMORE, C. (1988). The sensitive periods of the monkey visual cortex. In G. LENNERSTRAND, G. K. VON NOORDEN, AND E. C. CAMPOS (eds.). *Strabismus and Amblyopia: Experimental Basis for Advances in Clinical Management.* Vol. 49. New York: Plenum, pp. 219–234.

BLAKEMORE, C., AND VITAL-DURAND, F. (1981). Postnatal development of the monkey's visual system. In *The Fetus and Independent Life. Ciba Foundation Symposium.* Vol. 86. London: Pitman, pp. 152–171.

BLAKEMORE, C., VITAL-DURAND, F., AND GAREY, L. J. (1981). Recovery from monocular deprivation in the monkey. I. Recovery of physiological effects in the visual cortex. *Proc. R. Soc. Biol.* 213, 399–423.

BOOTHE, R. G., DOBSON, V., AND TELLER, D. Y. (1985). Postnatal development of vision in human and nonhuman primates. *Annu. Rev. Neurosci.* 8, 495–545.

BOOTHE, R. G., KIORPES, L., WILLIAMS, R. A., AND TELLER, D. Y. (1988). Operant measurements of contrast sensitivity in infant macaque monkeys during normal development. *Vision Res.* 28, 387–396.

BOWERING, E., MAURER, D., LEWIS, T. L., AND BRENT, H. P. (1991). Detection thresholds in the periphery of normal and visually deprived children [Abstract]. *Invest. Ophthalmol. Vis. Sci.* 32 (suppl.), 962.

BOWERING, E., MAURER, D., LEWIS, T. L., BRENT, P., AND BRENT, H. P. (1989). Development of the visual field in normal and binocularly deprived children [Abstract]. *Invest. Ophthalmol. Vis. Sci.* 30 (suppl.), 377.

BRADLEY, A., AND FREEMAN, R. (1982). Contrast sensitivity in children. *Vision Res.* 22, 953–959.

BRENT, H. P., LEWIS, T. L., AND MAURER, D. (1986). Effect of binocular deprivation from cataracts on development of Snellen acuity [Abstract]. *Invest. Ophthalmol. Vis. Sci.* 27 (suppl.), 151.

BURIAN, H. M., AND VON NOORDEN, G. K. (1985). *Binocular Vision and Ocular Motility: Theory and Management of Strabismus.* St. Louis: Mosby.

CATALANO, R. A., SIMON, J. W., JENKINS, P. L., AND KADEL, G. L.(1987). Preferential looking as a guide for amblyopia therapy in monocular infantile cataracts. *J. Pediatr. Ophthalmol. Strabismus* 24, 56–63.

CRAWFORD, M. L. J., DE FABER, J-T., HARWERTH, R. S., SMITH III, E. L., AND VON NOORDEN, G. K. (1989). The effects of reverse monocular deprivation in monkeys. II. Electrophysiological and anatomical studies. *Exp. Brain Res.* 74, 338–347.

CRAWFORD, M. L. J., PESCH, T. W., VON NOORDEN, G. K., HARWERTH, R. S., AND SMITH III, E. L. (1991). Bilateral form deprivation in monkeys: electrophysiologic and anatomic consequences. *Invest. Ophthalmol. Vis. Sci.* 32, 2328–2336.

CREWTHER, S. G., CREWTHER, D. P., AND MITCHELL, D. E. (1983). The effects of short-term occlusion therapy on reversal of the anatomical and physiological effects of monocular deprivation in the lateral geniculate nucleus and visual cortex of kittens. *Exp. Brain Res.* 51, 206–216.

DAVIES, P. D., AND TARBUCK, D. T. H. (1977). Management of cataracts in infancy and childhood. *Trans. Ophthalmol. Soc. UK* 97, 148–152.

DEREFELDT, G., LENNERSTRAND, G., AND LUNDH, B. (1979). Age variations in normal human contrast sensitivity. *Acta Ophthalmol. (Copenh.)* 57, 679–690.

DOBSON, V. (1990). Behavioral assessment of visual acuity in human infants. In M. A. BERKLEY AND W. C. STIBBINS (eds.). *Comparative Perception.* New York: Wiley, pp. 487–521.

DOBSON, V., AND SEBRIS, S. L. (1989). Longitudinal study of acuity and stereopsis in infants with or at-risk for esotropia. *Invest. Ophthalmol. Vis. Sci.* 30, 1146–1158.

DRUMMOND, G. T., SCOTT, W. E., AND KEECH, R. V. (1989). Management of monocular congenital cataracts. *Arch. Ophthalmol.* 107, 45–51.

ENOCH, J., AND RABINOWICZ, I. M. (1976). Early surgery and visual correction of an infant born with unilateral eye lens opacity. *Doc. Ophthalmol.* 41, 371–382.

ENOCH, J., RABINOWICZ, I. M., AND CAMPOS, E. C. (1979). Postsurgical contact lens correction of infants with sensory deprivation amblyopia associated with unilateral congenital cataract. *Doc. Ophthalmol.* 41, 371–382.

EVERETT, M. E., STAGER, D. R., WRIGHT, W. W., AND BIRCH, E. E. (1989). Management of unilateral cataracts. *Am. Orthoptic J.* 39, 106–111.

FANTZ, R., ORDY, J., AND UDELF, M. (1962). Maturation of pattern vision in infants during the first six months. *J. Comp. Physiol. Psychol.* 55, 907–917.

FRANCOIS, J. (1979). Late results of congenital cataract surgery. *Ophthalmology* 86, 1586–1598.

FRANCOIS, J. (1984). Surgical results of congenital cataracts: the Belgian experience. *Ophthalmic Forum* 7, 126–128.

FRANK, J., AND FRANCE, T. (1977). Visual acuity and binocularity in children with unilateral acquired aphakia. *J. Pediatr. Ophthalmol.* 14, 200–204.

FREEMAN, R. D., AND OHZAWA, I. (1988). Monocularly deprived cats: binocular tests of cortical cells reveal functional connections from the deprived eye. *J. Neurosci.* 8, 2491–2506.

GELBART, S. S., HOYT, C. S., JASTREBSKI, G., AND MARG, E. (1982). Long-term visual results in bilateral congenital cataracts. *Am. J. Ophthalmol.* 93, 615–621.

GWIAZDA, J., BAUER, J., AND HELD, R. (1989a). From visual acuity to hyperacuity: a 10-year update. *Can. J. Psychol.* 43, 109–120.

GWIAZDA, J., BAUER, J., THORN, F., AND HELD, R. (1989b). Stereoacuity development for crossed and uncrossed disparities in children [Abstract]. *Invest. Ophthalmol. Vis. Sci.* 30 (suppl.), 313.

HAINLINE, L., CAMENZULI, C., ABRAMOV, I., RAWLICK, L., AND LEMERISE, E. (1986). A forced-choice method for deriving infant spatial contrast sensitivity functions from optokinetic nystagmus [Abstract]. *Invest. Ophthalmol. Vis. Sci.* 27 (suppl.), 266.

HARRIS, L. R., AND SMITH, A. T. (1990). Plaids used to distinguish direct retinal and cortical contributions to horizontal optokinetic nystagmus [Abstract]. *Invest. Ophthalmol. Vis. Sci.* 31, 591.

HARRIS, L. R., LEPORÉ, F., GUILLEMOT, J. P., AND CYNADER, M. (1980). Abolition of optokinetic nystagmus in the cat. *Science* 210, 91–92.

HARRIS, L. R., LEWIS, T. L., AND MAURER, D. (1991). Plaids used to evaluate cortical and subcortical involvement in human optokinetic nystagmus (OKN) [Abstract]. *Invest. Ophthalmol. Vis. Sci.* 32 (suppl.), 1021.

HARWERTH, R., CRAWFORD, M., SMITH, E., AND BOLTZ, R. (1981). Behavioral studies of stimulus deprivation amblyopia in monkeys. *Vision Res.* 21, 779–789.

HARWERTH, R. S., SMITH III, E. L., CRAWFORD, M. L. J., AND VON NOORDEN, G. K. (1989). The effects of reverse monocular deprivation in monkeys. I. Psychophysical experiments. *Exp. Brain Res.* 74, 327–337.

HARWERTH, R. S., SMITH III, E. L., PAUL, A. D., CRAWFORD, M. L. J., AND VON NOORDEN, G. K. (1991). Functional effects of bilateral form deprivation in monkeys. *Invest. Ophthalmol. Vis. Sci.* 32, 2311–2327.

HELD, R., BIRCH, E., AND GWIAZDA, J. (1980). Stereoacuity of human infants. *Proc. Natl. Acad. Sci. USA* 77, 5572–5574.

HENDRICKSON, A., BOLES, J., AND MCLEAN, E. B. (1977). Visual acuity and behavior of monocularly deprived monkeys after retinal lesions. *Invest. Ophthalmol. Vis. Sci.* 16, 469–473.

HESS, R. F., AND HOWELL, E. R. (1977). The threshold contrast sensitivity function in strabismic amblyopia: evidence for a two type classification. *Vision Res.* 17, 1049–1055.

HESS, R. F., FRANCE, T. D., AND TULUNAY-KEESEY, U. (1981). Residual vision in humans who have been monocularly deprived of pattern stimulation in early life. *Exp. Brain Res.* 44, 295–311.

HILES, D. A., AND WALLAR, P. H. (1977). Visual results following infantile cataract surgery. *Int. Ophthalmol. Clin.* 17, 265–282.

HOFFMANN, K. P. (1981). Neuronal responses related to optokinetic nystagmus in the cat's nucleus of the optic tract. In A. FUCHS AND W. BECKER (eds.). *Progress in Oculomotor Research.* New York: Elsevier, pp. 443–454.

HOFFMANN, K. P. (1982). Cortical versus subcortical contributions to the optokinetic reflex in the cat. In G. LENNERSTRAND AND E. L. KELLER (eds.). *Functional Basis of Ocular Motility Disorders.* New York: Pergamon, pp. 303–310.

HOFFMANN, K. P. (1983). Control of the optokinetic reflex by the nucleus of the optic tract in the cat. In A. HEIN AND M. JEANNEROD (eds.). *Spatially Oriented Behavior.* New York: Springer-Verlag, pp. 135–153.

HOFFMANN, K. P. (1986). Visual inputs relevant for the optokinetic nystagmus in mammals. *Prog. Brain Res.* 64, 75–84.

HOFFMANN, K. P. (1989). Functional organization in the optokinetic system of mammals. In H. RAHMAN (ed.). *Progress in Zoology: Neuronal Plasticity and Brain Function.* New York: Gustav Fisher, pp. 261–271.

HOFFMANN, K. P., AND DISTLER, C. (1989). Quantitative analysis of visual receptive fields of neurons in nucleus of the accessory optic tract in macaque monkey. *J. Neurophysiol.* 62, 416–428.

HOFFMANN, K. P., AND SCHOPPMANN, A. (1981). A quantitative analysis of the direction-specific response of neurons in the cat's nucleus of the optic tract. *Exp. Brain Res.* 42, 146–157.

HOFFMANN, K. P., DISTLER, C., ERICKSON, R. G., AND MADER, W. (1988). Physiological and anatomical identification of the nucleus of the optic tract and dorsal terminal nucleus of the accessory optic tract in monkeys. *Exp. Brain Res.* 69, 635–644.

HOWARD, I. P., AND OHMI, M. (1984). The efficiency of the central and peripheral retina in driving human optokinetic nystagmus. *Vision Res.* 24, 969–976.

JACOBSON, S. G., MOHINDRA, I., AND HELD, R. (1981). Development of visual acuity in infants with congenital cataracts. *Br. J. Ophthalmol.* 65, 727–735.

JACOBSON, S. G., MOHINDRA, I., AND HELD, R. (1982). Visual acuity of infants with ocular diseases. *Am. J. Ophthalmol.* 93, 198–209.

KATO, I., HARADA, K., HASEGAWA, T., IGARASHI, T., KOIKE, Y., AND KAWASAKI, T. (1986). Role of the nucleus of the optic tract in monkeys in relation to optokinetic nystagmus. *Brain Res.* 364, 12–22.

KOCHER, L., AND PERENIN, M. (1983). La fonction de sensibilité au contraste dans l'amblyopie de privation. *J. Fr. Ophthalmol.* 6, 843–851.

LEGUIRE, L. E., ROGERS, G. L., AND BREMER, D. L. (1990). Amblyopia: the normal eye is not normal. *J. Pediatr. Ophthalmol. Strabismus* 27, 32–38.

LEHMKUHLE, S., KRATZ, K. E., AND SHERMAN, S. M. (1982). Spatial and temporal sensitivity of normal and amblyopic cats. *J. Neurophysiol.* 48, 372–387.

LEVI, D. M., AND HARWERTH, R. S. (1977). Spatio-temporal interactions in anisometropic and strabismic amblyopia. *Invest. Ophthalmol. Vis. Sci.* 16, 90–95.

LEVI, D. M., AND KLEIN, S. A. (1985). Vernier acuity, crowding and amblyopia. *Vision Res.* 25, 979–991.

LEWIS, T. L., AND MAURER, D. (1986). Preferential looking as a measure of visual resolution in infants and toddlers: a comparison of psychophysical methods. *Child Dev.* 57, 1062–1075.

LEWIS, T. L., AND MAURER, D. (1992). The development of the temporal and nasal visual fields during infancy. *Vision Res.* 32, 903–911.

LEWIS, T. L., MAURER, D., AND BLACKBURN, K. (1985a). The development of young infants' ability to detect stimuli in the nasal visual field. *Vision Res.* 25, 943–950.

LEWIS, T. L., MAURER, D., AND BRENT, H. P. (1985b). Optokinetic nystagmus in children treated for bilateral cataracts. In R. GRONER, G. W. MCCONKIE, AND C. MENZ (eds.). *Eye Movements and Human Information Processing.* Amsterdam: North Holland, pp. 85–105.

LEWIS, T. L., MAURER, D., AND BRENT, H. P. (1986). Effects on perceptual development of visual deprivation during infancy. *Br. J. Ophthalmol.* 70, 214–220.

LEWIS, T. L., MAURER, D., AND BRENT, H. P. (1989a). Optokinetic nystagmus in normal and visually deprived children: implications for cortical development. *Can. J. Psychol.* 43, 121–140.

LEWIS, T. L., MAURER, D., AND BRENT, H. P. (1990a). The development of visual resolution in infants and toddlers tested monocularly with optokinetic nystagmus. *Clin. Vis. Sci.* 5, 231–241.

LEWIS, T. L., MAURER, D., AND HOLMES, R. R. (1991). The development of OKN acuity for nasalward versus temporalward motion [Abstract]. *Invest. Ophthalmol. Vis. Sci.* 32 (suppl.), 961.

LEWIS, T. L., MAURER, D., SMITH, R. J., AND HASLIP, J. K. (1992). The development of symmetrical optokinetic nystagmus during infancy. *Clin. Vision Sci.* 7, 211–218.

LEWIS, T. L., MAURER, D., TYTLA, M. E., BOWERING, E., AND BRENT, H. P. (1989b). Vision in the "normal" eye of children treated for unilateral congenital cataract. *Invest. Ophthalmol. Vis. Sci.* 30 (suppl.), 376.

LEWIS, T. L., MAURER, D., AND VAN SCHAIK, C. S. (1990b). Monocular OKN acuity is asymmetrical in normal 3-month-olds [Abstract]. *Invest. Ophthalmol. Vis. Sci.* 31 (suppl.), 7.

MALACH, R., AND VAN SLUYTERS, R. C. (1989). Strabismus does not prevent recovery from monocular deprivation: a challenge for simple Hebbian models of synaptic modification. *Vis. Neurosci.* 3, 267–273.

MALACH, R., EBERT, R., AND VAN SLUYTERS, R. C. (1984a). Recovery from effects of brief monocular deprivation in the kitten. *J. Neurophysiol.* 51, 538–551.

MALACH, R., STRONG, N., AND VAN SLUYTERS, R. C. (1981). Analysis of monocular optokinetic nystagmus in normal and visually deprived kittens. *Brain Res.* 210, 367–372.

MALACH, R., STRONG, N. P., AND VAN SLUYTERS, R. C. (1984b). Horizontal optokinetic nystagmus in the cat: effects of long-term monocular deprivation. *Dev. Brain Res.* 13, 193–205.

MANNY, R., AND LEVI, D. (1982). Psychophysical investigations of the temporal modulation sensitivity function in amblyopia: uniform field flicker. *Invest. Ophthalmol. Vis. Sci.* 22, 515–524.

MARKNER, C., AND HOFFMANN, K. P. (1985). Variability in the effects of monocular deprivation on the optokinetic reflex of the non-deprived eye in the cat. *Exp. Brain Res.* 61, 117–127.

MAURER, D., AND LEWIS, T. L. (1991). The development of peripheral vision and its physiological underpinnings. In M. J. WEISS AND P. R. ZELAZO (eds.). *Newborn Attention.* Norwood, NJ: Ablex, pp. 218–255.

MAURER, D., JOBSON, S., AND LEWIS, T. L. (1986). The development of peripheral acuity [Astract]. *Infant Behav. Dev.* 9, 245.

MAURER, D., LEWIS, T. L., AND BRENT, H. P. (1983). Peripheral vision and optokinetic nystagmus in children with unilateral congenital cataract. *Behav. Brain Res.* 10, 151–161.

MAURER, D., LEWIS, T. L., AND BRENT, H. P. (1989a). Preferential looking and optokinetic nystagmus: concurrent and predictive validity [Abstract]. *Invest. Ophthalmol. Vis. Sci.* 30 (suppl.), 303.

MAURER, D., LEWIS, T. L., AND BRENT, H. P. (1989b). The effects of deprivation on human visual development: studies of children treated for cataracts. In F. J. MORRISON, C. LORD, AND D. P. KEATING (eds.). *Applied Developmental Psychology. Vol. 3. Psychological Development in Infancy.* San Diego: Academic Press, pp. 39–227.

MAYER, D. L. (1986). Acuity of amblyopic children for small field gratings and recognition stimuli. *Invest. Ophthalmol. Vis. Sci.* 27, 1148–1153.

MAYER, D. L., AND DOBSON, V. (1980). Assessment of vision in young children: a new operant approach yields estimates of acuity. *Invest. Ophthalmol. Vis. Sci.* 19, 566–570.

MAYER, D. L., AND DOBSON, V. (1982). Visual acuity development in infants and young children, as assessed by operant preferential looking. *Vision Res.* 22, 1141–1151.

MAYER, D. L., FULTON, A. B., AND HANSEN, R. M. (1985). Visual acuity of infants and children with retinal degenerations. *Ophthalmic Paediatr. Genet.* 5, 51–56.

MAYER, D. L., MOORE, B., AND ROBB, R. M. (1989). Assessment of vision and amblyopia by preferential looking tests after early surgery for unilateral congenital cataracts. *J. Pediatr. Ophthalmol. Strabismus* 26, 61–68.

McDONALD, M., DOBSON, V., SEBRIS, S. L., BAITCH, L., VARNER, D., AND TELLER, D. Y. (1985). The acuity card procedure: a rapid test of infant acuity. *Invest. Ophthalmol. Vis. Sci.* 26, 1158–1162.

MIOCHE, L., AND PERENIN, M. T. (1986). Central and peripheral residual vision in humans with bilateral deprivation amblyopia. *Exp. Brain Res.* 62, 259–272.

MITCHELL, D. E. (1988). The extent of visual recovery from early monocular or binocular visual deprivation in kittens. *J. Physiol. (Lond.)* 395, 639–660.

MITCHELL, D. E. (1991). The long-term effectiveness of different regimens of occlusion on recovery from early monocular deprivation in kittens. *Philos. Trans. R. Soc. Lond. [Biol.]* 333, 51–79.

MITCHELL, D. E., AND MURPHY, K. M. (1984). The effectiveness of reverse occlusion as a means of promoting visual recovery in monocularly deprived kittens. In J. STONE, B. DREHER, AND D. H. RAPAPORT (eds.). *Development of Visual Pathways in Mammals.* New York: Alan R. Liss, pp. 381–392.

MITCHELL, D. E., AND TIMNEY, B. (1982). Behavioral measurement of normal and abnormal development of vision in the cat. In D. J. INGLE, M. A. GOODALE, AND R. J. W. MANSFIELD (eds.). *Analysis of Visual Behavior.* Cambridge, MA: MIT Press, pp. 483–523.

MITCHELL, D. E., CYNADER, M., AND MOVSHON, J. A. (1977). Recovery from the effects of monocular deprivation in kittens. *J. Comp. Neurol.* 176, 53.

MOHINDRA, I., JACOBSON, S. G., AND HELD, R. (1983). Binocular vision form deprivation in human infants. *Doc. Ophthalmol.* 55, 237–249.

MOHN, G., SIRETEANU, R., AND VAN HOF-VAN DUIN, J. (1986). The relation of monocular optokinetic nystagmus to peripheral binocular interactions. *Invest. Ophthalmol. Vis. Sci.* 27, 565–574.

MOHN, G., AND VAN HOF-VAN DUIN, J. (1990). Development of spatial vision. In D. M. REGAN (ed.). *Vision and Visual Dysfunction. Vol. 10. Spatial Vision.* London: Macmillan, pp. 179–211.

MONTAROLO, P. G., PRECHT, W., AND STRATA, P. (1981). Functional organization of the mechanism subserving the optokinetic nystagmus in the cat. *Neuroscience* 6, 231–246.

MOVSHON, J., AND VAN SLUYTERS, R. (1981). Visual neural development. *Annu. Rev. Psychol.* 32, 477–522.

MURASUGI, C. M., HOWARD, I. P., AND OHMI, M. (1989). Human optokinetic nystagmus: competition between stationary and moving displays. *Percept. Psychophys.* 45, 137–144.

NAEGELE, J. R., AND HELD, R. (1982). The postnatal development of monocular optokinetic nystagmus in infants. *Vision Res.* 22, 341–346.

NAEGELE, J. R., AND HELD, R. (1983). Development of optokinetic nystagmus and effects of abnormal visual experience during infancy. In M. JEANNEROD AND A. HEIN (eds.). *Spatially Oriented Behavior.* New York: Springer-Verlag, pp. 155–174.

NORCIA, A. M., GARCIA, H., HUMPHRY, R., HOLMES, A., HAMER, R. D., AND OREL-BIXLER, D. (1991a). Anomolous motion VEPs in infants and in infantile esotropia. *Invest. Ophthalmol. Vis. Sci.* 32, 436–439.

NORCIA, A. M., JAMPOLSKY, A., HAMER, R., AND OREL-BIXLER, D. (1991b). Plasticity of human motion processing following strabismus surgery [Abstract]. *Invest. Ophthalmol. Vis. Sci.* 32 (suppl.), 1044.

NORCIA, A. M., TYLER, C. W., AND HAMER, R. D. (1990). Development of contrast sensitivity in the human infant. *Vision Res.* 30, 1475–1486.

O'DELL, C. D., GAMMON, J. A., FERNANDES, A., WILSON, J. R., AND BOOTHE, R. G. (1989). Development of acuity in a primate model of human infantile unilateral aphakia. *Invest. Ophthalmol. Vis. Sci.* 30, 2068–2074.

PACKER, O., HENDRICKSON, A. E., AND CURCIO, C. A. (1990). Developmental redistribution of photoreceptors across the *Macaca nemestrina* (pigtail macaque) retina. *J. Comp. Neurol.* 298, 472–493.

PASIK, P., AND PASIK, T. (1982). Visual functions in monkeys after total removal of visual cerebral cortex. In W. NEFF (ed.). *Contributions to Sensory Physiology.* Vol. 7. Orlando, FL: Academic Press.

PIRCHIO, M., SPINELLI, D., FIORENTINI, A., AND MAFFEI, L. (1978). Infant contrast sensitivity evaluated by evoked potentials. *Brain Res.* 141, 179–184.

PRATT-JOHNSON, J., AND TILLSON, G. (1981). Visual results in congenital cataract surgery performed under the age of one year. *Can. J. Ophthalmol.* 16, 19–31.

QUICK, M. W., TIGGES, M., GAMMON, J. A., AND BOOTHE, R. G. (1989). Early abnormal visual experience induces strabismus in infant monkeys. *Invest. Ophthalmol. Vis. Sci.* 30, 1012–1017.

ROBB, R. M., MAYER, D. L., AND MOORE, B. D. (1987). Results

of early treatment of unilateral congenital cataracts. *J. Pediatr. Ophthalmol. Strabismus* 24, 178–181.

ROGERS, G. L., TISCHLER, C. L., TSOU, B. H., HERTLE, R. W., AND FELLOWS, R. R. (1981). Visual acuities in infants with congenital cataracts operated on prior to 6 months of age. *Arch. Ophthalmol.* 99, 999–1003.

ROY, M. S., LACHAPELLE, P., AND LEPORÉ, F. (1989). Maturation of the optokinetic nystagmus as a function of the speed of stimulation in fullterm and preterm infants. *Clin. Vis. Sci.* 4, 357–366.

SCHILDER, P., PASIK, P., AND PASIK, T. (1972). Extrageniculostriate vision in the monkey. III. Circle vs. triangle and "red vs. green" discrimination. *Exp. Brain Res.* 14, 436–448.

SCHOR, C. M., AND LEVI, D. M. (1980). Disturbance of small-field horizontal and vertical optokinetic nystagmus in amblyopia. *Invest. Ophthalmol. Vis. Sci.* 19, 668–683.

SCOTT, W. E., DRUMMOND, G. T., KEECH, R. V., AND KARR, D. J. (1989). Management and visual acuity results of monocular congenital cataracts and persistent hyperplastic primary vitreous. *Aust. N.Z. J. Ophthalmol.* 17, 143–152.

SIMPSON, J. I., GIOLLI, R. A., AND BLANKS, R. H. I. (1988). The pretectal nuclear complex and the accessory optic system. In J. A. BÜTTNER-ENNEVER (ed.). *Neuroanatomy of the Oculomotor System.* New York: Elsevier, pp. 335–364.

SMITH, A. T., AND HARRIS, L. R. (1991). Use of plaid patterns to distinguish the corticofugal and direct retinal inputs to the brainstem optokinetic nystagmus generator. *Exp. Brain Res.* 86, 324–332.

SMITH, D. C. (1981). Developmental alterations in binocular competitive interactions and visual acuity in visually deprived cats. *J. Comp. Neurol.* 198, 667–676.

SMITH, D. C., AND HOLDETER, R. N. (1985). Binocular competitive interactions and recovery of visual acuity in long-term monocularly deprived cats. *Vision Res.* 25, 1783–1794.

SOKOL, S., MOSKOWITZ, A., AND MCCORMACK, G. (1988). Infant grating acuity is temporarily tuned. *Vision Res.* 28, 1357–1366.

SOKOL, S., MOSKOWITZ, A., AND MCCORMACK, G. (1992). Infant VEP and preferential looking acuity measured with phase alternating gratings. *Invest. Ophthalmol. Vis. Sci.* 22, 3156–3161.

SPARKS, D. L., MAYS, L. E., GURSKI, M. R., AND HICKEY, T. L. (1986). Long-term and short-term monocular deprivation in the rhesus monkey: effects on visual fields and optokinetic nystagmus. *J. Neurosci.* 6, 1771–1780.

STAGER, D. R., AND BIRCH, E. E. (1986). Preferential-looking acuity and stereopsis in infantile esotropia. *J. Pediatr. Ophthalmol. Strabismus,* 23, 160–165.

STRONG, N., MALACH, R., LEE, P., AND VAN SLUYTERS, R. C. (1984). Horizontal optokinetic nystagmus in the cat: recovery from cortical lesions. *Dev. Brain Res.* 13, 179–192.

SWANSON, W. H., AND BIRCH, E. E. (1990). Infant spatiotemporal vision: dependence of spatial contrast sensitivity on temporal frequency. *Vision Res.* 30, 1033–1048.

TAYLOR, M. M., AND CREELMAN, C. D. (1967). PEST: Efficient estimates on probability functions. *J. Acoust. Soc. Am.* 41, 782–787.

TAYLOR, D., VAEGEN, MORRIS, J. A., ROGERS, J. E., AND WARLAND, J. (1979). Amblyopia in bilateral infantile and juvenile cataracts: relationship to timing of current treatment. *Trans. Ophthalmol. Soc. UK* 99, 170–175.

TELLER, D. Y., MAYER, D. L., MAKOUS, W. L., AND ALLEN, J. L. (1982). Do preferential looking techniques underestimate infant visual acuity? *Vision Res.* 22, 1017–1024.

TELLER, D. Y., MCDONALD, M. A., PRESTON, K., SEBRIS, S. L., AND DOBSON, V. (1986). Assessment of visual acuity in infants and children: the acuity card procedure. *Dev. Med. Child Neurol.* 28, 779–789.

TYTLA, M. E., LEWIS, T. L., MAURER, D., AND BRENT, H. P. (in

press). Stereopsis following congenital cataract? *Invest. Ophthalmol. Vis. Sci.*

TYTLA, M. E., LEWIS, T. L., MAURER, D., AND BRENT, H. P. (1991). Peripheral contrast sensitivity in children treated for congenital cataract [Abstract]. *Invest. Ophthalmol. Vis. Sci.* 32 (suppl.), 819.

TYTLA, M. E., MAURER, D., LEWIS, T. L., AND BRENT, H. P. (1988). Contrast sensitivity in children treated for congenital cataract. *Clin. Vis. Sci.* 2, 251–264.

VAEGAN, AND TAYLOR, D. (1979). Critical period for deprivation amblyopia in children. *Trans. Ophthalmol. Soc. UK* 99, 432–439.

VAN DIE, G. C., AND COLLEWIJN, H. (1982). Optokinetic nystagmus in man. *Hum. Neurobiol.* 1, 111–119.

VAN DIE, G. C., AND COLLEWIJN, H. (1986). Control of human optokinetic nystagmus by the central and peripheral retina: effects of partial visual field masking, scotopic vision and central retinal scotoma. *Brain Res.* 383, 185–194.

VAN HOF-VAN DUIN, J. (1976). Early and permanent effects of monocular deprivation on pattern discrimination and visuomotor behavior in cats. *Brain Res.* 111, 261–276.

VAN HOF-VAN DUIN, J. (1978). Direction preference of optokinetic responses in monocularly tested normal kittens and light-deprived cats. *Arch. Ital. Biol.* 116, 471–477.

VAN HOF-VAN DUIN, J. (1979). Development of visuomotor behavior in normal and light-deprived cats. *Clin. Dev. Med.* 73, 112–123.

VAN HOF-VAN DUIN, J., AND MOHN, G. (1984). Vision in the preterm infant. In H. F. R. PRECHTL (ed.). *Continuity of Neural Functions from Prenatal to Postnatal Life.* Philadelphia: Lippincott, pp. 93–115.

VAN HOF-VAN DUIN, J., AND MOHN, G. (1985). The development of visual functions in preterm infants. *Ergeb. Exp. Med.* 46, 350–361.

VAN HOF-VAN DUIN, J., AND MOHN, G. (1986a). Monocular and binocular optokinetic nystagmus in humans with defective stereopsis. *Invest. Ophthalmol. Vis. Sci.* 27, 574–584.

VAN HOF-VAN DUIN, J., AND MOHN, G. (1986b). Visual field measurements, optokinetic nystagmus and the visual threatening response: normal and abnormal development. *Doc. Ophthalmol. Proc. Ser.* 45, 305–316.

WATKINS, D. W., WILSON, J. R., AND SHERMAN, S. M. (1978). Receptive-field properties of neurons in binocular and monocular segments of striate cortex in cats raised with binocular lid suture. *J. Neurophysiol.* 41, 322–337.

WILLIAMS, R. W., AND CHALUPA, L. M. (1983). Development of the retinal pathway to the pretectum of the cat. *Neuroscience* 10, 1249–1267.

WILSON, J., TIGGES, M., BOOTHE, R., AND QUICK, M. (1991). Correlations between anatomy, physiology, and behavior for monocular infantile aphakia in monkeys [Abstract]. *Invest. Ophthalmol. Vis. Sci.* 32 (suppl.), 819.

WYNGAARDEN, P. A., MAURER, D., LEWIS, T. L., HARVEY, P., AND ROSENBAUM, P. (1991). The relationship between developmental delay and grating acuity [Abstract]. *Invest. Ophthalmol. Vis. Sci.* 32 (suppl.), 961.

YAMAMOTO, M., BUN, J., AND OKUDA, T. (1983). Visual functions after traumatic cataract in children. In P. HENKIND (ed.). *Acta: XXIV International Congress of Ophthalmology.* Philadelphia: Lippincott.

ZEE, D. S., TUSA, R. J., HERDMAN, S. J., BUTLER, P. H., AND GÜCER, G. (1986). The acute and chronic effects of bilateral occipital lobectomy upon eye movements in monkey. In E. L. KELLER AND D. S. ZEE (eds.). *Adaptive Processes in Visual and Oculomotor Systems.* New York: Pergamon, pp. 267–274.

ZEE, D. S., TUSA, R. J., HERDMAN, S. J., BUTLER, P. H., AND GÜCER, G. (1987). Effects of occipital lobectomy upon eye movements in primate. *J. Neurophysiol.* 58, 883–907.

27 | Prematurity and visual development

ALISTAIR R. FIELDER, NIGEL FOREMAN, MERRICK J. MOSELEY, AND JUDITH ROBINSON

The statement, "Birth is sandwiched between pre- and postnatal events," although obviously correct, does not provide any clue to the significance of this event regarding subsequent development of the neonate. Teleologically, the timing of birth occurs at the end of the full gestational period, when maturation has reached an appropriate stage. What happens, though, when this event occurs prematurely? Exteriorization at term and before term are not strictly comparable. Preterm neonates are at different stages of development compared to their term counterparts, the environments into which they are placed and cared for are dissimilar, and the events that befall these two groups differ considerably.

There is ample evidence that visual experience during early life, including exposure to light, is vital for normal visual development (Barlow, 1975); and if it is abnormal during what is known as the sensitive period, it may adversely affect the immature visual system, resulting in amblyopia. To quote: "Visual input plays a role in activating the underlying plasticity mechanisms in the visual cortex" (Mower and Christen, 1985). It has been suggested that cortical plasticity and hence the sensitive period is dependent not on age and inherent maturational processes but on visual input; and it is activated by exposure to light and form (Cynader and Mitchell, 1980; Mower and Christen, 1985). Thus total dark rearing represents complete visual deprivation and produces an extension of cortical plasticity with prolongation of susceptibility to monocular deprivation beyond its normal limits. In contrast, bilateral suturing of the eyelids produces diffuse abnormal stimulation and disintegration of the cortical receptive fields' properties (Mower et al., 1981). Cortical orientation preferences in kittens have been altered by selective exposure (Leventhal and Hirsch, 1975), and constant electrical stimulation of rat visual cortex slices has produced long-term depression, long-term potentiation, or no change of activated synapses (Artola et al., 1990). These authors predicted that use-dependent synaptic modification depends on the balance between contingent excitatory and inhibitory neuronal influences.

The literature, however, also contains references indicating that the maturation of vision is governed predominantly by innately determined processes rather than environmental influences. For instance, a restricted environment did not alter cortical orientation bias in kittens (Stryker and Sherk, 1975); and Leehey and coworkers (1975), in a study on human infants, considered that orientational asymmetry depended on endogenous maturation rather than visual experience.

Clearly, this discussion on early visual experience and its relevance to the subsequent development of visual functions raises fascinating issues particularly for the infant born prematurely, whose gestational period may have been shortened by up to 40%. In only one study have monkeys been reared 3 weeks before term (Bourgeois et al., 1989). It is important to emphasize here the limitations of the experimental animal in this respect and to remind the reader that there is no adequate model for the preterm neonate, as only in the human is significant shortening of the gestational period compatible with survival.

The timing of premature birth and its significance for the immature visual system can therefore be considered under two headings:

1. The effects of premature exteriorization on the various systems and tissues with respect to: (a) shortening of the intrauterine period—removal from a milieu uniquely protective, suited to promote growth, and essentially devoid of external stimulation; and (b) exposure of immature tissues not to the environment experienced by the term or even the adult but to one that is not endured at any other stage of life.
2. The relative importance of environmental and innate influences on development.

Throughout this chapter the following issues are frequently addressed.

1. What is the effect of additional extrauterine experience consequent on premature birth? Is a particular sphere of development accelerated or retarded? If either, can it be accounted for by all, or only part, of the extrauterine experience?
2. Clinical associations. There is no normal preterm infant and consequently, for clinical studies, no control.

485

Therefore in any investigation on the preterm infant or ex-preterm child, it is important to attempt to differentiate factors that may influence outcome such as the etiology of preterm birth, clinical (systemic or ocular) associations/complications, and environmental hazards. The first of these factors is not considered, although the etiology of premature delivery may have implications for the infant that extend beyond the event of birth, as it may interfere with fetal development. For example, severe intrauterine growth retardation and preeclampsia probably share common etiological factors (Bennett and Elder, 1988). It is also important to attempt to determine whether visual pathway abnormalities are casually or causally related to coexistent systemic abnormalities. There is a dearth of information, and at present many of these issues cannot be resolved.

Before discussing the development of visual functions of the infant born prematurely four topics are considered: (1) the premature population; and (2) the environment; (3) the eye; and (4) ophthalmology of the neonate. Necessarily, only selected topics are discussed, and the emphasis throughout this chapter is on the environment and development of the healthy preterm infant. Clinical issues are briefly considered in later sections.

PREMATURE POPULATION

First, a clarification of terms is in order. *Gestation* is the period in utero and is calculated as commencing from the last menstrual period. Once birth has occurred the term gestational age (GA) is inappropriate and *postnatal age* (PNA), *postconceptual age* (PCA), or *postmenstrual age* (PMA) are used. The last is the preferred term here, as it is based, like gestation, on the date of the last menstrual period. The World Health Organisation's definition of *prematurity* is a gestational period of less than 37 weeks. The term *very immature neonate* refers to the infant born at a gestational age of less than 28 weeks.

There is a paucity of epidemiological data on the premature population, partly because birth notification data in many countries includes birth weight but not gestational age (Macfarlane et al., 1988). Most North American data present an additional problem, being hospital- rather than population-based. There is a close relation between birthweight and gestational age in infant groups, though in the case of multiple birth a correction factor is required, and on an individual infant basis discrepancies are not infrequent. Thus published tables relating gestational age to birth weight should be interpreted with caution, as most were produced before accurate assessment of gestational age was possible

(Macfarlane et al., 1988). To highlight the problem of obtaining accurate information, over the 10-year period starting in 1975 the quoted incidence of live births (in Scotland, the only U.K. country collecting both gestational age and birth weight data) at 20–27 weeks' gestation rose from 20.5% to 39.0%. These data relate to birth, not survival; and as suggested by Macfarlane et al. (1988), the increase may in part be due to greater reporting of low gestation births.

Because of advances in neonatal management, the survival rates for babies born before term have dramatically increased over the past three to four decades. Between 1942 and 1952, during the "first epidemic" of retinopathy of prematurity only about 8% of neonates with birth weight less than 1000 g survived the neonatal period (Silverman, 1980). By the two periods 1968–1972 and 1974–1978 the rate had increased to 35% and 48%, respectively (Mutch, 1986).

Data for the year 1979 in England and Wales show that among a total of 661,192 live births 45,754 were classified as low birth weight (< 2500 g), i.e., an incidence of 6.92%; and the incidence of very low birth weight infants (< 1500 g) was 0.92% (*OPCS Monitor*, 1988). Corresponding figures for low birth weight for Denmark, Norway, Sweden, and Romania were 5.8%, 4.5%, 4.3%, and 7.1%, respectively (Mutch, 1986). The survival rate for preterm neonates can be calculated using data collated by the U.K. Office for Population Censuses and Surveys for 1986 (*OPCS Monitor*, 1988), and for infants of less than 1500 g birth weight it was 64.5% during the perinatal period (first postnatal week), with 73.7% surviving the neonatal period (first postnatal 28 days). Although these figures suggest that more babies survive the neonatal than the perinatal period, differences in definitions explain this apparent anomaly: perinatal deaths are calculated to include live and stillbirths, whereas neonatal deaths are expressed as only a proportion of live births. According to a hospital-based study from Memphis, the immature neonate constitutes 3% of all live births but accounts for 50% of all perinatal deaths (Amon et al., 1987). Birth weight is a better predictor of survival than gestational age, although for infants less than 500 g birth weight and less than 25 weeks' gestation, it is still close to zero (Cooke, 1988).

These data demonstrate that survival of the very immature neonate is improving, particularly since the middle of the 1960s (Macfarlane et al., 1988). Hence there is now a new population for whom the gestational period has been shortened by up to 35–40%.

NEONATAL EYE

The relative weighting given to topics in this subsection may appear inappropriate; but as the retina and posterior visual pathway are dealt with in detail elsewhere in this book, a necessarily brief and superficial review at this juncture would be superfluous. In contrast, topics such as eyelid and pupillary function, which have previously received scant attention, are particularly relevant to the visual system of the preterm infant and are therefore considered in greater detail.

The eyelids have an obviously vital protective role for the eye and are fused until about 24–25 weeks GA (Jain et al., 1973). The blink reflex is modified by postconceptual age (Anday et al., 1990). Until recently the pattern of movement of the eyelids after eye opening has been virtually ignored. Berman et al. (1987) and Moseley et al. (1988b) estimated that eyelids of preterm neonates are closed 80% of the time, but neither of these studies covered a wide GA range. Eyelid opening has been studied in 49 preterm neonates (GA 24–35 weeks) in two neonatal units with observations spread over the 24-hour period (Robinson et al., 1989). Mean eyelid closure was 74%, but trends became apparent when infants were grouped according to gestational age. Infants less than 26 weeks PMA had closed eyelids for 55% of observations compared with 93% at 28 weeks PMA and 60% at 34 weeks PMA (Fig. 27-1). The degree of prematurity at birth neither hastened nor retarded the pattern of eyelid opening; thus at 34 weeks PMA the frequency of eyelid opening was similar for infants born at 25 and 32 weeks GA. Two responses to changes of illumination were noted: A transient opening (lasting about 2 minutes) in response to a sudden reduction in illumination and significantly greater periods of open-

ing when the dimmed lighting was maintained (77% versus 64%; $p < 0.002$).

When closed, the light transmission characteristics of the eyelids become important. This point has been investigated in both adults (Moseley et al., 1988a; Robinson et al., 1991) and infants (Robinson et al., 1991). In the study of Robinson et al. (1991) monochromatic light of known wavelength was transmitted along an optic fiber mounted on the surface of a modified opaque contact lens placed under the upper eyelid. Measurements were taken on the external lid surface at 10-nm intervals (20-nm for neonates) over the range of 400–700 nm. Both studies showed that the eyelids act as a red-pass filter, transmitting up to approximately 14.5% in adults and 21.4% in neonates at 700 nm. The amount of light transmitted declined with decreasing wavelength to less than 5% in both adults and neonates at 580 nm or less (Fig. 27-2). Broadly similar results have been obtained in the monkey by Crawford and Marc (1976). No significant difference between ethnic groups was detected in the nine preterm neonates investigated: four caucasian, two black, and three Indo-Pakistani infants (Robinson et al., 1991). The cumulative transmission of white light (400–700 nm) across the closed eyelid has been estimated by integration to be approximately 38%.

By term the eyeball is at a relatively advanced stage of development compared to the rest of the body, and it is implicit therefore that ocular growth is active during the gestational period. Globe dimensions during development have been measured using necropsy material

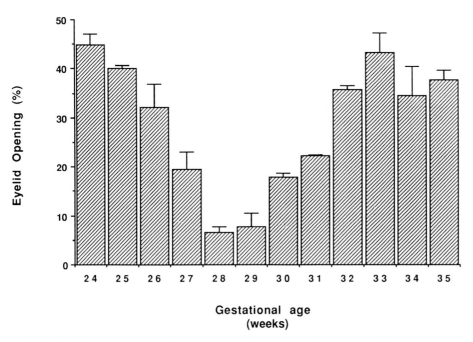

FIG. 27-1. Eyelid opening as a function of gestational age: observations over a 24-hour period during the first week of life. Each bar represents the mean ± SEM.

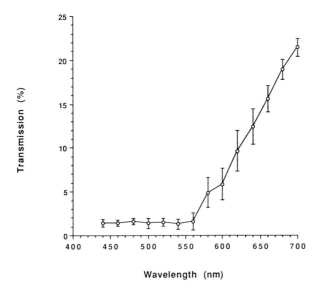

FIG. 27-2. Light transmission characteristics of the neonatal eyelid. Each point represents the mean ± SEM.

(Harayama et al., 1981; Robb, 1982) and in vivo using ultrasonography (Birnholz, 1985). In vivo recordings measure internal globe dimensions and thus underestimate the external dimensions by about 10% (Harayama et al., 1981; Robb, 1982). In contrast to previous workers who reported steady growth, Birnholz (1985) observed two spurts of activity, the first between 12 and 20 weeks GA and the second between 28 and 32 weeks GA. Transverse internal ocular diameters at 22.1, 26.8, and 37.8 weeks GA were 9.57, 11.74, and 15.82 mm, respectively (Birnholz, 1985). By term the external globe diameter is between 16 and 17 mm and reaches its adult size of 24 mm during the teens, with most of the postnatal increase seen during the first 3 years of life (Weale, 1982). Concurrent with these changes of globe size, the retinal surface area doubles between 28 weeks GA and term and increases another 50% over the first 2 years of life (Robb, 1982).

Most corneal growth occurs within the normal gestational period (Weale, 1982). Corneal diameter increases linearly (Robb, 1982; Weale, 1982) and has achieved adult dimensions within a few months of postnatal life. The pattern of change for corneal curvature is different, with flattening taking place rapidly during the last few weeks just before term, that is, during a stage when the preterm neonate has already been born. Up to about 27 weeks GA the cornea is hazy (Hittner et al., 1977).

R. J. Robinson (1966) investigated the development of 20 reflexes in order to produce an assessment battery that would enable the pediatrician to distinguish preterm from intrauterine growth-retarded neonates. The onset of the pupillary reflex to light was one of five reflexes that was highly correlated with gestational age and was noted in some babies at 29 weeks GA. In another study, Finnström (1971) reported the onset of the pupillary response between 29 and 31 weeks GA, and it was poorly correlated with GA. Both of these studies contained few very immature babies. The onset of this response has been investigated in 50 neonates (GA 26−34+ weeks) (Robinson and Fielder, 1990); and as shown in Figure 27-3, the response to light was absent before 30 weeks but was present in all by 35 weeks PMA. All infants who developed the reflex at 30 weeks PMA were born before 27 weeks, at an earlier PMA than the more mature, providing some evidence that early birth hastens its onset. The numbers, however, were insufficient for meaningful statistical analysis. Interestingly, iris color was gray before the onset of the reflex with other colors developing after this time. At each weekly observation session, pupil size was measured photographically (Robinson and Fielder, 1990). Mean horizontal and vertical pupil diameters, under standard neonatal unit illumination (560 lux), were, respectively, 3.46 mm (SD 0.78) and 3.49 mm (SD 0.72) before and 3.02 mm (SD 0.84) and 3.00 mm (SD 0.85) after the onset of the pupillary light reflex. These data correspond closely with values reported by Sindel et al. (1986) and Isenberg et al. (1989, 1990).

The hyaloid artery forms part of a transient vascular system that enters the eye at 6 weeks GA, fills the primary vitreous, and forms a network of vessels to nourish the lens (tunica vasculosa lentis) before regressing: the hyaloid artery by 28 weeks and the tunica vasculosa lentis by 34 weeks GA. The choriocapillaris is formed by 6 weeks GA, and by 22 weeks GA arteries are apparent (Sellheyer and Spitznas, 1988). The retina is avascular until 16 weeks of fetal life when mesenchymal cells grow out from the optic disc in sheets and later remodel to form the vascular network (Ashton, 1970). Retinal vascularization is complete in the nasal and temporal regions at around 32 weeks GA and just after term, respectively.

Visual pathway development is not considered here in detail, but a few points are pertinent. Retinal surface area increases by 50% during the first 2 years after birth at term; and because the growth of the anterior segment of the eye is at an advanced stage by term most of this growth of the eye must take place in its posterior segment, predominantly in the periphery rather than at its posterior pole. The retina has its full complement of cells by 6 months' gestation (Hollenberg and Spira, 1973), and the subsequent increase in retinal surface area is accommodated by shifts of distribution, rather than by cell division. At 22 weeks GA the fovea contains only one layer of cones, but by 24 weeks GA the foveolar depression is forming because of the peripheral migration of the inner retinal layers and rods. Subsequently there is a central movement of cones, but the process

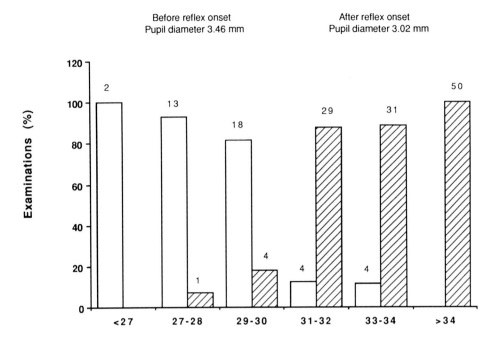

FIG. 27-3. Presence or absence of the pupil reflex to light according to postmenstrual age. Pupil diameter before and after the onset of the response is shown. The number of babies examined at each age is indicated by the number at the top of each bar. Clear and hatched bars indicate, respectively, the absence or presence of a pupillary reaction to light. One infant exhibited a reaction at 27 weeks but was subsequently nonreactive.

of foveal maturation is not complete until about 3–4 years of age (Yuodelis and Hendrickson, 1986). The peripheral retina is relatively well developed at term compared to the fovea (Abramov et al., 1982).

OPHTHALMOLOGY OF THE PRETERM INFANT

It is not the purpose of this chapter to discuss in detail neonatal clinical conditions. However, because retinopathy of prematurity (ROP) affects most very immature babies it cannot be ignored. ROP affects the advancing edge of the developing retinal vasculature. Thus close to term the process is observed in the peripheral retina, whereas in the most immature neonate in whom the retinal vessels have not progressed so peripherally, the retinopathy is located more posteriorly.

The incidence and severity of ROP rise with increasing immaturity. Birthweight-specific incidence figures for acute ROP are as follows.

<1000 g = 53.0% (Keith and Kitchen, 1984)
≤1300 g = 55.6% (Flynn et al., 1987)
≤1500 g = 48.1% (Schaffer et al., 1985)
≤1500 g = 34.9% (Reisner et al., 1985)

Corresponding figures from an epidemiological study in the United Kingdom (Ng et al., 1988) are as follows.

<1000 g = 88.5%
≤1300 g = 75.4%
≤1500 g = 60.1%
<28 weeks GA = 86.7%

Differences must be interpreted with caution; the higher incidence in the U.K. study can almost certainly be attributed to the intensive examination protocol rather than to the disease process itself, which is born out by the lower incidence of cicatricial disease in this study compared to any of the others listed (see Ng et al., 1988, for a discussion). For the purpose of this chapter, the essential point is that more very immature neonates than not develop acute ROP. That its onset appears to be governed more by the stage of development, probably at a retinal level, than by neonatal events (Fielder et al., 1986b, 1987, 1992a) suggests that for ROP to develop a certain stage of retinal maturation must have been reached. Although in most cases ROP resolves spontaneously and completely (to ophthalmoscopical evaluation) an appreciation of the sequence of events may be relevant to the future development of visual functions. Mintz-Hittner et al. (1990) reported in survivors of very low birth weight, after seemingly complete resolution of acute ROP, a retinovascular abnormality involving the central retina (reduced or absent foveal avascular zone) that was associated with reduced acuity. They postulated a cessation of vascular remodeling independent of ROP severity.

It is beyond the remit of this chapter to consider the pathogenesis of ROP, although it is interesting that environmental illumination, first suggested as a factor by Terry (1942), is again being implicated in its pathogenesis (Glass et al., 1985; Fielder et al., 1990, 1992b).

ENVIRONMENT

Babies born prematurely are nursed in an environment different from that experienced in utero. A considerable volume of research has been undertaken to investigate the physiological (e.g., temperature, humidity, and nutrition) and psychological requirements of the immature baby (e.g., stimulation, contact, and noise). One challenge of neonatology today is to create an environment which mimics that in utero more closely with regard to humidity and temperature, while permitting carers the access required to assist the immature respiratory, cardiac, and gastrointestinal systems to adjusting to life without the placenta (Whitelaw and Cooke, 1988).

Wolke (1987) considered that the frequency and types of stimulation provided by the sensory environment of neonatal units (NNUs) (i.e., light, noise, and handling) are inappropriate. Lucey (1973) proposed that the absence of cycling of noise and light may be detrimental to the development of infants born preterm, a hypothesis supported by Mann et al. (1986).

The amount of handling of neonates varies; thus during a typical 24-hour period those requiring intensive care were disturbed by a neonatologist on average 25 times, whereas for healthier infants it was 10 times. Overall, very immature neonates were handled by all staff and parents more than 100 times each day (Robinson et al., 1989), an incidence lower than the 234 times reported by Murdoch and Darlow (1984). Neonatal behavioral state may be affected by handling or medical interventions and often is associated with periods of crying or wakefulness (Apkarian et al., 1989; Robinson et al., 1989). Periods of wakefulness in high-dependency areas were associated with handling, and the maximum period of uninterrupted sleep was only 11 minutes (mean value); whereas in low-dependency areas it was a mean of 34 minutes (Robinson et al., 1989). Ignoring for this purpose the medical needs of the baby, neonatal units do not seem to provide the optimal environment for preterm neonates in this respect (Gabriel et al., 1981; Lawson et al., 1985; Wolke, 1987).

Thermoregulation is not fully developed in the term neonate; adult circadian rhythm of body temperature has yet to appear, although the swaddled baby can maintain thermal stability over the average environmental temperature range at home (Hull, 1988). The very immature preterm neonate, on the other hand, loses heat rapidly and has virtually no thermoregulatory control. Thus both fetus and preterm neonate require environmental heat to maintain homeostasis within a thermoneutral range designed to minimize energy expenditure. Infants kept in an environmental temperature of 36.5°C compared to 35.0°C grow faster (Glass et al., 1971), and temperature reduction retards head growth (Glass et al., 1975). Corneal temperature has been measured (Fielder et al., 1986a) using noncontact infrared radiation thermometry with means of 36.54°C and 36.80°C, respectively, for the right and left eyes (mean rectal temperature 36.80°C) of preterm infants, whereas for term babies the corresponding values were 36.40°C and 36.25°C (mean rectal temperature 37.03°C). Corneal temperature was higher when the neonate was placed in an incubator, although the rectal temperature remained constant. Normal fetal temperature at 38.1°C is above maternal core temperature (Walker et al., 1969); thus infants born prematurely suffer a temperature deficit of at least 1.5–2.0°C that is not regained throughout life. This deficit is, if anything, likely to be an underestimate, as this study (Fielder et al., 1986a) did not consider the temperature-lowering effects of eyelid opening and the environmental temperature when babies have been discharged to home, which is usually a few weeks before term. The effect, if any, of this temperature deficit is unknown, but it may retard the increase of corneal radius that occurs around term, at a time when the preterm infant has already been born (Fielder et al., 1986a). This fact raises the intriguing possibility that such persistence of a high radius of curvature could contribute to the myopia of ex-prematures (Fledelius, 1981a, 1982b), a type of myopia distinct from that occurring as a sequela of ROP.

Virtually no attention has been paid to the preterm infants' lighting environment; and in contrast to noise, there are no guidelines regarding the amount of light reaching the baby. While in utero a small amount of light is probably transmitted across the abdominal wall; the value of 2% reported by Jacques et al., (1987) is at a level where measurement error may exceed the absolute value.

Continuous illumination may have both physiological and biochemical effects on the developing infant (Gottfried et al., 1981). Mann and coworkers (1986) have shown that after discharge to home infants who had been exposed to a cyclic lighting regimen while in the NNU slept longer, fed better, and gained more weight than did their age-matched controls.

Neonatal units are illuminated 24 hours a day, typically by a mixture of daylight and overhead fluorescent lights. Several studies have reported on the levels of illumination within neonatal units (MacLeod and Stern, 1972; Hamer et al., 1984; R. J. Landry, 1985; Robinson et al., 1990a) and presented differing values. Unfortunately, data are difficult to compare because of methodological differences, including lack of a standard measurement location, absence of detail on measurement timing, and the uncertainties associated with instrumentation and its calibration, which can be of the order of ± 30–50%.

The ambient illumination within an NNU in the United States where sunlight can supplement the room illumination has been reported to exceed 10,000 lux (Hamer et al., 1984), a value above that known to cause retinal damage in animals. MacLeod and Stern (1972), in a survey of a single NNU designed to assess the effects of measurement position within the unit and the seasonal variations on illumination, found that the intensity of illumination ranged from 160 to 26,900 lux. The highest values were recorded near the windows on bright, sunny days. In general, this study indicated that there are natural variations in environmental lighting that are dependent on weather conditions, time of day, and location of the detector within the unit.

R. J. Landry and coworkers (1985), in a survey of eight American NNUs, reported mean levels of illumination ranging from 285 to 1485 lux. Both radiometric (i.e., spectral irradiance and irradiance at 455 nm) and simultaneous photometric (illuminance) measurements were recorded. Seven of the units were visited on only a single occasion, whereas the eighth was visited twice, once on a sunny day and then on a dull, overcast day. The results cite mean illuminances for each unit, obscuring variations within the units (i.e., between the high- and low-dependency areas). No details were provided as to the time of measurement (within the 24-hour period) or the season. The authors also noted that the total exposure of an infant in a study may depend on other factors such as those mentioned above, the use of eyeshields, and the frequency at which the fluorescent tubes are changed.

Lighting surveys have been performed in seven neonatal units in the United Kingdom with mean unit illuminance of 470 lux (range 192–890 lux). In four of the seven NNUs, the intensive care areas were significantly brighter than their corresponding low-dependency areas (890 lux versus 300 lux) (Robinson et al., 1990a). In two low-dependency areas where illumination was reduced at night, the mean illuminance was approximately 50 lux. Since the late 1960s NNU illumination has increased 5- to 10-fold, rising from 100 lux (Giunta and Rath, 1969) to about 560 lux (R. J. Landry et al., 1985; Robinson et al., 1990a), peaking to 10,000 lux if sunlight contributes (Hamer et al., 1984).

Not all environmental illumination reaches the eyelid. Preterm neonates are usually nursed prone, with the head turned to one side and the lower eyelid shielded by clothing, an arm, or the mattress. The effects of these postural changes on the illuminance reaching each eyelid have been monitored over the 24-hour period in 65 babies (J. Robinson, 1990; Robinson et al., 1990a,b). Illuminance was recorded by photodiodes placed at four sites: one above each eyebrow, one on the cot at face level, and one on the arm or leg covered by a blanket (the control). Readings were obtained every 10 seconds over the 24-hour period and the data then examined by time series analysis. The amount of light reaching the eyelid ranged from 30% to 100% (mean 47%); but owing to posturing, the lower eyelid received a mean of 25% (range 0–78%) of the available light in the environment and the upper eyelid a mean of 86% (range 57–100%).

In addition to general ward illumination, infants are exposed to light sources as part of their treatment and during examinations. Premature infants are often exposed to phototherapy (2400–3000 lux) for the treatment of neonatal jaundice. During such phototherapy, which may last for periods exceeding 24 hours, infants generally have their eyes shielded from the phototherapy lights by "patches," which transmit some of the light (Chin et al., 1987; Porat et al., 1988) ranging from less than 2% to 10% at 700 nm according to patch type (Robinson et al., 1991). These patches, however, are prone to slip away from the eyes—in one study for more than half of all observations (9,292 of 16,615) (Robinson et al., 1989).

Routine ophthalmoscopical examinations are performed on neonates of low gestational age to screen for ROP. Animal studies suggest that indirect ophthalmoscopy can cause retinal damage (Friedman and Kuwabara, 1968; Tso et al., 1972). Kirkness (1986) has evaluated the retinal hazard posed by this instrument by calculating the temperature rise that results from light absorption in the retina, correlating retinal irradiance values with safety guidelines, and comparing these figures with threshold values for retinal damage. These calculations suggest that indirect ophthalmoscopy poses no threat of retinal damage for the adult, provided exposure duration does not exceed 23–80 seconds per eye, depending on the power of the supplementary lens used.

Preterm babies are at risk of developing a variety of ocular problems in which early exposure to light has often been implicated (Moseley and Fielder, 1988), although as yet the adverse or even the beneficial effects of early light exposure to the human developing visual system are unknown. A prerequisite to this study is an understanding of the neonatal ocular light dose. Factors determining the dose can be divided into two broad categories: (1) environmental or physical factors, such as the intensity and spectral characteristics of the NNU lighting environment, and random shading effects; and (2) physiological factors such as the frequency of eyelid opening, light transmission characteristics of the closed eyelid, pupil area and reactivity, and the light transmission characteristics of the ocular media. Except for the last item, these factors have already been considered. The ocular media of neonates are highly transmissive, especially in the blue and ultraviolet regions of the spectrum (Boettner and Wolter, 1962; Lerman, 1985, 1988), and the lens at this time transmits more than 90% of light up to 420 nm (Barker, personal communication). Light does not enter the eye exclusively through the pupil, as the sclera and choroid transmit about 14%, again predominantly at the red end of the spectrum (Kopeiko et al., 1979; van den Berg et al., 1990). Using these data, the retinal irradiance received by a preterm neonate has been estimated (J. Robinson, 1990; Robinson et al., 1990b). As shown in Figure 27-4, it declines as a function of increasing postmenstrual age; but, for example, the immature neonate of 29 weeks PMA receives about 350 μW/cm^2, a level similar to that known to cause cone damage in the macaque monkey (Sykes et al., 1981).

Whether cone damage occurs in the human preterm infant is unknown, yet cone dysfunction has been reported in children who received stray light during phototherapy as neonates (Abramov et al., 1985); and low, but normal, acuity has been noted in ex-premature children (Sebris et al., 1984) and teenagers (Fledelius, 1981b). As mentioned, the dose-response relation for light damage and the immature visual system is not yet known, and currently data drawn from animal experimentation must be used (Kremers and van Norren, 1988; Moseley and Fielder, 1988). Finally, although light can undoubtedly damage the mature, and probably the immature, visual system, the possibility that it may be beneficial and accelerate visual development cannot be ignored. A variety of mechanisms could be invoked, such as hastening of myelination—although in the cat, this probably is not the case (Moore et al., 1976)—and the activation of cortical activity, to which we have already alluded.

ATTENTION

Research on visual attention in the healthy preterm infant has focused on two main issues: (1) whether the development of responses to a novel stimulus is accelerated or retarded by the extrauterine experience; and (2) if cognitive development is affected in the long term. If possible, both must be assessed independent of risk factors, such as the associations of prematurity (see above) and demographic factors. Preterm infants might benefit from all, some, or even none of their visual experience prior to term; conversely, premature exteriorization may adversely affect the immature visual pathways resulting in permanent disorganization of attention.

There is little information on the visual capacities of newly born preterm infants, as their fragile state often precludes formal behavioral testing. However, from as early as 30–32 weeks PMA there are periods of awareness, and visual fixation has been demonstrated at various periods using low spatial frequency patterned stimuli, including preferential looking (PL)-based tests (Miranda and Hack, 1979; Hack et al., 1981; Morante et al., 1982; Shepherd et al., 1985; Brown and Yamamoto, 1986). R. J. Robinson (1966) observed head-turning to a diffuse light by 32 weeks PMA, and by term there was no difference in this response between term and preterm neonates, although Ferrari et al. (1983) reported that, at term, preterm infants exhibit orientation less well than term neonates. Because the infant's visual attention (turning toward and fixating stimuli) provides the evidence for discrimination in PL tests, clearly even the 10-week premature neonate is capable of selectively attending to a novel source of stimulation. They also slowly track a moving stimulus, such as a red woollen ball (Dubowitz et al., 1980), although spontaneous scanning becomes evident only at around 35

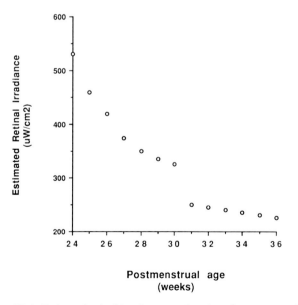

FIG. 27-4. Estimated retinal irradiance as a function of postmenstrual age (PMA). The reduction at 30–31 weeks PMA may partly be explained by the onset of the pupillary light reflex and the move from a high- to a low-dependency nursery. The latter is associated with lower luminance.

weeks (Hack et al., 1976). Preterm infants have been described as showing "visual capture," fixating particular stimuli for long periods before averting their gaze. Such an impression may have been gained from a subgroup of preterm infants who showed blank stares during infancy and who were later found to be retarded (Miranda and Hack, 1979); but it was not confirmed in a more recent study, in which no evidence of prolonged looking durations was noted in preterm neonates during this period (Foreman et al., 1991).

Reports of differences in responsiveness between preterm and term infants are ambiguous (Parmelee, 1975). In formal test situations, preterm neonates have been reported to spend longer than term infants fixating stimuli before averting their gaze (Spungen et al., 1985), although Kopp et al. (1975) noted this trait in only some preterm infants and others did not observe this effect at all (Fantz and Fagan, 1975; Friedman et al., 1981; Foreman et al., 1991). However, preterm neonates habituate slowly only to repeated stimulus presentations (Friedman et al., 1981; Rose, 1981b). Nevertheless, there are many reports of precocious development in preterm infants by their due date. Compared to term infants, they are said to (1) behave as if more experienced at relating to others (Avery and Litwack, 1983); (2) be "better organized" (St-Anne Dargassies, 1977); and (3) show advanced visual attentiveness (Gessell and Amatruda, 1945), more mature responses to three-dimensional faces (Fantz et al., 1975), and precocious maturity when focusing and when tracking moving stimuli (Dubowitz et al., 1980; Bloch, 1983). Electrophysiological and behavioral evidence of accelerated acuity development is considered in the section on acuity.

Assuming that the preterm infant possesses sufficient structural maturity in the visual system to be advantaged by the additional extrauterine experience, any aspect of behavioral development triggered or promoted by exposure to light or visual pattern (see above) may be expected to be accelerated in infants born before term. Scores on standardized developmental scales, which make extensive use of infants' visual responses, tend to be accelerated in the preterm infant but only during the first few months of life (Hunt and Rhodes, 1977), after which development largely follows a biological timetable (Fantz and Fagan, 1975; Fantz et al., 1975). It is doubtful whether behavioral acceleration during the immediate postterm period confers any long-term benefit, as it is of necessity greatest in infants having the shortest gestational periods (Hunt and Rhodes, 1977; Sigman et al., 1977), yet these infants are most at risk for later developmental delays (Caputo et al., 1979, 1981; Kitchen et al., 1980).

Components of the orienting response to peripheral targets have been separated experimentally by recording the turning response (phasic orienting) and subsequent duration of fixation response (tonic orienting, or "looking" time). These responses are also sometimes referred to as attention "getting" and attention "holding" (Cohen, 1972). Short attention getting and holding times are assumed to reflect greater maturity, as they characterize older infants (Fantz et al., 1962). Risk status is an important determinant of performance; preterm infants who have suffered intraventricular hemorrhage, respiratory distress syndrome, or other neonatal insults tend to exhibit lower arousal, lack of alertness, and longer looking durations than term or healthy preterm infants (Anderson et al., 1989). Although the latency of orienting toward a novel stimulus seems the obvious parameter of attention-getting, it has rarely been studied in infants; many authors have reported the number of separate fixations during a defined period as the dependent variable (Fantz et al., 1962; Hack et al., 1976; Vassella et al., 1977). However, Friedman and colleagues (1981) found that when stimuli consisting of red or green three-dimensional lighted translucent plastic boxes were waved 19 cm from their eyes, healthy premature infants responded at a slower rate (4.74 seconds versus 2.00 seconds) and habituated more slowly than term infants, implying a slower processing of visual information. Masi and Scott (1983) found that, at term, preterm infants took slightly longer than term infants to turn to a face. Foreman et al. (1991) studied the acquisition and maintenance of attention—the latency of phasic (attention "getting") and tonic (attention "holding") orientation in 38 preterm and 33 term infants. There was an initial plateau period before 44.7 weeks PCA (when latency is unrelated to age in preterm infants); thereafter, latency of phasic orientation decreased slowly in a linear fashion with increasing age in both groups of infants (Fig. 27-5). For all, tonic orientation also exhibited an initial plateau and fell abruptly at 53 weeks PCA. Despite the necessary integration of phasic and tonic orientation, during the early neonatal period the two appear to be independent. Around term, compared to term neonates the preterm neonates' latencies to turn were significantly shorter ($p < 0.02$) (Fig. 27-6), although tonic orientation times did not differ (Foreman et al., 1991). The former was not because term neonates had yet to recover from birth trauma; when data were plotted against postnatal age, during the first month of life preterm infants again exhibited significantly faster orienting responses. Observations that preterm infants show greater arousal and attention at term (Gessell and Amatruda, 1945; Sigman et al., 1977) and better organization (St-Anne Dargassies, 1977) may have been prompted by the infants' brisker responses to novelty.

With reduction of both latency of attention-getting and the duration of attention-holding during infancy, frequency of looking increases and fixation duration is

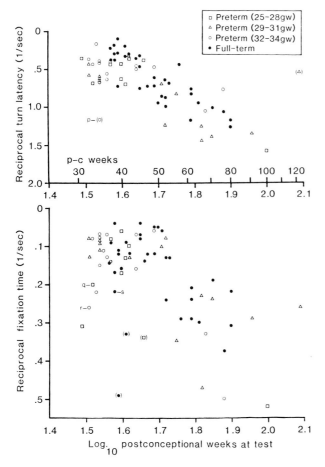

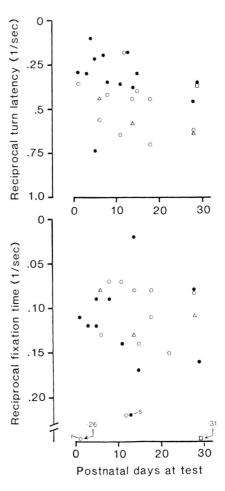

FIG. 27-5. (Top) Mean reciprocal turning latency (phasic orientation or attention-getting). (Bottom) Mean reciprocal fixation time (tonic orientation or attention-holding). Both are expressed as a function of postconceptual age. Both show a relative plateau in which latency is unrelated to age, followed by a decline. Turning during the first 30 postnatal days was significantly faster for preterm than term infants, although fixation times for these two groups were similar. Points in parentheses were not utilized for analysis. (From Foreman et al., 1991. By permission.)

FIG. 27-6. (Top) Mean reciprocal turning latency. (Bottom) Mean reciprocal fixation time. Both are plotted against postnatal age. Symbols are as for Figure 27-5. Preterm infants' turning latencies are significantly shorter than those for term infants; there is no difference for the duration of fixation.

reduced (obvious when performing PL tests). Similar trends have been observed in term neonates (Fantz et al., 1962; Sigman et al., 1977) and age-corrected preterm infants (Fantz and Fagan, 1975; Foreman et al., 1991), although there is a paucity of within-individual longitudinal data. Where differences are reported in visual behaviors between groups of term and age-corrected preterm infants, the latter are invariably delayed. Thus at 7 months looking durations have been found to be longer in preterm than in term infants, particularly if the former have suffered intraventricular hemorrhage or respiratory distress syndrome (S. H. Landry et al., 1985; Anderson et al., 1989), these infants being less responsive to novelty (Rose et al., 1988) and having poor visual orienting (Anderson et al., 1989). Preterm infants were found to pay less attention to toys, visually fixating them less frequently than term infants (Brach-

feld et al., 1980; Crawford, 1982; Landry and Chapieski, 1988).

The early development of attention in preterm infants adds yet another tier to the continuing debate on the nature and maturation of visual pathways during infancy. It is recognized that many of the ensuing comments are controversial and still speculative, but they nevertheless need to be raised. The division of labor within the visual system of the infant (Bronson, 1974; Maurer and Lewis, 1979) implies that extrageniculostriate (midbrain) systems guiding phasic orientation are relatively mature at term but that geniculostriate function emerges later, around 6–12 weeks after term (Atkinson, 1984; Braddick et al., 1986). The superior colliculus may have a role in the organization of eye movements including those used for scanning (Trevarthen, 1974; Karmel and Maisel, 1975) and for attentional redirection. There is little doubt that the midbrain develops earlier than cortical systems anatomically

(Cooper and Rakic, 1983) and neurophysiologically (Rose, 1981a).

Although early physiological models of visual development assumed an independence between cortex and midbrain (Bronson, 1974), it is now considered that this assumption is not so, although they are interactive in the organization of orienting behavior in the infant (Gardner and Karmel, 1983) and older subject (Foreman and Stevens, 1987), and that both systems are mature by 6–8 weeks after term (Bronson, 1982). However, the age at which cortical (geniculostriate) function emerges is still unknown. Karmel and Maisel (1975) suggested that during very early infancy the midbrain is responsible for all visual functions, and before around 2–3 months the cortex is virtually nonfunctional (Atkinson et al., 1988); although in view of the sophistication of term neonatal behaviors, Slater et al. (1988) considered this suggestion unlikely.

To investigate the possible interaction between sensory modalities when orienting, in this instance auditory and visual, a preliminary study was undertaken in preterm (14 infants, 26–32 weeks GA) and near term (12 infants, 33–40 weeks GA) infants aged 4.5–15.0 months corrected age (Foreman and Fielder, 1989). The latter, near-term comparison group was chosen in the absence

of a similarly treated but nonpremature group. Orientation was elicited to a peripheral stimulus for all infants irrespective of age at birth or at testing, but only when the stimulus consisted of a spatially coherent auditory-visual combination, i.e., where the light and sound occurred in the same point in space. Most (18 of 26) infants from both groups responded to a stimulus combination located 80–100 degrees in the periphery (Fig. 27-7). When the auditory and visual stimuli were presented in isolation, the former were generally preferred, as they were when stimuli were presented competitively—on opposite sides of the midline. The preliminary nature of this study has been mentioned, but three points nevertheless emerge. First, using a sound–light combination most infants, even if born prematurely, can respond to peripheral targets often seemingly beyond their supposed limits of effective visual field as measured by standard perimetry (Mohn and van Hof-van Duin, 1986). This topic is covered elsewhere in the book. Second, intersensory integration, intermodal enhancement, and stimulus localization ability develop relatively normally in infants born before term, and visual and auditory orienting systems are not topographically misaligned or otherwise greatly disrupted by premature birth. Third, as is mentioned later, these findings are

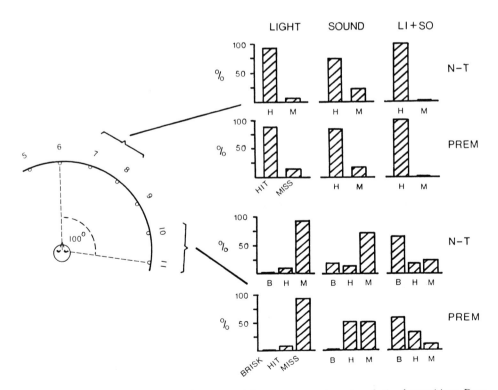

FIG. 27-7. Intermodal enhancement. Plane view of the apparatus and numbered stimulus positions. Data analyzed from central (7 plus 8) and peripheral (10 plus 11) positions. Subject groups: N-T = near term; PREM = preterm. Response type was recorded as brisk (B), hit (H), or miss (M). In both groups orientation nearly always occurred to light and usually to sound alone for central stimuli, whereas for peripheral stimuli a light-sound combination was considerably more effective. (From Foreman and Fielder, 1989. By permission.)

relevant to various aspects of the testing of visual functions of infants.

The link between early sensorimotor abnormalities and more subtle deficits on scholastic tasks is difficult to establish. The importance of maintaining an appropriate balance between turning and looking components of attention has been pointed out by Sigman (1983), as any disruption of this relation could have consequences for subsequent development. Developmental problems may be predicted from neonatal behaviors (Fagan and McGrath, 1981), although given the different nature of the tests used at the various periods of infancy and childhood it is seldom possible. Nevertheless, deficits in ex-preterms have been reported during early childhood (Meisels et al., 1987) and to persist in children of school age (Caputo et al., 1979, 1981), measured by a standard test battery on visual, visuomotor, and attentional scales. In another study (Foreman et al., submitted) a battery of visuospatial tasks were presented to ex-preterm children and compared with age-matched controls. Excluding those children with obvious neurological disorders, deficits remained only in eye-hand coordination and task perseverance, tasks that require, *inter alia*, the shifting and maintenance of attention. Thus although research to date indicates that preterms' neonatal attentional abnormalities are small and mainly temporary, they cannot be disregarded as causes of the more subtle cognitive deficits seen in school age preterm children that usually place them at the lower end of the normal ability range (Caputo et al., 1979, 1981).

The development of attention in preterm and term infants is of practical importance, as a variety of tests of visual functions involve the attentional responses of turning and fixating: the measurement of acuity using Acuity Cards and perimetry. Both require active and precise orienting responses in order to inform the observer that stimulus detection and discrimination have occurred. In both tests, sound often accompanies the presentation of the visual stimulus (e.g., the knocking sound of the Acuity Card). It is pertinent to recall that in perimetry combined sound–light presentation may induce a response even beyond the effective visual field. This topic also has theoretical implications, providing further clues to the neural substrates operative during infancy, before and after term, and offers yet another avenue for research into the possible beneficial or adverse effects of preterm birth.

ELECTRORETINOGRAPHY

The earliest measurement of any light-evoked responses is generally accredited to Zetterström (1952), who dem-

onstrated the presence of b-wave activity in a flash-elicited electroretinogram (ERG). The onset of ERG activity occurred mostly within the first week of life for neonates in the birth weight range 2000–2500 g, whereas for those with birth weights of 1000–1500 g, up to 9 weeks of postnatal development was required before an ERG could be demonstrated in all subjects. Winkelman and Horsten (1962) and Horsten and Winkleman (1962) were subsequently able to demonstrate both a- and b-wave activity on the first day of life, though in these investigations the youngest infant studied appeared to be 34 weeks GA.

Numerous authors have since confirmed the presence of ERG activity during early postnatal life (Alfieri et al., 1966; Rouher et al., 1967; Samson-Dollfus, 1968; Fogarty and Reuben, 1969) even in infants as young as 29 weeks of age (Ricci et al., 1983). Grose et al. (1989) have described the maturational changes in the ERG that occur within the period 30.5–53.0 weeks PMA. During this period both b-wave and, to a lesser extent, a-wave amplitudes were shown to increase and corresponding latencies to decrease. These authors were also able to identify the presence of oscillatory potentials in a number of recordings but only in infants older than 37 weeks PMA. Van Hof-van Duin and Mohn (1984) hinted at the possible use of the pattern electroretinogram (PERG) to estimate visual acuity, but to our knowledge this technique has yet to be applied to the preterm population. ERG investigations of ROP have also been undertaken (Bohár and Véli, 1977; Mets et al., 1990) but have yet to make an impact on clinical practice.

VISUALLY EVOKED POTENTIALS

Visually evoked potentials (VEPs) arising from flash stimulation have been recorded in infants as young as 24 weeks GA (Hrbek et al., 1973; Chin et al., 1985). At this age the response consists of a negative wave appearing after 300 ms, but by 34 weeks a positive wave develops at 200–250 ms (Mushin et al., 1986). Maturational changes underlying the development of the flash VEP have been attributed to the extent of dendritic formation (Purpura, 1976). Although acknowledging that latency changes in the flash VEP may predict developmental outcome, van Hof-van Duin and Mohn (1984) noted the limitations in the clinical utility of the flash VEP due to the wide intersubject variability and the apparent presence of a normal response in the absence of a functioning visual cortex. Another source of variability (Whyte et al., 1987; Apkarian et al., 1989) is that arousal state during testing may significantly influence both response amplitudes and latencies.

Some have considered the measurement of evoked responses to pattern stimulation to be impractical owing to the difficulty of ensuring adequate fixation (Placzek et al., 1985), but successful recordings evoked by phase-alternated gratings (Baraldi et al., 1981), pattern-reversal checkerboard stimuli (Sokol and Jones, 1979; Harding et al., 1989a,b), and swept sine-wave gratings (Norcia et al., 1987) have been achieved. Comprehensive investigations by Harding and colleagues (Grose et al., 1989; Harding, 1989a,b) have documented the maturation of the pattern reversal response between the ages of 30.5 and 53.0 weeks PMA. A single positive component was observed in the recordings obtained from the most immature infants having a mean latency of 320 ms at 32.5 weeks, which by 52 weeks PMA had significantly decreased to 125 ms (Harding et al., 1989a). Quantitative indices available from VEP recordings include not only response amplitudes and latencies providing information on visual pathway maturation but, in the case of sweep grating patterns, estimates of visual acuity (Norcia et al., 1987).

BEHAVIORAL TESTS

Behavioral testing has included a variety of qualitative and quantitative methods, including blink responses, fixation and following, optokinetic nystagmus, and visual field assessment. These subjects have been extensively reviewed elsewhere (Sokol and Jones, 1979; Fielder, 1988; Fielder et al., 1988); see also Attention (above). Here we consider only visual acuity as measured using pattern preferences for grating targets, as these responses provide a quantitative measure of spatial resolution that can be related to visual acuity recorded in older subjects. The advent of portable apparatus and simplified testing procedures such as the Acuity Card procedure (McDonald et al., 1985) permit rapid and reliable measurements on a routine basis.

Successful measurement of grating acuity in a younger premature population has been reported by several authors (Dobson et al., 1980; Manning et al., 1982; Morante et al., 1982; van Hof-van Duin and Mohn, 1984, 1986; Brown and Yamamoto, 1986; Birch and Spencer, 1989; Searle et al., 1989). Data provided by Brown and Yamamoto (1986) illustrate the improvement in resolution that occurs between 32 and 45 weeks GA in which mean acuity increased from 0.27 cycles/degree (cpd) to 0.75 cpd. These authors established the utility of the Acuity Card procedure for use within a young preterm population by achieving a successful test rate of 83%. Birch and Spencer (1991) have compared monocular acuities of preterm and term neonates, and Dob-

son et al. (1990) have employed Acuity Cards to document visual performance in the presence of ROP.

VISUAL FIELD AND COLOR VISION

The development of visual field and color vision are not considered here. The former subject is discussed in Chapter 7.

INNATE VERSUS ENVIRONMENTAL INFLUENCES

The preceding discussion has provided a brief overview of the progress made in documenting the early visual capacities of infants born prematurely. It is now time to return to questions posed earlier in the chapter: What is the effect of early exteriorization on the immature visual system? What is the relative importance of innate and environmental influences? A number of studies have shown that acuity development of preterm infants proceeds as though commencing from term; that is, when corrected for the degree of prematurity, both preterm and term infants exhibit the same maturational pattern (Fantz et al., 1975; Dobson et al., 1980; Baraldi et al., 1981; Morante et al., 1982; van Hof-van Duin et al., 1983; van Hof-van Duin and Mohn, 1984; Brown and Yamamoto, 1986). Contrasting with these reports, superiority of acuity in preterm subjects has been documented in several behavioral and electrophysiological studies (Sokol and Jones, 1979; Tyler and Norcia, 1985; Mohn and van Hof-van Duin, 1986; Norcia et al., 1987), indicating the possible beneficial effects of the environment. In these cases, where visual development appears to have been hastened by prematurity, the reported differences between groups are small. van Hof-van Duin and Mohn (1986) observed a mean difference of only 0.3 octave across the corrected age range 1–49 weeks. Most reports suggest that after 1 year of age the difference between postnatal and corrected age is negligible (van Hof-van Duin and Mohn, 1984), although there are two reports of acuities at the lower end of the normal range in ex-premature children at 3–4 years of age (Sebris et al., 1984) and 10–18 years of age (Fledelius, 1981b).

It is important, however, not to attribute any beneficial or adverse effect necessarily to the environment, as many other aspects may also be relevant; caution is required before correlating visual function to ocular or systemic pathology. Fetal development may be abnormal, as in intrauterine growth retardation (IUGR), which may be causally related to premature birth. Vernier acuity at 40 weeks after term in IUGR infants has been reported to be lower than in term infants (Stanley et al., 1989). Diet and intestinal absorptive capacity is another factor obviously affected by preterm birth, and Birch and coworkers (1990) accounted for observed superiority of both grating and VEP acuity in preterm infants compared to term infants by unspecified nutritional differences in human and commercially available formulas. More recent evidence by Uauy et al. (1990) has shown that ω-3 fatty acids, not present in commercial formulas, are essential for optimal function of the developing retina, as determined by ERG in low birth weight infants. Although deficiency of the aminosulfonic acid taurine is known to cause retinal and tapetal degeneration in developing animals, Harding et al. (1989a) were unable to identify differences in pattern VEPs obtained from preterm infants fed either taurine or taurine-free diets.

In summary, minor degrees of acceleration have been observed in various parameters; but, excluding those infants who have suffered complications of preterm birth, the development of visual acuity in the infant born before term appears to progress at a rate similar to his or her term counterpart—as though birth had occurred at term. Similar patterns of maturation have also been observed for eyelid opening, the onset of the pupil reflex to light, and orientation responses. Nevertheless, studies so far are relatively few, and more research is required to determine whether premature birth and its accompaniments either accelerate or retard any aspect of visual development.

REFRACTIVE STATUS

The association of prematurity and myopia is well known, but this topic must be subdivided into three areas: (1) myopia during the neonatal period; (2) myopia developing later; and (3) myopia associated, or not, with ROP.

During the neonatal period preterm infants are often myopic (Graham and Gray, 1963; Scharf et al., 1978; Dobson et al., 1981; Nissenkorn et al., 1983; Linfield and Davis, 1984; McCormick, et al., 1986), and its magnitude is probably inversely related to gestational age (Dobson et al., 1981). It follows that there is a trend toward emmetropia with increasing age (Scharf et al., 1978; Linfield and Davis, 1984; McCormick et al., 1986), and by the age of 1 year there is no difference between premature and term infants (Shapiro et al., 1980). Nissenkorn and coworkers (1983) reported a higher incidence of myopia during infancy; between myopia, acute ROP, and decreasing birth weight. As mentioned, there are many factors that could affect ocular growth, including temperature, visual experience, and, acute and cicatricial ROP. The association of myopia with cicatricial ROP is established (Nissenkorn et al., 1983;

Gordon and Donzis, 1986; Snir et al., 1988). The degree of myopia is positively correlated with the severity of the cicatricial disease but is not influenced by cryotherapy (Nissenkorn et al., 1983). Minor transient changes of acute ROP do not seem to affect subsequent refraction (Laws et al., 1992), although more myopia has been reported in association with regressed ROP than in the "normal" preterm infant (Kushner, 1982; Schaffer et al., 1984; Cats and Tan, 1989; Gibson et al., 1990). Infants stated to be without ROP have been noted to be less hyperopic than term infants (Koole et al., 1990). The mechanism of myopia associated with ROP is unknown, but it is in all probability multifactorial depending on the severity and duration of ROP; this process occurs at a period of rapid ocular growth that may be retarded by the acute phase and further restrained by the cicatricial phase. The following have also been reported: anomalies of corneal curvature (Hittner et al., 1979), corneal diameter (Kelly and Fielder, 1987), lens power (Gordon and Donzis, 1986), and axial length (Tasman, 1979; Gordon and Donzis, 1985). Astigmatism is particularly frequent in cases of resolved or cicatricial ROP. In a longitudinal study, Fledelius (1982a) demonstrated that low birth weight had a negative influence on eye size, interpupillary distance, and other anthropometric parameters. High corneal curvature persisted (Fledelius, 1982a,b), indicating an arrest of corneal development and causing the low myopia in ex-premature teenagers. This situation is probably distinct from the myopia associated with ROP.

CLINICAL ISSUES

So far the development of visual functions has concentrated on the premature infant who has had a relatively smooth passage through the neonatal period and did not suffer a significant ophthalmic or neurological complication—in other words, the healthy preterm. Unfortunately, this is not always the case, and clinical conditions of particular visual import are those with neurological involvement. ROP, although obviously a major cause of ophthalmic morbidity, having received considerable attention in the literature, is not considered further here. The developmental consequences of perinatal hypoxia have been examined using a battery of behavioral tests (Groenendaal et al., 1989). Neurologically abnormal preterm infants have been reported to exhibit maturational delays of acuity (Dubowitz et al., 1983; Placzek et al., 1985; van Hof-van Duin and Mohn, 1985; Norcia et al., 1987). We have suggested (Fielder et al., 1988) that these abnormalities could fall within the broad clinical spectrum of delayed visual maturation (DVM). It is probably not so, however, as those with DVM are usually totally unresponsive to any visual stimulus including a grating (Tresidder et al., 1990). The pathogenesis of this condition is unknown but raises again a fascinating question: Is acuity during early infancy subserved predominantly by subcortical/extrageniculostriate pathways (Bronson, 1974; Atkinson, 1984; Fielder and Evans, 1988)? Dubowitz et al. (1986), using cranial ultrasonography, observed that lesions near the thalamus, but not in the visual cortex, were likely to affect visual behavior. Roving eye movements (Dubowitz and Dubowitz, 1981) and tonic downgaze with convergence (Tamura and Hoyt, 1987), due to intraventricular hemorrhage, have been observed during the neonatal period; and, as mentioned, infants with intracranial hemorrhage exhibit poor orientation (Anderson et al., 1989).

Periventricular leukomalacia (PVL) is an ischemic neurological lesion that occurs as a complication of birth whether at term or before. Visual pathway involvement in this condition is frequent, particularly if the lesion is cystic and located posteriorly (Gibson et al., 1990). The neuroophthalmic associations of PVL include low acuity, delayed visual field development, strabismus, and supranuclear eye movement disorders (Weindling et al., 1985; Calvert et al., 1986; De Vreis et al., 1987; Lambert et al., 1987; Scher et al., 1989; Gibson et al., 1990). The mechanism of visual pathway involvement in PVL is unknown.

There have been a number of studies on the ophthalmic complications of preterm birth (Kitchen et al., 1980; Kushner, 1982; Keith and Kitchen, 1983; McCormick et al., 1986; Snir et al., 1988; Cats and Tan, 1989; Gibson et al., 1990). All report an increased incidence of refractive errors and strabismus (about 10–23%) and, less frequently, optic atrophy.

To conclude, the very immature infant is placed in a harsh environment and is at risk of developing a number of systemic and ophthalmic complications. Although the etiology of certain complications arising from this period can readily be determined, with our current dearth of knowledge it is not always possible. Finally, to emphasize this dilemma, a clinical example: We have undertaken a prospective study of ROP in the East Midlands of England of which a subcohort was used for epidemiological purposes (Ng et al., 1988). Among the original 572 infants of birth weight 1700 g or less, binocular vision was measured in 431 infants at around 6 months using the Acuity Card procedure (Laws et al., 1992). Despite all but eight infants falling within the normal range for age (Sebris et al., 1987), as can be seen in Figure 27-8 acuity declined according to the presence and severity of acute ROP. There was no significant difference between sequential ROP stages, but this effect persisted after correction for gestational age, age at testing, neurological complications, and excluding those with persistent retinal problems (Laws et al.,

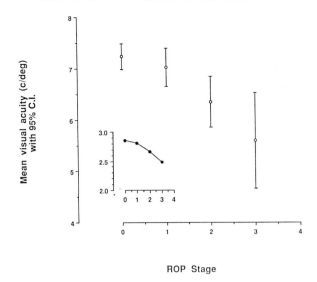

FIG. 27-8. Mean visual acuity by stage of ROP. Measured using the Acuity Card procedure on 431 infants of birth weight ≤ 1700 g around 6 months (corrected age). Each point represents mean acuity with 95% confidence intervals. (Inset) Same data with acuity plotted on a $\log_2$ axis.

1992). The question therefore arises: What is the basis of this slightly reduced, albeit still normal, acuity? The answer is not known. It is difficult to attribute it to the effects of ROP, a peripheral retinovascular disorder. The possibility of photoreceptor damage—by mechanism(s) as yet unknown—must be entertained.

Acknowledgments. The authors wish to acknowledge the support of the Medical Research Council of Great Britain, the Royal National Institute for the Blind, and the Wellcome Trust.

REFERENCES

ABRAMOV, I., GORDON, J., HENDRICKSON, A., HAINLINE, L., DOBSON, V., AND LA BOSSIERE, E. (1982). The retina of the newborn human infant. *Science* 217, 265–267.

ABRAMOV, I., HAINLINE, L., LEMERISE, E., AND BROWN, A. K. (1985). Changes in visual functions in children exposed as infants to prolonged illumination. *J. Am. Optom. Assoc.* 56, 614–619.

ALFIERI, R., SOLÉ, P., AND ROUHER, F. (1966). Dualité électrorétinographique chez le prématuré. *C. R. Soc. Biol.* 160, 2316–2317.

AMON, E., SIBAI, B. M., ANDERSON, G. D., AND MABIE, W. C. (1987). Obstetric variables predicting survival of the immature newborn (≤1000 gm): a five-year experience at a single perinatal center. *Am. J. Obstet. Gynecol.* 156, 1380–1389.

ANDAY, E. K., COHEN, M. E., AND HOFFMAN, H. S. (1990). The blink reflex: maturation and modification in neonate. *Dev. Med. Child Neurol.* 32, 142–150.

ANDERSON, L. T., COLL, C. G., VOHR, B. R., EMMONS, L., BRANN, B., SHAUL, P. W., MAYFIELD, S. R., AND OH, W. (1989). Behavioural characteristics and early temperament of premature infants with intracranial hemorrhage. *Early Hum. Dev.* 18, 273–283.

APKARIAN, P., MIRMIRAN, M., AND SPEKREIJSE, H. (1989). Luminance evoked potentials and neonatal temporal sensitivity: effects of maturation and behavioural state. *Invest. Ophthalmol. Vis. Sci.* 30 (suppl.), 314.

ARTOLA, A., BRÖCHER, S., AND SINGER, W. (1990). Different voltage-dependent thresholds for inducing long-term depression and long-term potentiation in slices of rat visual cortex. *Nature* 347, 69–72.

ASHTON, N. (1970). Retinal angiogenesis in the human embryo. *Br. Med. Bull.* 26, 103–106.

ATKINSON, J. (1984). Human visual development over the first few months of life: a review and hypothesis. *Hum. Neurobiol.* 3, 61–74.

ATKINSON, J., HOOD, B., WATTAM-BELL, J., ANKER, S., AND TRICKELBANK, J. (1988). Development of orientation discrimination in infancy. *Perception* 17, 587–595.

AVERY, M. E., AND LITWACK, G. (1983). *Born Early.* Boston: Little, Brown.

BARALDI, P., FERRARI, F., FONDA, S., AND PENNE, A. (1981). Vision in the neonate (full-term and premature): preliminary result of the application of some testing methods. *Doc. Ophthalmol.* 51, 101–112.

BARLOW, H. B. (1975). Visual experience and cortical function. *Nature* 258, 201–204.

BENNETT, P. R., AND ELDER, M. G. (1988). Extreme prematurity: the aetiology of preterm delivery. *Br. Med. Bull.* 44, 850–860.

BERMAN, J., HUTCHINS, R., GOLD, S., PELI, E., AND LINDSEY, P. (1987). Measurement of light exposure in infants at high risk of developing ROP. *Invest. Ophthalmol. Vis. Sci.* 28 (suppl.), 119.

BIRCH, E. E., AND SPENCER, R. (1989). Preferential-looking (PL) acuity of preterm infants with and without retinopathy of prematurity (ROP). *Invest. Ophthalmol. Vis. Sci.* 30 (suppl.), 318.

BIRCH, E. E., AND SPENCER, R. (1991). Monocular grating acuity of healthy preterm neonates. *Clin. Vis. Sci.* 6, 331–334.

BIRCH, E. E., BIRCH, D. G., AND UAUY, R. (1990). *Effects of Gestational Age at Birth and Diet on Visual Acuity Development. Noninvasive Assessment of the Visual System. Digest of Topical Meeting on Noninvasive Assessment of the Visual System.* Vol. 3. Washington, DC: Optical Society of America, pp. 14–17.

BIRNHOLZ, J. C. (1985). Ultrasonic fetal ophthalmology. *Early Hum. Dev.* 12, 199–209.

BLOCH, H. (1983). La poursuite visuelle chez le nouveau-né a terme et chez le premature. *Enfance* 1, 19–29.

BOETTNER, E. A., AND WOLTER, J. R. (1962). *Transmission of the Ocular Media.* Wright-Patterson Air Force Base, Ohio.

BOHÁR, A., AND VÉLI, M. (1977). Frühe ERG-Zeichen der retrolentalen Fibroplasie. *Klin. Monatsbl. Augenheilkd.* 170, 746–749.

BOURGEOIS, J. P., JASTREBOFF, P. J., AND RAKIC, P. (1989). Synaptogenesis in visual cortex of normal and preterm monkeys: evidence for intrinsic regulation of synaptic overproduction. *Proc. Natl. Acad. Sci. USA* 86, 4297–4301.

BRACHFELD, S., GOLDBERG, S., AND SLOMAN, J. (1980). Parent-infant interactions in free play at 8 and 12 months: effects of prematurity and immaturity. *Infant Behav. Dev.* 3, 289–305.

BRADDICK, O., WATTAM-BELL, J., AND ATKINSON, J. (1986). Orientation-specific cortical responses develop in early infancy. *Nature* 320, 617–619.

BRONSON, G. (1974). The postnatal growth of visual capacity. *Child Dev.* 45, 873–890.

BRONSON, G. W. (1982). *The Scanning Patterns of Human Infants: Implications for Visual Learning.* New York: Ablex.

BROWN, A. M., AND YAMAMOTO, M. (1986). Visual acuity in newborn and preterm infants measured with grating acuity cards. *Am. J. Ophthalmol.* 102, 245–253.

CALVERT, S. A., HOSKINS, E. M., FONG, K. W., AND FORSYTH, S. C. (1986). Periventricular leukomalacia: ultrasonic diagnosis and neurological outcome. *Acta Paediatr. Scand.* 75, 489–496.

CAPUTO, D. V., GOLDSTEIN, K. M., AND TAUB, H. B. (1979). The development of prematurely born children through middle childhood. In T. M. FIELD, A. M. SOSTEK, S. GOLDBERG, AND H. H. SHUMAN (eds.). *Infants Born at Risk.* New York: SP Medical and Scientific Books.

CAPUTO, D. V., GOLDSTEIN, K. M., AND TAUB, H. B. (1981). Neonatal compromise and later psychological development. In S. L. FRIEDMAN AND M. SIGMAN (eds.). *Preterm Birth and Psychological Development.* Orlando, FL: Academic Press.

CATS, B. P., AND TAN, K. E. W. P. (1989). Prematures with and without regressed retinopathy of prematurity: comparison of long-term (6–10 years) ophthalmological morbidity. *J. Pediatr. Ophthalmol. Strabismus* 26, 271–275.

CHIN, K. C., MOSELEY, M. J., AND BAYLISS, S. C. (1987). Light transmission of phototherapy eyeshields. *Arch. Dis. Child.* 62, 970–971.

CHIN, K. C., TAYLOR, M. J., MENZIES, R., AND WHYTE, H. H. (1985). Development of visual evoked potentials in neonates. *Arch. Dis. Child.* 60, 1166–1168.

COHEN, L. B. (1972). Attention-getting and attention-holding processes of infant visual preferences. *Child Dev.* 43, 869–879.

COOKE, R. W. I. (1988). Outcome and costs of care for the very immature infant. *Br. Med. Bull.* 44, 1133–1151.

COOPER, J. W., AND RAKIC, P. (1983). Gradients of cellular maturation and synaptogenesis in the superior colliculus of the fetal rhesus monkey. *J. Comp. Neurol.* 215, 165–186.

CRAWFORD, J. W. (1982). Mother-infant interaction in premature and full-term infants. *Child Dev.* 53, 957–962.

CRAWFORD, M. L. J., AND MARC, R. E. (1976). Light transmission of cat and monkey eyelids. *Vision Res.* 16, 323–324.

CYNADER, M., AND MITCHELL, D. (1980). Prolonged sensitivity to monocular deprivation in dark-reared cats. *J. Neurophysiol.* 43, 1026–1040.

DE VREIS, L. S., CONNELL, J. A., DUBOWITZ, L. M. S., OOZEER, R. C., PENNOCK, J. M., AND DUBOWITZ, V. (1987). Neurological electrophysiological and MRI abnormalities in infants with extensive cystic leukomalacia. *Neuropediatrics* 18, 61–66.

DOBSON, V., FULTON, A. B., MANNING, K., SALEM, D., AND PETERSEN, R. A. (1981). Cycloplegic refractions of premature infants. *Am. J. Ophthalmol.* 91, 490–495.

DOBSON, V., MAYER, D. L., AND LEE, C. P. (1980). Visual acuity screening of preterm infants. *Invest. Ophthalmol. Vis. Sci.* 19, 1498–1505.

DOBSON, V., QUINN, G. E., BIGLAN, A. W., TUNG, B., FLYNN, J. T., AND PALMER, E. A. (1990). Acuity card assessment of visual function in the cryotherapy for retinopathy of prematurity trial. *Invest. Ophthalmol. Vis. Sci.* 31, 1702–1708.

DUBOWITZ, L. M. S., LEVENE, M. I., MORANTE, A., PALMER, P., AND DUBOWITZ (1981). Neurologic signs in neonatal intraventricular haemorrhage: a correlation with real-time ultrasound. *J. Pediatrics* 99, 127–133.

DUBOWITZ, L. M. S., DE VRIES, L., MUSHIN, J., AND ARDEN, G. B. (1986). Visual function in the newborn infant: is it cortically mediated? *Lancet* 1, 1139–1141.

DUBOWITZ, L. M. S., DUBOWITZ, V., MORANTE, A., AND VERGHOTE, M. (1980). Visual function in the preterm and fullterm newborn infant. *Dev. Med. Child Neurol.* 22, 465–475.

DUBOWITZ, L. M. S., MUSHIN, J., MORANTE, A., AND PLACZEK, M. (1983). The maturation of visual acuity in neurologically normal and abnormal newborn infants. *Behav. Brain Res.* 10, 39–45.

FAGAN, J. F., AND MCGRATH, S. K. (1981). Infant recognition memory and later intelligence. *Intelligence* 5, 121–130.

FANTZ, R. L., AND FAGAN III, J. F. (1975). Visual attention to size and pattern details by term and preterm infants during the first six months. *Child Dev.* 46, 3–18.

FANTZ, R. L., FAGAN, J. F., AND MIRANDA, S. B. (1975). Early visual selectivity as a function of pattern variables, previous exposure, age from birth and conception and expected cognitive defect. In L. B. COHEN AND P. SALAPATEK (eds.). *Infant Perception from Sensation to Cognition.* Orlando, FL: Academic Press, pp. 249–345.

FANTZ, R. L., ORDY, J. M., AND UDELF, M. S. (1962). Maturation of pattern vision in infants during the first six months. *J. Comp. Physiol. Psychol.* 55, 907–917.

FERRARI, F., GROSOLI, M. V., FONTARA, G., AND CAVAZZUTI, G. B. (1983). Neurobehavioural comparison of low-risk preterm and fullterm infants at term at corrected age. *Dev. Med. Child Neurol.* 25, 450–458.

FIELDER, A. R. (1988). Disorders of vision. In M. I. LEVENE, M. J. BENNETT, AND J. PUNT (eds.). *Fetal and Neonatal Neurology and Neurosurgery.* Edinburgh: Churchill Livingstone, pp. 517–534.

FIELDER, A. R., AND EVANS, N. M. (1988). Is the geniculostriate system a prerequisite for nystagmus? *Eye* 2, 628–635.

FIELDER, A. R., LEVENE, M. I., RUSSELL-EGGITT, I. M., AND WEALE, R. A. (1986a). Temperature—a factor in ocular development. *Dev. Med. Child Neurol.* 28, 279–284.

FIELDER, A. R., MOSELEY, M. J., AND NG, Y. K. (1988). The immature visual system and premature birth. *Br. Med. Bull.* 44, 1093–1118.

FIELDER, A. R., NG, Y. K., AND LEVENE, M. I. (1986b). Retinopathy of prematurity: age at onset. *Arch. Dis. Child.* 61, 774–778.

FIELDER, A. R., NG, Y. K., LEVENE, M. I., AND SHAW, D. E. (1987). Retinopathy of prematurity: age at onset and the initial site of involvement; a preliminary report. In D. BENEZRA, S. J. RYAN, B. M. GLASER, AND R. P. MURPHY (eds.). *Ocular Circulation and Neovascularisation.* Dordrecht: Martinus Nijhoff/Dr W. Junk, 50, pp. 147–154.

FIELDER, A. R., ROBINSON, J., AND SHAW, D. E. (1990). ROP: Location a clue to its pathogenesis? *Invest. Ophthalmol. Vis. Sci.* 31 (suppl.), 584.

FIELDER, A. R., SHAW, D. E., ROBINSON, J., AND NG, Y. K. (1992a). Natural history of retinopathy of prematurity: a prospective study. *Eye* 6, 233–242.

FIELDER, A. R., ROBINSON, J., SHAW, D. E., NG, Y. K., AND MOSELEY, M. J. (1992b). Light and retinopathy of prematurity: does retinal location offer a clue? *Pediatrics* 89, 648–653.

FINNSTRÖM, O. (1971). Studies on maturity in newborn infants. III. Neurological examination. *Neuropadiatre* 3, 72–96.

FLEDELIUS, H. C. (1981a). Myopia of prematurity-changes during adolescence: a longitudinal study including ultrasound oculometry. *Doc. Ophthalmol. Proc. Ser.* 29, 217–222.

FLEDELIUS, H. C. (1981b). Ophthalmic changes from 10–18 years: a longitudinal study of sequels to low birthweight. II. Visual acuity. *Acta Ophthalmol. (Copenh.)* 59, 64–70.

FLEDELIUS, H. C. (1982a). Inhibited growth and development as permanent features of low birth weight. *Acta Paediatr. Scand.* 71, 645–650.

FLEDELIUS, H. C. (1982b). Ophthalmic changes from 10–18 years: a longitudinal study of sequels to low birthweight. III. Ultrasound oculometry and keratometry of the anterior eye segment. *Acta Ophthalmol. (Copenh.)* 60, 393–402.

FLYNN, J. T., BANCALARI, E., BACHYNSKI, B. N., BUCKLEY, E. B., BAWOL, R., GOLDBERG, R., CASSIDY, J., SCHIFFMAN, J., FEUER, W., GILLINGS, D., SIM, E., AND ROBERTS, J. (1987). Retinopathy of prematurity: diagnosis, severity, and natural history. *Ophthalmology* 94, 620–629.

FOGARTY, T. P., AND REUBEN, R. N. (1969). Light-evoked cortical and retinal responses in premature infants. *Arch. Ophthalmol.* 81, 454–459.

FOREMAN, N., AND FIELDER, A. (1989). Intermodal enhancement of stimulus localisation in infants born prematurely. *Percept. Motor Skills* 69, 43–50.

FOREMAN, N., AND STEVENS, R. (1987). Relationships between the superior colliculus and hippocampus: neural and behavioural considerations. *Behav. Brain Sci.* 10, 101–152.

FOREMAN, N., FIELDER, A., MINSHULL, C., HURRION, E., AND SERGIENKO, E. (submitted). Visual search, perception and visuomotor skill in children born at 27–32 weeks' gestation.

FOREMAN, N., FIELDER, A., PRICE, D., AND BOWLER, V. (1991). Tonic and phasic orientation in fullterm and preterm infants. *J. Exp. Child Psychol.* 51, 407–422.

FRIEDMAN, E., AND KUWABARA, T. (1968). The retinal pigment epithelium. IV. The damaging effects of radiant energy. *Arch. Ophthalmol.* 80, 265–279.

FRIEDMAN, S. L., JACOBS, B. S., AND WERTHMANN, M. W. (1981). Sensory processing in pre- and full-term infants in the neonatal period. In S. L. FRIEDMAN AND M. SIGMAN (eds.). *Preterm Birth and Psychological Development.* Orlando, FL: Academic Press, pp. 159–178.

GABRIEL, M., GRATE, B., AND JONAS, M. (1981). Sleep-wake pattern in preterm infants under two different care schedules during four-day polygraphic recording. *Neuropediatrics* 12, 366–373.

GARDNER, J. M., AND KARMEL, B. Z. (1983). Attention and arousal. In T. FIELD AND A. SOSTEK (eds.). *Infants Born at Risk: Physiological, Perceptual and Cognitive Processes.* Orlando, FL: Grune & Stratton.

GESSELL, A., AND AMATRUDA, C. S. (1945). *The Embryology of Behaviour.* New York: Harper & Row.

GIBSON, N. A., FIELDER, A. R., TROUNCE, J. Q., AND LEVENE, M. I. (1990). Ophthalmic findings in infants of very low birthweight. *Dev. Med. Child Neurol.* 32, 7–13.

GIUNTA, F., AND RATH, J. (1969). Effect of environmental illumination in prevention of hyperbilirubinemia of prematurity. *Pediatrics* 44, 162–167.

GLASS, L., LALA, R. A., JAISWAL, V., AND NIGAM, S. K. (1975). Effect of thermal environment and caloric intake on head growth of low birthweight infants during the late neonatal period. *Arch. Dis. Child.* 50, 571–573.

GLASS, L., SILVERMAN, W. A., AND SINCLAIR, J. C. (1971). Food, temperature, and head growth in neonates. *Lancet* 1, 1186–1187.

GLASS, P., AVERY, G. B., KOLINJAVADI, N., SUBRAMANIAN, S., KEYS, M. P., SOSTEK, A. M., AND FRIENDLY, D. S. (1985). Effect of bright light in the hospital nursery on the incidence of retinopathy of prematurity. *N. Engl. J. Med.* 313, 401–404.

GORDON, R. A., AND DONZIS, P. B. (1985). Refractive development of the human eye. *Arch. Ophthalmol.* 103, 785–789.

GORDON, R. A., AND DONZIS, P. B. (1986). Myopia associated with retinopathy of prematurity. *Ophthalmology* 93, 1593–1598.

GOTTFRIED, A. W., WALLACE-LANDE, B., SHERMAN-BROWN, S., AND HODGMAN, J. E. (1981). Physical and social environment of newborn infants in special care units. *Science* 214, 673–675.

GRAHAM, M. V., AND GRAY, O. P. (1963). Refraction of premature babies' eyes. *BMJ* 1, 1452–1454.

GROENENDAAL, F., van HOF-van DUIN, J., BAERTS, W., AND FETTER, W. P. F. (1989). Effects of perinatal hypoxia on visual development during the first year of (corrected) age. *Early Hum. Dev.* 20, 267–279.

GROSE, J., HARDING, G. F. A., WILTON, A. Y., AND BISSENDEN, J. G. (1989). The maturation of the pattern reversal and flash VEP and flash ERG in pre-term infants. *Clin. Vis. Sci.* 4, 239–246.

HACK, M., MOSTOW, A., AND MIRANDA, S. B. (1976). Development of attention in preterm infants. *Pediatrics* 58, 669–674.

HACK, M., MUSZYNSKI, S. Y., AND MIRANDA, S. B. (1981). State of awakeness during visual fixation in preterm infants. *Pediatrics* 68, 87–92.

HAMER, R. D., DOBSON, V., AND MAYER, M. J. (1984). Absolute thresholds in human infants exposed to continuous illumination. *Invest. Ophthalmol. Vis. Sci.* 25, 381–388.

HARAYAMA, K., AMEMIYA, T., AND NISHIMURA, H. (1981). Development of the eyeball during fetal life. *J. Pediatr. Ophthalmol. Strabismus* 18, 37–40.

HARDING, G. F. A., GROSE, J., WILTON, A. Y., AND BISSENDEN, J. G. (1989a). The pattern reversal VEP in short-gestation infants on taurine or taurine-free diet. *Doc. Ophthalmol.* 73, 103–109.

HARDING, G. F. A., GROSE, J., WILTON, A. Y., AND BISSENDEN, J. G. (1989b). The pattern reversal VEP in short-gestation infants. *Electroencephalogr. Clin. Neurophysiol.* 74, 76–80.

HITTNER, H. M., HIRSCH, N. J., AND RUDOLPH, A. J. (1977).

Assessment of gestational age by examination of the anterior vascular capsule of the lens. *J. Pediatr.* 91, 455–458.

HITTNER, H. M., RHODES, L. M., AND MCPHEARSON, A. R. (1979). Anterior segment abnormalities in cicatricial retinopathy of prematurity. *Ophthalmology* 86, 803–816.

HOLLENBERG, M., AND SPIRA, A. (1973). Human retinal development: ultrastructure of the outer retina. *Am. J. Anat.* 137, 357–386.

HORSTEN, G. P. M., AND WINKELMAN, J. E. (1962). Electrical activity of the retina in relation to histological differentiation in infants born prematurely and at full-term. *Vision Res.* 2, 269–276.

HRBEK, A., KARLBERG, P., AND OLSSON, T. (1973). Development of visual and somatosensory evoked responses in pre-term newborn infants. *Electroencephalogr. Clin. Neurophysiol.* 34, 225–232.

HULL, D. (1988). Thermal control in very immature infants. *Br. Med. Bull.* 44, 971–983.

HUNT, J. V., AND RHODES, L. (1977). Mental development of pre-term infants during the first year. *Child Dev.* 48, 204–210.

ISENBERG, S. J., DANG, Y., AND JOTTERAND, V. (1989). The pupils of term and preterm infants. *Am. J. Ophthalmol.* 108, 75–79.

ISENBERG, S. J., MOLARTE, A., AND VAZQUEZ, M. (1990). The fixed and dilated pupils of premature neonates. *Am. J. Ophthalmol.* 110, 168–171.

JACQUES, S. L., WEAVER, D. R., AND REPPERT, S. M. (1987). Penetration of light into the uterus of pregnant mammals. *Photochem. Photobiol.* 45, 637–641.

JAIN, K. K., BHANDARI, G. K., AND KORANNE, S. P. (1973). Histogenesis of the human eyelids. *East. Arch. Ophthalmol.* 3, 8–15.

KARMEL, B. Z., AND MAISEL, E. B. (1975). A neuronal activity model for infant visual attention. In L. B. COHEN AND P. SALAPATEK (eds.). *Infant Perception: From Sensation to Cognition.* Orlando, FL: Academic Press.

KEITH, C. G., AND KITCHEN, W. H. (1983). Ocular morbidity in infants of very low birthweight. *Br. J. Ophthalmol.* 67, 302–305.

KEITH, C. G., AND KITCHEN, W. H. (1984). Retinopathy of prematurity in extremely low birthweight infants. *Med. J. Aust.* 141, 225–227.

KELLY, S., AND FIELDER, A. (1987). Microcornea associated with retinopathy of prematurity. *Br. J. Ophthalmol.* 71, 201–203.

KIRKNESS, C. M. (1986). Do ophthalmic instruments pose a hazard of light-induced damage to the eye? In J. CRONLY-DILLON, E. S. ROSEN, AND J. MARSHALL (eds.). *Hazards of Light, Myths and Realities, Eye and Skin.* Oxford: Pergamon, pp. 179–186.

KITCHEN, W. H., RYAN, M. M., RICKARDS, A., MCDOUGALL, A. B., BILLSON, F. A., KEITH, E. H., AND NAYLOR, F. D. (1980). A longitudinal study of very low birthweight infants. IV. An overview of performance at eight years of age. *Dev. Med. Child Neurol.* 22, 172–188.

KOOLE, F. D., BAX, P. P., SAMSON, J. F., AND VAN DER LEI, J. (1990). Ocular examination in nine-month-old infants with very low birthweights. *Ophthalmic Paediatr. Genet.* 11, 89–94.

KOPEIKO, L. G., YU, M., KORETSKAYA, D. I., MITKOKH, O., AND CHENTSOVA, B. (1979). Spectral characteristics of eyeball coats. *Vest. Oftalmol.* Jan–Feb 1, 46–49.

KOPP, C. B., SIGMAN, M., PARMELEE, A. H., AND JEFFREY, W. E. (1975). Neurological organization and visual fixation in infants at 40 weeks conceptual age. *Dev. Psychobiol.* 8, 165–170.

KREMERS, J. J. M., AND VAN NORREN, D. (1988). Two classes of photochemical damage in the retina. *Lasers Light Ophthalmol.* 2, 41–52.

KUSHNER, B. (1982). Strabismus and amblyopia associated with regressed retinopathy of prematurity. *Arch. Ophthalmol.* 102, 256–261.

LAMBERT, S. R., HOYT, C. S., JAN, J. E., BARKOVICH, J., AND FLODMARK, O. (1987). Visual recovery from hypoxic cortical blindness during childhood. *Arch. Ophthalmol.* 105, 1371–1377.

LANDRY, R. J., SCHEIDT, P. C., AND HAMMOND, R. W. (1985).

Ambient light and phototherapy conditions of eight neonatal care units: a summary report. *Pediatrics* 75 (suppl.), 434–436.

LANDRY, S. H., AND CHAPIESKI, M. L. (1988). Visual attention during toy exploration in preterm infants: effects of medical risk and maternal interactions. *Infant Behav. Dev.* 11, 187–204.

LANDRY, S. H., LESLIE, N. A., FLETCHER, J. M., AND FRANCIS, D. J. (1985). Visual attention skills of premature infants with and without intraventricular hemorrhage. *Infant Behav. Dev.* 8, 309–321.

LAWS, D., SHAW, D. E., ROBINSON, J., JONES, H. S., NG, Y. K., AND FIELDER, A. R. (1992). Retinopathy of prematurity: a prospective study. Review at six months. *Eye* 6, 477–483.

LAWSON, K. R., TURKEWITZ, G., PLATT, M., AND MCCARTON, C. (1985). Infant state in relation to its environmental context. *Infant Behav. Dev.* 8, 269–281.

LEEHEY, S. C., MOSKOWITZ-COOK, A., BRILL, S., AND HELD, R. (1975). Orientational anisotropy in infant vision. *Science* 190, 900–902.

LERMAN, S. (1985). Ocular phototoxicity. In S. I. DAVIDSON AND F. T. FRAUNFELDER (eds.). *Recent Advances in Ophthalmology.* New York: Churchill Livingstone, pp. 109–136.

LERMAN, S. (1988). Ocular phototoxicity. *N. Engl. J. Med.* 319, 1475–1477.

LEVENTHAL, A. G., AND HIRSCH, H. V. B. (1975). Cortical effect of early selective exposure to diagonal lines. *Science* 190, 902–904.

LINFIELD, P. B., AND DAVIS, J. G. (1984). A study of the change in mean sphere refractive errors obtained from very low birthweight infants. In *First International Congress British College of Ophthalmic Opticians (Optometrists).* London, pp. 197–200.

LUCEY, J. F. (1973). The effects of light on the newly born infant. *J. Perinat. Med.* 1, 147–152.

MACFARLANE, A., COLE, S., JOHNSON, A., AND BOTTING, B. (1988). Epidemiology of birth before 28 weeks gestation. *Br. Med. Bull.* 44, 861–893.

MACLEOD, P., AND STERN, L. (1972). Natural variation in environment illumination in a newborn nursery. *Pediatrics* 50, 131–133.

MANN, N. P., HADDOW, R., STOKES, L., GOODLEY, S., AND RUTTER, N. (1986). Effect of night and day on preterm infants in a newborn nursery: randomised trial. *BMJ* 293, 1265–1267.

MANNING, K. A., FULTON, A. B., HANSEN, R. M., MAYER, D. L., PETERSEN, R. A., AND BARG, D. C. (1982). Preferential looking vision testing: application to evaluation of high-risk, prematurely born infants and children. *J. Pediatr. Ophthalmol. Strabismus* 19, 286–293.

MASI, W. S., AND SCOTT, K. G. (1983). Preterm and full-term infants' visual responses to mothers' and strangers' faces. In T. M. FIELD AND A. SOSTEK (eds.). *Infants Born at Risk: Physiological, Perceptual and Cognitive Processes.* Orlando, FL: Grune & Stratton.

MAURER, D., AND LEWIS, T. L. (1979). A physiological explanation of infants' early visual development. *Can. J. Psychol.* 33, 232–252.

MCCORMICK, A. Q., TREDGER, E. M., DUNN, H. G., AND GRUNAU, R. V. E. (1986). Ophthalmic disorders. In H. G. DUNN (ed.). *Sequelae of Low Birthweight: The Vancouver Study. Clinics in Developmental Medicine,* No. 95/96. Oxford: Blackwell, pp. 127–146.

MCDONALD, M., DOBSON, V., SEBRIS, S. L., BAITCH, L., VARNER, D., AND TELLER, D. Y. (1985). The acuity card procedure: a rapid test of infant acuity. *Invest. Ophthalmol. Vis. Sci.* 26, 1158–1162.

MEISELS, S. J., CROSS, D. R., AND PLUNKETT, J. W. (1987). Use of the Bayley infant behavior record with preterm and full-term infants. *Dev. Psychol.* 23, 475–482.

METS, M. B., PASS, A., SMITH, V. C., AND POKORNY, J. (1990). The electroretinogram in the first year of life in very low birthweight humans with retinopathy of prematurity. *Invest. Ophthalmol. Vis. Sci.* 31 (suppl.), 132.

MINTZ-HITTNER, H. A., MCGEE, J. K., KOGAN, A., MIRANDA, G., AND KRETZER, F. L. (1990). Abnormal foveal avascular zone in very, very low birthweight infants (< 750 grams) with or without severe retinopathy of prematurity. *Invest. Ophthalmol. Vis. Sci.* 31 (suppl.), 117.

MIRANDA, S. B., AND HACK, M. (1979). The predictive value of neonatal visual-perceptual behaviors. In T. M. FIELD, A. M. SOSTEK, S. GOLDBERG, AND H. H. SHUMAN (eds.). *Infants Born at Risk: Behavior and Development.* New York: SP Medical and Scientific Books.

MOHN, G., AND VAN HOF-VAN DUIN, J. (1986). Development of the binocular and monocular visual fields of human infants during the first year of life. *Clin. Vis. Sci.* 1, 51–64.

MOORE, C. L., KAHIL, R., AND WHITMAN, R. (1976). Development of myelination in optic tract of the cat. *J. Comp. Neurol.* 165, 125–136.

MORANTE, A., DUBOWITZ, L. M. S., LEVENE, M. I., AND DUBO-WITZ, V. (1982). The development of visual function in normal and neurologically abnormal preterm and fullterm infants. *Dev. Med. Child Neurol.* 24, 771–784.

MOSELEY, M. J., AND FIELDER, A. R. (1988). Light toxicity and the neonatal eye. *Clin. Vis. Sci.* 3, 75–82.

MOSELEY, M. J., BAYLISS, S. C., AND FIELDER, A. R. (1988a). Light transmission through the human eyelid: in vivo measurement. *Ophthalmic Physiol. Opt.* 8, 229–230.

MOSELEY, M. J., THOMPSON, J. R., LEVENE, M. I., AND FIELDER, A. R. (1988b). Effects of nursery illumination on frequency of eyelid opening and state in preterm neonates. *Early Hum. Dev.* 18, 13–26.

MOWER, G. D., AND CHRISTEN, W. G. (1985). Role of visual experience in activating critical period in cat visual cortex. *J. Neurophysiol.* 53, 572–587.

MOWER, G. D., BERRY, D., BURCHFIEL, J. L., AND DUFFY, F. H. (1981). Comparison of the effects of dark rearing and binocular suture on development and plasticity of cat visual cortex. *Brain Res.* 220, 255–267.

MURDOCH, D. R., AND DARLOW, B. A. (1984). Handling during neonatal intensive care. *Arch. Dis. Child.* 59, 957–961.

MUSHIN, J., DUBOWITZ, L. M. S., AND ARDEN, G. B. (1986). Visual function in the newborn infant: behavioural and electrophysiological studies. *Doc. Ophthalmol. Proc. Ser.* 45, 119–134.

MUTCH, L. M. M. (1986). Epidemiology, perinatal mortality and morbidity. In N. R. C. ROBERTON (ed.). *Textbook of Pediatrics.* Edinburgh: Churchill Livingstone, pp. 3–19.

NG, Y. K., SHAW, D. E., FIELDER, A. R., AND LEVENE, M. I. (1988). Epidemiology of retinopathy of prematurity. *Lancet* 1, 1235–1238.

NISSENKORN, I., YASSUR, Y., MASHKOWSKI, Y., SHERF, I., AND BEN-SIRA, I. (1983). Myopia in premature babies with and without retinopathy of prematurity. *Br. J. Ophthalmol.* 67, 170–173.

NORCIA, A. M., TYLER, C. W., PIECUCH, R., CLYMAN, R., AND GROBSTEIN, J. (1987). Visual acuity development in normal and abnormal preterm human infants. *J. Pediatr. Ophthalmol. Strabismus* 24, 70–74.

OPCS Monitor (1988). London: Office of Population Censuses and Surveys.

PARMELEE, A. H. (1975). Neurophysiological and behavioural organisation of premature infants in the first months of life. *Biol. Psychiatry* 10, 501–512.

PLACZEK, M., MUSHIN, J., AND DUBOWITZ, L. M. S. (1985). Maturation of the visual evoked response and its correlation with visual acuity in preterm infants. *Dev. Med. Child Neurol.* 27, 448–454.

PORAT, R., BRODSKY, N., AND HURT, H. (1988). Effective eye shielding during phototherapy. *Clin. Pediatr.* 28, 199–200.

PURPURA, D. P. (1976). Structure-dysfunction relations in the visual cortex of preterm infants. In M. A. B. BRAZIER AND F. COCEANI (eds.). *Brain Dysfunction in Infantile Febrile Convulsions.* New York: Raven Press, pp. 223–240.

REISNER, S. H., AMIR, J., SHOHAT, M., KRICKLER, R., NISSENKORN, I., AND BEN-SIRA, I. (1985). Retinopathy of prematurity: incidence and treatment. *Arch. Dis. Child.* 60, 698–701.

RICCI, B., FALSINI, B., VALENTINI, P., LACERRA, F., MOLLE, F., AND RUFI, L. (1983). Development of the main electroretinographic components in premature infants during the first weeks of life. *Arch. Soc. Oftalmol. Optom.* 17, 159–165.

ROBB, R. M. (1982). Increase in retinal surface area during infancy and childhood. *J. Pediatr. Ophthalmol. Strabismus* 19, 16–20.

ROBINSON, J. (1990). Light and the Eye of the Preterm Neonate. PhD thesis, University of Birmingham, United Kingdom.

ROBINSON, J., AND FIELDER, A. (1990). Pupillary diameter and reaction to light in preterm neonates. *Arch. Dis. Child.* 65, 35–38.

ROBINSON, J., BAYLISS, S. C., AND FIELDER, A. R. (1991). Transmission of light across the adult and neonatal eyelid in vivo. *Vision Res.* 31, 1837–1840.

ROBINSON, J., MOSELEY, M. J., AND FIELDER, A. R. (1990a). Illuminance of neonatal units. *Arch. Dis. Child.* 65, 675–682.

ROBINSON, J., MOSELEY, M. J., AND FIELDER, A. R. (1990b). Light and the eye of the preterm neonate. *Invest. Ophthalmol. Vis. Sci.* 31 (suppl.), 119.

ROBINSON, J., MOSELEY, M. J., FIELDER, A. R., AND BAYLISS, S. C. (1991). Light transmission measurements and phototherapy eyepatches. *Arch. Dis. Child.* 66, 59–61.

ROBINSON, J., MOSELEY, M. J., THOMPSON, J. R., AND FIELDER, A. R. (1989). Eyelid opening in preterm neonates. *Arch. Dis. Child.* 64, 943–948.

ROBINSON, R. J. (1966). Assessment of gestational age by neurological examination. *Arch. Dis. Child.* 41, 437–447.

ROSE, G. H. (1981a). Animal studies in developmental psychobiology: commentry on method, theory and human implications. In S. L. FRIEDMAN AND M. SIGMAN (eds.). *Preterm Birth and Psychological Development.* Orlando, FL: Academic Press, pp. 73–105.

ROSE, S. A. (1981b). Lags in the cognitive competence of prematurely born infants. In S. L. FRIEDMAN AND M. SIGMAN (eds.). *Preterm Birth and Psychological Development.* Orlando, FL: Academic Press.

ROSE, S. A., FELDMAN, J. F., McCARTON, C. M., AND WOLFSON, J. (1988). Information processing in seven-month-old infants as a function of risk status. *Child Dev.* 59, 589–603.

ROUHER, F., SOLÉ, P., AND ALFIERI, R. (1967). Le prématuré a-t-il une fonction photopique? *Bull. Soc. Ophtalmol. Fr.* 67, 27–31.

SAMSON-DOLLFUS, D. (1968). Dévlepement normal de l'ERG dépuis l'âge foetal de sept mois et demi jusqu'a l'âge de quatre mois après la naissance a terme. *Bull. Soc. Ophtalmol. Fr.* 68, 423–431.

SCHAFFER, D., QUINN, G., AND JOHNSON, L. (1984). Sequelae of arrested mild retinopathy of prematurity. *Arch. Ophthalmol.* 102, 373–376.

SCHAFFER, D. B., JOHNSON, L., QUINN, G. E., WESTON, M., AND BOWEN JR., F. W. (1985). Vitamin E and retinopathy of prematurity: follow up at one year. *Ophthalmology* 92, 1005–1011.

SCHARF, J., ZONIS, S., AND ZELTER, M. (1978). Refraction in premature babies: a prospective study. *J. Pediatr. Ophthalmol. Strabismus* 15, 48–50.

SCHER, M. S., DOBSON, V., CARPENTER, N. A., AND GUTHRIE, R. D. (1989). Visual and neurological outcome of infants with periventricular leukomalacia. *Dev. Med. Child Neurol.* 31, 353–365.

SEARLE, C. M., HORNE, S. M., AND BOURNE, K. M. (1989). Visual acuity development: a study of preterm and full-term infants. *Aus. N.Z. J. Ophthalmol.* 17, 23–26.

SEBRIS, S. L., DOBSON, V., McDONALD, M. A., AND TELLER, D. Y. (1987). Acuity cards for visual assessment of infants and children in clinical settings. *Clin. Vis. Sci.* 2, 45–58.

SEBRIS, S. L., DOBSON, V., AND HARTMANN, E. E. (1984). Assessment and prediction of visual acuity in 3- to 4-year old children born prior to term. *Hum. Neurobiol.* 3, 87–92.

SELLHEYER, K., AND SPITZNAS, M. (1988). Morphology of the developing choroidal vasculature in the human fetus. *Graefes Arch. Clin. Exp. Ophthalmol.* 226, 461–467.

SHAPIRO, A., YANKO, L., NAWRATZKI, I., AND MERIN, S. (1980).

Refractive power of premature children at infancy and early childhood. *Am. J Ophthalmol.* 90, 234–238.

SHEPHERD, P. A., FAGAN, J. F., AND KLEINER, K. A. (1985). Visual pattern detection in preterm neonates. *Infant Behav. Dev.* 8, 47–63.

SIGMAN, M. (1983). Individual differences in infant attention. In T. M. FIELD AND A. SOSTEK (eds.). *Infants Born at Risk: Physiological, Perceptual and Cognitive Processes.* Orlando, FL: Grune & Stratton.

SIGMAN, M., KOPP, C. B., LITTMAN, B., AND PARMELEE, A. H. (1977). Infant visual attentiveness in relation to birth condition. *Dev. Psychol.* 13, 431–437.

SILVERMAN, W. A. (1980). *Retrolental Fibroplasia: A Modern Parable.* Orlando, FL: Grune & Stratton.

SINDEL, B., BAKER, M., MAISELS, M., AND WEINSTEIN, J. (1986). A comparison of the pupillary and cardiovascular effects of various mydriatic agents in preterm infants. *J. Pediatr. Ophthalmol. Strabismus* 23, 273–276.

SLATER, A., MORISON, V., AND SOMERS, M. (1988). Orientation discrimination and cortical function in the human newborn. *Perception* 17, 597–602.

SNIR, M., NISSENKORN, I., SHERF, I., COHEN, S., AND BEN-SIRA, I. (1988). Visual acuity, strabismus and amblyopia in premature babies with and without retinopathy of prematurity. *Ann. Ophthalmol.* 20, 256–258.

SOKOL, S., AND JONES, K. (1979). Implicit time of pattern evoked potentials in infants: an index of maturation of spatial vision. *Vision Res.* 19, 747–755.

SPUNGEN, L. B., KURTZBERG, D., AND VAUGHAN, H. G. (1985). Patterns of looking behaviour in full-term and low birthweight infants at 40 weeks post-conceptual age. *Dev. Behav. Pediatr.* 6, 287–294.

ST-ANNE DARGASSIES, S. (1977). *Neurological Development in the Full-term and Premature Neonate.* Amsterdam: Elsevier.

STANLEY, O. H., FLEMING, P. J., AND MORGAN, M. H. (1989). Abnormal development of visual function following intrauterine growth retardation. *Early Hum. Dev.* 19, 87–101.

STRYKER, M. P., AND SHERK, H. (1975). Modification of cortical orientation selectivity in the cat by restricted visual experience: a reexamination. *Science* 190, 904–906.

SYKES, S. M., ROBINSON, W. G., WAXLER, M., AND KUWABARA, T. (1981). Damage to the monkey retina by broad-spectrum fluorescent light. *Invest. Ophthalmol. Vis. Sci.* 20, 425–434.

TAMURA, E. E., AND HOYT, C. S. (1987). Oculomotor consequences of intraventricular hemorrhages in premature infants. *Arch. Ophthalmol.* 105, 533–535.

TASMAN, W. (1979). Late complications of retrolental fibroplasia. *Ophthalmology* 86, 1724–1740.

TERRY, T. L. (1942). Extreme prematurity and fibroblastic overgrowth of persistent vascular sheath behind each crystalline lens. I. Preliminary report. *Am. J. Ophthalmol.* 35, 203–204.

TRESIDDER, J., FIELDER, A. R., AND NICHOLSON, J. (1990). Delayed visual maturation: ophthalmic and neurodevelopmental aspects. *Dev. Med. Child Neurol.* 32, 872–881.

TREVARTHEN, C. B. (1974). L'action dans l'espace et la perception de l'espace: mechanismes cerebraux de base. In F. BRESSON (ed.). *De l'Espace Corporel a l'Espace Ecologique.* Paris: Presses Universitaires de France.

TSO, M. O. M., FINE, B. S., AND ZIMMERMAN, L. E. (1972). Photic maculopathy produced by the indirect ophthalmoscope. *Am. J. Ophthalmol.* 73, 686–689.

TYLER, C. W., AND NORCIA, A. M. (1986). Plasticity of human acuity development with variations in visual experience. In E. L. KELLER AND D. S. ZEE (eds.). *Adaptive Processes in Visual and Oculomotor Systems.* Asolimar, CA: Pergamon, pp. 95–100.

UAUY, R. D., BIRCH, D. G., BIRCH, E. E., TYSON, J. E., AND HOFFMAN, D. R. (1990). Effect of dietary omega-3 fatty acids on retinal function of very-low-birth-weight neonates. *Pediatr. Res.* 28, 485–492.

VAN DEN BERG, T. J. T. P., DE WAARD, P. W. T., AND IJSPEERT, J. K. (1990). Light transmission through the ocular coats and retinal straylight distribution. *Invest. Ophthalmol. Vis. Sci.* 31 (suppl.), 412.

VAN HOF-VAN DUIN, J., AND MOHN, G. (1984). Vision in the preterm infant. In H. PRECHTL (ed.). *Continuity of Neural Functions from Prenatal to Postnatal Life. Clinics in Developmental Medicine,* No. 94. Philadelphia: Lippincott, pp. 93–114.

VAN HOF-VAN DUIN, J., AND MOHN, G. (1986). The development of visual acuity in normal fullterm and preterm infants. *Vision Res.* 26, 909–916.

VAN HOF-VAN DUIN, J., AND MOHN, G. (1985). The development of visual function in preterm infants. *Ergeb. Exp. Med.* 46, 350–361.

VAN HOF-VAN DUIN, J., FETTER, W. P. F., METTAU, J. W., AND BAERTS, W. (1983). Preferential looking acuity in preterm infants. *Behav. Brain Res.* 10, 47–50.

VASSELLA, F., GIAMBONINI, S., HEITS, B., KAUFMANN, R., KEHRLI, P., AND WALTI, U. (1977). Development of visual discrimination (pattern preferences) in normal infants. *Helv. Paediatr. Acta* 32, 319–329.

WALKER, D., WALKER, A., AND WOOD, C. (1969). Temperature of the human fetus. *J. Obstet. Gynaecol. Br. Commonw.* 76, 503–511.

WEALE, R. A. (1982). *Biography of the Eye: Development, Growth, Age.* London: H. K. Lewis.

WEINDLING, A. M., ROCHEFORT, M. J., CALVERT, S. A., FOK, T-F., AND WILKINSON, A. (1985). Development of cerebral palsy after ultrasonographic detection of periventricular cysts in the newborn. *Dev. Med. Child Neurol.* 27, 800–806.

WHITELAW, A., AND COOKE, R. W. I. (1988). The very immature infant: less than 28 weeks gestation. *Br. Med. Bull.* 44, 821–1151.

WHYTE, H. H., PEARCE, J. M., AND TAYLOR, M. J. (1987). Changes in the VEP in preterm neonates with arousal states, as assessed by EEG monitoring. *Electroencephalogr. Clin. Neurophysiol.* 68, 223–225.

WINKELMAN, J. E., AND HORSTEN, G. P. M. (1962). The ERG of premature and full-term born infants during their first days of life. *Ophthalmologica* 143, 92–101.

WOLKE, D. (1987). Environmental neonatology. *Arch. Dis. Child.* 62, 987–988.

YUODELIS, C., AND HENDRICKSON, A. (1986). A qualitative and quantitative analysis of the human fovea during development. *Vision Res.* 26, 847–855.

ZETTERSTRÖM, B. (1952). The electroretinogram in prematurely children. *Acta Ophthalmol. (Copenh.)* 30, 405–408.

28 | Visual factors in developmental delay and neurological disorders in infants

CREIG S. HOYT AND WILLIAM V. GOOD

When a baby is referred because the parents are worried about its vision, the cause is usually evident on the first examination. At the very least there is usually a strong suspicion about the site of the problem in the visual or neurological system. In some babies, no apparent cause can be found. Their vision just seems worse for their chronological age than it should be, and their estimated or measured visual function is worse than expected. In this group of infants, however, vision improves with time without specific treatment.

This phenomenon has been recognized for many years. Illingworth in 1961 first introduced the term "delayed visual maturation" to describe it. He described two children who had been visually unresponsive as infants but at 6 months of age began to be attentive to visual stimuli. It is noteworthy that one child was considerably late in walking. In all other regards, however, Illingworth's first two patients were not developmentally delayed except in regard to their visual function.

It should be noted that although Illingworth introduced the term, similar cases had probably been described previously under other terms. Beauvieux (1927, 1947) noted anomalous appearance of the optic discs in infants with what was referred to as "temporary visual inattention." With time, the discs appeared to assume a normal adult appearance, and visual function improved as well. Believing this problem to be due to a defect in myelination of the optic nerve, the author coined the terms *pseudoatrophie optique* and *dysgenesie myelinique*. Beauvieux (1947), however, appreciated that the situation could be more complex and can be compounded by neurodevelopmental or ocular anomalies that may influence eventual visual outcome. He considered that there were two distinct categories of affected infants. In the first, delayed visual maturation was an isolated anomaly, with rapid and complete recovery within 4–6 months. In the second, because of associated problems such as strabismus, high refractive errors, or mental retardation, visual improvement was slower and less complete.

Uemera and colleagues in 1981 presented a classification of developmentally delayed visual maturation in infants that included three separate categories. This classification had been prompted by the observation that many infants with apparent visual maturation delay were found to subsequently have other significant neurodevelopmental or visual problems. In their original classification, Uemera et al. suggested that type I should include patients who exhibit visual maturation delay with no other anomalies, type II should include infants with visual maturation delay who are mentally retarded or have a seizure disorder, and type III should include children with a primary visual abnormality and a superimposed visual maturation delay. These authors recognized that the simplistic notion that these infants simply had a temporarily delay in achieving normal visual milestones was often incorrect. It is not tenable to propose that infants with visual maturation delay are simply those whose visual attentiveness developed somewhat later than normal, just as some children walk relatively later than others despite the absence of any significant neurological problems.

Subsequently, several studies have emphasized that children with delayed visual maturation frequently have delays in other spheres of general development. Cole and coworkers (1984) reported that several children with delayed visual maturation were slow in learning to speak. Hoyt and coworkers (1983) noted general delays in the motor development of seven of eight children identified with delayed visual maturation. Lambert and coworkers (1989), in a study of nine children with delayed visual maturation, noted that four of the children were delayed by 3–5 months in achieving other developmental milestones, such as sitting and walking, compared with their unaffected siblings. One additional child was hypotonic and markedly developmentally delayed. They concluded that delayed visual maturation may be only one manifestation of global developmental delay in some children.

Fielder and coauthors (1985) attempted to clarify the problem of the associated neurodevelopmental problems seen in some of these infants. They reported 53 infants with delayed visual maturation. They divided them into three categories, as had Uemura, but they modified his classification slightly. Category I contained children in whom delayed visual maturation appeared as an isolated anomaly, category II those in whom obvious and persistent neurodevelopmental abnormalities were also noted, and category III those who had other ocular abnormalities presumably related to the delayed visual maturation. These authors went on to further subdivide group I. Group IA contained those children with a truly isolated problem, whereas group IB were children who had a history of perinatal medical complications. The authors, however, noted that it could not be entirely ruled out that some infants in group IA had suffered undetected neurological insults that might be responsible for their delayed visual maturation.

It has been our experience that longitudinal studies of our patients who would have been in Fielders' classification type IA have a disarming tendency to subsequently manifest evidence of neurodevelopmental problems that pediatric neurologists might in the past have referred to as "minimal brain damage." Many of these children, in our experience, are found later to have seizures, learning disabilities, attention deficit disorders, and other behavioral problems. This point is important to recall when reviewing the neuroradiological findings in these children.

The clinical profile of infants with visual maturation delay has evolved somewhat since the 1970s. All authorities would agree that these infants present with apparent poor visual function for their adjusted gestational age. There are, however, two striking discrepancies between the early reports of this syndrome [prior to that of Keiner (1951)] and the more recent literature [beginning with that of Illingworth (1961)]. Early reports emphasized that these children had poor or absent pupillary responses, and nystagmus was frequently reported. Subsequent reports have indicated that the pupillary response of these children is normal and that nystagmus is conspicuous by its absence unless there is coexisting anterior visual pathway disease that would ordinarily present with nystagmus (Uemura and Fielder's group III). For example, in the patient who has albinism and apparent visual maturation delay, the nystagmus is attributed to the albinism and not to the visual maturation delay.

ELECTROPHYSIOLOGICAL AND PSYCHOPHYSICAL STUDIES

Multiple diagnostic studies have been performed in these children in an attempt to ascertain the underlying patho-physiology of this phenomenon. It is fair to summarize by saying that these diagnostic studies have been relatively inconclusive and inconsistent. Nevertheless, a careful review of the electrophysical and psychophysical studies that have been performed as well as neuroradiographic investigations in these children are important if we are to understand the underlying abnormalities in these children.

Thus far there is consensus among the authorities who have performed electroretinography (ERG) on these infants that the ERG is entirely normal for the adjusted age of the children studied (Hoyt et al., 1983; Lambert et al., 1989; Tresidder et al., 1990). It should be noted that these ERG studies have been standard flash, nonfocal studies. No attempt to date has been made to study these infants with a focal stimulus or foveal-type ERG. Because of the mass response nature of flash ERG studies, the possibility that foveal maturation delay may play an important role in these children has not been convincingly ruled out. Nevertheless, the clinical behavior of infants with visual maturation delay appear to be too severe to be accounted for as the result of isolated foveal dysfunction.

In contrast to the agreement in the ERG studies, visual evoked potentials (VEPs) of these patients have produced variable and conflicting results. Regrettably, none of the VEP studies has been ideal, and each is marred by technological flaws. Mellor and Fielder (1980) reported that flash VEPs had delayed latencies as well as reduced amplitudes in four children with delayed visual maturation. All of these children were reported to have normal VEPs when tested after achieving normal visual behavior. Harel and coworkers (1983) described three infants with delayed visual maturation who had flash VEPs with delayed latencies that became normal by 1 year of age. Fielder et al. (1985) reported a large series of children with delayed visual maturation in which 78% had flash VEPs with prolonged latencies, abnormal waveforms, and decreased amplitudes. The nonspecific stimulus nature of flash VEPs and the multiple recording artifacts that have been noted in infant studies using these techniques suggest that flash VEP studies are probably not specific enough in their stimulus to be useful for evaluating this group of children (Bodis-Wollner et al., 1977).

Pattern VEPs have also been recorded in these children. Hoyt and coworkers (1983) reported a series of eight children with delayed visual maturation in which seven had pattern onset/offset VEPs with decreased amplitudes and delayed latencies. The authors unfortunately did not report if these patients were age-matched with normal visual attentive children. Lambert and coworkers (1989) reported the VEP results on nine children with the diagnosis of delayed visual maturation. They reported that there were no abnormalities of amplitude, waveform, or latency in these children compared to an age-matched population. This study unfortunately utilized a stimulus of 100-minute check size as the standard stimulus. This test of visual function and acuity is relatively coarse. Normal newborns easily respond to 30-minute checks, and babies 3–4 months of age respond to 7.5- or at least 15.0-minute checks (Moskowitz and Sokol, 1983). It is possible that had a smaller check size been used in this study significant abnormalities similar to those reported by Hoyt et al. would have been found. Indeed, in light of the results of Tresidder and coworkers (1990) using forced choice preferential looking (FPL) techniques, it seems almost certainly to be the case.

Tresidder and coworkers (1990) studied 26 infants with delayed visual maturation using the Acuity Card procedure with a portable apparatus as described by McDonald et al. (1985). Eighteen cards were used, ranging from 0.2 to 30.0 cycles/degree (cpd), at 1.0-octave intervals between 0.2 and 0.8 octave and at 0.5-octave intervals above that. Acuity data were compared with those of Sebris and coworkers (1987), who used the same technique for studying normal infants. All infants, regardless of the group, showed significant reduction in visual acuity on the initial examination with this technique. Visual improvement commenced as follows: Group 1A at 10–18 weeks; group 1B at 7–24 weeks; group 2 at 22–78 weeks; and group 3 at 13–28 weeks. All infants in group 1 (A and B) attained normal vision irrespective of a neurodevelopmental outcome. No patient in group 2 achieved normal acuity, and all in group 3 reached the lower end of the normal acuity range.

PATHOGENESIS OF DELAYED VISUAL MATURATION DURING INFANCY

Initially, when the entity of delayed visual maturation in infancy was considered to be an isolated, temporary phenomenon, attention was directed to the possible visual subsystems that undergo rapid and progressive maturation during the first few months of life that might account for this phenomenon. Indeed, the term "delayed visual maturation" implies that some subsystem shows an exaggerated prolongation of normal maturation to account for the poor visual behavior in these infants. As has already been noted, follow-up studies have indicated that a significant proportion of these children have evidence of neurological damage; and the notion that the pathophysiology of this disorder is an entirely temporary phenomenon cannot be invoked in these particular children (Hoyt et al., 1983; Cole et al., 1984; Fielder et al., 1985). On the other hand, there are children with delayed visual maturation who appear to be otherwise healthy and in whom normal visual function is established without evidence of other abnormalities (Fielder et al., 1985; Lambert et al., 1989; Tresidder et al., 1990). What subsystems within the visual system might be involved in the apparent delay in acquisition of normal visual function in these infants?

Several subsystems within the visual system account for the normal infant's delay in acquiring adult-like visual function. An exaggerated delay in the normal maturation of one or more of these systems might account for the phenomenon of delayed visual maturation in some of these infants.

The retina undergoes considerable structural and functional change postnatally. In 1986 Isenberg described the ophthalmoscopic appearance of the macula in 129 premature infants. He demonstrated that the macula does not appear adult-like until 42 weeks after conception. Histologically, rods and cones are distinguishable 15 weeks prior to birth (Hallingberg and Spira, 1973). At birth the cone inner and outer segments are short and thick, and many rods can still be found in the foveal region. Cones in the central retina do not attain adult-like dimensions until at least 4 months after birth (Abramov et al., 1982). On the other hand, there is considerable evidence from electrophysiological studies (Horstein and Winkelman, 1962; Winkleman and Horstein, 1962; Francois and De Rouk, 1964) and psychophysiological studies (Lewis et al., 1978; Lewis and Maurer, 1980) to suggest that central cones are functionally competent if not fully mature at birth. A longer than normal delay in foveal development might play a role in the apparently blind infants reported with visual maturation delay, as a normal flash ERG that is not focal does not rule out selective foveal underdevelopment. On the other hand, these infants present with what appears to be a far more extensive visual handicap than could be accounted for on the basis of foveal dysfunction alone.

Although it was early stated that the anterior visual pathway is completely myelinated within the first few months of life (Sattler, 1915; Cravioto, 1965), more recent studies contradict this view (Magoon and Robb, 1981). Magoon and Robb, in an autopsy study of myelination in human infants and young children, demonstrated that fibers in the optic nerve near the globe are beginning to become myelinated at birth, but the amount of myelin surrounding individual nerves increases dramatically during the ensuing months and may continue to increase until the age of 2 years. Using magnetic resonance imaging (MRI) studies, Barkovich and coworkers (1988) demonstrated that on T1-weighted images high signal intensity was present in the optic nerves, optic tracts, and optic radiations during the first month of life. This high signal intensity is thought to be due to progressive myelination (Holland et al., 1986; Lee et al., 1986; McArdle et al., 1987). It is noteworthy that Magoon and Robb's report was primarily a study of myelination of the optic nerve and chiasm and does not address the important question of myelination of the visual cortex and important subcortical structures involved in visual processing. This issue is addressed later in the chapter. There can be no question that this extended period of myelination of the anterior visual pathway plays some role in the normal maturation of visual function in the normal, healthy infant. However, Sokol (1979) has demonstrated with VEPs that by 3–5 months of age the latency of the major positive waveform to pattern stimulation with 60-minute checks reaches adult levels. This finding suggests that the functionally significant period of myelination of the anterior visual pathway is probably attained by this time. Moreover, although there is controversy among the VEP studies of infants with delayed visual maturation, a significant delay in the latency of the VEP has not been a principal feature of any of the studies that utilized check stimuli (Hoyt et al., 1983; Lambert et al., 1989). This finding again suggests that an abnormal delay in myelination of the anterior visual pathway is probably not a significant mechanism in the problem of delay of visual maturation during infancy.

Many authorities have directed their attention to the visual cortex to try to understand the problem of delayed visual maturation (Hoyt et al., 1983; Fielder et al., 1985; Lambert et al., 1989). Cortical neuronal dendritic growth and synaptic formation begin at 25 weeks' gestational age, are active around the time of birth, and continue during the first 2 years (Mellor and Fielder, 1980). There are conflicting reports of the proportion of visual cortical cells in experimental animals that have normal functional properties at birth. The presence of cells with adult types of function have been found in neonatal kittens (Hubel and Wiesel, 1963; Sherk and Stryker, 1976) and monkeys (Wiesel and Hubel, 1974). In human infants the maturity of the VEP has been correlated with the degree of dendrite formation, as shown by postmortem Golgi preparations from preterm infants of 25–33 weeks gestational age (Purpura, 1976). This study should be interpreted with some caution, however, as the origin of the VEP is still in some question. Moreover, the fact that a VEP can be generated in patients with little or no visual cortex seen on neuroradiographic studies calls into question whether the VEP should be used to correlate primary visual cortex neuronal activity (Bodis-Wollner et al., 1977; Spellman et al., 1977; Mohn and van Hof-van Duin, 1983).

Nevertheless, experimental studies of the role of excitatory amino acids in establishing the synaptic plasticity in the visual cortex provide additional suggestions for how visual cortex activity might be delayed without permanent damaging effects (Tsumoto et al., 1987). N-Methyl-D-aspartate receptors operate in the visual cortex of young kittens, so weak excitatory inputs to cortical neurons may be potentiated through immature non-N-methyl-D-aspartate receptors. It has been argued that these same receptors induce calcium entry into immature cortical neurons, thereby triggering the processes that underlie synaptic plasticity in the visual cortex (Kleinschmidt et al., 1987; Tsumoto et al., 1987). Could a delay in this process be responsible for the visual maturation delay seen in human infants?

Countering this proposal, Lambert and coworkers (1989) cited their normal VEP studies when arguing that a primary visual cortex site is unlikely to be the cause of visual maturation delay during infancy. They argued that delayed visual maturation in infants is more likely to occur secondary to an immaturity of the visual association areas that mediate visual attention. It should be recalled, however, that the check size used in their particular VEP study was relatively large, and this conclusion therefore may not be appropriate. Moreover, the FPL data of Tresidder et al. (1990) directly challenge this conclusion.

Tresidder and coworkers (1990) provided an alternative provocative thesis. They suggested that for the first few months of life vision may be subserved by the predominantly subcortical extrageniculostriate system (colliculus-pulvinar-parietal) concerned with detection, location, and orientation responses. After this time, the geniculostriate visual system (fovea, optic tracts, radiations, and occipital cortex) becomes functional. These authors cited the work of Dubowitz et al. (1986), who reported that lesions near the thalamus are more likely to affect visual behavior of neonates than those of the visual cortex. Dubowitz's contention is not supported by studies of visual loss in term infants with hypoxic-ischemic encephalopathy (Lambert et al., 1989) in whom visual responsiveness is often completely absent and a site of neurological insult is primarily cortical without brainstem involvement (Gillis, 1985).[1] Moreover, the precise role for the extrageniculostriate system in humans remains highly controversial (Campion et al., 1983). Nevertheless, Tresidder and coworkers suggested that delayed visual maturation during infancy is primarily due to a defect in the extrageniculostriate system. Their suggestion is that when the normal dominance of the geniculostriate system emerges after a few months the affected infants show their characteristic rapid visual improvement. This thesis is considered further when examining neuroradiological data in the following section.

NEURORADIOLOGICAL CONSIDERATIONS

It is obvious that clinical and electrophysiological studies have been unsuccessful in documenting the site or sites of alterations that account for delayed visual maturation during infancy. Advancements in the techniques of neuroimaging in infants have prompted us to reexamine the question of the origin of this phenomenon. In particular, the availability of high quality MRI scans in contrast to the previous computed tomography (CT) scans has provided us with initial evidence that imaging studies in these children may be important and revealing.

Normal Maturation Studies

Longitudinal MRI studies of changes in normal postnatal brain development have been completed (Barkovich et al., 1988) and correlate well with the myelination sequences determined by autopsy studies (Brody et al., 1987). The brain matures in an organized, predetermined pattern that correlates with the functions the newborn or infant performs at various stages of development. The myelination of white matter is an important component of brain maturation because it facilitates transmission of neural impulses through the central nervous system (CNS). Myelination patterns have therefore been considered markers for functional development.

We thought it would be interesting to examine the sequence of myelination in the geniculostriate system and contrast it to the extrageniculostriate system in normal infants of various ages. Our concern was to see if we could support or refute Tresidder and coworkers' thesis that the extrageniculostriate system is primarily responsible for visual function during the first months of life.

Brain maturation occurs at different rates and at different times on T1-weighted images than on the T2-weighted images. On short TR/TE images the appearance of the newborn brain is similar to that of long TR/TE images in adults. Thus white matter is of lower signal intensity than gray matter. With maturation the intensity of white matter increases relative to that of gray matter.

The following is a brief summary of the normal myelination maturation sequence during infancy as documented by Holland et al. (1986), Masmura (1987), and Barkovich et al. (1988): In the supratentorial region, the decussation of the superior cerebellar peduncles, the ventrolateral region of the thalamus, and the posterior limb of the internal capsule exhibit high signal intensity at birth. The development of high signal intensity proceeds rostrally from the pons along the corticospinal tracts into the cerebral peduncles, posterior limb of the internal capsule, and central portion of the centrum semiovale. The white matter of the pre- and postcentral gyri are of high signal intensity by about 1 month of age. The change to high signal intensity in the motor tracts is essentially complete by 3 months of age. In infants younger than 1 month, high signal intensity is present in the optic nerve, optic tracts, and optic ra-

diations. By 3 months the occipital white matter surrounding the calcarine fissure is of high signal intensity. The posterior limb of the internal capsule is of high signal intensity at birth. High signal intensity does not develop in the anterior limb until 2–3 months of age. The splenium of the corpus callosum shows high signal intensity in all infants by 4 months. Maturation of the subcortical white matter other than the visual and motor regions does not begin until 3 months. The deep white matter matures in a dorsal-to-rostral direction, with the deep occipital white matter maturing first and the frontal white matter last.

Similar longitudinal studies using T2-weighted images document the same stereotypical maturational changes (Barkovich et al., 1988). However, the overall appearance of the newborn brain on long TR/TE images is similar to that of the adult short TR/TE image in that white matter has a higher signal intensity than gray matter. Maturation sequences are seen as the reduction in the signal intensity of white matter relative to gray matter utilizing T2-weighted images. Barkovich's studies (1988, 1990) suggest that during the first 6 months of life T1-weighted images are most useful for assessing normal brain maturation, whereas after 6 months of age T2-weighted images are more useful.

If we now specifically examine those parts of the brain important to the extrageniculostriate system and those of the geniculostriate system, we can make some interesting observations. At birth the optic nerve, optic tracts, and radiations show ongoing myelination. However, the dorsal brainstem (in particular the area of the superior colliculus) and the thalamus, but not the pulvinar, also exhibit rapid myelination. (These areas are important in the extrageniculostriate system.) It is our belief that, after reviewing the MRI maturational studies published to date and those ongoing studies of our colleague, James Barkovich, no clear case can be made to either support or refute Tresidder's thesis regarding the importance of the extrageniculostriate system during early infancy.

Developmental Delay Studies

Dietrich and coworkers (1988) have performed similar maturational studies. They divided the appearance of the brain on T2-weighted spin-echo (SE) images into three patterns: (1) infantile, birth to 6 months of age; (2) isointense, 8–12 months; and (3) early adult, 10–12 months and onward. The infantile pattern is that of white matter being hyperintense relative to gray matter in the cerebral hemisphere, whereas the adult pattern shows hypointense white matter. These authors thought that isointense and early adult patterns are delayed in patients demonstrating neurological developmental delays (not visual). Barkovich (1990) reviewed 80 patients with moderate to severe developmental delays and suggested that MR imaging was useful for documenting delayed myelination in some of these patients. Harbord and coworkers (1990) investigated 30 developmentally delayed children with MRI scans. The results were divided into four categories based on the appearance of the white matter: (1) normal myelination; (2) global delayed myelination; (3) topographical distribution of myelin appropriate for age but white matter signal intensity more appropriate to a younger patient; and (4) patchy focal abnormalities. Of the 30 patients examined, 9 had delayed topographical distribution of myelination. One had signal intensity suggesting immaturity of the white matter, and one had patchy gray and white matter abnormalities. It seems clear that MRI studies can provide useful information on the myelination status of children with developmental delays, even when CT scans have been normal.

We thought that because there were good normative data for MRI maturational studies as well as evidence suggesting that delay in myelination in the studies that examined developmentally delayed infants (nonvisual studies), MRI studies might be useful for ascertaining the underlying pathophysiology of delayed visual maturation during infancy. To date, therefore, 14 patients with delayed visual maturation and no other visual or neurological problems have been studied (category 1A, Uemura and Fielder). We have been surprised and disappointed to find that no specific pattern of myelination abnormality on MRI studies could be identified in our children with visual maturation delay. However, three infants did show abnormal prolongation of the early infantile myelin pattern described by Dietrich et al. (1988). In the other 11 children, however, no such delayed pattern was identified. It was thought that in one patient the superior colliculus was poorly myelinated for age. Follow-up studies of all these patients are under way.

Of somewhat more surprise to us was the discovery that five of our patients with visual maturation delay revealed structural anomalies of various portions of the visual and motor areas. They included two patients with evidence of polymicrogyria, one with agyria-pachygyra, and two with mild forms of corpus callosum dysgenesis. Except for the one case of polymicrogyria involving the primary visual cortex (and in whom it could be shown later that the patient had an obvious congenital hemianopsia), the other four patients were considered to be neurologically normal by our pediatric neurological consultants. Thus it appears that a significant number of patients with presumed visual maturation delay without obvious clinical neurological deficits may in fact have nonspecific underlying structural anomalies of the CNS that apparently account for the initial clinical presentation. These patients should therefore be included in category 1B, rather than 1A. This point was emphasized in the clinical follow-up studies of Tresidder and coworkers (1990).

DISCUSSION AND CONCLUSIONS

At the present time, the clinical profile and pathophysiology of visual maturation delay during infancy require clarification. Should the term "maturational delay" be applied only to those children who appear to be entirely normal except for their apparent poor visual function for their adjusted gestational age? Or should we include under this heading children in whom known neurological and visual handicaps have been identified? As clinicians, we have all had the experience of examining patients with albinism during the first few months of life who appear to have little or no useful visual function. Parents of these children are understandably dismayed by the prospect of raising a blind child. Nevertheless, one reexamines these children at 2–3 years of age and commonly finds visual acuity of 20/80–20/100. In similar fashion, it is not unusual to examine children with a seizure disorder in whom little in the way of functional visual behavior can be identified during the first few months of life. If the seizure disorder is controlled, these children often show remarkable improvement in their apparent visual behavior. Are the same phenomena responsible for the apparent improvement of visual function in these children as those who were initially identified as otherwise entirely normal but simply delayed in their visual maturation?

Fundamental to the above clinical question is our continuing inability to identify a single underlying mechanism to explain the apparent delay in visual maturation in these children. The initial notion put forth by Illingworth (1961), when he first coined this term, is that these infants simply exhibit abnormal prolongation of normal maturation of visual function. There is reason to call into question this simplistic thesis. Indeed, if MRI studies similar to ours fail to identify a maturational delay pattern of myelination in the CNS and, in turn, frequently identify structural anomalies of the CNS, as we have, many of these children might be better included in the old terminology of "minimally neurologically damaged children," rather than "maturationally delayed." This point is, of course, corroborated by the longitudinal studies of children with the diagnosis of visual maturation delay in whom a high percentage are later found to have mild neurological and behavioral problems.

We suggest that a longitudinal study of infants considered to have maturational delay of vision is needed. Ideally, this study would include not only a clinical evaluation of these patients, but: (1) VEP studies using an appropriate small check size for the patient's age in an effort to examine latency and amplitude abnormalities; and (2) MRI studies at the time of diagnosis and at the time of apparent return of appropriate visual functions. Both T1- and T2-weighted images are required. Careful comparison of these studies with age-adjusted normal infants must then be carried out. Attention should be directed to examining the structures subserving both the geniculostriate and extrageniculostriate systems; (3) Long-term follow-up studies of these children is needed, including not only repeated ophthalmological examination but neurological and psychometric testing as well. It is our belief that the term "visual maturation delay" is often inappropriate and misleading. It fails to alert the clinician to the possibility that longitudinal studies can identify significant neurological and developmental problems in many of these patients. Moreover, the implied mechanism of delay in maturation of visual systems has not yet been documented, either with electrophysiological or neuroimaging studies. Until such studies are complete, the term "visual maturation delay" should be used with caution.

REFERENCES

ABRAMOV, I., GORDON, J., AND HENDRICKSON, A. (1982). The retina of the newborn human infant. *Science* 217, 265–267.

BARKOVICH, J. A. (1990). *Pediatric Neuroimaging*. New York: Raven Press, pp. 1–34.

BARKOVICH, J. A., KJOS, B. O., JACKSON, D. E., AND NORMAN, D. (1988). Normal maturation of the neonatal and infant brain: MR imaging at 1.5 T. *Radiology* 166, 173–1980.

BEAUVIEUX, J. (1927). La pseudo-atrophie optique des nouveau-nes. *Annal. Oculist.* 163, 881–921.

BEAUVIEUX, M. (1947). La cecite apparente chez le nouveau-ne la pseudo-atrophie grise du nerf optique. *Arch. Ophtalmol. (Paris)* 7, 241–249.

BODIS-WOLLNER, I., ATKIN, E., AND RAAB, E. (1977). Visual association cortex and vision in man: pattern evoked occipital potentials in a blind boy. *Science* 198, 629–631.

BRODY, B. A., KINNEY, H. C., KLOMAN, A. S., AND GILLES, F. H. (1987). Sequence of central nervous system myelination in human infancy. I. An autopsy study of myelination. *J. Neuropathol.* 46, 283–301.

CAMPION, J., LATTO, R., AND SMITH, Y. N. (1983). Is blind sight an effect of scattered light, spared cortex, and near-threshold vision? *Behav. Brain Sci.* 6, 428–461.

COLE, G. F., HUNGERFORD, J., AND JONES, R. B. (1984). Delayed visual maturation. *Arch. Dis. Child.* 59, 107–110.

CRAVIOTO, H. (1965). Electron microscopic studies of the developing human nervous system. II. The optic nerves. *J. Neuropathol. Exp. Neurol.* 24, 166–167.

DIETRICH, R. B., BRADLEY, W. G., AND ZAGAROZA, E. J. (1988). MR evaluation of early myelinization patterns in normal and developmentally delayed infants. *Am. J. Neuroradiol.* 9, 69–76.

DUBOWITZ, L., MUSHIN, I., DEVREIS, T., AND ARDEN, G. B. (1986). Visual function in the newborn infant: is it cortically mediated? *Lancet* 1, 1139–1141.

FIELDER, A. R., RUSSELL-EGGITT, I. R., DODD, K. L., AND MELLOR,

D. H. (1988). Delayed visual maturation. *Transactions of the Ophthalmological Societies of UK* 104(6), 653–661.

FRANCOIS, J., AND DE ROUCK, A. (1964). The electroretinogram in young children: single stimulus, twin flashes, and intermittent stimulation. *Doc. Ophthalmol.* 18, 330–343.

GILLIS, F. H. (1985). Neuropathological indicators of abnormal development. In I. M. FREEMAN (ed.). *Prenatal and Perinatal Factors Associated with Brain Disorders*. NIH Publ. No. 85. Washington, DC: Government Printing Office, p. 1149.

HALLINGBERG, M. J., AND SPIRA, A. W. (1973). Human retinal development: ultrastructure of the outer retina. *Am. J. Anat.* 137, 357–377.

HARBORD, M. G., FINN, I. P., HALL-CRAOGS, M. A., ROBB, S. A., KENDALL, B. E., AND BOYD, S. G. (1990). Myelination patterns on magnetic resonance of children with developmental delay. *Dev. Med. Child Neurol.* 32, 295–303.

HAREL, S., HOLTZMAN, M., AND FEINSOD, M. (1983). Delayed visual maturation. *Arch. Dis. Child.* 58, 298–299.

HOLLAND, B. A., HAAS, D. K., AND NORMAN, D. (1986). MRI of normal brain maturation. *Am. J. Neuroradiol.* 7, 201–208.

HORSTEIN, G. P. N., AND WINKLEMAN, J. E. (1962). Electrical activity of the retina in relation to the histologic differentiation in infants born prematurely and at full term. *Vision Res.* 2, 69–76.

HOYT, C. S., JASTRZEBSKI, G., AND MARG, E. (1983). Delayed visual maturation. *Br. J. Ophthalmol.* 67, 127–130.

HUBEL, D. H., AND WIESEL, T. N. (1963). Receptive fields of cells in striate cortex of very young, visually inexperienced kittens. *J. Neurophysiol.* 26, 994–1008.

ILLINGWORTH, R. S. (1961). Delayed visual maturation. *Arch. Dis. Child.* 36, 497–409.

ISENBERG, S. I. (1986). Macular development in the premature infant. *Am. J. Ophthalmol.* 101, 74–77.

KEINER, G. B. J. (1951). *New Viewpoints on the Origin of Squint*. The Hague: Martinus Nijhoff.

KLEINSCHMIDT, A., BEAR, M. F., AND SINGER, W. (1987). Blockade of "NMDA" receptors disrupts experience—dependent plasticity of kitten striate cortex. *Science* 238, 355–358.

LAMBERT, S. R., KRISS, A., AND TAYLOR, D. (1989). Delayed visual maturation. *Ophthalmology* 96, 524–529.

LEE, B. C., LIPPER, E., NASS, R., AND EHRICH, M. E. (1986). MRI of the central nervous system in neonates and young children. *Am. J. Neuroradiol.* 7, 605–616.

LEWIS, T. L., AND MAURER, D. (1980). Central vision in the newborn. *J. Exp. Child Psychol.* 29, 475–480.

LEWIS, T. L., MAURER, D., AND KAY, D. (1978). Newborn's central vision: whole or hole? *J. Exp. Child Psychol.* 26, 193–203.

MAGOON, E. H., AND ROBB, R. N. (1981). Development of myelin in the human optic nerve and tract. *Arch. Ophthalmol.* 99, 655–659.

MASUMURA, M. (1987). Proton relaxation time of immature brain. *Child. Nerv. Syst.* 3, 6–11.

McARDLE, C. B., RICHARDSON, C. J., AND NICHOLAS, D. A. (1987). Developmental features of the neonatal brain: MRI imaging; gray-white matter differentiation and myelination. *Radiology* 162, 223–229.

McDONALD, M. A., DOBSON, V., SEBRIS, S. L., BAITCH, L., VARNER, D., AND TELLER, D. Y. (1985). The Acuity Card procedure: a rapid test of visual acuity. *Invest. Ophthalmol. Vis. Sci.* 26, 1158–1162.

MELLOR, D. H., AND FIELDER, A. R. (1980). Dissociated visual development electrodiagnostic studies in infants who are slow to see. *Dev. Med. Child Neurol.* 22, 327–335.

MOHN, G., AND VAN HOF-VAN DUIN, J. (1983). Behavioral and electrophysiological measures of visual function in children with neurologic disorders. *Behav. Brain Res.* 10, 177–188.

MOSKOWITZ, A., AND SOKOL, S. (1983). Developmental changes

in the human visual system as reflected by the latency of the pattern reversal VEP. *Electroencephalogr. Clin. Neurophysiol.* 56, 1–15.

PURPURA, D. P. (1976). Structure dysfunction relations in the visual cortex of preterm infants. In N. A. B. BRAIZIER AND F. COCEANI (eds.). *Brain Dysfunction in Infantile Febrile Convulsions.* New York: Raven Press, pp. 223–230.

ROLAND, E. H., HILL, A., NORMAN, M. G., AND FLODMACK, O. (1988). Selective brainstem injury in an asphyxiated newborn. *Ann. Neurol.* 23, 89–92.

SATTLER, C. H. (1915). Uber die Marcheiden-entwickoung in Tractus opticus. *Graefes Arch. Klin. Ophthalmol.* 90, 271–298.

SEBRIS, S. L., DOBSON, V., MCDONALD, M. A., AND TELLER, D. Y. (1987). Acuity cards for visual assessment of infants and children in clinical settings. *Clin. Vis. Sci.* 2, 45–58.

SHERK, H., AND STRYKER, M. P. (1976). Quantitative studies of cortical orientation selectivity in visually inexperienced kittens. *J. Neurophysiol.* 39, 63–74.

SOKOL, S. (1978). Measurement of infant visual acuity from pattern reversal evoked potentials. *Vision Res.* 18, 33–39.

SPEHLMAN, R., GROSS, R. A., HO SU (1977). Visual evoked potentials and post-mortem findings in a case of cortical blindness. *Ann. Neurol.* 2, 531–534.

TRESIDDER, J., FIELDER, A. R., AND NICHOLSON, J. (1990). Delayed visual maturation: ophthalmic and neurodevelopmental aspects. *Dev. Med. Child Neurol.* 32, 872–881.

TSUMOTO, T., HAGIHARA, K., SATO, H., AND HATA, Y. (1987). NMDA receptors in the visual cortex of young kittens are more effective than those of adult cats. *Nature* 327, 513–514.

UEMERA, Y., AGUCCI, Y., AND KATSUMI, O. (1981). Visual developmental delay. *Ophthalmic Paediatr. Genet.* 1, 4–11.

WIESEL, T. N., AND HUBEL, D. H. (1974). Ordered arrangement of orientation columns in monkeys lacking visual experience. *J. Comp. Neurol.* 158, 307–318.

WILSON, E. R., MIRRA, S. S., AND SCHWARTZ, I. F. (1982). Congenital diencephalic and brainstem damage: neuropathologic study of three cases. *Acta Neuropathol. (Berl.)* 57, 70–74.

WINKLEMAN, J. E., AND HORSTEIN, G. P. N. (1962). The ERG of premature and full term grown infants during the first days of life. *Ophthalmologica* 143, 92–101.

VII. What Next in Infant Research?
Introduction*

KURT SIMONS

While the nature/nurture question is an old one, what might be considered the "golden age" of extensive empiric study of early visual development began in the 1960's, due in part to a zeitgeist-like confluence of three historical events: Hubel and Wiesel brought attention to developmental neurophysiology to an extent that had not previously been the case; Fantz demonstrated the preferential looking paradigm on which much of our current understanding of infant vision is based; and pediatric ophthalmology first emerged as a well-defined sub-specialty, bringing clinical attention to children's vision problems to a new level of sophistication. The subsequent decades have seen the accumulation of a large body of data, much of it summarized in the preceding chapters. These findings have gone a long way toward characterizing basic milestones in early visual development, in terms of both structural and functional status of a given modality at a given age. This work is not yet finished, certainly. For instance, much of our understanding of early visual acuity capability has been based on studies using redundant stimuli such as gratings, which may overestimate performance, especially in amblyopia, relative to linear Snellen acuity (Friendly et al. 1985, Mayer 1986, Simons 1983) or preferred eye fixation pattern (Birch et al. 1990, Wilcox & Sokol 1980) measures. Nonetheless, many of the broad quantitative structural and functional outlines of early vision are at this point at least sketched in. What then are some of the primary challenges confronting the upcoming "second generation" of studies of early visual development?

The formidable methodological obstacles to obtaining the basic "first generation" data, from the neurophysiologic to psychophysical visual levels, of necessity restricted many past investigations to, in effect, univariate measurement of maturational change of single functional components, whether a neuromodulator or nasal visual field size. It seems clear that one hallmark of the next generation of studies will be increasing attempts to study whole clusters of interacting variables simultaneously, both in human and primate infants. Familiar examples are the interaction between accommodation, vergence, central stereopsis and binocular fusion (Chapter 14) or between visual field configuration and fixational eye movements (Chapter 7). Less familiar, perhaps, are the opportunities being opened up by such developments as new imaging-based non-invasive windows on "real-time" brain function (Chapter 27, Demer et al. 1985) and the hardware and software computational means now available to evaluate output from multi-electrode arrays at the single-cell or noninvasive evoked potential level.

Interpretation of the results of such multivariate studies, it seems clear, will require more extensive use of quantitative modeling than has been the case to date, though the groundwork is already being laid (e.g., see Chapters 6, 9, 15, 23, 24, 29, 32). As Hood et al. and Wilson point out (Chapters 29 and 32), however, there remains a great deal to be done in the derivation of models of adult vision, which must precede adequate developmental variations.

In the drive to develop more comprehensive multivariate, model-based characterizations, it seems worth noting, there is a major intellectual resource that remains largely untapped by many laboratory researchers. That resource is the body of knowledge that might be termed clinical wisdom. It has long been conventional thinking by basic scientists to largely dismiss clinical reports as "anecdotal." Yet, ironically, in terms of multivariate thinking, the clinician is in some senses ahead of the basic scientist. Differential diagnosis requires consideration of many factors by the clinician, including the effects of a diversity of non-visual physiologic influences that are typically ignored by the focused research specialist. Furthermore, the clinician becomes intimately familiar in a multivariate way with the human "model" itself, through observation of how it

* This introduction incorporates ideas contributed by several individuals, whom the author thanks: Richard Aslin, Martin Banks, Eileen Birch, Alistair Fielder and Anne Fulton.

513

changes in the many variations of disease and dysfunction. This stands in contrast, sometimes dramatic, to such basic science standards as the relatively limited measurements made on laboratory animal models. The fact that the clinician may not always be able to provide a quantifiable statement of what he or she knows should not be allowed to distract attention from the great conceptual reach of that clinical "wisdom." More extensive efforts by basic scientists to tap into this heuristic clinical gold mine thus seem a theme worth pursuing in the "second generation" of visual development studies.

The advent of wider use of the multivariate/model approach will require in turn a rethinking of the measurements used to derive visual functional information. The idea of making a "judicious" (Chapter 30) choice of stimuli or deriving specialized "designer" (Chapter 10) stimuli will need to be expanded to take into account interactive aspects of the several modalities being stimulated. Thus, for instance, the traditional threshold measurement used for univariate studies may need to be replaced with a concept more akin to the aerospace concept of a performance "envelope" that expresses performance limits in terms of an interacting set of variables, which may individually be above or below their traditionally defined thresholds. Utility of the "envelope" approach has already been demonstrated in the ocular phototoxicity context (Chapter 25), for instance, and would seem equally applicable to the Donders' hypothesis (von Noorden 1990) of esotropia origin arising from hyperopia-induced excessive convergence (i.e. from accommodative demands outside the "envelope").

A "second generation" rethinking will also need to break new conceptual ground, looking beyond simply performance milestones and more closely considering the "why" and "how" of developing function. For instance, it has been traditional to assume that early visual function is a linearly or non-linearly decremented version of adult function, limited in resolution or sensitivity but qualitatively similar to adult vision. There are at least indications, however, that early visual experience may in fact be qualitatively different from adult vision, in keeping with what Tyler has characterized as a "larval" stage of vision (Chapter 16). Thus, there is evidence of a non-adult-like nonselective binocular combination of visual inputs from the two eyes early in life (Chapters 12 and 15), the infant exhibits refractive "errors" (i.e. they may in fact serve a deliberate developmental purpose) that disappear in the first year or so of life (Chapter 1) and there is reason to think the extrageniculostriate system may be more dominant in infant than in adult vision (Chapters 23, 26 and 28). If there is, then, a qualitative change involving these components in early visual development, what is the adaptive reason?

Finally, contemporary concerns about pediatric health care access, delivery and cost-effectiveness have given a new weight to the implications of visual development findings, such as with regard to the rationale for early vision screening (Fulton 1992, Lichter 1992). It seems clear that "second generation" thinking about such development will need to attempt some better formulations than currently available of the social and functional implications of visual deficit, and particularly prediction of the long-term effects of early deficits. The challenge of deriving an adequate formulation is compounded by the fact that it has not yet been satisfactorily achieved even for adults (Simons 1988). Here the question of what variables, or models, are chosen, and how they are interpreted, becomes particularly critical. Thus, for instance, a conventional measure of visual function, reading, or school performance based on reading, does not appear to be impaired by the presence of amblyopia when intelligence is controlled for (Helveston et al. 1985, Stewart-Brown et al. 1985). But suppose the amblyope is in a situation, such as manipulating a tool or avoiding falling or flying objects, where reduced depth localization performance "envelope" limitations come into play. A Scandinavian study found amblyopes more than 15 times as likely as the general population to lose vision in the healthy eye, due in more than half the cases to work-related trauma (Tommila & Tarkkanen 1981). (Public health statistics in the US on post-amblyopia blindness are unavailable since, under the Standard Classification of Causes of Blindness protocol, used by virtually all data collection agencies, individuals with blindness of different origin in each eye are classified on the basis of the blindness etiology of the most recently blind eye (Hillis et al. 1983)). And how can the psychological and social cost of the abnormal eye contact of uncorrected strabismus (Romano 1987) be adequately characterized in functional terms?

The four chapters in this section explore in some detail three aspects of "second generation" thinking about visual development. One (Chapter 31) reviews some important questions that are not new but remain unresolved, such as whether developmental status should be classified on the basis of best or most typical performance, and whether that performance should be compared to that of the traditional trained and motivated adult subject, or to that of uninstructed naive subjects. Another chapter (30), reviews the potential for application of sophisticated signal analysis techniques to evoked potential measurement of visual function, and the remaining two chapters (29, 32) are paradigmatic exercises in the derivation of models, complementing the models mentioned or derived in previous sections.

REFERENCES

BIRCH, E. E., STAGER, D. R., BERRY, P., AND EVERETT, M. E. (1990). Prospective assessment of acuity and stereopsis in amblyopic infantile esotropes following early surgery. *Invest. Ophthalmol. Vis. Sci.* 31, 758–765.

DEMER, J. L., VON NOORDEN, G. K., VOLKOW, N. D., AND GOULD, K. L. (1988). Imging of cerebral blood flow and metabolism in amblyopia by positron emission tomography. *Am. J. Ophthalmol.* 105, 337–347.

FRIENDLY, D. S., JAAFAR, M. S., AND MORILLO, D. L. (1990). A comparative study of grating and recognition acuity testing in children with anisometropic amblyopia without strabismus. *Am. J. Ophthalmol.* 110, 293–299.

FULTON, A. (1992). Screening preschool children to detect visual and ocular disorders. (editorial) *Arch. Ophthalmol.* 110, 1553–1554.

HELVESTON, E. M., WEBER, J. C., MILLER, K., ROBERTSON, K., HOHBERGER, G., ESTES, R., ELLIS, F. D., PICK, N., AND HELVESTON, B. H. (1985). Visual function and academic performance. *Am. J. Ophthalmol.* 99, 346–355.

HILLIS, A., FLYNN, J. T., AND HAWKINS, B. S. (1983). The evolving concept of amblyopia: A challenge to epidemiologists. *Am. J. Epidemiol.* 118, 192–205.

LICHTER, P. (1992). Vision screening and children's access to eye care. (editorial) *Ophthalmology* 99, 843–844.

MAYER, L. (1986). Acuity of amblyopic children for small field gratings and recognition stimuli. *Invest. Ophthalmol. Vis. Sci.* 27, 1148–1153.

Romano, P. (1987). The importance of binocular vision. (editorial) *Binoc. Vis.* 2, 176–178.

SIMONS, K. (1983). Visual acuity norms in young children. *Survey Ophthalmol.* 28, 84–92.

SIMONS, K. (1988). Visual acuity and the functional definition of blindness, Chapter 51, Vol. 5. In T. D. DUANE AND A. E. JAEGER (eds.), *Clinical Ophthalmology.* Philadelphia: Harper & Row.

STEWART-BROWN, S., HASLUMN, M. N., AND BUTLER, N. B. (1985). Educational attainment of 10-year-old children with treated and untreated visual defects. *Develop. Med. Child Neurol.* 27, 504–513.

TOMMILA, V., AND TARKKANEN, A. (1981). Incidence of loss of vision in the healthy eye in amblyopia. *Br. J. Ophthalmol.* 65, 575–577.

VON NOORDEN, G. K. (1990). Binocular vision and ocular motility (4th ed.). St. Louis: C. V. Mosby.

WILCOX, L. M., AND SOKOL, S. (1980). Changes in the binocular fixation patterns and the visually evoked potential in the treatment of esotropia with amblyopia. *Ophthalmology* 87, 1273–1281.

29 | Use of models to improve hypothesis delineation: A study of infant electroretinography

DONALD C. HOOD, DAVID G. BIRCH, AND
EILEEN E. BIRCH

Localizing the sites of developmental changes and describing their mechanisms are among the goals of research on the developing visual system. Attempting to identify sites and mechanisms of disease processes, Hood and Greenstein (1990) argued that these goals are best realized by specifying hypotheses within a model's framework. They illustrated this point with behavioral data from patients with retinal diseases and a model of rod system adaptation. Many patients with retinal disease show a large loss in sensitivity to a brief light presented in the dark. Some of these patients show a smaller loss in the presence of background lights than that measured in the dark. A variety of hypotheses had been advanced to explain these adaptation-dependent losses of sensitivity secondary to retinal diseases. To test these explanations, Hood and Greenstein (1990) argued that a model of adaptation of the normal visual system was required. Once this model was constructed, the alternative hypotheses could be specified in terms of the parameters of the model. A similar argument has been made for hypotheses about developmental processes (Hood, 1988). In short, testing hypotheses about developmental processes requires a model of the normal adult system for the behavior under study and hypotheses about sites and mechanisms specified within the context of this model. Here the use of models to improve the delineation of hypotheses about retinal development is illustrated by examining models of the electroretinogram (ERG).

NEONATAL ELECTRORETINOGRAM

An ERG can be recorded from the newborn. In fact, an ERG can even be recorded from preterm infants, 30–36 weeks postconception (Zetterstrom, 1952; Winkelman and Horsten, 1962; Mactier et al., 1988; Grose et al., 1989; Birch et al., 1990). The infant ERG responses, however, are smaller in amplitude and delayed in time even for the term infant (e.g., Zetterstrom, 1951; Barnet et al., 1965; Fulton and Hansen, 1982). The human ERG undergoes substantial change between 36 and 57 weeks postconception (Birch et al., 1990).

Figure 29-1 shows ERG records for an adult and for infants tested at either 36 or 57 weeks postconception. The stimulus was a 10-μs, short-wavelength Ganzfeld flash. The infants had their pupils dilated and were dark-adapted for 30 minutes. ERGs were recorded using a Burian-Allen lens; each record is the computer average of 20 responses to a flash of a single intensity. Other details can be found in Birch et al. (1990). The energy of the flash in log td-second is noted in the rightmost column. There are marked changes in the ERG between 36 and 57 weeks postconception. (Note in Figure 29-1 that the gain for the records for the 36-week infant is twice that for the 57-week infant and the adult.) Although the ERG from the 57-week-old is closer to that of the adult, there are still clear differences. There are a number of ways to quantify the changes in ERG waveform with development.

The vertebrate ERG shows two prominent peaks in potential, the a- and b-waves. The a- and b-waves of the ERG are labeled in Figure 29-2, where the solid curve is the adult ERG elicited by the most intense flash (2.0 log td-second) in Figure 29-1. Most of the work on the development of the ERG has focused on the trough-to-peak b-wave amplitude. This measure is taken as the vertical distance from the trough of the a-wave to the peak of the b-wave (shown by the solid vertical line in Figure 29-2). The data in Figure 29-3A are trough-to-peak b-wave amplitudes plotted on a logarithmic scale against the log of the flash energy. Shown in this figure are the data for three adults and 15 infants; 5 infants were tested at 57 weeks and 10 at 36 weeks postconception. These infants received optimal perinatal nutrition as part of a study (Uauy et al., 1990; Birch et al., 1992) that examined the effects of different formulas on the visual development of very low birth

517

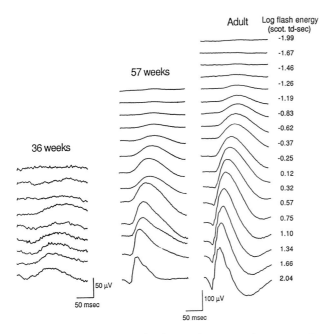

Adult Log flash energy
(scot. td-sec)

57 weeks

36 weeks

FIG. 29-1. Computer isolated rod ERGs from two infants (36 weeks and 57 weeks postconception) and an adult. Each record is the computer average of 20 responses to 10-μs flashes of a single intensity. The energy of the flash ranged from −2.0 to 2.0 log scot td-second. The calibrations for the 57-week infant and the adult is shown at the bottom right. The calibration for the 36-week infant is shown separately. See Birch et al. (1990) for more details.

weight (VLBW) infants. The data points in Figure 29-3B show the average trough-to-peak b-wave amplitudes from Figure 29-3A. There are clear differences among the adult, 57-week, and 36-week groups, and these differences can be quantitatively described.

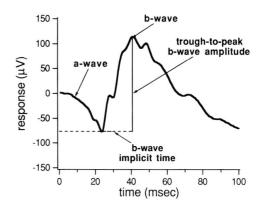

FIG. 29-2. Solid curve is a rod ERG response from a human eye. The stimulus was a short-wavelength, 10-μs flash of 2.0 log td-second. Two measures of the b-wave—trough-to-peak amplitude and implicit time—are shown by the solid vertical and dashed horizontal lines. (From Hood and Birch, 1992. By permission.)

Fulton and Hansen (1982, 1985) were the first to offer a quantitative analysis of the infant ERG. Following the analysis of Fulton and Rushton (1978), they fitted the so-called Naka-Rushton equation to infant ERG data. In particular, they fitted their data with the function

$$\frac{V}{Vm} = \frac{I}{I + K} \qquad (1)$$

where V = the trough-to-peak amplitude of the b-wave; Vm = the maximum value of the trough-to-peak amplitude; and I = the flash energy in td-second. The constant K = the semisaturation value; that is, when I = K, V is one-half of its maximum value Vm. For fits

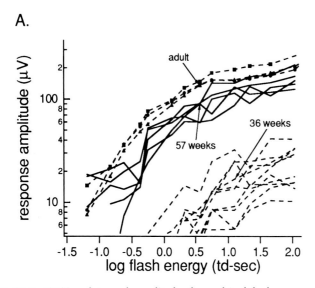

A.

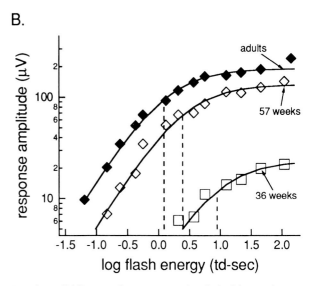

B.

FIG. 29-3. (A) Trough-to-peak amplitudes (log scale) of the b-wave are shown as a function of the log of the flash energy. Each curve was obtained from an intensity-response series as in Figure 29-1 from an individual subject. The data are shown for three adults (dashed lines and solid data points) and 15 infants; 5 infants were tested at

57 weeks (solid lines) and 10 at 36 weeks (dashed lines) after conception. (B) Data points are the average trough-to-peak b-wave amplitudes from (A). Smooth curves are the best fit of Eq. 1 to each set of data. See text for details.

to trough-to-peak b-wave amplitudes, these parameters are referred to as K_{bw} and Vm_{bw} to distinguish them from the parameters of fits of Eq. 1 to other measures of the ERG. The solid curves in Figure 29-3B are the best fit of Eq. 1 to the trough-to-peak b-wave amplitudes. The values of K_{bw} are shown by the interception of the dashed lines with the log intensity axis. Note that, in agreement with Fulton and Hansen (1982), the value of log K_{bw} decreases and the value of log Vm_{bw} increases as development progresses. The solid squares in Figure 29-4 show the changes in these parameters. Each axis is log of the ratio of the infants' parameters to the adults' parameters. Thus a value of 0 log relative K_{bw} or Vm_{bw} indicates an infant parameter that was equal to the adult value, and a log relative value of 0.3 (or −0.3) indicates an infant parameter that was twice (or one-half) the adult value. According to these data, between 36 and 57 weeks the maximum b-wave amplitude more than quadruples in size, and the value of K_{bw} decreases by about 0.8 log unit, or a factor of 6. In agreement with the Fulton and Hansen study, large changes are occurring after 36 weeks postconception, and these changes are affecting both the value of K_{bw} and the maximum trough-to-peak b-wave (Vm_{bw}) (Mets et al., 1989).

Attempts have been made to relate the changes in these parameters to sites or mechanisms of development. For example, any hypothesis that predicts an increase in quantal absorption during development predicts a decrease in K_{bw}, which follows from Eq. 1, as an increase in quantal absorption is equivalent to an increase in intensity. That is, $[aI/(aI + K)]$ is equivalent to $[I/(I + K/a)]$. It does not mean, of course, that a decrease in K_{bw} must be due to an increase in quantal absorption. In fact, different investigators have offered different interpretations of the changes in K_{bw} and Vm_{bw} (Arden et al., 1983; Massof et al., 1984; Birch and Fish, 1986; Fulton and Hansen, 1988; Birch et al., 1990). The best way to interpret changes in K_{bw} and Vm_{bw} in terms of changes in the retina is not clear. This confusion results from a lack of agreement on a model of the ERG.

SIMPLE, STATIC, TWO-STAGE MODEL OF THE ADULT ERG

To derive predictions for changes in K_{bw} and Vm_{bw} from alternative hypotheses requires a model of the adult ERG. A model of the ERG has been used with some success to identify the site of action of a retinal disease from changes in K_{bw} and Vm_{bw} (Hood, 1988; Johnson and Hood, 1988; Johnson and Massof, 1988). This model, based on a psychophysical model (Hood and Greenstein, 1990), has two sites: the receptors and the b-wave generators. Each site has a static nonlinear (SNL) response function described by Eq. 1. The model, shown in Figure 29-5A, is not specified in time and thus is referred to here as a static, two-site model. The output of the first site is the pooled rod receptor response and is given by a function of the form shown in Eq. 1. The response function of the second site, the b-wave generators, is also assumed to be of the same form, where the peak amplitude (P3) of the pooled receptor response is the input, and the peak amplitude (P_{bw}) of the b-wave mechanism's response is the output. The trough-to-peak b-wave amplitude of the ERG recorded at the electrode is V_{bw} and is equal to cP_{bw}. The constant of proportionality (c) varies among normal adults owing to factors unrelated to retinal function, such as differences in electrode resistance; c = 1.0 for the average adult. The effects of diseases such as retinitis pigmentosa that result in regional losses of receptors and thus decrease the number of P3 and P_{bw} generators can be represented by a value of c less than 1.0 (Hood and Birch, 1992). Although the infant has all its retinal cells by 36 weeks (Hollenberg and Spira, 1973), c could take on a different value if large areas of these cells were not functional or if the infant eyeball, for example, had a difference in resistance.

In this form, the model has five parameters: two semi-saturation constants (σ_{P3} and σ_{bw}), two maximum responses (Rm_{P3} and Rm_{bw}), and the constant c.[1] With

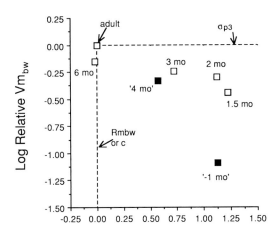

FIG. 29-4. Log relative Vm_{bw} versus log relative K_{bw} for ERG intensity-response functions recorded from infants. The open symbols are for infants 1.5–6.0 months of age (data from Fulton and Hansen, 1982). The filled symbols are from the fits to the data in Figure 29-3B. Vm_{bw} and K_{bw} values from fits as in Figure 29-3B are divided by the mean adult parameters. The 0 value represents adult values of Vm_{bw} and K_{bw}. The curves are the predictions for the static model. See text for details.

---

1. Here we use σ_{P3} rather than Ka as in the original formulation of Johnson and Hood (1988). The terms were changed to be consistent with the model to be presented below and with Granit's original assignment of the term PIII (called P3 here) as the receptor component of the ERG. Furthermore, the exponent $n = 1$ here.

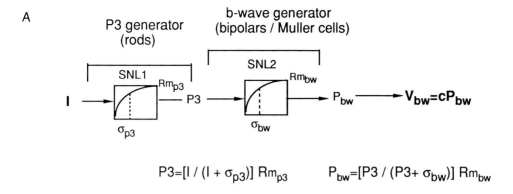

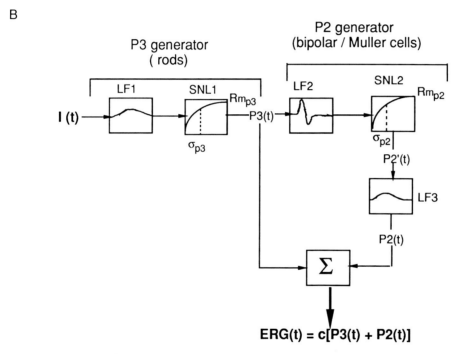

FIG. 29-5. (A) Static model. See text for details. (B) Dynamic model. See text and Hood and Birch (1992) for additional details.

the appropriate algebraic manipulations, the model predicts that the trough-to-peak b-wave amplitude (V_{bw}) varies with flash energy according to a function of the form of Eq. 1. In particular,

$$V_{bw} = \frac{I}{I + K_{bw}} Vm_{bw}$$

where

$$Vm_{bw} = \frac{cRm_{bw}}{1 + (\sigma_{bw}/Rm_{P3})} \quad (2)$$

and

$$K_{bw} = \frac{\sigma_{P3}}{1 + (Rm_{P3}/\sigma_{bw})} \quad (3)$$

Having made the static model explicit immediately illustrates the difficulty of differentiating among the hypotheses about sites of development with the trough-to-peak b-wave amplitudes. The model also makes it clear why there are competing explanations for the changes in the two parameters (K_{bw} and Vm_{bw}) estimated from the data. According to Eqs. 2 and 3, K_{bw} is affected by three of the five parameters in the model and Vm_{bw} by four. The data in Figures 29-3 and 29-4 indicate that retinal development is accompanied by large increases in Vm_{bw} and large decreases in K_{bw}. The model predicts that K_{bw} is decreased by decreases in the semisaturation value of either site (σ_{P3} or σ_{bw}) or increases in the maximum response of the first site (Rm_{P3}). The increase in Vm_{bw} can be produced by increases in the maximum response of either site (Rm_{P3} or Rm_{bw}), decreases in the semisaturation of the second site (σ_{bw}), or an increase in c. (Note that c and Rm_{bw} are equivalent in the model.) *Thus we cannot locate the retinal site of the changes in K_{bw} and Vm_{bw}.* As illustrated by the dashed lines in Figure 29-4, changing σ_{P3} only changes K_{bw}, and changing c or Rm_{P2} only changes Vm_{bw}. Thus we can say that the developmental process *cannot* involve *only* a change in one of these three parameters. For example, development cannot be simply attributed to either an increase in quantal absorption (σ_{P3}) or any single factor (e.g., a lower resistance attributable to a lower value of c). To say more, we must decrease the number of free parameters in the model or increase the information we extract from the data set. One approach to restricting the number of parameters in the model is to use the a-wave to obtain estimates of σ_{P3} and Rm_{P3}.

MEASURING THE PARAMETERS OF THE RECEPTORS (σ_{P3} and Rm_{P3})

For years, the a-wave has been used as an indicator of receptor sensitivity. According to Granit's classic analysis of the ERG, the leading edge of the a-wave is the sum of receptor activity P3 (Granit, 1933, 1947). We have shown that the a-wave of the human ERG can provide a measure of the parameters of P3, the human rod receptor activity (Hood and Birch, 1990a,b). In particular, the leading edge of the rod a-wave can be fitted with the same model used to describe the in vitro recordings from rod photoreceptors of the monkey. The solid curves in Figure 29-6 show ERGs recorded in response to relatively intense flashes (2.1–4.2 log td-second). The dashed curves are the fit of the receptor (P3) model to the leading edge of the ERG (Hood and Birch, 1990b).

The model fitted to the leading edge of the a-wave has among its four parameters σ_{P3} and Rm_{P3}. Thus our ability to distinguish between changes in these parameters can be tested by simulations of the model. The thin solid curves in Figure 29-7A,B show the first 25 ms of the model's P3 response to flashes of 2.0 (panel A) and 3.6 (panel B) log scot td-second. The bold dashed and solid curves show the effects of a fourfold increase in σ_{P3} or decrease in Rm_{P3} (or c). These curves

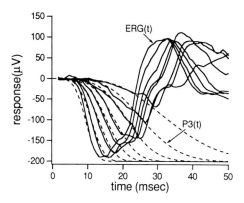

FIG. 29-6. Each solid curve is the computer average of rod ERG responses to 10-ms flashes of a single intensity. These are rod-driven responses isolated by computer-subtracting the cone contribution. The flash was of short wavelength light (W47A) and ranged in energy from 2.1 to 4.2 log td-second. The dashed curves are the predicted P3 responses from a model of the receptor response fitted to the leading edge of the a-wave. (Modified from Hood and Birch, 1990b).

are similar for the 2.0 log scot td-second flash. The a-wave cannot be used to distinguish among changes in σ_{P3}, Rm_{P3}, or c for flashes at or below 2.0 log scot td-second (Hood and Birch, 1990a).[2] A change in σ_{P3}, Rm_{P3}, or c has equivalent effects on the a-wave. With flashes that are more intense than those typically used in infant research, changes in σ_{P3} can be distinguished from a change in c or Rm_{P3} (Figure 29-7B).

Although we cannot estimate σ_{P3} and Rm_{P3} from the infants' ERGs available to us, we can use the a-wave to determine whether the receptor response is affected during development. Some investigators use the peak of the a-wave as a measure of relative receptor sensitivity. Hood and Birch (1990a) argued that it is not a good measure. First, the peak of the a-wave can be influenced by early oscillatory potentials. For processes such as development that may affect the oscillatory potentials differently from the a-wave (Birch et al., 1991), the peak amplitude is prone to error. More importantly, the peak a-wave could be influenced by the immaturity of the mechanisms generating the b-wave. For example, suppose an immaturity in the mechanisms generating the b-wave produced a delay in the appearance of the b-wave but left the a-wave unaltered in an immature state. Because the b-wave is delayed, a larger peak a-wave would be measured even though there was no change at the receptors. In fact, changing the mechanisms generating the b-wave and delaying its appear-

2. Hood and Birch (1990a) noted that because the first 25 ms of the receptor's response is an approximately linear function of flash energy for flash energies up to about 2.0 log td-second changes in σ_{P3} and Rm_{P3} cannot be distinguished.

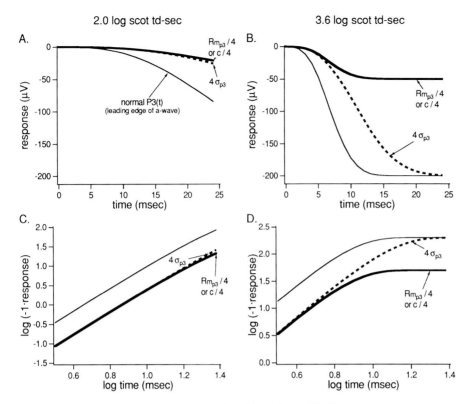

FIG. 29-7. (A) First 25 ms of the response predicted from the model of P3(t) to a 2.0 log scot td-second flash. The solid curve is the response for the adult. The interrupted curves show the effects on this response of increasing σ_{P3} or decreasing Rm_{P3} (or c) by a factor of 4. (B) As in (A) for a 3.5 log scot td-second flash. (C) Responses in (A) on log-log axes. The response amplitude was multiplied by -1 so that log response could be plotted. (D) Responses in (B) on log-log axes. The response amplitude was multiplied by -1 so that log response could be plotted. (Based on a figure from Hood and Birch, 1990a).

ance can markedly affect the estimate of the maturity of the receptors.[3]

Hood and Birch (1990a) suggested a procedure for avoiding these problems and for using more of the information in the a-wave. The theoretical curves in Figure 29-7C,D were obtained from the theoretical responses in Figure 29-7A,B by multiplying the curves by -1 to make them positive and then taking the log of the values. Note that for the 2.0 log td-second flash the predicted curves are of the same shape but displaced vertically on the log response axis, which is another way of showing that changes in the three parameters (σ_{P3}, Rm_{P3}, c) are equivalent to a multiplicative scaling of the response at each point in time. If $P3'(t)$ is the infant's response to the 2.0 log td-second flash and c', σ'_{P3} and $R'm_{P3}$ are the infant's parameters,

$$P3'(t) \cong P3(t)\cdot(c'/c)\cdot(\sigma'_{P3}/\sigma_{P3})^{-1}\cdot(R'm_{P3}/Rm_{P3})$$

and

$$\log[-1\cdot P3'(t)] \cong \log[-1\cdot P3(t)] + \triangle\log(c)$$
$$- \triangle\log(\sigma_{P3}) + \triangle\log(Rm_{P3}) \qquad (4)$$

where $P3(t)$ = the response for the normal adult, and $\triangle$ = the change in the log of the parameter.

Figure 29-8A shows the mean response to the 2.0 log td-second flash for the three groups. The a-waves are different. To display these a-waves on a log-log plot as in Figure 29-7C, the responses were multiplied by -1 and the log of these values taken. The data points in Figure 29-8B are the first 25 ms of the logged responses plotted against log time. Note that, as predicted by the model, the a-wave data for the three groups are approximately parallel on the log-log plot. The smooth curve is the mean of 10 adult observers from Hood and Birch (1990a). It was displaced vertically by -0.07, -0.55, and -1.07 log units to fit the three curves. As the theory suggests, these three sets of data can be fit by the same curve vertically displaced. The relative displacement tells us about the relative values of c, σ_{P3} and

---

3. To illustrate this point, consider the amplitude of the leading edge of the adult's a-wave in response to a 2.0 log td-second flash. According to the model of P3 (solid curve in Figure 29-7A), the response at 30 ms is more than twice as large as the response amplitude at 20 ms. Changing the mechanisms generating the b-wave to delay its appearance by only 10 ms can change by a factor of 2 the estimate of the size of the receptors' response.

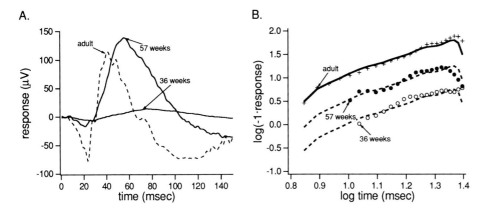

FIG. 29-8. (A) Averaged rod ERG response to the short-wavelength, 10-μs flash of 2.0 log td-second. The three curves are the averaged responses from the three adults (dashed curve), the 5 infants tested at 57 weeks (solid line), and the 10 infants at 36 weeks (solid line) after conception. (B) First 25 ms of the responses in (A) are plotted on log-log axes. The response amplitude was multiplied by −1 so that log response could be plotted. The solid smooth curve is the mean response for 10 normal observers from Hood and Birch (1990a). It was displaced vertically by −0.07 (solid), −0.55 (dashed), and −1.07 (dashed) log units to fit the three sets of data.

Rm_{P3}. Relative to the adult observers in this study, there is a change of about 1.0 log unit in one or more of these three parameters (σ_{P3}, Rm_{P3}, c) for the 36-week infants and a change of about 0.5 log unit in the case of the 57-week infants.

Thus the a-wave is smaller in the infant groups than in the adult, and the receptor (P3) model and the analysis above (Figure 29-8B, Eq. 4) indicate that some combination of change in c, σ_{P3}, and Rm_{P3} must be responsible. It still does not necessarily place the developmental process at the receptor. A change in c could be the result of a change in response size secondary to, for example, a different eye resistance. A change in c, however, makes a testable prediction. If the change in

the size of the ERG was entirely due to a smaller value of c, the infant ERG would resemble a scaled-down version of the adult ERG. Figure 29-9 shows the average response to the 2.0 log td-second flash from Figure 29-8A for the 36-week and 57-week groups. (The response scale is different from that in Figure 29-8A.) The dashed curve in each panel is the adult response to 2.0 log td-second scaled down by a multiplicative factor based on the vertical separations in Figure 29-8B. As expected, the leading edge of the a-waves coincide; smaller a-waves do not necessarily mean less sensitive (σ_{P3}) receptors. In this case, however, if the change in the ERG was entirely due to a change in c in Eq. 4, the rest of the responses should coincide; they do not.

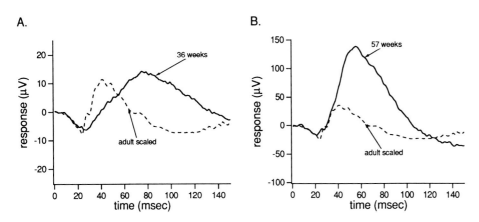

FIG. 29-9. (A) Averaged rod ERG response to the short-wavelength, 10-μs flash of 2.0 log td-second from Figure 29-8A for the 36-week (A) and 57-week (B) groups. (The response scale is different from that in Figure 29-8A.) The dashed curve in each panel is the adults response to 2.0 log td-second scaled down by a multiplicative factor based on the vertical separations in Figure 29-8B. [The multiplicative factors were equal to about 10 (A) and 3 (B), corresponding to separations in Figure 29-8B of 1.0 and 0.5 log unit.]

It is unlikely that much of the development process can be represented as a change in c. The maturation taking place between 36 and 57 weeks undoubtedly involves large changes at the receptors. We cannot, however, identify the cause of these changes as σ_{P3}, rather than Rm_{P3}. To further identify the sites of these changes requires more information. One approach would be to use more intense lights to distinguish between the receptor parameters (Figure 29-7B,D). A different approach is to improve our model to account for more of the ERG response.

NEED FOR A DYNAMIC MODEL OF THE ERG

There are two major problems with the static model of the b-wave described above. First, the model is not specified in time. The theoretical scheme advanced above, as well as attempts made by others to explain changes in K_{bw} and Vm_{bw}, assumes a static model of the b-wave (e.g., Fulton and Rushton, 1978; Arden et al., 1983; Hood, 1988, 1990; Fulton and Hansen, 1988; Johnson and Hood, 1988; Johnson and Massof, 1988). By static model we mean one in which the time course of the response is not specified.

The peak of the b-wave occurs sooner for more intense flashes. Figure 29-10 shows the time from flash onset to peak b-wave, called *implicit time* (Figure 29-2), for the data in Figure 29-3. The implicit time decreases as flash energy is increased. The longest implicit time for the adults is about 120 ms. This value is shorter than the time to the peak of the receptors' response, which is in the range of 150–200 ms (Penn and

Hagins, 1972; Baylor et al., 1984; Hood and Birch, 1990b). Thus it is not clear what is being assumed in the static model when the peak amplitude of P3 is described by Eq. 1; it cannot be the peak amplitude as in single cell physiology. Furthermore, the static model cannot predict changes in implicit times with increases in flash energy. The implicit times of the adult b-wave (filled symbols) vary by a factor of almost 3. A model is needed that predicts both the amplitude and the implicit time of the trough-to-peak b-wave. Once specified, this model can be used to test hypotheses about development.

Note in Figure 29-10 that the implicit time of the b-wave changes substantially during development (see also Fulton and Hansen, 1982; Grose et al., 1989). The infant data fall to the right of the adult data. To obtain a quantitative measure of this displacement, the means of the adult data were connected by solid lines and this mean adult curve was shifted horizontally by 0.35 and 1.20 log units to approximately coincide with the 57 and 36 week data, respectively. The horizontally displaced curves are shown as the dashed curves. The implication of this displacement is discussed below.

A second problem with the static model concerns the assumption of a b-wave generating mechanism. According to the static model, the parameters K_{bw} and Vm_{bw} extracted from the fit of Eq. 1 are the parameters of a "b-wave generating mechanism." According to the analysis of Granit and others, however, there is no b-wave generating mechanism (e.g., Granit, 1933, 1947; K. T. Brown, 1968; Heynen and van Norren, 1985). Figure 29-11 outlines Granit's model. In Granit's analysis (Granit, 1933, 1947) there is an inner nuclear layer mechanism(s) generating a potential PII (called here P2) that sums with PIII (called here P3) to produce the b-wave. (Not shown on this figure is PI, which is generated in the pigment epithelial layer and is too slow to influence our analysis.)

The ERG is more complicated than the simple model in Figure 29-11 suggests. We know, for example, that potentials such as the oscillatory potentials and slow PIII can influence the waveform. However, Granit's model offers a better approach to understanding changes in the ERG with development or disease processes than does use of the trough-to-peak b-wave amplitude (Hood and Birch, 1990b, 1992). According to Granit's analysis, to obtain a relatively uncontaminated measure of the inner nuclear layer activity from ERG records requires knowing the amplitude and time course of the receptor potential P3. The solid curves in Figure 29-12A are the adult ERGs as in Figure 29-1 shown on a single set of axes; the dashed curves are the predicted responses from the receptor (P3) model fitted to the leading edge of the a-wave in Figure 29-6. To replace trough-to-peak b-wave amplitude with Granit's esti-

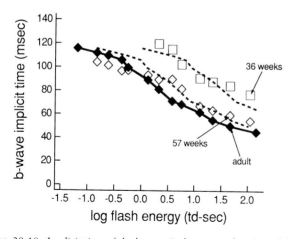

FIG. 29-10. Implicit time of the b-wave is shown as a function of the log of the flash energy. The data points are the average values for three adults (solid diamonds), 5 infants tested at 57 weeks (open diamonds), and 10 infants at 36 weeks (open squares) after conception. The solid curve is the mean of the data for the adults. The dashed curves are the mean normal curve displaced horizontally by 0.35 and 1.20 log units, respectively. See text for details.

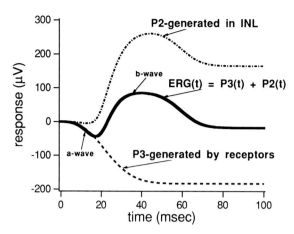

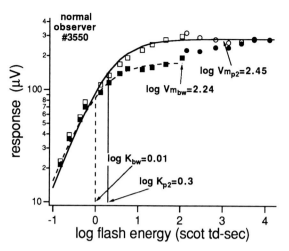

FIG. 29-11. Simplified version of Granit's model of the ERG. It was drawn to emphasize how the b-wave peak could underestimate the peak amplitude of P2. (From Hood and Birch, 1992. By permission.)

FIG. 29-13. For a normal adult observer, the amplitude of the derived P2 (open symbols) and the trough-to-peak b-wave amplitude (filled symbols) are plotted as a function of the log of the flash energy. The smooth curves are the fit of the Naka-Rushton function (Eq. 1) to all the derived P2 data (solid curve) and to the trough-to-peak b-wave amplitude data (dashed curve) up to flash energies of 2.0 log scot td-second. (Modified from Hood and Birch, 1992.)

mate of the peak amplitude of the inner nuclear layer activity (P2), Hood and Birch (1990b, 1992) derived P2 responses. The derived P2 responses are shown in Figure 29-12B for the records in Figure 29-12A. These P2 responses were derived by subtracting the dashed P3 curves from the solid ERG responses at each flash intensity. The peak of the responses in Figure 29-12B provides a measure of the peak amplitude for P2. The open squares in Figure 29-13 show the estimated peak amplitude of the inner nuclear layer activity (P2) and the filled squares the trough-to-peak b-wave amplitudes. The circles are the trough-to-peak b-wave amplitudes and P2 peak amplitudes for an extended series of flash intensities. Note that the trough-to-peak b-wave amplitude underestimates the peak amplitude of the response (P2) of the inner nuclear layer for flash intensities in the range of 0–3.0 log scot td-second. For flash intensities outside this range, the trough-to-peak b-wave amplitudes are approximately equal to the am-

plitude of the P2 response. It confirms Peachey et al.'s (1989) hypothesis that the trough-to-peak b-wave amplitude underestimates the peak amplitude of the response (P2) of the inner nuclear layer for intermediate flash intensities. [See also Breton and Montzka (1990) and Hood and Birch (1990b, 1992).]

If we assume Granit's model of the ERG, the procedure of fitting Eq. 1 to trough-to-peak b-wave data does not provide a veridical measure of inner nuclear layer activity. The solid curve in Figure 29-13 shows the fit of Eq. 1 to the P2 amplitude for the same range of intensities used for the fit shown by the dashed curve. The values of Vm_{P2} and K_{P2} are 60–100% larger than the corresponding parameters for the b-wave (Hood

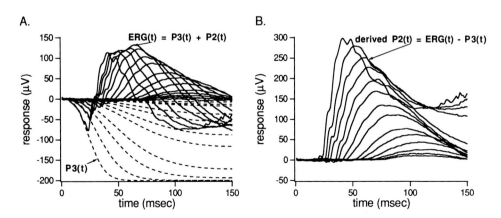

FIG. 29-12. (A) Solid curves are the ERG responses from an adult for the series of flash energies shown in Figure 29-1. Dashed curves are the theoretical rod receptor responses, P3(t). (B) Derived P2(t) responses. (From Hood and Birch, 1992. By permission.)

and Birch, 1990b, 1992). A model of the ERG must take into consideration the fact that the b-wave is the algebraic sum of two potentials of opposite sign.

DYNAMIC MODEL OF THE ERG

Hood and Birch (1992) have proposed a dynamic model of the ERG based on Granit's analysis. Figure 29-5B contains a representation of this model. The output, P3(t), of the rods (P3 generator) is described by the receptor (P3) model (Figure 29-6). The input to the P2 generator is P3(t), and the output is P2(t). The ERG is the sum of P3(t) and P2(t). The model differs from the static model in Figure 29-5A in two ways. First, the stimulus and the responses in the model are functions of time. The linear filters, labeled LF in Figure 29-5B, shape the time course of the P3 and P2 responses. Second, the ERG is the *sum* of two potentials P3(t) and P2(t) generated at different levels. A general form of the model should allow for differences in P3 and P2 generators across the retina. For now, we assume a homogeneous retina in which all rods and all P2 generators are identical, which allows us to represent the model's output as

$$ERG(t) = c[P3(t) + P2(t)] \qquad (5)$$

where c = 1.0 for the average adult retina. More detail can be found in Hood and Birch (1992).

The points in Figure 29-14 are the data from three normal observers for flashes up to 4.1 log td-second, or a factor of 100 above the range used with the infants. The dashed vertical line indicates the upper limit (2.0 log td-second) of the range of flash intensities used with the infants. The model's predicted trough-to-peak b-wave amplitudes (left panel) and b-wave implicit times (right panel) are shown by the solid curves. To fit these data the values of the time constants of the three linear

filters had to be estimated in addition to the five parameters shown in Figure 29-5B (Hood and Birch, 1992). The features of the data are reasonably well described. The dashed curves in Figure 29-14 are the predictions for the implicit times and amplitudes of P2. The model predicts that the b-wave measures differ from the measures of the INL potential, P2. These differences are due to the algebraic cancelation of P2 and P3. [See Hood and Birch (1992) for a discussion of this point.]

DYNAMIC MODEL AND HYPOTHESES ABOUT DEVELOPMENT

Having established that the model describes the b-wave data from the normal adult, predicted b-wave amplitude and implicit time functions can be derived for changes in the model's parameters. We temporarily assume that development does not affect the time constants of the retinal processes and we derive predictions for the changes in the five static parameters of the model. This simplifying assumption is discussed below. Figures 29-15 and 29-16 show the effects of changing five of the parameters: the receptor's semisaturation (σ_{P3}), the semisaturation of P2 (σ_{P2}), the maximum receptor response (Rm_{P3}), the maximum of the P2 response (Rm_{P2}), and c. The left-hand panels show the predicted trough-to-peak b-wave amplitudes and the right hand panels the b-wave implicit times. In every panel, the solid curve is the predicted response for the adult and the dashed curves show the effects of a change in the parameter of interest by a factor of 2 ($\times$), 4 (+), and 8 (*). The upper limit of the range of flash intensities (2.0 log td-second) used in the infant studies is marked by the vertical dashed line.

Considering the b-wave amplitude functions first. The predicted trough-to-peak b-wave amplitudes differ sub-

b-wave trough-to-peak amplitudes

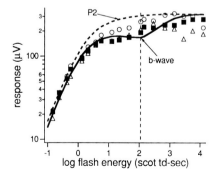

b-wave implicit times

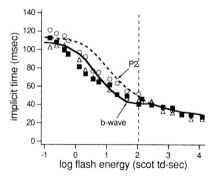

FIG. 29-14. Trough-to-peak b-wave amplitude (left) and b-wave implicit time (right) as a function of flash energy. The data points are for the three adult observers. The solid curves are the dynamic model's predicted trough-to-peak b-wave functions. The dashed curves are the dynamic model's predicted P2 functions.

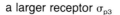

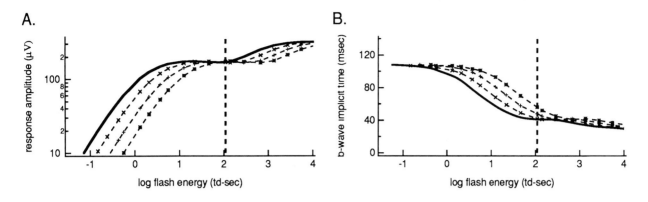

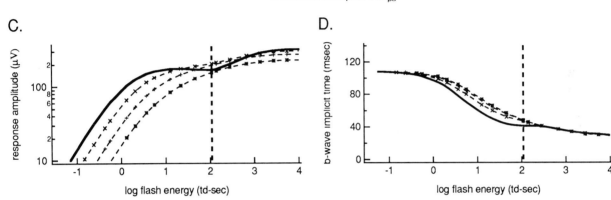

FIG. 29-15. Trough-to-peak b-wave amplitudes (A, C) and b-wave implicit times (B, D) predicted by the dynamic model. The solid curves are the predictions for the set of parameters used for fitting the data from the three adult observers (see Fig. 29-14). The three dashed curves are for increases in σ_{P3} (A, B) and decreases in Rm_{P3} (C, D) by factors of 2, 4, and 8.

stantially for changes in the five parameters. Changes in σ_{P3} and Rm_{P3} shift the position of the trough-to-peak b-wave amplitude function on a log intensity axis (increased K_{bw}) with little or no change in the maximum (Vm_{bw}). A change in c shifts the trough-to-peak b-wave amplitude function (Figure 29-16E) on a log response axis (decreased Vm_{bw}) with no change in the semisaturation (K_{bw}). The changes with σ_{P2} and Rm_{P2} are far more complicated. The unusual changes in the response-intensity curves for both INL changes of σ_{P2} and Rm_{P2} have a common cause, the algebraic combination of a normal receptor component (P3), with a diminished INL component (P2). [See Hood and Birch (1992) for more detail on this point.]

The changes in the model's parameters have different effects on the b-wave implicit time functions. The analysis of the implicit times and amplitudes clearly provides more information than either alone. Similar changes in the intensity-response functions do not correspond to similar changes in implicit times. For example, in Figure 29-15 the changes in the intensity-response functions

are similar, but the changes in the implicit times are different. These differences are useful for testing hypotheses about the sites and mechanisms of the developmental processes.

The dynamic model can help distinguish among the alternative hypotheses for changes in trough-to-peak b-wave amplitude (Figure 29-3) and b-wave implicit times (Figure 29-10) with development. The static model predicted similar effects for changes in σ_{P3}, σ_{P2}, and Rm_{P3}. The dynamic model produces different patterns of results if both amplitude and implicit time data are considered. Note that changes in only one of the five parameters, (σ_{P3}) produce a *large* lateral shift in the implicit time function. Recall that the dashed curves in Figure 29-10 through the data are the mean adult curve shifted on the log intensity axis by 0.35 and 1.20 log units to fit the data from the 57- and 36-week groups. According to the simulations of the dynamic model in Figures 29-15 and 29-16, the 1.2 log unit shift for the 36 weeks data could only result from a change in σ_{p3}. (Recall that we are temporarily assuming that devel-

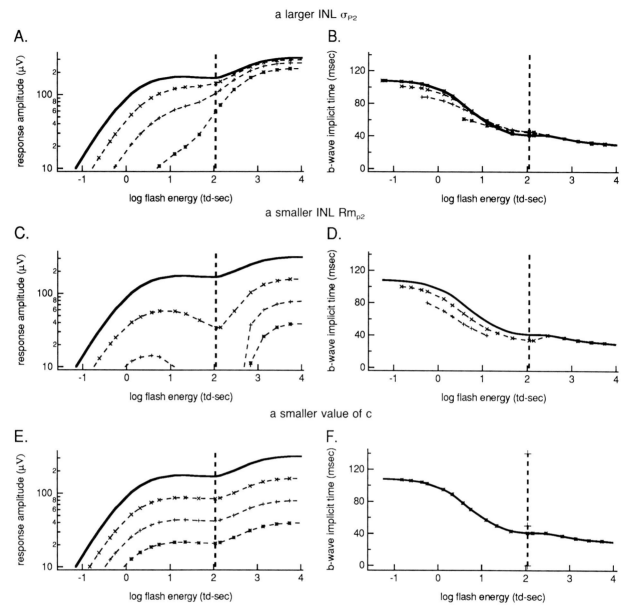

FIG. 29-16. Trough-to-peak b-wave amplitudes (A, C, E) and b-wave implicit times (B, D, F) predicted by the dynamic model. Solid curves are the predictions for the set of parameters used for fitting the data from the three adult observers (see Fig. 29-14). The three dashed curves are for increases in σ_{P2} (A, B), decreases in Rm_{P2} (C, D), or decreases in the c value (E, F) by factors of 2, 4, and 8.

opment does not change the time constants in the model.) Thus in the context of the dynamic model as articulated thus far, these data appear consistent with hypotheses that predict a large decrease in σ_{P3} with development. Increase pigment content, proper receptor alignment, and an increase in the gain of the receptor's transduction process are among the hypothesized changes that are represented by a decrease in σ_{P3}.

Can a change in σ_{P3} account for the b-wave data? The data from Figures 29-3 and 29-10 are presented again in Figures 29-17 and 29-18. The smooth curves are the model's predictions for different changes in the models parameters. The bold solid curve is the model's fit to the adult data seen in Figure 29-14. The dashed curves in Figure 29-17A,B show the model's fit to the data by changing only σ_{P3}. As expected, the model does a plausible job of fitting the implicit time data. Note, however, that the trough-to-peak b-wave amplitude data in Figure 29-17 show more of a decrease in amplitude than predicted by the σ_{P3} change. In fact, the infant

a larger σ_{p3}

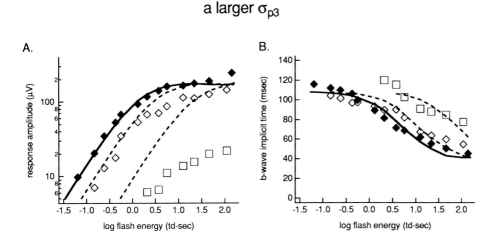

a smaller c and a larger σ_{p3}

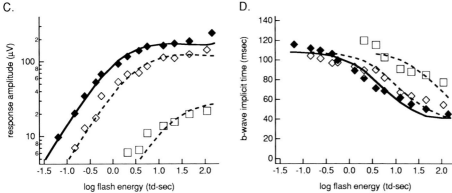

FIG. 29-17. Data points are the trough-to-peak b-wave amplitudes (A, C) and b-wave implicit times (B, D) for the data from Figures 29-3 and 29-10. The bold solid curves are the fit to the adult data from Figure 29-14. The dashed curves show the fit of the model to the infants' data. For these fits, the parameters of the model for the adult observers were changed in the following way. (A, B) For the 36-week group the log σ_{P3} was increased by 1.2 and for the 57-week group by 0.35. (C, D) For the 36-week group log σ_{P3} was increased by 1.2, and log c decreased by 0.8; and for the 57-week group log σ_{P3} was increased by 0.35, and log c decreased by 0.15.

data show small b-wave amplitudes that, according to the model, cannot be accounted for by changes at the receptor in either σ_{P3} or Rm_{P3}. One or more of the three parameters (c, σ_{P2}, Rm_{P2}) that produce marked decreases in response amplitude must be changing.

To illustrate the use of the model, a change in σ_{P3} was combined with each of the three parameters that could decrease Vm_{bw}. The dashed curves in Figure 29-17C,D show the model fitted by adding a change in c to the change in σ_{P3} described in panels A and B. This fit captures the general characteristics of the data. Of the other two parameters that could decrease Vm_{bw}, significant changes in σ_{P2} can be ruled out. Figure 29-18C,D illustrates that the 36-week data cannot be de-

scribed by a combined changes in σ_{P3} and σ_{P2}.[4] The dashed curves in Figure 29-18A,B show that changing Rm_{P2} in conjunction with σ_{P3} can approximate the data.

Thus the 36-week b-wave data can be fitted with a change in σ_{P3} combined with a change in either c or

---

4. The reason the 36-week data cannot be described by combined changes in σ_{P3} and σ_{P2} is the following. A decrease in σ_{P2} (Figure 29-16A,B) shifts the amplitude functions to the right (increases K_{bw}) without changing the position of the implicit time function. Thus adding an increase in σ_{P2} to the change in σ_{P3} described by the solid lines produces too large a shift (K_{bw}) in the b-wave amplitude function. Compensating for this shift by decreasing the amount by which we change σ_{P3} produces a misfit to the implicit time data.

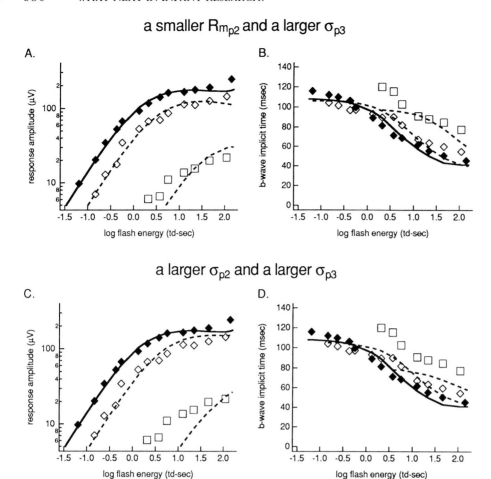

FIG. 29-18. Data points are the trough-to-peak b-wave amplitudes (A, C) and b-wave implicit times (B, D) for the data from Figures 29-3 and 29-10. Bold solid curves are the fit to the adult data from Figure 29-14. Dashed curves show the fit of the model to the infants' data. For these fits, the parameters of the model for the adult observers were changed in the following way. (A, B) For the 36-week group, log σ_{P3} was increased by 1.55, and log Rm_{P2} decreased by 0.5; and for the 57-week group, log σ_{P3} was increased by 0.35, and log Rm_{P2} decreased by 0.1. (C, D) For the 36-week group log σ_{P3} was increased by 1.2, and log σ_{P2} increased by 0.8; and for the 57-week group log σ_{P3} was increased by 0.35, and log σ_{P2} increased by 0.1.

Rm_{P2}. The analysis of the a-wave, however, indicates that neither fit is adequate when both the a- and b-wave amplitudes are considered. The analysis in Figure 29-8B and Eq. 4 indicated that the combined effects of the change in log c and log σ_{P3} cannot be greater than about 1.0 and 0.5 in the case of the 36- and 57-week data, respectively. For the 57-week data, either fit (σ_{P3} with c or Rm_{P2}) is in agreement with the a-wave analysis. For the 36-week data, however, neither fit of the model is consistent with the a-wave analysis in Figure 29-8. The fit in Figure 29-17C,D required a combined change in log c and log σ_{P3} of 2.0 log units, and the fit in Figure 29-18A,B required a change in σ_{P3} of 1.55 log units. In fact, no combination of changes in the five parameters provides for an adequate description of both the a- and b-wave data. In the context of the dynamic model, *we conclude that, in addition to receptor changes (σ_{P3}), the*

timing of the retinal processes is changing during development.

Figure 29-19 shows one possible fit of the model to the 36-week-old data. For this fit log σ_{P3} was increased by 1.0 log unit based on the a-wave analysis, and the parameters of the INL, including the timing represented by LF3 in Figure 29-5B, were changed. The dashed curve shows the fit of the model for a doubling of the time constant of LF3 and changes in log σ_{P2} and log Rm_{P2} of 0.4 and 0.5 log unit, respectively. No systematic attempt was made to obtain the best fitting combination of parameters, although numerous combinations were tried. Some of these other combinations did as well. However, all plausible fits had the following characteristics: (1) Large changes in σ_{P3} (up to 1.0 log unit) were always required. (Some of the change in σ_{P3} could be replaced with a change in c or Rm_{P3}). (2) The

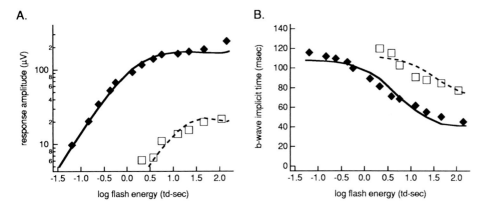

FIG. 29-19. Data points are the trough-to-peak b-wave amplitudes (A) and b-wave implicit times (B) for the data from Figures 29-3 and 29-10. Bold solid curves are the fit to the adult data from Figure 29-14. The dashed curves show the fit of the model to the 36-week infants' data. For these fits, the parameters of the model for the adult observers were changed in the following way. Log σ_{P3} was increased by 1.0, log Rm_{P2} decreased by 0.5, and log σ_{P2} was increased by 0.4. In addition, the time constant of LF3 was doubled.

INL changes had to include a smaller Rm_{P2} (including an increase in σ_{P2}, as in Figure 29-19, improved the fit). (3) The timing of the INL response P2 had to be changed (a slowing of LF3 in Figure 29-5B).

SUMMARY OF THE MODELING OF THE INFANT ERG

More precise localization of the magnitude of the developmental changes will be possible with both additional data and improvements in the model. ERGs to more intense stimuli would greatly aid the estimates of the parameters for the infant model. For example, the a-waves to relatively intense flashes would allow an estimate of the change in σ_{P3} (Figure 29-7) and the b-waves an estimate of the change in σ_{P2} versus Rm_{P2} (Figure 29-16). In addition, an improved model designed to capture the entire waveform of the ERG could also distinguish among various combinations of parameters.[5]

For now, we conclude that the infants' larger values of K_{bw} are mainly due to larger values of σ_{P3}, and that the markedly reduced Vm_{bw} in the case of the 36-week-olds is due to underdevelopment of the INL represented in the model as a reduced Rm_{P2} and probably a larger value of σ_{P2}. The longer implicit times of the b-wave are mainly due to larger values of σ_{P3} and, in the case of the 36-week infants, to immaturities of the INL mechanisms producing a slower response, P2.

---

5. Another simplification in the present version of the dynamic model is the assumption of an homogeneous retina. In particular, the model assumed that the P3 and P2 generators were identical across the retina. Given that there is evidence for a maturational gradient across the retina (Kretzer and Hitner, 1985; see also Chapter 17), this assumption needs further examination.

DELINEATING HYPOTHESES ABOUT MECHANISMS OF DEVELOPMENT AND A COMPARISON TO ANATOMICAL DATA

We earlier stated that to test hypotheses about developmental processes requires a model of the normal adult system for the behavior under study and hypotheses about sites and mechanisms specified within the context of this model. The dynamic model provides a good fit to the adult ERG data, which allows us to test any hypothesis about retinal development that can be phrased in terms of the parameters of the model. Because the model includes, in addition to the five parameters described above, parameters that set the time course of the receptor (P3) and INL (P2) responses, a wide range of hypotheses can be tested. Within the current limitations of the dynamic model, we concluded that development from 36 weeks on involves large changes in σ_{P3} as well as changes in the parameters of the INL. What are the possible mechanisms responsible for these changes?

The most obvious hypotheses consistent with a decrease in log σ_{P3} are those that predict an increase in the number of quanta absorbed. Less preretinal absorption of quanta with age would be an example of such a hypothesis. However, the infant probably has less, not more, light absorbed by preretinal media (Werner, 1982; Hansen and Fulton, 1989). Alternatively, the spacing between the receptors could be hypothesized to be greater in the infant. If there were more space between the rods of the 36-week-old infant, a smaller percentage of the quanta would be absorbed. This factor is unlikely to be substantial, as there is evidence that the receptor inner segments probably grow to keep the interstitial space approximately constant (Packer et al.,

1990). A third, more likely, hypothesis is that fewer quanta are absorbed in the infant's receptors because infants have less light-absorbing visual pigment in their rod outer segments. There is anatomical evidence to support this hypothesis. Drucker and Hendrickson (1989) reported that at about 36 weeks there was little or no evidence of rod outer segments in the area of the retina that probably dominates the adult ERG, the midperiphery. By 41 weeks the outer segments are 60% of adult length. Fulton et al. (1991) found photochemical evidence that there are large increases in rhodopsin content during early development. Thus there is photochemical and anatomical evidence that a large increase in pigment density is taking place during the developmental period covered in the present study. This evidence combined with the fit of the model above suggests that a major factor determining retinal sensitivity changes up to 57 weeks or more is an increase in pigment content. Furthermore, this hypothesis is consistent with the conclusion of Birch et al. (1992) that the fatty acid composition of an infant's formula affects the value of log K_{bw}. A determination of whether other developmental changes (e.g., larger receptors funneling more light or more efficient transduction) contribute to the decrease in σ_{P3} must await further improvements of both the model and the anatomical data.

The fits of the model also point to substantial changes taking place in the INL between 36 and 57 weeks. The improved fit obtained by changing LF3 of the model also suggests that P2 becomes faster with development. It is now clear that Granit's P2 potential is largely a response of the Müller cells that reflects an increase in extracellular potassium generated from the activity of the cells (e.g., bipolars) of the INL (e.g., Miller and Dowling, 1970; Newman and Odette, 1984; Karwoski and Proenza, 1987). Thus an increase in the size and the speed of P2 could be secondary to the development of the neuronal cells of the INL or their relation to the Müller cells.

COMPARISON TO PSYCHOPHYSICAL DATA AND CONSIDERATION OF GENERAL PROBLEMS WITH PSYCHOPHYSICAL MODELS

Large increases in sensitivity have been measured during the first few postnatal months using behavioral measures (Powers et al., 1981; Hamer and Schneck, 1984; Hansen et al., 1986). For example, Hansen et al. (1986) measured behavioral thresholds for infants at 4, 10, and 18 weeks postterm (about 44, 50, and 58 weeks, respectively, postconception). Thresholds were measured in the dark and on backgrounds of different intensities using a psychophysical procedure developed by Teller (1979). These behavioral data indicate that between 44

and 58 weeks dark-adapted threshold increases by about 1.0 log unit. Hood (1988) analyzed the Fulton and Hansen incremental threshold data obtained on background fields of different intensities within the context of a two-site model of the rod system (Hood and Greenstein, 1990). He concluded that the changes responsible for the increase in behavioral sensitivity were located in the retina, possibly at the receptors but certainly before the retinal site of adaptation. A comparison of the change in behaviorally measured thresholds to the changes in the ERG model's parameters estimated in this study supports this conclusion. The threshold of the ERG (the combined change in log K_{bw} and log Vm_{bw}) changes by 1.3 log units between 36 and 57 weeks and 0.7 log unit or so of this change is at the receptor. Thus it appears likely that the behavioral difference of 1.0 log unit between the 44 and 58 week groups is due to retinal development, partially of the INL but in large part at the receptoral level due to increased visual pigment.

For infants in the range of 48 to 52 weeks (2–3 months postterm), the behavioral thresholds are still 1.0–2.0 log units below the adults' sensitivity depending on the conditions used (Powers et al., 1981; Dannemiller and Banks, 1983; Hamer and Schneck, 1984; Schneck et al., 1984; Dannemiller, 1985; A. M. Brown, 1986, 1988; Hansen et al., 1986). The increase in behavioral sensitivity after 52 weeks or so is usually attributed to postretinal changes, as retinal anatomy is reasonably mature. Although the 48-week retina is said to resemble the adult retina (Mann, 1950; Abramov et al., 1982), the infant's ERG is clearly not an adult ERG. At 57 weeks, b-wave thresholds are elevated by 0.5 log unit, and oscillatory potentials and the maximum trough-to-peak b-wave amplitude (Vm_{bw}) are smaller than normal (Birch et al., 1990, 1991). Maximum trough-to-peak b-wave amplitude (Vm_{bw}) is below the adult value 1 year after birth (Mets et al., 1989). The general point, however, that there are large changes in sensitivity after 52 weeks that are unlikely to be due solely to retinal changes is still valid. It will be difficult to understand these differences between infant and adult behavioral sensitivities without a better model of the sensitivity of the adult to incremental lights. Some of the problems to be solved when developing behavioral models of adult visual functions are discussed in the next section.

COMMENTS ON BEHAVIORAL MODELS

Where Are the Sites of Sensitivity Changes?

One approach to identifying sites of development from behavioral data involves specifying the sites controlling sensitivity in the adult. Hypotheses yield different predictions depending on whether the developmental change is hypothesized to act before or after the site of sensitivity control (Hood and Greenstein, 1982, 1990; Greenstein and Hood, 1986). For example, by specifying that the primary site of sensitivity control for light adaptation in the adult is in the INL, Hood (1988) concluded that the Hansen et al. (1986) data were consistent with a developmental change acting before the site of adaptation, i.e., close to the receptors. Similar approaches can be applied to other paradigms. One weakness with this approach and most other attempts to establish sites of development based on behavioral data is a lack of understanding of the role of noise in the visual system.

Where Is the Noise and What Is the Detector?

Attempts to specify how development (or disease) alters the visual system can often uncover weaknesses in our models of normal adult vision. As an example, the observation that the sensitivity of the adult rod system decreases approximately as a square root of the background luminance has been accepted as evidence that quantal fluctuations in the physical stimulus limit detection over a range of low background luminances. Hood and Greenstein (1990), however, found they could not assume that quantal fluctuations limited sensitivity over any appreciable range of background intensities and still explain the behavioral data from patients with a disease (congenital stationary nightblindness) known to act after the generation of P3. Although the role of quantal fluctuations may be rescued by post hoc modifications of the decision rule or by adding other sources of noise, the role of extrinsic and intrinsic noise and their interaction with the detection process are far from understood (e.g., Cohn and Lasley, 1986; Graham and Hood, 1992).

Variations in the stimulus and in the neural response are physical (quantal) and biological facts of life. However, the way to incorporate quantal and biological noise into a quantitative model of the visual system has not been solved, which creates a difficult problem for those seeking to identify sites and mechanisms of development from behavioral data. First, the developmental process may alter the noise of the neural signal at one or more levels of the visual system. How does one handle this possibility without a model of the adult system that includes the sources and sites of noise? Furthermore, the nature of the assumptions about the detection process, as well as the nature and location of noise, are important.

Consider the results of a hypothetical experiment simulated by Graham and Hood (1992). An observer's task is to distinguish between a trial with a sinusoidally flickering light from a blank trail of the same mean luminance. They simulated the predictions for two commonly assumed detection mechanisms, a peak detector and an ideal (stimulus known exactly) detector. In their simulated system, a sensitivity change in the form of a temporal filter is placed before the detector and after an early noise source (e.g., quantal noise). The temporal filter had a frequency response function that simulated the temporal contrast sensitivity measured psychophysically in adult observers. With the ideal detector, the only noise that limits detection is at the frequency of the stimulus. That is, although quantal noise contains components at all temporal frequencies, the ideal detector knows the signal to be detected and thus is affected only by the noise at the signal frequency. Hence, because the filter decreases the amplitude of the signal and the noise by the same amount, the ideal detector being a signal-to-noise detector is unaffected by the temporal tuning of the filter. It is as if the filter were not present. The peak detector is affected by noise at other frequencies, and the effect of the temporal filter can be seen in the behavioral thresholds. Note that if this filter is altered by a developmental process, whether it is reflected in the behavioral data from infants depends on the type of detector assumed. In general, a developmental process that affects the signal but not the noise has different consequences depending on the detection assumptions and the nature of the noise. A developmental process affecting both signal and noise has uncertain effects, including no effect at all in the case illustrated above, depending on the assumptions about noise and detection.

In the absence of a model of the adult system with noise sources, the assumptions about noise and detection should be made clear. For example, Hood and Greenstein's (1990) model of the rod system adaptation assumes a peak detector and a constant amount of noise that is unaffected by disease and is located beyond the effects of retinal disease. In fact, without assumptions about noise and detection, existing attempts to identify sites and mechanisms of development from behavioral data probably implicitly assume a peak detector and a source of (late) noise occurring in the system beyond the location of the developmental changes.

SUMMARY

Large changes take place in retinal and postretinal function during the perinatal months. Within the context of a model of the adult ERG, we concluded that between 36 and 57 weeks a major portion of the change is at the receptoral level, although changes in the INL are also implicated. These retinal changes appear to account for most, if not all, of the increase in the behaviorally measured sensitivity to light during this period. Beyond 57 weeks, the large increase in behavioral sensitivity must reside mainly beyond the retina. Identifying the sites of these changes is currently hindered by the absence of a behavioral model of the adult system that incorporates sites and mechanisms of noise.

REFERENCES

ABRAMOV, I., GORDON, J., HENDRICKSON, A., HAINLINCE, L., DOBSON, V., AND LABOSSIERE, E. (1982). The retina of the newborn human infant. *Science* 217, 265–267.

ARDEN, G. B., CARTER, R. M., HOGG, G. R., POWELL, D. J., ERNST, W. K. J., CLOVER, G. M., LYNESS, A. L., AND QUINLAN, M. P. (1983). Rod and cone activity in patients with dominantly inherited retinitis pigmentosa: comparisons between psychophysical and electroretinographic measurements. *Br. J. Ophthalmol.* 97, 405–418.

BARNET, A. B., LODGE, A., AND ARMINGTON, J. C. (1965). Electroretinogram in newborn human infants. *Science* 148, 651–654.

BAYLOR, D. A., NUNN, B. J., AND SCHNAPF, J. L. (1984). The photocurrent, noise, and spectral sensitivity of rods of the monkey *Macaca fascicularis*. *J. Physiol. (Lond.)* 357, 575–607.

BIRCH, D. G., AND FISH, G. E. (1986). Rod ERGs in children with hereditary retinal degeneration. *J. Pediatr. Ophthalmol. Strabismus* 23, 227–232.

BIRCH, E. E., BIRCH, D. G., HOFFMAN, D. R., AND UAUY, R. D. (1992). Retinal development in very low-weight infants fed diets differing in omega-3 fatty acids. *Invest. Ophthalmol. Vis. Sci.* 33, 2365–2376.

BIRCH, E. E., BIRCH, D. G., PETRIG, B., AND UAUY, R. (1990). Retinal and cortical function of very low birthweight infants at 36 and 57 weeks postconception. *Clin. Vis. Res.* 5, 363–373.

BIRCH, E. E., BIRCH, D. G., AND UAUY, R. D. (1991). Maturation of the oscillatory potential of the human electroretinogram. *Opt. Soc. Am. Techn. Dig. Ser.* 1, 28–31.

BRETON, M. E., AND MONTZKA, D. (1990). Isolation of receptor photocurrent response in the gross electroretinogram. *Opt. Soc. Am. Techn. Dig. Ser.* 3, 58–61.

BROWN, A. M. (1986). Scotopic sensitivity of the two-month-old human infant. *Vision Res.* 26, 707–710.

BROWN, A. M. (1988). Saturation of rod initiated signals in 2-month-old human infants. *J. Opt. Soc. Am.* 5, 2145–2158.

BROWN, K. T. (1968). The electroretinogram: its components and their origin. *Vision Res.* 8, 633–678.

COHN, T. E., AND LASLEY, D. J. (1986). Visual sensitivity. *Annu. Rev. Psychol.* 37, 495–521.

DANNEMILLER, J. L. (1985). The early phase of dark adaptation in human infants. *Vision Res.* 25, 207–212.

DANNEMILLER, J. L., AND BANKS, M. S. (1983). The development of light adaptation in human infants. *Vision Res.* 23, 599–609.

DRUCKER, D. N., AND HENDRICKSON, A. E. (1989). The morphological development of extrafoveal human retina. *Invest. Ophthalmol. Vis. Sci.* 30 (suppl.), 226.

FULTON, A. B., AND HANSEN, R. M. (1982). Background adaptation in human infants: analysis of b-wave responses. *Doc. Ophthalmol.* 31, 191–197.

FULTON, A. B., AND HANSEN, R. M. (1985). Electroretinography: application of clinical studies in infants. *J. Pediatr. Ophthalmol. Strabismus* 22, 251–255.

FULTON, A. B., AND HANSEN, R. M. (1988). Scotopic stimulus/response relations of the b-wave of the electroretinogram. *Doc. Ophthalmol.* 68, 293–304.

FULTON, A. B., AND RUSHTON, W. A. H. (1978). The human rod ERG: correlation with psychophysical responses in light and dark adaptation. *Vision Res.* 18, 793–800.

FULTON, A. B., HANSEN, R. M., DODGE, J., SCHREMSER, J., ARMSTRONG, A., LANIER, F., DAWSON, W. W., AND WILLIAMS, T. P.

(1991). The relation of rhodopsin content and dark adapted sensitivity during human development. *Invest. Ophthalmol. Vis. Sci.* 32 (suppl.), 1043.

GRAHAM, N., AND HOOD, D. C. (1992). Quantal noise, other noise, and decision rules in dynamic models of light adaptation. *Vision Res.* 4, 779–787.

GRANIT, R. (1933). The components of the retinal action potential in mammals and their relation to the discharge in the optic nerve. *J. Physiol. (Lond.)* 77, 207–239.

GRANIT, R. (1947). *Sensory Mechanism of the Retina*. London: Oxford University Press.

GREENSTEIN, V., AND HOOD, D. C. (1986). Test of the decreased responsiveness hypothesis in retinitis pigmentosa. *Am. J. Optom. Physiol. Opt.* 63, 22–27.

GROSE, J., HARDING, G. F. A., WILTON, A. Y., AND BISSENDEN, J. G. (1989). The maturation of the pattern reversal VEP and flash ERG in pre-term infants. *Clin. Vis. Sci.* 4, 239–246.

HAMER, R. D., AND SCHNECK, M. E. (1984). Spatial summation in dark adapted human infants. *Vision Res.* 24, 77–85.

HANSEN, R. M., AND FULTON, A. B. (1989). Psychophysical estimates of ocular media density of human infants. *Vision Res.* 29, 687–690.

HANSEN, R. M., FULTON, A. B., AND HARRIS, S. J. (1986). Background adaptation in human infants. *Vision Res.* 26, 771–779.

HEYNEN, H. G. M., AND VAN NORREN, D. (1985). Origin of the electroretinogram in the intact macaque eye. I. Principle component analysis. *Vision Res.* 25, 697–707.

HOLLENBERG, M. J., AND SPIRA, A. W. (1973). Human retinal development: ultrastructure of the outer retina. *Am. J. Anat.* 137, 357–385.

HOOD, D. C. (1988). Testing hypotheses about development with ERG and incremental threshold data. *J. Opt. Soc. Am.* 5, 2159–2165.

HOOD, D. C. (1990). The ERG and sites and mechanisms of retinal disease, adaptation, and development. In *Advances in Photoreception*. Washington, DC: National Academy Press, pp. 41–58.

HOOD, D. C., AND BIRCH, D. G. (1990a). The a-wave of the human ERG and rod receptor function. *Invest. Ophthalmol. Vis. Sci.* 31, 2070–2081.

HOOD, D. C., AND BIRCH, D. G. (1990b). A quantitative measure of the electrical activity of human and photoreceptors using electroretinography. *Vis. Neurosci.* 5, 379–387.

HOOD, D. C., AND BIRCH, D. G. (1992). A computational model of amplitude and implicit time of the b-wave of the human ERG. *Vis. Neurosci.* 8, 107–126.

HOOD, D. C., AND GREENSTEIN, V. C. (1982). An approach to testing alternative hypothesis of changes in visual sensitivity due to retinal disease. *Invest. Ophthalmol. Vis. Sci.* 23, 96–101.

HOOD, D. C., AND GREENSTEIN, V. (1990). Models of the normal and abnormal rod system. *Vision Res.* 30, 51–68.

JOHNSON, M. A., AND HOOD, D. C. (1988). A theoretical interpretation of ERG abnormalities in central retinal vein occlusion. *Opt. Soc. Am. Techn. Dig.* 3, 84–87.

JOHNSON, M. A., AND MASSOF, R. W. (1988). Photoreceptor sensitivity loss in patients with central retinal vein occlusion and iris neovascularization. *Invest. Ophthalmol. Vis. Sci.* 29 (suppl.), 179.

KARWOSKI, C. J., AND PROENZA, L. M. (1987). Sources and sinks of light-evoked $D[K^+]_o$ in the vertebrate retina. *Can. J. Physiol. Pharmacol.* 65, 1009–1017.

KRETZER, F. L., AND HITTNER, H. M. (1985). Initiating events in the development of retinopathy of prematurity. In W. A. SILVERMAN AND J. T. FLYNN (eds.). *Retinopathy of Prematurity*. Oxford: Blackwell.

MACTIER, H., DEXTER, J. D., HEWLETT, J. E., LATHAM, C. B., AND WOODRUFF, C. W. (1988). The electroretinogram in preterm infants. *J. Pediatr.* 113, 607–612.

MANN, I. (1950). *The Development of the Human Retina.* Orlando, FL: Grune & Stratton.

MASSOF, R. W., WU, L., FINKELSTEIN, D., PERRY, D., STARR, S. J., AND JOHNSON, M. A. (1984). Properties of electroretinographic intensity-response functions in retinitis pigmentosa. *Doc. Ophthalmol.* 57, 279–296.

METS, M. B., PASS, A., SMITH, V. C., POKORNY, J., AND NEILSEN, J. (1989). The electroretinogram in the first year of life in very low birth weight humans. *Invest. Ophthalmol. Vis. Sci.* 30 (suppl.), 317.

MILLER, R. F., AND DOWLING, J. E. (1970). Intracellular responses of the Müller (glial) cells of the mudpuppy retina: their relation to b-wave of the electroretinogram. *J. Neurophysiol.* 33, 323–341.

NEWMAN, E. A., AND ODETTE, L. L. (1984). Model of electroretinogram b-wave generation: a test of the K^+ hypothesis. *J. Neurophysiol.* 51, 164–183.

PACKER, O., HENDRICKSON, A. E., AND CURCIO, C. A. (1990). Developmental redistribution of photoreceptors across the *Macaca nemestrina* (pigtail macaque) retina. *J. Comp. Neurol.* 298, 472–494.

PEACHEY, N. S., ALEXANDER, K. R., AND FISHMAN, G. A. (1989). The luminance-response function of the dark-adapted human electroretinogram. *Vision Res.* 29, 263–270.

PENN, R. D., AND HAGINS, W. A. (1972). Kinetics of the photocurrent of retinal rods. *Biophys. J.* 12, 1073–1094.

POWERS, M. K., SCHNECK, M. S., AND TELLER, D. Y. (1981). Spectral sensitivity of human infants at absolute visual threshold. *Vision Res.* 21, 1005–1016.

SCHNECK, M. E., HAMER, R. D., PACKER, O. S., AND TELLER, D. Y. (1984). Area threshold relations at controlled retinal locations in 1-month-old human infants. *Vision Res.* 24, 1753–1763.

TELLER, D. Y. (1979). The forced choice preferential looking method: a psychophysical technique for use with human infants. *Infant Behav. Dev.* 2, 135–153.

UAUY, R. D., BIRCH, D. G., BIRCH, E. E., TYSON, J. E., AND HOFFMAN, D. R. (1990). Effect of dietary omega-3 fatty acid on retinal function of very-low-birth-weight neonates. *Pediatr. Res.* 28, 485–492.

WERNER, J. S. (1982). Development of scotopic sensitivity and the absorption spectrum of the human ocular media. *J. Opt. Soc. Am.* 72, 247–258.

WINKELMAN, J. E., AND HORSTEN, G. P. M. (1962). The ERG of premature and full-term born infants during their first days of life. *Ophthalmologica* 143, 92–101.

ZETTERSTROM, B. (1951). The clinical electroretinogram. IV. The electroretinogram in children during the first days of life. *Acta Ophthalmol. (Copenh.)* 29, 295–304.

ZETTERSTROM, B. (1952). The electroretinogram in prematurely born children. *Acta Ophthalmol. (Copenh.)* 30, 405–408.

30 | Improving infant evoked response measurement

ANTHONY M. NORCIA

One of the major challenges facing researchers in the field of infancy has been the development of appropriate and effective methodologies for the objective assessment of visual function. It goes without saying that the limited response repertoire of the infant precludes the wholesale importation of methodology from traditional psychophysics, electrophysiology, or the clinic. The difficulty of the situation becomes worse in the face of visual impairment and is particularly forbidding in the case of infants who present with multiple handicaps, including neurological impairment.

This chapter outlines a number of ways of improving the production, recording, and analysis of the steady-state visual evoked potential as it is applied to the study of normal and abnormal infant development. We first outline several new signal processing methods that are anticipated to yield substantial improvements in the signal-to-noise ratio (SNR): the application of modern time-domain filtering techniques, multichannel recording, and robust statistical estimation procedures. Improving SNR—or the ability to detect the response—is of vital importance to any application of evoked potential recording. The visually evoked potential (VEP) is, after all, a small signal buried in a large amount of electroencephalographic (EEG) noise- and movement-related artifact. SNR plays a dominant role in determining both systematic and statistical errors of measurement. Systematic errors involve either the consistent under- or overestimation of visual performance. This type of error is of importance to both the visual theorist and the visual diagnostician/therapist. What is the grating acuity of a 4-month-old infant? What is the absolute loss associated with a particular infant's congenital cataract? Statistical errors define the precision with which a given measurement can be made. Statistical errors limit the theorist's ability to discriminate among competing models of visual performance and limit the diagnostician's ability to discriminate normal function from subtly (or not so subtly) abnormal function.

A second theme of this chapter is the interaction between theoretical and clinical questions and the design of the experimental paradigm for making the appropriate measurements. Depending on the intended application, different forces guide the choice of visual stimulus and the particular analysis of the response. The questions here are both "what" to measure and "how" to measure it. In some instances, one might know in advance that a particular threshold measurement is appropriate. One must then determine what aspects of the response reflect that threshold and design the experimental procedure and analysis so as to provide sufficient SNR to make the measurement. In other cases one might be interested in whether a particular neuronal interaction is present in infants or what the degree of selectivity for a visual feature might be. Several experimental paradigms that show promise in each of these areas but that have not yet been fully explored in infants are presented.

SPECIAL CHALLENGES OF PEDIATRIC LOW-VISION ASSESSMENT

Abnormal visual development can result from a host of factors. Genetic abnormalities cause a number of inherited retinal degenerations (Lambert et al., 1989) and some forms of congenital cataract (Merin and Crawford, 1971). Abnormalities can develop as the result of intrauterine infection (toxoplasmosis, cytomegalovirus), maternal systemic disease or substance abuse, hydrocephalus, or failures of embryogenesis of ocular structures (Buncic, 1987). Perinatal complications such as birth asphyxia produce cortical blindness (Lambert et al., 1987). Premature birth is associated with a wide range of visual complications, most notably retinopathy of prematurity (Keith and Kitchen, 1983; Ben Sira et al., 1988). During the postnatal period, abnormal refractive errors and strabismus can cause impairment through the development of amblyopia (Cuiffreda et al., 1990). Trauma, either accidental or through battering, can cause impairment (Frank et al., 1985).

For each of these conditions accurate information regarding the level of visual function of an individual infant would be of benefit when settling on a diagnosis, for providing parents with accurate functional information, for designing and monitoring treatment, rehabilitation, or an educational program, and in some cases for family genetic counseling.

Even normal infants fixate a test pattern for only short periods. Infants with visual loss typically have shorter fixation bouts and often present with erratic eye movements, or nystagmus. If vision loss is unilateral, an occlusive eye patch must be used to isolate each eye's response. Patches are generally well tolerated except in cases with severe unilateral visual impairment. In these cases it is often possible to obtain only limited data from the nonpreferred eye.

Many infants with severe visual impairment also have other developmental disabilities. It is not uncommon for visual loss to coexist with disorders that cause seizures. These infants are often medicated with drugs that, although controlling seizure activity, also reduce evoked potential activity. Systemic disease or medications can also alter the VEP (Hoyt, 1984). A significant number of infants who are referred for visual function testing are spastic and have uncontrollable muscle spasms that produce significant electromyographic artifacts. Many infants with severe visual impairment have nystagmus, which produces retinal image motion that reduces VEP amplitude. It also goes without saying that visual impairment per se can have profound effects on the amplitude of VEP activity.

The need for accurate measures of sensory function in visually impaired infants is critically important, as the developing visual system is most vulnerable to disease during infancy and is at the same time most amenable to treatment. During the first months of life, visual function improves dramatically; and the anatomy of the retina, lateral geniculate nucleus (LGN), and cortex take on more adult-like form. Grating acuity reaches one-half the adult level by 8 months of age (Norcia and Tyler, 1985) and contrast sensitivity by 10 weeks of age (Norcia et al., 1990). These functional changes parallel anatomical development: Foveal cone density and morphology change dramatically during the first year of life and are markedly advanced from the neonatal state by 15 months of age (Hendrickson and Youdelis, 1984). The dendritic morphology of the LGN relay nucleus becomes indistinguishable from that of the adult by 9 months of age (deCourten and Garey, 1982), and the volume of striate cortex reaches adult levels by 8 months of age (Huttenlocher et al., 1982). During the early phase of visual development, synapses are overproduced until a peak number is reached at 8 months of age (Huttenlocher et al., 1982). After this point, synapses are selectively eliminated until the adult density is reached by about 11 years of age (Huttenlocher et al., 1982). The formation of effective synapses in cortex and the subsequent elimination of ineffective synapses

occurs only during early development, and both these processes are critically dependent on the pattern of activity generated by visual stimulation. If a disease process is present during the early developmental period, both synapse formation and subsequent synapse elimination may be dramatically altered (so-called cortical plasticity).

The severity of visual loss accompanying disease during infancy depends not only on the severity of the disease per se (e.g., the density of a cataract) but also on its timing during development: the earlier the insult, the more profound the debility. On the other hand, the plasticity of cortical connections, although making the developing visual system vulnerable to disease, also confers on it a remarkable ability to regain normal function through properly timed and applied therapeutic interventions.

Despite the inherent difficulties of testing infants, infant vision researchers have had considerable success in acquiring information regarding the visual developmental status of infants and young children with a wide range of disorders. We believe, however, that significant improvements in technique are needed for widespread application of the VEP as a measure of function in visually impaired infants.

Higher SNR techniques would increase the probability of successful detection of responses made during shorter, less demanding presentations. The small signals of the severely visually impaired infant would be recorded with greater regularity and higher accuracy. Shortened presentation time would allow the examiner to conduct multiple tests, either to replicate important results or to examine different aspects of visual function within a single recording session. Advanced instrumentation and methodology will also provide a more complete description of the evoked response, which may yield increased diagnostic value in and of itself.

QUANTITATIVE ASSESSMENT OF VISION USING THE SWEEP VEP

In the past our approach to the problem of visual function assessment in infants has been to measure a variety of visual thresholds in infants using the "sweep VEP." The sweep VEP is based on Fourier analysis of the steady-state VEP (SSVEP). SSVEPs are produced whenever a periodic, time-varying stimulus is presented to the visual system. The SSVEP response consists of a series of harmonically related, narrow-band components that are integer multiples of the stimulation frequency [see Regan (1989) for a review of contemporary steady-state methodology].

Using Fourier analytical methods, the SNR of the SSVEP is usually sufficiently high to allow detection of

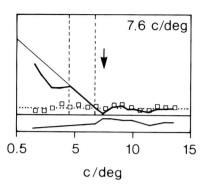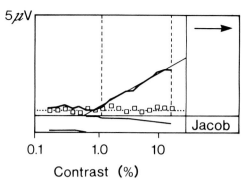

FIG. 30-1. Examples of spatial frequency (left) and contrast (right) sweep VEP records obtained from human infants. Thresholds are estimated by extrapolation of the high SNR portion of the curve to zero amplitude (cessation of visually driven cortical activity).

the VEP response while the experimenter "sweeps" or continuously changes the stimulus value. By sweeping the size of a bar pattern from coarse to fine, the VEP can be used to measure visual acuity (Regan, 1977; Tyler et al., 1979; Norcia and Tyler, 1985). Our emphasis on threshold measurement is different from the traditional analysis of waveform shape (peak amplitude and latency) that has been more widely used, especially in clinical investigations (Regan, 1989; Skarf, 1989).

Spatial frequency and contrast sweep VEP records are shown in Figure 30-1. The upper panels plot the amplitude of the second harmonic pattern reversal response as a function of spatial frequency (left) or contrast (right). The lower panels plot the response phase. Threshold is estimated by extrapolation of the amplitude versus spatial frequency or the amplitude versus contrast function to zero amplitude. The use of steady-state stimulation coupled with Fourier analysis affords sufficiently high SNR to be able to recover the response in near real time; in the top records of Figure 30-1 the analysis was conducted over a running 2-second data window. Each 10-second trial presents patterns spanning the full range of spatial frequencies (or contrasts) appropriate for the infant's developmental status. Using this technique in normal infants, we have routinely made 15–20 threshold determinations in single recording sessions lasting 20–45 minutes. Our usual practice is to acquire three to six 10-second replications of a given stimulation condition. In normal infants the repeatability of the acuity measures is about 0.5 octave (Hamer et al., 1989). We can routinely measure contrast thresholds of less than 1% in infants older than 10 weeks of age (Norcia et al., 1990).

THRESHOLD ASSUMPTION

The extrapolation to zero amplitude technique for assigning threshold values implicitly assumes that the

evoked response amplitude actually goes to zero at a nonzero value of the stimulus—that is, that there truly is a threshold below which there is no stimulus-related activity in visual cortex. The experimenter can never observe this threshold directly because the visually driven signals arriving from cortex are obscured by a large amount of electrical noise from the EEG and muscle electrical activity. The stimulus–response relation assumed by our analysis is illustrated in Figure 30-2. We plotted response amplitude (R) as a function of stimulus intensity (on a log axis). This stimulus/response relation—a linear increase of amplitude as a function of log stimulus intensity—is believed to hold for luminance contrast (Campbell and Maffei, 1970). The effect of

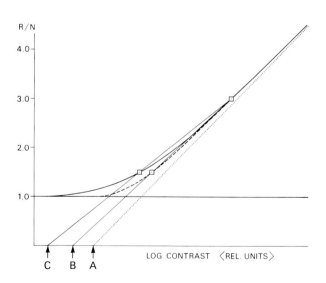

FIG. 30-2. Stimulus/response function from Norcia et al. (1989). The evoked response is modeled as a linear increase in amplitude as a function of log contrast, starting at a threshold value, below which there is no stimulus-related activity. The presence of additive noise distorts the true shape of the stimulus/response function and can lead to small systematic overestimates of sensitivity. (From Norcia et al., 1989. Measurement of spatial contrast sensitivity with the swept contrast VEP. *Vision Res.* 29, 627–637. By permission.)

noise is to distort the shape of the "stimulus–response function" by varying amounts depending on the SNR. At high SNRs, the distortion by noise is negligible. At low SNRs, the apparent amplitude of the signal is inflated by noise, and there is a tendency toward systematic overestimation of sensitivity. In practice, the overestimate is small when the extrapolation is based on a contrast response function with "reasonable" SNR. However, when all of the available measurements are of low SNR, the variability can be large. In any situation where a relation of this kind is found, it is of considerable importance to attain the highest possible SNR. It can be done by increasing the signal strength through appropriate stimulus design or by decreasing the noise level by careful signal analysis and through control of the infant's behavior.

MODERN SIGNAL PROCESSING METHODS APPLIED TO THE SSVEP

The current use of Fourier analytical techniques has gone a long way toward providing high SNR recordings based on the SSVEP. However, there are a number of limitations of the Fourier-based methods that make them less than ideal for the sweep VEP. Use of the swept parameter technique necessitates calculating the spectrum over short time windows (0.25–4.00 seconds) that are continuously shifted over longer data records (10–40 seconds). One consequence of the short data records needed to resolve time-varying sweep responses is that frequency resolution is poor and SNR is modest with the currently applied methods. Spectral leakage through window side lobes is a significant problem. It has not been fully appreciated by workers in the field of evoked potentials that the discrete Fourier transform (DFT) method is an overly general procedure that is optimum only for detecting sine waves of *unknown* frequency and phase in Gaussian white noise. We are just now beginning to use methods designed to achieve improved SNR by fully exploiting the experimenter's prior knowledge of the exact frequency of the response and that utilize modern methods that are both data-adaptive and optimal for non-Gaussian and nonstationary noise distributions, such as the EEG.

Numerous "high-resolution" spectrum estimators have been developed since the 1970s that provide better frequency resolution than is possible with the Fourier transform method. Our work exploits both high resolution spectrum estimation and modern adaptive filtering techniques. Both the spectrum estimation and adaptive filter techniques are based on parametric models of the signal and noise distributions. There are literally hundreds, if not thousands, of reports on high resolution estimators and adaptive filters for use in the fields

of radar, sonar, image processing, radio astronomy, biomedicine, speech analysis and synthesis, geophysics, seismology, and oceanography. This revolution has largely bypassed the evoked potential community, although a few applications of modern spectrum analysis to the VEP have been presented in the literature. A high resolution spectrum analysis procedure, linear predictive coding, has been applied to the analysis of transient VEPs (Norcia et al., 1986). The technique was sufficiently powerful to be able to detect single-trial responses. Similar results had been obtained previously for electroretinographic (ERG) recordings (Gur and Zeevi, 1980). Other workers have developed adaptive filters for the transient evoked potential (Thakor, 1987), but there is only one brief report on modern filtering techniques applied to the SSVEP (Eizenmann et al., 1989).

Because steady-state stimulation forces the response to occur at a known frequency, we can use this prior knowledge to eliminate a large proportion of the EEG noise by first band-pass filtering the EEG over a narrow band centered on the frequency of interest. Because we know in advance which frequencies are signal frequencies and which are noise, we can virtually eliminate the potential for leakage by applying a prefilter that passes only the regions of the spectrum around the response-component frequencies. This operation by itself is effective in improving the SNR of the conventional Fourier-based method (Fig. 30-3). We are also working with an additional step where the resulting time domain waveform with its "improved" SNR is then submitted to a new high-resolution spectrum analysis procedure (mean forward/backward prediction, or MFBP) (Tang, 1990; Tang and Norcia, 1990).

Figure 30-3 compares the conventional DFT method with two variants of our two-stage procedure: (1) bandpass filter followed by DFT; and (2) bandpass filter followed by MFBP. The data are from a simulation study in which known amplitude sine waves were buried in prerecorded samples of human EEGs. In the left panel we plotted a measure of phase coherence (Rayleigh statistic) (Mardia, 1982) as a function of the SNR of a sine wave in EEG noise, and in the right panel we plotted the estimated amplitude of a known sine wave of unit amplitude, again in EEG noise. The first point of interest is that comparable levels of phase coherence are obtained at SNRs that are a factor of about 5 db lower with the new methods. The middle panel plots the accuracy of each of the three methods for determining the amplitude of a known sinusoid. At high SNRs, each of the techniques produces a nearly correct amplitude measurement. This region of the curve is comparable to the rightmost portion of Figure 30-2. As SNR decreases, all of the measures increasingly overestimate the amplitude of the test signal, a natural consequence of the addition EEG noise to the signal, as

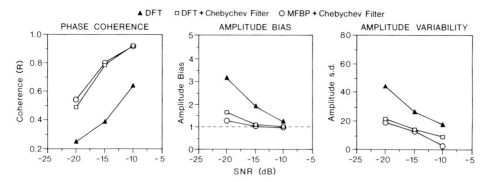

FIG. 30-3. Comparison of the phase coherence, amplitude bias, and amplitude variability of the DFT and MFBP methods as a function of the SNR of a unit amplitude, 10 Hz sine-wave in high-alpha activity EEG noise. The MFBP and prefiltered DFT methods have higher coherence, lower amplitude bias, and variability at all signal levels, particularly at the lowest signal levels. MFBP consistently outperforms either DFT procedure. ▲ = DFT; □ = DFT + Chebychev filter; ○ = MFBP + Chebychev filter.

illustrated in Figure 30-2. It is clear, however, that over-estimation of true signal amplitude is substantially less with the newer methods. Comparable accuracies are attained at about 6- to 10-db-lower SNRs with the new methods than with the DFT alone. The variability of the amplitude measure is shown in the right-hand portion of Figure 30-3. Again the newer methods provide significantly less variable measures of the true signal values. These methods thus provide less biased and less variable estimates of the parameters of the signal. The MFBP results in further improvements, particularly for short data records.

How do the new methods perform for human VEP data? We have begun to look at this question in adults using an experimental protocol designed to mimic our simulation results. We varied the SNR of the VEP by systematically varying stimulus contrast. Each of five observers viewed a series of pattern-reversing gratings that ranged in contrast from 0.5% to 80.0% (none of the observers could detect the 0.5% contrast gratings under the conditions of the test). The gratings were presented for 10 seconds at each contrast, and the record was broken into forty 0.25-second records. Each of the three methods was used to calculate the amplitude and phase of the VEP for each record. The experiment thus compared the ability of the different methods to operate on short data records, such as those that might be used in a swept parameter experiment.

The upper panel of Figure 30-4 shows the estimated amplitude of the VEP as a function of contrast for one of the observers. The first point to observe is that the estimated noise level for the lowest contrast pattern is about a factor of 2 lower for the newer methods than for the conventional DFT. The amplitude estimates con-

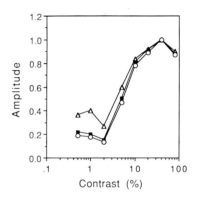

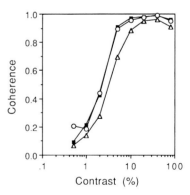

FIG. 30-4. Human VEP contrast response functions. (Top) Amplitude of the pattern reversal response plotted as a function of stimulus contrast. The raw data were processed using three methods: △ = data processed with the DFT; ■ = data first passed through a digital bandpass filter before the DFT was calculated; ○ = digital filter followed by the MFPB procedure. The DFT-processed data shows about twofold less overall improvement in SNR between the threshold region and 80% contrast compared to the two new methods. (Bottom) Coherence of the VEP phase across repeated response epochs plotted as a function of contrast for each of the three methods. Both of the newer methods achieve higher coherence at lower response levels.

verge with one another at high SNR. This situation is exactly analogous to our simulation results in Figure 30-3. The first several points of the DFT amplitude versus contrast response function represent systematic overestimates of the true VEP amplitude. The lower panel of the figure plots response coherence. It can be seen that the response is more detectable with the newer methods and that detectability increases more rapidly at low contrasts with the new methods than it does for the DFT.

An improvement in SNR of 6 dB (factor of 2) should allow an experimenter to attain the same SNR as previously possible with four times less looking time on the part of the infant. Put another way, one should be able to attain the same level of statistical error with half as many trials of one-half the duration of a conventional DFT analysis. Conversely, for the same looking time, measurements should be obtainable with significantly improved statistical and systematic errors.

IMPROVING MEASUREMENTS THROUGH MULTICHANNEL RECORDING

Clinical and developmental studies using the steady-state VEP have almost always used only one or two recording channels (see reviews in Skarf, 1989; Regan, 1989), largely because of technical limitations of the available hardware. However, such an analysis presupposes that the response amplitude is always optimal at the chosen electrode site(s) for all stimuli and all individuals regardless of age or diagnostic category. That this assumption may be overly simple is illustrated in Figure 30-5, which presents 21-channel topographical maps of the SSVEPs recorded from one observer using pattern on/off and pattern reversal presentation modes. These maps come from a larger set recorded in a group of 14 observers (Baseler et al., 1991).

With steady-state topographical mapping, one forms an amplitude (and phase) map for each integer har-

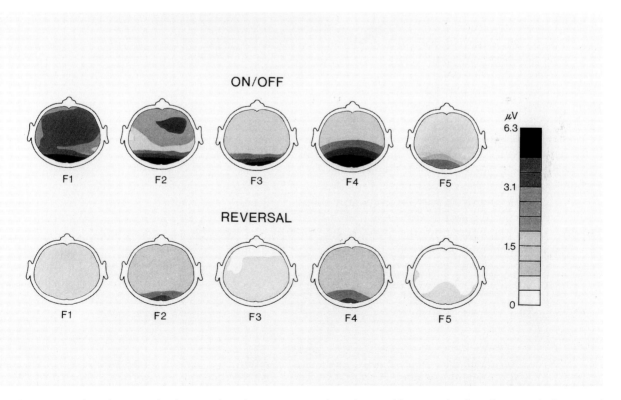

FIG. 30-5. Twenty-one channel topographical maps of steady-state evoked potentials evoked by two stimuli in the same observer. Stimulus frequency was 3 Hz; response frequencies were F1 = 3 Hz; F2 = 6 Hz; F3 = 9 Hz; F4 = 12 Hz; F5 = 15 Hz. On/off modulated responses, represented in the top panel are more widely distributed over the scalp, are of larger amplitude, and occur at both even and odd harmonies of the input frequency. Pattern reversal responses (bottom panel) occur only at the even harmonic of the input frequency and are concentrated over a smaller region of the scalp.

monic multiple of the stimulation frequency. In this experiment, the stimuli were all modulated at a base rate of 3 Hz. A number of characteristic features are apparent. The first is that the reversal stimuli produce responses only at even-numbered harmonics of the stimulus frequency, whereas the on/off stimuli produce responses at both even- and odd-harmonic multiples. The second is that the pattern of activity over the scalp is different for the two stimuli. The pattern on/off response shows activity over widely distributed regions of the scalp, some of them far forward of the occipital leads. The functional significance, if any, of these more anterior regions of activity is an interesting question for future research. It is certainly suggestive of widespread activation of more than just primary visual cortex.

We have also noted that not only do different stimuli produce different topographical distributions of potential over the scalp, but that there is nontrivial, interindividual variation in topography within a given stimulus condition. These two observations make it unlikely that a single recording channel, or even two channels, is sufficient to consistently tap the location of largest response amplitude, let alone to describe adequately the topography of the response. Having more electrodes ensures that the highest amplitude region is sampled in each observer, improving SNR by an unknown, but possibly large, amount in a worse case situation (see Fig. 30-6 below). A second point is that information from multiple electrodes with signal on them can be averaged or combined in a number of ways to increase the detectability of the response. Finally and perhaps most importantly, the changes in scalp topography that no doubt occur during development or in different diseases may be of substantial theoretical/diagnostic value.

There are several possible schemes for combining data across channels to more effectively measure the VEP stimulus/response function. One procedure involves calculating response amplitude as a vector quantity based on the Pythagorean Sum of all electrode sites for a given response harmonic. That is, for the jth harmonic, we can form both a *coherent* average

$$|\vec{A_j}| = \frac{\left[\left(\sum_{i=1}^{n} A_{ij} \sin \phi_{ij} \right)^2 + \left(\sum_{i=1}^{n} A_{ij} \cos \phi_{ij} \right)^2 \right]^{1/2}}{n}$$

where n = the total number of channels and A_{ij} and ϕ_{ij} = the amplitude and phase, respectively, for the ith channel, jth harmonic. It is also possible to form an *incoherent* average across channels:

$$\langle A_j \rangle = \frac{\sum_{i=1}^{n} A_{ij}}{n}.$$

The simplest multi-channel detection scheme involves always taking the single channel that has the largest amplitude. This scheme will always outperform a single channel scheme because it guarantees that the largest amplitude location on the scalp is sampled. Beyond this, additional gains may be accrued by averaging responses across channels, to the extent that several channels contain significant signals and that are contaminated by uncorrelated noise. If, however, only one channel has a strong signal, or if many "superfluous" channels are included, multichannel averaging schemes founder. The primary guard against this problem is to focus the recording sites in regions that map the most probable location of the peak response. Averaging channels over the high response region reduces the likelihood of including channels that do not have signals. The SNR improvement obtainable by averaging multiple channels depends on the absolute signal values at each channel and the extent of correlation of the background noise across all channels in the average.

Instead of the "all or one" procedures described above, one can select a subset of channels for analysis using a "jack-knife" or "bootstrap" approach to combining information across channels. This procedure is adapted from the field of robust statistical estimation (Efron, 1979). In the jack-knife method, a measure (e.g., the multichannel SNR) is computed, first, from all the data at hand and, second (and repeatedly), from each combination of channels—less one. The usual use of the jack-knife method is to provide a robust estimate of the measure being computed and an error term for the measure that is not dependent on the underlying noise distribution. The jack-knife method can also be used to detect "outliers"—those channels that produce the largest increments and decrements to the multichannel average. In this way one can rank order the channels in terms of their contribution to the multichannel average and then apply a channel weighting factor that emphasizes the positive contributions and deemphasizes or eliminates the negatively contributing channels. A further advantage of the jack-knife procedure is that it can provide robust amplitude and phase estimates as well as error variance measures for the multichannel average and any regressions derived from it (Norcia et al., 1985a).

These schemes have yet to be tried in adults, let alone in infants, but it is manifestly clear from Figure 30-5 that the current practice of characterizing the evoked response at one or two electrodes is unlikely to represent the response adequately. In addition to the relatively mundane concern of always finding the region of largest amplitude, there is a great deal of information in the scalp topography produced by each kind of stimulation. At the most basic level, one can conclude that if the scalp topography produced by two different stimuli that fall on the same retinal locations is different, different mechanisms have been engaged by the different stimuli.

IMPROVED DETECTION OF SMALL VEPS BY RECORDING MULTIPLE RESPONSE HARMONICS

A common practice for measuring steady-state VEPs has been to record at relatively high stimulation rates and to measure only a single harmonic of the response (at one or two electrodes). Absolute EEG noise levels vary considerably at different response harmonics; and although it is generally true that the second harmonic is the largest amplitude component of the steady-state reversal response, higher harmonics sometimes have larger SNRs owing to the rapid falloff of EEG (noise) amplitude at high frequencies. When lower stimulation frequencies are used, the higher harmonics of both the pattern reversal on pattern on-off responses can be large. In Figure 30-5, the fourth harmonic was actually the largest component of the pattern on/off response.

Examples of the complex harmonic structure of steady-state reversal and pattern on/off responses are shown in Figure 30-6. In this experiment, the stimulation frequency was 4 Hz and the spatial frequency of the grating 3.0 cycles/degree (cpd). Two channels were recorded symmetrically about the midline. First it should be noted that each stimulus produces a response that consists of many harmonics, including significant activity up to the 10th harmonic at 40 Hz (upper right panel, on/off stimulation). Second, for this observer, the largest component of the on/off response was nearly four times larger than the largest component of the reversal response. We return to this finding in a later section. Third, the on/off spectrum contains more components than does the reversal response; and finally, the particular component patterns observed depend strongly on the electrode placement. The second harmonic of the reversal response (lower right) was nearly three times larger than at the mirror symmetrical recording site (lower left).

One of the main features of the on/off VEP that should be exploited is the fact that the response spectrum for these stimuli contains both odd and even harmonics, whereas the spectrum resulting from reversing stimuli contains predominantly even harmonics. With on-off stimuli one therefore has approximately twice the number of frequencies at which the response can be detected compared to reversing stimuli. In the data set presented in Figure 30-5, it was possible to record six harmonics with on-off stimulation in a situation where only three harmonics were recordable with pattern reversal.

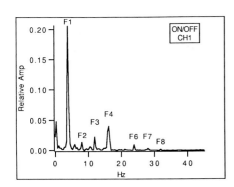

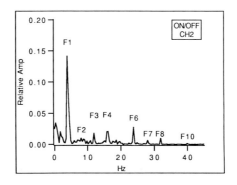

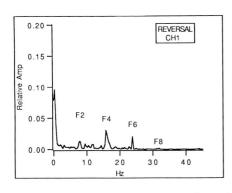

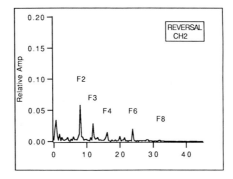

FIG. 30-6. FFT spectra for pattern on/off stimulation (top panels) and pattern reversal (bottom panels). Left panels are for a derivation of Oz versus O1, right panels for a derivation of Oz versus O2. The on/off response has the largest single component and also has more components, making it easier to detect in noise.

FREQUENCY DIVERSITY METHODS FOR VEP DETECTION

A common practice in modern communication systems is to broadcast a message simultaneously over multiple frequency bands in hopes that the SNR in one or more of the noisy communications "channels" is high enough to allow the message to be received. It is known as "frequency diversity transmission." We suggest a somewhat analogous procedure VEP recording that combines information across multiple response harmonics.

A simple example illustrates how one such detection scheme that uses multiple response harmonics can afford detection of smaller evoked responses than when a single harmonic is used. We assume that the noise at each harmonic is uncorrelated. (Preliminary work indicates that this condition is substantially the case.)

For each harmonic, we select a threshold such that the probability of noise being higher than the threshold is p_h. If our criterion for the acceptance of a signal is that *each* of n individual harmonics is above its respective threshold, the probability that noise will pass this criterion is $p = p_h^n$. That is, if we want the overall probability for noise to pass the criterion to be p, the threshold for each harmonic can be set $p_h = \sqrt[n]{p} > p$. For example, if we desire to maintain an overall 1% probability that noise will pass the criterion ($p = 0.01$), and if we have two independent observations at different harmonics, the threshold for each harmonic can be set such that $p_h = \sqrt[2]{p} = 0.10$. If three independent harmonics are available, an overall 1% probability of noise to pass the criterion can be attained with a 0.215 level in each channel.

It is not necessary, as in this example, to use equal, fixed thresholds at each channel; rather, a joint probability can be calculated. In either case, a larger number of harmonics allows lower thresholds for each harmonic with the same overall probability of noise passing the criterion.

The exact gain to be expected from this particular scheme depends on the degree of cross-harmonic correlation, the SNR of each of the harmonics used, and the form of the underlying EEG noise distribution. In Figure 30-5, the first four harmonics of the pattern on/off response had comparable amplitudes. In Figure 30-6, the first harmonic amplitude was larger than the rest, but its SNR was nearly matched by a number of the higher harmonics that had lower noise levels.

A more direct analogy to the communications example is simply to monitor multiple harmonics and say that there is signal present if any one of the harmonics is above threshold. In this case the individual harmonic thresholds must be *raised* because multiple tests are being conducted.

The foregoing discussion of the signal processing of the SSVEP applies to any stimulus one might choose, as it is always of use to obtain the highest possible SNR. It is also advantageous to describe the response completely, both as an aid to improving one's ability to measure small responses and to be able to understand the processes underlying the response, some of which might change with development or disease.

IMPROVING MEASUREMENTS THROUGH JUDICIOUS CHOICE OF STIMULI

There are several factors that govern the choice of the visual stimulus used for both clinical and basic science studies that utilize the VEP: (1) The responses to that stimulus must be affected in a consistent and preferably dramatic way by the disease under study or by normal development; (2) the response generated must be large enough to be consistently recorded; (3) the form of the response versus stimulus intensity function should be well behaved, easy to characterize, and consistent across patients with the same disease or across normals of the same age; and (4) the stimulus must allow the investigator sufficient control to rule out contributions of confounding stimulus variables.

This section begins by considering a number of issues related to the interplay of stimulus design and response analysis. The measurement of grating acuity is used as a paradigm case to illustrate each of the factors listed at the beginning of this section. Grating acuity was chosen as a paradigm case, as much of the experimental work on normal visual development during infancy has concerned itself with the growth of acuity and contrast sensitivity and because most clinical studies have also focused on this type of acuity development.

The pattern reversal response is easily recorded in normal infants with the sweep VEP method. Reliable acuity estimates can be obtained in a high percentage of infants, and several thresholds can be measured within the attention span of the infant (Hamer et al., 1989). VEP acuity shows considerable development in normal infants (Marg et al., 1976; Sokol, 1978; Norcia and Tyler, 1985), and VEP acuity measured with pattern reversing gratings is consistently affected by the common childhood disorder amblyopia, although not to the same degree as conventional letter acuity (Orel-Bixler and Norcia, 1986). VEP grating acuity, although not optimally sensitive, is still a valid indicator of visual loss in a wide variety of visual disorders in infants (Orel-Bixler et al., 1989).

When thinking of how to improve clinical acuity measures, one has a choice of making more accurate and robust measurements of grating acuity or finding a more sensitive acuity test. The ultimate definition of success boils down to how well each of the two acuities can be measured in visually impaired infants. A test that is highly sensitive to the disease process but that cannot be quantified is not useful. Ideally, one would like to have it both ways—to be able to obtain the most sensitive functional measure (e.g., stereo or Vernier acuity) at high SNR, even in impaired infants.

Because measures of grating acuity have played the dominant role in both normal developmental and clinical studies, the case of improving the grating acuity measure is considered first. A number of the principles illustrated for the grating acuity case may also apply to studies of other stimulus dimensions. Measurement of Vernier acuity with the sweep VEP is then illustrated. The second part of this section deals with a number of relatively novel visual stimulation techniques that have yet to be widely applied in infancy research.

IMPROVING GRATING ACUITY MEASUREMENT

Previous investigators have reported that the transient pattern on/off response is larger than the reversal response recorded from the same pattern (Spekreijse et al., 1973). We have evidence that it may also be true for the SSVEP. In Figure 30-5 the on/off response was considerably larger than the reversal response recorded at the same spatial and temporal frequency. The first five harmonics of the on/off response peaked at 6.3, 6.4, 5.9, 6.6, and 3.0 μV. The second and fourth harmonics of the reversal response were only 3.9 and 3.7 μV, respectively. The 60–80% greater amplitude of the on/off response at the second and fourth harmonics alone would translate into a factor of 2.5–3.2 times reduction in recording time for this subject. In Figure 30-6, another subject showed a fourfold larger amplitude of the dominant response component for on/off as opposed to reversal stimulation, which translates to a 16-fold reduction in recording time to attain the same SNR. It thus stands to reason that it should be possible to obtain higher SNR measures of grating acuity through the use of pattern on/off rather than pattern reversal stimulation.

It has also been reported that the spatial frequency tuning function of the on/off SSVEP has a simple inverted-U shape, much like the contrast sensitivity function (Remky and Strasburger, 1990). This finding contrasts with the notoriously complex spatial tuning of the pattern reversal response, which often differs widely among individuals (Tyler et al., 1978). Accurate determination of acuity from this function requires finely spaced sampling of a wide range of spatial frequencies spanning the acuity limit (Norcia and Tyler, 1985). The simpler form of the pattern on/off spatial tuning function may make it possible to perform more reliable

threshold estimates based on extrapolations and to obtain accurate estimates on coarser sampling of tuning function obtained from brief recording sets.

Second, Remky and Strasburger (1990) also reported that on/off pattern stimulation produces a constant response phase as a function of spatial frequency, unlike pattern reversal stimulation. A number of authors have noted the latter phenomenon and have indicated that it rules out the use of phase-sensitive detection of the response. Phase-sensitive detection offers a theoretical SNR advantage over phase-insensitive detection such as that afforded by the Fourier transform method (Peli et al., 1988). If an SSVEP can be produced with a constant or nearly constant phase, it is possible to estimate the response phase at high spatial frequency (where response amplitude is low) from estimates made at lower spatial frequencies (where the response amplitude is considerably higher). This information can then be used to aid in the decision as to whether portions of the evoked response amplitude function near threshold are signal or noise.

Can reliable pattern on/off responses be measured using the sweep method? Do all the harmonics contribute over the high spatial frequency range needed to estimate acuity? We have made preliminary measurements of the first four harmonics of the pattern on/off spatial tuning function in adults using the sweep method and a 4-Hz stimulation rate (Fig. 30-7). Spatial tuning functions are shown for the first four harmonics of the response. It should first be noted that each harmonic produces a significant response that extends to high spatial frequencies near the acuity limit. The spatial tuning functions for the first two harmonics are simple low-pass functions. We thus expect that more than one harmonic of the response can be used to form an estimate of threshold.

It thus appears that a relatively minor change in the temporal modulation of a grating pattern may produce a response that is substantially easier to detect on several counts and one in which the evoked potential amplitude versus spatial frequency tuning function may be less complex. It is of interest to see if different components of the on/off response (or the reversal response, for that matter) show different developmental sequences when considered separately. A question here is whether a response component—defined analytically—has any *functional* identity as a physiological component.

ALTERNATIVE VEP RESOLUTION MEASURES

There are of course many ways to define the resolution capabilities of the developing visual system. Developmentalists are interested in charting the development of each of these abilities in order to understand underlying

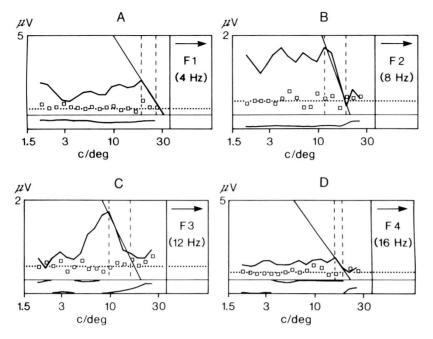

FIG. 30-7. Spatial frequency tuning function for the first, second, third, and fourth harmonics of the 4-Hz pattern on/off VEP. Acuity estimates can be made independently at each of the four harmonics.

visual mechanisms. Clinically, a different approach to acuity measurement is to abandon grating acuity and to seek a test with greater intrinsic sensitivity to pathology. Vernier acuity has been preferred by many as a particularly important measure of fine pattern vision. Vernier acuity is known to be more severely affected than is grating acuity in strabismic amblyopia, one of the most common childhood disorders and one of the disorders where grating acuity tests are known to underestimate the full loss associated with amblyopia (Gstalder and Green, 1971; Levi and Klein, 1982; Mayer et al., 1984). Stereo acuity, on the other hand, is regarded by many as a particularly sensitive test of binocular vision.

Vernier acuity has been measured using both transient VEPs and sweep SSVEPs. The transient VEP studies found that the Vernier-related response was small and difficult to distinguish objectively from confounding motion-related response (Levi et al., 1983; Zak and Berkeley, 1986). The reason for the difficulty is that in order to produce an evoked response elements of the stimulus must be moved to introduce Vernier offsets. The introduction of the Vernier offset and the target motion are simultaneous and thus produce temporally overlapping responses. A given deflection of the transient VEP waveform may thus contain contributions from both movement and Vernier mechanisms. Frequency domain analysis affords rather good SNR and an objective analytical method for separating Vernier-related from motion-related response components (Norcia et al., 1988a). The frequency domain technique

takes advantage of the substantial amplitude asymmetry in the Vernier VEP to the two phases of the stimulus. Levi et al. (1983) observed that the breaking of co-linearity produces a larger response than does the transition from non-co-linearity to co-linearity. Such an asymmetry manifests as the presence of odd-harmonic response components.

A paradigm data set, illustrating the Fourier components of the Vernier VEP is shown in Figure 30-8. The left-hand panels plot the first (odd symmetrical) and second (even symmetrical) harmonics of the Vernier alignment/misalignment response. They are both prominent and have similar thresholds (on the order of 15 arc seconds). The stimulus for the data in the middle panels had an identical set of moving elements—all that differed was the spatial relation between the moving and static elements. In this case, both phases were spatially offset, and the pattern had mirror symmetry. As can be seen in the center panels, the first (odd) harmonic component of the Vernier VEP disappears when neither phase of the stimulus is co-linear. The unique occurrence of odd harmonic components based on co-linearity is consistent with the presence of mechanisms that accurately code the spatial position of features adjacent to one another in the visual field. Although motion-related and Vernier-related response components occur simultaneously in time, they appear to be distinct in the frequency domain because of a fortuitous neuronal response asymmetry. It should be noted that the steady-state Vernier VEP situation is a subclass of the windmill/dartboard stimulus developed by Zemon and Ratliff

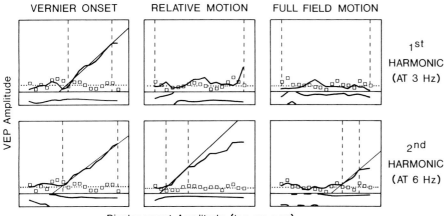

VERNIER ONSET   RELATIVE MOTION   FULL FIELD MOTION

1st HARMONIC (AT 3 Hz)

2nd HARMONIC (AT 6 Hz)

VEP Amplitude

Displacement Amplitude (log arc sec)

FIG. 30-8. Comparison of stimulus response functions for Vernier onset/offset, relative motion, and full-field motion stimuli. (Top) VEP amplitude is plotted versus displacement function for the first harmonic response; only the Vernier stimulus produces a measurable first harmonic. (Bottom) Second harmonic response function plotted for each of the three stimuli; the Vernier and relative motion response function differ slightly from each other and are distinctly different from the full-field response in this observer.

(1982), and our analysis of the Vernier VEP is based on theirs. The right-hand panels of Figure 30-8 plot data from an absolute motion condition in which the whole grating was simply "jittered" back and forth at 3 Hz. Little response is observed at the second harmonic, and none is present at the first harmonic. The fact that the second harmonic is attenuated relative to the alignment/misalignment conditions suggest that there may be response components that are selective for relative (rather than absolute) motion. Separation of these two components is difficult, except in fortuitous cases such as this one, as both relative and absolute motions produce even-order response spectra.

Another VEP amplitude versus Vernier offset response function for an adult is shown in Figure 30-9. In the context of our "design criteria," this response has several desirable features. The first is that the threshold is very low: 14 arc seconds. It is thus well in the range of the visual hyperacuities (Westheimer, 1975). We found that Vernier VEP thresholds are comparable to thresholds for left/right discrimination of the position of the offset measured psychophysically, and we also noted that the Vernier VEP thresholds have an eccentricity dependence similar to that observed for position discrimination (Norcia et al., 1988b). The Vernier VEP response is of reasonable amplitude in adults, as illustrated by the high SNR of the recording in Figures 30-8 and 30-9. The response phase in nearly constant, and the response function is simple in form. These two factors suggest that a relatively coarse sampling of the Vernier stimulus/response function may still yield reliable Vernier acuities. As noted before, the complexity of the pattern reversal amplitude versus spatial-frequency tuning function necessitates a detailed sampling strat-

egy. If the level of detail can be lowered without loss of accuracy, the time saved can be applied toward increasing the SNR.

Another measure of wide interest to both developmentalists and clinicians is stereo acuity. Stereo acuity has been measured behaviorally in infants (Held et al., 1980; Birch et al., 1982) but has been measured in adults only using the VEP (Norcia et al., 1985b). Stereopsis and stereo acuity can be measured using dynamic random-dot stereograms (DRDSs) and the VEP (Norcia et al., 1985b). DRDSs represent what are among the

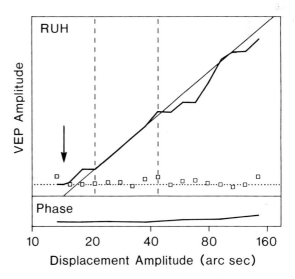

FIG. 30-9. Sweep VEP measurement of Vernier acuity. VEP amplitude versus Vernier offset size function in this observer is a monotonically increasing function with a nearly constant phase. Extrapolation of the suprathreshold portion of the response function to zero amplitude yields a Vernier acuity estimate of 14 arc seconds.

most highly selective visual stimuli in use today: Responses to these targets can arise only after the sight of binocular combination. They are thus ideal from the standpoint of stimulus control and specificity. Unfortunately, the responses generated by these stimuli are small and are thus difficult to detect (Norcia et al., 1985b).

MULTIINPUT STIMULATION/ANALYSIS PARADIGMS

Most applications of the VEP to infant research have measured the response to a single, spatially extended target. It is possible, however, to present two or more targets simultaneously and to measure a response to each of them. The only requirement is that each target has its own temporal signature, which is orthogonal or independent of each of the other targets. Orthogonality is accomplished easily in the SSVEP through the use of different temporal modulation frequencies for each of the targets. Orthogonality can also be achieved through the use of specialized noise sequences (Sutter, 1987).

There are several paradigms that arise with multiple input stimulation. The first to be discussed is the case where the targets are nonoverlapping in space. This technique was utilized by Regan and Milner (1978) as part of an evoked potential perimetry test, and Allen et al. (1989) used the technique to study the development of foveal and peripheral acuity. The stimulus arrangement is illustrated in Figure 30-10. Infants were induced to fixate a small 4 degrees diameter field that contained

a swept spatial frequency or swept contrast grating. A second, peripheral field extended in an arc in the lower field spanning eccentricities of 8–16 degrees. This field was swept simultaneously but at a different temporal frequency. Because the foveal and peripheral targets produced responses that were, in effect, "labeled," they could be distinguished from one another by Fourier analysis. This paradigm allowed the foveal and peripheral acuities and contrast sensitivities to be measured in half the time that would be required if they were measured successively. Second, the paradigm also controls for many state variables, such as level of arousal, fixation stability, or muscle activity that might otherwise be free to vary among successive trials.

A second variation of the multiinput stimulation techniques involves presenting two (or more) stimuli simultaneously to the same retinal areas. Such stimuli may be processed by mechanisms that interact with one another and can be used to measure the selectivity characteristics of visual mechanisms in a variety of masking studies. Several examples of two input masking studies have been presented in the adult VEP literature. Regan and Regan (1987) studied orientation selectivity in adults using a two-input paradigm. Their study exploited a number of the features of multiinput stimulation, each of which is of interest in studies of infants. Regan and Regan employed a vertical test grating that was reversed in contrast at 8 Hz. The response to this grating was observed as a function of the orientation of a second, superimposed grating modulated at 7 Hz. The masker was systematically varied in orientation. The authors

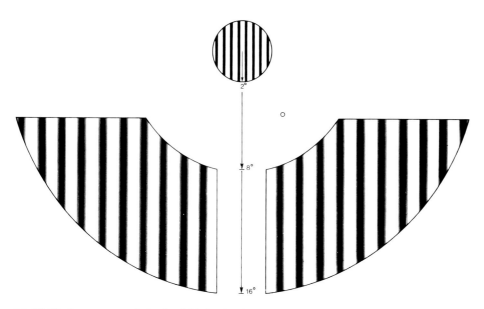

FIG. 30-10. Arrangement of stimulus fields for simultaneous measurement of foveal and peripheral VEPs in infants (Allen et al., 1989). The central field is modulated at one temporal frequency and the peripheral field at another. The two frequencies should not be multiples of one another. Spectrum analysis separates the responses from each field.

then measured response components that were harmonic multiples of the test and mask frequencies. They noted that the amplitude of the response to the test grating went through a minimum over a narrow range of masker orientations centered on the orientation of the test (Fig. 30-11).

Regan and Regan (1987) also measured evoked responses at a number of nonlinear combination frequencies. Responses at nonharmonic combination frequencies occur when the neural mechanisms responding to the different inputs interact in a nonlinear fashion. These authors observed that a nonlinear interaction peaked precisely at the same orientations at which the response to the test grating went through a minimum and vice versa. They also observed a peak in the interaction terms at orthogonal orientations, which is consistent with the presence of cross-orientation inhibition. This paradigm could easily be extended to studies of infant orientation bandwidth and to studies of the development of cross-orientation inhibition (Morrone and Burr, 1986).

The steady-state masking paradigm could of course be extended to a whole host of other stimulus dimensions. Regan (1983) had first used two-component stimulation to study spatial and temporal channel bandwidths using the VEP. Fiorentini et al. (1983) applied the technique to study of spatial channel bandwidth in infants. Masking functions can also be obtained quickly using the sweep VEP, an example of which is illustrated in Figure 30-12. An adult observer was presented with a 4 cpd test grating modulating at 9 Hz. Superimposed on the test was a second masking grating modulated at 7 Hz. The mask was swept logarithmically in spatial frequency between 2 and 8 cpd. The figure plots the amplitude of the response to the test grating as a function of mask spatial frequency. When the mask is within less than 1.0 octave of the spatial frequency of the test, the response to the test is attenuated. From this function a spatial channel bandwidth of 1.0 octave, full width, can be derived. The two curves represent repeated measures in which the direction of the spatial sweep either started at low spatial frequency and swept to high spatial frequency or vice versa. Orientation bandwidths could be measured in a similar fashion.

There are several particularly attractive features of the test/mask paradigm from the point of view of experimental design. The use of a constant test stimulus controls for a host of factors known to affect the evoked response. Unlike studies in which the test is varied parametrically, all parameters of the test here are constant: The retinal area being stimulated does not change, and the spatial and temporal parameters and contrast re-

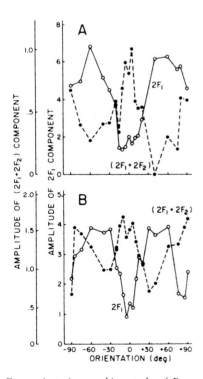

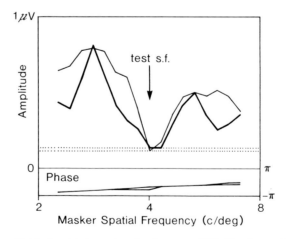

FIG. 30-11. Cross-orientation masking study of Regan and Regan (1987). Open symbols plot the response to a vertical test grating as the function of the orientation of a masking grating; filled symbols plot a response due to nonlinear interaction between the test and the variable orientation mask. The two curves mirror one another: The response to the test is smallest when the interaction term is largest and vice versa. The curves also show evidence of cross-orientation masking. (From Regan and Regan, 1987. Nonlinearity in human visual responses to two-dimensional patterns and a limitation of Fourier methods. *Vision Res.* 27, 2181–2183. By permission.)

FIG. 30-12. Spatial channel tuning by sweep VEP. The figure plots the amplitude of the response from a test grating of 4 cpd modulated at 7 Hz as a function of the spatial frequency of a masking grating modulated at 9 Hz. The spatial frequency of the mask was swept either from low to high or high to low spatial frequency in 10-second trials. The response to the test stimulus is attenuated over a narrow range of masker spatial frequencies, in this case centered on the test frequency.

main constant. All parametric changes in the test response that occur as the mask is changed can therefore be unambiguously attributed to neuronal interaction between the test and the mask. Interestingly, in this context it should be possible to study masking by stimuli that themselves do not even produce evoked potentials, two important examples being static patterns and continuously drifting patterns. In these cases it may be possible to measure indirectly at least some of properties of the mechanism(s) responding to the mask by their influence on the mechanism(s) responding to the test.

A second attractive feature of the masking paradigm is the availability of the nonlinear interaction terms. At the most basic level the simple presence of such terms provides direct evidence that the two inputs interact neuronally. In normal adults, for example, stimulation of one eye with luminance flicker of one frequency and the other eye with another frequency produces a response at the difference frequency that is indicative of the presence of binocular interaction in visual cortex (Baitch and Levi, 1988). This technique has been applied to normal infants (Baitch and Srebro, 1990) and to infants and children with binocular abnormalities (Schmeisser and Baker, 1990).

Nonlinear interactions produce complex patterns of response at many of the possible combination frequencies (Regan and Regan, 1987, 1988). Interpretation of these patterns of response is at present a difficult proposition. In principle, the pattern of nonlinear terms contains a great deal of information about the dynamics of visual processing and the kinds of nonlinear transformations being performed by the visual system. Interpretation of these nonlinear components, however, requires that one have a nonlinear model of the pathway under test. Such models are beginning to appear and may prove fruitful in the future (Regan and Regan, 1988).

CONCLUSION

It should be clear from the foregoing that current and past VEP techniques have tapped only a small proportion of the information available on the scalp that is related to visual processing. In the past, our description of the response has been incomplete. To the extent that VEPs reflect the activity of underlying visual mechanisms, a more extensive descriptive analysis adds significantly. More complete descriptions of the response involve the analysis of all the components of the response and a more thorough analysis of the scalp topography of the response.

A second central issue in improving response measurement in infants is the development of maximally effective signal processing and stimulation procedures for use with short data records. Until better methods of fixation control for infants are developed, measurements of infant evoked responses will, of necessity, be derived from much shorter recordings than are possible with adults. The use of the swept parameter technique also explicitly requires methods that are maximally effective with short data records. Fourier analytical methods lose much of their effectiveness when short data records are used. It appears that a number of procedures developed since the 1970s in such diverse areas as seismology, antenna design, speech processing, and radar may be of great utility in the study of infant evoked potentials. If one cannot make accurate measurements in the first place, all other intended uses of the VEP information become moot.

Greater precision and completeness of the analysis of the SSVEP will contribute to several more general issues in visual physiology as understood by the evoked response. The ultimate goal in evoked potential studies is to relate the patterns of electrical activity recorded on the scalp to the mechanisms of visual processing. In this effort, the completeness with which we analyze the response is an obvious limiting step. Detailed descriptive analysis of the evoked response is a precursor to the formal analysis of the recordings into functional components that can be identified across individuals and that can be shown to reflect aspects of visual processing. Component identification studies are common in the area of transient and event-related potential studies in adults. However, techniques such as prinicipal components analysis and related procedures have only rarely been applied to the SSVEP (Gutowitz et al., 1986). Frequency domain analysis such as that shown in Figure 30-5 represents a first step on the way to future analyses of the SSVEP into components consisting of particular harmonic structures, each with their characteristic topographical distributions. These physiological components can then be correlated with visual function in normal and abnormal observers and across age.

The use of selective stimulation techniques are of paramount importance to VEP recording, as they are in any experimental analysis of the visual system. Unlike psychophysical studies in which the output variable from the infant is essentially a yes/no decision, evoked potential studies can be designed to obtain continuous output measures, complete with timing information related to response dynamics and scalp topography information that is intimately tied to the anatomy of the visual projection. As we saw in the case of the Vernier acuity paradigm, selective stimulation coupled with selective analysis allows one to break the response into functionally related components—in this case the response to Vernier alignment versus the response to motion. In infants one cannot direct the subject to respond to specific aspects of the stimulus. One must remove all the confounds in the stimulus before proceeding. In the case of the Vernier VEP, the responses to the confounded motion and Vernier-related cues can be separated in the analysis owing to the fortuitous nature of nonlinear processing in the visual system.

All this is not to say the evoked potential represents a complete method for analyzing the visual system. In present practice, however, the potential power of the steady-state paradigm for visual systems analysis has been greatly underutilized.

REFERENCES

ALLEN, D., TYLER, C. W., AND NORCIA, A. M. (1989). Development of grating acuity and contrast sensitivity in the central and peripheral field of the human infant. *Invest. Ophthalmol. Vis. Sci.* 30 (suppl.), 311.

BAITCH, L., AND LEVI, D. (1988). Electrophysiological evidence for nonlinear binocular interactions in the human visual cortex. *Vision Res.* 28, 1139–1143.

BAITCH, L., AND SREBRO, R. (1990). Binocular interactions in sleeping and awake human infants. *Invest. Ophthalmol. Vis. Sci.* 31 (suppl.), 251.

BASELER, H., NORCIA, A. M., WONG, P., CARNEY, T., AND KLEIN, S. (1991). VEP topography of perceptually diverse stimuli. *Invest. Ophthalmol. Vis. Sci.* 32 (suppl.), 1273.

BEN SIRA, I., NISSENKORN, I., AND KREMER, I. (1988). Retinopathy of prematurity. *Surv. Ophthalmol.* 33, 1–16.

BIRCH, E. E., GWIAZDA, J., AND HELD, R. (1982). Stereoacuity development for crossed and uncrossed disparities. *Vision Res.* 22, 507–513.

BUNCIC, J. R. (1987). The blind infant. *Pediatr. Clin. North Am.* 34, 1403–1413.

CAMPBELL, F. W., AND MAFFEI, L. (1970). Electrophysiological evidence for the existence of orientation and size detectors in the human visual system. *J. Physiol. (Lond.)* 207, 635–652.

CUIFFREDA, K. J., LEVI, D. M., AND SELENOW, W. (1990). *Amblyopia: Basic and Clinical Aspects.* New York: Butterworth-Heinemann.

DECOURTEN, C., AND GAREY, L. J. (1982). Morphology of the neurons of the human lateral geniculate nucleus and their normal development. *Exp. Brain Res.* 47, 159–171.

EFRON, B. (1979). Bootstrap methods: another look at the jackknife. *Statistician* 7, 1–26.

EIZENMANN, M., McCOLLOUGH, D., HUI, R., AND SKARF, B. (1989). Detection of threshold visual evoked potentials (VEPs). In; Non-invasive assessment of the visual system. *Opt. Soc. Am. Techn. Dig. Ser.* 7, 88–91.

FIORENTINI, A., PIRCHIO, M., AND SPINELLI, D. (1983). Electrophysiological evidence for spatial frequency selective mechanisms in adults and infants. *Vision Res.* 23, 119–127.

FRANK, Y., ZIMMERMAN, R., AND LEEDS, N. M. D. (1985). Neurological manifestations in abused children who have been shaken. *Dev. Med. Child Neurol.* 27, 312–316.

GSTALDER, R. J., AND GREEN, D. G. (1971). Laser interferometric acuity in amblyopia. *J. Pediatr. Ophthalmol.* 8, 251–256.

GUR, M., AND ZEEVI, Y. (1980). Frequency-domain analysis of the human electroretinogram. *J. Opt. Soc. Am.* 70, 53–59.

GUTOWITZ, H., ZEMON, V., VICTOR, J., AND KNIGHT, B. W. (1986). Source geometry and dynamics of the visual evoked potential. *Electroencephalogr. Clin. Neurophysiol.* 64, 308–327.

HAMER, R. D., NORCIA, A. M., TYLER, C. W., AND HSU, C. (1989). The development of monocular and binocular VEP acuity. *Vision Res.* 29, 397–408.

HELD, R., BIRCH, E. E., AND GWIAZDA, J. (1980). Stereoacuity of human infants. *Proc. Natl. Acad. Sci. USA* 77, 5572–5574.

HENDRICKSON, A., AND YOUDELIS, C. (1984). The morphological development of the human fovea. *Ophthalmology* 91, 603–612.

HOYT, C. S. (1984). The clinical usefulness of the visual evoked response. *J. Pediatr. Ophthalmol. Strabismus* 21, 231–234.

HUTTENLOCHER, P. R., deCOURTEN, C., GAREY, L., AND VAN DER LOOS, D. (1982). Synaptogenesis in human visual cortex—evidence for synapse elimination during normal development. *Neurosci. Lett.* 33, 247–252.

KEITH, C. G., AND KITCHEN, W. H. (1983). Ocular morbidity in infants of very low birth weight. *Br. J. Ophthalmol.* 67, 302–305.

LAMBERT, S. R., HOYT, C. R., JAN, J. E., BARKOVITCH, J., AND FLODMARK, O. (1987). Visual recovery from hypoxic cortical blindness in childhood: CT and MRI predictors. *Arch. Ophthalmol.* 105, 1371–1377.

LAMBERT, S. R., TAYLOR, D., AND KRISS, T. (1989). The infant with nystagmus, normal appearing fundi, but an abnormal ERG. *Surv. Ophthalmol.* 34, 173–186.

LEVI, D. M., AND KLEIN, S. (1982). Differences in vernier discrimination for gratings between strabismic and anisometropic amblyopia. *Invest. Ophthalmol. Vis. Sci.* 23, 398–407.

LEVI, D. M., MANNY, R. E., KLEIN, S., AND STEINMAN, S. B. (1983). Electrophysiological correlates of hyperacuity in the human visual cortex. *Nature* 306, 468–470.

MARDIA, J. (1982). *Statistics of Directional Data.* New York: Wiley.

MARG, E., FREEMAN, D. N., PELTZMAN, P., AND GOLDSTEIN, P. J. (1976). Visual acuity development in human infants: evoked potential measurements. *Invest. Ophthalmol.* 15, 150–153.

MAYER, D. L., FULTON, A. B., AND RODIER, D. (1984). Grating and recognition acuities of pediatric patients. *Ophthalmology* 91, 947–953.

MERIN, S., AND CRAWFORD, J. S. (1971). Etiology of congenital cataracts. *Can. J. Ophthalmol.* 6, 178–184.

MORRONE, M. C., AND BURR, D. C. (1986). Evidence for the existence and development of visual inhibition in humans. *Nature* 321, 235–237.

NORCIA, A. M., AND TYLER, C. W. (1985). Spatial frequency sweep VEP: visual acuity during the first year of life. *Vision Res.* 25, 1399–1405.

NORCIA, A. M., CLARKE, M., AND TYLER, C. W. (1985a). Digital filtering and robust regression techniques for estimating sensory thresholds from the evoked potential. *IEEE Eng. Med. Biol. Magazine* 4, 26–32.

NORCIA, A. M., MANNY, R. E., AND WESEMANN, W. (1988a). Vernier acuity measured using the sweep VEP. Non-invasive assessment of the visual system. *Opt. Soc. Am. Techn. Dig. Ser.* 3, 151.

NORCIA, A. M., SATO, T., SHINN, P., AND MERTUS, J. (1986). Methods for the identification of evoked response components in the frequency and combined time/frequency domains. *Electroencephalogr. Clin. Neurophysiol.* 65, 212–226.

NORCIA, A. M., SUTTER, E. E., AND TYLER, C. W. (1985b). Electrophysiological evidence for the existence of coarse and fine disparity mechanisms in human. *Vision Res.* 25, 1603–1611.

NORCIA, A. M., TYLER, C. W., AND HAMER, R. D. (1990). Development of contrast sensitivity in the human infant. *Vision Res.* 30, 1475–1486.

NORCIA, A. M., TYLER, C. W., HAMER, R. D., AND WESEMANN, W. (1989). Measurement of spatial contrast sensitivity with the swept contrast VEP. *Vision Res.* 29, 627–637.

NORCIA, A. M., WESEMANN, W., AND MANNY, R. (1988b). Sweep VEP vernier acuity and its cortical magnification. *Invest. Ophthalmol. Vis. Sci.* 29 (suppl.), 370.

OREL-BIXLER, D., AND NORCIA, A. M. (1986). Subjective and VEP acuity for normal and abnormally sighted children. *Invest. Ophthalmol. Vis. Sci.* 27 (suppl.), 152.

OREL-BIXLER, D., HAEGERSTROM-PORTNOY, G., AND HALL, A. (1989). Visual assessment of the multiply handicapped patient. *Optom. Vis. Sci.* 66, 530–536.

PELI, E., McCORMACK, G., AND SOKOL, S. (1988). Signal to noise ratio considerations in the analysis of sweep visual-evoked potentials. *Appl. Opt.* 27, 1094–1098.

REGAN, D. (1977). Speedy assessment of visual acuity in amblyopia by the evoked potential method. *Ophthalmologica* 175, 159–164.

REGAN, D. (1983). Spatial frequency mechanisms in human vision investigated by evoked potential recording. *Vision Res.* 23, 1401–1408.

REGAN, D. (1989). *Human Brain Electrophysiology: Evoked Potentials and Evoked Magnetic Fields in Science and Medicine.* New York: Elsevier.

REGAN, D., AND MILNER, B. A. (1978). Objective perimetry by evoked potential recording: limitations. *Electroencephalogr. Clin. Neurophysiol.* 44, 393–397.

REGAN, D., AND REGAN, M. P. (1987). Non-linearity in human visual responses to two-dimensional patterns, and a limitation of fourier methods. *Vision Res.* 27, 2181–2182.

REGAN, D., AND REGAN, M. P. (1988). A frequency domain technique for characterizing nonlinearities in biological systems. *J. Theor. Biol.* 133, 293–317.

REMKY, A., AND STRASBURGER, H. (1990). Steady-state on-off VEP closely related to suprathreshold contrast perception. *Invest. Ophthalmol. Vis. Sci.* 31 (suppl.), 256.

SCHMEISSER, E. T., AND BAKER, R. S. (1990). Amblyopia, binocularity and dichoptic VEPs. *Invest. Ophthalmol. Vis. Sci.* 31 (suppl.), 605.

SKARF, B. (1989). Clinical use of visual evoked potentials. *Ophthalmol. Clin. North Am.* 2, 499–518.

SOKOL, S. (1978). Measurement of infant visual acuity from pattern reversal evoked potentials. *Vision Res.* 18, 33–41.

SPEKREIJSE, H., VAN DER TWEEL, L. H., AND ZUIDEMA, T. (1973). Contrast evoked responses in man. *Vision Res.* 13, 1577–1601.

SUTTER, E. E. (1987). A practical nonstochastic approach to nonlinear time-domain analysis. In V. MARMARELIS (ed.). *Advanced Methods of Physiological System Modelling.* Vol. 1. Los Angeles: Biomedical Simulation Resource, University of Southern California, pp. 303–315.

TANG, Y. (1990). Improving the accuracy of the parameter estimation for real exponentially damped sinusoids in noise. *IEE Proc. Radar Signal Processing* 157F, 256–260.

TANG, Y., AND NORCIA, A. M. (1990). Improved parameter estimation of steady-state visual evoked potentials. *Proc. IEEE Eng. Med. Biol. Soc.* 12, 903–905.

THAKOR, N. V. (1987). Adaptive filtering of evoked potentials. *IEEE Trans. BME* 34, 6–14.

TYLER, C. W., APKARIAN, P., AND NAKAYAMA, K. (1978). Multiple spatial-frequency tuning of electrical responses from the human brain. *Exp. Brain Res.* 33, 538–550.

TYLER, C. W., APKARIAN, P., LEVI, D. M., AND NAKAYAMA, K. (1979). Rapid assessment of visual function: an electronic sweep technique for the pattern visual evoked potential. *Invest. Ophthalmol. Vis. Sci.* 18, 703–713.

WESTHEIMER, G. (1975). Visual acuity and hyperacuity. *Invest. Ophthalmol. Vis. Sci.* 14, 570–572.

ZAK, R., AND BERKELEY, M. A. (1986). Evoked potentials elicited by brief vernier offsets: estimating vernier thresholds and properties of the neural substrate. *Vision Res.* 26, 439–451.

ZEMON, V., AND RATLIFF, F. (1982). Visual evoked potentials: evidence for lateral interactions. *Proc. Natl. Acad. Sci. USA* 79, 5723–5726.

31 | Whither infant psychophysics?

ISRAEL ABRAMOV

My topic cuts a wide swath across the field of infant vision: It deals with the ways and means we use to ask infants what they see, discriminate, distinguish with their visual sense. I shall not try to analyze each method in detail, but shall concentrate on general themes that intersect with all these topics. Some of my comments will seem critical. But I, too, am a practitioner of infant psychophysics, and the comments are aimed as much at my own work as at that of others.

WHO ARE THE SUBJECTS?

It is an obvious point that, as with the related species of "adults," all infants are not the same. In particular, the question is: What is a "normal" infant, and what are her or his visual capacities? A goodly amount of work on infants simply states the ages and sexes of the subjects without careful attention to deciding if all are comparably normal. I argue that, at the least, all subjects should be screened to see that they meet some minimal visual criteria for being able to perform the task in question. For example, in studies of spatial resolution it might be appropriate to screen for obvious defects in optical quality of the retinal images: The various forms of photorefraction provide the means for doing so (see Chapter 1). These considerations are particularly important for clinical work, as abnormal individuals can be identified only by reference to those accepted as normal for a given age.

It may not be enough just to screen subjects with something like photorefraction. The state of alertness of the infant during a test can also greatly affect performance. For example, it has been said that 1-month-old infants do not show good accommodative behavior—they do not readily refocus for targets presented at different distances. This point is true only if the data are averaged across all the infants who were tested. When we eliminate data from individuals who show no evidence of attending to any of the stimuli, even very young infants vary accommodation appropriately and reasonably accurately over distances up to 2 meters (Banks, 1980; Hainline et al., 1992). This raises an interesting question: What is normal for a 1-month-old? These

infants are typically less alert and attentive than older infants and for this reason alone can be expected not to accommodate well at all times. I hold, however, that it is important to know what they *can* do, rather than what they *usually* do.

The populations from which we choose infants may also affect outcomes. A few examples can make the point. Male and female infants are not interchangeable: Young female infants are more likely to show stereopsis than are males of the same age (Gwiazda et al., 1989). There may be ethnic differences in the amount of pre-retinal ocular pigmentation (as discussed earlier), which can affect photorefraction measures by reducing the fundal reflection; we have also observed, anecdotally, that the image of a light source formed by reflection from the cornea is larger in dark-skinned individuals (adults and infants) than in more lightly pigmented individuals. The against-the-rule astigmatism that has been widely reported for infants may not be completely general; Chinese infants are also astigmatic, but their astigmatism follows the rule (Thorn et al., 1987).

Because vision develops across infancy, we often lump subjects into cohorts by age to specify average performance. We do it to reduce one source of noise (between-subject variability) in infant data, and because we may be overly conditioned to employ standard statistical tests such as the ANOVA. However, if the thing in which we are interested changes rapidly with age or the rate of change is not constant, we can reach radically different conclusions depending on where we choose to place the boundaries between the age groups. There is no necessary logic that says we must group infants by months or even weeks—or what to do with an infant whose age is midway between two groups. It might be preferable not to group infants by age but to treat age as a continuous variable and to describe the tested capacity by regression (possibly nonlinear) of that dependent measure on age.

A related problem is the amount of time it takes to test an infant: If it takes several sessions to measure a 2-week-old infant's capacity accurately, what then is the "age" associated with that datum?

Thus immaturity of some infant function could be due to genuine immaturity, to inattention, or to use of an insensitive response measure. However, an infant's capacities can be deemed immature only by reference to the endpoint of maturation, the adult. But which adult? Traditionally, psychophysicists have reported findings from highly trained, motivated, "world-class" observers. By their nature, infants cannot be instructed in the same way as adults. Relatively little attention has been paid to testing adults with the same apparatus used for infants; and even with minimal instructions about the task, it is not easy to find adults whose data could serve as the endpoint for infants' data. For example, in our investigations of the age changes in spatial contrast sensitivity, we measured eye movements elicited by drifting sinusoidal gratings (Hainline and Abramov, 1992). Our comparison adults were simply told to look at the stimulus screen, but we later learned that some of them thought that the moving gratings were there to distract them and so they deliberately tried to hold their eyes still (Hainline et al., 1987)!

STIMULUS VARIABLES

Much of the literature suggests that we believe the only thing affecting subjects' responses is the variable we have chosen to study. Many relevant factors are rarely controlled, however, and may not even be separable from the variable of interest. The problem is especially acute with an unknown and rapidly developing organism. In my mind the most glaring example is the general lack of control of temporal factors for the stimuli designed to study other visual dimensions. It is, of course, tedious to vary systematically the temporal attributes of everything we choose to study in infants. Yet our conclusions about visual capacities at different ages may depend on the precise temporal values used. For example, to record VEPs, stimuli must vary in time, yet the optimum temporal rates are not the same for recording an orientation-reversal VEP or an appearance/disappearance VEP; the existence of the orientation-reversal VEP is thought to indicate cortical function, but its time of onset is pushed to ever younger ages when the temporal rate is reduced (see Chapter 10).

Spatial resolution is particularly open to this lack of control. Spatial and temporal resolution are not separable: The values obtained for one function depend on the values for the other, and resolution is best described by a three-dimensional spatiotemporal surface (Kelly, 1979). Data exist for adults, but as yet we have nothing comparable from infants. Moreover, it is not easy to control temporal factors. Even when stimuli are static, as in forced-choice preferential looking (FPL) tests of acuity, there is no guarantee that they are static on the retina—unfortunately we have motile eyes. We tend to forget that even adults who are casually looking at a

scene do not have stable fixations; fixational drifts can be as high as 1–2 degrees/second (e.g., Murphy, 1978; Skavenski et al., 1979). This is enough to introduce significant temporal modulation, thereby reducing sensitivity to high spatial frequencies and increasing it for low spatial frequencies. One way of dealing with this, but at the cost of considerable instrumentation, is to use drifting gratings as stimuli and to monitor the eye movements elicited during each trial. When the grating is above threshold, the following movements reduce or eliminate the drift on the retina; when the grating approaches threshold, the following movements are themselves reduced, so retinal velocity approaches external stimulus velocity (Hainline et al., 1987; Hainline and Abramov, 1992).

Retinal inhomogeneity, which exists even in infants (Abramov et al., 1982; Yuodelis and Hendrickson, 1986), must also be considered, as it can change the proximal values of a stimulus. A telling example is the effect on spatial resolution of differences in cone morphology across the retina and the changes in this with age: Infants' foveal cones sample the retinal image quite coarsely and, additionally, are relatively poor at catching photons, which may be enough to account for infants' poor acuity (Brown et al., 1987; Banks and Bennett, 1988). However, in order to calculate such effects one must assume specific values for the relevant aspects of the anatomy. The outcomes can change dramatically even when parameter valves are varied within "acceptable" ranges (for more detail, see Chapter 6). And yet it is sometimes possible to make a virtue of retinal inhomogeneity and use it to bolster the validity of a new procedure: The visual fields of infants are not as extensive on the nasal side (i.e., imaged on temporal retina), which agrees well with anatomical measures of a nasotemporal asymmetry (see Chapter 7). More usually, however, retinal variations pose problems: The immaturity of the fovea at birth suggests that infants may respond more to peripheral than central stimulation, but the weighting is unknown, as is the timing of the change over to the adult's preferred use of the fovea for most visual tasks. Also, stimulus fields are typically large so responses represent some unknown average of different receptors, cells, preretinal filtering, and so on.

The interplay of retinal factors and stimulus size may account for some of the difficulties in interpreting the development of scotopic vision (see Chapter 8). The scotopic increment thresholds of young infants are proportional not to background intensity (Weber's law) but to the square root of that intensity (De Vries-Rose law). The argument is made that Weber's law in adults is due to rod–cone interactions, and that these interactions may be immature in infants. Even adults, however, show the square root relation when stimuli are small. Stimuli presented in the periphery of infants' visual fields may seem large by adult standards (e.g., 10 degrees in diameter when shown at 20 degrees eccentricity from the center of the field) but may be small for infants at such eccentricities because neurons with small receptive fields are not yet fully operational: Would infants obey Weber's law if the stimuli were larger?

Scotopic tests have also been used with infants to investigate the clarity of the ocular media which can modify the retinal illuminance: Deviations of the short-wavelength limb of the scotopic function, derived either psychophysically or electrophysiologically, from the absorption spectrum of rhodopsin can be attributed to selective light losses in the ocular media. From such comparisons, it has been reported that infants are approximately 0.5–0.8 log units more sensitive than young adults at 400 nm (Werner, 1982; Hansen and Fulton, 1989). Other studies, however, have found that infants' scotopic sensitivity agrees closely with the Commission Internationale de l'Eclairage's (CIE) standard scotopic function (Powers et al., 1981), implying the same preretinal absorption spectrum for infants and the young adults from whom the CIE standard was obtained; even at photopic levels, infants and adults seem equally sensitive to short wavelengths when tested with moving gratings (see Chapter 9). Are these studies sampling from the same population? The answer affects any additional analyses. One study (see Chapter 8) used the preretinal differences to correct the spectral luminosity functions; the resulting functions were narrower than those of adults, leading to the interpretation that infants' rods have lower absorptance, thereby producing the narrower spectral functions, but this conclusion is warranted only if a correction for preretinal factors is warranted.

METHODS FOR TESTING INFANTS

Those who study infant vision move as easily among techniques as do those who study adults. How are we then to compare findings across techniques—are the findings comparable? When comparing findings from behavioral and electrophysiological methods, everyone acknowledges that the linkages deserve careful scrutiny. However, the differences among some of the behavioral techniques are often glossed over. Even though my points are probably known by all practitioners, I think we all need a reminder.

The currently preeminent method is FPL, but there are at least two major variants in common use whose properties have not been compared fully. As originally conceived by Teller and her colleagues, the infant is first faced with as large and as uniform a visual field as possible. A stimulus is then presented on one side or the other. The underlying assumption is that the infant prefers to look at something rather than at nothing and so orients toward the stimulus when it is above threshold. Creating the necessary display is not easy. To measure acuity with fine gratings of high contrast, the luminance of the field as a whole must match the space average of the grating; the stimulus must be insertable seamlessly at each possible test location; and the boundaries of the stimulus field should not themselves aid in detection. With the advent of computer-generated displays, an alternative technique became popular: Two cathode ray tubes (CRTs) are placed on either side of a visual field that is usually dark; on each trial the stimulus is presented on one CRT while the other has "nothing"; for acuity tests, it would be unpatterned and at the mean luminance of the other. The assumption seems to be that the infant prefers to look at a just visible stimulus over an equally salient, albeit blank, field. This assumption is no longer as compelling as in the one in the original case. Additionally, the original procedure is more akin to finding an absolute threshold, whereas the latter is more like a classical discrimination procedure.

It has also been noted that in the second version of FPL infants sometimes show a negative preference; as stimuli approach threshold, subjects show a positive preference for the blank field (Held et al., 1979; but see also Banks et al., 1982). It may be that they find barely visible stimuli aversive, which reminds us that both versions depend on *preference*. Procedural details obviously can affect preference behavior and become important when screening individuals for visual abnormalities compared with a normative population; the exact procedure is as much a part of the norm as is the sample of infants. Furthermore, an infant may detect a stimulus according to one measure but "fail" to orient toward it (e.g., heart rate deceleration, but no change in orientation; Finlay and Ivinkis, 1984; see below).

More generally, when working with adults we assume that the ability to perform the required responses remains relatively stable, and that the major variable is the visibility of the stimulus. It is not so with infants, whose motoric and sensory capacities are both changing, and it may be difficult to tell which is more important in a particular case. For example, in dynamic perimetry a stimulus is moved in from the edge of the field until the infant looks at it. At an early age, however, the latency to initiate a saccade may be long, so that when the response is made the stimulus is already well past the point at which it first became visible, and the field may be underestimated. The problem is even more acute in clinical cases in which field deficits are often associated with oculomotor problems (see Chapter 7). A related issue is that the retina is far from uniform. With adults, most tests are confined to the central retina, but with FPL stimuli are first presented in the periphery. Thresholds from FPL may be heavily influenced by peripheral sensitivity, but it is not usual to compare infant data to adult data from peripheral loci or to adults tested in the same apparatus as the infants.

We may need to develop and refine psychophysical methods that are alternatives to the great workhorse of FPL. Some of the work on methods that use eye-movements and drifting stimuli seem promising both for spatial resolution (Hainline et al., 1987; Hainline and Abramov, 1992) and for some aspects of color vision (see Chapter 9). While some of the optical systems for monitoring eye-movements are complex and costly, simpler procedures (e.g., electro-oculograms) may be adequate, and new forms of eye-tracker that require less rigid restraint of the subject could be developed. But we must be cautious about excessive enthusiasm for one response measure: Infants presented with targets in the periphery of the visual field may not "detect" the target by measures of eye movements—they may not make a saccade to that target or orient toward it. However, other measures, such as a change in heart rate may show that the target was seen (Finlay and Ivinkis, 1984). Nonetheless, eye-movement techniques have the virtue that they can, in principle, specify where on the subject's retina the stimulus was presented, thereby ameliorating some of the problems stemming from retinal inhomogeneities. Of course, to do so one must solve the knotty problem of calibrating the eye-tracker (e.g., Harris et al., 1981).

Adults can be instructed about what to do and can be cajoled into cooperating for lengthy testing sessions. Infants must have their interest engaged by the procedure, which must also lead them into the task—"instruct" them. To maintain alertness, many of us include procedures between trials such as bouncing the infant up and down, presenting clearly visible and "interesting" stimuli on the test screens, and so on. However, there are virtually no investigations of the effects of these added manipulations. Many of these problems seem to me to stem from the general methodology that currently dominates infant psychophysics: reliance either on reflexive responses (e.g., OKN) or on the infants' interest in the procedure. These are essentially passive procedures, and yet infants are not "laid-back" (except in a literal sense) individuals—casual observation is enough to show that they want to interact actively with their surroundings. There is another domain that has similar problems of conveying to the subjects what they are supposed to do and keeping them at it: animal psychophysics, many of whose methods rely on well-established principles of operant conditioning requiring active participation by the subject (e.g., Stebbins, 1970). Operant techniques have the advantage that they can be used to shape subjects' behavior so that they attend to the relevant aspects of the stimuli—the procedure brings responses under control of the stimulus, rather than relying on something, such as preference for certain stimuli, that is built into the subject. Furthermore, the reinforcers that are used also serve to maintain attentiveness.

There is a tradition of operant procedures with infants, but it has not been extensively followed in the area of basic visual psychophysics. One paradigm is habituation/dishabituation: A response is specified that can be elicited by a "novel" stimulus; that stimulus is then presented until the infant "habituates" to it as indexed by a reduction in the response; the original stimulus is then replaced by another one, which will renew the initial level of responding provided the infant detects that it is different. The designated responses have ranged from "looking time" (e.g., Colombo and Horowitz, 1985) to "high-amplitude sucking" (HAS; see Jusczyk, 1985). In HAS the infant sucks on a nipple connected to a pressure transducer; sucks of greater force than some criterion (estimated from baseline measures for each infant) turn on the stimulus; when sucks drop below criterion, the stimulus disappears to be revived only if sucks again increase. Infants soon learn that their sucking controls the stimulus, but if the same thing keeps appearing, they seem to lose interest—at least, sucking diminishes; if a discriminably different stimulus appears, suck amplitude increases markedly. The advantage of such a method is that the infant directly controls the stimulus and hence must be attending to it. The disadvantage is that each "trial" is long. Furthermore, some infants, especially those who have not been used to a pacifier, refuse to cooperate. A related procedure is one in which rather than measuring sucking, a ribbon is attached to the infant's leg to record leg-kicks; during the habituation phase, the leg kicks also activate the stimuli—for instance, shaking a mobile above the crib. This has been successfully used to study infants' memories of previously seen objects attached to such mobiles (e.g., Rovee-Collier and Fagen, 1981). Clearly, such methods could be readily adapted to control any sort of visual stimulus. Although, like FPL, these habituation methods rely on the infant's presumptive liking for novelty, there may be also a reinforcement associated with the infant's ability to control the immediate environment.

In order to bring a response under complete control of a discriminative stimulus, a clear reinforcer must follow each response only when the designated stimulus is present. In the above methods, the reinforcer is implicit. Explicit reinforcers are the rule in animal psychophysics, but have only rarely been used with infants. One example is from an adaptation of classical FPL for use with older infants (usually 6 months to 1 year), in which orientation by the infant towards the side with the stimulus is followed by the appearance of a dancing musical toy (canonically, a bear; Mayer and Dobson, 1980). This seems to work well with this recalcitrant age group, but still the reinforcer seems to lack the basic, elemental character of the sorts of reinforcers used with animals: food, water, and so on. There are obvious problems associated with using such oral rewards, ranging from dietary to sanitary considerations. Nonetheless, there is a successful example in which toddlers were rewarded for correct responses in a psychophysical task with food pellets (a.k.a., "Cheerios"; Birch and Hale, 1989).

While I do not recommend placing potential infant subjects on diets to maintain body weight at 75% of normal so that food can be used as a reinforcer, I do argue that many of the problems we find working with infants may be reduced if we develop operant methods with their powerful abilities to activate and maintain behaviors directed toward the stimuli. Together with this we also must develop psychophysical algorithms that yield acceptable estimates of thresholds in time spans tuned to the infants' attention spans. We cannot simply import adult procedures with their reliance on unrealistically large numbers of trials; with infants, variances may actually increase as trials are increased. Unfortunately, however, reducing the number of trials may introduce biases into the estimates of threshold. On this point, there is a promising alternative to staircase procedures which is based on a modified binary search (MOBS); it seems relatively insensitive to response errors and requires far fewer trials (10–12) for good threshold estimates (Tyrrell and Owens, 1988). It is also heartening that some of the methods that use eye movements as the response measure can "get away with" only about 5 repetitions per data point (Hainline et al., 1987; see also Chapter 9).

PSYCHOPHYSIOLOGICAL LINKING HYPOTHESES

Many popular experimental procedures are aimed at relating behavioral and physiological development, but the hypotheses that link these domains are not always analyzed or stated explicitly (Teller, 1984). A common way is to choose stimuli that can segregate responses attributed to different portions of the nervous system. However, in each case the logic should be examined carefully to see whether the "excluded" pathways have really been excluded or their responses have simply been reduced by some unknown amount.

The best known of these approaches is probably the use of isoluminant stimuli to isolate responses driven only by the parvocellular pathways. Accepting that the magnocellular neurons are indeed the sole basis for spectral luminosity (e.g., Lee et al., 1990), isoluminant stimuli merely ensure that these neurons respond *equally*

to all stimuli and not that they fail to respond at all. Isoluminant stimuli cannot be discriminated by these cells, but they still may respond strongly to them; this strong, albeit constant, response can affect sensation. One is not necessarily studying responses driven by everything other than the magnocellular pathways. A more subtle point is that luminosity is defined according to some criterion response. Unfortunately, the resulting spectral sensitivity function can change markedly for different criteria; even "canonical" heterochromatic flicker photometry does not have a canonical flicker rate, and the curves differ drastically as rate is varied. This fact could present problems, for example, when luminance equations are derived from dynamic stimuli (flicker or motion) and are then used to control static stimuli.

Another example is the widely held assumption that orientation selectivity is a property of cortical units, and therefore the emergence of such selectivity in psychophysical tests is an index of the emergence of functional neuronal units in the cortex (e.g., see Chapter 10). Even retinal ganglion cells, however, may have receptive fields that differ sufficiently from the popular picture of radially symmetrical, circular fields. The ratio of major to minor diameters of fields in cats and macaques is about $1.3:1$ (Kaplan, 1991). If the only orientations that are tested differ by 90 degrees, then even the ganglion cells may have fields that are sufficiently elongated to permit discrimination.

Motion selectivity is also taken as a mark of cortical activity. This capacity does not seem to be present before about 2 months. Even so, some kind of motion selectivity must be present earlier to provide the basis for optokinetic nystagmus (OKN), which can be elicited readily in younger infants. It is ascribed to a parallel pathway (existing at birth) to the nucleus of the optic tract, however, and so this selectivity is not cortical in origin. Thus the motion detection that marks cortical function must be one that is a property only of cortical units, which has an air of circularity about it. A candidate cortical marking function is smooth pursuit, which is taken to require the cortex, and so if at some young age cortical units are not yet functional, smooth pursuit should not be apparent. This point is contentious, but there seems to be enough evidence that very young infants can show episodes of good smooth pursuit, provided they are alert and the stimulus velocity is low (Hainline, 1985). Additionally, it might be noted that we do not really know the sequence in which cortical and subcortical pathways develop in primates. In current models, there is an early subcortical pathway that, in very young infants, subserves optokinetic nystagmus together with its well-known monocular asymmetry (e.g., Atkinson and Braddick, 1981; Naegele and Held, 1982); descending inputs from the cortex develop later and serve to obscure the asymmetry. But this model derives largely from analyses of the cat's visual system (e.g., Hoffmann, 1983). Its direct applicability to the human case could be questioned, given the many differences between cat and human visual systems.

There may be no simple procedure to ensure that some pathway is or is not involved in some behavior. However, this general approach can still be valuable, especially if results add to lines of evidence converging on a particular interpretation. A good example is the development of color vision as tested by a novel technique measuring the eye movements elicited by drifting chromatic gratings (see Chapter 9). Luminosity is measured by adjusting the relative intensities of stripes of different spectral content so as to minimize following eye movements. It presumably equates stimuli for the magnocellular pathway to the cortex. (However, if cortical areas are not fully operational in young infants, the procedure may be studying brainstem color vision.) And if motion-detecting units are driven only by magnocellular pathways, there should not be any visible motion in a purely chromatic grating. However, even at equiluminance, gratings whose stripes differ in hue still elicit some following from infants as well as from adults. This factor complicates the possible interpretations, as color discrimination is presumed to be derived from the activity of spectrally opponent parvocellular neurons projecting to the cortex; the optokinetic movements elicited by purely chromatic gratings should be due to cortical projections to the brainstem, which are thought not to be operative in young infants who still show directional asymmetries in horizontal OKN. Despite the difficulties with interpretation, the technique is useful: Infants respond well in this situation, providing unusually precise psychophysical function measurements. The method also deals elegantly with the problem of matching chromatic and luminance contrasts: The following of a drifting grating of fixed luminance contrast is titrated by varying the chromatic contrast of an equiluminant grating drifting in the opposite direction.

CONCLUSIONS

"You've come a long way, baby!"—but we should not be smug about it.

Acknowledgments. I thank Drs. Louise Hainline and Patricia Riddell for very helpful comments. The work was supported, in part, by NIH grant EY03957.

REFERENCES

ABRAMOV, I., GORDON, J., HENDRICKSON, A., HAINLINE, L., DOBSON, M. V., AND LaBOSSIERE, E. (1982). The retina of the newborn human infant. *Science* 217, 265–267.

ATKINSON, J., AND BRADDICK, O. (1981). Development of optokinetic nystagmus in infants: an indicator of cortical binocularity? In D. F. FISHER, R. A. MONTY, AND J. W. SENDERS (eds.). *Eye Movements, Cognition and Visual Perception.* Hillsdale, NJ: Erlbaum, pp. 53–64.

BANKS, M. S. (1980). The development of visual accommodation in early infancy. *Child Dev.* 51, 646–666.

BANKS, M. S., AND BENNETT, P. J. (1988). Optical and photoreceptor immaturities limit the spatial and chromatic vision of human neonates. *J. Opt. Soc. Am.* [A]5, 2059–2079.

BANKS, M. S., STEPHENS, B. R., AND DANNEMILLER, J. L. (1982). A failure to observe negative preference in infant acuity testing. *Vision Res.* 22, 1025–1031.

BIRCH, E. E., AND HALE, L. A.(1989). Operant assessment of stereoacuity. *Clin. Vision Sci.* 4, 295–300.

BROWN, A. M., DOBSON, V., AND MAIER, J. (1987). Visual acuity of human infants at scotopic, mesopic and photopic luminances. *Vision Res.* 27, 1845–1858.

COLOMBO, J., AND HOROWITZ, F. D. (1985). A parametric study of the infant control procedure. *Infant Behav. Dev.* 8, 117–121.

FINLAY, D. C., AND IVINKIS, A. (1984). Cardiac and visual responses to stimuli presented foveally and peripherally as a function of speed of moving stimuli. *Dev. Psychol.* 18, 692–698.

GWIAZDA, J., BAUER JR., J. A., AND HELD, R. (1989). Binocular function in human infants: correlation of stereoptic and fusion-rivalry discriminations. *J. Pediatr. Ophthalmol. Strabismus* 26, 128–132.

HAINLINE, L. (1985). Oculomotor control in human infants. In R. GRONER, G. W. McCONKIE, AND C. MENZ (eds.). *Eye Movements and Human Information Processing.* Amsterdam: Elsevier-North Holland, pp. 71–84.

HAINLINE, L., AND ABRAMOV, I. (1992). Assessing visual development: is infant vision good enough? In C. ROVEE-COLLIER AND L. P. LIPSITT (eds.). *Advances in Infancy Research.* Vol. 7. Norwood, NJ: Ablex, pp. 39–102.

HAINLINE, L., DE BIE, J., ABRAMOV, I., AND CAMENZULI, C. (1987). Eye movement voting: a new technique for deriving spatial contrast sensitivity. *Clin. Vision Sci.* 2, 33–44.

HAINLINE, L., RIDDELL, P., GROSE-FIFER, J., AND ABRAMOV, I. (1992). Development of accommodation and convergence in infancy. *Behav. Brain Res.* 49, 33–50.

HANSEN, R. M., AND FULTON, A. B. (1989). Psychophysical estimates of ocular media density of human infants. *Vision Res.* 29, 687–690.

HARRIS, C. M., HAINLINE, L., AND ABRAMOV, I. (1981). A method for calibrating an eye-monitoring system for use with infants. *Behav. Res. Meth. Instrum. Comput.* 13, 11–17.

HELD, R., GWIAZDA, J., BRILL, S., MOHINDRA, J., AND WOLFE, J. (1979). Infant visual acuity is underestimated because near threshold gratings are not preferentially fixated. *Vision Res.* 19, 675–683.

HOFFMANN, K. P. (1983). Control of the optokinetic reflex by the nucleus of the optic tract in the cat. In A. HEIN AND M. JEANNEROD (eds.). *Spatially Oriented Behavior.* New York: Springer-Verlag.

JUSCZYK, P. W. (1985). The high-amplitude sucking technique as a methodological tool in speech perception research. In G. GOTTLIEB AND N. A. KRASNEGOR (eds.). *Measurement of Audition and Vision in the First Year of Postnatal Life.* Norwood, NJ: Ablex.

KAPLAN, E. (1991). The receptive field structure of retinal ganglion cells in cat and monkey. In A. G. LEVENTHAL (ed.). *The Neural Basis of Visual Function.* Vol. IV. *Vision and Visual Dysfunction.* Boca Raton, FL: CRC Press, pp. 10–40.

KELLY, D. H. (1979). Motion and vision. II. Stabilized spatio-temporal threshold surface. *J. Opt. Soc. Am.* 69, 1340–1349.

LEE, B. B., POKORNY, J., SMITH, V. C., MARTIN, P. R., AND VALBERG, A. (1990). Luminance and chromatic modulation sensitivity of macaque ganglion cells and human observers. *J. Opt. Soc. Am.* [A]7, 2223–2236.

MAYER, D. L., AND DOBSON, M. V. (1980). Assessment of vision in young children: A new operant approach yields estimates of acuity. *Invest. Ophthalmol. Vis. Sci.* 19, 566–570.

MURPHY, B. J. (1978). Pattern thresholds for moving and stationary gratings during smooth eye movements. *Vision Res.* 18, 521–530.

NAEGELE, J. R., AND HELD, R. (1982). The post-natal development of monocular optokinetic nystagmus in infants. *Vision Res.* 22, 341–346.

POWERS, M. K., SCHNECK, M., AND TELLER, D. Y. (1981). Spectral sensitivity of human infants at absolute visual threshold. *Vision Res.* 21, 1005–1016.

ROVEE-COLLIER, C., AND FAGEN, J. W. (1981). The retrieval of memory in early infancy. In L. P. LIPSITT (ed.). *Advances in Infancy Research. Vol. 1.* Norwood, NJ: Ablex.

SKAVENSKI, A. A., HANSEN, R. M., STEINMAN, R. M., AND WINTERSON, B. J. (1979). Quality of retinal image stabilization during small natural and artificial body rotations in man. *Vision Res.* 19, 675–683.

STEBBINS, W. C. (ED.) (1970). *Animal Psychophysics: the Design and Conduct of Sensory Experiments.* New York: Plenum Press.

TELLER, D. Y. (1984). Linking propositions. *Vision Res.* 24, 1233–1246.

THORN, F., HELD, R., AND FANG, L-L. (1987). Orthogonal astigmatic axes in Chinese and caucasian infants. *Invest. Ophthalmol. Vis. Sci.* 28, 191–194.

TYRRELL, R. A., AND OWENS, D. A. (1988). A rapid technique to assess the resting states of the eyes and other threshold phenomena: the Modified Binary Search (MOBS). *Behav. Res. Meth. Instrum. Comput.* 20, 137–141.

WERNER, J. S. (1982). Development of scotopic sensitivity and the absorption spectrum of the human ocular media. *J. Opt. Soc. Am.* 72, 247–258.

YUODELIS, C., AND HENDRICKSON, A. (1986). A qualitative and quantitative analysis of the human fovea during development. *Vision Res.* 26, 847–855.

32 | Theories of infant visual development

HUGH R. WILSON

The neonatal visual system is characterized by low acuity, reduced contrast sensitivity, and the absence of a variety of functional capabilities, such as stereopsis (Dobson et al., 1978; Gwiazda et al., 1980; Birch et al., 1982; Banks and Salapatek, 1983). Until recently no theoretical explanation of these visual immaturities was possible, as there were simply no relevant anatomical or physiological data on which to base developmental theories. This situation changed dramatically with the publication of quantitative data documenting two key aspects of infant foveal immaturity (Hendrickson and Yuodelis, 1984; Yuodelis and Hendrickson, 1986). In particular, the density of infant foveal cones is much lower than in adults, and the length of infant cone outer segments is greatly reduced. These immaturities appear to be largely limited to the central retina, as infant peripheral retina appears normal (Abramov et al., 1982).

What aspects of visual development can be explained by anatomical immaturity of the infant fovea? Two theories have emerged to answer this question. In the first, I (Wilson, 1988) used infant anatomical data to transform a quantitative model of adult spatial vision (Wilson and Bergen, 1979; Wilson et al., 1983) back into a model for infant vision. In the second, Banks and Bennett (1988) developed an infant ideal observer model. Both models agree that infant foveal immaturity has the effect of reducing infant acuity and depressing contrast sensitivity, but there are important quantitative differences between the two approaches as well. Accordingly, the first goal of this chapter is to summarize and extend my 1988 model (Wilson, 1988). This model comes tantalizingly close to predicting the development of acuity and contrast sensitivity as measured at the cortical level using visual evoked potentials (VEPs) (Norcia and Tyler, 1985; Norcia et al., 1988, 1990). Similarities and differences between the two theories are highlighted where appropriate.

Infant retinal anatomy cannot, of course, provide an explanation for the absence of higher visual functions, such as stereopsis, in neonates (Birch et al., 1982). However, there is documentation of anatomical immaturity in the striatic cortex of neonates, particularly with respect to the density of synaptic connections (Conel, 1939;

Huttenlocher et al., 1982). The development of synaptic connections correlates well with the advent of stereopsis, orientation selectivity, and other cortical functions. However, there is as yet no theoretical framework for interpreting postnatal cortical synapse formation, so this chapter ends with a few relevant speculations.

INFANT RETINAL ANATOMY

Hendrickson and Yuodelis (1984; Yuodelis and Hendrickson, 1986) observed that the infant fovea was immature in several key respects (see Chapter 17). First, the ganglion cell layer covered the entire central retina, and thus there was no true foveal pit. Second, the foveal cone density was much lower than in adults. Finally, the outer segments of foveal cones were much shorter than in the adult. During the course of postnatal development, therefore, cone migration into the foveal region increases the cone density, and migration of central ganglion cells toward the periphery concurrently produces the foveal pit. In addition, outer segments grow in length, thus increasing the number of layers of photopigment-containing membrane. These developments are limited to about the central 5.0 degrees of the retina (Abramov et al., 1982).

From a theoretical perspective, the two crucial aspects of foveal immaturity are decreased outer segment length and reduced cone density. Yuodelis and Hendrickson (1986) have published quantitative data on both factors for four retinas aged 5 days, 15 months, 45 months, and 37 years. With the caveat that only one retina of each age has been studied, let us examine the data on the assumption that they are representative.

Before delving into the implications of infant foveal anatomy, a brief digression on the relevance of theory to visual development may be warranted. It is obvious that reduced foveal cone density and outer segment length must have detrimental effects on infant spatial vision. Can these factors alone account for empirical infant acuity and contrast sensitivity deficits? This question can be answered only by developing a quantitative theory of the effects of these two factors on spatial vision. If such a theory does predict infant data accurately, we may conclude that foveal immaturity is indeed the limiting factor in contrast sensitivity function (CSF) and acuity development. In any event, we shall fully understand development only when we have a quantitative theory that accurately predicts infant visual function based on differences between infant and adult anatomy and physiology.

EFFECT OF REDUCED OUTER SEGMENT LENGTH

Data on cone outer segment dimensions are plotted in Figure 32-1. Although the width remains constant at about 1.2 μm, the length growth from 3.1 μm at 5 days to about 45.5 μm in the adult. This length increase by a factor of 14.7 suggests that the adult outer segment should capture a much greater percentage of the incident photons than the infant. This difference in quantum catch may be easily calculated if it is assumed that the density of photopigment per unit length is constant across development. Photon capture is essentially a Poisson process in which each photopigment-containing membrane has the same probability of capturing the photons that reach it. Given this fact, it is a simple matter to determine that the probability p of photon capture for an outer segment of length x is

$$P = 1 - e^{-x/L} \qquad (1)$$

where L = the characteristic length of the Poisson process. Based on data indicating that adult foveal cones capture about 84% of the incident quanta (Pokorny and Smith, 1976; Pokorny et al., 1976), L is calculated to be 24.8 μm (Wilson, 1988). On the assumption that the photopigment density per unit length is the same in infants (which implies that L has the same value for infants), infant foveal cones capture only about 11.8% of the incident quanta—a reduction from the adult value

TABLE 32-1. *Anatomical data on foveal development.*[a]

Age	Outer segment length (μm)	Sensitivity reduction	Cone spacing (arc min)	Calculated acuity (cpd)
5 Days	3.1	2.7×	2.18	8.0
15 Months	22.5	1.2×	1.19	16.0
45 Months	29.5	1.1×	0.70	25.9
37 Years	45.5	1.0×	0.47	35.5

[a]Summary of the implications of the anatomical data of Yuodelis and Hendrickson (1986) for infant visual development. The sensitivity reduction factors (C) are square roots of values calculated from Eq. (1) using the listed outer segment lengths. They are reported relative to the adult value. Foveal cone spacing (M in the text is the ratio to the infant value) has been corrected for growth in the axial length of the eye using the data of Larsen (1971). Acuities were calculated using these factors in Eq. (8).

by a factor of 7.2. As the signal-to-noise ratio for a Poisson process grows with the square root of the signal strength, infant contrast sensitivity would be reduced by $\sqrt{7.2}$, or 2.7. CSF reduction factors at other ages are listed in Table 32-1. Kelly (1972) has demonstrated that the CSF varies with the square root of the mean luminance at most spatial frequencies, and this evidence provides direct support for the present approach to infant contrast sensitivity. Bennett and Banks (1988) arrived at essentially the same result regarding the effects of reduced outer segment length on infant contrast sensitivity.

EFFECT OF REDUCED FOVEAL CONE DENSITY

Yuodelis and Hendrickson (1986) reported that neonate foveal cones were spaced about 3.34 times farther apart on the retina than were cones in the adult fovea. To convert this distance to cone spacing in arc minutes it is necessary to compensate for growth of the eye during development. Larsen (1971) has reported that axial length increases from an average of 16.5 mm at birth to 23.0 mm during adulthood, which is a factor of 1.39. Combining these factors results in the estimate that infant cones are spaced about 4.64 times farther apart than are those in the adult. Values of foveal cone spacing in arc minutes corrected for eye growth are plotted in Figure 32-2 and listed in Table 32-1. From these figures it may be concluded that the Nyquist limit for the neonate fovea is about 13.8 cycles/degree (cpd) (Wilson, 1988).[1]

The effect of increased foveal cone spacing on infant vision depends on additional anatomical assumptions.

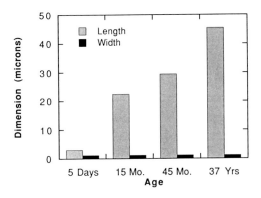

FIG. 32-1. Length and width of foveal cone outer segments as a function of age. The data are from Yuodelis and Hendrickson (1986). Although outer segment width remains constant, the length grows by a factor of about 15 from birth to adulthood. Anatomical data at each age are based on just one retina.

---

1. This figure is simply obtained from the reciprocal of twice the foveal cone spacing. At the optimal orientation in an hexagonal lattice the Nyquist frequency would increase to 15.8 cpd.

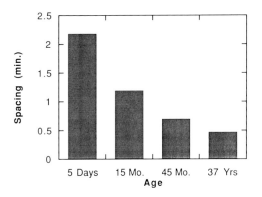

FIG. 32-2. Variations in foveal cone spacing with age. In order to express the results in terms of visual angle (min. arc), the anatomical data of Yuodelis and Hendrickson (1986) have been corrected for the axial growth of the eye using the data of Larsen (1971). Infant foveal cones are initially spaced about 4.6 times further apart than adult cones but migrate inward over at least four years of life to achieve adult levels. Note that this spacing difference implies an adult/ infant density ratio of about 21.2.

I have made the following assumption (Wilson, 1988, p. 616): "If each cortical cell receives information from a fixed set of foveal cones throughout development, its receptive field would necessarily be larger in the infant due to the increased cone spacing." The implications of this assumption are illustrated in Figure 32-3. On the left are portions of the hexagonal cone array (black circles) with the cones closely spaced for the adult and more widely spaced for the infant. If, via intervening circuitry (e.g., bipolars, ganglion cells, lateral geniculate nucleus, or LGN), the set of cones within the gray region provided input to a cortical unit in the adult, the assumption above requires that this unit must have had a much larger receptive field at birth. Based on this assumption, therefore, the effect of increased foveal cone spacing in the infant is to introduce a *spatial scale change* that shifts spatial frequency tuning toward lower spatial frequencies by a factor equal to the relative increase in cone spacing. The response of these receptive fields to a cosine grating is illustrated in one dimension on the right side of Figure 32-3. The five cones depicted (gray rectangles) lie close together in the adult but farther apart in the infant. However, these cones fall at the same points under a cosine grating in both adult and infant if that grating if shifted toward lower spatial frequencies in the infant by an amount proportional to the increased foveal cone spacing. For the gratings shown, therefore, the adult and infant cones receive identical stimulation, which demonstrates that the assumption above implies a scale shift toward lower spatial frequencies.

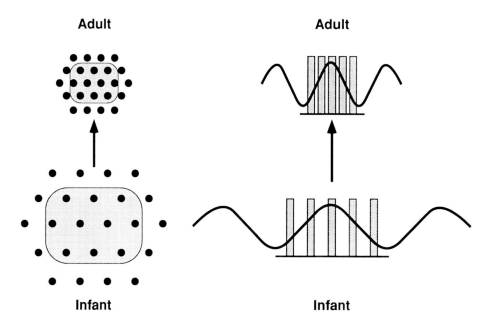

FIG. 32-3. Spatial scale change caused by cone migration. On the lower left a portion of the hexagonal cone mosaic of an infant is accentuated in gray. Assume that this group of cones provides (via bipolar cells, ganglion cells, and the LGN) the input to a cortical unit. If this cortical unit remains connected to the same group of cells throughout life, then foveal cone migration will result in this unit receiving input from a much smaller retinal region in the adult (upper left). The effect of this migration on the response to cosine gratings is illustrated in one dimension on the right. Imagine that each vertical rectangle here is a single cone seen in profile. (Differences in outer segment length have been ignored in the diagram to emphasize the spatial aspects of cone migration.) Superimposed on each set of cones is the luminance profile of a cosine grating. Although the infant cones are further apart (lower right), each receives stimulation identical to the adult cones (upper right) when the spatial frequency of the grating is reduced as shown. (The fixed width of the cones leads to a minor correction to this as discussed in the text.) Thus, increased infant cone spacing produces a spatial scale shift toward low spatial frequencies.

Two modifications must be made to the spatial scale change hypothesis, one trivial and one more substantial. First, it is apparent from the right of Figure 32-3 that as foveal cone diameter is constant during development (Fig. 32-1), each adult cone captures quanta over a larger fraction of a grating cycle than each infant cone. In regions where the luminance profile of the grating is linear (e.g., near the nodes), it makes absolutely no difference. However, for cones positioned at the 0- and 180-degree phases of the cosine, infant cones receive a slightly higher mean quantum flux in view of the slower spatial variation of the lower frequency cosine. Calculations assuming a 0.5 arc minute diameter circular collection area for foveal cones show that the effect would be to increase infant sensitivity by about 4% at the acuity limit.[2] This minute correction, ignored previously (Wilson, 1988), makes virtually no difference in the predictions below.

The more substantial modification of the spatial scale shift hypothesis is due to the role of the optics. Psychophysically measured spatial mechanism sensitivity curves (Wilson and Bergen, 1979; Wilson et al., 1983) are a product of both neural and optical stages. Therefore simply using the increased infant cone spacing to produce a spatial scale shift factor (Wilson, 1988) implicitly shifts the optical contribution as well.[3] The correct way to introduce the spatial scale shift is the following. As psychophysically measured functions are the result of convolution by the optics followed by neural interactions or pooling, one must first deconvolve the sensitivity curve with the adult optical line spread function to remove the optical contribution. The resulting neural function is then shifted by the factor estimated from infant retinal anatomy, and the result is finally convolved with the infant optical function. Deconvolution is normally a complex business, but if both the psychophysical filters and the optical line spread function are represented by Gaussian functions, deconvolution may be accomplished analytically. This is done in the next section.

With this correction for the optics, the increased infant cone separation produces a shift of the CSF toward lower spatial frequencies. The situation is diagrammed in logarithmic coordinates on the left of Figure 32-4. Here the adult CSF is shifted downward by the factor C, representing the loss of sensitivity due to decreased outer segment length in the infant; and this function is then shifted toward lower spatial frequencies by the factor M, reflecting increased infant cone spacing. With C = 2.7 and M = 4.6, this curve predicts a relatively small sensitivity loss at low spatial frequencies in the infant but a rather large acuity loss (A). With the exception of the optical correction, this analysis of infant foveal data is the one developed previously (Wilson, 1988).

Banks and Bennett (1988) incorporated the sensitivity change (C) due to decreased outer segment length in the same fashion as I did (Wilson, 1988), but they analyzed the effect of increased cone separation differently. Recall that the spatial scale shift is based on the assumption that cortical units receive input from the same set of cones throughout development (Wilson, 1988). As an alternative, Banks and Bennett (1988) modified the ideal observer model (Geisler, 1984, 1989) to restrict processing to a fixed number of cycles of each spatial frequency in both infant and adult; which means that any given grating can be detected based on the responses of far fewer cones in the infant than in the adult. In consequence, the signal-to-noise ratio in infants should be reduced by the square root of the ratio of infant to adult cone density. This alternative analysis therefore leads to the conclusion that the increase in infant foveal cone spacing should result in a further downward shift of the CSF toward reduced sensitivities, as is shown by M on the right of Figure 32-4. Note that this approach predicts a large sensitivity loss (S) at low spatial frequencies but a much smaller acuity reduction than when using my approach (Wilson, 1988).

Two points should be emphasized concerning the difference between the two forms of analysis illustrated in Figure 32-4. First, they depend on different assumptions concerning changes in anatomical connections during development. My 1988 approach assumes that connections to cortical units are constant during development, whereas the Banks and Bennett (1988) approach assumes that each cortical unit incorporates more and more cones within a fixed retinal area as development proceeds. These assumptions clearly lead to different quantitative predictions, so it is possible to ask which one provides the better explanation of the data. As discussed below, data by Norcia et al. (1990) favor my 1988 hypothesis. Second, by choosing to restrict analysis to a fixed number of cycles for each spatial frequency, the Banks and Bennett (1988) model is no longer strictly an ideal observer model. Thus it is not "atheoretical" but, rather, entails a process of changing anatomical connections during development.

MATHEMATICAL DEVELOPMENT

This section provides a concise quantitative treatment of retinal development derived from a psychophysical

---

2. This calculation involves evaluation of the two-dimensional integral of a patch of cosine grating over a circular aperture 0.5 arc minute in diameter. In this instance an adult grating frequency of 30 cpd was compared with an infant frequency of 6 cpd. It indicated that infant cones at the peaks (and troughs) of the luminance profile would receive 8% more quanta. Because of the signal-to-noise ratio of Poisson processes, it would increase infant sensitivity by the square root of this value, or 4%.

3. I am indebted to M. Banks for pointing out this problem with my original formulation of the spatial scale shift.

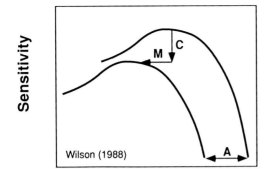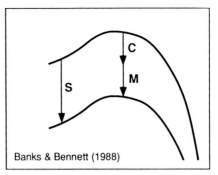

Spatial Frequency

FIG. 32-4. Effects of infant foveal anatomy on the CSF. The two illustrations contrast the hypotheses proposed by Wilson (left) and Banks and Bennett (right). Relative to the adult CSF (upper curve in both panels), reduced outer segment length uniformly reduces sensitivity by a factor **C** in both models. On logarithmic coordinates this is a simple downward shift. The effect of increased foveal cone spacing is modeled as a spatial scale shift by factor **M** towards lower spatial frequencies on the left, but as a further reduction in sensitivity on the right. Quantitatively, the spatial scale shift hypothesis on the left produces a larger acuity reduction **A**, while the assumption that increased cone spacing simply reduces sensitivity produces the larger sensitivity reduction **S** (right). Data by Norcia et al. (1990) support the spatial scale shift hypothesis shown on the left.

model for adult spatial vision (Wilson et al., 1983; Wilson and Gelb, 1984; Wilson, 1986, 1991). Readers not interested in mathematical details may skip to the next section, where the model is compared with developmental data.

Results of psychophysical and physiological research have clearly demonstrated that the CSF represents the envelope of a number of mechanisms, each tuned to a 1.0- to 2.0-octave range of spatial frequencies (DeValois and DeValois, 1988; Graham, 1989; Wilson et al., 1990). Spatial frequency sensitivity curves for the underlying mechanisms have been estimated from masking data (Wilson et al., 1983) and can be accurately fit by a difference of three Gaussian functions (Wilson and Gelb, 1984):

$$F(x,y) = A\{e^{-x^2/\sigma_1^2} - Be^{-x^2/\sigma_2^2}$$
$$+ Ce^{-x^2/\sigma_3^2}\} e^{-y^2/\sigma_y^2} \quad (2)$$

The first term in brackets produces the excitatory center of the filter; the second represents the inhibitory surround; and the third reflects a weak secondary excitatory zone. These psychophysical filters have the characteristics of simple cell receptive fields in striate cortex (Wilson et al., 1990). As written, $F(x,y)$ describes a vertically oriented filter; but other orientations may be easily obtained through rotation of coordinates. All of the parameters associated with these filters have been measured psychophysically and published elsewhere (Wilson and Gelb, 1984; Wilson, 1991). As we shall be dealing with one-dimensional cosine gratings, it will be convenient to consider only the x variation of this function and to deal with its Fourier transform:

$$S(\omega) = A\sqrt{\pi}(\sigma_1 e^{-\pi^2\sigma_1^2\omega^2} - B\sigma_2 e^{-\pi^2\sigma_2^2\omega^2}$$
$$+ C\sigma_3 e^{-\pi^2\sigma_3^2\omega^2}) \quad (3)$$

Here ω = the spatial frequency in cycles per degree. Plots of Eq. 3 for the six mechanisms measured by Wilson et al. (1983) are shown in Figure 32-5. The relative heights of the mechanisms are appropriate for temporal frequencies including 6.0 Hz, the frequency used in the VEP measurements to be discussed. The CSF is given by the envelope of these six functions and is shown in Figure 32-7 (see below).

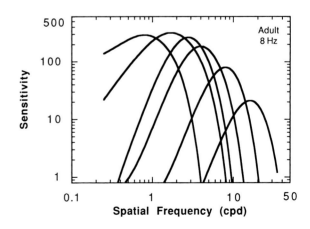

FIG. 32-5. Spatial frequency tuned mechanisms measured in adults (Wilson et al., 1983). The six frequency sensitivity curves are plotted at the correct heights for 6–8 Hz temporal modulation. Maximum sensitivity for the group of curves was adjusted to fit adult VEP sensitivities in the Norcia et al. (1990) study. The adult CSF is predicted by the sensitivity envelope of these six curves.

Adult spatial mechanisms must now be transformed to reflect infant retinal immaturity. As discussed above, the effect of reduced outer segment length is to decrease contrast sensitivity by a factor $C = 2.7$, which is easily incorporated into Eq. 3 by replacing A with A/C.

The spatial scale shift occasioned by decreased foveal cone density requires a somewhat more complicated modification. The simplest approach is to replace the space constants σ_1, σ_2, σ_3, and σ_y with $M\sigma_1$, etc., where M = the scale change factor (Wilson, 1988).[4] As pointed out by Banks (personal communication), however, this implicitly scales the optical contribution to Eq. 3 by the same factor. To deal with the optics more effectively, it is necessary to first deconvolve $S(\omega)$ with the optical line spread function (LSF). To perform this exercise, the optical LSF is approximated by a single Gaussian function of unit area. Geisler (1984) approximated the optical line spread function data of Campbell and Gubisch (1966) with a sum of two Gaussians. As the narrower Gaussian is the only one affecting the high-frequency portion of the CSF and grating acuity, it is used for our present purposes. Geisler (1984) estimated its space constant to be $\sigma_0 = 0.0104$ degrees.[5]

Consider for the moment just one of the Gaussians in Eq. 3. Its space constant is the result of convolution of the optical LSF with the following neural connectivity function. In the Fourier domain the optical convolution becomes multiplication, so we have:

$$Ae^{-\pi^2\sigma_1^2\omega^2} = Ae^{-\pi^2\sigma_0^2\omega^2}e^{-\pi^2\sigma_N^2\omega^2}$$

$$= Ae^{-\pi^2(\sigma_0^2+\sigma_N^2)\omega^2} \quad (4)$$

where σ_N = the space constant of the neural interactions. Given that σ_1 and σ_0 are known, the equation can easily be solved for σ_N:

$$\sigma_N = \sqrt{\sigma_1^2 - \sigma_0^2} \quad (5)$$

Now the increased infant cone spacing can be incorporated through multiplication of σ_N by M. There remains only the detail of convolving with the LSF of the infant optics. If the space constant of this LSF is σ_{IO}, the resulting infant space constant is given by:

$$\sigma_{1I} = \sqrt{M^2(\sigma_1^2 - \sigma_0^2) + \sigma_{IO}^2} \quad (6)$$

This expression allows us to consider infant optics that may be poorer than those of the adult as well as those for which $\sigma_{IO} = \sigma_O$. For example, note that if $\sigma_{IO} = M\sigma_O$, then $\sigma_{1I} = M\sigma_1$. This situation is the one case in which the simple scale transformation I used (Wilson, 1988) is fully valid. Analogous expressions are obtained relating infant space constants to adult values of σ_2 and σ_3.

The fully transformed infant mechanism sensitivity function may now be obtained from Eq. 3 by replacing the space constants with Eq. 6 and analogous expressions. Note, however, that for a pure spatial scale change this replacement occurs only in the exponents. For example, the first term in Eq. 3 becomes in the infant:

$$\frac{A}{C}\sqrt{\pi}\sigma_1e^{-\pi^2[M^2(\sigma_1^2-\sigma_0^2)+\sigma_{IO}^2]\omega^2} \quad (7)$$

This expression represents the narrowest Gaussian in infant spatial filters, so it determines the acuity limit. As acuity is simply the spatial frequency at which sensitivity drops to unity, infant acuity can be predicted by equating expression 7 to one and solving for ω. The result is:

$$\omega = \sqrt{\frac{\ln(A\sigma_1\sqrt{\pi}/C)}{\{\sigma_{IO}^2 + (\sigma_1^2 - \sigma_0^2)M^2\}\pi^2}} \quad (8)$$

For the highest frequency filter measured in adults $\alpha_1 = 0.019$ degree, A = 2704/degree (Wilson and Gelb, 1984; Wilson, 1991), and $\sigma_0 = 0.0104$ degree (Geisler, 1984). The acuities in Table 32-1 were calculated from Eq. 8 using these values plus the assumption that infant and adult optics are identical ($\sigma_O = \sigma_{IO}$).

INFANT ACUITY AND CONTRAST SENSITIVITY

The previous section provided a quantitative description of the effects of infant outer segment length and cone spacing on underlying visual mechanisms. These theoretical results are first compared with infant grating acuity data. It is well known that forced choice preferential looking (FPL) acuities fall significantly below VEP acuities for at least the first year of life. Accordingly, the predictions are compared primarily with VEP data. The open circles in Figure 32-6 represent mean VEP acuities over the first 13 months of life (Norcia and Tyler, 1985). The VEP acuities of four infants at 5 weeks of age from a subsequent study are also shown (open squares) (Norcia et al., 1990). Mean acuity increases from 4.5 cpd at 1 month up to about 18 cpd at 8 months. Norcia et al. (1990) reported comparable data from another group of infants. From 8 to 13 months, however, acuity remains roughly constant.

Infant retinas were available only at 5 days and 15 months age, and the calculated acuities of 8.0 cpd and

---

4. Multiplication of all space constants by M in the Fourier transform of Eq. 2 or 3 has the effect of shifting the function a distance M to the left on logarithmic spatial frequency coordinates. When this function is inverse Fourier transformed in two dimensions to recover the spatial filter, a factor of $1/M^2$ multiplies the gain A. It reflects reduced cone density per unit area caused by the scale change. This point was correctly described previously but was not adequately explained (Wilson, 1988).

5. Geisler (1984) reported his space constant in minutes of arc and defined his Gaussians to have a factor of 2 in the denominator of the exponent, in keeping with the conventions of statistics.

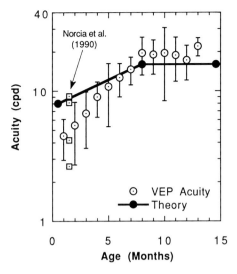

FIG. 32-6. Development of infant acuity measured using VEPs. Open circles plot means and standard deviations for ages 1–13 months as reported by Norcia and Tyler (1985). The four open squares on the left show VEP acuities at 5 weeks as reported by Norcia et al. (1990). Theoretical predictions are indicated by the solid circles and heavy line. Although infant retinas have only been examined at 5 days and 15 months of age, it was hypothesized that the 15 month retina reflected characteristics of a developmental plateau (evident in the VEP acuity data) beginning at age 8 months. Although the predicted acuity lies above the mean VEP acuity at one month, note that the prediction agrees almost perfectly with two of the four acuities plotted as squares.

16.0 cpd, respectively, are plotted appropriately in Figure 32-6 (solid circles). Although no anatomical data are yet available at intervening ages, it may be conjectured that infant foveal cone spacing and outer segment length remain roughly constant during the period 8–13 months when VEP acuity has plateaued. Accordingly, the 15-month acuity has been reproduced at 8 months and the three points connected with straight lines. It is apparent that the calculated 15-month acuity agrees well with average VEP acuities over the 8- to 13-month period. The calculated acuity for the 5-day-old fovea, however, falls more than 1 standard deviation (SD) above the means for 1- to 2-month-old infants. Note, however, that acuities for two of the four 1-month-old infants studied by Norcia et al. (1990) are virtually identical to the theoretical value of 8.0 cpd (open squares). Thus it is plausible that the anatomical factors calculated from the one 5-day retina provide a complete explanation of VEP acuity for a subset of infants who are above the average. In this context it is worth remembering that normal adult acuities vary over 1.0 octave (20/20–20/10), and the foveal cone density in four adult eyes has been reported to vary by a factor of 3.3 (Curcio et al., 1987). This cone density difference translates into a factor of 1.8 in adult cone spacing, so it is likely that a similar range occurs in neonates.

As mentioned above, behavioral FPL acuities are much lower than VEP acuities at birth. As the VEP reflects activity in striate cortex, the much lower FPL acuities are presumably the result of immaturities at higher stages of the visual system. Certainly, FPL acuities of 1–2 cpd in neonates (Gwiazda et al., 1980; Mayer and Dobson, 1982) are too low to be explained by peripheral vision, as infant peripheral retina appears normal (Abramov et al., 1982). For example, adult acuity at 45 degrees eccentricity is about 3.0 cpd, which is about twice as high as neonate FPL acuity. However, the approach developed above does provide a reasonably accurate description of FPL acuities from 15 months to adulthood (Wilson, 1988).

As illustrated in Figure 32-4, the two major aspects of infant retinal immaturity can be used to predict the infant CSF given the adult CSF. As the adult CSF is known to be the envelope of a number of more narrowly tuned mechanisms, such as those in Figure 32-5, it is only necessary to compensate these mechanisms for infant foveal cone spacing and outer segment length and then calculate their sensitivity envelope. The relative heights of the individual mechanisms in Figure 32-5 are those reported previously for these temporal conditions (Wilson and Gelb, 1984). However, the peak sensitivity of the envelope was set at 315, which is the peak adult VEP sensitivity reported by Norcia et al. (1990). This adult sensitivity shift reflects the fact that Norcia et al. (1990) used a mean luminance of 220 candelas (cd)/m², whereas Wilson et al. (1983) conducted their masking studies at 17.5 cd/m². As shown by Kelly (1972), the sensitivity shift may be calculated as the square root of the luminance ratio.

The calculated adult CSF at a temporal frequency of 6–8 Hz is plotted as the higher solid curve in Figure 32-7. The remaining two curves in Figure 32-7 show CSFs predicted for the neonate and 15-month-old infant. Although not shown, the 45-month CSF falls about half way between the adult and 15-month curves. They were derived from the adult function by first shifting it to lower sensitivities to reflect reduced outer segment length and then shifting it toward lower spatial frequencies to reflect increased foveal cone spacing (left panel of Fig. 32-4).

The predicted adult (dashed line) and infant (solid line) CSFs are compared with VEP contrast sensitivity data (Norcia et al., 1990) in Figure 32-8. The good fit to the adult data was expected, as the model was developed to fit adult psychophysical sensitivities. The predicted infant CSF is compared with average VEP data at 5 weeks and 9 weeks of age. The theory clearly provides a good fit to the average 9-week-old infant, although it is systematically too high at 5 weeks. The discrepancy between theoretical and empirical CSFs at 5 weeks is by an average factor of 3.16. As with the

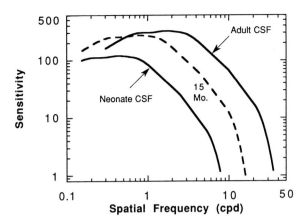

FIG. 32-7. Theoretical CSFs for neonate (5 day), 15 month, and adult. The adult CSF represents the envelope of the mechanisms in Figure 32-5. The neonate and 15 month CSFs were derived from the adult by introducing a sensitivity loss due to reduced cone outer segment length plus a spatial scale shift due to decreased foveal cone density as illustrated on the left side of Figure 32-4. Although not shown, the predicted CSF at 45 months lies about halfway between the 15-month and adult curves.

acuity data in Figure 32-6, however, there are individual infants who show sensitivities at least as high as those predicted. For example, the open square in Figure 32-8 plots the 0.25 cpd sensitivity of Jacob (from Fig. 3 of Norcia et al., 1990). Thus it is possible that the one neonatal eye examined by Yuodelis and Hendrickson (1986) had characteristics placing it toward the more sensitive end of the normal range.

Given the excellent fit between the neonate theory and the 9-week data, however, it seems most likely that

an additional maturation process occurs between 1 and 2 months of age. As cone spacing and decreased outer segment length cannot account for the reduced sensitivity at 5 weeks compared to 9 weeks (assuming the one neonate retina to be average), a further sensitivity reduction factor must be sought. The calculations above have assumed that the photopigment density per unit length of the outer segment is the same in infants and adults. If, however, the density in neonates were about 10 times lower, it would shift the theoretical curve downward by the observed factor of 3.16. A rapid increase of photopigment densities to adult levels between 5 and 9 weeks could then explain the data. This hypothesis, of course, requires anatomical evaluation.

The theoretical CSF derived from the 15-month-old retina is compared with VEP data in Figure 32-9. As the oldest data available were obtained at 31 weeks of age (Norcia et al., 1990), they have been plotted for comparison with predictions (solid curve). Partial justification for this comparison between 8 and 15 months is provided by the observed plateau in VEP acuity evident in Figure 32-6 (Norcia and Tyler, 1985). The agreement between theory and data is reasonably good, although the mean VEP sensitivity at 31 weeks is slightly lower than predicted. There are, however, individual infants whose CSFs fit the theory well. For example, the open squares in Figure 32-9 show data for David at 21 weeks of age (Norcia et al., 1990). As these data agree with the theory so well, we may tentatively conclude that foveal immaturity can predict contrast sen-

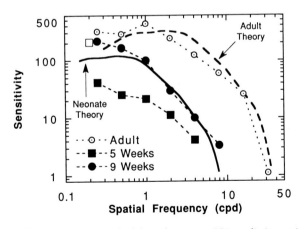

FIG. 32-8. Comparison of adult and neonate CSF predictions with VEP data (Norcia et al., 1990). Agreement between adult theory (dashed curve) and data (open circles) was expected, as the theory was developed from adult psychophysics. The neonate prediction (solid curve) lies above average sensitivities at 5 weeks (solid squares), but it accurately fits infant data at 9 weeks (solid circles). However, at least one 5 week infant (Jacob et al., 1990) recorded a sensitivity even higher than the neonate prediction (open square at 0.25 cpd). See text for discussion.

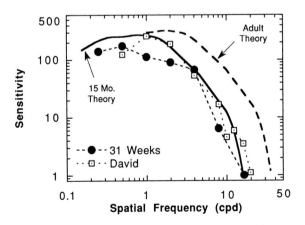

FIG. 32-9. Comparison of CSF predictions and VEP data (Norcia et al., 1990) for older infants. The solid curve is the CSF predicted from data on one 15-month-old retina. Compared with the average CSF at 31 weeks (solid circles), the theory is reasonably accurate in shape and only slightly high in sensitivity. However, data for individual infants, such as David (open squares), fit the theory almost perfectly. The adult CSF (dashed curve) is plotted for reference. Note that at this age peak infant sensitivities are almost equal to those of adults. However, the high spatial frequency limb of the CSF is shifted toward lower spatial frequencies in infants. These VEP data therefore support the spatial scale change hypothesis.

sitivity in the 5- to 8-month age range. Corroboration of this point requires anatomical data on retinas at these ages.

Given the caveat that theoretical predictions have been based on one retina at each age, it appears that foveal immaturity does predict both VEP acuity and the CSF from about 9 weeks to 31 weeks of age. As predictions based on the 45-month retina fall between the 15-month and adult curves in Figure 32-9, it is also likely that the 45-month predictions will prove accurate when the data become available. The discrepancy between the neonate theory and 5-week VEP data in Figure 32-8 clearly requires further study. Either the one 5-day retina examined by Yuodelis and Hendrickson (1986) has anatomical features falling toward the high acuity and sensitivity ends of the infant distribution, or an additional maturational factor must be involved. One candidate for this additional factor would be reduced photopigment density in the outer segment.

Two anatomical factors have led to the predictions here: reduced outer segment length and increased infant foveal cone spacing. As emphasized by Figure 32-4, these factors have been utilized differently in the two available theories of infant development. The key issue is whether increased foveal cone spacing produces a spatial scale shift (Wilson, 1988) or simply causes a further decrease in sensitivity (Banks and Bennett, 1988). A spatial scale shift follows from the hypothesis that cortical mechanisms are connected to the same array of neighboring cones throughout development (Fig. 32-3). The CSF data of Norcia et al. (1990) provide clear evidence in favor of the spatial scale shift hypothesis. As they noted, peak contrast sensitivity has almost reached adult levels by 9 weeks of age (Fig. 32-8). Thereafter, the primary change is a progressive shift toward higher acuity with almost no increase in sensitivity. This empirical pattern of results is impossible on the hypothesis diagrammed on the right of Figure 32-4, as acuity improvement here can be produced only by large sensitivity increases. With the spatial scale change hypothesis, however, the developmental effects of outer segment growth and increasing foveal cone density are orthogonal: The former causes an upward shift of the CSF, whereas the latter shifts the CSF toward higher spatial frequencies. These two factors are graphed as a function of age in Figure 32-10. The gray bars plot sensitivity at each age relative to the adult and have been derived from outer segment length data as discussed above. Note that the sensitivity is more than 84% of the adult value by 15 months of age. The black bars plot the ratio of adult to infant foveal cone spacing, a figure proportional to the development of acuity toward adult levels. Even with only four ages represented, it is clear that this spatial scale shift takes a much longer time to approach adult levels. As shown above, this is

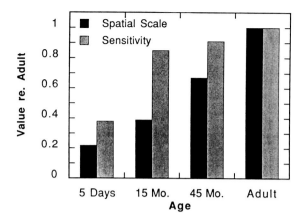

FIG. 32-10. Two foveal factors affecting infant spatial vision. The light gray bars indicate the development of peak CSF sensitivity as limited by cone outer segment length. Black bars indicate the spatial scale change of infant foveal vision relative to the adult. Thus, these values are reciprocals of relative cone spacing. Note that the sensitivity factor has reached 85% of adult values by 15 months of age, while the spatial scale shift has only attained 67% of adult levels by 45 months. Thus, infant retinal anatomy is consistent with the two developmental time courses observed in VEP measurements of the CSF (Norcia et al., 1990).

in reasonable quantitative agreement with infant VEP data (Norcia and Tyler, 1985; Norcia et al., 1990), which support the spatial scale shift hypothesis (Wilson, 1988).

FLICKER SENSITIVITY

The approach developed here can also be used to predict infant temporal frequency sensitivity. Sensitivity to uniform flickering fields is known to be mediated by transient mechanisms tuned to low spatial frequencies (Watson and Nachmias, 1977; Lehky and Wilson, 1984; Bergen and Wilson, 1985; Lehky, 1985). As the response to uniform fields is not affected by increased foveal cone spacing, only the sensitivity decrease by a factor of 2.7 due to decreased outer segment length affects flicker sensitivity. Kelly (1971; Kelly and Wilson, 1978) has shown that the high frequency portion of the temporal sensitivity curve falls along an asymptote determined by the diffusion equation. Thus the critical flicker frequency (CFF) is just that frequency α for which

$$Ke^{-\sqrt{2\pi\tau\alpha}} = 1 \qquad (9)$$

The time constant τ has been estimated to be about 0.50 (Kelly, 1971).

Regan (1981) has reported that 4-week-old infants have CFFs averaging 40.7 Hz. By 12 weeks this figure had improved to 51.5 Hz, which was not significantly different from adult foveal values. If one assumes an adult CFF of 51.5 Hz and uses it to obtain an adult value of K, Eq. 9 predicts that a reduction of K by a factor of 2.7 would reduce the infant CFF to 43.8 Hz, which is close to the observed value. Even if K were reduced by a further factor of 3 in accord with the sensitivity data in Figure 32-8, it would reduce the predicted CFF only to 36.3 Hz. Thus the relatively high infant CFF can be predicted fairly well from reduced quantum catch by the shorter infant cone outer segments. This conclusion is important, as it suggests that the time constant τ for infant foveal cones is identical to that for adult cones.

CORTICAL DEVELOPMENT

The foregoing has shown that infant retinal immaturity provides the major and perhaps only limitation on infant acuity and contrast sensitivity as measured by the VEP. However, many cortical functions such as stereopsis and orientation selectivity have been shown to be absent at birth and to develop during the first year of life. Development of these functions obviously cannot be attributed to retinal factors.

It has been known for a long time that axonal and dendritic arbors in human striate cortex continue to develop during the first year of life (Conel, 1939). Huttenlocher et al. (1982) have quantified this development by measuring the density of synapses in human striate cortex as a function of age. As shown in Figure 32-11, synaptic density remains constant for the first 2 months of life and then increases to more than double this value by 8 months of age. Synaptic density subsequently slowly decreases to adult levels over about a decade. During the period of synaptic proliferation from 2 to 8 months, a number of visual capabilities appear. For example, the solid horizontal bar indicates the period during which adult-like orientation selectivity develops as determined by VEP techniques (Morrone and Burr, 1986). Similarly, the solid circles plot percentages of infants showing stereopsis at each age (Birch et al., 1982), and it is striking how this function parallels the increase in synaptic density. Finally, the first evidence of binocular rivalry has been reported at about 3.5 months (arrow at bottom) (Shimojo et al., 1986).

From these observations it seems apparent that at least orientation selectivity and stereopsis are dependent on postnatal cortical synapse formation for their normal development. There is physiological evidence that orientation selectivity is dependent on inhibitory cortical circuits (Sillito, 1975, 1979), so it is plausible to suggest that cortical synapse formation from 2 to 8 months of life reflects development of cortical inhibitory circuits (Wilson, 1988). Similarly, binocular rivalry clearly requires some form of interocular inhibition (Blake, 1989),

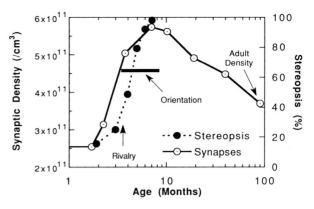

FIG. 32-11. Development of cortical synaptic density compared with age of onset of various cortical functions. Density of synapses in human striate cortex is plotted as a function of age in months (open circles, left ordinate). Data are from Huttenlocher et al. (1982). Note that density remains constant for the first two months of life and then rapidly more than doubles between 2 and 8 months. Following this period of synaptic proliferation there is a slow decrease to adult levels over about a decade. Solid circles (right ordinate) plot the percentage of infants displaying stereopsis (Birch et al., 1982). It is striking that the population averaged development of stereopsis shows almost the same time course as the increase in cortical synaptic density. The heavy horizontal line marked "Orientation" indicates the time window during which cortical orientation selectivity has first been observed in VEP studies (Morrone and Burr, 1986). Finally, the arrow marked "Rivalry" shows the onset of binocular rivalry (Shimojo et al., 1986). Both orientation selectivity and rivalry first appear during the period of synaptic proliferation.

so here again cortical synapse proliferation may reflect inhibitory circuit development.

Stereopsis is a more complex issue. Certainly, infant visual experience can dramatically alter binocular aspects of cortical anatomy (Movshon and VanSluyters, 1981; Wiesel, 1982). However, the critical period for these developmental effects seems to occur mainly after 8 months of age, at a time when cortical synaptic density is decreasing. In the absence of adequate models for adult stereopsis (Blake and Wilson, 1991), it is probably best to be content with the empirical correlation between cortical synapse formation and the emergence of stereopsis in Figure 32-11.

CONCLUSIONS AND CONJECTURES

If it is assumed that cortical units receive input originating from a fixed array of neighboring cones throughout development, the increased spacing of infant foveal cones produces a spatial scale shift toward lower spatial frequencies (Wilson, 1988). This shift plus the decrease in contrast sensitivity caused by reduced outer segment length come tantalizingly close to providing an explanation for the development of VEP acuity and the CSF. With the caveat that predictions are based on anatomy from one 5-day-old and one 15-month-old retina (Yu-odelis and Hendrickson, 1986), the theory provides a reasonable fit to VEP data (Norcia et al., 1990) from 9 weeks through 13 months of age and probably on into adulthood.

The one 5-day-old fovea produces predictions of both contrast sensitivity (Fig. 32-8) and acuity (Fig. 32-6) somewhat above the means for 1-month-old infants. One possibility is that the anatomy of this retina falls toward one end of the typical human range. Two lines of evidence support this idea. First, foveal cone densities in the four adult human retinas studied vary by a factor of 3.3 (Curcio et al., 1987), which translates into a 1.8 : 1.0 range of normal adult cone spacings. Second, VEP acuities for two of the four 1-month-old infants in the Norcia et al. (1990) study are virtually identical to the theoretical value (Fig. 32-6), and the contrast sensitivity of at least one infant in that study was some-what above the theoretical value (Fig. 32-8). The other possibility is that additional immaturity is involved. One hypothesis is that photopigment density per unit length of the outer segment is lower in neonates than in adults. To account for a 5-week CSF that is more than three times lower than predicted would require a 10-fold reduction in pigment density. A decision between these possibilities must clearly await further anatomical data.

The ideal observer approach adopted by Banks and Bennett (1988) was based on different assumptions that interpret reduced outer segment length *and* decreased cone spacing as producing decreases in contrast sensitivity (see right side of Fig. 32-4). This approach fares less well with the data than does the spatial scale change hypothesis. In particular, Norcia et al. (1990) have discovered that development is characterized by an initial rapid increase in contrast sensitivity. After this point, peak sensitivity remains almost constant, whereas acuity and the entire high spatial frequency side of the CSF march toward higher frequencies. This change cannot occur on the Banks and Bennett (1988) hypothesis, as the only shift in the CSF is a uniform sensitivity loss. It should be stressed that this ideal observer model is not "atheoretical" but, rather, contains implicit hypotheses about changing neural connectivity during development (see above).

The spatial scale change hypothesis and the data of Norcia et al. (1990) definitively reject the "dark glasses" hypothesis of infant visual development. This hypothesis states that the only difference between infant and adult vision is decreased infant sensitivity resulting from a lower quantum catch (due to the metaphoric presence of dark glasses in the infant visual system). If it were true, a simple increase in mean luminance should be able to transform infant into adult vision. It is impossible, however, for a spatial scale change to be com-pensated by an increase in luminance, as a scale change can be compensated only by magnification of the image (Fig. 32-3).

There is one final consequence of foveal cone migration that warrants mention. As cones migrate during development, not only the dimensions of cortical filters but also their locations must change. The distances over which it occurs can be substantial. For simplicity, suppose that infant foveal cone spacing is uniformly greater by a factor of M out to eccentricity E. During development, cones at E migrate inward until adult foveal cone densities are achieved, at which time these cones are located at eccentricity E/M. Thus the cumulative migration distance is $E(1 - 1/M)$. For M = 4.64 (Table 32-1), and E in the range 1–2 degrees, this distance is 0.8–1.6 degrees (Wilson, 1988), which is a large distance for an adult visual system that can localize lines in hyperacuity tasks to about 5.0 arc seconds (West-heimer, 1979). Cortical plasticity must clearly compensate for this position shift during development.

Little has been said here about FPL measures of infant acuity and contrast sensitivity. FPL data fall far below VEP meausres during the first year of life, and the theory developed here cannot explain it (Wilson, 1988). As the VEP is a measure of activity in striate cortex, and as VEP data are reasonably well explained by retinal immaturity, the only plausible conclusion is that FPL measurements reflect immaturities beyond the striate site of the VEP.

At this juncture it seems clear that the definitive theoretical treatment of CSF and acuity development must await further anatomical data. In particular, retinas at a range of ages between birth and 15 months must be analyzed. Furthermore, it is necessary to obtain some measure of anatomical variability, at least at birth and during the 8- to 15-month acuity plateau. The appropriate way to analyze these data as they become available is within a theoretical framework incorporating a sensitivity loss resulting from shortened outer segments and a spatial scale shift caused by reduced foveal cone density (Wilson, 1988).

Where should developmental theories go from here? Even if we assume that the analysis above ultimately proves fully capable of predicting CSF and acuity development, these analyses comprise a modest set of measurements of human visual function. Consider the postnatal development of stereopsis. As shown in Figure 32-11, it is strongly correlated with the period of cortical synapse proliferation. This observation, however, is empirical, not theoretical. One problem besetting potential theories of stereoscopic development is that there are as yet no fully adequate models of adult stereopsis (Blake and Wilson, 1991). Nevertheless, a few conjectures may be useful here to suggest directions in which such a model might evolve.

What advantages are there in developmental modification in contrast to genetic specification of the visual system? At least two are obvious. First, development can fine-tune the system to compensate for cone migration, increasing interocular distance, and so on. Second, the greater the extent to which anatomical connections can be acquired during development, the less the amount of genetic information needed to specify the system. Connectionist learning models are currently in vogue, and studies such as that by Lehky and Sejnowski (1988) and Miller et al. (1989) have shown that a surprising amount of visual structure can arise through stimulus-driven synaptic change. For useful learning to occur, however, connectionist nets require a significant amount of a priori structure: they are never totally random.

How might a minimum of genetic structure be used to constrain the postnatal development of stereopsis? It has been established that low spatial frequency (coarse scale) mechanisms can process much larger disparities than fine-scale mechanisms tuned to higher spatial frequencies (Schor et al., 1984). Furthermore, disparity processing on low spatial frequency scales has been shown to constrain disparity analysis on higher frequency scales (Wilson et al., 1991). The largest and smallest foveal mechanisms in adults have peak spatial frequencies estimated to differ by a factor of 20 (Wilson and Gelb, 1984). From the sampling theorem, it follows that in two dimensions 400 times as many cells and connections are necessary for processing on the highest in contrast to the lowest frequency scale, suggesting a *coarse-to-fine scale developmental hypothesis*. Suppose that the coarsest spatial frequency scale is genetically prewired to process large disparities. Subsequently, activity on the coarse scale serves to constrain and guide development of stereopsis on successively finer scales, which could reduce the necessary genetic information to less than 1/400 of that otherwise required. Furthermore, it would permit the processing of small disparities on fine resolution scales to be fine-tuned during development. Finally, disparity processing on the coarse scale would provide the a priori framework for developing connections on finer scales.

Although the coarse-to-fine scale stereoscopic developmental hypothesis is purely conjectural at present, it immediately suggests new experiments on infant vision. In particular, infant stereopsis should develop first at spatial frequencies that are low relative to infant acuity, and stereopsis should only appear at higher spatial frequencies later. In addition, the range of disparities that can be fused by infants should be similar to or larger than the fusion range for adults. These cases are examples of the way in which even crudely articulated models can help to guide experimentation. Exploration of this and other strategies for the development of stere-

opsis and other higher visual functions remains a challenge for future developmental theories.

Acknowledgment. This research was supported by NIH grant EY02158 to the author.

REFERENCES

ABRAMOV, I., GORDON, J., HENDRICKSON, A., HAINLINE, L., DOBSON, V., AND LABOSSIERE, E. (1982). The retina of the newborn human infant. *Science* 217, 265–267.

BANKS, M. S., AND BENNETT, P. J. (1988). Optical and photoreceptor immaturities limit the spatial and chromatic vision of human neonates. *J. Opt. Soc. Am.* [A] 5, 2059–2079.

BANKS, M. S., AND SALAPATEK, P. (1983). Infant visual perception. In M. HAITH AND J. CAMPOS (eds.). *Biology and Infancy*. New York: Wiley, pp. 435–471.

BERGEN, J. R., AND WILSON, H. R. (1985). Prediction of flicker sensitivities from temporal three-pulse data. *Vision Res.* 25, 577–582.

BIRCH, E. E., GWIAZDA, J., AND HELD, R. (1982). Stereoacuity development for crossed and uncrossed disparities in human infants. *Vision Res.* 22, 507–513.

BLAKE, R. (1989). A neural theory of binocular rivalry. *Psychol. Rev.* 96, 145–167.

BLAKE, R., AND WILSON, H. R. (1991). Theories of stereoscopic vision. *Trends Neurosci.* 14, 445–452.

CAMPBELL, F. W., AND GUBISCH, R. W. (1966). Optical quality of the human eye. *J. Physiol. (Lond.)* 186, 558–578.

CONEL, J. L. (1939). *The Postnatal Development of the Human Cerebral Cortex*. Cambridge, MA: Harvard University Press.

CURCIO, C. A., SLOAN, K. R., PACKER, O., HENDRICKSON, A. E., AND KALINA, R. E. (1987). Distribution of cones in human and monkey retina: individual variability and radial asymmetry. *Science* 236, 579–582.

DEVALOIS, R. L., AND DEVALOIS, K. K. (1988). *Spatial Vision*. New York: Oxford University Press.

DOBSON, V., TELLER, D. Y., AND BELGUM, J. (1978). Visual acuity in human infants assessed with stationary stripes and phase-alternated checkerboards. *Vision Res.* 18, 1233–1238.

GEISLER, W. S. (1984). Physical limits of acuity and hyperacuity. *J. Opt. Soc. Am.* [A] 1, 775–782.

GEISLER, W. S. (1989). Sequential ideal-observer analysis of visual discriminations. *Psychol. Rev.* 96, 267–314.

GRAHAM, N. (1989). *Visual Pattern Analyzers*. New York: Oxford University Press.

GWIAZDA, J., BRILL, S., MONINDRA, I., AND HELD, R. (1980). Preferential looking acuity in infants from two to fifty-eight weeks of age. *Am. J. Optom. Physiol. Opt.* 57, 428–432.

HENDRICKSON, A. E., AND YUODELIS, C. (1984). The morphological development of the human fovea. *Ophthalmology* 91, 603–612.

HUTTENLOCHER, P. R., DECOURTEN, C., GAREY, L. J., AND VAN DER LOOS, H. (1982). Synaptogenesis in human visual cortex—evidence for synapse elimination during normal development. *Neurosci. Lett.* 33, 247–252.

KELLY, D. H. (1971). Theory of flicker and transient responses. I. Uniform fields. *J. Opt. Soc. Am.* 61, 537–546.

KELLY, D. H. (1972). Adaptation effects on spatio-temporal sine wave thresholds. *Vision Res.* 12, 89–101.

KELLY, D. H., AND WILSON, H. R. (1978). Human flicker sensitivity: two stages of retinal diffusion. *Science* 202, 896–899.

LARSEN, J. S. (1971). The sagittal growth of the eye. IV. Ultrasonic measurement of the axial length of the eye from birth to puberty. *Acta Ophthalmol. (Copenh.)* 49, 873–886.

LEHKY, S. R. (1985). Temporal properties of visual channels measured by masking. *J. Opt. Soc. Am.* [A] 2, 1260–1272.

LEHKY, S., AND SEJNOWSKI, T. J. (1988). Network model of shape-from-shading: neural function arises from both receptive and projective fields. *Nature* 333, 452–454.

LEHKY, S. R., AND WILSON, H. R. (1984). Temporal characteristics of visual channels measured by masking. *J. Opt. Soc. Am.* [A] 1, 1272.

MAYER, D. L., AND DOBSON, V. (1982). Visual acuity development in infants and young children, as assessed by operant preferential looking. *Vision Res.* 22, 1141–1151.

MILLER, K. D., KELLER, J. B., AND STRYKER, M. P. (1989). Ocular dominance column development: analysis and simulation. *Science* 245, 605–615.

MORRONE, M. C., AND BURR, D. C. (1986). Evidence for the existence and development of visual inhibition in humans. *Nature* 321, 235–237.

MOVSHON, J. A., AND VANSLUYTERS, R. C. (1981). Visual neural development. *Annu. Rev. Psychol.* 32, 477–522.

NORCIA, A. M., AND TYLER, C. W. (1985). Spatial frequency sweep VEP: visual acuity during the first year of life. *Vision Res.* 25, 1399–1408.

NORCIA, A. M., TYLER, C. W., AND HAMER, R. (1988). High visual contrast sensitivity in the young human infant. *Invest. Ophthalmol. Vis. Sci.*

NORCIA, A. M., TYLER, C. W., AND HAMER, R. D. (1990). Development of contrast sensitivity in the human infant. *Vision Res.* 30, 1475–1486.

POKORNY, J., AND SMITH, V. C. (1976). Effect of field size on red-green color mixture equations. *J. Opt. Soc. Am.* 66, 705–708.

POKORNY, J., SMITH, V. C., AND STARR, S. (1976). Variability of color mixture data. II. The effect of viewing field size on the unit coordinates. *Vision Res.* 16, 1095–1098.

REGAN, D. M. (1981). Development of critical flicker frequency in human infants. *Vision Res.* 21, 549–555.

SCHOR, C., WOOD, I., AND OGAWA, J. (1984). Binocular sensory fusion is limited by spatial resolution. *Vision Res.* 24, 661–665.

SHIMOJO, S., BAUER, J., O'CONNELL, K. M., AND HELD, R. (1986). Per-stereoptic binocular vision in infants. *Vision Res.* 26, 501–510.

SILLITO, A. M. (1975). The contribution of inhibitory mechanisms to the receptive field properties of neurones in the striate cortex of the cat. *J. Physiol. (Lond.)* 250, 305–329.

SILLITO, A. M. (1979). Inhibitory mechanisms influencing complex cell orientation selectivity and their modification at high resting discharge levels. *J. Physiol. (Lond.)* 289, 33–53.

WATSON, A. B., AND NACHMIAS J. (1977). Patterns of temporal integration in the detection of gratings. *Vision Res.* 17, 893–902.

WESTHEIMER, G. (1979). Spatial sense of the eye. *Invest. Ophthalmol. Vis. Sci.* 18, 893–912.

WIESEL, T. N. (1982). Postnatal development of the visual cortex and the influence of environment. *Nature* 299, 583–591.

WILSON, H. R. (1986). Responses of spatial mechanisms can explain hyperacuity. *Vision Res.* 26, 453–469.

WILSON, H. R. (1988). Development of spatiotemporal mechanisms in infant vision. *Vision Res.* 28, 611–628.

WILSON, H. R. (1991). Psychophysical models of spatial vision and hyperacuity. In D. REGAN (ed.). *Spatial Form Vision*. New York: Macmillan.

WILSON, H. R., AND BERGEN, J. R. (1979). A four mechanism model for threshold spatial vision. *Vision Res.* 19, 19–32.

WILSON, H. R., AND GELB, D. J. (1984). Modified line element theory for spatial frequency and width discrimination. *J. Opt. Soc. Am.* [A] 1, 124–131.

WILSON, H. R., BLAKE, R., AND HALPERN, D. L. (1991). Coarse spatial scales constrain the range of binocular fusion on fine scales. *J. Opt. Soc. Am.* [A] 8, 229–236.

WILSON, H. R., LEVI, D., MAFFEI, L., ROVAMO, J., AND DEVALOIS, R. L. (1990). The perception of form: retina to striate cortex. In L. SPILLMAN AND J. S. WERNER (eds.). *The Neurophysiological Foundations of Visual Perception*. Orlando, FL: Academic Press.

WILSON, H. R., MCFARLANE, D. K., AND PHILLIPS, G. C. (1983). Spatial frequency tuning of orientation selective units estimated by oblique masking. *Vision Res.* 23, 873–882.

YUODELIS, C., AND HENDRICKSON, A. (1986). A qualitative and quantitative analysis of the human fovea during development. *Vision Res.* 26, 847–855.

Index

Note: Page numbers followed by t refer to tables, page numbers followed by f refer to figures.

Accommodation, 30–33
  accuracy measurement and, 30–31
  attentional factors and, 32
  dynamics of, 33
  in esotropia, 335–336
  motor factors and, 32
  near triad eye movements and, 42
  refractive development and, 20
  sensory deficits and, 32
  stimulus-response functions, 31f, 32f
  vergence and, 36, 43
Acuity. *See* Visual acuity
Acuity card procedure, 312, 319–331
  amblyopes and, 328
  delayed visual maturation and, 507
  limitations of, 329–330
    accuracy of measurement, 329
    bias, 329–330
    myopic refractive errors and, 330
  nonverbal adults and, 329
  premature infants and, 328–329, 497
  quality assurance with, 331
  research base for, 319–321
    gestational age and, 321
    grating orientation and, 321
    monocular versus binocular acuity, 321
    stimulus luminance and, 320
    target distance and, 320–321
  scrambled cards, 330
  testability rates, 325–326
  validation studies, 321–325
    construct validity, 322–323, 322f
    content validity, 323
    criterion-related validity, 323–325, 324t
  variational effects, 326–328
    stimulus configuration, 326–327
    stimulus orientation, 327
    testing procedure, 327–328
Albinism
  screening procedures and, 337
  strabismic amblyopia and, 416–418
Albino heterozygote optomotor miswiring, 426
Amblyopia, 391–405
  acuity and, 395–396
  acuity card procedure and, 328
  cataract, infant, and, 454
  color vision and, 392
  contrast sensitivity and, 393, 396, 466
  developmental period and, 398–399
  eccentricity and, 403–405, 403f, 404f, 405f
  effective age and, 399–401, 399f, 400f
  electroretinography in, 419
  environmental factors and, 300, 376
  fixation preference in, 314f, 315
  fluorescein angiography in, 419
  hyperacuity and, 394–395, 396

light sense and, 391–392
  luminance increment thresholds and, 392
  maternal birth posture and, 438–439
  meridional, 344–345, 345f
  natural history and, 401–402
  occlusion therapy for, 339, 456
  photoprotection for, 442
  preferential looking in, 313f
  pupillary light reflex in, 419
  pursuit asymmetries and, 371
  refraction and, 343, 439–441
  retinal involvement in, 418–423
  risk factors for, 415
  screening procedures and, 336–340
  spatial mapping distortions in, 415–426, 415f
  spatial vision in, 393–394
  stereopsis and, 255, 430, 472
  Stiles-Crawford effect in, 392, 419
  temporal processing in, 392–393, 425
  time encoding defects and, 425–426
  treatment of, 339, 438, 454
  Vernier acuity and, 396–398, 397f
  visual evoked potentials in, 314f, 315
Amblyopiagenesis, 301, 431–433, 432f, 454; *See also* Amblyopia
Amino acids, excitatory, and eye growth, 25
Aminosulfonic acid taurine, 498
Aniseikonia
  and infantile cataracts, 480
  and longitudinal horopter, 241
Angle kappa, and eye alignment, 241, 350, 438
Angle lambda, 241
  and change in the horopter with development, 243
Anisometropia, 10–11. *See also* Anisometropic amblyopes
  axial length and, 10
  and later development, 11
  and visual development, 301
Anisometropic amblyopes, 391
  and developmental timing, 399–402
  eccentricity and, 403–405
  hyperacuity and, 395
  visual acuity and, 393
Anisotropy, of orientation visual-evoked potentials, 166–167
Anomalous retinal correspondence, 414, 431, 433
Anticonvulsants, and pursuit, 65
Aperture, receptor, age-related changes in, 102, 102f, 293–294, 299, 560
Area PG, and conjugate eye movements, 52–53
Astigmatism
  changes in with age, 8, 15, 342–343, 343f
  consequences of, 9, 344

during early infancy, 7
  later development, 11
  and off-axis refractions, 7
  one to five years, 10
  and prematurity, 8, 498
Atropine, and accommodation, 20
Attentional factors
  and accommodation, 32
  and convergence, 34
  and premature infants, 492–496, 494f, 495f
Autofluorescence, and retinal light scatter, 424–425
Autorefraction, and accommodation measurement, 31, 32, 32f
Axial length, 242–243
  and refractive state, 10

Background adaptation, and scotopic sensitivity, 136–139
Balint syndrome, 58
Barrel distortion, of retinal images, 241
Bathopsis, 356–357
Beer-Lambert relation, 180
Behavioral measurement. *See also* Behavioral models
  of orientational discrimination, 168–169
  in premature infants, 497
Behavioral models
  problems with, 532–533
Bias, and acuity card procedure, 329–330
Binocular processing, 267–278, 381
  dichoptic mechanisms, 270–272
    dichoptic summation, 271–272, 272f
    interocular rivalry and suppression, 271
    luster, 270–271
  dynamic stereomechanisms, 274–276
    chromatic stereomotion perception, 274–276, 275f
    real stereomotion perception, 274
  fusion, 201, 229, 250
  global interactions and, 276
  heterarchical model, 267–270, 268f
    model structure, 269–270
    specialized disparity mechanisms, 268–269, 269f
  hypercyclopean perception and, 276–278
    object constancy, 278
    orientation specificity, 277
    spatial frequency specificity, 277
    stereomotion perception, 277–278
  static stereomechanisms, 272–274
    coarse disparity, 272–273
    depth tilt from diffrequency, 273–274
    fine disparity, 272
    orientational disparity, 273
Binocular rivalry
  discrimination of in infants, 201

Binocular summation of brightness, 252–253, 253f
Binocular vision. *See also* Binocular processing; Convergence; Stereopsis
  acuity measurement and, 230–231, 321
  basics of, 197–199
  binocular beats, 214, 252
  binocular deficit cascade, 427–430
  binocular processing modes, 267–278
  catabolism and, 430–431, 433
  disparity, 197, 225, 237–238
  function onset, 201–202, 225, 250
  interocular visual development, 201–222
  mature, 254–255
  versus monocular vision in development, 413–415
  nasal motion bias and, 367, 371
  neural mechanisms and development of, 231–232
  and optokinetic nystagmus, 85
  orthoptic examination of, 338
  sensorimotor adaptation and horopter development, 237–248
  sensory threshold and, 258–261
  two-stage developmental model, 250–256
  visually evoked potentials and, 252
  visual fields, 123–124, 123f
Biochemical pathways, and growth response, 24–26
Birth posture, maternal, 438–439
Birth trauma
  and amblyopia, 421–423
  and strabismus, 426–427
Bleaching adaptation, and scotopic sensitivity, 139, 140f
Botulinum toxin chemodenervation, 358–359
Brain damage, and strabismus, 426–427
Brightness summation, binocular, 252–253, 253f
Bruckner test, 358, 358f, 360f
b-wave sensitivity, 132–133, 132f, 133f
  and background adaptation, 138–139, 138f, 139f

Cambridge Crowding Cards, 338
Catabolism, binocular, 430–431, 433
Cataract, infant, 455–480
  accommodation after surgery, 480
  aniseikonia and, 480
  competition between eyes and, 478–479
  contrast sensitivity and, 466–472
  cortical projections and, 477–478
  deprivation and, 478–479
  fusion and, 472–474
  grating acuity and, 455–463
  linear letter acuity and, 463–466
  optokinetic nystagmus and, 459–463, 478–480
    symmetry of, 474–477
  preferential looking and, 455–459, 478–480
  sensitive periods and, 478
  stereopsis and, 473–474, 478
  strabismus and, 479
Cell development, retinal, 287
Centripetal cone migration, and horopter, 245–246, 246f
Cerebellum, and conjugate eye movements, 52

Choriocapillaris, in neonates, 488
Chromatic aberration, 26
Chromatic channels, 145
Chromatic discrimination, 150, 151–152, 558
  stereomotion and, 274–276, 275f
Coarse disparity processing, 278–279
Color vision, infant, 143–160, 182
  amblyopia and, 392
  contrast discrimination and, 187–192
  discrimination ellipsoids and motion nulls, 157–160
  isoluminant plane and, 155–157
  moving stimuli and, 152–154
    motion nulling, 153–154
    motion photometry, 153
    optokinetic nystagmus and, 154
  rod dominance hypothesis, 160
  three-dimensional color spaces, 144–152
    discrimination ellipsoids and, 149–152
    null plane analysis and, 144–149
  uniform loss hypothesis, 160
Concurrent validity, and acuity card procedure, 323–325
  interobserver reliability, 323–325, 324t
  intraobserver reliability, 323
Cones, foveal, and visual development. *See* Fovea
Cone excitation space, 144–145, 145f
Conjugate eye movements
  classes of, 40, 47–48
  fixation. *See* Fixation
  measurement, methodological considerations, 70–75
    corneal reflection trackers, 71–75
    direct observations, 70
    electrooculogram, 70–71
  neural mechanisms controlling, 48–53
    area PG, 52–53
    cerebellum, 52
    frontal eye fields, 52
    parietal cortex, 52–53
    superior colliculus, 50–51
  oculomotor interactions, 42, 66–67
  pursuit. *See* Pursuit
  reflex, 41–42, 81
  saccades. *See* Saccades
  study of infant, critique, 75
Construct validity, and acuity card procedure, 322–323
Content validity, and acuity card procedure, 323
Contrast discrimination, and intrinsic noise, 187–192
  contrast-dependent noise, 190, 191, 191f
  contrast increment threshold functions, 188–189, 189f
  contrast noise, 190, 191f
  detection threshold measurement, 187
  difference signals, 190, 192f
  discrimination threshold measurement, 187, 193–196
  Minkowski function, 190, 191f
  psychometric functions, 188, 188f
Contrast sensitivity, 97, 187
  and amblyopia, 393–394, 396, 466
  and foveal anatomy, 293–294, 299, 563–568, 564f
  and ideal observer theory, 92, 184, 186–187
  and infantile cataract, 466–472
    animal study comparison, 471

bilateral cases, 467–469, 468f–470f
  comparison to normal infants, 469, 471
  peripheral sensitivity, 469
  unilateral cases, 467
  in normal adult, 466f
  peripheral, 121, 469
  visual evoked potentials in, 540, 566–568, 567f
Convergence, 33–37
  accommodation interactions, 36–37
  attentional factors and, 34
  corneal reflection photography in, 33–34
  estimated binocular alignment in newborns, 33f
  resting position and, 35
  retinal disparity and, 34, 34f
  spatial resolution and, 34–35, 35f
Corneal growth, in neonates, 488
Corneal reflection photography
  in accommodation-convergence interactions, 36–37
  and convergence, 33–34
Corneal reflection trackers, 71–75
  calibration and, 72–74
  elements of, 72f
  problems with, 72
  techniques, 71–72
Corpus callosum, and fusion/stereopsis development, 436–437
Cortical development, 299; *See also* Visual cortex
  binocular, 231–232
  and stereopsis, 227, 569, 569f
Cortical neurons, orientation selectivity of, 169–170
Cortical projections, and cataract, 477–478
Critical fusion frequency, and amblyopia, 392–393
Cross-orientation masking, and visual evoked potentials, 549, 549f
Cycloplegic refraction, 5
  in neonates, 6
  one to five years, 9
  and prematurity, 7–8
  three months to one year, 8

Dark-adapted sensitivity measurements, 130–133. *See also* Scotopic sensitivity
  reliability of, 316
  for retinal degenerations, 314f, 315
da Vinci stereopsis, 217, 218f–220f, 221, 222, 265–266
Defect screening, visual field, 122
Delayed visual maturation, 505–511. *See also* Premature
Density, optical, and infant rods, 179–181
Deprivation, visual, 15, 300, 401, 454, 477
Depth tilt, from diffrequency, 273–274
"Detroit model", and abnormal visual input, 398–399
Developmental models. *See* Models, developmental
De Vries-Rose law, 554
Dichoptic mechanisms, and binocular processing, 201, 229, 264–265, 270–272, 409
Diet, and preterm birth, 498

Difference-of-Gaussian luminance profile, 270, 272
Diffrequency, depth tilt from, 273–274
Directional selectivity. *See* Motion processing
Direct observation, in research, 70
Discrimination ellipsoids, 149–152, 149f
  and color experimentation, 157–160, 158f, 159f
  and cone contrast sensitivity, 182–183
  infant discrimination thresholds, 150
  MacAdam, 182–183, 183f
  pancake and cigar effects, 149f, 150
  Russian doll models, 149–150, 149f, 150–152
Disinhibition, subcortical, 436
Disparity. *See also* Binocular processing; Binocular vision; Stereopsis
  detection and binocular vision, 254, 254f
  nonconventional cues, and stereopsis, 280
  sign biases and hemiretina, 437–438
  and stereoscopic processing
    coarse, 272–273
    fine, 272
    orientational, 273
Distortion. *See* Mapping distortion
Dorsal terminal nucleus, and optokinetic nystagmus, 475–476, 477f
Drift velocity, and fixation, 59–60, 60f

Eccentricity, and amblyopia, 403–405
  and resolution/Vernier ratio, 403, 404f
Ecological optics, 215–216
Eigengrau, in light adaptation models, 137–139, 138f, 139f
Electrooculography, 70–71
  and color vision experimentation, 155
  and stereograms, 225
Electrophysiological methods, and visual field assessment, 122
Electroretinography, 122, 517–534
  in amblyopia, 419
  in background adaptation, 138–139
  in dark-adapted sensitivity measurement, 132–133
  in delayed visual maturation, 506
  dynamic model, 526, 526f
    and hypothesis about development, 526–531
    need for, 524–526, 524f–525f
  Granit's model of, 524–526, 525f
  infant and adult compared, 517, 518f
  measuring receptor parameters, 521–524, 521f–523f
  Naka-Rushton equation, 518–519
  in premature infants, 496
  static model, 519–521, 520f
    problems with, 524
  trough-to-peak b-wave amplitudes, 517–518, 518f
  vertebrate, 517, 518f
Emmetropization, 11, 17, 340
  and chromatic aberration, 26
  under closed-loop conditions, 17–19
    lens experiment results, 18–19, 19f
    refractive error recovery, 17
  local control of, 19–20
  mathematical model for, 20, 21f
Environmental influences, on visual development, 300–301

ERG. *See* Electroretinography
Escape from rivalry, and occlusion constraints, 217, 217f, 220–221, 220f–221f, 222
Esotropia, 349–360
  accommodative, 335–336
  binocularity and, 232, 254, 255, 350, 436
  detection of, 335, 349–353
  early screening and, 442
  environmental factors and, 376, 479
  and fusion/stereopsis development, 254, 436
  genetic factors in, 376
  monofixation syndrome and, 353
  and motion processing deficits, 375
  as a motor adaptation to a visual bias, 376
  onset and, 351–353, 352f
  orthotropization and, 254, 350–351
  screening for, 335, 349–350
  sensory testing, 356–357
  stereopsis and, 232–234, 233f, 254, 374
  surgery for, 353–356
    early surgery benefits, 357
    long-term results, 355–356
    refinements and, 356
    selective approach, 355
    before six months, 357–358
    specifics of, 353–354
    surgical dose-response curve, 354–355
    uniform approach, 355
  treatment of, 353–359
    botulism toxin chemodenervation, 358–359
  visual motion pathway in, 375–376, 375f
Ethnic differences
  and infant screening, 553
  and strabismus, 417
Examination of visual status, 309–315. *See also* Vision screening
  acuity cards. *See* Acuity card procedure
  clinical measures, 312–315
    infant test evaluation, 312–314, 313f–314f
    longitudinal measures, 315
    short-cut procedures, 312
  fixation preference, 311
  office examination, 311–312
  patient population data, 309–311
    age of first visit, 309, 310f
    referral data, 309–311, 310f
  prism displacement, 311
  pupillary responses, 311
  refraction measurement, 311–312
  test sensitivity and specificity, 312–315
    dark adapted threshold and retinal degeneration, 314f
    fixation preference and amblyopia, 314f
    ideal test, 313f
    interocular differences of preferential looking, 313f
    scotopic b-wave amplitudes, 314f
    visual evoked potentials and amblyopia, 314f
Exotropia, 355
  and photophobia, 433
Eye alignment. *See also* Strabismus
  codevelopment with fusion and stereopsis, 225, 254, 374–375, 410
  onset of during first year, 225, 254, 350, 364–365, 365f, 410

Eyelids, in neonates, 487
  light transmission characteristics, 488f
  opening and gestational age, 487f

Family history, and infant examination, 311
Feedback loops
  emmetropization and, 17–19, 20
  eye alignment and. *See* Eye alignment; Orthotropization
  and refractive errors, 14–15, 20–24
    accommodative loops, 21–24, 24t
    local loop, 21, 22f
Filtering, in the front-end of visual system, 91–92
Finite focus refraction, 5
Fixation, 39–40, 48
  and amblyopia, 314f, 315
  binocular, 40, 413
  defined, 48
  image slippage and, 59–60, 60f
  interpretation of infant, 62
  monocular, 39–40, 413
  motion detection and, 60
  preference evaluation, 311
  refixation accuracy, 61–62, 61f
  and vision loss, 537
Flicker sensitivity, 568–569
Fluorescein angiography, in amblyopia, 419
Fogged refraction, 5
Forced-choice method of constant stimuli procedure, 312
Forced-choice preferential looking technique. *See also* Acuity card procedure; Preferential looking technique
  importance of, 320
  in interocular acuity differences, 263
  refining methodology, 556
  variants of, 555–556
Fourier analysis, and visual evoked potentials, 537–538, 539–541
Fovea
  development of, 98, 287–291, 289t, 290f, 560
    comparative in monkey and human, 288t, 289t
    cone, 100–101, 100f–101f, 289t, 290t, 537
    and contrast sensitivity development, 98, 299
    and stereopsis development, 226, 243
    and visual acuity development, 293–294
  disc distance from, 438
  ideal observer theory and, 91, 185–187, 186f
Frequency diversity transmission, and visual evoked potentials, 544
Frontal eye fields, 117
  and conjugate eye movements, 49, 52
  and saccades, 57–58, 58f
Fusion
  binocular, 201, 250, 270, 410
  corpus callosum and, 436–437
  dichoptic, 264–265
  and infantile cataract, 472–474
  and stereopsis, 250
    developmental asynchrony and, 436–437
    in normal binocular vision, 229
  and vergence, 33, 43

Genetic factors
  and binocular vision, 442–443
  and refractive errors, 14–15
  screening procedures and, 337
  and strabismus, 376, 416–418, 442
Gestational versus post-natal, post-
      conceptual, and post-menstrual age,
      486
Globe, ocular
  changes with age and horopter, 243
  flexing, in accommodation, 438
  in neonates, 487–488
  retinal structure maturation and,
      419–421
  and stereoscopic processing, 276
Grating acuity. See also Acuity card
      procedure; Visual acuity
  and amblyopia, 395
  cataract and, 455–462
  improving measurement of, 545
  and infant retinal immaturity, 566–568
  orientation of, 163, 321
  in premature infants, 497, 498
Growth retardation, intrauterine, 497

Handling of neonates, in neonatal units,
      490
Harmonics, and visual evoked potentials,
      543
Heart-rate index of orienting, and
      peripheral vision, 122
Hemiretina, 412
  and disparity sign biases, 437–438
  nasal, 412, 437
  and strabismus, 372
  temporal, 412, 437
Hemorrhages, retinal, and amblyopia, 421
Heredity. See Genetic factors
Hering-Hillebrand deviation, 240
Hering's law of yoked eye movements, 40,
      246–248, 247f
Heterarchial model of binocular processing,
      267–270
Heterochromatic flicker photometry, 146
  infant, 148
Horopter development, 237
  and centripetal cone migration, 245–246,
      246f
  and interpupillary distance, 244–245,
      244f, 245f
  sensorimotor adaptation and, 237–248
    binocular disparity, 237–238
    development of ocular parameters,
      242–243, 243f
    empirical longitudinal horopter,
      240–242, 240f, 241f
    empirical vertical horopter, 242, 242f
    growth parameters and empirical
      horopter, 243–246
    Hering's law of yoked eye movements,
      246–248
    theoretical longitudinal horopter, 238,
      238f
    theoretical vertical horopter, 238–240,
      239f
Hyaloid artery, 488
Hybrid static-kinetic perimetry method,
      119–121, 120f
  and visual field defect screening, 122
Hyperacuity, 228–229. See also Vernier
      acuity

  and amblyopia, 394–395, 396
  and stereopsis, 228
Hypercyclopean perception, and
      stereoscopic processing, 276–278
Hypercyclopean processing, development of,
      280
Hyperopia
  in infancy, 6, 342
  later development, 11
  and neonates, 6
  and prematurity, 7

Ideal observer theory, and visual
      development, 92, 183, 560
Identical visual directions, and horopter,
      240
Illiterate E test, 338
Illumination, in neonatal nurseries,
      490–491
Image velocity, and horopter, 244, 244f
Increment threshold spectral sensitivity, and
      amblyopia, 392
Infrared photography, in accommodation-
      convergence interactions, 36
Interocular vision, 201–222. See also
      Binocular processing; Binocular
      vision
  acuity differences and stereopsis,
      263–264
  and occlusion constraints, 214–221
  prestereoptic visual function, 202–214,
      251
  rivalry and, 279
  stereopsis and, 221, 263–264
  suppression, and 279
Interpupillary distance, 242–243, 438
  and horopter, 244–245, 244f, 245f
Intestinal absorptive capacity, and preterm
      birth, 498
Intrauterine growth retardation, 497
Intrinsic noise
  cone contrast sensitivity and color vision,
      182–183
  and contrast discrimination, 187–192
  ideal observer theory and, 183–187
  and infant rod stimulation, 179–182
  and response variability, 178–179, 179f
  Weber fraction and, 181
Isoluminance
  and color vision, 145, 146–148, 147f,
      148f, 155–157, 156f
  stimuli and, 557
  visual losses at, 153
Isomerization rate, and spatial vision, 93t
Isotropic photorefraction. See
      Photorefraction

Jittered stereogram, 434f, 435
Joint null line, 145, 145f

Kinetic perimetry method, 117–118, 118f.
      See also Visual fields

Lateral geniculate nucleus
  and conjugate eye movements, 49

  development of, 537
  and orientation selectivity, 169
  and visual development, 299–300,
      302–303
Leukomalacia, periventricular, 499
Levodopa, in amblyopia, 419
LH-test, 338
Light adaptation models, and scotopic
      sensitivity, 137–138, 138f
Lighting environment, and preterm infants,
      490–491
Light losses, and scotopic sensitivity, 130,
      131f
Light scatter, interocular, and amblyopia,
      424–425
Light sensitivity
  and amblyopia, 392
  photopic peripheral, 121
Light transmission, ocular, in neonates,
      488
Linear letter acuity, and infantile cataract,
      463–466, 465f, 465t, 466f
Linear predictive coding, and visual evoked
      potentials, 539
Longitudinal horopter, 238, 238f,
      240–241, 240f, 241f. See also
      Horopter development
Low birthweight infants. See also
      Premature infants
  screening procedures and, 337
  and strabismus, 376
Luminance channel, and color vision, 145
Luminance contrast, in color vision
      experimentation, 157–160, 158f,
      159f
Luminance increment thresholds, and
      amblyopia, 392
Luster, binocular, 270–271

MacAdam ellipses, 182–183, 183f
Magnetic resonance imaging, in delayed
      visual maturation, 509–510
Magnocellular pathways, and conjugate eye
      movements, 49
Manifest refraction, 5
Mapping distortions
  cortical topographical, in strabismus, 372,
      415
  neurontropy model, 427–435
  retinocorticals in strabismic amblyopia,
      415–426, 415f
    albinotic mapping error, 416–418
    retinal origins and, 418–423
Mean forward/backward prediction, and
      visual evoked potentials, 539–540,
      540f
Measurement accuracy, and acuity card
      procedure, 329
Media, ocular, transmittance, 92–93, 130
  developmental changes in, 93t, 98
Meridional amblyopia, 344–345, 345f
Meridional magnification, of visual images,
      242f
Mesencephalic reticular formation, 50
Metamers, 145
Microdetachments, retinal, and amblyopia,
      421–423
Midbrain binocularity deficits, 436
Minimally distinct border matches, 146
  infant, 148
Minkowski function, 190, 191f

Models
    binocular vision, heterarchical, 267
    color discrimination, Russian doll, 149
    developmental, 513
        Banks and Bennett, 98–104, 563
        binocular vision, 250
        "Detroit model," of deprivation
            susceptibility, 398
        infant acuity and contrast sensitivity,
            98, 178, 226, 293, 563
        infant color vision, 150
        infant electroretinography, 517
        infant oculomotor, 67
        infant refraction, 19
        motion processing abnormalities, and
            esotropia, 377
        neurontropy, of amblyopia origins, 427
        Wilson, 104–115, 563
    light adaptation, 137
    oculomotor, 51, 58
Monocular vision
    acuity and, 230–231
        testing, 321
    versus binocular vision in development,
        413–415
    eccentric fixation and, 414
    neurons and presstereoptic visual system,
        213
    and ocular constraints, 218f
    and optokinetic nystagmus, 84–85
    pattern deprivation and, 231–232
    visual fields, 124–125, 124f, 125f
Monofixation syndrome, 233
    and esotropia, 335, 356
Motion detection, 59, 172–173
Motion nulling technique, 153–154
    color experimentation, 157–160, 158f,
        159f
Motion pathway, visual
    development of, 376–377, 377f
    and esotropia, 375–376
    maldevelopment of, 377–379, 378f
    neurons and, 374f
    topographical distortions in strabismus,
        372–374
Motion photometry, 153
Motion processing. See also Stereomotion
        perception
    codevelopment with stereopsis and eye
        alignment, 374–375
    and fixation, 60
    and infant testing, 557
    mechanisms of, 170–175
        behavioral discrimination of differential
            motion, 172–173
        directionality and optokinetic
            nystagmus, 173–174
        directional visual-evoked potential
            responses and, 171–172, 171f
        motion and other visual selectivities,
            175
        motion-dependent perceptual
            capabilities, 174–175
        nasotemporal biases and, 366–367,
            369f
    and perceptual capabilites, 174–175
Motion selectivity, 170
Movement, detection model, for nasally
        directed bias, 379–380, 379f, 380f
Multichannel recording, and visual evoked
        potentials, 541–543, 541f
Multiinput stimulation, and visual evoked
        potentials, 548–550, 548f, 549f

Multiple response harmonics, and visual
        evoked potentials, 543
Multiple sclerosis, and pursuit, 65
Multiply handicapped visually impaired
        children, 339
Muscle spasms, and vision loss, 537
Myelination
    and delayed visual maturation, 507–508
    normal maturation sequence, 509
    and stereopsis time encoding, 425
Myopia
    acuity card insensitivity to, 330
    axial length and, 10
    deprivation
        accommodation and, 15–16
        biochemical correlates of, 25–26
        chickens as model for, 16–17, 17f
        comparison between human and animal
            models, 15
        recovery from, 16
        visual signal and, 16
    and prematurity, 7, 498

Naka-Rushton equation, 518
Nasal field extent, and monocular visual
        fields, 124–127, 124f, 125f, 126f
Nasal hemiretina, 412, 437
Nasotemporal biases
    and binocularity, 367, 371
    motion processing and, 366–367, 369f
    movement detection and, 379–382, 379f,
        380f, 382f
    topographical distortions and, 373–374
Nasotemporal development, of primary
        visual cortex, 371–372, 372f
Near refraction, 5
Near triad eye movements, 42–43
    accommodation and, 42
    pupillary reflex and, 42
    vergence and, 42–43
Neonatal nurseries, environmental factors
        and, 490–492
Neural development, visual, 67–68, 296,
        364, 505
Neural mechanisms
    and conjugate eye movements, 48–53
    and normal visual development, 299–300
    and presstereoptic visual system, 211–214
    and visual deprivation, 301–303, 302f,
        303f
Neural transfer function, 92, 95–97, 97,
        102, 109–110, 113–115
Neuroglia cells, and eye growth, 25–26
Neurological disability, screening
        procedures and, 337
Neurological neonatal discharge
        examination, 338
Neuronal model, of stereopsis onset,
        250–251, 251f
Neuronal pathways, and presstereoptic visual
        system, 212–213, 213f
Neurontropy, binocular, model
        amblyopiagenesis and, 431–432
        binocular catabolism and, 430–431
Neurotransmitters, retinal, and deprivation
        myopia, 25
Night vision. See Scotopic vision
Nodal distance, developmental changes in,
        93t
Noncycloplegic refraction
    in neonates, 6

one to five years, 9–10
    three months to one year, 8
Nonfixing eye, habitual suppression of, 232
Nonselective convergence hypothesis. See
        Presstereoptic visual system
Nonverbal adults, and acuity card
        procedure, 329
Nucleus of optic tract, and optokinetic
        nystagmus, 475–476, 477f
Nulling metric, 154
Nulling techniques. See Motion nulling;
        Null plane analysis; Optokinetic
        nystagmus
Null plane analysis, and three dimensional
        color spaces, 144–149
    cone excitation space, 144–146, 145f
    infant null planes, 148–149
    spectral sensitivity curves, 144, 144f
    tilt of isoluminant plane, 146–148, 147f,
        148f
Nyquist frequency, 95

Object constancy, hypercyclopean, 278
Occlusion, and depth perception, 265–267,
        266f
Occlusion constraints, and interocular
        vision, 214–221
    da Vinci stereopsis, 217, 218f–220f, 221,
        222
    escape from rivalry effect, 217, 217f,
        220–221, 220f–221f
    slit-motion effects, 214–217, 215f, 216f,
        221, 222
Occlusion therapy, of amblyopia, 339, 456
Ocular dominance, and presstereoptic visual
        system, 212, 212f, 214
Ocular light dose, neonatal, 490–492
Oculomotor function
    conjugate eye movements, 47–76; See
        also Conjugate eye movements;
        Saccadic eye movements
    disjunctive eye movements, 42–43; See
        also Convergence; Vergence
    fixation, 39–40, 48
    near triad eye movements, 42–43
    reflex conjugate eye movements, 41–42
    vestibuloocular reflex. See
        Vestibuloocular reflex
Off-axis refraction, and astigmatism, 7
OKN. See Optokinetic nystagmus
Operant techniques, in infant testing, 556
Opsoclonus, 62
Optical eye trackers. See Corneal reflection
        trackers
Optical immaturities, and visual
        development, 94–98. See also
        Development analysis models
Optical transfer functions, 94f, 98, 102,
        105–106, 109, 113–115
Optokinetic after-nystagmus, 84, 86
Optokinetic nystagmus. See Optokinetic
        reflex
Optokinetic reflex, 41–42, 83
    binocular, 122, 412
    and color vision testing, 155–160
        discrimination ellipsoids and motion
            nulls, 157–160
        tilts of isoluminant plane, 155–157
    developmental comparisons, 86
    function of, 85
    gain and, 84

Optokinetic reflex (Continued)
  and infantile cataract, 459–463, 460f,
      461f, 478–480
    bilateral, 459
    symmetry studies, 474–477, 476f
    testing success with, 460t
    unilateral, 459–461
  monocular asymmetries, 84–85, 371
  motion selectivity and, 173–174
  nulling techniques, 154, 154f
  pursuit versus reflexive, 84
  stare- versus look-optokinetic nystagmus,
      83
  visual evoked potentials and, 537
Optotype matching test, 338
Orbital axes, angular relation in
    development, 410, 410f
Orientation sensitivity
  hypercyclopean specificity, 277
  tuning, 167–168
  and visual-evoked potentials, 163–170
    age as factor, 165, 165f
    anisotropy of, 166–167, 167f
    behavioral measures, 168–169
    orientation tuning, 167–168, 167f
    phase-reversal compared, 164–166,
        165f
    and preterm infants, 166, 166f
    selectivity mechanisms, 169–170
    and spatial frequency, 165, 166f
    stimulus sequence, 164f
    temporal and spatial determinants,
        164–166
Orthogonal photorefraction, 31
Orthotropization, 254–255, 350–351, 352f

Pancake model, and discrimination
    ellipsoids, 149f, 150
Panum's fusional areas, 245
Parafovea, development of, 292–293, 292f
Parietal cortex, and conjugate eye
    movements, 52–53
Patching, See Occlusion therapy
Perceptual capabilities, motion-dependent,
    174–175
Perimetry. See Visual fields
Peripheral acuity development, 121, 261,
    403
  versus foveal acuity, 263
Peripheral contrast sensitivity, in infant
    cataract, 469
Peripheral field sensitivity, 121
Peripheral retina development, 291–293
Periventricular leukomalacia, 499
Persistent hyperplastic primary vitreous,
    456, 458, 464
Phase reversal visual-evoked potentials,
    164–166, 165f, 170
Photoisomerization, 178
Photometry. See Heterochromatic flicker
    photometry; Minimally distinct
    border matches; Motion photometry
Photon absorption, and infant rods, 180
Photon catch, and ideal contrast sensitivity,
    93f
Photon noise, 178
Photophobia, 433, 435
Photoprotection, 442
Photoreceptors, 287. See also Fovea; Retina
  directional forces in accommodation and,
      420, 420f

efficiency, 92–93
electroretinographic measurement of
    function, 521
in normal visual development, 94, 287,
    299, 560
parafoveal, 293, 293f
Photorefraction
  in accommodation-convergence
      interactions, 36–37
  and accommodation measurement, 31
  and accommodative accuracy in infants,
      31
  isotropic, 31, 339
  in screening, 340
Phototoxic insult, and amblyopia, 423–425
Phototropism, cone, and amblyopia,
    424–425
Poisson processes, and intrinsic noise, 178
Pontine paramedian reticular formation, 50
Postconceptional age, defined, 486
Postmenstrual age, defined, 486
Postnatal age, defined, 486
Postreceptoral processsing, 95, 145–146,
    146f, 569
Postreceptoral pooling, and scotopic
    sensitivity, 136
Predictive validity, and acuity card
    procedure, 325
Preferential looking technique. See also
    Acuity card procedure; Forced-choice
    preferential looking technique
  and infantile cataract, 455–459, 456t,
      461–462, 478–480
    bilateral cases, 455, 457, 457f
    duration of deprivation, 458t
    testing success with, 457t
    unilateral cases, 456, 457–459, 458f
  and visual acuity, 319–320
Premature infants, 485–499. See also Low
    birthweight infants
  and acuity card procedure, 328–329
  and astigmatism, 8, 498
  behavioral tests of vision in, 497
  electroretinography in, 496
  environmental influences, 490–492,
      497–498
  epidemiological data, 486
  handling of, 490
  lighting environment and, 490–492
  and myopia, 498
  neonatal eye characteristics, 486–489
    corneal growth, 488
    eyelids, 487, 487f
    globe, 488
    pupillary reflex to light, 488, 489f
    vascular system, 488
    visual pathway development, 488–489
  net spherical refractions of, 10
  ocular light dose and, 492, 492f
  ophthalmology of, 489–490
  and orientation response, 166
  refractive studies in, 7, 498
  and retinopathy of prematurity,
      489–490, 498
  screening procedures and, 337
  thermoregulation and, 490
  visual attention and, 492–496
  visual evoked potentials in, 496–497
Prestereoptic visual function, 202–214
  binocular inputs during, 201–202
  model of, 250–252
  nonselective convergence hypothesis,
      202–211

and color, 208, 211, 212f
and contrast, 204–206, 207f–208f,
    208
interocularly combined grids
    experiment, 202–204, 203f–204f,
    205f
and spatial frequency, 208, 210f–211f
underlying neuronal mechanisms,
    211–214, 250
columnar segregation of ocular
    dominance, 214
neuronal pathways, 212–213, 213f
ocular dominance distributions, 212,
    212f
Preterm infants. See Premature infants
Primates, visual development in, 296–304.
    See also Retina, development of
environmental influences, 300–301
limits and visual deprivation, 301–303
neural mechanisms, 299–300
normal visual development, 297–300
optics, 297–299
photoreceptors, 299
spatial vision, 296–297
Prisms
  and compression of visual space, 240
  in evaluation of fixation preference, 311
  and strabismus, 442
Probability summation at threshold, 253
Progressive supranuclear palsy, and pursuit,
    65
Psychophysiological linking hypothesis, and
    infant testing, 557–558
Pupil
  developmental changes in, 92–93, 93t,
      98
  light reflexes
    in amblyopia, 419
    and near triad eye movements, 42
    in neonates, 488
  measurement of response, 311
  as response indicator, 122
Pursuit eye movements, 41, 62
  alternative forms of, 63–64, 65f
  asymmetry of
    in amblyopia, 371
    in strabismus, 365–366, 366f–368f
  interpretation of infant, 64–65

Quantal catch, and scotopic sensitivity, 133,
    133f

Racial factors, in strabismus incidence, 417
Reaching responses, and stereopsis, 228
Receptive field profiles, 96, 96f
Referral, 309–311, 310f
Refixation, 61–62, 61f
Reflexive eye movements. See Conjugate eye
    movement; Optokinetic reflex;
    Vestibulo-ocular reflex
Refraction, 3, 5
  accommodation and, 30–33, 36–37
  anisometropia, 10–11
  axial length, globe, and, 10
  changes in with age, 5, 342–343, 342f
  convergence and, 33–37
  early detection of strabismus and,
      340–342, 341f
  emmetropization and, 11, 17, 340

Refraction (*Continued*)
    implications of early for later visual
        development, 11
    measurement of, 5, 311–312
    neonate
        normal development, 5–7
        prematurity, 7–8, 498
    one to five years, 9–10
    and strabismus, 343, 439
    three months to one year, 8–9
    values of screening for, 343
    visually guided control of, 14–27
Reinforcement, in infant testing, 556–557
Resolution, spatial. *See* Visual acuity
Resolution/Vernier acuity ratio, 395,
    400–401
Response variability, and intrinsic noise,
    178–179, 179f
Resting position, in accommodation-
    convergence interaction, 37
Reticular formation, mesenecephalic, 50
Retina. *See also* Fovea; Photoreceptor
    in amblyopia, 418–423
        hemorrhages, 421
        microdetachments, 421–423
        structure maturation and globe growth,
            419–421
    barrel distortion and, 241
    degenerations of, 314f, 315
    and delayed visual maturation, 507
    development of, 98–102, 99f, 100f,
        287–294, 560–565
        cell populations in primate, 287
        fovea, 287–291
        in neonates, 488
        peripheral retina, 291–293
        and spatial visual acuity, 293–294
    disparity of and convergence, 34, 34f
    illuminance, and scotopic sensitivity, 130,
        131f
    inhomogeneity and, 554
    maturation of and stereopsis, 226, 226f
    mosaic, density of, 242–243
    pigment epithelium melanin abnormality
        in, 337, 417
    retinal coverage, 94
    retinopathy of prematurity, 121–122,
        489–490
    retinoscopy, 6–7, 338–339
Retinitis pigmentosa, 337, 417
Retinopathy of prematurity, 121–122,
    489–490. *See also* Premature infant
    and myopia, 498
Retinoscopy, 338–339
    artifact of, 6–7
Rhodopsin, and scotopic sensitivity,
    133–135, 134f
Rivalry
    discrimination of, 201
    interocular, 271, 279
    and occlusion constraints, 217, 220–221,
        222
Rod dominance hypothesis, and color
    vision, 143
Rod null planes, 148
Rod ring, midperipheral, development of,
    292–293, 293f
Rods, and intrinsic noise, 179–182
    absolute and intrinsic thresholds and,
        181–182, 182f
    night vision sensitivity, 180–181, 180f
    optical density and, 179–181
    photon absorption and, 180

spectral sensitivity and, 180
    thermal isomerization and, 180
R4 test, 338
Russian dolls model, and discrimination
    ellipsoids, 149–150, 149f
    and infant color vision, 150–152, 152f

Saccades, 40–41. *See also* Conjugate eye
    movements
    accuracy and, 53–55
    brain center control, 58f
    defined, 48–49
    examples of, 54f
    latencies and, 55–56
    morphology of, 53
    possible interpretations, 56–59
Scotopic b-wave amplitudes, for pediatric
    retinal degenerations, 314f, 315
Scotopic vision, development of, 130
    axial density of rhodopsin and, 133–135,
        134f
    background adaptation, 136–139
        and b-wave, 138–139, 138f, 139f
        light adaptation models, 137–138,
            138f
        psychophysics, 136–137, 137f
    bleaching adaptation, 139
    dark-adapted sensitivity measurement,
        130–133
        electroretinogram b-wave results,
            132–133, 132f
        psychophysics, 130–131
    light losses in ocular media, 92, 130, 131f
    quantal catch and, 133, 133f
    spatial summation and, 136, 136f
    specification of retinal illuminance, 130,
        131f
    temporal summation functions, 135–136,
        135f
Seizures, and vision loss, 537
Selectivity, in clinical test evaluation, 312
Sensitive period, 300
    and cataract, 478
    and visual development, 231, 300
Sensitivity, in clinical test evaluation, 312
Sensorimotor adaptation, and horopter
    development, 237–248. *See also*
    Horopter development
Sensory deficits, and accommodation, 32
Sensory factors, and conjugate eye
    movements, 69–70
Sensory testing, 312, 318, 338, 356–357,
    455
Sensory threshold, 258–261
    threshold behavior in infant cortical
        evoked potentials, 259–261
    true threshold model, 259
Sequential ideal-observer analysis approach,
    92f
Shape distortion, of retinal images, 241
Sheridan-Gardiner Test, 338
Signal processing methods, and visual
    evoked potentials, 539–541
Signal-to-noise ratio
    modern signal processing methods and,
        539–541
    and visual evoked potentials, 536
Simultaneous perception, and stereopsis,
    229
Sinewave luminance gratings, in visual
    processing experiments, 261–263,
    262f

Slit motion, and ocular constraints,
    214–217, 215f, 216f, 221, 222
Smooth pursuit. *See* Pursuit
Space perception, stereoscopic, model for,
    267–270
Spatial determinants, of orientation visual-
    evoked potentials, 164–166
Spatial vision. *See also* Contrast sensitivity;
    Visual acuity
    intrinsic noise and, 178–196
    motion selectivity and, 173–175
    orientation selectivity and, 163–173
    scotopic retinal sensitivity and, 130–139
    summation and scotopic sensitivity, 136,
        136f
    visual field development and, 117–127
Spectral sensitivity. *See also* Color vision,
    infant
    and amblyopia, 392
    and infant rods, 180
Spherical refractive error. *See* Refraction
Square-root law, in developmental analysis
    models, 108–109
Square-wave jerks, in eye movements, 62,
    65
Static perimetry. *See* Visual fields
Stereoacuity, 228. *See also* Stereopsis
Stereograms. *See* Stereopsis
Stereograting, 277
Stereomechanisms, and binocular processing
    dynamic, 274–276
    static, 272–274
Stereomotion detection, and binocular and
    monocular vision, 414
Stereomotion perception
    chromatic, 274–276, 275
    cyclopean, 276
    hypercyclopean, 277–278
    real, 274
Stereopsis, 197–198, 224–234, 263–267.
    See also Binocular processing;
    Binocular vision; Prestereoptic visual
    function
    acuity and, 229–232
        interocular acuity differences and,
            229–230, 230f
        monocular versus binocular acuity and,
            230–231, 231f
        stereoacuity development, 228, 228f
    amblyopia and, 255, 427, 472
    assessment stimuli
        line stereograms, 224
        random dot stereograms, 224–225
    binocular optomotor alignment and, 253,
        374, 412–413
    binocular versus monocular vision in,
        413–415
    classes of, 411–412, 411t
    codevelopment with motion processing
        and eye alignment, 374–375
    corpus callosum and, 436–437
    cortical maturation and, 227, 251, 569
    da Vinci, 217, 218f–220f, 221, 222,
        265–266
    depth from occlusion and, 265–267,
        266f
    development of, 225, 280, 409–413
    dichoptic fusion and, 264–265
    esotropia and, 232–234, 233f, 254, 255,
        374
    fusion and, 229, 229f
        developmental asynchrony, 436–437
    global versus local, 427

Stereopsis (*Continued*)
  hyperacuity and, 228–229
  infant cataract and, 472–474, 478
  interocular differences and, 263–264
  local versus global, 427
  motion processing and, 374
  nonconventional disparity cues and, 280
  onset of, 225, 225f, 250, 374, 410
    factors determining, 225–227
    neuronal model, 250–251, 251f
    prestereoptic vision, 201,251–252, 409
  orbital axes and, 410, 410f
  retinal maturation and, 226, 226f
  simultaneous perception and, 229
  time encoding defects, 425–426
  vergence and, 227, 253–254
Stiles-Crawford effect, and amblyopia 392,
    419
Stimulus
  sequence for orientation-reversal visual-
    evoked potentials, 164f
  variables in infant testing, 554–555
  and visual acuity testing, 320
    acuity card procedure, 326–327
Storage mechanisms, and optokinetic
    response, 86
Strabismogenesis, 435–438
Strabismus. *See also* Esotropia; Exotropia;
    Eye alignment; Orthotropization
  albino misrouting and, 426
  and amblyopia. *See* Amblyopia
  and binocular versus monocular vision
    predominance, 414–415
  birth trauma-based defects, 426–427
  and brain damage, 426–427
  congenital cataract and, 472
  cycle of visual cortex maldevelopment
    and, 375–376
  early detection of refractive errors and,
    340–342, 341f
  experimental validation and, 382–384
  genetic factors and, 376, 416–418
  historical notions of, 384–386, 385f
  infantile cataract and, 479
  maternal birth posture and, 438–439
  motion pathway in visual cortex and,
    365–366, 372
  nasal motion bias and binocularity, 367,
    371
  nasotemporal development of visual
    cortex and, 371–372
  and postnatal age, 365f
  prism treatment and, 442
  referral for examination and, 310
  refraction and, 343, 439–441
  screening procedures for, 336–340
  surgery and, 353, 441–442
  topographical abnormalities, cortical,
    and, 372, 378f, 415
  visual development and, 301
Summation, dichoptic, 271–272, 272f
Superior colliculus
  and conjugate eye movements, 50–51
  and saccades, 57, 58f
Suppression, interocular, 271, 279
Surgical treatment of strabismus, 353–356,
    441–442
Sweep visual evoked potentials. *See* Visual
    evoked potentials
Synapses
  and cortical density, 569, 569f
  and visual development, 537

Target distance, and visual acuity testing,
    320–321
Teller Acuity Cards; See Acuity card
    procedure
Temporal determinants, of orientation
    visual-evoked potentials, 164–166
Temporal field extent, and monocular visual
    fields, 124–127, 124f, 125f, 126f
Temporal hemiretina, 412, 437
Temporal processing, and amblyopia,
    392–393, 425–426
Temporal summation functions, and
    scotopic sensitivity, 135–136, 135f
Testability rates, and acuity card procedure,
    325–326
Thalamus, lesions of, and delayed visual
    maturation, 508
Thermal isomerization, and infant rods, 180
Thermoregulation, and neonates, 490
Threshold assumption, and visual evoked
    potential, 538–539
Time encoding defects, and amblyopia,
    425–426
Titmus test, 356–357
Tonic vergence, 43
Tranquilizers, and pursuit, 65
Transfer function, optical, 94
Tritan channels, and color vision, 145
Two-stage model of binocular development,
    250–256

Uniform loss hypothesis, and color vision,
    143, 150

Validation studies. *See also* Acuity card
    procedure; Sensitivity; Selectivity
  concurrent validity, 323–325
  construct validity, 322–323
  content validity, 323
  predictive validity, 325
Vascularization, in neonates, 488
Vasointestinal polypeptide, and deprivation
    myopia, 25
Vergence. *See also* Convergence
  binocular and monocular vision and, 414
  near triad eye movements and, 42–43
  premotor neuron pool in, 383f
  stereopsis and, 227, 253–254
Vernier acuity
  amblyopia and, 395, 395f, 396–398,
    397f, 398f
  in binocular and monocular vision, 413
  visual evoked potentials and, 546–548,
    547f
Versional eye movements. *See* Conjugate
    eye movements
Vertical disparity, and interpupillary
    distance, 245, 245f
Vertical fusional vergence amplitude,
    442–443
Vertical horopter, 238–240, 239f, 242,
    242f. *See also* Horopter development
Vestibuloocular reflex, 41
  compared to adult, 85–86
  gain and, 82
  phase and, 81–82
  storage mechanisms, 86
  time constants and, 81
  visual-vestibular interactions, 82–83, 83f

Vieth-Muller circle, 238f
  longitudinal horopter and, 238, 240,
    240f, 241
  vertical horopter and, 238, 239
Vision screening, 335–346
  accommodative ability and refractive
    errors, 345–346
  albinism and, 337
  amblyopia and, 336–340
    meridional, 344–345
  esotropia and, 349–350
  ethnic differences and, 553
  genetic disorders and, 337
  infant alertness and, 553
  initial age and, 309, 310f
  low-birth rate infants and, 337
  neurological disability and, 337
  predictive value of, 343
  premature infants and, 337
  procedures, review of, 336–338
  refractive errors and strabismus, 340
  retinitis pigmentosa and, 337
  stimulus variables and, 553–555
  strabismus and, 336–340
Visual acuity. *See also* Acuity card
    procedure; Contrast sensitivity
  and accomodation, 32
  and amblyopia, 301, 313, 349, 354
  and eye movements, 69, 83
  and optical development, 92, 297
  and optokinetic response, 83
  and retinal development, 91, 293, 298,
    560
  and stereopsis, 229–232, 263
  and visual deprivation, 301, 455
  visual evoked potential measurement of,
    315, 395, 537
  and vision screening, 338
Visual cortex. *See also* Cortical development
  and delayed visual maturation, 508
  nasotemporal development of, 371–372,
    372f
  strabismus and maldevelopment of,
    375–376
Visual evoked potentials, 536
  alternative measures of, 545–548, 546f,
    547f
  in amblyopia, 314f, 315, 395
  binocular, 252
  contrast sensitivity function in, 540,
    566–568, 567f
  in delayed visual maturation, 506–507
  and dichoptic fusion, 264–265
  frequency diversity methods for, 544
  and infant retinal immaturity, 566–568
  and interocular acuity differences, 264
  linear predictive coding and, 539
  mean forward/backward prediction and,
    539–540, 540f
  motion selective mechanisms in, 171–173
  multichannel recording in, 541–543,
    541f
  multiinput stimulation/analysis paradigms
    in, 548–550, 549f
  multiple response harmonic and, 543,
    543f
  and orientation. *See* Orientation
  in premature infants, 496–497, 498
  stimuli choice and, 544–545
  sweep visual evoked potential, 537
  threshold assumption and, 538–539,
    538f

Visual evoked potentials (*Continued*)
Vernier acuity and, 546–548, 547f
and visual field assessment, 122
Visual fields, 117–127
assessment of
clinical applications and, 121–122
electrophysiological methods, 122
hybrid static-kinetic perimetry and, 119–121, 120f
kinetic perimetry and, 117–118, 118f
peripheral field sensitivity and, 121
psychophysiological methods, 122
static perimetry and, 119
defect, screening for, 122
distortions and strabismus, 373–374, 373f
maturation of, 123–125

binocular field extent, 123–124, 123f
monocular visual field extent, 124–125, 124f, 125f
primate, 410f
rabbit, 410f
Visual pathways
and delayed visual maturation, 507–508
development in neonates, 488–489
and oculomotor control, 49–50
Visual status, examination of. *See* Examination of visual status
Visual-vestibular interactions, 82–83, 83f
Volitional oculomotor mechanisms, 68–69

Weber's law, 181–183, 554
Wheatstone stereopsis, 221

White sphere kinetic method, 118, 121–122. *See also* Visual fields
Worth 4-dot test, 356

Yoking ratio, of vertical eye movements, 247f, 248

Zero amplitude technique, and visual evoked potentials, 538